MEDICAL-SURGICAL
CARE PLANNING

Third Edition

MEDICAL-SURGICAL CARE PLANNING

Third Edition

Nancy M. Holloway, RN, MSN
Critical Care Educator
Nancy Holloway & Associates
Orinda, California

Springhouse Corporation
Springhouse, Pennsylvania

Staff

Executive Director
Matthew Cahill

Clinical Director
Judith Schilling McCann, RN, MSN

Editorial Director
Donna O. Carpenter

Design Director
John Hubbard

Managing Editor
David Moreau

Acquisitions Editors
Patricia Fischer, RN, BSN; Louise Quinn

Senior Editor
Karen Diamond

Clinical Consultant
Lori Neri, RN, MSN

Copy Editors
Cynthia C. Breuninger (manager), Karen C. Comerford, Stacey A. Follin, Brenna H. Mayer, Pamela Wingrod

Designers
Arlene Putterman (associate art director), Mary Ludwicki

Manufacturing
Deborah Meiris (director), Patricia K. Dorshaw (manager), Otto Mezei

Editorial Assistant
Beverly Lane

Printed in the United States of America.

MSCP3-010798

℞ A member of the Reed Elsevier plc group

Library of Congress Cataloging-in-Publication Data

Medical surgical care planning / [edited by] Nancy M. Holloway. — 3rd ed.
   p.   cm.
   Includes bibliographical references and index.
   1. Nursing care plans. 2. Nursing. 3. Surgical nursing. 4. Diagnosis related groups. I. Holloway, Nancy M.
   [DNLM: 1. Patient Care Planning. 2 Nursing Diagnosis. 3. Diagnosis-Related Groups. WY 100 M4877 1999]
RT49.M45 1998
610.73—dc21

DNLM/DLC   98-17557
ISBN 0-87434-925-7 (alk. paper)   CIP

Contents

Consultants and contributors

Consultants

Janice M. Beitz,
RN, PhD, CS, CNOR, CETN
Director, Graduate Nursing Program
LaSalle University School of Nursing
Philadelphia

Mary Kay Flynn,
RN, DNSc, CCRN
Professor in Nursing
Mesa Community College, Boswell Center
Sun City, Ariz.

Latrell P. Fowler,
BSN, MN, PhD
Assistant Professor
Medical University of South Carolina Satellite at
Francis Marion University
Florence, S.C.

Cathy A. Machacyk,
RN, BSN
Regional Rehabilitation and Subacute Director
UPC Health Network
Orlando, Fla.

Contributors

Sandra Allen,
RN,C
Nutrition Support–I.V. Nurse Specialist
Doctors Hospital
Columbus, Ohio
(Total parenteral nutrition)

Gerene S. Bauldoff,
RN, MSN
Project Director, LV Function & Duration of
Mechanical Ventilation Study
University of Pittsburgh School of Nursing
(Myasthenia gravis)

Nancy Newell Bell,
RN, MN, MDiv, CCRN
Assistant Clinical Professor
University of California
San Francisco
(Fractured femur, Multiple trauma)

Diane Sadler Benson,
RN, MS, MEd
Lecturer, Department of Nursing
Humboldt State University
Arcata, Calif.
(Diabetes mellitus, Diabetic ketoacidosis, Disseminated
intravascular coagulation, Hyperosmolar hyperglycemic
nonketotic syndrome, Hypoglycemia, Pain)

Audrey J. Berman,
RN, MSN, PhD, AOCN
Associate Dean, Nursing Academic Affairs
Samuel Merritt College
Oakland, Calif.
(Hysterectomy, Lymphoma)

Claudia J. Beverly,
RN, PhD
Associate Director, Center on Aging
University of Arkansas for Medical Sciences
Little Rock
(Total joint replacement in a lower extremity)

Ruth Brewer,
APRN, BSN, MN, PhD
Professor of Nursing-Family Nurse Practitioner
McNeese State University
Lake Charles, La.
(Femoral-popliteal bypass, Inflammatory bowel disease)

Karen T. Bruchak,
RN, MSN, MBA
Assistant Administrator, Cancer Clinical Programs
University of Pennsylvania Cancer Center
Philadelphia
(Lung cancer, Radical neck dissection)

Nancy E. Casali,
RN, BSN
Clinical Services Manager
University of Arkansas for Medical Sciences
Little Rock
(Total joint replacement in a lower extremity)

Patricia C. Cloud,
RN, MSN
Associate Professor, Graduate and Undergraduate
Nursing
McNeese State University
Department of Nursing
Lake Charles, La.
(Mastectomy)

Karen L. Cooper,
RN, MSN, CCRN, CNA
Administrative Supervisor
Kaiser Permanente San Francisco
Managed Care Specialist
Zurich Insurance
San Francisco
(Abdominal aortic aneurysm repair, Cholecystectomy)

Dorothy B. Doughty,
RN, MN, CETN
Program Director, Wound Ostomy Continence Nursing
Education Program
Emory University
Atlanta
(Colostomy)

Phyllis R. Easterling,
RN, EdD, FNP
Associate Professor, Nursing
Samuel Merritt College
Oakland, Calif.
(Acute renal failure, Anorexia, Major burns, Retinal detachment, Skin grafts, Thoracotomy, Urolithiasis)

Gayle Flo,
ARNP, RN, MN, CCRN
Critical Care Clinical Nurse Specialist
Good Samaritan Hospital
Puyallup, Wash.
(Cerebrovascular accident)

Ellie Franges,
RN, MSN, CNRN, CCRN
Director, Neuroscience Services
Sacred Heart Hospital
Allentown, Pa.
(Alzheimer's disease)

Joanne Soldano Garcia,
RN, MS, CCRN
Administrative Director, Medical Cardiology and
Transplant Services
Rush-Presbyterian-St. Luke's Medical Center
Chicago
(Heart failure)

Patricia F. Henry,
RN, MS, CCRN
Critical Care Clinical Nurse Specialist
Summit Medical Center
Oakland, Calif.
(Duodenal ulcer, Gastrointestinal hemorrhage, Liver failure, Pancreatitis)

Mel Herman,
RN, BA, CCRN
Patient Care Coordinator
Summit Medical Center
Oakland, Calif.
(Adult respiratory distress syndrome, Mechanical ventilation)

Kathleen Hester,
RN, BSN, CCRN
Director
Critical Care, Telemetry, Emergency Nursing Service
Mt. Diablo Medical Center
Concord, Calif.
(Acute MI: Critical care unit, Acute MI: Telemetry unit)

Margaret Hodge,
RN, EdD
Clinical Instructor
California State University
Sacramento
Clinical Nurse Scientist
University of California, Davis Health System
(Drug overdose, Seizures)

Katherine Purgatorio Howard,
RN,C, MSN
Staff Educator
Bayonne (N.J.) Hospital
(Angina, Leukemia)

Beth Colvin Huff,
RN, MSN, CS
Consultant, Women's Health Nursing
Nashville, Tenn.
(Radioactive implant for cervical cancer)

Lauren M. Isacson,
RN,C, BSN, MPA, PHR
Human Resources Development Coordinator
Meridian Health Systems
Neptune, N.J.
(Peritoneal dialysis)

Philip A. John,
CCS
Health Information Consultant
Contract Health Information Services
Palm Desert, Calif.
(The role of DRGs in delivering quality care; DRG information on clinical plans)

Donna M. Knisely,
RN, MSN, CDE
Diabetes Educator, Clinical Specialist–Medical-Surgical
Columbia Arlington (Va.) Hospital
(Multiple sclerosis)

Larry E. Lancaster,
RN, MSN, EdD
Professor
Vanderbilt University - School of Nursing
Nashville, Tenn.
(Chronic renal failure)

Shirley L. Lewis,
RN, MSN, OCN
Head Nurse Manager
Columbia Arlington (Va.) Hospital
(Dying)

Wendy M. Mancini,
RN, MSN, CCRN, CNA, CNS
Clinical Nurse Specialist
Jersey Shore Medical Center
Neptune, N.J.
(Cardiogenic shock)

Barbara Martin,
RN, PhD
Unit Director
Rush-Presbyterian-St. Luke's Medical Center
Chicago
(Permanent pacemaker implantation)

Kate McClure,
RN, MS, CCRN
Adjunct Assistant Professor
Samuel Merritt College
Oakland, Calif.
(Esophagitis and gastroenteritis, Hypovolemic shock,
Nephrectomy, Pulmonary embolism, Septic shock)

Molly J. Moran,
RN, MS, CS, ANP, OCN
Hematology-Medical Oncology Clinical Nurse
Specialist
The Arthur G. James Cancer Hospital and Research
Institute
The Ohio State University Medical Center
Columbus
(Anemia)

Scarlott K. Mueller,
RN, MPH
Vice President-Chief Nursing Officer
Columbia North Florida Regional Medical Center
Gainesville
(Grieving, Prostatectomy)

Carolyn E. Munroe,
RN,C, BS, ADN
Director of Program Development
Columbia Homecare - North Florida Division
Gainesville
(Thrombophlebitis)

Christine E. Ortiz,
RN, MS, PhDc
Hospice Nurse
Visiting Nurses and Hospice of San Francisco
(Acquired immunodeficiency syndrome)

Elizabeth Poulson,
RN, MS, MA
Instructor, College of Nursing
Rush University
Chicago
(Permanent pacemaker insertion)

Ellene Rifas,
RN, EdD
Vice President
Alliance for Learning
Sacramento, Calif.
(Asthma, Chronic obstructive pulmonary disease,
Pneumonia)

Terry C. Rodriguez,
RN,C, CETN
Clinical Nurse Educator
SGS Surgical Associates
Oakland, Calif.
(Geriatric care; Ileal conduit urinary diversion)

Dennis G. Ross,
RN, MAE, PhD
Professor of Nursing
Castleton (Vt.) State College
(Osteomyelitis)

LuAnn E. Sanderson,
ARNP, MSN, CNS
Assistant Professor of Nursing
Fort Hays State University
Department of Nursing
Hays, Kans.
(Ineffective family coping: Compromised, Ineffective
individual coping)

Patricia C. Seifert,
RN, MSN, CNOR, CRNFA
Manager, Open Heart Surgery
Halifax Medical Center
Daytona Beach, Fla.
(Cardiac surgery, Surgery)

Debra Lynn Thelen,
RN, MS, ACRN
Clinical Research Nurse
Community Consortium
San Francisco
(Acquired immunodeficiency syndrome)

M. Susan Theodoropoulos,
RN,C, MSN
Director of Education and Research
Arlington (Va.) Hospital
(Amputation)

Charlene Thomas,
RN, PhD
Associate Director of Nursing
Rush-Presbyterian-St. Luke's Medical Center
Chicago
(Permanent pacemaker insertion)

Nancy C. Thomas,
RN, BSN, CCRN
Staff Nurse, Critical Care Center
Good Samaritan Hospital
Puyallup, Wash.
(Cerebrovascular accident)

Cindy Wagner,
RN,C, MS
Gerontological Clinical Nurse Specialist
Doctors Hospital
Columbus, Ohio
(Nutritional deficit)

Patricia Harvey Webb,
RN,C, MS, EdD
Assistant Professor, Nursing
Samuel Merritt College
Oakland, Calif.
(Carotid endarterectomy, Craniotomy, Critical care
transfer criteria guidelines,Glaucoma, Guillain-Barré
syndrome, Increased intracranial pressure,
Laminectomy, Monitoring standards)

Acknowledgments

Publishing a book is never a sole creative endeavor. I extend a special thank you to our contributors and consultants, acknowledged by name in a separate section, and the talented publishing team at Springhouse Corporation.

Dedication

This book is dedicated to D. Michael Holloway, my husband, for championing my dreams, and to Jason and Willow Holloway, my son and daughter, for making it all worthwhile.

Preface

Medical-Surgical Care Planning, Third Edition, is essential. Why? Because it integrates three major factors in nursing — care planning, nursing diagnoses, and diagnosis-related groups (DRGs) — and provides information nurses need to meet the 1992 Joint Commission on the Accreditation of Healthcare Organizations (JCAHO) Nursing Care Standards. Focusing on care of the adult medical-surgical patient, this book:
• distinguishes clearly between nursing's collaborative functions (those shared with medicine) and its independent functions (those unique to nursing)
• offers the bedside nurse, nursing student, and nursing educator comprehensive, realistic clinical plans to meet their educational needs.

Why are plans of care important?
Clinically, plans of care offer a way to plan and communicate appropriate patient care. Legally, they offer a framework for establishing the standard of care for a given situation. Financially, they can validate the appropriateness of care and justify staffing levels and patient-care charges.

If plans of care are so important, why don't more nurses use them?
Most nurses are first exposed to plans of care as students. They soon learn that writing out individual plans can be frustrating and time consuming. After graduation, most nurses practice in a hectic, complex environment that allows little time for thoughtful care planning.

Even nurses who would like to use written plans of care may be at a loss when trying to integrate nursing diagnoses into their planning. Overwhelmed, they may turn to previously published books for guidance, only to find the information too general or too theoretical, that common medical problems are renamed in nursing diagnosis terminology, or that nursing diagnoses are not matched to medical disorders.

Yet *clinically relevant* plans of care can help nurses answer many of the questions they ask daily:
• "What are the most important points to cover during a physical assessment when I haven't got time to check everything?"
• "Which laboratory tests and diagnostic procedures should I anticipate, and what do they typically show?"
• "What are this patient's nursing priorities?"
• "Which problems is this patient most likely to experience?"
• "Why are certain interventions important?"
• "Which complications can occur with this disorder?"

• "How long is this patient likely to be in the hospital?"
• "Realistically, how much patient teaching can I accomplish?"
• "From a nursing standpoint, how will I know when this patient is ready for discharge?"

The solution: This book
Medical-Surgical Care Planning, Third Edition, provides clinically relevant answers to common questions about patient care because it targets the needs of the "hands-on" nurse clinician through standardized plans of care. Distinguishing features include:
• 11 general plans of care covering conditions nurses encounter daily, such as impaired physical mobility and knowledge deficit
• 71 plans of care, organized by body system, covering various medical-surgical conditions and procedures (including critical care disorders)
• 8 clinical pathways
• nursing diagnoses (using selected terminology from the North American Nursing Diagnosis Association) and collaborative problems (using familiar medical terminology such as shock) arranged in order of importance.

This approach will help you see the total picture of patient care; differentiate between collaborative and independent nursing responsibilities; apply the latest official nursing diagnoses; and avoid forcing all planning under nursing diagnoses, a process that only renames medical diagnoses and fosters confusion between nursing and medicine.

Each plan presents the latest clinically relevant DRG information, including DRG numbers, principal diagnoses, and mean length of stay, to help you understand the reimbursement system responsible for today's cost-conscious health care environment and to help you anticipate the patient's recovery and plan patient teaching. Common historical and subjective findings are presented according to Gordon's functional health patterns, a widely accepted format that blends both traditional and contemporary methods of nursing assessment; objective findings are listed by body system. This assessment information will help you recognize pertinent signs and symptoms and understand how the nursing diagnoses and collaborative problems were identified.

The plans of care build on a goal-directed, action-oriented approach to care planning that ranks problems and interventions in order of importance and identifies specific outcome criteria. This approach will help you determine the most important patient problems, decide what to do first, and recognize when a problem has been resolved.

JCAHO standards' impact on nursing

The 1992 update represents the first major revision of the Nursing Care Standards since 1978. The JCAHO Nursing Standards Task Force, which included 23 representatives from various nursing services and educational programs, adopted the new standards after circulating two drafts and considering feedback from more than 50,000 nurses.

Where the former Nursing Services Standards focused on the process of care to determine if the nursing organization could provide quality care, the new Nursing Care Standards focus more on the patient and the outcomes of care to determine the quality of care provided. In addition, the new standards emphasize patient-family education and discharge planning. Consequently, nurses will play an even more important role in helping hospitals maintain accreditation. Such accountability is likely to *increase* interest in care planning.

The revised standards also place increased emphasis on documentation, requiring that nursing information involving assessment, nursing diagnoses or patient needs, interventions, and outcomes become a permanent part of the medical record. Care may be documented directly in the patient's record or indirectly through references to other documents. However, this documentation does not have to be the handwritten, complex, case-study approach to care planning that educators find helpful, or the routine, repetitive handwritten plan that many hospital nurses rightly dismiss as irrelevant and time consuming. Instead of being required to provide handwritten plans of care for all patients, nursing departments now have more flexibility in documenting care. Nurses may now choose to document care planning through standards of care, clinical practice guidelines, critical paths, or preprinted plans of care.

When individualized as recommended, the standardized plans in this book can help nurses meet all of the JCAHO's requirements. The plans cover all the elements required for documentation of care planning and also include useful information about patient outcomes, patient-family education, and discharge planning.

Standardized vs. individualized plans

Major differences of opinion exist in nursing concerning standardized and individualized plans of care. Opponents of standardization argue that it equals depersonalization. Advocates argue that standardization promotes efficiency, by limiting planning time without sacrificing quality, and fosters quality assurance. This disagreement cannot be resolved easily; however, this book combines the advantages of standard plans of care

with unusual features that help minimize their disadvantages:
• The plans blend standardized and individualized aspects of care. Standardization works better in some areas of care planning than others: problems, priorities, and interventions usually can be standardized, but outcome criteria, timing of interventions, and discharge criteria require significant individualization. This book takes these factors into account and encourages flexibility in areas that vary significantly among patients.
• Space is provided at the end of each problem for the nurse to add additional interventions and rationales specific to the individual patient's needs.

These unusual features challenge the nurse to think creatively. Because the resulting plan is pertinent and individualized, its clinical usefulness is ensured.

However, the most important point to remember in the debate over standardized versus individualized plans of care is that a plan of care does not cause depersonalized care; rather, the nurse's attitude is the culprit. The nurse who appreciates patients as individuals will use a standard plan as a starting point, staying attuned to the individual patient's responses while applying the art and science of nursing.

Why nurses will continue to use plans of care

Plans of care provide a valuable way to organize care, meet JCAHO's requirements for documentation, and prepare for site visits. In addition, many institutions have invested substantial time and money to develop systems of care planning appropriate for their patients. Before abandoning such systems, they would need to identify a better one and find the funds, time, and expertise to implement it—a difficult undertaking in this era of scarce resources. Finally, instructors in schools of nursing will continue to use plans of care as a method for teaching patient care because of the plans' comprehensiveness.

Ultimately, any plan of care is only as good as the nurse who provides the care. Conscientious nurses find plans of care a resource for learning new information quickly, refreshing their knowledge, and focusing their energy on the most important problems their patients may encounter. The contributors to *Medical-Surgical Care Planning,* Third Edition, have based their plans on a blend of clinical expertise, nursing diagnosis, and care planning — always keeping in mind the nurse on the front line. This book will provide welcome help for nurses facing the daily challenge of providing quality patient care.

Nancy M. Holloway

Part 1

Introduction

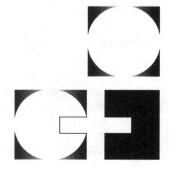

Trends and issues in health care and nursing

Major developments in American society and the health care industry are producing revolutionary changes in health care delivery. The most significant developments include our aging population (also known as the "graying of America"), chronic care, and restricted access to care. Other critical issues include the evolution of health care, its impact on the patient and on nursing, and opportunities for advanced practice.

POPULATION TRENDS: THE GRAYING OF AMERICA

By the year 2000, about 35 million Americans will be age 65 or older, with those age 85 or older constituting the fastest growing age-group. The percentage of elderly patients with disabilities is declining, partly due to the decline in diseases that cause disability in the elderly, such as stroke and heart disease. Despite this decline, however, the sheer number of people who are aging means that long-term disability will continue to be a major problem in our health care system.

Only about 5% of elderly citizens live in nursing homes; patients are usually discharged to their homes from the acute care hospital. Unfortunately, shorter hospital stays mean the nurse often doesn't have enough time to educate caregivers. Additionally, a patient over age 85 may have an elderly caregiver who also requires medical care or assistance with daily living.

Elderly patients require a range of services; the most important include home health care, homemaker or chore services, transportation, assistance with activities of daily living, nutrition services, and an emergency response system. Integration of these services is important but in many cases doesn't exist; nurses could help bridge this gap. The Program of All-Inclusive Care for the Elderly (PACE) is a good example of a program that delivers comprehensive care for the elderly. With 11 sites nationwide, PACE focuses on preventive care and maintaining function to avoid the need for costly inpatient care.

CHRONIC CARE

The intersection of an aging population and a health care system focused on acute care creates another trend: the increasing importance of chronic care. Chronic care consists of medical care, rehabilitation, and assistance with activities of daily living.

Several factors affect the health status of older Americans. These patients commonly have multiple chronic disorders. According to the American Association of Retired Persons, the most common disorders in those over age 50 are hypertension, arthritis, heart disease, hearing disorders, cataracts, sinusitis, orthopedic disorders, and diabetes — all chronic conditions that last for years. In addition, older people are at risk for receiving inadequate medical care because of poverty, forgetfulness, hearing or vision impairments, and transportation problems, among other factors. Finally, older people are at risk for experiencing unexpected adverse effects associated with complex drug regimens.

ACCESS TO CARE

About 41 million Americans (17.4% of the population) are uninsured, making access to care a major issue in our current health care system. Our nation's economic restructuring means that many higher-paying manufacturing jobs have been replaced by low-paying service sector jobs that don't offer benefits. Of all uninsured children, about 89% are in working families. Over the next 3 to 5 years, the working poor probably will have less access to care, and the safety net will continue to deteriorate.

"The whole issue of the uninsured is the Achilles' heel of the reshaping of our health care system by market forces," says Kathryn Duke, a researcher from the University of California, San Francisco, Institute for Health Policy Studies. The uninsured are less likely to seek care, so they are usually seriously ill when they finally do. Although some steps have been taken to achieve wider access to health care, the goals of universal coverage, a single-payer system, and a national health insurance plan will remain unrealized.

Doctors and nurse practitioners will increasingly control access to the health care system. However, their efforts to refer patients for specialized services will be hampered by spending caps and a limited number of specialists participating in insurance plans.

EVOLUTION OF HEALTH CARE

The evolution of health care will be characterized by reduced spending, increased governmental regulation, and changes in the site of health care delivery.

Reimbursement issues

Enrollment in managed care plans will continue expanding, especially among Medicaid recipients. Health care providers and plan administrators will continually seek the most cost-effective ways to deliver care. Prevention, case management, and rehabilitation will be emphasized.

The health care system will continue to reel from the reduced rate of Medicare and Medicaid spending. Medicare spending will be reduced by $115 billion over the next 5 years, with most of the savings coming from reduced payments to providers, hospitals, and health maintenance organizations (HMOs). Even more troublesome is the change in the payment system for home health care, until recently a fee-for-service system. As of January 1, 1998, Medicare (and to a lesser extent Medicaid) began using a prospective payment system to pay for home care. In response to this system, the home care field is likely to experience the same belt-tightening that has become common in many hospitals.

Government regulation

Government regulation will play an increasing role in the health care field. Already, state regulators are becoming more involved in policing managed care organizations (for example, by citing hospitals for violating federal laws against patient dumping). Pressure from lawmakers and consumer groups will continue to eliminate objectionable practices, such as excluding benefits for preexisting conditions or canceling the policies of patients with catastrophic illnesses. Managed care organizations will likely respond to consumer backlash and temper their approach primarily to avoid more restrictive legislation. Ongoing consolidation and mergers among health care facilities will form large hospital chains that will be monitored closely by the federal government for violations of antitrust laws. Vigorous federal prosecution of Medicare fraud will continue.

Site of care

Outpatient care and community programs — as opposed to inpatient acute care — have become popular sites of care. In the largest survey ever conducted of nurses' views on health care and nursing practice, the *American Journal of Nursing (AJN)* polled more than 7,000 nurses nationwide about patient care. This survey provides the best picture so far of the state of health care and nursing practice. More than half of the respondents reported that their health care organization had reduced the number of beds or closed units in the last year. Managed care is the major factor driving down hospital stays, with HMOs using an average of 34% less inpatient care. More community hospitals are likely to close, and job prospects for RNs in hospitals across the country are dwindling.

Outpatient services are taking greater responsibility for complex care regimens previously managed by inpatient services. For example, AIDS patients today receive more of their care in ambulatory facilities. The trend toward same-day and outpatient surgery — driven by managed care, improved anesthesia, and advances in pain management — means that patients are commonly back home a few hours after a procedure or treatment.

Professionals caring for these patients need a different approach and greater range of skills than they did a few years ago. The demands of maintaining quality care within a shorter period of time present a daunting challenge for nurses. These conditions require more critical thinking; the nurse needs an ability to establish relationships quickly as well as excellent patient assessment skills.

A patient's satisfaction with his care is directly related to his expectations of the experience. Preparation is one of the keys to achieving patient satisfaction. As one nurse notes, "Patients need to know that they're going to move through quickly. Patients think they're there for a day, but it's really a piece of a day; rarely is someone there 8 to 12 hours. That's information patients need to know up front — that they are being moved through not because we're rushing them but rather because criteria have been met and they are ready for discharge."

Consumers also are likely to see increased growth of long-term facilities. According to a survey by the National Center for Health Care Statistics, there has been a significant drop in the proportion of elderly people entering nursing homes.

"What we're seeing now is the diversification of long-term care," says David Kyllo, a spokesman for the American Health Care Association, which represents two-thirds of the nation's nursing homes. "Twenty-five years ago you had nursing homes doing the lighter care as well as the heavier care. Today, nursing homes have evolved to become the provider of more complex medical care. Lighter care has gone to assisted living or in-home care."

Nurses are likely to see an explosion of community-based programs, which are popular because most people want to live at home and because home care is cost-effective. Most nursing jobs will be in the community because of the increased need for health professionals in ambulatory care, home health, schools, and prisons. According to the American Medical Association, more than 80% of all health care takes place in the home. This shift in the site of health care requires a corresponding shift in the attitudes of health care professionals.

"Our hospital system in the past several decades has been built on an illness model: If you're sick, you go to the hospital," says Susan Odegaard Turner, a nurse who helped develop a guide for health care providers to assist nurses in making the transition to the new characteristics of health care. "Managed care is based on a wellness concept: You try to keep somebody out of the hospital and manage them in an off-site environment — an alternative site."

The shift of focus to ambulatory facilities is having a great impact on nurses, especially critical care nurses. Gloria McNeal, a critical care RN who has studied the role of critical care nurses in caring for patients beyond traditional institutional boundaries, found that "about 2 years ago…it became very clear to me that critical care was going to expand into the realm of high-tech home care." Patients are either bypassing the intensive care unit or leaving more quickly; the average length of stay is down from $3\frac{1}{2}$ days to $1\frac{1}{2}$ days.

Other opportunities for nurses are expanding. Nurses have more opportunities to provide care in nontraditional settings such as nurse advice lines; as independent contractors or employees of case management firms, such as workers' compensation, disability, or health insurance carriers; or as legal consultants for attorneys.

IMPACT ON THE PATIENT

Reduced spending, increased governmental regulation, and shifts in the site of care will impact the patient. Health care providers will need to focus more attention on patient satisfaction and patient education. The alternative health care trend will continue as patients seek relief from stress and pain.

Patient satisfaction

Paul Schyve, a senior vice president of the Joint Commission for the Accreditation of Health Care Organizations (JCAHO), says that "ten years ago, JCAHO based its assessments of the quality of care on standards like staffing and a facility's resources. Now JCAHO looks at other things, such as how healthy and satisfied patients are and how much their care costs." Patient satisfaction was evaluated in the American Hospital Association's "Eye on Patients," which surveyed 37,000 patients about the care they received in 1996 at 120 hospitals, clinics, or doctor offices. Among the significant concerns patients mentioned were having little say in their treatment, receiving inadequate information, and experiencing posthospital "abandonment." As Sharon Ostwald, director of the Center on Aging at the University of Texas-Houston Health Science Center, commented, "The focus is on getting the patient out of the hospital, and we've sort of lost track of who's going to take care of them the day they walk out the door."

Patient education

The last decade has brought three major changes in patient education: the increasing impact of technology,

change in the site of health education, and the increasing sophistication of health care consumers.

The Internet has improved access to health information for millions of people and is bringing together people with similar health issues in forums and chat rooms. Hospital-associated learning centers are providing "one stop" education for patients and family. One example, the Beth Israel Learning Center in Boston, provides printed material, videotapes, a consumer health database, and free access to the Internet. A growing number of hospitals now have web sites on the World Wide Web, delivering health care information through cyberspace. Ask-A-Nurse at St. Francis Hospital and Medical Center in Topeka, Kansas, allows users to E-mail questions to RNs.

Technology also is impacting the way care is delivered. Increasingly, phone-nursing experts are providing patients with information, advice, coaching and referrals to specialists, and in some cases providing care similar to case management. Employee Managed Care Corporation (EMC[2]) in Seattle, Washington, provides several types of nurse phone services:
• CareWise, a 24-hour-a-day service that covers decision support in areas of health and medicine
• CareSupport, which provides detailed teaching and support for those with chronic disorders
• Living Wise, which provides lifestyle management support
• CareWise Stat, which provides triage services.

State-of-the-art telemedicine systems (which use ordinary phone lines to transmit video, audio, and diagnostic information), such as the Personal Telemedicine System developed by American Telecare in Eden Prairie, Minnesota, allow nurses in an office to check a patient's blood pressure, pulse, and temperature; evaluate heart or lung sounds; and examine wound sites of a patient at home.

In many cases, the site of patient education has changed dramatically. Whereas most patient education previously occurred in the hospital, education now is occurring in doctors' offices, patients' homes, and cyberspace.

"Most hospitals are seeing 50% to 60% actual outpatients (those staying less than 23 hours). Another 20% of patients stay in the hospital a few days, and many of those are admitted following surgery," says operating room nurse Denise Geuder, Director of Cardiovascular and Surgery Services for St. Francis Hospital in Tulsa, Oklahoma. Because of the shortened stays, almost all preoperative teaching has to be done on an outpatient basis. Most nurses use a combined approach of a preadmission phone call or visit, instruction before and after the procedure, and a follow-up call 24 hours after discharge. The teaching process now begins earlier, in many cases in the doctor's office.

Because of increased media coverage and increased public awareness, patients now are beginning to take more responsibility for their health care choices. Most consumers, however, don't have the knowledge or skills to evaluate available information about health care facilities, for example, report cards that contain complicated information. The Agency for Health Care Policy and Research (AHCPR) is now sponsoring several studies to determine how consumers make health care decisions.

Alternative care
One intriguing development in health care is the widespread use of alternative health care. Millions of patients are turning to herbalists, acupuncturists, homeopaths, and chiropractors; over $13 billion is spent annually on such care. Among the reasons for its popularity is its ability to offer chronically ill patients relief from stress or pain that traditional Western medicine has not treated successfully. In addition, the growing multiculturalism of American society introduces health care practices that are mainstream in their culture of origin such as the use of acupuncture in Chinese medicine.

IMPACT ON NURSING
Changes in the health care system offer nurses both challenges and opportunities. Challenges include changes in the nurse-patient relationship and in job expectations and increased emphasis on collaboration. Nursing education and advanced practice nursing programs will provide additional opportunities for nurses.

Change in the nurse-patient relationship
"Nurses across the nation, in every setting and specialty, report that they're taking care of more patients, have been cross-trained to take on more nursing responsibilities, and have substantially less time to provide all aspects of nursing," according to the *AJN* survey. This reduction probably is due to a combination of factors, including cuts in the overall number of RNs, more patients assigned to each RN, shorter lengths of stay, and increased complexity of patient care. Nurses report having less time to teach patients, less continuity of care, an increase in unexpected readmissions (especially in emergency and psychiatric or mental health care), an increase in complications (especially in gerontology), and an increase in job-related injuries. The nurse's role has changed from providing direct care to managing nursing care and resources for a patient, according to Rita Turley, Regional Vice President of Patient Services for the Sisters of Charity of Leavenworth Health Services Corp., Montana Region. Clinicians need to be more adept at managing care rather than simply delivering services.

Change in job expectations
Nurses increasingly are expected to provide more services with fewer resources. They must be flexible and take on more supervisory responsibility. The increased responsibility for supervision is the result of two trends: the increased substitution of part-time or temporary RNs for full-time RNs and the substitution of unlicensed assistive personnel (UAP) for RNs. Of *AJN* survey respondents, about 87% reported that the introduction of UAPs has not improved the quality of patient care. (For more information, see *Pros and cons of the emerging nurse-patient relationship,* page 6.)

Increased emphasis on collaboration
A nationwide demonstration project, "Strengthening Hospital Nursing: A Program to Improve Patient Care," has given 20 health care institutions $1 million each over 5 years to show how collaboration can improve care. Collaboration among nurses and other professionals — rather than working in isolation or attempting to solve problems within a single discipline — is critical for success. Because nursing is too complex, and systems and technology change so quickly, old ways have to be modified — but they need to be modified in collaboration with other professionals, according to Sandra Robinson, acting director for the Center for Quality Measurement and Improvement at the AHCPR. This project also shows that nurses must articulate their contributions and communicate across disciplines. Overall, nursing's contribution to patient outcomes and hospital performance has not been well understood or documented. As a result, nursing is gradually refocusing its approach on outcomes.

Opportunities for advanced practice nursing
The shifting sands of the health care system offer many opportunities for nursing. An increased number of advanced practice programs are preparing nurse practitioners for new roles and new settings. The greatest opportunities involve promoting health, preventing disease, and managing patients through the entire continuum of care. In the area of health promotion, programs aimed at reducing lifestyle risk factors, such as those on obesity, smoking, exercise, nutrition, and family planning, will be areas of major growth. Other likely areas of growth include home health care, hospice nursing, and independent nurse clinics, particularly in rural and underserved areas. "Right now, people who have chronic problems have to integrate the care they receive from different providers themselves," points out Regina Herzlinger, Harvard Business School professor. Nurses could play a pivotal role in integrating patient care.

Pros and cons of the emerging nurse-patient relationship

According to most nurses, the nurse-patient relationship continues to evolve under managed care. One readily apparent change is the more vigorous role a patient plays, such as assuming responsibility for improving his condition by becoming an active partner in the collaborative efforts of the health care team.

Nurses, too, have witnessed changes in their roles. With family members commonly serving as the patient's primary caregiver, more and more nurses are seeing themselves as coordinators, coaches, patient advocates, and supervisors of others — including unlicensed assistive personnel — who provide some of the hands-on care that nurses once performed.

Nurses cite the following advantages and disadvantages of this emerging relationship.

Pros

• Greater emphasis on assessment, planning, educating, and co-ordinating

• Less task-based responsibility

• Opportunities to be more directly available to patients such as by phone

• Greater patient knowledge of and active participation in their care

Cons

• Less opportunity for direct, hands-on care

• More emphasis on delegation and supervision

• Less time for casual interaction with patients

• Fewer immediate rewards

Adapted with permission from Gray, B.B. "Issues at the Crossroads, Part 2: Managed Care Gives Rise to a New Nurse-Patient Relationship," *Nurseweek* 8(20):1, 22-23, October 1, 1995.

Nursing practice and education

Changes in health care practice will result in tremendous opportunities for nursing education. For example, nurses in acute care need immediate education about delegation and supervisory skills, stress management, and case management. Ambulatory care nurses need skills in assessment, prioritizing, and critical care. There could be a greater role for professional organizations to help the nurse adapt to health care restructuring. One forward-looking organization, the American Association of Critical Care Nurses, has put together a program, "Transitions in Health Care Program," to provide transition training to nurses.

Nurses also need to develop familiarity with federal, state, and local laws governing health care delivery. This is especially important as facilities experiment with various staffing mixes, some of which may endanger patients, such as using more UAPs than RNs can safely supervise during a shift. Also, because some nurses have been terminated for whistle-blowing over patient endangerment and free-speech activities, there must be a drive for laws to protect whistle blowers.

The nursing profession also must develop continuing education programs to allow nurses to move from acute care to ambulatory care. One idea involves developing "continuous learning centers" to allow 2-year graduates and others to obtain the training and preceptorships they will need to take on the emerging new roles in the profession, according to Judy Martin-Holland, president of the American Nurses Association-California. Nurses need to become computer literate, too, particularly if they are involved in teaching. Computer-assisted instruction is used in 90% of programs surveyed by the American Association of Colleges of Nursing, though computerization has barely begun in the care setting; an estimated 90% of health care information is still paper-based.

CONCLUSION

The next decade promises to be exciting for health care professionals. Major changes in American society and in the health care arena will offer professionals extraordinary opportunities for professional growth. Nurses can greatly improve their chances of success by becoming aware of and preparing for these major changes.

REFERENCES

Chalfant, A. "Are You Prepared for the Alternative Therapy Craze?" *Nurseweek* 10(8):1,6, April 14, 1997.

Chriss, L. "Video Calls Connect Home Care Nurses with Patients," *Nurseweek* 9(6):7, March 18, 1996.

"Congress Approves Budget with Drastic Medicare Cuts," *Nurseweek* 10(16):2, August 4, 1997.

Dunham-Taylor, J., et al. "Surviving Capitation," *AJN* 96(3): 26-29, March 1996.

Federwisch, A. "Caring for a Graying America," *Nurseweek* 10(8):1,7, April 14, 1997.

Gray, B. "Issues at the Crossroads, Part 2," *Nurseweek* 8(20):1, 22-23, October 1, 1995.

Gray, B. "Phone Nurses Go Beyond Triage," *Nurseweek* 9(23):1, 6, November 11, 1996.

Gray, B. "Which Way Now? Columbia's Woes Signal Big Changes," *Nurseweek* 10(19):1, 24, September 15, 1997.

Gray, B., and Federwisch, A. "Experts in Their Own Words: Health Care Leaders Predict the Future," *Nurseweek* 10(1): 22-23, January 6, 1997.

"Hospital Care Under Attack by Patients in AHA Report," *Nurseweek* 10(4):20, February 17, 1997.

Hudson, S. "Faster Surgical Care Demands Planning," *Nurseweek* 10(6):1, 24, March 17, 1997.

Hudson, S. "Gathering Hard Data on How Nurses Affect Quality," *Nurseweek* 10(19), September 15, 1997.

Mahlmeister, L. "What's Ahead for Health Care, Professional Practice," *Nurseweek* 8(1):26-27, January 1995.

Nelson, V. "Chronic Care Problems Will Grow as U.S. Ages," *Nurseweek* 10(15):1, 6, July 21, 1997.

Nelson, V. "Innovations Have Far-Reaching Effects," *Nurseweek* 10(1):1, 7, January 6, 1997.

Nelson, V. "Insurance and Health: What's the Link?" *Nurseweek* 10(10):1, 22, May 12, 1997.

"Nursing Home Admissions Drop While Population Ages," *Nurseweek* 10(4):19, February 17, 1997.

Paladichuk, A. "Gloria McNeal: Breaking Down the Walls: Critical Care at Home and on the Road," *Critical Care Nurse* 17(2): 94-99, April 1997.

Paladichuk, A. "Susan Odegaard Turner: Managing Transitions: A Proactive Approach," *Critical Care Nurse* 17(3):94-99, June 1997.

"Researchers Say Percentage of Elderly Who Have Disabilities Is on the Decline," *Nurseweek* 10(8):3, April 1997.

Shindul-Rothschild, J., et al. "10 Keys to Quality Care," *AJN* 97(11):35-43, November 1997.

Shindul-Rothschild, J., et al. "Where Have All the Nurses Gone? Final Results of Our Patient Care Survey," *AJN* 96(11):25-44, November 1996.

Sponselli, C. "Health Care Enters Cyberspace with Hospital Sites on the Web," *Nurseweek* 9(21):1, 23, October 14, 1996.

Sponselli, C. "Patient Education Meets Technology," *Nurseweek* 9(10):1, 24, May 13, 1996.

Wann, M. "Are Patients Ready to Shop for Their Health Care?" *Nurseweek* 10(1):1, 6, January 6, 1997.

Wann, M. "Searching for Quality Health Care," *Nurseweek* 10(3):1, 7, February 3, 1997.

Role of DRGs in delivering quality care

Medicare's prospective payment system (PPS) has dramatically altered the U.S. health care system. Faced with new restrictions and regulations affecting delivery of care, nurses increasingly have been confronted by twin challenges: sicker patients and shorter hospital stays. Nurses also play a key role in maintaining a hospital's financial viability in this competitive, market-driven health care environment. To maintain quality patient care under PPS, nurses have become increasingly sophisticated and innovative.

EVOLUTION OF PPS

Charges for hospital care used to be based on a retrospective method of payment. Hospital charges reflected what the market would bear and commonly were arbitrary, unrelated to the actual costs of delivering services. For the most part, nursing has been a nonbillable direct service that was bundled under room and board charges in the hospital bill. However, in recent years, third-party payers have demanded more explicit accounting for all services and appropriate charges for every area of health care delivery. In response, hospitals have begun to unbundle all units of service, including nursing.

As one of the nation's primary insurers, Medicare was the first to change its reimbursement method. PPS was an attempt to conserve the dwindling dollars in the Medicare trust fund set up in the 1960s to ensure health care access for America's elderly citizens.

Under Medicare's PPS, diagnosis-related groups (DRGs) were developed to identify clinically homogeneous groups of diagnoses that use similar tests, treatments, and services and therefore could be reimbursed at similar rates. This federal system is now mandatory for Medicare recipients at all acute care hospitals. Besides standardizing payment, this classification system was designed to put acute hospitalized patients into groups that could be used to predict resource consumption.

At present, 503 DRGs are grouped into 25 major diagnostic categories based on anatomic organ systems such as the respiratory system. The predetermined rate of reimbursement for each DRG is based on such factors as principal diagnosis, patient age, presence of complications or comorbidities, occurrence of an operating room procedure, and discharge type. All these factors are combined to determine which DRG will be assigned when the patient is discharged.

The DRG system is incongruous in many ways, the most important of which is that it does not consider the severity of the patient's illness. Thus, for two patients with the same illness (and therefore the same assigned DRG), a hospital would be reimbursed at the same rate even though one patient may be severely ill and need more services and a longer length of stay (LOS). DRGs are, in effect, an averaging system: A hospital loses money on cases whose cost of care exceeds the amount paid for the assigned DRG, and it makes money on cases in which costs are less than the DRG payment. Many patients who would have been hospitalized in the past are now treated as outpatients and, conversely, only patients who meet strict criteria may be admitted to acute care facilities. Hospitals, therefore, typically have sicker patients to care for than in the past, and patient care must be managed as efficiently as possible for a hospital to remain financially viable.

HOW DRGs ARE ASSIGNED

After discharge, a patient is assigned a DRG based on the following factors:
• principal diagnosis — the diagnosis that necessitated admission to the hospital
• secondary diagnosis — all secondary conditions that exist at the time of admission or that develop during hospitalization and affect the treatment or LOS
• operative procedures — any surgical procedures performed for definitive treatment rather than for diagnostic or exploratory purposes
• age — for some conditions, a different reimbursement rate applies for patients under age 17 than for those age 17 and over
• discharge status — whether the patient was discharged home or transferred to another hospital
• complications — any conditions arising during hospitalization that may prolong the LOS at least 1 day in approximately 75% of patients (such as diabetes)
• comorbidity — a preexisting condition that will increase the LOS at least 1 day in about 75% of patients.

All these factors need to be considered and the presence or absence of each factor determined to identify the correct DRG.

HOW DRGs ARE USED

Once the DRG has been determined, the administrator can identify further statistical measures affecting reimbursement, such as geometric mean LOS, relative weight, and outliers.

Geometric mean LOS

Each DRG has an assigned geometric mean LOS. The terms *geometric mean LOS* and *mean LOS* in this book refer to specific DRG statistical data for *groups* of patients. (The unqualified term *LOS* is a general abbreviation referring to an *individual* patient's LOS.) The geometric mean LOS is a statistical measure used in cost accounting solely to determine when a patient becomes a "day outlier" (see "Outliers" later in this entry).

The geometric mean LOS is an average derived from data that indicated the mean LOS for patients with specific diagnoses or undergoing specific procedures at the time the DRG system was updated. This has four important implications:

• The geometric mean LOS should be understood as an indicator of when most patients within each DRG *were* discharged during the period of data collection. It was never intended as a guide to determine when a specific patient *should* be discharged.

• Current hospital stays are significantly shorter than the geometric mean LOS. Since 1984, the actual LOS across the country for nearly every DRG has decreased dramatically as more patients receive treatment in outpatient facilities, in doctors' offices, and within a much shorter length of time in the hospital.

• The geometric mean LOS has nothing to do with the point after which a hospital loses money on a case. That point can be determined only after studying each case.

• In most cases, a hospital begins losing money before the geometric mean LOS is reached because actual costs of caring for the patient usually exceed the reimbursement rate before this point. This is partly because hospital costs have continued to increase as the actual LOS has continued to decrease.

Relative weight

Relative weight, a statistical term used in DRG reimbursement, determines the actual dollars a particular hospital is paid for a given DRG. Among other factors, it is based on categorizing the hospital as acute or chronic, teaching or nonteaching, and urban or rural. The weight assigned each DRG is reevaluated and revised regularly. Because relative weights vary greatly from hospital to hospital and area to area and because of periodic revisions, they are not specified in this book.

Outliers

An outlier is a case that uses more than its assigned resources. Two types of outliers exist — day outliers and cost outliers. A day outlier is a case that exceeds the geometric mean LOS by at least 17 days, on average. Although hospitals receive an additional payment for day outliers, payment never covers the costs or charges incurred during an extended LOS.

Day outliers were predicted to account for 5% of all Medicare discharges when PPS began. The latest data

suggest only 1.5% of discharges become day outliers. In most instances, day outliers are severely ill patients with multisystem failure. Preventing a patient from becoming a day outlier is rarely under the nurse's control.

A cost outlier is a case that doesn't exceed the allowed number of days but does exceed the expected cost. Cost outliers are even rarer than day outliers. This book doesn't include information on cost outliers.

KEYS TO SUCCESS UNDER DRGs

Several major factors affect a hospital's financial success under DRGs:

• accurate coding of all medical record data upon the patient's discharge. A medical records professional must choose the diagnosis that was chiefly responsible for the admission and take into account all of the factors, such as complications and comorbidities, that will place the diagnosis in the highest-paying category. The coder depends on the documentation in the medical record when assigning the DRG.

• effective and efficient management of the "products" of hospitals, such as hours of nursing care, laboratory tests, medications, supplies, and other services. The more efficiently care is delivered, the greater the hospital's profit.

• an appropriate "case mix" (a hospital's mixture of patients, defined by the severity of illness and assigned DRGs). A hospital must maintain a mixture of patients with various DRGs to plan and manage resource allocation within defined reimbursement parameters.

• using the appropriate site of care and LOS. Care will be reimbursed only if it's provided in the appropriate setting. For example, hospitals won't be reimbursed for care that could have been appropriately provided in an outpatient setting. LOS also must be appropriate. Although patients can be discharged only when medically stable, the hospital must ensure that only necessary costs are incurred.

• preventing complications. Because complications increase the likelihood that care costs will exceed reimbursement, their prevention is a key factor in maintaining fiscal control.

NURSE'S ROLE IN A PPS

The overall impact of government regulations and third-party payers on the health care delivery system presents the nurse with challenges and opportunities. Nurses are instrumental in ensuring both the quality of care and the hospital's financial success under any PPS. They can take several steps, as outlined in this section, to exert a positive impact on a hospital's bottom line while maintaining the quality of patient care.

Care planning

The nurse must be able to prioritize and deliver care within the projected LOS — which means establishing and following an explicit plan of care. Care planning is an essential means for determining goals and desired outcomes of care. Only through planning can care be managed effectively and efficiently. This book is designed to help the nurse provide quality care within the constraints of cost containment. Caring for a patient without a plan of care is like starting an unfamiliar trip without a road map. You may eventually reach the desired destination, but most certainly it will involve many unnecessary detours and increased time, effort, and money. This book identifies the "destination" of care — the patient outcome criteria — as well as the most direct routes for getting there.

Early discharge planning

The nurse must be involved in discharge planning from the moment of patient admission, whenever possible. By beginning early, the nurse can help ensure that the patient is ready for discharge. For example, the nurse can emphasize patient and family education, maximize the patient's self-care abilities, and arrange for continued care when indicated, such as through home care nursing or nursing home placement.

Patient education

Patient and family education is a key element in preventing readmissions. The patient's perception of quality care is also enhanced when the nurse promotes self-care and describes how to manage health problems after discharge.

Documentation

Accurate documentation promotes communication among caregivers, maximizing the benefits of hospitalization while minimizing the LOS. Also, documentation is crucial to receiving appropriate reimbursement for services. Documenting complications and comorbidities is particularly important because they have even greater significance now than in the past.

Quality assurance

Quality assurance is a mandatory element that should include establishing specific nursing standards and monitoring adherence to those standards.

Economics of health care

The nurse also needs to be aware of how the new economics of health care affects the professional status of nursing. This is a good time to advance the function and image of nurses as independent health care practitioners who can be judged not only on how they benefit patients but also on how they contribute to a hospital's economic viability.

RETROSPECTIVE REVIEW

Besides DRGs, other changes in health care delivery continue to increase the pressure to provide care in the most efficient manner possible. Health maintenance organizations (HMOs) and other competitive medical plans, now a major source for health care reimbursement, have been particularly important.

The nurse should be aware of the complexity of reimbursement methods. Most third-party payers (not just Medicare) use a prospective payment mechanism to reimburse hospitals. For example, many HMOs currently pay hospitals on a negotiated rate not unlike DRGs. Also, all third-party payers are negotiating discounted rates for services provided in acute care facilities in return for guaranteeing that their subscribers will use specific facilities for their acute care needs. Such arrangements are important for hospitals because they ensure a constant source of admissions. With LOSs much shorter than they were before PPS, hospitals must count on a stable census to ensure maximum efficiency and a constant cash flow.

For patients, incentives from PPSs to hospitals mean shorter stays and possibly fewer services. Because of perceptions of premature patient discharges and underuse of necessary services, state peer review organizations (PROs) were mandated to increase review of care provided in acute care facilities.

This mandate has led PROs to establish explicit review criteria for medical care. Within the DRG system, however, the Health Care Financing Administration and state PROs are developing and using generic and disease-specific criteria retrospectively to determine the appropriateness of admission and discharge and of the quality of care. Such information could be useful to nurses in care planning. Although PROs are reviewing only Medicare cases now, in the near future all hospital admissions, outpatient procedures, home care services, and care in doctors' offices and long-term facilities will be reviewed in a similar manner.

NURSING CHALLENGE

Today, the nurse faces greater challenges than ever with sicker patients requiring more complex care during shorter hospital stays. This book features the expertise of professional colleagues who understand the complexities of those challenges and who offer powerful help in meeting them.

REFERENCES

Health Care Financing Administration. "Rules and Regulations," Prospective Payment System, *Federal Register,* June 2, 1997.
St. Anthony's DRG Guidebook 1998. Reston, Va.: St. Anthony's Publications, 1997.

Nursing diagnosis

The American Nurses Association Social Policy Statement (1980) defines *nursing* as "the diagnosis and treatment of human responses to actual or potential health problems." The North American Nursing Diagnosis Association (NANDA) defines *nursing diagnosis* as "a clinical judgment about individual, family, or community responses to actual and potential health problems or life processes. Nursing diagnoses provide the basis for selection of nursing interventions to achieve outcomes for which the nurse is accountable." Although nurses have been diagnosing patient problems for years, the term *nursing diagnosis* is relatively recent.

CREATING A COMMON LANGUAGE

Past diagnostic efforts have been hampered by the lack of a common language for labeling nursing problems. To overcome this barrier, the National Conference Group on the Classification of Nursing Diagnoses began identifying and classifying health problems that nurses treat. That organization, formed at the first National Conference on Classification of Nursing Diagnoses in 1973, became NANDA. Periodically, NANDA releases a list of diagnoses accepted for study and clinical testing. The current list appears in Appendix D.

However, nurses have had difficulty with NANDA terminology. Many are frustrated by the categories' complexity, esoteric language, vagueness, wordiness, and differing levels of abstraction; some NANDA diagnostic labels are not clinically useful. Because the clinical experts who wrote the plans of care in this book found some NANDA diagnoses useful and others not, the editor made the following decisions:
• This book identifies nursing diagnoses using NANDA terminology whenever possible. If a diagnosis couldn't be found on the list to fit a patient problem that nurses treat independently, a new diagnosis was created.
• The official list is alphabetized by basic concept first, followed by modifiers, if any (for example, "airway clearance, ineffective"). In this book, diagnoses are modified to reflect usual conversational sequences.
• Because of its wordiness, "Alteration in nutrition: less than body requirements" has been replaced with "Nutritional deficit."

Two related issues have provoked substantial controversy and major differences of opinion within the nursing diagnosis community — the scope of nursing diagnosis and the possible renaming of medical diagnoses with nursing diagnostic language. This controversy stems, in part, from the continued difficulty nurses face in articulating the dimensions of their practice and, particularly, in differentiating it from medical practice.

Many nurses believe that nursing diagnoses should describe only the independent domain of nursing, the area of clinical judgment in which the nurse functions in a self-directed way to prescribe definitive therapy for human responses to health problems, achieving outcomes for which the nurse is accountable. Others believe that nursing diagnoses should address all areas in which nurses make clinical judgments, including those in which the nurse carries out medical treatments.

This book uses nursing diagnoses for the independent domain of nursing only. Several accepted nursing diagnoses, such as "Decreased cardiac output" and "Altered tissue perfusion," do rename medical problems; these are pathophysiologic manifestations of disease.

Renaming problems already defined by other disciplines simply perpetuates the confusion between nursing and medicine. In this book, such problems are clearly identified as *collaborative* problems requiring both medical and nursing interventions. They are named with familiar terminology, such as "cardiogenic shock" instead of "Decreased cardiac output," "ischemia" instead of "Impaired tissue perfusion," and "hypoxemia" instead of "Altered gas exchange."

In some cases, a nursing diagnosis fits a nonacute problem but not a related acute problem, such as "Fluid volume deficit." In a nonacute fluid volume deficit, independent nursing interventions, such as providing preferred fluids and encouraging fluid intake, are paramount. In an acute fluid volume deficit, however, medical interventions, such as ordering the insertion of an I.V. catheter and prescribing specific I.V. solutions, are paramount. In this book, "Fluid volume deficit" is used in the first situation and "hypovolemia" in the second for diagnostic clarity. The distinction between acute and nonacute may prove a fruitful path for exploration in further attempts to increase the clinical usefulness of nursing diagnoses.

REFERENCES

American Nurses Association, Congress for Nursing Practice. *Nursing: A Social Policy Statement.* Kansas City, Mo.: American Nurses Association, 1980.

Gordon, M. *Manual of Nursing Diagnosis 1997-1998.* St. Louis: Mosby–Year Book, Inc., 1997.

Gordon, M. *Nursing Diagnosis: Process and Application*, 3rd ed. St. Louis: Mosby–Year Book, Inc., 1994.

North American Nursing Diagnosis Association. *Nursing Diagnoses: Definitions & Classification 1997-1998.* Philadelphia: NANDA, 1996.

Using the plans of care

This book is intended as a guide for providing quality hands-on nursing care to patients, not as a substitute for the broad clinical knowledge found in more exhaustive nursing references. Consequently, these plans of care are designed to give you the maximum amount of clinically relevant information within a minimal number of pages. Every plan of care is divided into sections, each presenting a different type of information. Becoming familiar with the plans' basic format will enable you to use their practical information efficiently. Explanations of each section follow, along with specific recommendations for using the plans of care in practice.

DRG INFORMATION

Immediately after the title of each complete clinical plan, abbreviated *DRG information* appears, including:
• relevant DRG numbers (Some clinical disorders, such as myasthenia gravis, always have the same DRG. Others, such as circulatory disorders, are divided into several DRGs.)
• mean LOS for the disorder
• comments, if appropriate, designed to put the DRG into perspective.

Ideally, each plan of care would include the average LOS for the disorder to guide patient and family teaching and to provide a benchmark against which the nurse could assess the patient's progress toward discharge. Unfortunately, such information isn't available. However, this book provides the best substitute: the geometric mean LOS, a statistical measure used in cost accounting. Use this information to anticipate when teaching and discharge planning should be well under way and when maximum hospital benefit usually has been reached. Don't use the mean LOS as a target for discharge; doing so will almost certainly ensure that the hospital loses money. Instead, when the patient's needs permit, plan for an LOS shorter than the mean LOS. Remember that the mean LOS relates to discharge from the hospital, not transfer from one unit to another. Mean LOS information is updated periodically and published in the *Federal Register*.

INTRODUCTION

In *Definition and time focus,* the disease, surgical procedure, or patient problem on which the plan focuses is briefly discussed within a specific time frame. Surgical plans of care usually cover the immediate preoperative and postoperative phases of care. Medical plans of care focus on the most acute phase of the illness, the period in which the patient is most likely to be hospitalized in an acute care unit.

Etiology and precipitating factors lists factors that directly or indirectly contribute to the condition's development, grouped according to pathophysiologic mechanism when possible.

FOCUSED ASSESSMENT GUIDELINES

The assessment guidelines list specific findings common to most patients with the identified condition. The intent is to give you a vivid picture of the typical patient presentation.

The first assessment section, *Nursing history (functional health pattern findings),* presents subjective and historical data organized by Gordon's functional health patterns framework. (See *Functional health patterns.*) The health patterns represent 11 broad categories within the holistic wellness-illness system. Each of the health patterns provides useful parameters for assessing any patient. Because the emphasis of this section is on definitive or common findings, only those patterns with data relevant to the condition are included in the discussion of a specific disorder.

The second assessment section, *Physical findings,* presents typical objective findings for a patient with the identified condition. Physical findings are organized by body system, an option familiar to most nurses.

Diagnostic studies, the next assessment section, provides information regarding laboratory and diagnostic tests usually performed for the diagnosis and treatment of the specified condition. Not all the tests listed may be performed on a particular patient; individual factors affect what is actually ordered. However, the astute nurse is aware of the significance of studies and tests pertaining to the patient's condition and, when indicated, collaborates with the doctor to select such studies.

Finally, *Potential complications* lists the condition's most common complications. Because promoting wellness and preventing illness are now a significant part of nursing practice, the nurse must be aware of potential complications in order to intervene appropriately on the patient's behalf.

NURSING DIAGNOSES AND COLLABORATIVE PROBLEMS

This section begins with a feature new to this edition, called *Clinical snapshot,* that provides a sharp, concise

Functional health patterns

The following health patterns represent broad categories within the wellness-illness continuum. These categories focus on a person's functional abilities.

1. Health perception–Health management pattern
   - Perceived pattern of health and well-being
   - How health is managed

2. Nutritional-metabolic pattern
   - Food and fluid consumption relative to metabolic need
   - Pattern indicators of local nutrient supply

3. Elimination pattern
   - Patterns of excretory function

4. Activity-exercise pattern
   - Exercise, activity, leisure, and recreation

5. Sleep-rest pattern
   - Pattern of sleep, rest, and relaxation

6. Cognitive-perceptual pattern
   - Sensory-perceptual pattern
   - Cognitive pattern

7. Self-perception–Self-concept pattern
   - Self-concept pattern
   - Perceptions of self

8. Role-relationship pattern
   - Role engagement – family, work, social
   - Relationships

9. Sexuality-reproductive pattern
   - Patterns of satisfaction
   - Dissatisfaction with sexuality pattern
   - Reproductive pattern

10. Coping–stress tolerance pattern
    - General coping pattern and effectiveness
    - Effectiveness of the pattern in terms of stress tolerance

11. Value-belief pattern
    - Values, beliefs (including spiritual), and goals

Adapted with permission from Gordon, M. *Nursing Diagnosis: Process and Application,* 3rd ed. St. Louis: Mosby–Year Book, Inc., 1994.

picture of patient problems and the actions needed to resolve them. In the left column, it lists *Major nursing diagnoses and collaborative problems,* a brief itemization of key health problems that the nurse is likely to find in patients with the designated medical condition. Next, in the right column, it lists the corresponding *Key outcomes.* These outcomes, developed by clinical experts, provide specific guidelines for assessing the patient's readiness for discharge from the unit. They are particularly helpful when a rapid discharge or transfer decision must be made such as when the unit is full and a critically ill patient must be admitted from the emergency department. For critically ill patients, the criteria in this section supplement those in Appendix E, Critical Care Transfer Criteria Guidelines. The criteria are intended as a guide only; if a patient doesn't meet them, the health care team must make appropriate arrangements to fulfill any remaining needs.

Each clinical snapshot is then followed by the main body of the plan of care: the predictable patient health problems caused by the pathophysiology. Patients may have problems or be at risk for developing them. A problem is a condition with identifiable signs and symptoms that are present in all or most patients with the disorder. If the patient doesn't have signs and symptoms, but is at risk for developing a disorder, the problem is labeled "risk" (formerly called a "potential problem" in nursing diagnosis terminology).

Because nursing practice is based on both nursing and medical diagnoses, a patient problem is identified as either a *Nursing diagnosis* or a *Collaborative problem.*

Nursing diagnoses are those human responses the nurse identifies and treats independently. The nurse can prescribe nursing interventions that don't require other professionals' approval and can assume accountability for the patient's response. Plans of care that focus only on nursing diagnoses are indicated by an icon showing a circle in a box, symbolizing independent action.

Independent action

Collaborative problems are those that require the doctor and nurse to work together to meet desired patient outcomes. Although the doctor is accountable for definitive interventions, the nurse may initiate monitoring, implement medical orders, act under medically approved protocols, or institute measures to prevent complications. Disease-related plans of care are indicated by an icon showing two boxes joined to form a plus sign, symbolizing collaboration.

Collaboration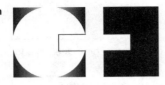

In most plans, the most important patient problems are presented first. However, some surgical procedure plans present preoperative problems first to provide logical flow.

After problem identification, the *Nursing priority* indicates the focus for the nursing interventions that follow.

Each priority is followed by specific *Patient outcome criteria,* defined as ideal expected patient responses to the interventions and grouped according to ideal time periods for achievement. These criteria, based on the clinical expertise of the nurses who contributed to this book, focus on specific, measurable patient responses that can guide the nurse in evaluating care. However, these criteria are intended only as a guide; individual variation is to be expected because outcomes depend on many factors.

Interventions and *Rationales* are presented in two columns. Interventions are based on clinical experience and nursing literature and thus represent a blend of practice and theory. The rationales are purposefully brief but incorporate relevant physiologic mechanisms whenever possible, along with other helpful data.

The most important interventions usually appear first. Interventions may be interdependent or independent in nature. Another health care provider, typically a doctor, initiates interdependent functions. However, whether acting under direct or indirect supervision or according to protocol, the nurse must use sound nursing judgment when carrying out an interdependent function. The nurse may initiate independent functions according to the terms of professional licensure and the particular state's nurse practice act.

Nurses have long recognized that patients respond best to care that takes personal characteristics and preferences into consideration. Consequently, space is provided at the end of each problem section for additional individualized interventions.

DISCHARGE PLANNING

The next section of the plan of care includes three guides for planning discharge and documenting care: *Discharge checklist, Teaching checklist,* and *Documentation checklist.*

The *Discharge checklist,* developed by clinical experts and a discharge planning expert, provides a brief summary of items that should be considered when planning for discharge.

The *Teaching checklist* ensures that the patient's and family's learning needs related to the condition have

been considered. Ideally, teaching should begin on or before admission and continue throughout the patient's hospital stay and convalescence. Because the plans focus on inpatient care, teaching interventions reflect only what may be reasonable to accomplish on the unit. Interventions related to teaching are interwoven throughout the plans or included in a special "Knowledge deficit" problem. (Refer to the "Knowledge deficit" plan for general teaching information.) The nurse can expect that various health care professionals, such as dietitians, doctors, clinical specialists, and social workers, will be responsible for different aspects of patient teaching, in addition to what the nurse provides.

Finally, the *Documentation checklist* provides a summary of items that should appear in the patient record. Changes in health care payment systems and Joint Commission on the Accreditation of Healthcare Organization requirements make thorough documentation more essential than ever. Accurate documentation also helps protect the nurse in the event of case-related litigation. However, now, as always, the best way to avoid legal problems is to maintain high standards of care, impeccable professionalism, and warm, caring relationships with patients.

ASSOCIATED PLANS OF CARE AND REFERENCES

Finally, each plan of care concludes with a list of *Associated plans of care,* which refers you to related plans found elsewhere in this book, and *References,* which can be helpful if you seek further information.

ORGANIZATION OF THE BOOK

This book presents two types of plans: general plans of care and plans of care for specific disorders. The general plans provide detailed interventions for common patient problems, such as pain, knowledge deficit, grieving, and dying. They're designed to be used with the diagnosis- or procedure-based comprehensive plans that constitute the main portion of the book. The plans for specific disorders contain the depth of detail appropriate for education and reference.

When using any of these plans of care in clinical practice, you may benefit from closely reading the plan first. Thereafter, you can refer to the plan each shift, addressing problems and documenting interventions in the nurse's notes. Before the patient is discharged, you can review the appropriate sections and evaluate all teaching and documentation, using the checklists as a guide.

Clinical pathways

The last decade has introduced far-ranging changes in the health care delivery system. Factors affecting health care delivery include the proliferation of PPSs, decreased financial resources for hospitals, an increasing number of elderly people, a shift from inpatient to outpatient care, and the AIDS crisis. As a result, health care has changed its focus from the process of delivering care to cost-effective patient outcomes. Interdisciplinary collaboration is critical to providing optimal care while conserving financial resources. The clinical pathway system is one approach to providing outcome-driven, interdisciplinary health care. The pathway documents the plan of care and expected patient outcomes within a given time frame. Providers can track variances from the planned outcome and make needed adjustments to improve future outcomes.

First introduced as a case management tool in the mid-1980s, it's known by a variety of names: critical paths, practice guidelines, clinical guidelines, clinical protocols or algorithms, practice guidelines, among others. This book uses the term *clinical pathway*.

BENEFITS OF CLINICAL PATHWAYS

A clinical pathway tracks patient progress in a managed-care system and outlines the typical course of care for patients with similar, uncomplicated problems. It functions as a blueprint or map of the key events a patient may experience during care, organized according to time and tailored to a particular facility. This approach focuses on patient outcomes and includes only the most important steps in care. It serves as a clear, compact practice pattern, reminding clinicians of the most current guidelines for care. It promotes critical thinking, enhances collaboration among disciplines, provides optimal patient outcomes, and saves money.

COMPLEMENT TO PLANS OF CARE

The clinical pathway is a logical evolution of the nursing plan of care because it integrates traditional plans of care with a focus on outcomes and interdisciplinary collaboration. Clinical pathways may include nursing diagnoses, but many don't, so independent nursing interventions may not be included (dependent and interdependent nursing actions are included). In addition, by definition a clinical pathway for a clinical population doesn't reflect comorbidities (coexisting clinical problems). To reflect clinical problems not included in the pathway, the nurse can use a standard pathway plus individualized nursing

diagnoses. According to Spath, a pathway can thus complement or replace the nursing plan of care.

BEST CARE, LOWEST COST

The goal of a clinical pathway system is to plan for the best care at the lowest cost by increasing collaboration and efficiency among clinicians and across disciplines, promoting timely use of hospital resources, reducing system breakdowns, and focusing the health care team's attention on important aspects of care and the most current interventions likely to have a positive impact on patient outcomes. According to Beyea, this system improves collaboration by improving communication and helping team members understand the intricacies of patient care and the pattern of progress for specific groups of patients. This outcomes-driven system helps health care providers offer consistent patient care and collect data for continuous quality improvement. The pathway can also serve as a streamlined documentation tool.

CONTENTS

The contents of clinical pathways are similar among institutions nationwide, but the organization of the contents may differ. Typically, the clinical pathway format consists of a time frame across the top of the page, with categories of data in a column along the left margin. The time frame may be measured in hours, days (the most common), weeks, or stages of care. The categories usually include assessments, tests, medications, other treatments, nutrition, activity, teaching, and discharge planning. Hydo states that some plans may include "decision points" at key periods in the plan. Typically, the decision points occur at the end of particular phases of care (such as the diagnostic phase) when different options may be considered. The intersection of these two frames provides activities sequenced in the most logical order and interventions specific for each day.

The clinical pathway for a particular patient is kept in a convenient location for all health care team members to use. One of the benefits of the clinical pathway is that it can be used on every shift to plan and monitor care. Specifically, the pathway can answer ongoing questions the nurse or other clinician has, including:
• What should be happening this shift?
• What is really happening?
• What isn't being done and why?
• How should the problem be fixed?
• Who will do it and when?

For peak effectiveness, a clinical pathway is used as part of the overall system of patient care. This shift from activities to outcomes in providing care requires a long-term commitment to improve patient care. (See *Elements of clinical pathway–based patient care.*)

The clinical pathway can serve as a streamlined interdisciplinary documentation tool; activities can be checked off as they are performed. Aronson and Maljanian state that the pathway also serves as the basis for documentation by exception. Documentation by exception is a method that emphasizes abnormal findings, which eliminates repetitive narrative notes about normal findings. Variances from the projected pathway can then be summarized for quality reviews.

DEVELOPING A PATHWAY

The process of developing a clinical pathway begins with the formation of a health care team, made up of professionals from all disciplines involved in a particular area of care. The team identifies the types of patients who require significant resources. Usually, this population is characterized by high cost, high volume, or high risk. The team may also target such populations to decrease variability in practice. Note that the clinical pathway approach isn't used for patients with comorbidities, complex medical issues, or unpredictable outcomes.

Pathway-related software and other products are commercially available. The committee needs to decide whether the cost of research, development, and implementation outweighs the purchase price and availability of packaged programs. If the team decides to proceed, it either creates pathways itself according to the following procedure or selects ready-made pathways based on a similar procedure.

Next, the team gathers information from such sources as professional literature, chart analysis, insurance reimbursement tables, and doctor practice patterns.

Ideally, the team uses benchmarks, "criteria... derived from organizations or communities which have been identified as models of the most effective and efficient practices," according to Aspling and Lagoe. Major types of benchmark data include community-based practice, research literature (especially useful because it summarizes a range of expert opinions), information from professional associations, and health care vendor studies. With these resources, team members identify desirable outcomes that represent realistic and measurable patient behaviors, and together the team determines the best way to manage that type of patient.

EVALUATING A PATHWAY'S EFFECTIVENESS

After piloting the pathway (typically for 6 months), the team evaluates and revises it and then implements it systemwide. Many factors are used to evaluate a pathway's effectiveness. An effective plan's organizational outcomes include a decrease in LOS and patient charges. Postdischarge complications, as measured by emergency department visits or hospital readmissions for the same disorder, should decrease or at least remain

---

Elements of clinical pathway–based patient care

Make sure the following statements describe your clinical pathway patient management strategy.

• Our clinical pathways are designed by a multidisciplinary team of health care professionals representing all the disciplines involved in caring for the patient for whom the pathway is being designed.

• Our clinical pathways aren't considered standards of care; they're considered a description of the important interventions of care the health care team believes will achieve the optimal outcomes (maximum quality and minimum cost).

• Variances from the pathway are expected and considered desirable when warranted by the patient's clinical condition.

• Our clinical pathways are used by all clinicians to guide patient management decisions and are readily accessible to them throughout the episode of care.

• Our clinical pathways are integral to the process of patient care and add value to the patient care experience for caregivers and patients.

• Our clinical pathway–based patient care process includes:

(1) a concurrent mechanism that affects changes in the process of care when a patient's response to care varies from the pathway without valid cause or (2) a system that allows the process of care to be revised when pathway variances are warranted.

• Pathway variance data aren't used in evaluating the competency of individual doctors or other caregivers.

• Pathway variance data are used in the aggregate to identify system breakdowns that require improvement to constantly improve patient care activities.

• Pathway variance data are correlated with patient outcome data and are used in the aggregate to support the clinical pathway "best care" hypothesis or to modify the pathway to reflect improvements in the "best care" hypothesis.

• Clinical pathways are regularly updated with the publication of new clinical practice guidelines, research studies, and other relevant practice parameters to ensure that they reflect the best available knowledge about patient management practices.

Adapted with permission from Spath, P. *Clinical Paths: Tools for Outcomes Management.* Chicago: American Hospital Publishing, 1994, p.15.

the same. Finally, patient and clinician satisfaction should increase. If a pathway is accepted by the medical community, it will help standardize doctor practices.

PATIENT TEACHING

Patient teaching is a crucial aspect of a clinical pathway. Ideally, the patient and family receive a simplified version of the pathway, which the nurse reviews with the patient daily. Standardized teaching protocols, described in the pathway, give the nurse detailed guides to teaching for both current needs and discharge needs. The nurse should review printed handouts with the patient and his family before discharge. Shorter LOSs make patient-teaching aids especially important because the patient may not be recovered enough at discharge to be ready for teaching. The nurse can review the handouts with family members, and the handouts can serve as a reference once the patient returns home.

VARIANCES

A variance is a deviation from the clinical pathway that causes a delay in achieving an expected outcome. It's detected when the patient doesn't progress as expected or when an expected outcome isn't achieved. Because documenting and analyzing every single variance is time-consuming and not cost-effective, significant variances — such as those that will prolong LOS, increase cost of care, or interfere with achieving expected outcomes — must be tracked.

Three different types of variance exist: patient, clinician, and system. A patient variance is a complication that affects care or discharge, such as a patient on a ventilator who develops pneumonia. A clinician variance is an intervention that isn't ordered (for example, a doctor's failure to discontinue oxygen when it's no longer needed). A system variance usually is an interdepartmental problem that prolongs stay such as lack of diagnostic testing on weekends.

It is important to detect, analyze, and correct variances, both for individual patients and for groups of patients. A three-step system is used to record and analyze variances, according to Esler, et al. The bedside nurse first identifies and documents the variance, either on the clinical pathway or, more commonly, on a separate variance form. This allows for prompt intervention in the clinical setting. Next, analyzing the clinical pathways variance helps providers find and eliminate system breakdowns. The person in charge of the pathway system analyzes problems for groups of patients, providing management with data to correct system problems. Finally, the interdisciplinary team that developed the pathway examines periodic reports and may revise the pathway if needed. Pathways also are updated regularly to incorporate developments in medical knowl-

edge. In this way, the data serves as the basis for continual quality improvement. Variance analysis is the key for fine-tuning the pathway and the system.

IMPLEMENTATION

To date, nursing literature has focused on the benefits of using pathways and the steps taken to construct them. Relatively little information is available on the issues involved, critical items to include in the pathway, the process of defining outcomes, variance measures, or implementation difficulties, according to Little and Whipple.

Spath provides one useful categorization of the causes of breakdown in an organization's efforts to implement a clinical pathway system. Acceptance of the pathway system by doctors is crucial. Other potential causes of breakdown include lack of interdisciplinary acceptance, lack of leadership (especially failure to define clear goals), and unrealistic time frames for designing and implementing pathways. Spath estimates that the time necessary to produce one well-designed, interdisciplinary clinical path ranges from 1 month to 1 year.

CONCLUSION

Clinical pathways are in a state of evolution. Their widespread use in hospitals nationwide marks a growing awareness that health care delivery has changed dramatically in the last decade. Clinicians' acceptance of patient care systems based on clinical pathways highlights their growing awareness that collaboration is the keystone of optimal patient care.

REFERENCES

Aronson, B., and Maljanian, R. "Critical Path Education: Necessary Components and Effective Strategies," *The Journal of Continuing Education in Nursing* 27(5):215-19, September-October 1996.

Aspling, D., and Lagoe, R. "Benchmarking for Clinical Pathways in Hospitals: A Summary of Sources," *Nursing Economics* 14(2): 92-97, March-April 1996.

Beyea, S. *Critical Pathways for Collaborative Nursing Care.* Menlo Park, Calif.: Addison-Wesley-Longman Publishing Co., 1996.

Esler, R., et al. "Patient-Centered Pneumonia Care: A Case Management Success Story," *AJN* 94(11):34-38, November 1994.

Hydo, B. "Designing an Effective Clinical Pathway for Stroke," *AJN* 95(3):44-51, March 1995.

Little, A., and Whipple, T. "Clinical Pathway Implementation in the Acute Care Hospital Setting," *Journal of Nursing Care Quality* 11(2):54-61, December 1996.

Mosher, C., et al. "Upgrading Practice with Critical Pathways," *AJN* 92(1):41-44, January 1992.

Spath, P., ed. *Clinical Paths: Tools for Outcomes Management.* Chicago: American Hospital Publishing, 1994.

Villaire, M. "Jill Ley: Putting Critical Pathways on the Map," *Critical Care Nurse* 15(3):106-13, June 1995.

Part 2

General plans of care

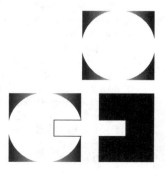

Dying

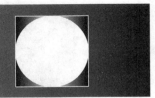

INTRODUCTION

Definition and time focus
Death, according to Dr. Elisabeth Kübler-Ross, is "the key to the door of life." An awareness of death's inevitability and the contemplation of our fears and feelings about it can lead to a heightened appreciation for life and a more courageous and thoughtful response to its challenges. Nurses deal with death daily and thus have repeated opportunities to assist dying patients and their families.

More than any other professional, the nurse has close and continuing contact with patients, direct experience with those who die, and concern for meeting the emotional and physiologic needs of patients and their families. Death remains the "great unknown," but the patient and loved ones have the right to continue sharing life until the end; the nurse can help. This plan focuses on the needs of the dying patient and the bereaved family in the hospital setting.

Etiology and precipitating factors
Death may result from:
• disease (or, occasionally, complications of the treatment of disease)
• injury or accident
• debilitation
• suicide or homicide.

FOCUSED ASSESSMENT GUIDELINES

Nursing history (functional health pattern findings)
Because etiologic factors vary so widely in dying persons, no typical findings exist. Thus, this section presents an assessment guide to assist the nurse in planning care for the patient who is admitted with a diagnosis suggesting impending death. However, no such guide is appropriate for all patients. The answers to the following questions may help the nurse intervene effectively on behalf of the dying and their families, but the nurse must use professional judgment in deciding what, when, and how much to ask a patient.

Health perception–health management pattern
• Is the patient aware of the prognosis? If so, for how long? If not, whose decision was it not to tell him?
• If not aware of the prognosis, what does the patient believe is the reason for hospitalization?

• What measures were taken to help support or improve the patient's physical or emotional condition before this hospitalization? Does the patient believe they have helped? If so, how?
• What are the patient's expectations about this hospital admission and the proposed treatment?

Nutritional-metabolic pattern
• Does the patient have any dietary preferences or intolerances?
• Has the patient been anorexic, vomiting, or dysphagic?

Elimination pattern
• What is the patient's present elimination status and pattern?
• Are any elimination aids currently used?

Activity-exercise pattern
• What is the patient's current activity level and tolerance?

Sleep-rest pattern
• What are the patient's present sleeping habits?
• Does the patient feel rested? If not, why?

Cognitive-perceptual pattern
• Does the patient have pain? If so, how severe is it?
• Is the patient's pain controlled? If so, by what?

Self-perception–self-concept pattern
• Which events or achievements have brought the patient the most satisfaction?
• What does the patient most want to accomplish before dying?

Role-relationship pattern
• Who are the patient's significant others?
• Among these, has the patient any long-standing, unresolved conflicts or other "unfinished business"?
• Has the patient been able to talk about dying and death with loved ones?
• How are loved ones handling the situation?

Coping–stress tolerance pattern
• If aware of the prognosis, how is the patient coping?
• What resources are available to help the patient cope?

Value-belief pattern
• What is the patient's religious or spiritual orientation?
• What does the patient believe about death?

Physical findings
Physical findings in dying patients vary widely, depending on the cause of impending death; see the plan related to the patient's specific disease or condition.

Diagnostic studies
See the plan related to the patient's specific disease or condition.

CLINICAL SNAPSHOT

DYING

Major nursing diagnoses	Key patient outcomes
Fear	Identify specific fears.
Powerlessness	Participate in decisions related to care.
Personal identity disturbance	Maintain preferred coping behaviors.
Risk for spiritual distress	Maintain personally meaningful spiritual practices, if desired.
Risk for pain	Describe pain level as being less than the goal level (typically less than 3 on a 0 to 10 pain rating scale).
Risk for fluid volume deficit	Experience minimum discomfort related to dehydration.
Altered family processes	(The family will) share concerns with the patient and each other.
Family coping: Potential for growth	(The family will) make contact with support persons.

NURSING DIAGNOSIS

Fear related to potential pain, loss, emotional upheaval, and the unknowns of dying

Nursing priority

Promote identification of and confrontation with specific realistic fears.

Patient outcome criteria

According to individual readiness, the patient will:
• identify specific fears
• express feelings, as desired
• use appropriate resources.

Interventions

1. Examine personal fears and feelings about death. Before involvement with the dying patient and the family, identify previous experiences with death, and be aware of personal emotions, religious or spiritual beliefs, and fears. If talking about death is too uncomfortable, refer the patient and family to another professional with the necessary skills.

Rationales

1. A caregiver's personal feelings about and experiences with death affect the ability to promote healthy emotional responses. While most health care providers feel some anxiety over discussing dying and death with their patients, nurses who have difficulty with issues of death are less able to empathize with the patient and family. Appropriate referral allows emotional needs to be addressed.

2. Assess the patient's coping style and previous experience with deaths of relatives or friends. Observe patient behaviors, and confer with the family and other caregivers as needed.

2. Each person responds differently to the threat of death. When threatened, most people initially revert to familiar coping mechanisms, and caregivers must be aware of these in establishing therapeutic communication. Previous experiences with death do much to shape behavioral responses and may contribute significantly to the patient's overall ability to cope.

3. Use role modeling to facilitate expression of feelings, as appropriate: "If I were facing what you face right now, I think I might feel scared (or 'angry' or 'depressed')."

3. The patient may need "permission" to discuss fears. Opening discussion by focusing on the caregiver's feelings allows the patient the option of responding with an expression of personal feelings (if ready) and reassures the patient that such feelings are normal and acceptable. For some patients, expression of fears reduces their impact.

4. Support coping mechanisms. Avoid forcing the patient to confront emotional issues.

4. Each patient moves through various stages, at various times, in coping with death's ultimate threat to individuality. Forcing issues is counterproductive and may damage the therapeutic relationship. Showing respect for the individual promotes trust.

5. As indicated by the patient's responsiveness to role modeling, help the patient identify specific fears and prioritize them. Acknowledge the unknowns.

5. Identification of specific fears helps reduce the sense of overwhelming threat. Pain, loss of control, and being a burden to others are common fears of dying patients; identifying fear-causing factors allows a patient to begin making specific plans to cope with them. Acknowledging unknowns reassures the patient that the caregiver recognizes the enormity of the questions faced.

6. Identify the patient's support system and resource base. Coordinate involvement of patient, family, and other members of the health care team in making plans to deal with anticipated problems and needs.

6. Coordination of resources and support for the patient is essential in reducing the sense of isolation, which contributes to fear. The nurse's "in-between" position can help facilitate teamwork.

7. As needed, provide appropriate referrals, such as to a psychiatric liaison nurse, social worker, hospice, chaplain, or support group related to the specific disorder.

7. The patient and family may not be aware of available resources. Even if referrals aren't used, knowledge of their availability can be comforting.

8. Provide companionship when possible.

8. Simply sitting quietly beside the patient communicates concern and may decrease the sense of isolation.

9. If the patient is confronting imminent unexpected death (for example, as a result of trauma), provide brief, clear explanations and offer to call a member of the clergy. Provide a support person for the family, and — if at all possible — allow a family member to see the patient before death.

9. Even in the emergency care setting, patients have the right to caring communication, which may help reduce fear. Survivors of near-death experiences report hearing conversation and being aware of activity around them even when they appeared unresponsive. Surviving spouses of victims of sudden death list their need to see their spouse during resuscitation or before death as the concern that produced the most anguish for them.

10. Additional individualized interventions: _____

10. Rationales: _____

Nursing diagnosis

Powerlessness related to inevitability of death, lack of control over body functions, and dependence on others for care

Nursing priority

Increase the patient's sense of personal power while promoting acceptance of the condition.

Patient outcome criteria

According to individual readiness, the patient will:
• participate in decisions related to care
• verbalize inner strengths
• set realistic goals
• initiate activity to put affairs in order.

Interventions

1. Encourage personal decision making whenever possible. Allow maximum flexibility for scheduling activities, treatments, or visitors. Include the dying patient in making care-related decisions, as appropriate.

2. Recognize and support courageous attitudes.

3. Accept personal powerlessness to alter the fact that the patient is dying.

4. Help the patient identify inner strengths. Ask the patient to recall past losses: How did the patient deal with them? What did the patient learn from them?

5. Encourage the patient to establish realistic goals for the remainder of life.

6. Know the wishes of the patient in regard to end-of-life treatment decisions. Ensure that a copy of formal documents (living will or durable power of attorney for health care) is placed in the patient's medical record.

7. Assist the patient, as needed, to put affairs in order — for example, planning the funeral and memorial, writing a will, settling economic affairs, and making arrangements for survivors.

8. Additional individualized interventions: _____

Rationales

1. Patients relinquish many freedoms, regardless of the reason for their hospitalization. Allowing as many choices as possible promotes a sense of control and increases the patient's coping ability. "Taking over" by caregivers diminishes the patient's self-esteem and should be avoided unless absolutely necessary.

2. Regardless of external circumstances, individuals maintain the freedom to choose their attitude and approach to life and death. Acknowledgment of courageous attitudes reinforces feelings of self-worth.

3. Health care professionals usually are anguished when they can't save their patients. Realistic self-assessment is essential to prevent caregiver burnout and to maintain the potential for effective intervention in areas that can be altered.

4. Recalling other losses may help the patient build on previously learned coping skills. Losses throughout life may have uniquely provided the individual with qualities that can be used in facing death.

5. Establishing goals provides a focus for energy and reduces helplessness. Realistic evaluation of capabilities helps acceptance.

6. Patients have the right to decide that cardiopulmonary resuscitation, mechanical respirators, or any other life-prolonging procedures that would only artificially prolong the dying process be withheld. If unable to make these decisions, the patient may have appointed an agent (family or friend) to make these health care decisions.

7. Putting affairs in order increases the patient's sense of control and may help soften the anticipated effects of the death on loved ones. "Unfinished business" may interfere with the patient's ability to move through coping stages.

8. Rationales: _____

General plans of care

NURSING DIAGNOSIS
Personal identity disturbance related to imminent threat of death

Nursing priority
Help the patient maintain and enrich personal identity throughout the remainder of life.

Patient outcome criteria
According to individual readiness, the patient will:
• maintain preferred coping behaviors
• recall and review life experiences
• participate in creative activity (as able)
• touch family members freely, if desired.

Interventions

1. Use active listening skills, paying special attention to nonverbal or symbolic communication. Use reflective statements and open-ended observations to offer an opportunity for discussion of difficult issues.

2. Accept and respect the patient's right to use denial or avoidance behavior. Whatever the patient's response, try to communicate your understanding.

3. Be honest with the patient in answering questions, but don't force discussion of issues the patient hasn't introduced or to which he hasn't responded. Take care to maintain hope for meaningful experiences.

4. Encourage reminiscence and review of life experiences.

5. Promote creative expression. Encourage family and friends to provide materials the patient can use for drawing, painting, writing or other creative pursuits, or obtain materials from the occupational therapy department.

6. Explore the option of preparing audiotaped or videotaped messages or mementos for family and friends to share after the patient's death (or earlier, if the patient wishes).

Rationales

1. A patient facing death may use nonverbal or symbolic communication to describe experiences and to test another person's willingness to talk about them. Rushed or distracted behavior from caregivers may distance the dying patient and contribute to feelings of alienation. Active listening and sharing show concern and respect for the patient as an individual.

2. The patient may choose to use denial or avoidance to the end; if so, respect this choice. In addition, denial correlates with longer survival, according to research.

3. Honesty, even when truths are painful, reflects respect for the patient as an individual. However, the patient has the right to choose which issues to discuss. Research suggests that hopelessness correlates with poorer prognosis.

4. Life experiences have helped to shape the patient's unique identity. Reminiscence helps the patient remain connected to important core experiences and provides the caregiver with additional information that may aid in understanding the patient's behavior and response to family needs.

5. Creative activity gives voice to individual expression, helping the patient maintain a sense of uniqueness. Also, drawings, paintings, or other original work may provide clues to the patient's state of acceptance.

6. The patient may feel more comfortable expressing feelings in this way. The process of recording helps achieve acceptance of impending death. Such mementos may offer the patient comfort in sensing that some aspect of individual identity will endure. These records may also be valued by families in preserving the memory of the loved one.

7. Use touch generously when providing care, unless it makes the patient uncomfortable. Encourage family affection, including holding, rocking, and even lying next to the patient.

7. Illness and hospitalization may reduce the frequency of physical contact with others, which normally helps provide body image self-definition. Encouraging family affection helps maintain physical contact. Also, touch provides comfort and communicates genuine caring more effectively than almost any other measure.

8. Additional individualized interventions: _____
_____

8. Rationales: _____
_____

NURSING DIAGNOSIS

Risk for spiritual distress related to confrontation with the unknown

Nursing priority

Help the patient savor the remaining period of life and identify meaning in impending death.

Patient outcome criteria

Throughout the remainder of life, the patient will:
• maintain personally meaningful spiritual practices, if desired
• find pleasure in some activities.

Interventions

1. Support the patient's personal spiritual beliefs, even if they seem unusual or unfamiliar.

2. Recognize that facing death and dealing with separation are developmental tasks for all humans. Promote a focus on growth and learning, rather than on disease or injury.

3. Acknowledge what dying patients have to teach others, and express this to the patient and family, when appropriate.

4. Provide privacy according to the patient's wishes.

5. Offer to call the spiritual adviser of the patient's choice — for example, a member of the clergy, counselor, or friend. Obtain and provide religious texts and other inspirational readings if requested.

Rationales

1. Spiritual beliefs provide comfort based on specific personal meaningfulness to the patient. Attempting to alter such beliefs or supplant them with others shows lack of respect for the patient's choices and may precipitate undue conflict and distress.

2. Because our culture places such emphasis on youth, we lack the societal integration of death as part of life that many other cultures take for granted. To help a patient accept impending death, caregivers must acknowledge it as a stage of development and validate its importance. Non-disease-related interventions (discussed throughout this plan) help redirect coping efforts toward positive life closure.

3. Nurses can learn much from dying patients that may help in caring for others. In this way, dying patients may touch the lives of others they will never meet. Recognition of the lessons a dying person may pass on to others can help the patient find meaning in death and a sense of connectedness with life.

4. The hospital environment may allow the patient minimal time to be alone. A patient struggling with spiritual issues may need uninterrupted time for prayer or meditation.

5. A spiritual adviser may provide guidance or perform rituals the patient views as essential. Religious readings may be satisfying to a patient with a traditional religious orientation, although others may find comfort in nonreligious literature that has special personal significance.

General plans of care

6. Explore the possibility of organ donation, if appropriate, with the patient and family. Be familiar with hospital and regional policy and procedures for arranging donation of organs. Consider the underlying disease before discussing donation of specific organs.

6. Patients and families can find meaning and consolation in knowing others may benefit from organ donation. Many programs now have broad interlinking systems for identification of donors and transplantation of donated organs. Underlying disease may make some organs unsatisfactory for donation, but others (such as skin) typically are usable and may not require immediate transplantation.

7. Address the patient while providing care, even if the patient appears unresponsive or comatose. Encourage family members to continue talking to the patient.

7. Survivors of near-death experiences and persons who recover from deep or prolonged coma have reported remembering conversation that took place around them while they were apparently unconscious.

8. Worry less about saying the "wrong thing" than about being afraid to communicate caring. In this way, set an example that family members may follow.

8. Because of prolonged close contact with dying patients and interaction with their families, nurses are uniquely suited to help facilitate dialogue about dying between the patient and family. In many cases, patients and families are afraid to raise the subject directly, out of concern that they may cause emotional upset. The nurse may be able to act as a liaison to help communication, thereby reducing guilt and anxiety and further preparing the patient and family for separation.

9. Maintain a positive attitude. Promote activities that provide even a few moments of enjoyment. Avoid generalizations that attempt to explain the patient's suffering.

9. The caregiver's positive attitude may help the patient maintain hope and find pleasure in living even while approaching death. Small pleasures may be extremely meaningful when the patient's world view is narrowed by illness. Generalizations or attempts to provide simplistic explanations (for example, "It may be a blessing") indicate shallow appreciation for the patient's situation and may be interpreted as dismissal of real concerns.

10. Additional individualized interventions: _____
_____

10. Rationales: _____
_____

Nursing diagnosis

Risk for pain related to underlying disease or injury

Nursing priority

Relieve pain, if present, while allowing the patient to remain as alert as possible.

Patient outcome criteria

Throughout the hospital stay, the patient will:
• participate in decisions regarding pain control (to the extent possible)
• describe his pain level as being less than the goal level (typically less than 4 on a 0 to 10 pain rating scale).

Interventions

1. See the "Pain" plan, page 88.

Rationales

1. This plan provides interventions useful for any patient in pain.

2. Assess the patient's level of discomfort frequently. Use pain scales as a concrete means for the patient to describe the pain. Compare his current level of pain with the goal level (typically less than 4 on a 0 to 10 pain rating scale). Urge calling for medication before the pain becomes severe.

3. To the extent possible, include the patient in decisions regarding pain medications.

4. When possible, control pain with oral medication, rather than with intramuscular (I.M.) injections. If the patient is unable to tolerate oral medications, consider arranging for I.V. injections or infusions or subcutaneous injections or infusions. Investigate analgesic combinations, such as long- and short-acting medications or narcotics and nonsteroidal anti-inflammatory drugs (NSAIDs).

5. Recognize that the usual safe dose levels may not apply to the terminally ill patient. Consult the doctor if the ordered dosage no longer seems effective.

6. Assess for psychological factors that may exacerbate pain, and intervene to treat them.

7. If abdominal distention causes pain, consider using return-flow enemas. Ensure that routine stool softeners or laxatives have been prescribed, as indicated by the patient's condition.

8. Additional individualized interventions: _____

2. A patient's level of discomfort has a significant impact on the emotional adjustment to limited life expectancy: Patients with poorly controlled pain tend to have more difficulty coping with other issues. Pain scales, used with other modes of subjective and objective assessment, can provide valuable confirmation or suggest the need to reevaluate assumptions about the patient's pain. Medication given early in the pain cycle is more effective.

3. Ability to control pain allows the patient to use limited energy for other, more rewarding, purposes.

4. Repeated I.M. injections, particularly in the debilitated patient, traumatize skin and gradually become less effective as areas of scarring develop and inhibit absorption. Analgesic combinations may achieve better control over chronic and acute pain episodes. NSAIDs may be effective for bone pain. Around-the-clock medication administration may be required for effective pain control.

5. A patient maintained on narcotic analgesics for an extended period may develop significant tolerance and require amounts of medication considerably larger than the usual dosage to achieve comparable effects.

6. The pain threshold may be lowered by boredom, anxiety, and loneliness.

7. Narcotic analgesics, lack of activity, and resultant slowing of peristalsis may cause painful abdominal distention and constipation. Gentle return-flow enemas may reduce discomfort. Medications can contribute further to constipation, and stool softeners or laxatives may be required regularly.

8. Rationales: _____

Nursing diagnosis

Risk for fluid volume deficit related to anorexia and dehydration associated with imminent death

Nursing priority

Promote patient comfort during the dying process.

Patient outcome criterion

During the final phase of the dying process, the patient will experience minimum discomfort related to dehydration.

Interventions

1. Avoid vigorous fluid replacement for terminally ill patients. Respect patient wishes regarding hydration and artificial feeding.

Rationales

1. Dehydration is normal in terminal illnesses. I.V. hydration or artificial feeding may unnecessarily prolong discomfort. Patient wishes regarding hydration and artificial feeding must be honored.

General plans of care

2. Offer frequent mouth care, ice chips, sips of water, or hard candy, as indicated by the patient's condition.

3. Provide meticulous skin care. Use soap sparingly and lotion generously if dry skin is present. Turn the patient carefully to prevent shearing.

4. Additional individualized interventions: _____
_____

2. These measures may help reduce discomfort related to mouth dryness and minimal oral intake.

3. Dehydration and debilitation contribute to poor skin turgor and increased risk of skin breakdown. Soap dries skin, increasing irritation. Gentle massage with lotion and careful turning demonstrate care and help prevent complications.

4. Rationales: _____
_____

Nursing diagnosis

Altered family processes related to imminent death of a family member

Nursing priority

Promote family integrity by facilitating healthy coping, mutual support, and communication with the dying person.

Patient outcome criteria

- Throughout the patient's hospital stay, the family will:
  - participate in care
  - share concerns with the patient and each other
  - appear well rested most of the time.
- Throughout the hospital stay, the patient will exhibit minimal anxiety over the family's well-being.

Interventions

1. See the "Ineffective family coping: Compromised" plan, page 63.

2. Assess the family's level of acceptance and coping by observing behaviors and interactions of individuals with the patient and by providing time for private discussions with family members, as needed. Be alert to differences among individual family members and clues to the family's previous experiences with death, if any.

3. Liberalize visiting policies, as needed. Allow private time for the family to be with the patient. Encourage family members to participate in care, remaining alert for signs of possible anxiety or discomfort.

4. When possible, facilitate family dialogue, remaining aware of established family roles and expectations. Offer to introduce topics, as appropriate; strive to promote face-to-face communication when possible.

Rationales

1. This plan provides guidelines for helping families at risk for crisis.

2. Effective intervention must be appropriately correlated with the stage of acceptance. Each member of the family may respond differently to the threat of loss. Previous family deaths may affect members' ability to cope in mutually supportive ways.

3. Family integrity is more likely to be maintained when members are able to continue their usual level of contact with one another. Helping with patient care reduces the family's sense of helplessness and provides special comfort to the patient. However, this shouldn't substitute for the nurse's cultivation of close involvement with the patient and family. The nurse must avoid giving the impression of dismissing or neglecting the patient.

4. Discussing issues surrounding death is difficult for most families and may be compounded by unresolved conflicts, guilt, or role demands. The nurse may be able to open up communication about sensitive issues. Family stability is related to long-standing patterns of behavior, so interventions that are at odds with these will be unsuccessful. Direct communication promotes maximum understanding and helps minimize later guilt over things left unsaid.

5. Be aware of cultural attitudes that may affect family response.

5. Every culture views death in a different way. Some observe specific rituals for the occasion; some emphasize withdrawal from others. Being aware of such differences helps the nurse plan interventions to support the family's cultural heritage.

6. Help the family identify and mobilize external resources, such as friends, clergy, counselors, and financial resources. Provide referrals to a psychiatric clinician or social worker or for pastoral care, as needed.

6. A family coping with death, especially if the dying is prolonged, may require added support to deal with stresses. Other professionals may offer such assistance as spiritual or psychological counseling, temporary housing placement, and guidance in identifying programs to help with the financial burden of care.

7. Encourage family members to maintain their physical and emotional strength. Emphasize the importance of adequate rest, food, and exercise. Suggest that family members take turns at the bedside if they are reluctant to leave the patient unattended.

7. Maintenance of physical and emotional well-being is essential if family members are to continue providing support for the patient and each other. "Break times" help the family maintain contact with external resources and reduce the emotional strain of constant attendance to the dying person's needs.

8. Additional individualized interventions: _____

8. Rationales: _____

General plans of care

NURSING DIAGNOSIS

Family coping: Potential for growth related to bereavement and mourning

Nursing priority

Facilitate the initiation of healthy grieving after death.

Patient outcome criteria

Before survivors leave the hospital, they will:
• view and touch the body, if desired
• express initial grief or disbelief
• make contact with support persons.

Interventions

1. See the "Grieving" plan, page 44.

2. If not already acquainted with the family, introduce yourself, identify your relationship as the patient's caregiver, and express sympathy.

3. Allow family members to see and touch the body. If death was sudden and unexpected, prepare them for the appearance of the body in advance, explaining that all measures were tried in an attempt to restore life. Ensure that the body is respectfully covered. Don't remove all indications of emergency intervention before allowing the family into the room, but leave side rails down and face and hands visible.

Rationales

1. This plan contains general interventions helpful in caring for bereaved families.

2. If the family arrives after the patient has died, or if the family doesn't know caregivers from previous contact, such an introduction serves to reassure them that the patient died with concerned caregivers at hand.

3. Seeing and touching the body of the loved one helps the family accept the reality of death. Advance preparation may help reduce distress. The face and hands invite touch if accessible; if not, the family may be reluctant to disturb coverings. Gross blood or other secretions should be removed before the family enters, but putting away all supplies and cleaning the room before the family sees the body may create doubts that "everything possible was done" for the patient.

4. Use direct, simple sentences, avoiding use of euphemisms, to describe the death. Provide comforting observations when possible — such as, "He died quietly and appeared to have no pain" or "She told me last night about the good times you used to have, and she seemed very happy."

5. Acknowledge the family's loss by gently reorienting them to the reality of death with such statements as "It must be hard to accept that he's really dead." Avoid overly sentimental statements.

6. Avoid recommending or encouraging sedation of a family member unless severely dysfunctional behavior is present.

7. Offer to call a friend, member of the clergy, or counselor to help with immediate arrangements. If the family does not designate such a person, offer the services of the hospital chaplain, a liaison nurse, or another in-house professional skilled in dealing with grief.

8. Prepare the family for the work of grieving. Emphasize the normality of a wide range of emotional responses (such as anger, guilt, sadness, frustration, resentment, fear, and depression) and behaviors (such as crying, laughing, withdrawal, and confusion) in response to loss of a loved one.

9. Listen patiently to retellings of the story of the death, especially if it was unexpected. Avoid statements that might be interpreted as judgmental.

10. Reemphasize the need for health-promoting self-care behaviors during the grieving period.

11. Ensure that significant others will be available to be with survivors after they leave the hospital.

12. If possible, provide a follow-up call to surviving family members 1 to 3 months after the death. Keeping a callback calendar on the unit can help in organizing this task.

13. Additional individualized interventions: _____
_____

4. Most family members are too anxious at this time to comprehend complex explanations. Euphemisms such as "passed on" may offend some family members and can interfere with reality orientation. Sharing selected, specific observations with family members may help minimize guilt and promote healthy grieving.

5. Shock and disbelief are normal initial responses to sudden death and, to a certain degree, even to expected death. Gentle reorientation aids in integrating death into reality. Overly sentimental utterances may be inappropriate to the family's actual relationship with the deceased.

6. Sedation may delay initiation of the normal grieving process.

7. During the initial stages of grieving, family members may exhibit indecision, disorganization, and disorientation. Providing an advocate helps reduce the family's distress while they are making necessary arrangements, such as for disposition of the body.

8. Family members are sometimes unprepared for the various feelings experienced in the grieving process; some may feel they are "going crazy" when unexpected feelings occur. Understanding that such emotional disorganization is a normal and healthy response to loss can help the family deal with these feelings.

9. Retelling of events by survivors is an essential part of reality acceptance and coping. Judgmental utterances may provoke severe guilt reactions in family members.

10. Grieving places additional stress on survivors, who are at increased risk for developing physical illness during mourning. Health-promoting behavior such as exercise can help release emotional energy and reduce the effects of stress.

11 Grieving is facilitated by sharing feelings with others. Few cases of loneliness are as profound as that of a bereaved person, newly alone.

12. Follow-up from caregivers to survivors is the final step in care of the dying patient and provides the family with added assurance that their loved one was special and received care accordingly. This call also provides an opportunity to identify dysfunctional grieving and make appropriate referrals, if needed.

13. Rationales: _____
_____

DISCHARGE PLANNING

Discharge checklist
If the patient is discharged home before death occurs, the patient should have:
- ❐ referral to a hospice or to a home health care agency
- ❐ adequate support system for family members.

Teaching checklist
If the patient is discharged home before death, document that the patient and family demonstrate an understanding of:
- ❐ support and resources available
- ❐ what to do when death is imminent
- ❐ what the family should do after death occurs
- ❐ what to expect in normal mourning and grieving.

Documentation checklist
If the patient is discharged home before death, using outcome criteria as a guide, document:
- ❐ fears
- ❐ feelings expressed
- ❐ goals
- ❐ preferred coping behaviors
- ❐ spiritual or religious practices
- ❐ pain-control measures
- ❐ family members' behaviors
- ❐ patient and family teaching
- ❐ discharge planning.

If death occurs in the hospital, document:
- ❐ time and circumstances of death
- ❐ request for autopsy
- ❐ request for organ and tissue donation
- ❐ disposition of body and effects
- ❐ family support measures implemented.

ASSOCIATED PLANS OF CARE

Geriatric care
Grieving
Ineffective family coping: Compromised
Ineffective individual coping
Pain
(See also the plan for the specific disease or disorder.)

REFERENCES

Frankl, V.E. *Man's Search for Meaning.* New York: Pocket Books, 1995.

Hoff, L.A. *People in Crisis: Understanding and Helping,* 4th ed. San Francisco: Jossey-Bass, 1995.

Jung, C.G. *Modern Man in Search of a Soul.* New York: Harcourt, Brace, Jovanovich, 1996.

Kalish, R.A., ed. *The Final Transition.* Farmingdale, N.Y.: Baywood Publishing Co., 1985.

Kübler-Ross, E., ed. *Death: The Final Stage of Growth.* Englewood Cliffs, N.J.: Prentice-Hall, 1975.

Kübler-Ross, E. *Living with Death and Dying.* New York: Simon and Schuster, 1997.

Tatelbaum, J. *The Courage to Grieve: Creative Living, Recovery, and Growth through Grief.* New York: Harper & Row Publishers, 1984.

General plans of care

Geriatric care

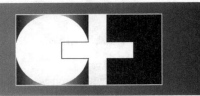

INTRODUCTION

Definition and time focus
The geriatric patient is defined as a person age 75 or older who is admitted into an acute care hospital setting. This plan focuses on care needs specific to aging and to the sudden impact of hospitalization.

Etiology and precipitating factors
The geriatric patient is prone to health problems because of the following changes associated with aging:
• increased susceptibility to infection
• decreased muscle strength and generalized debility
• increased potential for chronic disease because of genetic flaws that appear with advancing age
• psychosocial isolation
• limited income and earning ability.

FOCUSED ASSESSMENT GUIDELINES

Nursing history (functional health pattern findings)
Health perception–health management pattern
• Various presenting problems, depending on the underlying disease
Nutritional-metabolic pattern
• Decreased appetite resulting from trauma or disease and impact of hospitalization
• Preference for usual dietary pattern of frequent, small meals
• Appetite greatest during morning hours
• Chewing problems due to ill-fitting or lost dentures
Elimination pattern
• Constipation
• Regular use of laxatives or enemas
• Urinary incontinence or urine retention related to prostatic hyperplasia (males), relaxation of perineal support (females), immobility, or environmental changes
Activity-exercise pattern
• Stiffness resulting from bed rest and decreased activity
• Fear of falls because of general weakness
Sleep-rest pattern
• Shorter sleep cycles and early morning awakening

Cognitive-perceptual pattern
• Difficulty remembering or comprehending events that led to hospitalization
• Discomfort from forced confinement and limited physical activity
• Visual or sensory deficits
Self-perception–self-concept pattern
• Lack of self-confidence in maintaining independent activities
• Sense of despair because of inability to provide personal self-care (if ability is curtailed by disease or health problem)
Role-relationship pattern
• Social isolation
• Fear of uselessness and of becoming a family burden with increased care needs arising from health problem
Coping–stress tolerance pattern
• Anticipatory grief over loss of personal independence caused by chronic disease
• Dependence on others and loss of interest in living because of helplessness caused by illness
Value-belief pattern
• Mourning of loss of meaningful religious practices such as church attendance
• Anger at God, directed toward others or self, reflecting depression
• Inability to find meaning or purpose in existence
• Strong ethnic identity that may conflict with values of hospital and staff

Physical findings
General physiologic differences associated with aging are noted here. Specific physical findings related to particular disease or illness aren't discussed.
Gastrointestinal
• Decreased saliva and ptyalin secretion
• Decreased esophageal nerve function
• Decreased gastric and intestinal motility
• Decreased hydrochloric acid production
• Delayed gastric emptying
• Decreased fat and calcium absorption
Cardiovascular
• Increased systolic pressure
• Increased pulse rate
• Orthostatic hypotension
• Arterial insufficiency
• Narrowing of vessels
• Decreased blood flow to organs
• Increased systemic vascular resistance

Neurologic
• Decreased sense of smell, taste, vision, touch, and hearing
• Decreased deep tendon reflexes
• Reduced nerve conduction time
• Generally slower responses
• Reduced speed of fine motor movements
• Alteration in sleep patterns (3- to 4-hour sleep periods)

Integumentary
• Increased wrinkles
• Loss of skin turgor and elasticity
• Thinning skin (from reduced subcutaneous fat)
• Reduced sebaceous and sweat gland function
• Skin dryness
• Changes in nail thickness
• Brown or black wartlike areas of skin (seborrheic keratosis)
• Red-purple overgrowth of dilated blood vessels (cherry angioma)

Musculoskeletal
• Decreased bone mass, possible osteoporosis
• Decrease in height
• Flexed posture
• Calcified cartilage and ligaments
• Decreased muscle tone and strength
• Gait changes
• Decreased range of motion (may be due to osteoarthritis, rheumatoid arthritis, or gout)

Respiratory
• Decreased lung tissue compliance (elasticity)
• Calcification of vertebral cartilage, with reduced rib mobility and chest expansion
• Decreased vital capacity
• Decreased coughing efficiency

Genitourinary
• Enlarged prostate in male
• Decrease in number of renal nephrons
• Decrease in urine concentration ability
• Increased nocturia
• Reduced vaginal lubrication in female
• Stress incontinence in female due to decreased muscle tone, uterine prolapse, and decreased bladder capacity

Endocrine
• Thyroid — increased nodularity
• Parathyroid — decreased hormone release
• Pancreas — delayed insulin release from beta cells
• Adrenals — decreased aldosterone and ketosteroid levels

Eye
• Decreased light permeability of lens (cataracts) and cornea
• Decreased speed of adaptation to darkness
• Decreased accommodation
• Increased astigmatism

• Less efficient intraocular fluid absorption (can lead to glaucoma)
• White lipid deposit at edge of iris (arcus senilis)
• Drying of conjunctivae
• Increased nystagmus on lateral gaze

Ear
• Pure tone loss
• High-frequency loss
• Impacted cerumen
• Significant hearing loss in one-third of those over age 65 and in one-half of those over age 80

Nose
• Increase in coarse hairs

Mouth and throat
• Decreased saliva
• Increased dryness
• Loss of teeth
• Receding gums
• Atrophy of taste buds
• Slowed gag reflex

Diagnostic studies
Tests ordered depend on the particular disease or on presenting pathophysiology or symptoms.

Potential complications
• Mental confusion
• Contractures
• Fecal impaction
• Falls and fractures
• Urine retention and cystitis
• Pulmonary emboli
• Depression
• Hopelessness
• Loneliness
• Grief

General plans of care

GERIATRIC CARE

Major nursing diagnoses and collaborative problems	Key patient outcomes
Risk for altered thought processes: Slowed or diminished responsiveness	Adapt to hospital routine without agitation.
Risk for altered thought processes: Confusion	Maintain orientation at or above baseline.
Risk for nutritional deficit	Eat 50% or more of items on food tray.
Risk for impaired physical mobility	Show no new evidence of reddened skin areas.
Sleep pattern disturbance	Report sleeping at least 5 to 6 hours at a time.
Social isolation	Maintain social contacts.
Spiritual distress	Verbalize or display satisfaction with provisions for spiritual needs.

NURSING DIAGNOSIS

Risk for altered thought processes: Slowed or diminished responsiveness related to cerebral degeneration

Nursing priority

Allow ample time for all behaviors and responses.

Patient outcome criteria

Throughout the hospital stay, the patient will:
• perform self-care activities (to the degree possible) without evidence of feeling rushed
• adapt to hospital routine without agitation.

Interventions

1. Assess mental status: Note orientation, remote and recent memory, ability to interpret and abstract, and general rapidity of response.

2. Depending on deficits identified, institute appropriate measures:

• Allow increased response time when speaking with an older person.
• Give information concisely and slowly.

• Allow ample time for activities of daily living and care-related procedures.
• Avoid shouting at the patient or using baby talk when communicating.

Rationales

1. Mental status may be altered because of cerebral degeneration or other factors such as medications but must be assessed individually. Many elderly patients retain full alertness.

2. Compensation for any deficits can allow an older person to maintain dignity and active participation in daily activities.
• Thought processing may be slower in an older adult.

• Concise, slowed speech helps prevent information overload and decreases the risk of misunderstanding.
• Slower thinking may be accompanied by slower performance of tasks.
• Slowed responses don't necessarily imply a hearing deficit. Shouting may increase the patient's anxiety, further impairing performance of tasks. Use of baby talk is demeaning and may erode self-esteem already compromised by disability and dependence on others for care.

3. Once hospital activities are established, maintain a routine as much as possible.

3. Adaptation to change may be slower in an older patient. Routines provide security and reassurance. Major environmental alterations, particularly when accompanied by physiologic changes, may precipitate depression, confusion, or psychosis.

4. Additional individualized interventions: _____

4. Rationales: _____

_____

_____

Nursing diagnosis

Risk for altered thought processes: Confusion related to diminished perception of sensory data

Nursing priorities
- Promote increased clarity of sensory-perceptual stimuli.
- Decrease agitation related to confusion.

Patient outcome criteria
Throughout the hospital stay, the patient will:
- perform self-care activities (to the degree possible) without evidence of feeling rushed
- participate in prescribed therapy (such as physical therapy or occupational therapy)
- adapt to hospital routine without agitation.

Interventions

1. When confusion is evident, attempt to identify the cause, such as a change in hearing, visual ability, or mental status (see previous diagnosis). Be aware of other factors that can cause confusion, such as metabolic alterations, hypoxemia, electrolyte imbalances, or medications. If possible, plan time to sit with the patient, engage in conversation, and provide reorientation to surroundings. If the patient is amenable, use touch often during communications.

2. Before speaking, alert the patient by touch; speak only when clearly in the patient's line of vision. Keep your face in the light.

3. Speak in a low tone. (If the patient's hearing is greatly impaired and no hearing aid is available, place a stethoscope into the patient's ears, then speak into the bell.) Provide a telephone amplifier.

4. Provide the patient's own glasses for reading, as needed.

5. Allow extra time for adjustment to changes in light levels. Turn on lights slowly if there are several in the room.

6. Provide adequate illumination during the day and at night.

Rationales

1. Confusion may be related to misunderstanding because of deafness or to disorientation from visual impairment. Confusion may also be a symptom of more serious problems. Assuming that confusion is the normal mental state of a patient may leave unresolved problems that have physical or physiologic causes. Touching and engaging in conversation can reduce the depersonalizing effects of hospitalization that may increase confusion.

2. If information is not heard clearly, it may be misperceived and increase confusion. Older persons may compensate for hearing deficits by lipreading and must see your facial features to do so.

3. Loss of high-frequency hearing ability usually occurs first.

4. Distance accommodation decreases with aging.

5. Light accommodation also decreases with aging.

6. Sundowning is a condition in which the older patient tends to become confused at the end of the day, when fading light causes loss of visual cues. Commonly marked by wandering, it is reduced when the available lighting allows clear visualization of persons, objects, and surroundings.

General plans of care

7. Use restraints only as necessary to prevent injury when the patient is unattended. Explain the reasons for using restraints to both patient and family.

8. Provide environmental cues to orient the patient — for example, a clock, a calendar, or pictures of loved ones.

9. Encourage the use of audiotaped or videotaped messages from family members if disorientation persists.

10. Additional individualized interventions: _____

7. Confusion may contribute to falls and accidents, but restraints should not be used as a substitute for adequate care and supervision. Use of restraints may damage the patient's self-esteem and promote dependence on others for meeting basic needs. Restraints may actually cause injury, such as falls or decreased circulation if restraints become too tight.

8. Confusion and disorientation are reduced by familiar objects in the immediate environment.

9. Taped messages provide the comfort of familiar voices (or voices and faces) when the family isn't able to visit and may decrease agitation and restlessness associated with disorientation.

10. Rationales: _____

COLLABORATIVE PROBLEM

Risk for renal impairment related to physiologic degeneration of nephrons and glomeruli

Nursing priority

Compensate for decreased renal function.

Patient outcome criteria

Throughout the hospital stay, the patient will show:
• no medication-induced confusion or stupor
• no toxic adverse effects from medications
• no medication overdose from cumulative effect of reduced renal function
• no signs or symptoms of fluid overload.

Interventions

1. Monitor the patient for toxic adverse effects.

2. Administer narcotics and sedatives judiciously.

3. Collaborate with the doctor to adjust fluid intake.

4. Monitor for signs of fluid overload, such as neck vein distention, increased central venous pressure readings, crackles, dependent edema, increased pulse rate, and rapid weight gain.

5. Additional individualized interventions: _____

Rationales

1. Altered and erratic renal function caused by aging may affect the drug excretion rate, causing toxicity at lower doses.

2. Normal doses of these drugs may create an overdose for the older person because of the cumulative effect of reduced renal excretion.

3. Impaired renal function may cause heart failure. In addition, the aging heart is less efficient, further contributing to the risk of heart failure.

4. Impaired renal function may cause fluid retention.

5. Rationales: _____

NURSING DIAGNOSIS

Risk for nutritional deficit related to taste bud atrophy, poor dentition, decreased saliva and ptyalin secretion, economic limitations, or poor dietary habits

Nursing priority

Promote optimal nutritional intake.

Patient outcome criteria

- Within 1 day of admission, the patient will:
  - verbalize dietary habits and preferences
  - identify factors interfering with adequate nutritional intake
  - eat 50% or more of items on food tray, if appropriate.
- By the time of discharge, the patient will:
  - list dietary recommendations and specific foods to avoid or increase in diet, on request
  - identify resources and referrals for assistance with meals, shopping, or financial needs (if appropriate).

Interventions

1. With the dietitian, assess the patient's dietary habits and history. Note the adequacy of protein, calorie, vitamin, and mineral intake. Assess the levels of saturated fat and sodium in the usual diet. Note special dietary preferences.

2. Plan, with the patient and dietitian, to meet therapeutic dietary needs during hospitalization, providing foods according to the patient's usual pattern if the diet is nutritionally adequate. If the diet isn't adequate, teach the patient about dietary recommendations. Allow family members to bring food from home if appropriate.

3. Ensure that the diet plan is compatible with the patient's chewing capability. Arrange for a dental consultation if poor dentition is a factor.

4. Encourage liberal seasoning of food with herbs and spices, observing dietary limitations required for underlying conditions.

5. Serve all meals with the patient out of bed and seated in a chair, preferably in the company of others.

6. Assess for environmental, physical, and emotional factors that may contribute to poor nutritional intake at home. Examples include:
- inadequate income
- lack of transportation for shopping
- lack of space or equipment for food preparation or storage
- lack of energy for preparing food
- loneliness and depression.

Rationales

1. Nutritional deficits place the patient at increased risk for infection, skin breakdown, and other complications. A high intake of saturated fats and salt may contribute to coronary artery disease and hypertension—two factors associated with mortality in elderly patients. Preferences must be considered, however, because an older patient may be reluctant to alter established dietary patterns.

2. Including the patient in diet planning promotes a sense of control and may improve compliance. Familiar foods are more likely to be eaten. Maintaining usual patterns whenever possible helps provide a sense of security—particularly important to the elderly person in an unfamiliar environment.

3. Chewing difficulty may compromise adequate nutritional intake.

4. Because taste bud sensitivity diminishes with age, bland foods may be left uneaten.

5. Eating meals in bed in a semi-Fowler's position can lead to aspiration. Socialization can help to increase the patient's dietary intake.

6. An elderly patient may be reluctant to verbalize reasons for poor nutrition unless questioned specifically.

General plans of care

7. Before discharge, make appropriate referrals to alleviate or eliminate any identified problems.

8. Additional individualized interventions: _____
_____

7. Careful predischarge assessment, problem solving, and referral are essential to prevent exacerbation of nutritional problems after discharge.

8. Rationales: _____
_____

Nursing diagnosis

Risk for impaired physical mobility related to general weakness, calcification around joints, arthritis, or debilitation from underlying disease

Nursing priority

Maintain healthy skin, optimal activity pattern, and bowel functions.

Patient outcome criteria

Throughout the hospital stay, the patient will:
• show no new evidence of reddened skin areas
• show no new dry skin areas
• show no pruritus
• show no new skin lesions or infections
• have no crackles, fever, or other evidence of pneumonia
• establish regular bowel elimination
• have stool normal in amount, color, and consistency.

Interventions

1. Provide appropriate skin care, as follows.

• Omit soap during bathing.

• Apply oil to dry skin areas.

• Maintain the patient's usual bathing pattern — for example, every other day.

• Inspect the patient's skin twice daily for tissue breakdown.

2. Promote appropriate activity, as follows.

• Take the patient's history to identify activities of daily living (ADLs) and the need for special exercises. Encourage maintenance of usual pattern of activity, keeping patient out of bed most of day.
• Institute active or passive exercise, or both, as soon as medical protocol permits.

• Maintain all parts of the patient's body in functional anatomic alignment.

Rationales

1. The stated measures will help ensure proper skin care.
• Soap is drying, and older persons have decreased function of sebaceous glands.
• Oil may prevent increasing dryness, which can lead to tissue breakdown.
• Increasing the frequency of baths may reduce normal skin flora and increase irritation and dryness.

• Pressure on bony prominences may produce pressure ulcers because older adults have less elastic body tissue and less fatty tissue.

2. Implementing the stated measures helps ensure adequate activity.
• Maintaining normal activity and exercise patterns is essential for optimal physiologic function. Special exercises may be required to maintain the tone of particular muscle groups.
• Exercise helps prevent thrombophlebitis, contractures, footdrop, and external rotation of the legs — complications associated with impaired mobility.
• Functional alignment prevents contractures and external rotation.

• If the patient is on bed rest, turn from back to side according to nursing protocol or at least every 2 hours during the day and every 4 hours at night.
• Encourage deep-breathing exercises hourly while the patient is awake. Each shift, assess breath sounds. Report decreased breath sounds, crackles, or other abnormal findings promptly.

• Seek order for occupational therapy (OT) or physical therapy evaluation.

3. Promote normal bowel function.

• Identify the patient's typical bowel care regimen. If the patient is dependent on enemas or laxatives, discuss more appropriate alternatives.
• Add bran, prune juice, or other acceptable roughage to meals, as the patient's medical condition allows.
• Maintain adequate fluid intake.

• Administer and document the use of stool softeners or laxatives, as ordered.
• Provide bedpan or commode assistance, following the patient's schedule as closely as possible.

4. Additional individualized interventions: _____

• Regular movement reduces the risk of hypostatic pneumonia and pressure ulcers.

• Decreased elasticity in lung tissue, commonly associated with aging, places these patients at increased risk for stasis of pulmonary secretions and resultant pulmonary infection. In this population, pneumonia is associated with higher mortality.

• OT can maximize independence in ADL function and the therapist can recommend valuable assistive devices. Physical therapists may recommend walkers or other safety devices to increase strength, mobility, safety, and independence.

3. Implementing the stated measures helps ensure normal bowel function.
• Individualized care is essential for normal bowel function and a sense of emotional well-being.

• Decreased physical mobility contributes to constipation. Adding roughage to the diet stimulates peristalsis.
• Adequate fluid intake is essential to prevent drying of stool in the rectal vault, which can lead to fecal impaction.
• If unable to assume a normal position on the toilet, the older person may need medicinal assistance.
• Maintaining routine timing facilitates bowel evacuation.

4. Rationales: _____

NURSING DIAGNOSIS

Sleep pattern disturbance related to reduction in exercise, stress arising from concern with illness, anticipation of personal losses, unfamiliarity of surroundings, or discomfort associated with illness

Nursing priority

Minimize sleep disturbance during hospital stay.

Patient outcome criteria

Within 2 days of admission, the patient will:
• appear rested
• report sleeping at least 5 to 6 hours at a time.

Interventions

1. Provide frequent rest and sleep periods.

Rationales

1. Older persons have less stage IV sleep and frequently awaken spontaneously. Shorter, more frequent sleep and rest periods are, in many cases, more appropriate than one long sleep period.

General plans of care

2. Visit patient frequently during the day; encourage participation in activities.

3. Assess for and document factors that may cause sleep disruption. Treat causes appropriately—for example, if pain causes wakefulness, administer analgesics before bedtime or provide other comfort measures. Group procedures to avoid interrupting sleep cycles.

4. Adapt the hospital environment to simulate the patient's home setting whenever possible.

5. Provide as quiet an environment as possible (for example, turn off the radio or television if this reflects the usual home situation).

6. "Shorten" the night by arranging activities around late bedtime and checking in early in the morning with food and conversation.

7. Additional individualized interventions: _____

2. Boredom and inactivity contribute to sleep pattern disturbance.

3. Sleep deprivation may result in confusion, irritability, short-term memory loss, or other neuropsychiatric manifestations

4. Moving the bed into a position similar to that at home or modifying other room details (such as the position of the radio or television) can produce a sense of security and familiarity and promote environmental comfort, inducing rest and sleep.

5. Similarity of environmental sounds enhances relaxation.

6. Because older people sleep for shorter periods, their night's sleep may be only 4 to 5 hours.

7. Rationales: _____

NURSING DIAGNOSIS

Self-esteem disturbance related to dependent patient role, anxiety over loss of physical or mental competence, powerlessness to alter the aging process, societal emphasis on youth, or sense of purposelessness

Nursing priority

Promote a positive self-image while providing opportunities to demonstrate competence.

Patient outcome criteria

Throughout the hospital stay, the patient will:
• participate in decision making
• participate in self-care to the extent possible
• set realistic goals and pursue them
• initiate involvement with others.

Interventions

1. Whenever possible, offer choices and include the patient in decision making related to care.

2. Involve the patient in self-care activities as much as possible, paying special attention to grooming and hygiene needs.

3. Affirm positive qualities (for example, "You have a good sense of humor"). Help the patient identify and use coping behaviors learned in dealing successfully with earlier situations.

Rationales

1. Participating in decision making increases the patient's sense of personal competence and promotes independence.

2. "Taking over" by caregivers devalues the patient's abilities and may lead to dependence and depression. A neat personal appearance contributes to feelings of self-worth.

3. Expressing appreciation of positive attributes helps reinforce associated behaviors. Examining coping skills learned from previous experiences may help the patient build strengths in dealing with the current situation.

4. Move the conversation away from constant repetition of bodily problems.

5. Review life activities that reflect accomplishments.

6. Allow time for verbalization of feelings, such as sadness and powerlessness. Avoid overoptimistic responses.

7. Encourage realistic goal setting.

8. Facilitate behavior that is considerate of others.

9. Provide diversionary activity appropriate to the patient's abilities, allowing opportunities for creative expression whenever possible. Refer the patient to the occupational therapist, as indicated.

10. Additional individualized interventions: _____
_____

4. Repetition of negative thoughts only reinforces their impact.

5. Achievements and their recognition bolster a sense of societal usefulness.

6. Aging entails dealing with multiple losses, and feelings of sadness are a part of normal coping. Active listening and acceptance show respect for the patient as an individual and promote a sense of self-worth.

7. Goal achievement fosters feelings of self-mastery

8. Focusing on others' needs reduces dependence and increases feelings of usefulness.

9. Emotional well-being is enhanced by diversionary activities. Creative activities allow another avenue for expression of feelings and demonstration of unique abilities. The occupational therapist can help the patient select diversionary activities appropriate to functional capabilities.

10. Rationales: _____
_____

NURSING DIAGNOSIS

Social isolation related to decreased physical capacity, effects of illness, fear of burdening others, death or disability of peers, or sense of personal uselessness

Nursing priority

Promote social interaction and provide opportunities for positive feedback from others.

Patient outcome criteria

• Within 3 days of admission, the patient will:
 – maintain social contacts
 – make no comments reflecting loneliness.
• Within 3 days of the patient's admission, family members will approach nurses freely with care suggestions and questions.

Interventions

1. Include ethnicity in initial and ongoing assessment of adaptation to hospitalization.

2. Assess the patient's social resources and the willingness and ability of family, friends, and other caregivers to participate in care.

3. Involve family members in the planning — and, when possible, the provision — of care. Ask family members to identify specific needs or preferences the patient may have.

Rationales

1. Culturally sensitive care is essential to prevent social isolation.

2. Social isolation results from numerous factors. For example, the patient may hesitate to verbalize needs because of pride and independence; tactful intervention by the nurse may help link the patient with untapped social contacts.

3. Involvement of family members in care helps reduce isolation related to unfamiliar surroundings and prevents a sense of abandonment, which can occur in a hospitalized elderly patient. Participation in care while the patient is hospitalized also allows family members to practice care techniques and ask questions in a "safe" setting. Family members are most attuned to the patient's special needs.

General plans of care

4. Encourage generous use of touch in care provision and as affectionate gestures, unless the patient appears uncomfortable with physical contact.

5. Encourage family members to help the patient maintain previously established roles and functions in the family as much as possible.

6. Ensure telephone access. Discuss bedside telephone costs with the family or social worker, explaining the critical need for the patient to maintain communication with family and friends.

7. Initiate a social services referral, as needed, to arrange transportation for visitors — such as a senior citizens' or church group's van.

8. Present socialization concerns and problems to other members of the hospital staff, including the chaplain, dietitian, and housekeepers.

9. Additional individualized interventions: _____

4. Older adults have diminished sensory capacities. Touch reduces "skin hunger" (the desire for human tactile contact) and communicates caring.

5. Maintaining roles — for example, as wise counselor or confidante — helps the older person maintain a sense of belonging and decreases feelings of uselessness.

6. For many elderly patients with impaired mobility, the telephone provides an essential link to the outside world. Also, elderly friends may be unable to visit, so the telephone may be their only means of offering support to the patient.

7. The patient and family may be unaware of available transportation resources.

8. Interaction with all members of the hospital staff may serve as a temporary replacement for the patient's normal social contacts.

9. Rationales: _____

Nursing diagnosis

Spiritual distress related to inability to maintain usual religious and spiritual practices (if any) or loss of sense of life's meaning and purpose

Nursing priority

Provide for participation in meaningful religious and spiritual practices, if desired.

Patient outcome criteria

Throughout the hospital stay, the patient will:
• verbalize or display satisfaction with provisions for spiritual needs (if appropriate)
• express an ability to endure crisis (if appropriate).

Interventions

1. Identify the patient's normal preference and pattern for religious activities, if appropriate. Encourage participation in formal services if available. Arrange for visits by clergy as permitted, or suggest that the family provide a tape of the religious service. See the "Dying" plan, page 20.

2. If the patient wishes to read religious literature but can't do so, read it, get a volunteer to read it, or obtain it on a cassette tape.

3. Provide privacy for personal prayer time, when desired.

4. Keep religious articles such as rosary beads conveniently available.

Rationales

1. Maintenance of usual spiritual support increases coping ability. The "Dying" plan contains other specific interventions for patients experiencing spiritual distress.

2. Maintaining continuity in religious experience provides special comfort.

3. Encouraging expressions of trust and faith in God or a supreme being provides solace and a sense of providential care during crises.

4. Religious articles may provide reassurance and serve as a reminder of spiritual resources.

5. Additional individualized interventions:_____

5. Rationales: _____

DISCHARGE PLANNING

Discharge checklist
Before discharge, the patient should show evidence of:
❏ meeting discharge criteria for the specific disease or condition
❏ appropriate referrals made for home care assistance as needed, or for care facility placement, if indicated
❏ special attention to age-related needs, such as a hearing aid, eyeglasses, and assistive devices.

Teaching checklist
Document evidence that the patient and family demonstrate an understanding of:
❏ details specific to the patient's disease or condition
❏ all discharge medications' purpose, dosage, administration schedule, and adverse effects requiring medical attention
❏ care needs arising from illness
❏ dietary needs
❏ feeding assistance needs
❏ mental status changes: thought processing, insight, judgment, or confusion
❏ toileting needs
❏ mobility and transfer needs
❏ hygiene needs
❏ social and emotional needs to reduce loneliness and isolation
❏ need for relationships with family and friends
❏ family and friends' access to care facility, if placement planned
❏ resources available for older persons
❏ how to contact the doctor
❏ use of durable medical equipment.

Documentation checklist
Using outcome criteria as a guide, document:
❏ clinical status on admission
❏ significant changes in status
❏ patient and family teaching
❏ discharge planning
❏ other data pertinent to specific disease or condition.

ASSOCIATED PLANS OF CARE

Dying
Grieving
Ineffective family coping: Compromised
Ineffective individual coping
Knowledge deficit

Pain
(See also the plan for the patient's specific disease or condition.)

REFERENCES

Chenitz, W., et al. *Clinical Gerontological Nursing.* Philadelphia: W.B. Saunders Co., 1991.
Leuckenotte, A. *Gerontologic Nursing.* St. Louis: Mosby–Year Book, Inc., 1996.
Miller, C. *Nursing Care of Older Adults: Theory and Practice,* 2nd ed. Philadelphia: Lippincott-Raven Pubs., 1995.

General plans of care

Grieving

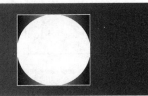

INTRODUCTION

Definition and time focus
Grief is the normal response to an actual or potential loss. It is a natural, necessary, and dynamic process. Anticipatory grieving occurs before an actual loss. Dysfunctional grieving is the ineffective, pathologic, delayed, or exaggerated response to an actual or potential loss. Theoretical phases of the grieving process have been outlined by various authors (see *The grieving process*). As in all theoretical models, the phases are overlapping and may or may not be sequential; that is, the patient or family may fluctuate between phases during the process.

This plan focuses on the patient and family members coping with impending or actual losses.

Etiology and precipitating factors
• Loss of body image or some aspect of self (such as social role or body part due to amputation or mastectomy)
• Loss of loved one or significant other through separation, divorce, or death
• Loss of material objects (such as income or belongings)
• Loss through a maturational or developmental process (such as aging or weaning an infant)

The grieving process

Lindeman (1944)
Shock or disbelief → Acute mourning → Reentry into daily life → Decreased image of deceased

Engel (1964)
Denial → Developing awareness → Restitution

Kübler-Ross (1969)
Denial → Anger → Bargaining → Depression Acceptance

Rando (1981)
Avoidance → Confrontation → Reestablishment

FOCUSED ASSESSMENT GUIDELINES

Nursing history (functional health pattern findings)
Health perception–health management pattern
• Real or imagined loss
Nutritional-metabolic pattern
• Nausea and vomiting, weight loss, or anorexia
• Increased food, drug, or alcohol intake as means of coping
Elimination pattern
• GI upset, diarrhea, or constipation
Activity-exercise pattern
• Shortness of breath
• Exhaustion, weakness, inability to maintain organized activity patterns, or restlessness
Sleep-rest pattern
• Insomnia caused by disruption of normal sleep pattern or frequent crying episodes
Cognitive-perceptual pattern
• Guilt
• Sorrow, emptiness, or "heaviness"
Self-perception–self-concept pattern
• Worthlessness
• Decreased ability to fulfill personal life expectations
Role-relationship pattern
• Episodes of withdrawal or social isolation (especially with dysfunctional grieving)
Sexuality-reproductive pattern
• Loss of sexual desire or hypersexuality
• Menstrual irregularity in female
Coping–stress tolerance pattern
• Difficulty expressing feelings about the loss
• Rationalization or intellectualization of the loss to make it less painful, especially during bargaining phase
• Frequent crying episodes, usually associated with shock or with denial or depression phases
• Hostility during anger phase in attempt to resist the impact of the loss
• Avoidance of any discussion of the loss (especially with dysfunctional grieving)
• Previous experiences with depression
• "Rehearsal" of events surrounding the loss
• Preoccupation with lost object or image
Value-belief pattern
• Need for increased spiritual or pastoral support
• Increased use of prayer or meditation
• Doubts in religious beliefs
• Reports of specific cultural beliefs, rituals, or traditions

Physical findings

Loss is a body stressor that can trigger physiologic as well as psychological stress and can decrease the immune system's resistance to infection and illness.

Cardiovascular
- Palpitations
- Hypertension
- Arrhythmias

Pulmonary
- Increased respirations
- Deep sighing

Gastrointestinal
- Vomiting
- Diarrhea or constipation

Neurologic
- Irritability
- Anxiety
- Agitation
- Paresthesia

Integumentary
- Diaphoresis
- Cold, clammy skin
- Flushed skin

Musculoskeletal
- Decreased muscle tone
- Weakness

Diagnostic studies

Physical debilitation and illness resulting from grieving may require studies, but these will vary widely, depending on the signs and symptoms exhibited. For example, palpitations and pulse irregularities may indicate the need for an electrocardiogram to rule out significant cardiac problems.

Potential complications
- Crisis state
- Major depression with suicidal or homicidal potential
- Physical deterioration
- Dysfunctional grieving

CLINICAL SNAPSHOT

GRIEVING

Major nursing diagnoses	Key patient outcomes
Grieving	Demonstrate positive coping behaviors.
Risk for dysfunctional grieving	Verify the absence of suicidal or homicidal thinking.

NURSING DIAGNOSIS

Grieving related to impending or actual physical or functional loss

Nursing priority

Facilitate a healthy grieving process.

Patient outcome criteria

According to individual readiness, the patient will, on request:
- identify the meaning of the loss
- communicate feelings, especially anger, guilt, or sorrow
- identify strategies to cope with the loss
- identify role and relationship changes
- identify and use spiritual support and resources
- perform self-care
- make decisions about care.

Interventions

1. Provide the patient with accurate information before any procedure or treatment that may affect appearance, physical or sexual functioning, or role performance.

2. Assess and document the patient's response to information about the disease, implications, and treatment. Include responses to past experiences with loss.

3. Discuss meaning of the loss with the patient.

4. Assess and discuss any cultural issues that relate to the patient's or family's grief experience.

5. Discuss changes in social roles or relationships that may result from the loss.

6. Provide time to be with the patient and family.

7. Assess and document the patient's current phase of grief. Recognize that fluctuations among phases may occur.

8. Support and facilitate the expression of feelings associated with anger, guilt, sorrow, and sadness during any phase of grieving. Listen nonjudgmentally. Recognize and accept any feelings of anger directed toward the health care team.

9. Encourage the release of emotion through crying. If the patient is receptive, hold the patient's hand and use touch liberally.

10. Assess for and promote positive coping mechanisms — for example, building and sharing close relationships, engaging in creative activities and exercise, and openly expressing feelings related to loss and readjustment. See the "Dying" plan, page 20.

11. Provide spiritual support as needed by the patient throughout grieving, or suggest appropriate resources.

12. Encourage participation in daily self-care activities.

13. Provide positive reinforcement and realistic hope about the patient's progress.

14. Allow the patient to make decisions whenever possible.

15. Assess and assist activation of personal support systems.

16. Additional individualized interventions: _____

Rationales

1. Accurate information prevents misconceptions and may decrease fears related to the loss.

2. Past experiences and values influence the current loss experience.

3. Establishing the significance of the loss enhances the person's ability to identify and release feelings related to the loss

4. Cultural beliefs, rituals, or traditions may influence the response to the grief process.

5. Physical or functional loss may cause social changes associated with income, career, and relationships. Discussing these changes helps identify the impact of the loss and alternatives for lifestyle adjustments.

6. The nurse's time spent with the patient and family can encourage the necessary review and processing of the loss. Feelings of loneliness or social isolation may also be decreased, reassuring the patient that caregivers perceive the loss as significant.

7. Identifying unresolved issues facilitates the grieving process.

8. Expressing feelings openly may enable the patient to move more easily through the phases of grieving. The nurse's nonjudgmental listening enables the patient to express feelings without fear of rejection.

9. The nurse's encouragement reassures the patient (and family, if indicated) that crying is a normal response to loss. Hand-holding and use of touch provide reassurance and help the patient relax.

10. Coping with loss is a developmental task. Losses increase in occurrence and intensity throughout life. Adaptive coping methods are derived from previous losses. The "Dying" plan contains general interventions helpful to those coping with loss.

11. Spiritual support assists with fostering a sense of meaning, hope, love, and satisfaction with life.

12. Self-care promotes feelings of self-control and independence, increasing self-esteem.

13. Reinforcement and reassurance build self-confidence.

14. Decision making enables the person to maintain control.

15. The patient may need gentle guidance to identify resources. Sharing feelings with closest friends or family aids in adjustment to loss.

16. Rationales: _____

NURSING DIAGNOSIS

Risk for dysfunctional grieving related to unresolved feelings about physical or functional loss

Nursing priority

Identify dysfunctional grieving and make appropriate referrals.

Patient outcome criteria

According to individual readiness, the patient will, on request:
• acknowledge the loss
• discuss the experience realistically
• report using healthy coping strategies
• understand and accept his own and other's responses to the loss
• express and accept personal feelings
• identify resources within the family and community
• verify the absence of suicidal or homicidal thinking.

Interventions

1. Assess and document the patient's responses to the loss. Identify feelings of unresolved guilt or anger. Recognize avoidance of discussing the loss. Be alert to possible use of alcohol or recreational drugs as an escape.

2. Assess and document the patient's daily activity level and ability to perform roles.

3. Assess the patient's physical well-being and initiate a medical referral as indicated. Teach the importance of maintaining physical health.

4. Monitor and document the administration of tranquilizers, antidepressants, and sedatives.

5. Observe the patient for signs and symptoms of potential suicide or homicide: increased agitation, insomnia, self-incrimination, and feelings of worthlessness, helplessness, and hopelessness.

6. Assess suicide risk by talking with the patient (see *Assessment of suicide potential,* page 48). Consult with the patient's doctor regarding referral or intervention.

7. Involve other resource persons, such as social workers, chaplains, or psychiatrists, as indicated or requested by the patient and family.

8. Provide follow-up referral for the patient after discharge.

9. Additional individualized interventions: _____

_____

Rationales

1. Accurate assessment allows understanding of the dynamics of the grieving process. Unresolved guilt and anger are common symptoms of pathologic grief and may result in major depression. Avoidance of discussing the loss may indicate delayed grief. Drug or alcohol abuse contributes to dysfunctional resolution of loss.

2. Withdrawal and social isolation commonly occur with chronic grieving.

3. Grieving requires emotional and physical energy. Prolonged grieving may result in physical illness and debilitation. Somatic symptoms may mask a depression resulting from delayed or absent grief.

4. Tranquilizers, antidepressants, and sedatives may occasionally be helpful; however, overmedication may result in prolonging the grieving.

5. Anxiety and depression may be exaggerated during chronic grieving states.

6. Frank discussion of suicide potential with the patient helps identify and define stressors and may relieve anxiety; it won't cause a suicide attempt.

7. Such referrals help identify financial, social, spiritual, and community resources. Psychiatric care identifies unhealthy responses and promotes healthy grieving.

8. Follow-up visits by nurses, chaplains, social workers, and other support persons should be based on patient need. During early grieving, weekly visits are likely to be helpful. Support groups may be helpful.

9. Rationales: _____

_____

General plans of care

Assessment of suicide potential

The alert nurse is aware of suicide risk factors and specifically assesses patients at risk by asking direct questions.

Major risk factors	Questions	Additional risk factors
Intent Contrary to popular myth, asking patients directly about suicide doesn't cause attempts. Patients tend to answer truthfully and are typically relieved that someone has acknowledged their distress.	"Are you thinking about killing yourself?" or "Are you considering suicide?"	**Resources** Lack of social and personal resources to deal with external or internal crises, or a perception by the patient that such resources are unavailable, increases the likelihood of suicide. **Recent loss or life changes** Loss or the threat of loss increases suicide risk. Even other kinds of change (a promotion, household move, or changes in roles or responsibilities) can increase stress and overwhelm the patient's coping abilities.
Plan Patients who verbalize clearly defined, detailed plans for suicide are at greater risk than those who vaguely want to die.	"Do you have a plan to do it?"	**Physical illness** Physical illness may increase suicide risk, particularly if the illness involves major life changes or a threat to essential aspects of self-image.
Lethality of method Highly lethal methods (such as firearms, hanging, or jumping from a height) greatly increase risk.	"How would you do it?"	**Alcohol or drug abuse** Substance abuse may increase impulsive behavior and contribute to depression, thus increasing suicide risk. Additionally, alcohol or drugs may increase risk by potentiating other drugs or decreasing a person's overall level of awareness.
Availability of means Patients who have the means readily available are at higher risk.	"Do you have a gun at home?"	**Sudden behavior change** Any abrupt change in behavior may signal suicidal intent. **Isolation** Physical or emotional isolation greatly increases suicide risk.
Personal and family history Most people who succeed at suicide have made previous attempts. If previous attempts used highly lethal means or were unsuccessful only by accident (that is, if the plan didn't allow for rescue), risk is increased. Those who have lost loved ones to suicide are at greater risk.	"Have you tried to kill yourself before?" "How? What happened?" "Has anyone in your family committed suicide?"	**Age, sex, marital status** Older males have a higher rate of successful suicide, possibly because they tend to choose more certain means. Risk of suicide may be increased for separated, widowed, or divorced persons. These parameters, however, are less reliable predictors than those above.
Goals If the patient is unable to envision or articulate future goals or plans, suicide potential is increased.	"Where do you see yourself next month? In 1 year? In 5 years?"	

DISCHARGE PLANNING

Discharge checklist
Before discharge, the patient should show evidence of:
- ❏ acknowledgment of the loss and its meaning
- ❏ demonstration of positive coping behaviors
- ❏ identification of social and community support systems
- ❏ no display of suicidal or homicidal thinking.

Teaching checklist
Document evidence that the patient and family demonstrate an understanding of:
- ❏ normal grief responses
- ❏ phases of the grieving process
- ❏ information concerning role changes and physical loss
- ❏ importance of maintaining physical health and well-being of the patient and family
- ❏ information about the patient's illness and medical treatment
- ❏ need to be understanding and accepting of those who are grieving
- ❏ community resources including support groups and interagency referral.

Documentation checklist
Using outcome criteria as a guide, document:
- ❏ past experiences and responses to loss
- ❏ current perception and meaning of loss
- ❏ changes in role relationships, body image, and self-esteem
- ❏ positive or maladaptive coping behaviors
- ❏ cultural influences
- ❏ support systems
- ❏ level of activity and participation in self-care
- ❏ medication with tranquilizers, antidepressants, or sedatives
- ❏ signs and symptoms of suicidal or homicidal potential
- ❏ interdisciplinary referrals
- ❏ patient and family teaching
- ❏ discharge planning.

ASSOCIATED PLANS OF CARE
Dying
Ineffective family coping: Compromised
Ineffective individual coping

REFERENCES

Cowles, K. "Cultural Perspectives of Grief: An Expanded Concept Analysis," *Journal of Advance Nursing* 23(2):287-94, February 1996.

Groenwald, S., et al. *Cancer Nursing Principles and Practice.* Sudbury, Mass.: Jones & Bartlett Pubs., Inc., 1997.

McNally, J., et al. *Guidelines for Oncology Nursing Practice,* 2nd ed. Philadelphia: W.B. Saunders Co., 1991.

Valente, S.M., et al. "Responding Therapeutically to Bereavement and Grief," *Nurseweek* 9(8):10-11, 15, April 15, 1996.

Worden, J. *Grief Counseling and Grief Therapy: A Handbook for the Mental Health Practitioner.* New York: Springer Publishing Co., 1991.

General plans of care

Impaired physical mobility

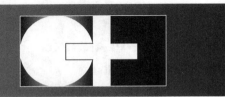

INTRODUCTION

Definition and time focus

Impaired physical mobility is a condition in which an individual has limited ability for independent physical movement. Acutely ill or injured patients are physically unable to engage in normal activities; physical recovery itself may demand activity limitations. Rest is essential for healing and should be encouraged; however, prolonged bed rest can result in well-documented physical and emotional disabilities that can add to the patient's problems. The effects of decreased mobility must be addressed early in the planning of care and reviewed frequently throughout the patient's hospital stay. This plan focuses on the care of the patient whose condition causes impairment or requires restriction of physical mobility.

Etiology and precipitating factors

- Injury that prevents weight bearing (such as trauma)
- Illness that causes activity intolerance (such as cardiopulmonary disorders)
- Acute injury that causes paralysis or paresis (such as cerebrovascular accident [CVA] or spinal cord injury)
- Chronic or acute disabling conditions (such as severe arthritis or Guillain-Barré syndrome)
- Sensory-perceptual alterations (as in CVA)
- Therapeutic restrictions
- Reluctance to attempt movement

FOCUSED ASSESSMENT GUIDELINES

Nursing history (functional health pattern findings)

Because the patient's subjective responses to immobility may vary widely, depending on the underlying condition, this section presents a guide to assessing the patient with a mobility impairment.

Health perception–health management pattern
- Is the patient's mobility problem new, or does it reflect long-standing disability?
- What is the extent of the patient's activity limitation?
- Does the patient normally use any mobility aids at home (such as a walker, cane, or wheelchair)?
- Does the patient have a cast, splint, traction, or other immobilizing device?

- Does the patient have equipment that interferes with normal mobility, such as a ventilator or multiple I.V. lines?
- Does the patient have preexisting conditions that affect mobility, such as CVA or amputation, or a progressive debilitating disease, such as multiple sclerosis or acquired immunodeficiency syndrome?
- Does the patient have a history of blood disorders, integumentary problems, pulmonary disease, or cardiac disease?

Nutritional-metabolic pattern
- What is the patient's baseline nutritional status? (See the "Nutritional deficit" plan, page 80.)
- Is the patient able or permitted to take oral nourishment?
- Is the patient receiving artificial nutrition, such as total parenteral nutrition or nasogastric or gastric tube feedings?

Elimination pattern
- When was the patient's last bowel movement?
- Does the patient normally use elimination aids, such as laxatives or enemas?
- Does the patient have a preexisting condition requiring a bowel regimen that includes removal of impacted feces?
- Does the patient have a history of calculi, renal disease, or recurrent urinary tract infections?
- If the patient has an indwelling urinary catheter, when was it placed?

Activity-exercise pattern
- Is the patient able to perform any self-care activity?
- What was the patient's baseline activity tolerance before hospitalization?
- Are all joints capable of full range of motion?

Cognitive-perceptual pattern
- Is the patient conscious and alert?
- Does the patient have any sensory deficits (such as blindness, deafness, or hemiparesis)?

Self-perception–self-concept pattern
- What is the patient's attitude toward resuming physical activity?

Role-relationship pattern
- Does the patient's occupation require full mobility?
- Does the patient have a supportive social network?
- Are family members involved in care of the patient at home?

Sexuality-reproductive pattern
- Does the patient's mobility impairment potentially affect sexual function?

Coping–stress tolerance pattern
• Has the patient used physical activity as a primary coping behavior or stress-relieving measure?

Physical findings
Because physical findings vary widely in patients with reduced mobility depending on their underlying condition, this section has been refocused to outline some of the major physiologic effects of immobility on body systems.

Cardiovascular
• Orthostatic hypotension (related to reduced autonomic neurovascular reflex response)
• Reduced stroke volume
• Gradually increasing tachycardia (related to deconditioning effects)
• Decreased oxygen uptake
• Venous pooling (related to lack of muscle activity)
• Plasma volume loss
• Blood volume loss
• Reduced cardiac reserve

Respiratory
• Restricted diaphragmatic and costal excursion
• Reduced ciliary activity
• Reduced vital capacity
• Reduced gas exchange (related to gravitational effects)
• Reduced production of surfactant

Gastrointestinal
• Decreased peristalsis
• Increased sphincter tone
• Abdominal distention
• Anorexia

Neurologic
• Decreased sensorium
• Paralysis or paresis related to CVA or spinal cord injury

Integumentary
• Reduced skin turgor
• Impaired wound healing
• Dependent edema

Musculoskeletal
• Reduced muscle mass
• Decreased strength and endurance
• Bone demineralization (at increased rate)
• Fibrosis or ankylosis
• Calcium deposition in soft tissue

Renal
• Hypercalciuria and precipitation of calcium salts (related to bone demineralization)
• Increased renal blood flow
• Initial diuresis (related to decreased antidiuretic hormone [ADH] release)
• Bladder distention
• Urinary stasis

Metabolic
• Increased rate of catabolism
• Decreased basal metabolic rate
• Increased excretion of electrolytes

Diagnostic studies
Because no diagnostic studies specifically apply to all patients with impaired mobility, only the usual laboratory test findings related to the physiologic changes described in the preceding section are presented here. Laboratory tests may include:
• serum protein level — usually decreased from accelerated catabolism
• serum and urine calcium and phosphate levels — increased from bone demineralization
• arterial blood gas (ABG) measurements — may show reduced partial pressure of arterial oxygen (PaO_2) and increased partial pressure of arterial carbon dioxide, indicating hypoventilation and impaired gas exchange
• blood urea nitrogen level — may be elevated from catabolic activity
• urine pH — may be elevated from decreased levels of acid end products released by muscle activity
• hematocrit — may be increased from plasma and blood volume losses and diuresis.

Potential complications
• Thromboembolic phenomena
• Atelectasis
• Pneumonia
• Infections
• Skin breakdown, potential pressure-ulcer formation
• Constipation
• Contractures
• Osteoporosis
• Muscle wasting
• Urinary calculi
• Difficulty coping

CLINICAL SNAPSHOT

IMPAIRED PHYSICAL MOBILITY

Major nursing diagnoses and collaborative problems	Key patient outcomes
Risk for ineffective airway clearance	Maintain a clear airway.
Risk for pulmonary embolism	Display no signs of pulmonary embolism.
Risk for impaired skin integrity	Maintain clear, intact skin.
Risk for altered urinary elimination	Maintain urine output of at least 60 ml/hour.
Risk for constipation	Maintain normal bowel elimination.
Risk for disuse syndrome: Muscle atrophy and joint contractures	Perform exercises as taught, if condition permits.
Situational low self-esteem	Express feelings related to losses, if desired.

NURSING DIAGNOSIS

Risk for ineffective airway clearance related to reduced diaphragmatic and costal excursion, stasis of secretions, decreased ciliary activity, weakness, and underlying disease process

Nursing priorities

- Maintain a clear airway.
- Prevent pulmonary complications.

Patient outcome criteria

Throughout the hospital stay, the patient will:
- maintain a clear airway
- change position (or be turned) at least every 2 hours
- perform pulmonary hygiene measures at least every 2 hours while awake, as the patient's condition permits
- exhibit no evidence of pneumonia, atelectasis, or pulmonary embolus.

Interventions

1. Assess pulmonary capabilities at least every 2 hours while the patient is awake, as appropriate. Evaluate level of alertness, ability to cough and deep breathe, respiratory rate and effort, and breath sounds.

2. Evaluate for risk factors that affect pulmonary status, such as obesity, lung disease, incisions, abdominal distention, neuromuscular dysfunction, chest wall pathology, and medications that depress respirations.

Rationales

1. Initial and ongoing assessments provide direction for planning care. The factors listed are crucial determinants of the patient's ability to counteract the effects of bed rest on pulmonary function.

2. The risk factors listed are associated with increased incidence of serious pulmonary complications.

3. Monitor vital signs, fluid intake and output, hemodynamic pressures, and electrocardiogram findings according to Appendix A, Monitoring Standards, or unit protocol. Report changes or abnormal findings promptly.

4. Obtain and monitor ABG measurements as ordered. Monitor vital capacity and other pulmonary function studies, as ordered, and report any abnormal findings promptly.

5. Initiate measures to promote effective breathing:

• Place the patient in Fowler's or semi-Fowler's position, as condition permits, and change position at least every 2 hours while awake.

• Encourage deep breathing at least every 2 hours while awake, and assist the patient using an incentive spirometer, as ordered. Check with the doctor about including coughing with deep breathing.

• Teach the patient to splint incisions, if present, and provide assistance, if necessary.
• Reduce abdominal distention, when possible, through use of gastric suction, return-flow enema, or other measures, as ordered.

6. Initiate measures to promote airway clearance:

• Provide humidification of inspired air.

• Encourage an adequate fluid intake, typically eight to twelve 8-oz (240-ml) glasses a day as the patient's condition allows.
• Suction, as needed, providing supplemental oxygen before and after the procedure.

• Perform chest physiotherapy every 4 hours while the patient is awake (or more frequently, as indicated).

3. Bed rest has significant effects on cardiovascular function, including a reduction in stroke volume (which may induce tachycardia), redistribution of blood flow (which may contribute to orthostatic hypotension), and decreased cardiovascular reserve (resulting in reduced exercise tolerance and general deconditioning). Careful monitoring of cardiovascular parameters aids in early detection of preventable complications.

4. ABG measurements provide direct evaluation of ventilatory status. Pulmonary function studies aid further classification and evaluation of the effects of bed rest on the lungs (bed rest is associated with decreased ventilatory capacity).

5. Maintaining an effective breathing pattern reduces the risk of developing pulmonary complications.
• Patients on bed rest commonly assume a slumped position, decreasing the adequacy of chest expansion. Frequent repositioning helps facilitate drainage of secretions by gravity.
• Deep breathing and incentive spirometry may increase inspiratory reserve volume, promote maximum alveolar inflation, and improve ventilation-perfusion ratios. Deep breathing may actually reverse microatelectasis related to hypoventilation. The incentive spirometer also provides a goal for the patient. The effectiveness of coughing as an airway clearance measure is controversial because its direct effects on small airways haven't been shown, and coughing may increase intrathoracic pressure and lead to alveolar microatelectasis. Some clinicians believe coughing may result in a "milking" effect from smaller to larger airways. If coughing is used, it should always be followed by several deep breaths to help reinflate alveoli.
• Splinting may decrease the fear of pain and promote deeper breathing and fuller chest wall expansion.
• Abdominal distention exerts upward pressure on the diaphragm, reducing chest excursion.

6. Pulmonary hygiene measures help reduce the risk of developing pulmonary complications.
• Humidification may help decrease the viscosity of secretions and helps minimize upper airway irritation if constant supplemental oxygen is required.
• Rehydration of dehydrated patients can promote increased mucociliary clearance.

• Suctioning may be necessary for airway clearance, especially in persons with weak or absent cough or artificial airways. Supplemental oxygen is essential because suctioning can cause significant reduction in PaO_2.
• Chest physiotherapy may help prevent pooling of secretions and loosen mucus plugs. When used in combination with postural drainage, it can help bring secretions into larger airways for easier expectoration.

General plans of care

7. Monitor for pulmonary complications associated with bed rest, as follows:
• pneumonia — crackles, rhonchi, chest pain, fever, productive cough, tachypnea, tachycardia, whispered pectoriloquy, infected sputum specimen and increased white blood cells (WBCs), or consolidation or effusion on chest X-ray

• atelectasis — bronchial or decreased breath sounds, dull percussion note over affected side, tachypnea, tachycardia, restlessness, tracheal shift toward affected side on chest X-ray, or cyanosis (in advanced macroatelectasis)
• pulmonary embolus — see the "Risk for pulmonary embolism" problem below.

8. Additional individualized interventions: _____

7. Pulmonary insult complicates treatment and increases mortality risk in the acutely ill patient.
• Prompt detection and treatment of pulmonary infections is essential because their presence exacerbates ventilatory compromise. Purulent sputum is more tenacious because it contains viscous leukocyte deoxyribonucleic acid. In addition, proteolytic enzymes released from destroyed leukocytes can increase inflammation, resulting in bronchoconstriction.
• Bed rest aids the development of atelectasis because of reduced chest expansion, ventilatory capacity, and secretion clearance. Microatelectasis is common and may appear on chest X-ray. When atelectasis occurs, ventilatory capacity is reduced because inspired air can't reach the affected areas.
• Pulmonary embolus is the most immediately life-threatening complication associated with bed rest.

8. Rationales: _____

COLLABORATIVE PROBLEM

Risk for pulmonary embolism related to venous pooling, loss of vasomotor tone, lack of skeletal muscle contraction, and increased blood viscosity

Nursing priority

Prevent or promptly detect and treat thromboembolic complications.

Patient outcome criteria

Throughout the hospital stay, the patient will:
• perform leg exercises at least every 2 hours during waking hours as instructed or receive passive range-of-motion exercises
• increase activity to maximum level permitted
• display no signs of pulmonary embolus or thrombophlebitis.

Interventions

1. Evaluate the patient for factors that increase the risk of thromboembolism, including:
• previous history of deep vein thrombosis
• abdominal, pelvic, or orthopedic surgery
• trauma
• history of varicosities, cancer, smoking, CVA, or bleeding disorders
• use of oral contraceptives or other medications that affect clotting
• dehydration
• obesity
• hypertension, diabetes mellitus, or renal disease
• paralysis
• decreased alertness
• age (over 40 years).

Rationales

1. Any factor that contributes to venous stasis, hypercoagulability, trauma, or degeneration of blood vessels increases the risk of thromboembolism. Because bed rest can cause thromboembolism, noting any additional contributing factors will help in identifying the highest-risk patients and planning their care.

2. Initiate measures to promote venous return and decrease venous pooling:
• Teach the patient to perform leg exercises every 1 to 2 hours while awake, such as flexion and extension of the feet and quadriceps setting. Elevate legs 15 degrees.
• Avoid using the gatch bed, crossing legs, or placing pillows directly under the popliteal area.
• Apply graded antiembolism stockings, taking care to remove them at least three times daily for 30 to 60 minutes, or according to unit protocol. Discuss use of pneumatic devices, such as special boots, with the doctor.

• Increase activity to permit ambulation as soon as the patient's condition allows. Use caution when first getting the patient out of bed.

3. For high-risk patients, administer prophylactic anticoagulants, if ordered (typically low-dose heparin or warfarin sodium [Coumadin]). Monitor clotting studies (prothrombin time [PT], international normalized ratio [INR], or activated partial thromboplastin time [PTT]) daily for these patients, as ordered. Question anticoagulant orders for trauma patients and others with possible cardiovascular instability or bleeding problems. Monitor for signs and symptoms of occult bleeding, such as a positive test for hemoglobin in stool or urine, in patients receiving anticoagulant therapy.

4. Monitor for evidence of thromboembolic complications, including:
• pulmonary embolism—tachypnea, sudden dyspnea, pleuritic chest pain, restlessness, feelings of impending doom, diaphoresis, hypotension, pallor, or cyanosis. If these signs and symptoms occur, elevate the head of the bed, administer oxygen, obtain a specimen for ABG study, and notify the doctor immediately.

• thrombophlebitis—erythema, edema, tenderness, venous patterning or engorgement, positive Homans' sign, cording, or calf pain. Avoid deep palpation of the affected area. If swelling is suspected, initiate daily measurements of leg circumference at a designated point (make an indelible mark on the patient for subsequent measurement). If these signs and symptoms occur, notify the doctor immediately and elevate the affected extremity.

5. Additional individualized interventions: _____
_____

2. Venous stasis is associated with increased incidence of thromboembolic complications.
• Leg exercises cause muscle contraction, promoting venous return toward the heart. Leg elevation promotes gravity drainage from peripheral vessels.
• These measures may cause venous compression or occlusion, increasing the risk of complications.
• Antiembolism stockings "squeeze" superficial vessels and may promote venous return. Removal permits skin examination and allows drying of accumulated moisture. Pneumatic devices may also promote venous return; their use is particularly desirable if heparin is contraindicated.
• Weight bearing increases muscle contraction and also decreases bone demineralization associated with immobility. Clots from immobility are most likely to embolize when the patient first resumes activity.

3. Heparin inactivates fibrin, thus preventing fibrin clot formation and reducing the risk of enlargement of existing clots. Warfarin interferes with vitamin K production, thus decreasing production of clotting factors. Monitoring PT, INR, or PTT permits dosage adjustment as needed. Anticoagulants may induce bleeding in susceptible patients.

4. Early detection and treatment of thromboembolic phenomena may minimize their effects.
• Pulmonary embolism is the blockage of a pulmonary artery by a thrombus. As a result, alveoli are ventilated but not perfused, resulting in increased alveolar dead space in the affected lung tissue. A large embolus may significantly increase pulmonary vascular resistance, which may lead to right-sided heart failure. Pulmonary infarction may also occur if the embolus is large. ABG findings guide intervention.
• Thrombophlebitis may occur in superficial or deep veins; the leg veins are usually affected. Superficial thrombophlebitis, although not dangerous, can cause significant discomfort; deep vein thrombophlebitis, however, may lead to life-threatening movement of clots to the lung. Initial erythema, swelling, and tenderness are related to inflammatory changes, while later signs (such as cording and a positive Homans' sign) represent actual thrombus formation. Deep palpation may cause dislodgment of clots. Measuring leg circumference provides an objective evaluation of swelling. Elevating the affected extremity helps minimize venous stasis.

5. Rationales: _____
_____

General plans of care

NURSING DIAGNOSIS
Risk for impaired skin integrity related to impeded capillary flow, possible altered sensation, or venous stasis

Nursing priority
Prevent skin breakdown.

Patient outcome criteria
Throughout the hospital stay, the patient will:
- maintain clear, intact skin
- exhibit no evidence of skin breakdown
- maintain adequate nutritional intake.

Interventions

1. On the patient's admission to the unit, and at least daily thereafter, inspect the skin carefully, evaluating color, texture, turgor, dryness, sensation, and capillary refill.

2. Evaluate for factors that increase the risk of skin breakdown, such as nutritional deficit, obesity, diabetes mellitus (or other conditions affecting vascular status), incontinence, decreased sensation, infection, excessive moisture, old age, decreased alertness, and paralysis.

3. Initiate measures to prevent skin breakdown, including:
- turning and repositioning every 1 to 2 hours, massaging areas of pressure and bony prominences

- careful turning technique

- judicious use of lotion, avoidance of harsh soaps, and careful cleaning, especially for the incontinent patient, followed by gentle but thorough drying

- use of convoluted foam mattress, flotation pad or water bed, sheepskins, air mattress, air-fluidized bead system (Clinitron therapy bed), low-air-loss bed, or kinetic (RotoRest) bed, as available and indicated

- adequate nutrition.

Rationales

1. Initial and ongoing assessment is the first step in providing individualized care. Abnormal findings may provide clues to problems and can be used to guide care planning.

2. Bed rest alone places any patient at increased risk for skin problems because pressure areas may develop rapidly if motion is restricted or impossible. The patient with one or more of the conditions listed should be considered at extremely high risk. Early evaluation of such factors allows for preventive measures.

3. Preventing skin breakdown is much easier than treating a problem after it develops.
- Repositioning allows redistribution of pressure. Massage stimulates circulation and promotes comfort; bony prominences are the most common sites of skin breakdown.
- Rapid or overly vigorous turning may cause delicate skin to shear.
- Dry skin is more prone to cracking and peeling, but excessive moisture provides a medium for bacterial growth and may lead to maceration. Soaps may be irritating. Urine and feces, if left in contact with skin, may cause chemical irritation and contribute to rapid breakdown of tissue.
- Special bedding or beds may help improve patient comfort, distribute pressure more evenly, and reduce the deleterious effects of impaired mobility. Special beds don't eliminate the need to turn and reposition the patient.
- Immobility contributes to increased catabolism and tissue breakdown; also, using stored fats as an energy source may reduce adipose tissue that provides cushioning. Protein is essential for maintaining and rebuilding tissue.

4. Monitor for evidence of impending skin breakdown: edema, blanching, coldness, tenderness, redness, or blistering. Brief reactive hyperemia of the skin is normal following relief from pressure. If reactive hyperemia doesn't resolve after 15 minutes, institute additional protective measures for the affected area.

4. Early detection of impending problems permits treatment before skin breakdown occurs. The signs and symptoms listed result when pressure and immobility diminish perfusion. Pressure ulcers can result from as little as 1 hour of pressure and immobility, if the pressure is great enough to impede capillary flow. Additionally, subcutaneous tissue and muscle have usually suffered ischemia before the ulcer becomes apparent on the skin surface, so early detection and treatment are vital.

5. If a pressure ulcer develops, institute a therapeutic regimen immediately, according to the doctor's orders or unit protocol.

5. Treatment of pressure ulcers varies among practitioners and institutions. Prompt treatment is essential to avert development of additional complications, such as osteomyelitis

6. Additional individualized interventions: _____

6. Rationales: _____

NURSING DIAGNOSIS

Risk for altered urinary elimination related to diuresis, stasis of urine, positioning, or bone demineralization

Nursing priorities
• Promote normal urine elimination.
• Prevent urinary system complications.

Patient outcome criteria
Throughout the hospital stay, the patient will:
• maintain urine output of at least 60 ml/hour
• maintain fluid intake of at least eight 8-oz (240-ml) glasses daily, unless contraindicated
• exhibit no signs of urinary tract infection or calculi.

Interventions

1. Assess the patient's normal urine elimination pattern, if possible, by noting the following:
• frequency, time, and amount of voidings
• any change in the usual pattern
• continence
• special measures used to initiate or control voiding; note color, odor, and appearance (including inspection for increased sedimentation).

2. Evaluate factors that may increase the risk of urinary complications, such as:
• dehydration
• incontinence
• indwelling catheters
• narcotics, sedatives, diuretics, or other medications that affect renal function or alertness
• diabetes
• neurogenic bladder dysfunction
• pregnancy
• immunosuppression
• shock
• altered acid-base or electrolyte status.

Rationales

1. Assessment of the patient's normal elimination status is the first step in planning individualized care.

2. Immobility has several effects on urinary elimination. Bed rest increases the solute load of the kidneys because tissue breakdown and bone demineralization both occur at an increased rate. The increased thoracic blood volume associated with the supine position triggers decreased ADH release, resulting in diuresis. The supine position also contributes to urinary stasis, because downward urine flow is normally enhanced by gravity. Additionally, complete bladder emptying may be harder to achieve in the supine position. Any additional factors, such as those listed, contribute further to the risk of complications and must be considered in care planning.

General plans of care

3. Initiate measures to promote normal urine elimination:

• Have a female patient sit on a bedside commode and allow a male patient to stand to urinate, condition permitting.

• Encourage adequate fluid intake (eight to twelve 8-oz [240-ml] glasses daily), unless contraindicated.

• Promote as much activity as the patient's condition permits — turning, sitting, leg dangling, standing, walking, or range-of-motion exercises.
• Provide privacy during attempts to void.

• Use measures to promote full emptying of the bladder, as needed, such as running water nearby, pouring warm water over the perineum, and applying manual pressure over the bladder.
• Use urinary catheterization only as needed to prevent distention and stasis. Exercise strict aseptic technique during insertion and care of catheters.

4. Measure urine output hourly and report values less than 60 ml/hour for 2 hours. Assess for bladder distention at least every 8 hours. Measure urine pH every 8 hours and report levels greater than 6. Monitor routine urine cultures, as ordered.

5. Monitor for indications of urinary tract complications, as follows:
• infection — burning, frequency, and urgency (if voiding voluntarily); cloudy, foul-smelling urine; hematuria; fever; low back pain; or increased white blood cell count
• calculi — severe flank pain, lower abdominal pain, hematuria, nausea, or altered urine stream (if a calculus lodges in the bladder neck or urethra).

6. If indications of urinary complications are detected, notify the doctor promptly and collaborate in treatment.

7. Additional individualized interventions: _____
_____

3. Measures to promote normal elimination may help reduce the risk of developing urinary system complications.
• The upright position facilitates improved urine flow from the ureters and bladder and usually is more comfortable for the patient. In addition, studies report no significant differences in oxygen consumption and cardiovascular response between in-bed and out-of-bed toileting. Weight-bearing exercise of any kind, including the effort to sit or stand, may also help reduce deleterious orthostasis and bone demineralization.
• Calcium precipitation and resultant calculi formation are less likely to occur in dilute urine. Also, an adequate quantity of dilute urine increases frequency of urination, reducing the likelihood of infection from stasis.
• Position changes promote urine drainage, minimize stasis, and reduce protein breakdown associated with immobilization.
• The sphincter relaxation necessary for voiding may be difficult to achieve unless privacy is ensured.
• Bladder distention may cause back pressure and eventual nephron damage. Incomplete bladder emptying is also associated with increased risk of infection.

• Urinary catheterization is associated with a high incidence of nosocomial infections. Placement of a catheter in the normally sterile urinary tract exposes the patient to pathogens that may cause infection.

4. Urine output of less than 60 ml/hour may indicate impending renal failure or other complications. Bladder distention and resultant urinary stasis may occur even in a catheterized patient if the tube becomes obstructed by sediment, blood clots, or calculi. Alkaline urine contributes to the formation of calcium calculi. Routine urine cultures allow early detection of infection.

5. Urinary tract complications usually result from several interrelated factors.
• Urinary tract infection may be related to stasis, dehydration, bladder distention, or any factor that damages the protective mucosal lining of the bladder, such as calculi or catheterization.
• Calcium excretion is increased in a patient on prolonged bed rest because of increased bone breakdown. Most calculi are composed of calcium salts. Such factors as stasis, infection, and decreased urine volume contribute to calculi formation. Also, because of low levels of muscle contraction, a smaller-than-normal quantity of acid end products is excreted, and the urine becomes increasingly alkaline, a condition that favors calculi formation.

6. Treatment of urinary pathology in acutely ill patients must be carefully coordinated with treatment of the patient's primary condition to avoid further complications.

7. Rationales: _____
_____

NURSING DIAGNOSIS

Risk for constipation related to weakness of abdominal muscles, loss of defecation reflex, slowed peristalsis, altered nutritional intake, or psychological inhibition

Nursing priority

Promote normal bowel elimination.

Patient outcome criteria

Throughout the hospital stay, the patient will:
• maintain normal bowel elimination
• perform abdominal exercises as taught, if the condition permits
• exhibit no signs of constipation.

Interventions

1. Assess the patient's normal bowel elimination pattern, if possible, noting the frequency, times, color, and consistency of stools; any change in the usual pattern; continence; use of laxatives or enemas; date and time of last bowel movement; and bowel sounds. Monitor bowel status daily.

2. Evaluate the patient for factors that may increase the risk of constipation, including dehydration; narcotics, iron intake, anticholinergics, or other medications affecting peristaltic function; paralysis; age (because of reduced colon tone); cachexia; emphysema (because of reduced ability to increase intra-abdominal pressure); abdominal surgery; abdominal tumors; pregnancy; ascites; hemorrhoids; nothing-by-mouth status; and trauma.

3. Initiate measures to promote normal bowel elimination:
• Allow the use of a bedside commode or toilet, if the condition permits. Encourage the patient to attempt defecation at usual times or when the urge arises.
• Encourage the patient to contract abdominal muscles while exhaling during defecation attempts. Instruct the patient to avoid Valsalva's maneuver.

• As the patient's condition permits, teach exercises to maintain or strengthen abdominal muscles, such as contracting and relaxing abdominal muscles several times per hour and performing leg lifts.
• Encourage adequate fluid intake, unless contraindicated.
• Encourage natural laxatives and high-fiber foods, as permitted and tolerated.
• Provide privacy and comfort measures during toileting, such as ensuring warmth and providing air freshener.

Rationales

1. Assessment of the patient's normal elimination status is the first step in planning individualized care. Daily monitoring helps in early identification of potential problems.

2. Because normal bowel motility depends in part on abdominal muscle contraction and physical activity, immobility predisposes the patient to constipation. Any additional factors, such as those listed, contribute further to the risk of complications and must be considered in care planning.

3. Maintaining normal bowel elimination reduces the risk of developing bowel complications.
• The normal defecation position facilitates evacuation. If defecation is suppressed despite impulses from rectal distention, colon motility eventually may be inhibited.
• Contraction of abdominal muscles increases intra-abdominal pressure and aids in evacuation. Valsalva's maneuver causes a vagal response and, in susceptible patients, may result in bradycardia, heart block, or other cardiovascular complications.
• Bed rest results in generalized muscle atrophy. Weakness of the abdominal muscles may render the patient unable to assist with evacuation.

• Inadequate fluid intake may cause dry, hard stools that are more difficult to expel.
• Whole-grain cereals, fruits and vegetables, and prune juice help promote natural elimination.
• Bowel activity may be inhibited if the patient is anxious, embarrassed, or uncomfortable.

General plans of care

4. Assess for indications of constipation, such as absence of bowel movements; hard, dry, small stools; sensation of rectal fullness; abdominal distention or mass; headache; decreased appetite; hard stool felt in rectal vault on digital examination; or ribbonlike diarrhea.

5. As necessary, collaborate with the doctor to select appropriate elimination aids, such as laxatives, suppositories, enemas, or stool softeners.

6. Additional individualized interventions: _____
_____

4. In the absence of normal bowel elimination, water continues to be reabsorbed from the stool that remains in the bowel, and the stool becomes harder, dryer, and more compacted. As softer stool collects behind it, increasing peristaltic pressure may result in a forceful expulsion of diarrhea past the hard stool mass.

5. Laxatives, suppositories, and enemas may be necessary occasionally, but their frequent use may disrupt normal bowel functioning. Stool softeners may help in the natural expulsion of stool and are not habit-forming.

6. Rationales: _____
_____

NURSING DIAGNOSIS

Risk for disuse syndrome: Muscle atrophy and joint contractures related to disuse, nonfunctional positioning, and reduced muscle tone

Nursing priority

Maintain maximum functional integrity of bone and muscle.

Patient outcome criteria

Throughout the hospital stay, the patient will:
• perform exercises as taught, if the condition permits
• maintain functional alignment of all joints.

Interventions

1. Evaluate the patient for factors that increase the risk of significant muscle, bone, and joint complications, including preexisting conditions that reduce mobility (such as arthritis, paralysis, paresis, or debilitation), decreased level of alertness, spinal injury or surgery, major burns, and trauma.

2. Initiate measures to preserve motor function and strength:
• weight bearing, as the condition permits, even if only standing at the bedside or on a tilt table several times daily

• active exercise, as the condition permits, including hourly ankle rotation and flexion and extension of the feet and quadriceps during waking hours
• complete range of motion to all joints at least four times daily, as the condition permits

Rationales

1. Normal bone and muscle function depend on activity, which maintains and increases muscle strength, maintains balanced muscle tone, and promotes normal bone formation. When a muscle is immobilized, 10% to 15% of its strength may be lost in as little as 1 week, and it may atrophy to half its size within 1 month. Disuse atrophy leads to shortening of muscle fibers and reduces joint motion. Immobilization decreases osteoblastic deposition of bone matrix, but normal osteoclastic destruction continues, depleting calcium and other minerals essential for bone stability. The other factors listed may add to the risk of significant bone- and muscle-related complications.

2. Maintaining healthy bone and muscle function is easier than restoring function after disability.
• Weight-bearing exercise stimulates osteoblastic activity by providing normal stress to bones. Lack of weight bearing is the primary contributor to osteoporosis, a condition in which the bones are so weakened that the patient is prone to fractures.
• Active exercises promote maximum muscle contraction and help maintain strength and endurance.

• Putting the joint through its full range of motion stretches the surrounding muscle fibers and maintains the coordinated function of joint structures.

• careful positioning to maintain functional alignment, using such devices as trochanter rolls, hand rolls, splints, footboards, and padding between thighs (if hip adduction is a problem); alternating flexion and extension of extremities when turning; and repositioning at least every 2 hours.

3. Additional individualized interventions: _____

• If functional alignment isn't maintained, serious joint contractures may result, requiring surgical intervention or prolonged corrective physical therapy.

3. Rationales: _____

NURSING DIAGNOSIS

Situational low self-esteem related to dependent patient role

Nursing priority

Promote positive self-image.

Patient outcome criteria

Throughout the hospital stay, the patient will:
• express feelings related to losses
• participate in decision making related to care
• exercise healthy coping behaviors.

Interventions

1. Assess the effects of reduced mobility on self-concept. Encourage expression of feelings and identification of primary losses.

2. Encourage the patient's participation in self-care and decision making, as the condition permits.

3. Anticipate such behaviors as regression, withdrawal, aggression, apathy, and crying. Try to help the patient interpret these normal responses to loss.

4. See the "Sensory-perceptual alteration" plan, page 96.

5. See the "Ineffective individual coping" plan, page 67.

6. Additional individualized interventions: _____

Rationales

1. Identifying what the loss of normal mobility means to the individual is the first step in care planning. A patient's reaction to immobility can vary enormously, depending on baseline activity level and the importance of physical function to identity.

2. Participating in self-care, even in small ways, preserves a patient's sense of identity and integrity.

3. Immobility may cause disorganization of the psyche as the individual attempts to cope with the profound loss of usual roles, stimulation, and independence. Helping the patient to understand the normalcy of his reactions may reduce psychic disequilibrium and facilitate healthy coping strategies.

4. Immobility results in significant reduction in normal sensory stimulation. This can contribute to decreased motivation, reduced ability to learn and solve problems, sleep disturbances, and other problems that may compound the patient's distress. The "Sensory-perceptual alteration" plan contains detailed information on preventing, detecting, and treating this problem.

5. The "Ineffective individual coping" plan contains further interventions that may be helpful in caring for the patient with low self-esteem.

6. Rationales: _____

General plans of care

DISCHARGE PLANNING
Discharge checklist
Before discharge, the patient should show evidence of no life-threatening or disabling complications of immobility.

Teaching checklist
Document evidence that the patient and family demonstrate an understanding of:
❑ activity recommendations, restrictions, and limitations
❑ measures to avert orthostatic hypotension and activity intolerance
❑ indicators of clinically significant activity intolerance
❑ signs of complications related to impaired mobility
❑ use of mobility aids.

Documentation checklist
Using outcome criteria as a guide, document:
❑ clinical status on admission
❑ significant changes in status
❑ pertinent laboratory and diagnostic test findings
❑ protective measures initiated
❑ response to resumption of activity
❑ complications of immobility, if any
❑ patient and family teaching
❑ discharge planning.

ASSOCIATED PLANS OF CARE

Geriatric care
Ineffective individual coping
Nutritional deficit
Sensory-perceptual alteration

REFERENCES

Alessi, C., and Henderson, C. "Constipation and Fecal Impaction in the Long-Term Care Patient," *Clinics in Geriatric Medicine* 4(3):571-88, August 1988.

Daley, J., et al. "Use of Standardized Nursing Diagnoses and Interventions in Long-Term Care," *Journal of Gerontological Nursing* 21(8):29-36, August 1995.

Holloway, N. *Nursing the Critically Ill Adult,* 3rd ed. Menlo Park, Calif.: Addison-Wesley-Longman Publishing Co., 1993.

Kozier, B., et al. *Fundamentals of Nursing: Concepts, Process and Practice.* Menlo Park, Calif.: Addison-Wesley-Longman Publishing Co., 1995.

Olson, E.V., et al. "The Hazards of Immobility," *AJN* 90(3):43-48, March 1990.

Oullet, L., and Rush, K. "A Study of Nurses' Perception of Client Mobility," *Western Journal of Nursing Research* 18(5):565-79, October 1996.

Roberts, B., et al. "The Congruence of Nursing Diagnoses and Supporting Clinical Evidence," *Nursing Diagnosis* 7(3):108-15, July-September 1996.

Ineffective family coping: Compromised

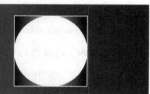

INTRODUCTION

Definition and time focus
Family coping becomes compromised when a usually supportive family member provides insufficient, ineffective, or compromised support, comfort, assistance, or encouragement that the patient may need to adapt to his health challenge. A patient's hospitalization can cause a crisis within the family because usual coping and support mechanisms may be overwhelmed. This plan focuses on the family's ability to manage the stressors that affect them during the patient's hospital stay.

Etiology and precipitating factors
• Illness or injury of family member
• Disruption of usual family activities and routines
• Family disunity
• Loss of control by patient or family
• Role changes within the family
• Unfamiliar hospital environment
• Restricted visitation of loved ones
• Loss of income, cost of medical care
• Poverty

FOCUSED ASSESSMENT GUIDELINES

Nursing history (functional health pattern findings for family)
Nutritional-metabolic pattern
• Neglect of nutritional intake while family member is hospitalized
Sleep-rest pattern
• Inadequate sleep or rest while family member is hospitalized
Cognitive-perceptual pattern
• Inaccurate understanding of the patient's condition
• Failure to request clarification of information about the patient's situation
• Tendency to pay attention to only some aspects of the information given
• Lack of skills or education to understand complex medical information
Self-perception–self-concept pattern
• Inability to cope with current situation
• Anxiety, fear, or anger
• Unresolved guilt or hostility

• Unawareness of feelings or perceptions of other family members
• Discomfort with emotional reactions of other family members
Role-relationship pattern
• Lack of interaction among family members
• Difficulty communicating feelings and perceptions to other family members
• Difficulty reaching decisions
• Rigidly established roles within the family structure
• Inability to provide emotional support for each other
• Anger or disagreement over the plan of care
Coping–stress tolerance pattern
• Use of inappropriate coping methods
• Use of non-growth-promoting methods (denial, depression, violence, or substance abuse) to handle past crises
• Failure to identify all coping strategies available within the family system
• Regression or increased dependence characterized by reliance on others to solve problems
Value-belief pattern
• Value conflicts among family members
• Unrealistic beliefs about health, disease, or roles and abilities of other family members

Physical findings
Not applicable

Diagnostic studies
Not applicable

Potential complications
• High anxiety levels among family members
• Transfer of anxiety from family to patient
• Unrealistic expectations of patient — for example, expecting full recovery of neurologic function in a brain-damaged person
• Unrealistic expectations of other family members — for example, expecting uncommunicative member to become emotionally supportive in crisis
• Inattention to family members' physical and psychosocial needs
• Inadequate preparation for the patient's discharge or death
• Disintegration of the family unit

NURSING DIAGNOSIS

Ineffective family coping related to illness and hospitalization of family member

Nursing priority

Help the family identify, develop, and use healthy coping skills.

Patient outcome criteria

- Within 2 days of the patient's admission, family members will:
  - verbalize feelings to the nurse, if desired
  - recognize their physical needs for food and rest.
- By the time of the patient's discharge, family members will:
  - verbalize feelings appropriately to each other
  - participate actively in caring for the ill family member
  - use healthy coping mechanisms
  - demonstrate listening and supportive behaviors to each other
  - identify resources within and outside the family
  - develop a plan or strategy to provide necessary care and support for the ill family member after discharge.

Interventions

1. Assess and document the origins of the crisis and the family members' responses to it. Identify factors contributing to vulnerability in a crisis state. Observe nonverbal behaviors, such as eye contact and body posture.

2. Demonstrate interest and concern for the patient's family members. Acknowledge their feelings about the situation — for example, "This must be very difficult for you."

3. Take measures to minimize the family members' level of anxiety: Provide a quiet, private place for discussion; avoid elaborate information or unnecessary questions; and remain available to the family. Document the family's initial status and response to nursing interventions.

4. Provide accurate, timely information about the patient's treatment and care. Give explanations in lay terms, encourage questions, and introduce topics likely to be of interest. Reinforce information given by the doctor. Document the information given to the family.

Rationales

1. Situational factors (such as illness or death), transitional states (developmental turning point or life-cycle phase), and sociocultural factors all can contribute to a crisis. Families in which several of these factors are present are at higher risk for crisis development. Nonverbal behaviors, such as clenched fists or lack of eye contact, provide valuable clues about the family's emotional state.

2. Approaching the family with a warm and respectful attitude lays the groundwork for developing a trusting relationship.

3. In states of heightened anxiety, the ability to think clearly, handle new information, and make appropriate decisions is impaired. Minimizing distractions reduces anxiety and helps family members regain control of their thinking processes.

4. Family members must be well informed to develop an accurate perception of the patient's illness or injury. Medical jargon may increase anxiety in some individuals. Clear, simple explanations will be understood best. Encouraging questions dispels possible discomfort over not knowing answers, while suggesting topics reduces possible discomfort over not knowing what to ask. Anxiety and misunderstanding can be minimized by giving explanations in lay terms and by reinforcing or clarifying information given by the doctor. Family members who understand their own problems as well as the patient's can recognize their needs and identify appropriate solutions.

5. Clarify family members' perceptions of the information given to them. Don't assume that what was stated was what the family heard and understood. Document the family's level of understanding.

6. Reduce the stress associated with the hospital environment. Individualize visitation privileges. Orient the family to hospital facilities. Arrange for a quiet place for the family to meet with the doctor. Provide pillows and blankets for family members spending the night at the hospital.

7. Assist family members in caring for their own physical and psychosocial needs. Encourage adequate rest periods. Reinforce the need for adequate dietary intake.

8. Encourage family members to express their feelings about the impact of the patient's illness. Ask open-ended questions. Listen carefully to each person. Support communication among family members. Observe how feelings are expressed and how family members behave. Document the family's response and behavior. Identify, when possible, the family member who is the primary health and illness resource for the family, and include that person in all teaching. Also, make sure that person has an adequate support system.

9. Promote awareness of family strengths by identifying areas in which the members work well together. Document identified family strengths and weaknesses. Direct nursing interventions toward encouraging family strengths — for example, support family efforts to learn care techniques or to bring in special items from home, as permitted.

10. Facilitate family communication when dysfunctions are present. Encourage verbalization and recognition of feelings. Provide referrals to other professionals (mental health liaison nurse, social worker, clinical specialist, clinical psychologist, or member of the clergy) when family problems lie outside the role of the staff nurse.

11. Focus on immediate, concrete problems.

12. Help the family develop a realistic appraisal of the situation and an action plan. Explore coping skills and support systems available to the family. Help them identify resources, such as friends, other family members, self-help groups related to the diagnosis, home health care nurses, or homemaking assistance. Ensure that the plan is appropriate to the family's functional level, dependence needs, and lifestyle.

5. Asking for feedback and clarification allows the nurse to determine the family members' actual level of understanding.

6. Manipulating the hospital environment decreases the family's physical distress in adjusting to the patient's hospitalization.

7. Development of problem-solving skills and effective coping strategies is impaired when family members are physically exhausted, malnourished, or stressed by unmet emotional or psychosocial needs.

8. Awareness of feelings and the ability to express them clearly and appropriately are important elements of healthy coping behaviors. Help-seeking behaviors are aided by intrafamily communication and realistic discussion of how the patient's illness may affect family functioning. By using open-ended questions, the nurse can guide the family's communication. Listening to the family and helping them clarify their feelings and perceptions will help the nurse identify areas where additional support is needed. Most families have one member who is the informed "health liaison person" who may act as caregiver, teacher, and interpreter. Acknowledgment of this role facilitates therapeutic intervention.

9. Acknowledging family strengths, such as closeness, open communication, or willingness to help each other, aids the family in identifying their resources for coping with the crisis.

10. The nurse's role is to listen, support, and clarify — not solve — the family's problems. The nurse helps the family to identify available resources and to make informed decisions about using them.

11. A primary nursing focus is to reduce the family members' anxiety so they can think constructively and make use of problem-solving skills. In many cases, anxiety can be decreased by attending to easily removable stressors; for example, refer an out-of-town family to the social services department to arrange for housing while the patient is hospitalized.

12. In establishing a plan of action, family members need to match their own needs and the patient's with available resources. By providing such information, the nurse helps the family develop a plan to meet their needs.

General plans of care

13. Encourage independent decision making by family members.

14. With the patient and family, follow up and evaluate the implementation of the plan of action.

15. Avoid imposing personal values or codes of behavior on family members.

16. Additional individualized interventions: _____

13. Allowing family members to make decisions promotes their independence.

14. Evaluation of the plan of action reinforces successful strategies and may suggest additional or alternate interventions. Evaluation done with the family is an excellent way to provide positive feedback and acknowledge their new coping skills.

15. In order to intervene effectively with a family in crisis, the nurse must develop an awareness of personal value systems and beliefs related to cultural norms. This allows the nurse to view the family's problems without imposing personal values on the family system.

16. Rationales: _____

DISCHARGE PLANNING

Discharge checklist
Before discharge, the patient should show evidence of:
❏ identification of the impact of the patient's illness on family function
❏ plans for dealing with changes within the family
❏ identification of internal and external resources available to family members
❏ initial contact with selected external resources.

Teaching checklist
Document evidence that the patient and family demonstrate an understanding of:
❏ extent and implication of the patient's illness and limitations
❏ changes in family roles and function such as new responsibilities each member must assume to facilitate care of the patient at home
❏ resources and referrals available to the family.

Documentation checklist
Using outcome criteria as a guide, document:
❏ family's initial emotional status
❏ precipitating factors in crisis and the meaning of crisis to family members
❏ changes in emotional status related to nursing interventions
❏ treatment and care information given to family members
❏ family's level of understanding of information provided
❏ family members' ability to express feelings
❏ identified family strengths and weaknesses
❏ referrals to community resources.

ASSOCIATED PLANS OF CARE

Dying
Grieving
Ineffective individual coping
Knowledge deficit

REFERENCES

Carpenito, L. *Nursing Diagnosis: Application to Clinical Practice,* 7th ed. Philadelphia: Lippincott-Raven Pubs., 1997.
Hickey, M. "What Are the Needs of Families of Critically Ill Patients? A Review of the Literature since 1976," *Heart & Lung* 19(4):401-15, July 1990.
Kleeman, K.M. "Families in Crisis due to Multiple Traumas," *Critical Care Clinics of North America* 1(1):23-31, March 1989.
Miller, C.A. *Nursing Care of Older Adults,* 2nd ed. Glenview, Ill.: Scott Foresman, 1995.
Tinstman, C.F., and Crimlisk, J. "Infantile Alpha I Antitrypsin Deficiency: A Case Report," *Gastroenterology Nursing* 18(1): 20-26, January-February 1995.
Wong, D.L. *Essentials of Pediatric Nursing,* 3rd ed. St. Louis: Mosby–Year Book, Inc., 1995.

Ineffective individual coping

INTRODUCTION

Definition and time focus
Ineffective coping is the impairment of a person's adaptive behaviors and ability to meet life's demands and roles. This plan focuses on the patient who is hospitalized for an acute illness or an exacerbation of a chronic condition and whose usual coping mechanisms aren't effective in maintaining psychological equilibrium.

Etiology and precipitating factors
- Stimuli likely to cause ineffective coping in illness
  - Pain and incapacitation
  - Lack of sleep
  - Stressful hospital environment and treatment procedures
  - Loss of control over what is happening to self
  - Loss of hope
  - Lack of meaningful contact with loved ones
  - Uncertain future
- Conditions necessary for a stimulus to cause ineffective coping
  - Perception of a harmful stimulus or cues that a harmful stimulus is imminent
  - Perception that the harmful stimulus threatens the individual's goals or values
  - Perception that the patient's resources are not equal to coping with the threat

FOCUSED ASSESSMENT GUIDELINES

Nursing history (functional health pattern findings)
Health perception–health management pattern
- Perception of illness and hospitalization as a loss of control that threatens fulfillment of usual roles or threatens life itself
- Drastically reduced ability to solve problems effectively
  - Selecting course of action without weighing alternatives
  - Feeling overwhelmed by alternatives and being unable to select a course of action
- Failure to follow plan of treatment

Nutritional-metabolic pattern
- Anorexia, nausea, or vomiting
- Weight loss from anorexia
- Frequent overeating to deal with stress

Elimination pattern
- Diarrhea or constipation from dietary changes or stress

Activity-exercise pattern
- Occasional hyperactivity and inability to rest
- Occasional withdrawal, listlessness, or fatigue

Sleep-rest pattern
- Sleep disturbance
  - More than usual amount of sleep
  - Difficulty falling asleep
  - Early awakening followed by inability to return to sleep (early morning insomnia)
  - Frequent night-time awakening

Cognitive-perceptual pattern
- Diminished ability to view the world objectively
- Decreased ability to take in information
- Lack of information necessary to make decisions
- Suspicion surrounding intentions of caregivers

Self-perception–self-concept pattern
- Feeling that the threat is greater than available internal resources to combat it
- Inability to control events affecting the situation

Role-relationship pattern
- Decreased ability to communicate needs
- Feelings of isolation and inability to respond to caring from others
- Occasional inability to control impulsive behavior, possibly leading to hostility, aggression, or suicidal behavior

Sexuality-reproductive pattern
- Loss of libido, impotence, or orgasmic dysfunction

Coping–stress tolerance pattern
- Physiologic responses related to sympathetic nervous system stimulation such as tachycardia
- Increased number of infections related to alteration in the immune system
- Denial of symptoms and delay in seeking treatment
- Various negative coping behaviors, depending on individual and environmental factors
  - Anger and hostility
  - Anxiety and hyperactivity
  - Depression and withdrawal
  - Suicidal ideation
- Behavior that alienates caregivers and removes a source of support
- History of ineffective coping mechanisms, such as drug or alcohol abuse, nicotine addiction, or overeating

Value-belief pattern
- Loss of faith related to feelings of hopelessness and abandonment

Physical findings
General appearance
- Anxious facial expression
- Flat affect
- Poor eye contact
- Slumped posture
Cardiovascular
- Elevated blood pressure
- Increased heart rate
- Increased ventricular arrhythmias (occasionally)
Pulmonary
- Increased rate and depth of respirations
Gastrointestinal
- Vomiting
- Diarrhea
- GI bleeding (if stress ulcer develops)
Neurologic
- Dilated pupils, as sympathetic nervous system response (occasionally)
- Restlessness
- Lethargy
Integumentary
- Diaphoresis (occasionally)
Musculoskeletal
- Increased muscle tension and pain

Diagnostic studies
In the clinical setting, laboratory tests aren't normally done to identify ineffective coping. Remember, however, that physiologic responses to stress can mimic disease.
- Arterial blood gas measurements may reveal respiratory alkalosis from an increased rate and depth of respiration (hyperventilation).
- White blood cell count may be increased.
- Mental status examination
  – Appearance may yield clues about self-perception (patients coping ineffectively may not care about their appearance).
  – Behavior (body movements, tone of voice) is an indicator of the person's self-expression ability, an important coping skill; behavior may vary, depending on the patient's expressive style. The relationship of the patient with caregivers is also important to assess: Is the patient controlling, passive, aggressive, suspicious, or uncooperative?
  – Impaired cognitive function (orientation, memory, and judgment) may be demonstrated by the inability to problem-solve.
  – Feelings shown indicate which emotions the patient expresses and their appropriateness to the situation; wide variety of feelings possible, ranging from anxiety to anger to depression and typically including isolation and hopelessness
  – Perceptions indicate the patient's view of the situation; perceptions of threat are based on previous experi-

ence, values, and beliefs along with perception of inadequate resources in relation to the magnitude of the threat. Which coping mechanisms were used in the past? Which were useful? Which are potentially harmful—for example, smoking, alcohol use, or drug use?
- Suicide assessment—a patient who feels hopeless and helpless needs to be asked about presence of suicidal thoughts; this question doesn't cause a patient to think about suicide but instead provides an opportunity to talk about these disturbing feelings. Factors associated with high risk include:
  – high level of anxiety or panic
  – severe depression
  – minimal ability to perform activities of daily living
  – few or no sources of support or significant others
  – continued abuse of alcohol or drugs, or both
  – negative view of previous psychiatric help (if applicable)
  – one or more previous suicide attempts
  – marked hostility
  – frequent or constant thoughts of suicide
  – suicide plan that is specific in method and timing
  – possession of means to carry out the plan, such as physical capacity and weapon.
(See also *Assessment of suicide potential,* page 48, in the "Grieving" plan.)

Potential complications
- Physiologic
  – Increased risk of falls and accidents
  – Ventricular arrhythmias
  – Increased susceptibility to infections
- Psychological
  – Suicide or homicide
  – Major depression
  – Reactive psychosis
  – Disintegration of family unit

NURSING DIAGNOSIS

Ineffective individual coping related to illness and hospitalization

Nursing priorities

- Establish rapport and trust.
- Accurately identify threat and coping resources.
- Intervene to optimize coping skills.
- Evaluate the effectiveness of interventions.

Patient outcome criteria

Within 2 days of identification of ineffective coping, the patient will:
- express an accurate understanding of the current situation and plan of treatment
- state that any pain is within tolerable limits
- participate in developing a plan of care
- use support offered by caregivers.

Interventions

1. Form a positive relationship with the patient.
- Convey a sense of caring and concern for what happens to the patient.
- Use appropriate eye contact.
- Convey feelings of comfort and relaxation by approaching the patient calmly, including the patient in all bedside conversations, and speaking in a well-modulated tone.
- Identify personal reactions to the patient's coping style that could interfere with formation of a helping relationship. Avoid judging the patient's behavior.

2. Rule out organic causes for such behavioral changes as decreased alertness, impaired memory, confusion, restlessness, or depression.

3. Provide factual information about the illness and plan of treatment. Reinforce information the patient has received from the doctor. Be prepared to repeat information in clear, concise language.

4. With the patient, identify the source of the threat.

Rationales

1. Patients report that feelings of being uncared for interfere with their recovery and contribute to feelings of hopelessness. An ineffective relationship with caregivers drains energy that could be better used for healing. Conversely, patients who feel positive about their nurses say this gives them an energy that helps with healing, decreases isolation, and increases coping ability. People express anxiety, pain, and needs for privacy and intimacy in various ways, depending on their cultural and personal biases. For example, if the patient who feels comfortable expressing pain openly is cared for by a nurse who believes that pain should be tolerated in silence, an ineffective nurse-patient relationship may result. Recognizing one's cultural and personal biases is the first step in avoiding prejudicial responses to the patient's behavior, which is a unique pattern used to decrease anxiety.

2. Behavioral changes that appear to be signs of ineffective coping may actually represent such physiologic problems as hypoxia, electrolyte imbalance, or drug toxicity. Assuming that all behavioral responses are related to psychological mechanisms may delay needed medical treatment.

3. For problem solving to begin, the patient needs accurate information. Patients who are coping ineffectively have a decreased ability to hear and assimilate information.

4. Whether or not a stimulus is felt as threatening depends on values, beliefs, and the perception of available resources. The patient may not perceive an obvious, identifiable threat (such as a diagnosis of cancer) as the primary threat. Conversely, what seems routine to the nurse may be frightening to the patient.

General plans of care

5. Help the patient be specific about what seems threatening.

6. With the patient, identify modifiable components of the threat.

7. Help the patient identify personal strengths and external resources, such as family, friends, and economic means.

8. Identify external resources and make appropriate referrals — for example, for social services, spiritual counseling, or psychiatric interventions.

9. Keep pain at a tolerable level.

10. Ensure adequate nutrition and sleep.

11. Control environmental stimuli that drain adaptive energy needed to maintain psychological equilibrium: Provide privacy for all invasive procedures and for nursing and self-care activities; eliminate conversation around the bedside that doesn't include the patient; and decrease environmental noise.

12. Offer alternative strategies to counteract the effects of the threat — for example, guided imagery, relaxation techniques, or back rubs.

13. Give choices related to the patient's care and situation whenever possible.

14. Provide opportunities for loved ones to interact with the patient in meaningful ways.

15. Assess responses to nursing interventions, and collaborate with the doctor to determine if pharmacologic intervention would be helpful.

16. Additional individualized interventions: _____
_____

5. Patients may have misconceptions about what is happening to them. If they can specify their fears, the nurse can plan specific actions such as providing information that helps the patient see the situation realistically.

6. In many cases, people coping ineffectively are unable to separate their situation into manageable parts; instead, they view the problem as overwhelming and unmanageable. If they can view the problem in its component parts, their anxiety may be reduced and effective coping behaviors become more possible.

7. People in crisis may not identify their strengths. They will need assistance in assessing resources and identifying ways to activate them.

8. Expansion of the patient's base of support helps decrease the perceived magnitude of the specific threat.

9. Pain is a common source of fear. Uncontrolled pain increases anxiety and decreases the energy available for coping.

10. Inadequate diet and lack of sleep are stressors themselves and, as such, decrease the amount of energy available for coping and adaptation.

11. Every stimulus in the environment is a potential threat. Stimuli not normally viewed as threatening may, in combination, create more stress and decrease coping ability.

12. The relaxation response is the physiologic opposite of anxiety. Relaxation techniques may help the patient cope with stress and regain control.

13. Maintaining some ability to control one's life helps to combat feelings of helplessness.

14. A positive response from loved ones encourages a more positive response to treatment and decreases the sense of isolation.

15. Antianxiety medications may be helpful in decreasing potentially harmful physiologic and psychological effects of anxiety. Antidepressants may be useful in patients with signs of severe depression.

16. Rationales: _____
_____

DISCHARGE PLANNING

Discharge checklist
Before discharge, the patient should show evidence of:
- ❏ perception of increased ability to cope with the situation
- ❏ ability to name resources appropriate to the situation
- ❏ increased ability to manage the current situation by defining the problem and reasonable solutions.

Teaching checklist
Document evidence that the patient and family demonstrate an understanding of:
- ❏ diagnosis, plan of treatment, and prognosis
- ❏ expected physiologic responses during recovery
- ❏ community resources appropriate to perceived problems
- ❏ appropriate alternative coping strategies
- ❏ how to contact the doctor.

Documentation checklist
Using outcome criteria as a guide, document:
- ❏ coping status on admission
- ❏ significant changes in appearance, affect, behavior, perception, and cognitive function
- ❏ psychological responses to hospitalization and interventions
- ❏ significant physiologic stress responses
- ❏ sleep patterns
- ❏ nutritional intake
- ❏ pain control
- ❏ response to caregivers
- ❏ response to interventions designed to increase coping skills
- ❏ suicide risk
- ❏ referrals made
- ❏ patient and family teaching
- ❏ discharge planning.

ASSOCIATED PLANS OF CARE

Dying
Grieving
Ineffective family coping: Compromised
Knowledge deficit
Pain

REFERENCES

Bates, B. *A Pocket Guide to Physical Examination and History Taking,* 2nd ed. Philadelphia: Lippincott-Raven Pubs., 1995.

Ferguson, J.S., and Smith, A. "Aggressive Behavior on an Inpatient Geriatric Unit," *Journal of Psychosocial Nursing* 34(3):27-32, March 1996.

Kaplan, H.I., and Sadock, B.J. *Pocket Handbook of Clinical Psychiatry,* 2nd ed. Baltimore: Williams & Wilkins Co., 1996.

Twibell, R.S., et al. "Spiritual and Coping Needs of Critically Ill Patients: Validations of Nursing Diagnoses," *Dimensions of Critical Care Nursing* 15(5):245-53, September-October 1996.

Unguarski, P.J., and Hurley, P.M. "Nursing Research in HIV/AIDS Home Care, Part 2," *Home Healthcare Nurse* 13(4):9-13, July-August 1995.

General plans of care

Knowledge deficit

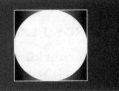

INTRODUCTION

Definition and time focus
A knowledge deficit is an absence or deficiency of cognitive information related to a specific topic. This teaching plan focuses on the acutely ill patient and family. Although a major teaching program during hospitalization is inappropriate for most patients, you can capitalize on unexpected teaching opportunities to meet immediate learning needs as well as to identify long-range learning needs. The latter are usually addressed after the patient has been discharged or transferred to an environment more conducive to learning.

Through expert teaching, the nurse can provide a context for the patient and family to understand the rationale for therapeutic interventions. Teaching is most effective when it pervades all phases of patient care.

Because of the importance of knowledge deficit as a patient problem and the number of possible interventions, problems in this plan are subdivided by cause.

Etiology and precipitating factors
- Unfamiliar diagnostic procedure
- New diagnosis
- Alteration in existing health problem
- Unfamiliar or altered treatment plan
- Complex treatment regimen
- Denial
- Anxiety

FOCUSED ASSESSMENT GUIDELINES

Nursing history (functional health pattern findings)
Because each patient's knowledge deficit will be individual, this section presents a guide for assessment of teaching and learning factors.

Health perception–health management pattern
- Did the patient delay seeking medical attention?
- Does the patient lack knowledge about the disorder?
- Does the patient express lack of confidence in managing the condition?
- Does the patient express misconceptions about health status?
- Has the patient failed to comply with recommended health practices?
- Does the patient fail to carry out self-care, even though physically able?

Nutritional-metabolic pattern
- Does the patient express concerns about the effects of the disorder on nutrition and eating habits?
- Has the patient had difficulty staying on a prescribed dietary regimen?

Activity-exercise pattern
- Does the patient express concerns about life-changing physical limitations because of the disorder?

Cognitive-perceptual pattern
- Does the patient express concerns about specific details of a diagnostic or therapeutic procedure?
- Does the patient have sensory deficits, such as visual or hearing impairments?
- Does the patient lack psychomotor skills needed to maintain a home treatment regimen?
- Has the patient experienced confusion or changes in thought processes from the disorder?
- Has the patient shown signs of misinterpreting information such as by asking inappropriate questions?

Self-perception–self-concept pattern
- Does the patient express concerns about an inability to maintain the treatment regimen?
- Does the patient report anxiety about changes in body image from the disorder?

Role-relationship pattern
- Does the patient want a family member present or available during procedures?
- Does the patient express concerns about job, income, family responsibilities, or the family's response to lifestyle changes because of the disorder?

Sexuality-reproductive pattern
- Does the patient report concern about the disorder's impact on sexual activity?
- Does the patient express concern about the impact of changes in sexual activity on a spouse or partner?

Coping–stress tolerance pattern
- Does the patient display an unusual amount of anxiety?
- Does the patient display denial of the disorder?
- Does the patient report depression because of lifestyle changes caused by the disorder?
- Does the patient express concerns about coping behaviors and motivation?

Physical findings
Not applicable

Diagnostic studies
Not applicable

Potential complication
- Exacerbation of disorder

CLINICAL SNAPSHOT

KNOWLEDGE DEFICIT

Major nursing diagnoses	Key patient outcomes
Risk for knowledge deficit related to lack of readiness to learn	Be physiologically stable.
Risk for knowledge deficit related to teaching program inappropriate for current needs	Have learning needs documented in chart.
Risk for knowledge deficit related to inadequate or ineffective implementation of teaching plan	Have teaching accomplished during stay documented in chart.
Risk for knowledge deficit related to lack of needed modification in teaching	Express satisfaction with teaching plan.

NURSING DIAGNOSIS

Risk for knowledge deficit related to lack of readiness to learn

Nursing priority

Determine readiness to learn.

Patient outcome criteria

Before initiation of teaching, the patient will:
• be physiologically stable
• discuss current knowledge of the disorder when asked
• identify primary perceived learning needs
• display motivation to learn such as by asking appropriate questions.

Interventions

1. Assess the impact of the patient's disorder on lifestyle.

2. Determine the patient's stage of adaptation to the disorder: shock and disbelief, developing awareness, or resolution and reorganization. Consider psychological issues when planning teaching objectives and content during each phase.

3. Assess the patient's physical readiness to learn: Is the patient physiologically stable, rested, and pain-free? If not, defer a formal teaching program.

Rationales

1. The degree of impact determines the extent of teaching necessary. Areas of impact provide foci around which learning experiences should be structured.

2. Different psychological work occurs in each of these phases. Attempting to provide teaching inappropriate for a particular phase results in increased learner anxiety or irritation and inability to absorb information.

3. Teaching is most effective when the patient is ready to learn. Readiness to learn depends on physical as well as psychological factors. Determining readiness to learn requires weighing the interaction of numerous variables. Learning requires energy that won't be available if the patient is unstable, tired, or in pain. Because of shortened hospital stays, few patients reach physical or emotional readiness to learn extensive amounts of information before discharge.

General plans of care

4. Determine the patient's motivation to learn. For example, has the patient asked appropriate questions about status or care? Is the patient preoccupied, distracted, or emotionally labile?

4. Motivation is the crucial variable in learning and may be absent initially because of anxiety or preoccupation with personal needs. Prolonged absence of interest in learning about the condition may be a clue to an underlying emotional disorder requiring treatment before the patient can assume independent self-care. Motivation may be developed through teaching by linking relevant information to the patient's particular concerns.

5. Determine the general pattern of health maintenance; for example, has the patient sought regular medical checkups, followed previous health recommendations, eaten a balanced diet, and exercised regularly?

5. The general pattern can provide clues to overall acceptance of responsibility for self-care and receptivity to teaching.

6. Assess the patient's current knowledge of the disorder and its implications, the likelihood of complications, and the likelihood of cure or disease control. Specifically ask about the doctor's explanations, the patient's past experiences, and information received from family, friends, and the media.

6. Adults learn best when teaching builds on previous knowledge or experience. Assessing recall of the doctor's explanations as well as the patient's past experiences and exposure to health information provides an opportunity for evaluating attitudes and the accuracy and completeness of knowledge.

7. Ask how much the patient wants to know, if possible. Consider the patient's preference for information in planning teaching.

7. Research suggests that the common assumption that teaching reduces anxiety or otherwise helps the patient isn't always true; people vary in the degree of detail they find helpful. Those who cope with a threatening experience by avoiding it generally want to know relatively little about impending experiences, whereas those who cope by learning as much as possible about the threatening experience want to know a great deal. Providing the first type of patient with detailed information increases anxiety, whereas withholding it from the second type of patient increases stress. When possible, match preference and teaching appropriately to respect individual differences and support the patient's preferred learning style.

8. Determine learning needs. Consider needs expressed by the patient and family; predictable disorder-related concerns and responses; and activities necessary to monitor health status, prevent disease, implement prescribed therapy, and prevent complications or recurrence.

8. Learning needs determine appropriate content. Learning occurs most rapidly when it's relevant to current needs and past experiences. Responding to expressed needs displays sensitivity to the patient's and family's concerns. Identifying predictable concerns and responses and necessary self-care activities helps the nurse fulfill learning needs of which the patient and family may be unaware.

9. Estimate learning capacity. Assess the patient's age; language skills; ability to read, write, and reason; and educational, religious, and cultural background.

9. Sociocultural factors affect the speed and degree of learning. Awareness of the patient's age, background, and general capacity for logical thought and self-expression helps the nurse present material at an appropriate learning level.

10. Additional individualized interventions: _____

_____

10. Rationales: _____

_____

NURSING DIAGNOSIS

Risk for knowledge deficit related to teaching program inappropriate for current needs

Nursing priority

Plan an individualized teaching strategy.

Patient outcome criteria

Before discharge, the patient will:
• identify priority learning needs
• have learning needs documented in chart.

Interventions

1. Determine realistic goals for learning while the patient is in the hospital. Work with the patient and family to ensure that goals are mutually acceptable.

2. Determine what to teach by assessing what is essential from the patient's viewpoint. Set priorities for content by dividing it into "need to know now" and "need to know later" categories.

3. Provide a logical sequence to the information presented. In general, teach the acutely ill patient only:
• information about expressed concerns

• high-priority information—specific teaching without which the patient's condition may be seriously jeopardized.

4. Select appropriate teaching methods, such as individual bedside instruction, discussions, and demonstrations.

5. Be creative in choosing appropriate teaching materials, such as booklets, instruction sheets, films, videotapes, models or dolls, slides, and audiotapes. Consider the educational level, advantages, availability, patient's learning style, and the learning environment.

Rationales

1. Goals determine content. Goal-directed learning is more efficient than fragmented, unfocused learning. Active participation in goal setting increases the likelihood that the patient and family will understand goals and support them.

2. Because the patient's attention span may be limited and the hospital stay may be short, set priorities for content. Content largely determines the appropriate teaching method.

3. Proper sequencing allows the patient to build on current knowledge and experience.
• Learning is strongest when it fulfills perceived needs. Dealing with initial concerns displays sensitivity to the patient, helps establish rapport and trust, and frees the patient's energy to focus on further learning. In general, only crucial questions are answered for the acutely ill patient; the remainder are deferred.
• Presenting essential information early in the teaching period helps ensure that all the critical information will have been covered by the time of discharge.

4. Although various teaching methods exist (see *Teaching strategies,* page 76), individual instruction, discussion, and demonstration are most appropriate in the hospital because of constraints imposed by the patient's condition and the environment.

5. The more senses involved in learning, the more likely the patient will retain the information. Printed materials provide consistency, reinforce orally presented information, and provide a source to which the patient can refer as needed. Models (for example, of the heart or a pacemaker) help the patient visualize how something works. Dolls may be useful adjuncts for teaching. Slides, audiotapes, films, and videotapes can vividly present an experience—for example, by showing a diagnostic procedure from the patient's viewpoint. These audiovisuals may not be suitable, however, unless the patient is stable enough to focus attention on them and the learning environment is conducive to using them. If used, they should be supplemented by a one-on-one follow-up discussion.

General plans of care

Teaching strategies

Method	Characteristics	Appropriate uses	Disadvantages
Individual bedside instruction	• One-on-one interaction between teacher and patient • Immediate feedback • Informal	• Acute phase • Sensitive topics • "Private" patient • Emotionally labile patient • Patient with language difficulties • Patient with limited education	• Time consuming
Group session	• Small or large number of patients • Informal • Interchange of ideas	• General content • Patients at similar readiness levels	• Lack of individualization
Lecture	• Highly structured • Efficient	• Large amount of factual content • Rehabilitation program	• Lack of opportunity for teacher-patient interaction • Possible failure to engage the patient's interest (Disadvantages may be overcome by alternating lectures with interactive learning opportunities, such as question-and-answer periods or skill demonstrations.)
Discussion	• Interchange of ideas • More informal than lecture • More opportunity to adapt content and evaluate patient comprehension	• Acute phase • Sensitive topics • When attitudinal change is desired • Highly verbal patient	• Time consuming • Possibly uncomfortable for some patients because of cultural norms that discourage expression
Demonstration and return demonstration	• Observation and supervised practice • Immediate feedback	• Teaching psychomotor skills	• Requires actual equipment

6. Determine how best to teach the content to an individual patient at a particular time. Consider the advantages and disadvantages of various teaching methods, the appropriateness and availability of educational materials, and the patient's personality.

7. Decide who should teach what: Consider the primary nurse, a nurse with special related expertise, and other health care professionals. Mention the availability of visitors from community or self-help groups when the patient is more stable physiologically.

8. Decide when to teach.

6. In many cases, combinations of teaching methods and educational materials can achieve a desired goal. Selecting the combination most appropriate to this patient makes learning "come alive."

7. Depending on the content and patient preferences, different teachers may be necessary or appropriate to reinforce learning. Support groups may provide especially relevant information based on personal experience with the patient's disorder. In many cases, their credibility makes them invaluable in helping the patient accept the need for long-term education and rehabilitation. Their visits may need to be deferred until after the patient has stabilized and can benefit from their insights and competencies. Knowing that others have coped productively with similar experiences may provide the patient with hope that facilitates the necessary learning.

8. Choosing appropriate times to teach capitalizes on learning readiness. Appropriate sequencing builds on previously presented material and enhances integration of learning.

9. Plan evaluation strategies based on goals and objectives, such as observing, questioning, and having the patient demonstrate new skills.

9. Evaluation commonly is interwoven with the presentation. Clear evaluation plans help ensure measurable goals and increase the likelihood that the nurse will recognize spontaneous opportunities for evaluation and respond appropriately to them.

10. Communicate the teaching strategy to other professionals involved in the patient's care.

10. Communication enhances consistency of information provided by caregivers, permits appropriate reinforcement, and minimizes unnecessary repetition.

11. Identify and document long-range learning needs. If the patient is transferred to another unit, communicate learning needs to colleagues on the receiving unit and arrange for continuation of the teaching plan.

11. The patient's condition, extensiveness of learning needs, and the busy unit atmosphere may complicate the patient's learning before transfer. Documentation and communication of long-range learning needs allow personalization of ongoing educational efforts.

12. Additional individualized interventions: _____

12. Rationales: _____

NURSING DIAGNOSIS

Risk for knowledge deficit related to inadequate or ineffective implementation of the teaching plan

Nursing priority

Implement an individualized teaching plan that maximizes learning, retention, and compliance.

Patient outcome criterion

According to individual readiness, the patient will indicate interest in learning during care activities.

Interventions

1. Incorporate teaching into other nursing activities. Be alert for unexpected teaching opportunities; for example, use symptomatic episodes (such as an insulin reaction in a newly diagnosed diabetic) to help the patient and family learn to identify symptoms.

Rationales

1. The hectic pace of most units allows little time for extended teaching sessions. Incorporating teaching into other activities increases the likelihood of accomplishing it and contributes to an atmosphere of naturalness and informality. Activity-related teaching (for example, teaching stoma care whenever the stoma is visible) also reinforces learning. The immediacy of a symptomatic episode makes it a powerful teaching tool for establishing the importance of the patient's and family's active involvement in learning

2. Present yourself as enthusiastic, knowledgeable, and approachable.

2. Enthusiasm is contagious. Presenting yourself as knowledgeable increases credibility, and maintaining approachability allows the patient to feel comfortable capitalizing on your expertise.

3. Present manageable amounts of information at any one time.

3. Too much information at one time causes confusion. The patient may lose sight of key points.

4. Provide simple explanations, using easy-to-understand terminology.

4. Medical and nursing jargon distances the patient and family members. Intricate explanations may confuse or overwhelm them.

5. Use review and repetition judiciously, considering individual factors.

5. Physiologic changes, pain medications, anxiety, the unit environment, and the patient's age may contribute to a short attention span and poor retention. (Elderly persons commonly have difficulty remembering details.)

General plans of care

6. Before planned teaching, assess for physiologic needs (such as thirst or an urge to void) and intense emotions. Meet any physiologic needs first, and encourage the patient to express any strong emotions.

6. Unmet physiologic needs and strong emotions interfere with the ability to concentrate on learning.

7. Provide opportunities for immediate application of learning. For example, after you have taught pulse taking, have the patient count your radial pulse while you take your carotid pulse for comparison.

7. Immediate application improves retention.

8. Ask for feedback: Were the words understandable? Was the presentation too fast, too slow, too detailed, or too scant? Adjust terminology, pace, and amount of information accordingly.

8. The patient may be reluctant to reveal lack of understanding. Soliciting feedback demonstrates respect for the learner and permits adjustments before the patient becomes lost, overwhelmed, or bored.

9. Be alert for signs of pain, fatigue, confusion, or boredom, such as grimacing, fidgeting, yawning, agitation, or lack of eye contact.

9. These nonverbal signs may provide clues to the need for modification or conclusion of the teaching session.

10. Promote a positive outlook; solicit feelings and convey confidence in the patient's ability to learn.

10. The patient may initially feel overwhelmed and insecure about learning because of the magnitude, urgency, or unfamiliarity of necessary adaptations to illness.

11. Encourage active participation. Use interactive teaching methods.

11. Adults learn best when actively involved. Active participation also facilitates changes needed to allow recovery from or adaptation to the patient's disorder.

12. Document teaching sessions. Communicate progress to appropriate caregivers.

12. Documentation provides a teaching record for legal purposes and enhances continuity of teaching among caregivers.

13. Additional individualized interventions: _____

13. Rationales: _____

Nursing diagnosis
Risk for knowledge deficit related to lack of needed modification in teaching

Nursing priorities
• Evaluate learning.
• Modify teaching when appropriate.

Patient outcome criteria
According to individual readiness, the patient will:
• demonstrate learning
• display minimal anxiety about self-care
• express satisfaction with teaching plan
• display realistic appraisal of continuing learning needs
• identify appropriate learning resources.

Interventions

1. During and after teaching, determine what learning has occurred. For example, observe the patient, ask questions, or have the patient demonstrate a new skill.

Rationales

1. Determining learning accomplishment permits resolution of some learning needs and provides guidance for meeting others.

2. With the patient, compare learning to date against previously identified goals.

3. Modify the teaching plan as indicated by unmet goals or new learning needs.

4. Refer the patient and family to health care and community agencies, as appropriate, before discharge.

5. Additional individualized interventions: _____

2. Comparison indicates whether goals have been achieved or whether their appropriateness should be reevaluated.

3. Frequent evaluation and modification of the teaching plan ensures that the teaching is tailored to individual learning capabilities and ongoing learning needs.

4. Needs not met by the time of discharge require follow-up.

5. Rationales: _____

DISCHARGE PLANNING

Discharge checklist
Before discharge, the patient should show evidence of:
- ❏ identification of learning needs
- ❏ teaching accomplished during the stay.

Teaching checklist
Document evidence that the patient and family demonstrate an understanding of:
- ❏ key pathophysiologic aspects of the disorder
- ❏ signs and symptoms requiring medical attention
- ❏ dietary modifications, if appropriate
- ❏ medications
- ❏ other therapies
- ❏ community resources for adjustment to lifestyle changes.

Documentation checklist
Using outcome criteria as a guide, document:
- ❏ assessment of readiness for learning
- ❏ identification of factors that may inhibit learning
- ❏ identification of learning goals
- ❏ response of the patient and family to the teaching plan
- ❏ problems encountered in teaching
- ❏ evaluation of learning.

ASSOCIATED PLANS OF CARE

Ineffective family coping: Compromised
Ineffective individual coping
Pain
(Also see the plan for the specific disorder.)

REFERENCES

Coenen, A., et al. "Use of the Nursing Minimum Data Set to Describe Nursing Interventions for Selected Nursing Diagnoses and Related Factors in an Acute Care Setting," *Nursing Diagnosis* 6(3):108-14, July-September 1995.

Gordon, M. *Manual of Nursing Diagnosis, 1997-1998.* St. Louis: Mosby–Year Book, Inc., 1997.

Gordon, M. *Nursing Diagnosis: Process and Application,* 3rd ed. St. Louis: Mosby–Year Book, Inc., 1994.

Katz, J. "Back to Basics: Providing Effective Patient Teaching," *AJN* 97(5):33-36, May 1997.

Smith, A., and Chang, B. "Nursing Diagnoses for Hospitalized Patients with AIDS," *Nursing Diagnosis* 7(1):9-18, January-March 1996.

General plans of care

Nutritional deficit

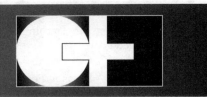

INTRODUCTION

Definition and time focus
A nutritional deficit exists when a patient doesn't ingest or absorb the nutrients necessary to meet metabolic needs. Adequate nutrition is vitally important in recovering from critical illness. Besides glucose needs for cellular metabolism and energy production, many other nutritional needs exist. For example, calories, protein, and potassium are necessary to rebuild injured tissue; proteins, fatty acids, and phosphate are necessary to fight infection; and trace elements are necessary for optimal functioning of enzyme systems. This plan focuses on the acutely ill patient whose survival and recovery may be threatened by inadequate nutrition. (*Note:* The official NANDA wording for this disorder is "Alteration in nutrition: Less than body requirements.")

Etiology and precipitating factors
• Contraindications to eating, as with peptic ulcer or pancreatitis
• Decreased appetite
• Nothing by mouth for more than 4 days
• Inability to chew, as with jaw wiring or poor dentition
• Impaired swallowing, as with stroke, coma, or obstruction
• Preexisting malnutrition, as with cancer or anorexia nervosa
• Decreased GI motility, as with paralytic ileus
• Failure to absorb nutrients, as with malabsorption syndrome, ulcerative colitis, or acquired immunodeficiency syndrome
• Hypermetabolic state, as with burns or trauma
• Protein loss from wounds (pressure sores, surgical wounds)
• Insufficient finances or transportation to obtain food
• Depression, dementia, delirium

FOCUSED ASSESSMENT GUIDELINES

Nursing history (functional health pattern findings)
Health perception–health management pattern
• History of chronic GI disorder
• Preexisting debility
Nutritional-metabolic pattern
• Anorexia, indigestion, nausea, or vomiting
• Difficulty or pain on swallowing
• Refusal to eat
Activity-exercise pattern
• Weakness or lack of energy
Cognitive-perceptual pattern
• Abdominal pain
Coping–stress tolerance pattern
• Depression

Physical findings
General appearance
• Emaciation (if preexisting malnutrition exists)
• Weakness
• Recent unintentional weight loss
Gastrointestinal
• Weak mastication or swallowing muscles
• Inflamed oral cavity or tongue
• Vomiting
• Absent bowel sounds
• Diarrhea
• Hepatomegaly
Neurologic
• Lethargy
• Decreased level of consciousness
• Paresthesia
• Confusion
• Disorientation
Integumentary
• Subcutaneous fat loss
• Dry, scaly skin
• Poor skin turgor
• Sparse, lackluster, or easily plucked hair
• Dry, cracked lips; red cracks at corners of mouth
• Thin, brittle nails
Musculoskeletal
• Weakness
• Body weight at least 20% below ideal weight for height and frame
• Poor muscle tone
• Muscle wasting

Diagnostic studies
See *Diagnostic studies in nutritional deficit.*

Potential complications
• Reduced immunocompetence
• Electrolyte imbalances
• Poor wound healing

Diagnostic studies in nutritional deficit

Various diagnostic studies may be performed in the care of a patient with a nutritional deficit. These studies can be used to assess weight loss, muscle protein stores, or visceral protein stores; estimate body fat reserves; or obtain additional information on the patient's nutritional status.

To assess weight loss and significance
Use the following calculations along with midarm muscle circumference and skin-fold measurements.

Calculating usual body weight
To calculate the patient's usual body weight percentage, use this formula:
    current weight ÷ usual body weight x 100
Malnutrition is rated as mild (85%), moderate (75% to 84%), or severe (less than 74%).

Calculating weight loss
To calculate the patient's weight loss as a percentage, use this formula:
    ([usual weight – current weight] ÷ usual weight) x 100
Weight loss is considered severe if the percentage is more than 5% over 1 month, more than 7.5% over 3 months, or more than 10% over 6 months.

Calculating body mass index (BMI)
To calculate the patient's BMI, use this formula:
    BMI = weight in kilograms ÷ height in square meters
The normal range is 20 to 25 kg/m^2.

To assess muscle protein stores
Height-weight ratio
About 85% or less of the expected value indicates significant protein-calorie malnutrition. (Height and weight are the most significant factors in determining malnutrition.) In the Harris-Benedict equation, the patient's height-weight ratio predicts calorie expenditure. The height-weight ratio is compared with the patient's historical height-weight ratio to determine the severity of malnutrition and the preferred method of feeding the patient.

Midarm circumference (MAC) and midarm muscle circumference (MAMC)
These tests estimate fat and skeletal muscle mass. Measurements are compared to a standard table: 35% to 40% of normal indicates mild depletion of muscle and fat; 25% to 34%, moderate depletion; and less than 25%, severe depletion. MAMC is calculated using MAC and skin-fold measurements and evaluated in comparison with standard tables.

24-hour urine urea nitrogen excretion
This test indicates the severity of protein catabolism. The normal range is 4 to 10 g/day; greater than 10 g/day in a patient with major injuries or sepsis indicates hypermetabolism and a need for increased calories or nitrogen for tissue repair. In a patient who is stable, has no injuries, and is gaining weight, a 24-hour urine urea greater than 10 g/day can indicate overfeeding. (To ensure a positive nitrogen balance in the catabolic patient, approximately 4 to 6 g of nitrogen is given in excess of the amount excreted in the urine.)

Creatinine height index
This shows the relationship between creatinine level and the patient's height and indirectly measures depletion of muscle mass. A range of 60% to 80% of normal represents moderate protein depletion; less than 60% indicates severe depletion. (Creatinine excretion varies directly according to loss of skeletal muscle mass; creatinine height index is obtained by comparing creatinine and height-weight ratio with charts listing normal creatinine excretion for height and weight. Increased creatinine excretion indicates skeletal muscle breakdown.)

Nitrogen balance
The value is obtained by comparing urine urea nitrogen excretion with nitrogen intake (calculated from protein intake). In malnutrition, negative nitrogen balance reveals a catabolic state. A positive nitrogen balance of 2 to 3 g is ideal; in severe illness, zero nitrogen balance may be the realistic maximum attainable.

To assess visceral protein stores
These include plasma proteins, hemoglobin, clotting factors, hormones, antibodies, and enzymes.

Total lymphocyte count (TLC)
This study helps evaluate immunocompetence; a value of 1,200 to 2,000/mm^3 indicates mild lymphocyte depletion; 800 to 1,199/mm^3, moderate depletion; and less than 800/mm^3, severe depletion. (Severe depletion indicates inadequate antibody production and an impaired ability to fight infection. Nutritional repletion is indicated to improve the body's defense mechanisms. TLC is not an accurate indicator of nutritional status in patients on immunosuppressive therapy.)

Albumin
A serum level of less than 3 g/dl correlates with increased severity of illness. A value of 2.8 to 3.5 g/dl indicates mild visceral protein depletion; 2.1 to 2.7 g/dl, moderate depletion; and less than 2.1 g/dl, severe depletion. Because the albumin level falls slowly, it isn't a reliable early indicator of malnutrition. Prealbumin (PAB) is more responsive than albumin to changes in nutrition because of its short half-life (2 days) and small body pool. It increases 1 mg/dl/day with nutritional support. Levels can be affected by stress, liver and renal dysfunction, or acute inflammation. A PAB level below 8 mg/dl indicates severe malnutrition; levels of 10 to 16 mg/dl indicate moderate malnutrition.

Transferrin
This study measures the level of a protein synthesized in the liver. A serum level of 150 to 200 mg/dl indicates mild visceral protein depletion; 100 to 149 mg/dl, moderate depletion; and less than 100 mg/dl, severe depletion. Serum concentration levels fall rapidly with starvation and stress over approximately 8 days. Serial serum transferrin levels indicate response to nutritional therapy.

(continued)

Diagnostic studies in nutritional deficit *(continued)*

Skin-test antigens
This study evaluates cell-mediated immunity, which can decrease with severe malnutrition. This may be assessed using skin-test antigens, such as mumps, *Candida*, streptokinase, or streptodornase. If a negative reaction occurs, malnutrition may be the cause, and the body lacks defense mechanisms to fight infection. A positive reaction is induration exceeding 5 mm, in response to at least two antigens, within 24 to 48 hours.

To estimate body fat reserves
Skin-fold measurements (such as triceps skin fold)
These measurements help estimate the patient's body fat reserves. Measurements are compared with a standard table of values: 35% to 40% of normal indicates mild fat depletion; 25% to 34%, moderate depletion; and less than 25%, severe depletion. The measurements are difficult to evaluate if the patient has edema or can't sit. Serial measurements made by the same observer are more accurate.

Other studies
Total iron-binding capacity (TIBC)
This measures the ability of iron to bind with transferrin transported in the blood. Followed serially, TIBC indicates if nutritional support is correcting the patient's nutritional state.

Serum electrolyte levels
Levels are obtained to serve as baseline values and to guide replacement therapy; in patients with malnutrition, they typically reveal hyponatremia, hypokalemia, hypomagnesemia, and hypophosphatemia.

Serum cholesterol
Levels below 150 mg/dl can indicate malnutrition. Evaluate with other tests.

CLINICAL SNAPSHOT

NUTRITIONAL DEFICIT

Major nursing diagnoses and collaborative problems	Key patient outcomes
Nutritional deficit related to difficulty chewing or swallowing, sore throat after endotracheal intubation, or dry mouth	Swallow without choking.
Nutritional deficit related to anorexia	Eat and retain at least three-quarters of prescribed diet, if able.
Nutritional deficit related to inability to digest nutrients or hypermetabolic state	Tolerate enteral or parenteral feedings, if any, without adverse effect.

NURSING DIAGNOSIS

Nutritional deficit related to difficulty chewing or swallowing, sore throat after endotracheal extubation, or dry mouth

Nursing priority

Compensate for eating difficulties.

Patient outcome criteria

According to individual readiness, the patient will:
• eat the prescribed diet without difficulty
• swallow without choking.

Interventions

1. Assess and document causes. Initiate referrals as appropriate — for example, to a dentist or speech pathologist.

2. Assess level of consciousness and ability to chew and swallow, and check for gag reflex. Observe for coughing or moist voice after eating.

3. In collaboration with the dietitian or nutritional support nurse and as ordered, provide a diet appropriate to the patient's abilities — for example, liquids, soft foods, or food requiring little cutting.

4. If the patient has a sore mouth or throat, obtain an order for viscous lidocaine (Xylocaine). If the patient has been extubated recently, explain that the sore throat usually resolves spontaneously within a few days.

5. Place the patient sitting upright for meals, with the head flexed forward about 45 degrees, unless contraindicated.

6. Have suction equipment available nearby but out of the patient's sight. Suction food, fluids, and accumulated saliva, as needed.

7. Provide assistance, as needed. If the patient has had a stroke, place food in the unaffected side of the mouth.

8. Document feeding technique and food intake.

9. Additional individualized interventions: _____

Rationales

1. Some eating difficulties call for diagnosis or interventions beyond the scope of nursing. For example, a dentist may be able to diagnose jaw pain or a speech pathologist may be able to teach swallowing technique.

2. Alertness, ability to chew and swallow, and a gag reflex determine if the patient can safely ingest nutrients orally.

3. An appropriate diet minimizes patient frustration when eating.

4. Use of viscous lidocaine, a topical anesthetic, reduces discomfort. Knowing that the sore throat, common after extubation, will probably disappear after extubation may increase the patient's tolerance of the discomfort.

5. This position maintains esophageal patency, facilitates swallowing, and minimizes the risk of aspiration.

6. If the patient has sudden difficulty swallowing, prompt suctioning prevents aspiration. Keeping the equipment out of sight creates a more pleasant eating environment.

7. Providing assistance increases food intake. Placing the food in the unaffected side facilitates use of the tongue to move food toward the back of the mouth.

8. Documenting the technique provides for continuity of care; records are necessary to monitor the adequacy of food intake.

9. Rationales: _____

NURSING DIAGNOSIS

Nutritional deficit related to anorexia

Nursing priority

Promote appetite.

Patient outcome criterion

According to individual readiness, the patient will eat and retain at least three-quarters of the prescribed diet.

Interventions

1. Assess possible causes of anorexia, such as nausea and vomiting, unpleasant sights and odors, depression, and medications. Determine food preferences.

Rationales

1. Accurate identification of anorexia's cause facilitates selection of appropriate interventions.

2. Provide a pleasant eating environment. For example, place an emesis basin nearby but out of direct sight (if someone will be staying at the bedside); remove tissues containing sputum.

3. Before meals, promote rest; administer analgesics or antiemetics, as needed and ordered; avoid painful procedures; and provide oral hygiene.

4. Emphasize the importance of eating. Use positive terms when presenting food; for example, "Here's a milkshake to help you regain your strength," rather than "Do you think you'll be able to keep this down?"

5. Provide social interaction during meals, preferably with family and friends.

6. Offer small, frequent feedings of highly nutritious foods, including the patient's preferences whenever possible.

7. Limit fluid intake at mealtimes.

8. If the patient begins to feel nauseated, encourage slow, deep breathing. If vomiting occurs, document the amount and type of emesis. Provide oral hygiene afterward.

9. Praise the patient for signs of increased appetite.

10. Additional individualized interventions: _____

2. Removal of noxious sights and smells may decrease anorexia, nausea, and vomiting.

3. Adequate rest conserves the energy necessary to eat. Analgesics, antiemetics, and avoidance of painful procedures remove the influences of pain, nausea, and emotional stress. Oral hygiene removes unpleasant tastes.

4. Emphasizing the importance of eating encourages the patient to eat despite anorexia. Positive terms capitalize on the power of suggestion to influence the subconscious mind.

5. Social interaction increases food intake by providing a pleasant distraction from anorexia. Involving family and friends strengthens interpersonal bonds.

6. Small meals promote prompt gastric emptying, lessening anorexia and nausea. When food intake is low, every mouthful must count toward meeting nutrient needs.

7. Large amounts of fluid distend the stomach, causing early satiety and promoting nausea.

8. Deep breathing helps to diminish the vomiting reflex. Documentation of emesis is necessary to maintain accurate intake and output records and to evaluate the adequacy of oral nutrition. Oral hygiene removes unpleasant tastes.

9. Praise acknowledges the patient's efforts to overcome anorexia and reinforces desired behavior.

10. Rationales: _____

COLLABORATIVE PROBLEM

Nutritional deficit related to inability to digest nutrients or hypermetabolic state

Nursing priority

Provide nutrients in a form that can be assimilated.

Patient outcome criteria

Within 7 days of admission, the patient will:
• tolerate enteral or parenteral feedings (if ordered) without adverse effects
• gain up to 2½ lb (1 kg) per week.

Interventions

1. Stay alert for increased nutrient needs, such as from trauma, burns, infection, surgical wounds, and fever. Also observe the patient for indicators (such as diarrhea) of possible inability to absorb nutrients.

Rationales

1. Early recognition of the patient's decreased absorptive ability or increased needs helps provide adequate nutrition before debilitation occurs.

2. Collaborate with the dietitian, nutritional support service, and doctor to obtain a comprehensive nutritional assessment.

3. Assess and document bowel sounds and abdominal distention every 4 hours.

4. Collaborate with nutritional experts to establish nutrient requirements, depending on whether the following exist:
• starvation

• hypermetabolism.

5. Provide the appropriate nutritional replacement, as ordered. Options include the following:
• enteral feeding (via nasogastric, gastrostomy, or jejunostomy tubes), such as:
  – meal replacements

  – nutrient supplements

  – defined-formula diets.

• parenteral nutrition

  – peripheral parenteral nutrition (PPN)

  – total parenteral nutrition (TPN), also known as central venous nutrition or total nutrient admixture.

2. A comprehensive assessment includes anthropometric and laboratory measurements performed by colleagues with special nutritional expertise. These measurements document the type and degree of nutritional deficit and provide guidelines for selecting appropriate nutritional interventions.

3. Bowel sounds indicate whether the patient can tolerate enteral feedings or whether parenteral feedings are necessary. Abdominal distention suggests paralytic ileus.

4. Nutrient requirements vary depending on whether the patient is merely nutritionally depleted or is experiencing a hypermetabolic state.
• Early starvation is characterized by various compensatory mechanisms, including glycogenolysis, lipolysis, proteolysis, and gluconeogenesis. Rapid catabolism produces rapid weight loss, osmotic diuresis, and urinary nitrogen loss. After approximately 10 days, the metabolic rate slows and weight loss continues at a slower rate while the body uses fat as its primary energy source. After several months, exhaustion of fat stores causes the body to use visceral protein for energy.
• The release of catecholamines, glucocorticoids, and mineralocorticoids in response to stress cause the traumatized or infected patient to develop greater glucose mobilization than the starved patient. Rapid weight loss and osmotic diuresis are delayed for approximately 24 to 48 hours after trauma.

5. Nutritional replacement methods depend on the patient's needs.
• Enteral feeding is preferred for the patient with a functioning GI tract.
  – Meal replacements are nutritionally complete but require digestive and absorptive abilities.
  – Supplements, although nutritionally incomplete, can replace one or more specific nutrients.
  – Defined-formula diets are nutritionally complete and require little digestion.
• Parenteral nutrition is appropriate for patients who cannot meet nutritional needs through GI absorption. It's administered peripherally or centrally.
  – PPN may be prescribed if calorie needs are relatively low, relatively short-term GI dysfunction is anticipated, and peripheral veins are adequate.
  – TPN is appropriate for patients with relatively high calorie needs because TPN solutions have greater calorie and protein content than peripheral venous solutions.

General plans of care

6. Perform these interventions if the patient is receiving tube feedings:
• Check tube placement before each feeding.

• Monitor bowel sounds, bowel movements, residual amounts, abdominal girth, intake and output, and weight.
• Keep the head of the bed elevated during and for 1 hour after feedings.
• Begin with small amounts (25 to 50 ml/hr) of full strength isotonic solution; dilute hypertonic (greater than 300 mOsm/kg) solutions. Increase the amount and concentration as tolerated (usually 25 ml every 12 hours). Don't increase the concentration and rate at the same time.
• Use a bolus, intermittent, or continuous method as ordered.

7. If the patient is receiving TPN, ensure delivery of the prescribed solutions and monitor for complications. Refer to the "Total parenteral nutrition" plan, page 527, for details.

8. Additional individualized interventions: _____

6. Nursing measures for tube feedings are designed to facilitate absorption and prevent complications.
• Checking tube placement confirms that the tube is in the stomach or jejunum, as appropriate. With a nasogastric tube, checking ensures that it hasn't migrated upward into the trachea.
• Monitoring promotes early identification of complications, such as ileus or obstruction.

• Elevation prevents reflux of solution into the esophagus.
• Large amounts of concentrated solution may provoke osmotic diarrhea. Gradual increases allow time for the GI system to adapt to the increased volume and solute load.

• The method of delivery can depend on the patient's disease and ability to tolerate feedings. Intermittent or continuous methods are less likely to cause adverse GI effects such as nausea or diarrhea.

7. TPN is a complex therapy with numerous nursing considerations.

8. Rationales: _____

DISCHARGE PLANNING

Discharge checklist
Before discharge, the patient should show evidence of:
❐ assessment of nutritional status
❐ implementation of appropriate nutritional support.

Teaching checklist
Document evidence that the patient and family demonstrate an understanding of:
❐ importance of nutrition to recovery
❐ rationale for selection of a specific nutritional support method.

Documentation checklist
Using outcome criteria as a guide, document:
❐ clinical status on admission
❐ significant changes in status
❐ pertinent diagnostic test findings
❐ specific nutritional support method
❐ tolerance of method
❐ complications, if any
❐ daily nutritional intake
❐ medications administered, if any
❐ attitude toward eating

❐ patient and family teaching
❐ discharge planning.

ASSOCIATED PLANS OF CARE

See the plan for the specific disorder.

REFERENCES

Antonelli, I., et al. "Nutritional Assessment: A Primary Component of Multidimensional Geriatric Assessment in the Acute Care Setting," *Journal of the American Geriatrics Society* 44(2):166-74, February 1996.

Barrocas, A., et al. "Assessing Health Status in the Elderly: The Nutrition Screening Initiative," *Journal of Health Care for the Poor and Underserved* 7(3):210-18, August 1996.

Cotton, E., et al. "A Nutritional Assessment Tool for Older Patients," *Professional Nurse* 11(9):609-12, June 1996.

Davis, C., and Stables, I. "Audit of Nutrition Screening in Patients with Acute Illness," *Nursing Times* 92(8):35-37, February 1996.

Dudek, S. *Nutrition Handbook for Nursing Practice,* 3rd ed. Philadelphia: Lippincott-Raven Pubs., 1997.

Eschleman, M. *Introductory Nutrition and Nutrition Therapy,* 3rd ed. Philadelphia: Lippincott-Raven Pubs., 1996.

Flanigan, K. "Nutritional Aspects of Wound Healing," *Advances in Wound Care* 10(2):48-52, May-June 1997.

Groff, J. *Advanced Nutrition and Human Metabolism,* 2nd ed. Minneapolis-St. Paul: West Publishing Co., 1995.

Lutz, C. *Nutrition and Diet Therapy.* Philadelphia: F.A. Davis Co., 1997.

Manning, E.M., and Shenkin, A. "Nutritional Assessment in the Critically Ill," *Critical Care Clinics* 11(3):603-34, July 1995.

Mitchell, M. *Nutrition Across the Life Span.* Philadelphia: W.B. Saunders Co., 1997.

Nightingale, J.M., et al. "Three Simple Methods of Detecting Malnutrition on Medical Wards," *Journal of the Royal Society of Medicine* 89(3):144-48, March 1996.

Norton, B. "Nutritional Assessment," *Nursing Times* 92(26):71-76, June 26, 1996.

Phaneuf, C. "Screening Elders for Nutritional Deficits," *AJN* 96(3):58-60, March 1996.

Robshaw, V., and Marbrow, S. "Raising Awareness of Patients' Nutritional State," *Professional Nurse* 11(1):41-42, October 1995.

Strauss, E.A., and Margolis, D.J. "Malnutrition in Patients with Pressure Ulcers: Morbidity, Mortality, and Clinically Practical Assessments," *Advances in Wound Care* 9(5):37-40, September-October 1996.

Totosian, M., ed. *Nutrition for the Hospitalized Patient: Basic Science and Principles of Practice.* New York: Dekker, 1995.

Whitney, E. *Nutrition for Health and Health Care.* Minneapolis-St. Paul: West Publishing Co. 1996.

Wilson, J. "Nutritional Assessment and Its Application," *Journal of Intravenous Nursing* 19(6):307-14, November-December 1996.

Worthington-Roberts, B., and Rodwell, S., eds. *Nutrition Throughout the Life Cycle,* 3rd ed. St. Louis: Mosby–Year Book, Inc., 1996.

General plans of care

Pain

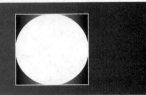

INTRODUCTION

Definition and time focus

Pain represents neurologic or emotional suffering in response to a noxious stimulus. It's best prevented or relieved when the nurse continually anticipates it. Although individuals experience pain differently, pain's symbolic meaning as a danger and threat commonly heightens a patient's perceptions of it. Sophisticated pain management demands patience, sensitivity, compassion, and a repertoire of pain-control techniques. Because of individual factors and the availability of the various pain-control techniques to choose from, the nurse must exercise keen judgment in selecting the best strategy for a particular patient at a particular time. This plan focuses on the care of a patient experiencing acute pain, lasting minutes to days. Because many patients in today's acute care settings also experience chronic pain from such conditions as arthritis, neuropathy, and cancer, the plan also includes an intervention section highlighting the differences in chronic pain management.

Etiology and precipitating factors
• Surgical or accidental trauma
• Inflammation
• Musculoskeletal disorders such as muscle spasm
• Neuropathies secondary to such conditions as diabetes mellitus, acquired immunodeficiency syndrome, or multiple sclerosis
• Visceral disorders such as myocardial infarction
• Vascular disorders such as sickle cell anemia
• Invasive diagnostic procedures
• Excessive pressure, such as with immobility
• Cancer

FOCUSED ASSESSMENT GUIDELINES

Nursing history (functional health pattern findings)
Health perception–health management pattern
• Acute physical discomfort, typically described as pain, pressure, tightness, soreness, or a crushing or burning sensation
Nutritional-metabolic pattern
• Anorexia, nausea, or vomiting
Activity-exercise pattern
• Intense fatigue and decreased ability to perform activities of daily living

Sleep-rest pattern
• Inability to rest or sleep
Cognitive-perceptual pattern
• Inability to concentrate
Self-perception–self-concept pattern
• Anxiety or depression
Role-relationship pattern
• Concern that others discount pain
• Decreased desire to interact with others
Coping–stress tolerance pattern
• Decreased ability to deal with frustration or other stress
Value-belief pattern
• Belief that suffering is punishment for wrongdoing or bad deeds
• Reluctance to take medication for pain relief because of religion, belief system, or fear of addiction

Physical findings
General appearance
• Tense, guarded posture
• Facial grimacing
• Crying
• Moaning
Musculoskeletal
• Muscle spasms
• Unnatural stillness
• Increased physical activity (uncommon)
Integumentary
• Diaphoresis
• Pallor
Neurologic
• Impaired concentration
• Irritability
• Restlessness
Cardiovascular
• Hypertension and tachycardia
• Hypotension and bradycardia (uncommon)
Respiratory
• Tachypnea
• Gasping

Diagnostic studies

No specific studies indicate the presence or degree of pain. Various procedures may be indicated in the differential diagnosis of pain. For example, for chest pain, the patient may undergo a 12-lead electrocardiogram, chest X-ray, creatine kinase level measurements, and pulmonary ventilation scan to differentiate acute myocardial infarction from pulmonary embolism. See plans of care on specific disorders for details.

Potential complications
• Exhaustion
• Intractable pain
• Suicide

Nursing diagnosis

Pain from tissue injury, ischemia, infarction, inflammation, edema, tension, or spasm

Nursing priority

Prevent or ameliorate pain.

Patient outcome criteria

Within 1 hour after the onset of pain, the patient will:
• rate pain as less than the goal level (typically less than 3 on a 0 to 10 pain rating scale)
• have a relaxed posture and facial expression
• have vital signs within normal limits.

Interventions

1. Monitor continually for possible indicators of pain, including verbalization, grimacing, diaphoresis, tense posture, splinting, restlessness, irritability, emotional withdrawal, and changes in vital signs.

2. Analyze and document pain characteristics systematically; for example, use the PQRST mnemonic:
• P = precipitators
• Q = quality
• R = region and radiation
• S = severity
• T = time (frequency and duration).
Use a pain rating scale; the standard is the 0 to 10 Pain Intensity Scale with 0 indicating no pain and 10 indicating the worst possible pain. Have the patient choose a goal pain level and then ask him to rate his current level of pain. For information on assessing adults with language difficulty, see *Wong-Baker Faces Pain Rating Scale,* page 90. Promptly report any new or increased pain to the doctor.

3. Prepare the patient for brief, unavoidably painful experiences such as percutaneous skin puncture for arterial blood gas sampling. State clear expectations for behavior, such as "If it hurts, squeeze your wife's hand but hold your other arm still."

Rationales

1. The acutely ill patient may not be fully conscious because of the underlying disease or medications that blunt perception. As a result, verbal reports alone may not adequately indicate the presence and degree of pain. Astute observation may provide ongoing protection against unreported or underreported pain.

2. Careful analysis of pain characteristics aids in the differential diagnosis of pain. Systematic analysis prevents hasty and possibly inaccurate conclusions about the quality or probable cause of pain. Standardized pain rating provides a benchmark reference. Pain ratings are used as a baseline and as an indicator of treatment effectiveness. The patient-selected goal is the pain level that allows him to eat, sleep, and perform other required physical activities (such as ambulation and coughing after surgery). Patient self-report is the most reliable indicator of the existence and intensity of adult pain. New or increased pain requires prompt medical evaluation.

3. The psychological assault of unexpected pain can unnerve even the most stoic person and make coping with the pain needlessly stressful. Brief explanations decrease fear of the unknown and help the patient prepare for the experience. Positive suggestions provide an appropriate way to cope with the pain.

General plans of care

Wong-Baker Faces Pain Rating Scale

The Wong-Baker Faces Pain Rating Scale, used for pediatric patients ages 3 and older, can also be used for adult patients with language difficulties. Explain to the patient that each face shows either a person who feels happy because he has no pain or a person who feels sad because he has some or a lot of pain. Ask the patient to choose the face that best describes how he is feeling.

Face 0 is very happy because he doesn't hurt at all. Face 2 hurts just a little bit. Face 4 hurts a little more. Face 6 hurts even more. Face 8 hurts a whole lot. Face 10 hurts as much as you can imagine, although you don't have to be crying to feel this bad.

| 0 | 2 | 4 | 6 | 8 | 10 |

Source: Wong, D.L. *Whaley & Wong's Nursing Care of Infants and Children.* St. Louis: Mosby–Year Book, Inc., 1995.

4. When preparing the patient for a painful experience, try to find out how much the patient wants to know. If possible, tailor the degree of detail to the patient's preference for information and the procedure's extensiveness.

5. During painful procedures, provide ongoing support and positive reinforcement:

• Use brief, simple directions, as needed. Use therapeutic touch, if accepted by the patient.

• When the experience is over, encourage the patient to express feelings, if desired. Convey acceptance for the way the patient handled pain, using praise generously when appropriate.

6. Reduce factors that may increase pain, such as anxiety that reports of pain won't be believed, a sense of isolation, and fatigue. Accept the patient's description of pain. Convey the sense that the patient isn't alone. Encourage the patient to rest sufficiently. Control environmental factors, such as noise, temperature, and lighting, when possible.

4. Patient teaching doesn't necessarily reduce anxiety; people vary in the degree of detail they find helpful. Some individuals seek information to reduce their anxiety, while others find detailed information increases their stress about impending situations. When possible, match teaching detail to the patient's preferred coping style.

5. Providing support and encouragement during the experience increases the patient's sense of security and control.
• Brief, simple directions are necessary because pain reduces comprehension and retention of information. Touch may convey comfort more profoundly than words.
• Discussing the pain experience afterward provides an opportunity for psychological integration and closure of the experience, which is necessary to "let go" of it. Conveying acceptance is particularly important for patients who scream or otherwise lose control because it reassures them and may relieve any residual feelings of shame.

6. Listening to the patient respectfully and implying an alliance against pain help reduce anxiety. Feeling well-rested increases tolerance of pain and the ability to cope with it. Environmental factors may exacerbate the pain. Constant, irritating noise, for example, may cause increased muscle tension and irritability.

7. For patients with ongoing pain, explicitly convey the goal of aggressive pain management. State the intent to prevent or "stay on top" of the pain. For acute or chronic pain that occurs most of the day, administer pain medication in "preventive" around-the-clock dosing. For acute pain, reevaluate dose and timing every 24 hours. Use a rating scale to compare the patient's current pain level to his chosen goal level as a measure of effectiveness. Once pain becomes intermittent, administer only as needed.
• The pain rating scale may be used to titrate dose and interval to keep rating as close to the patient goal as possible.
• Use regular pain assessment to ensure that pain is managed within "acceptable" levels, rather than allowed to become severe.

8. Work with the patient to identify the most effective ways to control pain. Explore various pain-control methods. Assess patient's usual pain relief measures at home. Use positive terms and the power of suggestion.

9. Collaborate with the doctor and clinical pharmacist as needed to determine an effective analgesic regimen. Administer and document analgesics as ordered. Analgesics may include:
• nonnarcotic analgesics or nonsteroidal anti-inflammatory drugs (NSAIDs), such as aspirin, acetaminophen, ibuprofen, ketorolac, and other NSAIDs

• opioids (narcotics), such as codeine, morphine, and meperidine (Demerol). *Note:* Meperidine shouldn't be used for more than 48 hours.

• adjuvant drugs, such as antidepressants, tricyclics (such as amitriptyline and desipramine) and selective serotonin reuptake inhibitors (such as fluoxetine [Prozac], sertraline [Zoloft], venlafaxine [Effexor]); anticonvulsants (such as carbamazepine [Tegretol]); skeletal muscle relaxants; or corticosteroids (for cancer-related pain).

7. Explicit goals imply that the situation is manageable, which is reassuring and reduces the fear of being overwhelmed by pain. Pain is more effectively controlled when a constant blood level is maintained. Less medication is needed to control pain when dosing is around-the-clock, rather than the peaks and valleys of dosing on an as-needed basis.

8. Involving the patient in pain-control strategies promotes a sense of mastery that reduces fears of helplessness or loss of control. Using positive terms interrupts the cycle of negativity, in which pain worsens negativity and negativity worsens pain. Capitalizing on the power of suggestion creates an expectation that interventions will be successful. It may also help trigger release of endorphins, opiate-like analgesic substances that the body releases in response to certain stimuli.

9. Personalizing the analgesic regimen recognizes individual differences in pain perception and provides the most effective control for a particular patient.

• Nonnarcotic analgesics work peripherally, inhibiting formation of prostaglandins and bradykinins (inflammatory mediators that increase pain). These drugs are used alone for mild pain and in combination with opioids for moderate and severe pain. Better pain control is achieved when drugs are combined, rather than when opioids are used alone. In many cases, ketorolac is given parenterally for postsurgical pain.
• Opioids work by occupying central receptor sites, decreasing the perception of pain. They're used for moderate or severe pain and cancer pain, and they may cause sedation, respiratory depression, nausea, vomiting, or constipation. Meperidine has an active metabolite that is a central nervous system stimulant. It accumulates due to a half-life (15 to 20 hours) longer than the parent drug (3 to 6 hours).
• Antidepressants are used for neuropathic pain. SSRIs appear to reduce pain transmission by changing the balance of neurotransmitters along pain pathways. See individual drug information for adverse effects. Anticonvulsants are used for neuropathic and "phantom" pain. Muscle relaxants reduce muscle spasm and steroids reduce swelling and pressure on nerves. Phenothiazines (Phenergan) have been found to be ineffective in potentiating analgesia and should be used only to control nausea (an opioid adverse effect).

10. Use a combination of nonpharmacologic pain-control strategies:

• positioning (Cushion and elevate the painful area, if possible. Avoid pressure or tension on it. Encourage the patient to rest in a comfortable position, but also to change position every hour while awake. Explain the rationale for position changes, provide gentle reminders, and assist with movement, as necessary.)

• cutaneous stimulation from massage or applications of heat, cold, or mentholated ointments

• contralateral stimulation, such as scratching or massage, when the injured area is not directly accessible (for example, under a cast).

11. Explore various behavioral pain-control strategies, including:

• distraction techniques, such as talking or listening to lively music

• relaxation techniques, such as rhythmic breathing, progressive muscle relaxation, listening to relaxation tapes or soothing music, or meditation

• use of relaxation, breathing, and guided imagery during painful procedures.

12. Minimize discomfort from adverse effects of narcotic analgesics.

10. Because various factors may cause or exacerbate pain, various techniques may bring relief. Trying a variety of pain-control measures allows for an individualized, multifaceted approach, which is more likely to be successful than a single strategy.
• Cushioning increases comfort, while elevation reduces edema. Avoiding pressure or tension eliminates additional painful stimuli to an already sensitive area. Rest increases pain tolerance. Position changes improve perfusion, helping remove chemical mediators of inflammation and bringing oxygen and other nutrients to healing tissue. Position changes also help prevent complications of immobility. Because moving the painful area may temporarily increase pain, patient education, gentle but firm reminders, and active assistance may be necessary to ensure attention to this important need.
• Pain impulses are believed to be transmitted along peripheral nerve fibers to ascending spinal cord pathways to the brain. Sharp, acute pain is transmitted along small-diameter, type A fibers, whereas dull, chronic pain is transmitted along smaller type C fibers. Stimulation of large sensory (nonpain) fibers inhibits these ascending pain pathways. In addition, massage increases perfusion and reduces muscle tension. Cold-induced vasoconstriction reduces edema and is especially helpful in the first 48 hours after injury. Cold can be used at any time. Heat increases circulation, mobility, and muscle relaxation, which is particularly helpful in decreasing painful reflex muscle spasms.
• Stimulation of the area opposite the painful one may provide relief, probably by triggering release of endorphins, opiate-like substances that relieve pain.

11. Behavioral strategies divert attention from the pain, promote a sense of self-control, encourage muscle relaxation, and may stimulate endorphin release.
• Distraction is especially helpful for brief episodes of pain, but may increase pain perception and fatigue after the distracting stimulus is removed.
• These techniques reduce muscle tension, enhance rest, and promote a sense of well-being by stimulating the "relaxation response," which counteracts the physiologic arousal of the stress response.
• The image of flying and looking down on a peaceful setting is especially helpful to detach the patient from the painful experience.

12. Narcotic analgesic use can result in constipation, nausea and vomiting, stomatitis, and injury. (See *Preventing adverse effects of narcotic analgesics.*)

Preventing adverse effects of narcotic analgesics

Complication	Interventions	Rationales
Constipation	• Encourage bowel evacuation as soon as the urge to defecate occurs.	• Bowel evacuation can be delayed by voluntary inhibition of the urge to defecate, leading to constipation. Learning to defecate as soon as the urge occurs avoids this problem.
	• Encourage intake of at least eight 8-oz (240-ml) glasses of fluids daily and a high-fiber, well-balanced diet.	• Fluids promote optimal stool consistency; a diet high in fiber increases peristalsis.
	• Encourage moderate exercise, unless contraindicated, with emphasis on increasing abdominal muscle tone.	• Voluntary contraction of abdominal wall muscles helps expel feces.
	• Administer and document medications for increasing bowel elimination, as ordered.	• Stool softeners retard reabsorption of water and coat the intestinal lining. Laxatives stimulate peristalsis or add bulk.
	• Evaluate and document the frequency of elimination and consistency of stool.	• Monitoring elimination patterns determines the effectiveness of and need for continued use of laxatives.
Nausea and vomiting	• Instruct the patient that nausea may decrease after a few doses.	• Information helps reduce anxiety, which can increase nausea.
	• Eliminate noxious sights and smells from the environment.	• Noxious stimuli can stimulate the vomiting center.
	• Encourage the patient to move and change position slowly.	• Movement may stimulate the vomiting center in the medulla.
	• Encourage the patient to deep-breathe and swallow.	• Deep breathing and swallowing decrease the strength of the vomiting reflex.
	• Consult with the doctor about changing the narcotic analgesic.	• The patient may have less nausea and vomiting in response to another narcotic.
	• Administer and document an antiemetic, as ordered, using nursing judgment.	• Antiemetics decrease stimulation of the vomiting center and usually potentiate narcotic effects.
	• Evaluate and document the effects of antiemetics in relieving nausea and vomiting.	• Monitoring the response to medication determines its effectiveness and the need for continued antiemetics.
Stomatitis	• Encourage or provide mouth care at frequent intervals, after meals and as needed.	• Narcotic-induced mouth dryness may cause discomfort and contribute to mucous membrane breakdown (stomatitis). Cleanliness and moisture maintain the integrity of the mucous membrane.
	• Encourage the patient to breathe through the nose, if possible.	• Dryness of the oral mucous membrane may cause breakdown.
	• Encourage fluid intake of at least eight 8-oz (240-ml) glasses daily.	• Adequate hydration reduces discomfort and helps maintain the integrity of the oral mucous membrane.
	• Tell the patient not to use mouthwash or other products containing alcohol.	• Alcohol has a drying effect on the oral mucous membrane.
Injury	• Orient the patient to time and place, verbally and with touch, and explain the call system.	• Information provides support and relieves anxiety.
	• Instruct the patient to request assistance when getting out of bed.	• Assistance with ambulation will help prevent falls.
	• Secure the side rails and keep the bed at its lowest level.	• These measures prevent injuries and avert the possibility of the patient's falling out of bed.
	• Instruct the patient and family regarding the hazards of sedation when driving, smoking in bed, and so forth.	• Information about specific hazards helps prevent accidents and injury.

General plans of care

13. Involve the family in pain-relief strategies. Help them understand the patient's behavior in the context of the pain. Explain the rationale for pain-control techniques. Correct misconceptions, if present. When possible, have family members participate in providing pain relief such as massage. Explicitly acknowledge the difficulty in observing a loved one's pain, and provide emotional support.

13. Capitalizing on family bonds can provide a level of interpersonal comfort that exceeds what concerned, supportive staff can provide. Understanding pain behaviors may help the family be more patient, and correcting misconceptions (such as the danger of addiction) may relieve unwarranted anxiety. Acknowledgment of family members' emotional suffering conveys respect and concern for them, and nurturing family members increases their coping skills and ability to support the patient.

14. If constant pain is present, collaborate with the patient, family, doctor, and pharmacist to optimize pain relief through such measures as:

14. Persistent pain may demoralize the patient and make suffering seem unbearable. A collaborative approach using several options increases the likelihood of finding the optimal pain-control regimen for a given patient.

• continuous I.V. or subcutaneous infusion or patient-controlled analgesia devices that use bolus and continuous administration

• Continuous infusions allow for more effective control by maintaining constant analgesic blood levels. Patient-controlled analgesia devices allow for immediate pain relief, increasing the patient's sense of control over pain and maintaining a constant blood level.

• spinal (epidural or intrathecal) narcotic administration

• These techniques deliver small doses of narcotics directly to endorphin receptor sites, allowing powerful pain control without the usual systemic effects of narcotics.

• transcutaneous electrical nerve stimulation (TENS) or acupuncture

• TENS transmits an electrical stimulus to the painful area, and acupuncture uses needles to stimulate sensitive areas. These techniques are thought to stimulate endorphin and enkephalin release, thus providing analgesia, and block ascending pain transmission pathways.

• hypnosis, guided imagery, and biofeedback.

• These techniques alter pain perception but require motivation and training, so they may not be appropriate for some patients.

15. Exert particular caution with spinal (epidural or intrathecal) narcotic administration. Follow agency protocol for monitoring adverse effects.

15. These techniques are used for long-term pain control in cancer and postoperative patients (such as after thoracotomy, orthopedic surgery, or abdominal surgery). They allow potent pain control with fewer adverse effects than systemic analgesics by delivering small doses of analgesic agents, such as morphine and local anesthetics, close to endogenous endorphin receptor sites.

• Double-check the dosage.

• Narcotic overdoses delivered by this route can be lethal.

• Reduce or discontinue the parenteral dosage, as ordered.

• Central narcotic administration is so potent that continuation of normal parenteral dosage will result in narcotic overdose.

• Use preservative-free narcotics, such as morphine, meperidine, or fentanyl (Sublimaze).

• The preservative in most commercial preparations causes meningeal irritation.

• Maintain the catheter as prescribed by unit protocol.

• Specific catheter care varies but includes maintenance of catheter patency and observation for catheter displacement.

16. Evaluate and document the patient's response to pain-relief measures hourly and as needed. Use the pain-rating scale to assess effectiveness. If the patient rates his pain higher than the goal he selected, medicate as needed. Be alert for "clock watching" for the next analgesic dose.

16. Monitoring the effectiveness of pain relief determines the appropriateness of methods used. The main reason for "clock watching" behavior is inadequate pain relief.

17. For chronic pain, use all appropriate interventions in this plan.
• For chronic nonmalignant pain, use around-the-clock dosing of nonnarcotic analgesics and adjuvant drugs. Individualize dosing and intervals to achieve pain control.
• For chronic malignant cancer pain, use all three drug groups. Don't use combination products. Reassure the patient that "addiction" isn't a consideration and that pain control is the goal. Once dose is determined, nonparenteral administration is used; usually, oral and transdermal narcotics can control pain. Tolerance is developed to most narcotic adverse effects, except constipation. Monitor for respiratory depression with dosage increases.

18. Additional individualized interventions: _____

17. Most nonmalignant pain can be managed by a combination of nonnarcotic drugs and nondrug interventions.
• Use of antidepressant drugs is effective in many cases of chronic pain management.

• Morphine is the standard narcotic for cancer pain control because it comes in many different dosage forms and there is no upper-end dose limit. Tolerance and physical dependence do develop; these don't indicate addiction (psychological dependence). Tolerance generally requires dosage increases; addiction is rare. Because malignant pain ends with death, physical dependence isn't an issue. Many health care professionals inappropriately fear addiction and undermedicate patients with cancer pain.

18. Rationales: _____

DISCHARGE PLANNING

Discharge checklist
Before discharge, the patient should show evidence of:
❏ pain-relief measures effective in reducing pain to tolerable level
❏ vital signs within normal limits.

Teaching checklist
Document evidence that the patient and family demonstrate an understanding of:
❏ anticipated course of pain in relation to the medical condition
❏ all discharge medications' purpose, dosage, administration schedule, and adverse effects requiring medical attention (usual discharge medications are oral analgesics)
❏ nonpharmacologic relief strategies
❏ symptoms and severity of pain warranting medical care
❏ dates, times, and location of follow-up appointments
❏ how to contact the doctor.

Documentation checklist
Using outcome criteria as a guide, document:
❏ clinical status on admission
❏ significant changes in status
❏ pertinent laboratory and diagnostic test findings
❏ pain characteristics
❏ analgesic administration
❏ nonpharmacologic strategies
❏ behavioral strategies
❏ effectiveness of measures
❏ patient's and family's response to pain
❏ patient and family teaching
❏ discharge planning.

ASSOCIATED PLANS OF CARE

Dying
Grieving
Impaired physical mobility
Ineffective family coping: Compromised
Ineffective individual coping
Sensory-perceptual alteration

REFERENCES

Agency for Health Care Policy and Research. *Acute Pain Management: Operative or Medical Procedures and Trauma. Clinical Practice Guideline No. 1.* Rockville, Md.: U.S. Department of Health and Human Services (AHCPR Publication No. 92-0032), 1992.

Agency for Health Care Policy and Research. *Management of Cancer Pain. Clinical Practice Guideline No. 9.* Rockville, Md.: U.S. Department of Health and Human Services (AHCPR Publication No. 94-0592), 1994.

Gordon, D.B., and Ward, S.E. "Correcting Patient Misconceptions about Pain," *AJN* 95(7):43-45, July 1995.

http://www.healthtouch.com/level1/leaflets/ahcpr. Agency for Health Care Policy and Research, U.S. Public Health Service.

McCaffery, M., and Beebe, A. *Pain: Clinical Manual for Nursing Practice.* St. Louis: Mosby–Year Book, Inc., 1989.

Pasero, C.L., and McCaffery, M. "Managing Postoperative Pain in the Elderly," *AJN* 96(10):38-46, October 1996.

Principles of Analgesic Use in the Treatment of Acute Pain and Cancer Pain, 3rd ed. Skokie, Ill.: American Pain Society, 1992.

Seely, S.K., et al. "Acute Pain in the High Acuity Patient," in *High Acuity Nursing,* 2nd ed. Stamford, Conn.: Appleton & Lange, 1996.

Stannard, D., et al. "Clinical Judgment and Management of Postoperative Pain in Critical Care Patients," *American Journal of Critical Care* 5(6):433-41, November 1996.

Wong, D.L. *Whaley & Wong's Nursing Care of Infants and Children.* St. Louis: Mosby–Year Book, Inc., 1995.

General plans of care

Sensory-perceptual alteration

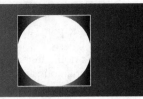

INTRODUCTION

Definition and time focus
A sensory-perceptual alteration is a state in which a person experiences a change in the amount or patterning of oncoming stimuli, accompanied by a diminished, exaggerated, distorted, or impaired response to such stimuli. Such alterations may affect a patient's overall well-being in numerous ways. The hospital unit environment, the physiologic manifestations of illness, and the psychological stress caused by hospitalization may have a severe cumulative effect unless the nurse initiates astute anticipatory intervention. Most nurses are familiar with the phenomenon of a patient's environmental disorientation. This distressing response may be averted or minimized by careful assessment and attention to modifiable aspects of the patient's environment. Family members may be a particularly helpful resource for nursing care planning for this problem because they can provide information about the patient's usual home environment and sensory-perceptual abilities. Nursing intervention for this problem, perhaps more than for any other nursing diagnosis, must be individually tailored to the patient's subjective view of the situation. When using this diagnosis, specify the type of alteration (visual, auditory, kinesthetic, gustatory, tactile, or olfactory).

The interventions for sensory-perceptual alteration have been grouped into problems according to cause.

Etiology and precipitating factors
• Unfamiliar, complex environment
• Monotonous environment
• Perceptual deficits, such as uncompensated deafness
• Chemical alterations (endogenous or exogenous)
• Psychological stress
• Bed rest
• Medications

FOCUSED ASSESSMENT GUIDELINES

Nursing history (functional health pattern findings)
The patient with a sensory-perceptual alteration may be unable to provide meaningful subjective data for assessment purposes. The patient's family may be especially helpful in providing information about baseline mental status and normal activities and interests. Although findings may vary widely among individuals, the following are common findings associated with sensory-perceptual alteration.

Health perception–health management pattern
• Unrealistic ideas regarding condition

Nutritional-metabolic pattern
• Reduced appetite or apathy toward food

Activity-exercise pattern
• Insomnia or fatigue
• Wandering behavior
• Hyperactivity

Cognitive-perceptual pattern
• Impaired judgment
• Loss of sense of time
• Memory impairment
• Reduced attention span
• Misidentification of familiar persons
• Increased need for pain medications

Self-perception–self-concept pattern
• Assumption that all external stimuli have reference to self (ideas of reference)
• Verbalization of paranoid ideas
• Expression of suicidal thoughts

Coping–stress tolerance pattern
• Withdrawal from others in response to perceived threat
• Demanding behavior; repeated requests to satisfy minor needs
• Obsessive or compulsive behavior such as constant rearrangement of familiar items
• Inability to make decisions
• Aggressive behavior; verbal or sexual overtures
• Crying or rage in response to minor frustration or annoyance

Physical findings
Physical manifestations of sensory-perceptual alteration may vary widely, depending on the patient's underlying condition and other factors. The findings listed below, however, may indicate such an alteration is present, and the astute nurse will be alert to such cues.

General appearance
• Nervous mannerisms
• Anxious facial expression
• Flat affect

Neurologic
• Restlessness
• Irritability
• Combativeness
• Confusion or disorientation
• Nystagmus
• Delusions or hallucinations

- Psychosis
- Depression

Cardiopulmonary
- Cardiac arrhythmias (associated with sleep deprivation)

Respiratory
- Hyperventilation or other physiologic manifestations of tension or anxiety
- Reduced ventilatory response to hypoxia and hypercapnia (associated with sleep deprivation)

Musculoskeletal
- Increased muscle tension
- Hand tremors

Diagnostic studies
No laboratory tests or diagnostic procedures exist specifically for patients with sensory-perceptual alteration; however, any patient with altered mental status for any reason should be evaluated for possible toxic, endocrine, or metabolic causes for symptoms.

Potential complications
- Acute brain syndrome
- Physical injury from confusion
- Crisis state

CLINICAL SNAPSHOT

SENSORY-PERCEPTUAL ALTERATION

Major nursing diagnoses	Key patient outcomes
Sensory-perceptual alteration related to excessive or insufficient environmental stimuli	Remain oriented.
Sensory-perceptual alteration related to altered sensory reception, transmission, or integration	Have documented identification of specific sensory-perceptual alterations, if present.
Sensory-perceptual alteration related to endogenous or exogenous chemical alterations	Display a clear sensorium.
Sensory-perceptual alteration related to psychological stress	Display relaxed posture and facial expression.

NURSING DIAGNOSIS

Sensory-perceptual alteration related to excessive or insufficient environmental stimuli

Nursing priorities

- Promote normal processing and integration of environmental cues.
- Control stimuli for maximum therapeutic effect.

Patient outcome criteria

Within 24 hours of admission, the patient will:
- remain oriented (if applicable)
- experience at least one uninterrupted sleep cycle of 2 hours or more.

General plans of care

Interventions

1. Assess the unit environment. Evaluate the type, quantity, duration, frequency, and clarity of auditory, visual, olfactory, tactile, and gustatory stimuli. To maintain alertness to the unit environment, the staff might periodically role-play as patients, as unit census permits.

2. Assess the patient's normal routines, including the general home environment, activity, diet, and sleep patterns. Ask the patient or family to provide information regarding specific personal habits or preferences, such as reading before bedtime or leaving the television or radio on during waking hours. Ask the patient or family to describe a typical 24-hour period. As feasible, modify care routines and the unit environment to resemble the patient's home surroundings. If possible, provide food that is familiar.

3. Orient the patient and family to the unit, explaining structure and routines. At the same time each day, review with them the day's activity plan and instruct them regarding special procedures or changes that are anticipated. As much as possible, prepare the patient and family in advance for change of any kind. Attempt to provide continuity in staffing.

4. Provide cues to orientation and reinforce them frequently while providing care. Ensure, for example, that a large clock and calendar are placed within the patient's visual field; wear name tags that are easy to read and introduce yourself to the patient at least once a shift until familiarity is established. For patients with visual deficits, always introduce yourself when approaching the bedside and before touching the patient. For a patient without visual impairment, encourage the family to bring in photographs or other small items from home to place on the wall or at the bedside.

5. Control environmental stimuli, as possible, to provide an environment that is secure and meaningful for the patient. Pay particular attention to the type and level of unit noise, ensuring that extraneous conversation is kept to a minimum. Encourage questions and provide interpretation of unfamiliar sensory stimuli as part of the patient's orientation to the unit — for example, "That beeping sound is an alarm on a patient's I.V. monitor," or "The hissing you hear is a machine that helps another patient to breathe."

Rationales

1. The patient in the hospital unit is subjected to a dramatic reduction in some types of stimuli (visual, gustatory, tactile) and an increase in other types (auditory). Such changes, particularly when the patient's ability to perceive, integrate, and cope with new information is impaired by physiologic stress, may result in significant mental status alterations. Staff awareness of the environment to which most patients are constantly exposed is essential for effective intervention on the patient's behalf. Nurses may become so habituated to the work environment that their sensitivity to its effects on patients is reduced. Role-playing as a patient may increase awareness.

2. Careful assessment of the patient's usual prehospitalization surroundings is essential to making appropriate adjustments. A description of the customary 24-hour routine provides valuable information about interrelationships and the significance of various aspects of the patient's life. Modification of routines, surroundings, and food may promote a sense of security.

3. Structure and routine aid the patient in interpreting and processing unfamiliar environmental cues. Reviewing plans at the same time each day reinforces the routine and increases security. Advance preparation allows the patient and family to integrate and cope with change more effectively. Continuity of staffing adds to the patient's repertoire of familiar information.

4. Reality testing requires input of familiar, predictable, and meaningful external informational cues. Without such orientation guides, internal and external events may become confused. Studies have shown that even normal, healthy individuals experience sensory-perceptual alterations when subjected to bed rest and its attendant sensory-perceptual deprivation. Even a few familiar items from home, particularly photographs of loved ones, may help the patient maintain orientation and reduce the alienation patients experience in the strange environment of the hospital unit.

5. Studies have shown that ambient noise in hospital units distresses the patient, increasing muscle tension and diastolic pressure and contributing to sleep disturbances. Nurse, staff, and visitor conversations may be even more disruptive to normal rest and sleep than the steady noise from equipment. Without normal sensory stimulation, the patient commonly interprets all overheard conversations as self-pertaining. For example, the patient who overhears a staff conversation about a surgical procedure may assume he is to undergo such a procedure. By interpreting unfamiliar stimuli and answering all questions, the nurse can increase the patient's security and promote adaptation to the unit environment.

6. As the patient's condition permits, encourage family participation in care. Explain the potential benefits of family-patient contact even when the patient is unresponsive. Speak to the patient when providing care, using touch generously unless the patient appears uncomfortable with physical contact.

6. Family contact decreases the strangeness of the environment and promotes orientation. Even patients who appear unconscious may continue to process environmental input, particularly sounds. Familiar verbal and tactile stimuli reduce sensory deprivation and provide reassurance. Touching the patient is one way of acknowledging the human dimension of care, which the patient may otherwise perceive as secondary in the high-technology setting.

7. Schedule care to provide uninterrupted patient sleep cycles of 2 hours or more by:

7. The function of sleep is unknown, but it may help maintain central nervous system control of various homeostatic mechanisms. Some theories postulate that sleep is essential for normal processing and integrating of information. Studies have shown a decrease in the mental status of sleep-deprived patients. The procedures listed help minimize these effects.

• grouping necessary procedures

• Grouping procedures minimizes interruption of normal sleep cycles, which usually last 90 to 120 minutes.

• using continuous monitoring devices to check routine vital signs and other parameters

• Monitoring devices don't require waking the patient.

• scheduling planned sleep times, as possible, to coincide with usual home pattern

• When the patient's usual rhythm is disrupted, an effective sleep pattern may be difficult to reestablish.

• minimizing noise (especially sudden, loud sounds), setting alarms as low as safety allows, and turning off equipment when not in use

• Even sounds that don't cause the patient to awaken completely may disrupt the normal sleep cycle. Abrupt loud sounds are more likely to cause awakening, though even continuous, low-level noise may alter the normal pattern.

• evaluating for possible effects of medications on the sleep pattern and discussing their probable benefits and risks with the doctor, as appropriate

• Many medications, including morphine, phenobarbital, and diazepam (Valium), may decrease rapid eye movement (REM) sleep. REM sleep is considered essential to normal psychological functioning. The greatest amount of REM sleep occurs toward the end of a sleep period.

• assessing for pain

• Pain management can prevent restlessness and promote relaxation and sleep.

• providing eyeshades, earplugs, extra blankets or pillows, and other comfort measures

• Most people find sleeping in lighted areas difficult. Reducing stimulation and providing comfort measures help achieve sleep.

• teaching relaxation techniques, such as imagery, progressive muscle relaxation, massage, and deep breathing, or administering sedatives, as ordered.

• Relaxation can induce sleep. If it's insufficient, sedatives may help the patient obtain much-needed sleep, even in a disturbing environment.

8. Assess the patient's mental status daily, noting particularly any alteration in orientation or memory. Be especially observant for indications of sensory-perceptual alteration in elderly patients and in children.

8. Early detection allows for preventive intervention. Older and younger patients are most susceptible to the effects of significant sensory-perceptual changes.

9. When leaving the bedside, always explain to the patient where you're going and approximately when you'll return, and make sure the call bell is within reach.

9. Knowing what to expect from the nurse decreases the patient's anxiety and provides a time reference. Leaving the call bell within reach helps ensure that the patient can obtain assistance when needed.

10. Additional individualized interventions: _____

10. Rationales: _____

NURSING DIAGNOSIS

Sensory-perceptual alteration related to altered sensory reception, transmission, or integration

Nursing priority

Minimize or compensate for sensory-perceptual deficits.

Patient outcome criterion

Within 8 hours of admission and then daily, the patient will repeat baseline reality orientation information when asked, if appropriate.

Interventions

1. Assess for conditions in which sensory reception, transmission, or integration is likely to be impaired, such as old age, neurologic abnormalities, use of neuromuscular blocking agents, vision or hearing problems, immobilization, endotracheal intubation, tracheostomy and mechanical ventilation, altered level of consciousness, depression, or anxiety. If such conditions are present, identify the type and level of dysfunction, if possible, and note it in the plan of care or post a notice near the patient's bed — for example, "Deafness in right ear, full hearing in left" or "Speak slowly."

2. Consult the medical history for additional pertinent data regarding specific deficits, such as the anatomic site and physiologic effects of cerebrovascular accident. Tailor care accordingly.

3. Ensure reading glasses or a hearing aid is available to the patient who needs either. Consider using mirrors to expand vision field if immobilization restricts movement.

4. For any patient with altered mentation or consciousness, except Alzheimer's disease, provide reality orientation at regular, planned intervals (at least every 8 hours). Include the time, day, date and year, location, and a brief explanation of the patient's immediate circumstances. Even if the patient is unresponsive, continue to provide such information regularly until the patient can repeat it on request.

5. Additional individualized interventions: _____

Rationales

1. Evaluation for risk factors permits early intervention to avert severe sensory deprivation and its distressing aftereffects.

2. Attempting to implement interventions that are inappropriate to the patient's functional level may increase frustration and reduce the patient's motivation to communicate.

3. Accurate visual and auditory perceptions are the patient's primary connections to the external world and enhance reality orientation.

4. Reality orientation provides an essential anchor and a sense of security for patients recovering from altered consciousness, who commonly are uncertain whether they are dead or alive. In Alzheimer's disease, reality orientation may increase agitation. Numerous case studies reveal that even unresponsive patients are receptive to auditory stimuli and many remember conversations of others even after a prolonged coma.

5. Rationales: _____

NURSING DIAGNOSIS

Sensory-perceptual alteration related to endogenous or exogenous chemical alterations

Nursing priority

Identify and treat possible causes of biochemical alteration.

Patient outcome criteria

Throughout the hospital stay, the patient will:
• display a clear sensorium
• make verbal statements congruent with reality.

Interventions

1. Assess for conditions that may contribute to chemically induced sensory-perceptual alterations, such as the therapeutic medication regimen, drug intoxication, diabetes or other metabolic disorders, or electrolyte and acid-base imbalances. Collaborate with the doctor to treat the underlying cause.

2. Provide appropriate, accurate explanations to the patient and family about the effects of psychotropic medications or other chemical causes of sensory-perceptual alteration.

3. Additional individualized interventions: _____

Rationales

1. Appropriate intervention to decrease the effects of sensory-perceptual changes depends on accurate identification of their cause.

2. The patient and family may be alarmed or ashamed about chemically induced behavior. Providing explanations and displaying an attitude of acceptance promotes trust and open communication.

3. Rationales: _____

NURSING DIAGNOSIS

Sensory-perceptual alteration related to psychological stress

Nursing priority

Promote effective coping.

Patient outcome criteria

Throughout the hospital stay, the patient will:
• express feelings regarding stressors, on request
• display relaxed posture and facial expression.

Interventions

1. Be aware of the patient's needs for personal space. Ask permission and provide explanations before performing procedures. Provide effective screening to protect the patient's privacy.

2. See the "Ineffective individual coping" plan, page 67.

3. Additional individualized interventions: _____

Rationales

1. Everyone is protective of unconsciously defined personal boundaries, which help an individual maintain ego integration. For the acutely ill patient, these boundaries are constantly assaulted by invasive tubing, procedures, and noise the patient can't control. Even small measures to acknowledge these boundaries may reduce stress from loss of control.

2. The "Ineffective individual coping" plan contains detailed interventions for the patient experiencing psychological stress.

3. Rationales: _____

General plans of care

DISCHARGE PLANNING

Discharge checklist

Before discharge, the patient shows evidence of:
- ❏ identification of specific sensory-perceptual alterations, if present
- ❏ successful resolution or ongoing treatment of sensory-perceptual problems.

Teaching checklist

Document evidence that the patient and family demonstrate an understanding of:
- ❏ signs and symptoms of sensory-perceptual alteration
- ❏ causes of sensory-perceptual alterations
- ❏ reality orientation measures
- ❏ stress-reduction measures
- ❏ measures to promote sleep.

Documentation checklist

Using outcome criteria as a guide, document:
- ❏ clinical status on admission
- ❏ significant changes in status
- ❏ pertinent diagnostic test findings
- ❏ reality orientation measures
- ❏ sleep status
- ❏ family participation in care
- ❏ patient and family teaching
- ❏ potential discharge needs
- ❏ safety measures.

ASSOCIATED PLANS OF CARE

Impaired physical mobility
Ineffective individual coping
Knowledge deficit
Pain

REFERENCES

Granberg, A., et al. "Intensive Care Syndrome: A Literature Review," *Intensive and Critical Care Nursing* 12(3):173-82, June 1996.

Laitinen, H. "Patients' Experience of Confusion in the Intensive Care Unit Following Cardiac Surgery," *Intensive and Critical Care Nursing* 12(2):79-83, April 1996.

Wilson, L. "Sensory-Perceptual Alteration: Diagnosis, Predictors, and Interventions in the Hospitalized Adult," *Nursing Clinics of North America* 28(4):741-47, December 1993.

Surgery

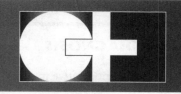

Introduction

Definition and time focus
Surgery is an important medical therapy used for diagnostic, curative, restorative, palliative, or cosmetic reasons. This plan focuses on care of surgical patients.

Etiology and precipitating factors
Precipitating factors aren't applicable in this general plan of care.

Focused assessment guidelines
Nursing history and physical findings aren't applicable in this general plan of care.

Diagnostic studies
• Urinalysis
• Complete blood count (CBC)

• Prothrombin time and partial thromboplastin time
• Electrolyte panel
• Blood urea nitrogen and creatinine levels
• Blood typing and cross-matching.
• Chest X-ray
• 12-lead electrocardiogram (ECG)
• Special studies depending on the disorder

Potential complications
• Shock
• Atelectasis
• Pulmonary embolism
• Thrombophlebitis
• Wound infection, dehiscence, and evisceration
• Paralytic ileus
• Acute renal failure
• Urine retention
• Aspiration
• Malignant hyperthermia
• Hypothermia

General plans of care

CLINICAL SNAPSHOT

Surgery

Major nursing diagnoses and collaborative problems	Key patient outcomes
Knowledge deficit: Perioperative routines	Demonstrate ability to cough, deep-breathe, use incentive spirometer, and perform leg exercises.
Risk for postoperative shock	Have a pulse rate of 60 to 100 beats/minute, a systolic blood pressure of 90 to 140 mm Hg, and a diastolic blood pressure of 50 to 90 mm Hg.
Pain	Rate pain as less than the chosen goal level (typically less than 3 on a 0 to 10 pain rating scale).
Risk for postoperative atelectasis	Manifest clear breath sounds in all lobes.
Risk for postoperative thromboembolic phenomena	Show no signs of thromboembolic phenomena.
Risk for postoperative injury	Ambulate without injury.
Risk for infection	Perform wound care.
Risk for postoperative urinary retention	Show no signs of urine retention.
Risk for postoperative paralytic ileus	Have normal bowel sounds.
Risk for malignant hyperthermia	Show no signs of malignant hyperthermia.
Nausea or vomiting	Be free from nausea or vomiting.

NURSING DIAGNOSIS

Knowledge deficit: Perioperative routines, related to lack of familiarity with hospital procedures

Nursing priority

Prepare the patient for perioperative routines.

Patient outcome criteria

Before surgery, the patient will:
• verbalize understanding of perioperative routines
• demonstrate ability to cough, deep-breathe, use the incentive spirometer, and perform leg exercises.

Interventions

1. See the "Knowledge deficit" plan, page 72.

2. Instruct the patient in the various aspects of perioperative routines, such as time of surgery, food or fluid restrictions, type of anesthesia, insertion of I.V. and intra-arterial lines, personnel, the environments of the operating and recovery rooms and surgical intensive care unit, type of wound and dressing, tubes, drains, and postoperative respiratory care. Include demonstrations and return demonstrations of coughing, deep breathing, spirometry, splinting the incision, and leg exercises.

3. Additional individualized interventions: _____

Rationales

1. Generalized interventions regarding patient teaching are included in the "Knowledge deficit" plan.

2. Patients will be more likely to remember and comply with preoperative, intraoperative and postoperative procedures if they understand the rationale for them, have been instructed before surgery, and have practiced activities where appropriate.

3. Rationales: _____

COLLABORATIVE PROBLEM

Risk for postoperative shock related to hemorrhage or hypovolemia

Nursing priority

Detect shock.

Patient outcome criteria

• Within 12 hours after surgery, the patient will:
 – have a pulse rate of 60 to 100 beats/minute, a systolic blood pressure of 90 to 140 mm Hg, and a diastolic blood pressure of 50 to 90 mm Hg
 – display minimal bloody drainage on dressing and in wound drains
 – maintain a urine output greater than 60 ml/hour.
• Within 2 days after surgery, the patient will display balanced fluid intake and output.

Interventions

1. Monitor and document vital signs on admission to the nursing unit and every 4 hours. If vital signs have changed significantly from recovery room findings, monitor and document every 15 to 30 minutes until stable. Report abnormalities. Estimate intraoperative blood loss from the surgical record and laboratory blood studies.

2. Assess the surgical dressing on admission to the unit, every hour for 4 hours, then every 4 hours. Mark any drainage, and note on the dressing the date and time it occurred. Document and report excessive drainage.

3. Assess the amount and character of drainage from wound-drainage tubes when assessing the surgical dressing. Report bright red bloody drainage.

4. Reinforce the surgical dressing as needed. Don't change the original surgical dressing unless specifically ordered to do so.

5. Assess the surgical area for swelling or hematoma. Document and report abnormalities.

6. Monitor for changes in mental status. Be alert for restlessness and a sense of impending doom. Document and report such signs.

7. Assess and maintain I.V. line patency. Maintain I.V. fluids at the ordered rate.

8. Monitor urine output every hour for 4 hours, then every 4 hours, during the immediate postoperative period. Report urine output of less than 60 ml/hour and, in such cases, measure urine specific gravity. Administer I.V. fluids and diuretics as ordered, to maintain urine output at greater than 60 ml/hour and specific gravity at 1.010 to 1.025.

9. Monitor hemoglobin level and hematocrit, as ordered. Determine availability of blood and blood products.

10. Monitor fluid intake and output every 8 hours with an accumulated total every 24 hours for at least 3 to 4 days after surgery.

11. Additional individualized interventions: _____

Rationales

1. Hypotension and tachycardia may indicate hemorrhage. Estimated blood loss guides fluid and blood replacement.

2. Hemorrhage typically occurs within the first several hours after surgery. Frequent assessments allow for its prompt detection. Marking the extent of drainage permits objective serial measurements.

3. Bright red blood from drainage tubes may indicate arterial hemorrhage.

4. Changing the surgical dressing may disrupt the wound edge, cause bleeding, and introduce bacteria.

5. Swelling or hematoma may indicate internal bleeding.

6. Changes in mental status may reflect cerebral hypoxia, indicating decreased cerebral perfusion from hemorrhage or hypovolemia.

7. A patent I.V. line is essential to fluid replacement. Fluids will be ordered according to the surgeon's preference. At times, fluid replacement is the only treatment necessary for hypovolemic shock.

8. Urine output decreases if the patient is bleeding or is hypovolemic. The kidneys retain fluid to maintain intravascular pressure. Urine specific gravity will reveal urine concentration as the body attempts to conserve fluid. Additionally, blood flow to the kidneys is reduced if the patient is in shock, thereby decreasing the glomerular filtration rate and urine output. I.V. fluids and diuretics help maintain the glomerular filtration rate to prevent acute tubular necrosis.

9. Hemoglobin level and hematocrit don't drop immediately with excessive blood loss because plasma is lost along with red blood cells. If bleeding persists, the blood remaining in the vessels will become more dilute as kidneys conserve water and as fluid shifts from interstitial to intravascular spaces; then hemoglobin level and hematocrit will drop. Rapid administration of blood and blood products may be necessary; confirming their availability avoids delays in initiating therapy.

10. For the first 48 hours after surgery, intake may exceed output because of fluid loss (from hemorrhage, vomiting, or diaphoresis) and increased secretion of antidiuretic hormone and aldosterone.

11. Rationales: _____

General plans of care

NURSING DIAGNOSIS

Pain related to surgical tissue trauma, positioning, and reflex muscle spasm

Nursing priority

Relieve pain.

Patient outcome criterion

Within 1 hour of reporting pain, the patient will rate pain as less than the chosen goal level (typically less than 3 on a 0 to 10 pain rating scale).

Interventions	Rationales
1. See the "Pain" plan, page 88.	**1.** The "Pain" plan contains detailed information on pain assessment and management.
2. Additional individualized interventions: _____	**2.** Rationales: _____

COLLABORATIVE PROBLEM

Risk for postoperative atelectasis related to immobility and ciliary depression from anesthesia

Nursing priority

Prevent atelectasis.

Patient outcome criteria

Throughout the postoperative period, the patient will:
- display a respiratory rate of 12 to 20 breaths/minute
- have nonlabored, deep respirations
- manifest clear breath sounds in all lobes.

Interventions

1. Elevated temperature may indicate atelectasis, which can lead to pneumonia. Respirations may be shallow after anesthesia.

2. Auscultate for breath sounds every 4 hours on the first postoperative day, then once per shift. Document and report abnormalities.

3. Instruct and coach the patient in diaphragmatic breathing and chest splinting.

4. Assist the patient in using the incentive spirometer — 10 breaths every hour during the day, every 2 hours at night. In the first 24 hours, coach the patient on its use; then, once the patient is alert, encourage independent use and assess its effectiveness.

Rationales

1. Assess vital signs according to unit protocol for the first day after surgery, then every 4 hours. Note the characteristics of respirations. Monitor the amount and characteristics of sputum. Document and report abnormalities.

2. Breath sounds may be diminished postoperatively because air exchange is decreased in atelectatic areas.

3. Diaphragmatic breathing increases lung expansion by allowing the diaphragm to descend fully. Chest splinting reduces pain and facilitates breathing.

4. Use of the incentive spirometer promotes sustained maximal inspiration, which inflates alveoli as fully as possible.

5. Help the patient turn at least every 2 hours unless contraindicated.

6. Help the patient progressively increase ambulation.

7. Encourage adequate fluid intake.

8. Additional individualized interventions: _____

5. Position changes provide for better ventilation of all lobes of the lungs and promote drainage of secretions.

6. Ambulation promotes adequate ventilation by increasing the respiratory rate.

7. Respiratory secretions will be thinner and more easily expectorated if the patient is well hydrated.

8. Rationales: _____

COLLABORATIVE PROBLEM

Risk for postoperative thromboembolic phenomena related to immobility, dehydration, and possible fat particle escape or aggregation

Nursing priority

Prevent thromboembolism.

Patient outcome criteria

• Throughout the postoperative period, the patient will show no signs of thromboembolic phenomena.
• By the time of discharge, the patient will be able to identify an appropriate postdischarge activity schedule.

Interventions

1. Instruct and coach the patient to do leg exercises hourly while awake: foot flexion and extention, ankle rotation, knee flexion and extention, and quadriceps setting.

2. Assess twice daily for signs of thromboembolic phenomena. If any of these signs or symptoms is present, alert the doctor promptly:

• thrombophlebitis (redness, swelling, increased warmth along the vein, possibly a positive Homans' sign, and pain)
• pulmonary thromboembolism (sharp, stabbing chest pain, worsening on deep inspiration or coughing; hemoptysis; pleural friction rub; and tachypnea)
• fat embolism (dyspnea, restlessness, and petechiae)

• peripheral vascular thromboembolism (pallor, weak pulse, loss of sensation).

3. Administer heparin as ordered; monitor and report increased bleeding.

4. Encourage early ambulation after surgery.

5. Avoid using the gatch bed or placing pillows under the patient's knees.

Rationales

1. Leg exercises promote blood flow in the legs. Muscle contractions compress the veins and help prevent venous stasis, a major cause of clot formation.

2. Systematic observations aid in prompt detection of thromboembolic phenomena. Prompt treatment reduces the risk of clot extension, pulmonary infarction, or pulmonary arrest.
• Vessel wall inflammation and clot formation produce signs and symptoms of thrombophlebitis.

• Pulmonary thromboembolism occurs when a clot detaches from a vessel and lodges in the lungs.

• Fat embolism is a risk after orthopedic trauma or surgery (such as femoral fractures or sternum-splitting incisions). It may result from the escape of fat particles from bone marrow or from an aggregation of fat particles in the bloodstream.
• Blood clots and sclerotic plaques can detach and lodge in the peripheral vascular bed.

3. Heparin is an anticoagulant that can prevent thrombus formation.

4. Ambulation promotes blood flow in the legs.

5. Pressure on the popliteal blood vessels can slow blood circulation to and from the legs. Appropriate positioning also decreases venous stasis.

General plans of care

6. Encourage adequate fluid intake (in the initial postoperative period, I.V. fluids will be administered).

6. Inadequate fluid intake causes dehydration, which leads to increased blood viscosity — another major contributor to clot formation.

7. Apply antiembolism stockings, if ordered. Remove them twice daily for 1 hour.

7. Antiembolism stockings compress the leg veins and prevent venous stasis. Stockings should be removed periodically to allow for thrombophlebitis assessment and skin inspection.

8. Before discharge, teach the patient and family about guidelines for resuming normal activity.

8. Patients and families probably will have specific questions or concerns about the type and progression of allowable activity after discharge. Providing guidelines promotes the resumption of activity at an appropriate pace, which in turn lessens immobility-related complications and promotes a sense of well-being.

9. Additional individualized interventions: _____

9. Rationales: _____

NURSING DIAGNOSIS

Risk for postoperative injury related to possible changes in mental status caused by anesthesia and analgesia

Nursing priority

Prevent injury.

Patient outcome criteria

Within 24 hours after surgery, the patient will:
• be free from injury
• seek appropriate assistance with activity from the nurse.

Interventions

1. Assess the patient's level of consciousness, orientation, and ability to follow directions every 30 to 60 minutes in the first 8 to 10 hours postoperatively. Compare to preoperative level of consciousness and mental status.

2. Position the drowsy patient in a side-lying position; have suction equipment available.

3. Keep side rails up in the initial postoperative period, until the patient is awake and alert.

4. Keep the call cord within the patient's reach.

5. Keep the bed in the low position.

Rationales

1. A greater risk of injury exists if the patient is drowsy or disoriented. Frequent observation allows prompt detection of injury risk factors, if present. Preoperative status provides a baseline for comparison.

2. In a side-lying position, the patient has less risk of aspirating secretions or vomitus. Suction equipment at bedside facilitates prompt airway clearance of secretions or vomitus.

3. Side rails help prevent falls.

4. If the call cord is within reach, the patient is more likely to ask the nurse for assistance.

5. The low bed position is safer for the patient.

6. Monitor postural vital signs and assist the patient with initial postoperative activity. Observe for a pulse rate increase of more than 20 beats/minute, a systolic blood pressure decrease of more than 10 mm Hg, a decreased level of consciousness, diaphoresis, and cyanosis. If present, discontinue activity and alert the doctor.

7. Additional individualized interventions: _____
_____

6. When first ambulating, the patient may feel dizzy or have an unsteady gait from orthostatic hypotension. This occurs because immobility compromises the ability of peripheral vessels to constrict when the patient assumes an upright position. Orthostatic hypotension can also occur if the patient is hypovolemic, producing the more alarming signs listed and requiring medical evaluation and I.V. fluid replacement.

7. Rationales: _____
_____

NURSING DIAGNOSIS

Risk for infection related to surgical intervention

Nursing priority

Promote wound healing.

Patient outcome criteria

- Within 3 days after surgery, the patient will:
  - be afebrile
  - show healing wound with no signs of infection.
- Within 7 days after surgery, the patient will have a clean, dry, and well-approximated surgical wound.

Interventions

1. Identify risk factors for surgical wound infection:

- obesity

- extremes of age

- immunosuppression
- poor nutritional status
- diabetes mellitus.

2. Assess the surgical wound and other invasive sites once per shift for:
- evidence of normal healing, such as approximation of wound margins and absence of purulent or foul-smelling drainage

- signs of dehiscence, such as poorly approximated wound edges and serous drainage from a previously nondraining wound (If dehiscence occurs, cover with a dry sterile dressing and notify the doctor immediately.)
- signs of evisceration, such as disruption of the surgical wound with protrusion of the viscera. (If evisceration occurs, cover the viscerated organs with sterile saline-soaked gauze and notify the doctor immediately.)

Rationales

1. Knowledge of risk factors enables the nurse to individualize patient care.
- Adipose tissue is poorly vascularized, retarding healing.
- The very young and the very old have less physiologic reserve.
- A compromised host is at greater risk for infection.
- A catabolic state retards wound repair.
- Impaired glucose metabolism delays healing.

2. Regular assessment promotes early detection of suboptimal healing.
- The normally healing wound is well approximated and without evidence of infection. (The surgical wound, however, may be reddened in the first 3 postoperative days — the normal inflammatory response.)
- Wound dehiscence most commonly occurs 3 to 11 days after surgery. Application of a sterile dressing reduces the risk of infection.

- Eviscerated organs must be kept moist and surgical intervention must be prompt because blood supply to tissues is compromised when organs herniate.

General plans of care

3. Determine wound classification:

• clean — minimal endogenous contamination present (such as with breast biopsy)

• clean-contaminated — possible endogenous bacterial contamination present (such as with appendectomy)

• contaminated — contamination present (such as with trauma)
• dirty — infected tissue present (such as with abscess).

4. Monitor temperature every 4 hours. Document and report elevations.

5. Maintain a clean, dry incision. Teach patient and family to perform wound care as ordered.

6. Use strict aseptic technique when performing wound care. Instruct the patient and family in hand-washing technique; aseptic technique; and wound care, including dressing change and application, irrigations and cleaning procedures, proper disposal of soiled dressings, and bathing by shower (not tub) until the wound is healed.

7. Instruct the patient and family in signs and symptoms of infection: elevated temperature, abdominal pain, and purulent or foul-smelling wound drainage.

8. Encourage adequate nutritional intake every shift. Document intake every shift.

9. Additional individualized interventions: _____
_____

3. Wound classification is a predictor of surgical wound infection.
• In this wound class, the respiratory, alimentary, or genitourinary tract isn't entered during surgery so the likelihood of contamination is minimal.
• In this wound class, the respiratory, alimentary, or genitourinary tract is entered under controlled conditions, but infection isn't noted and the risk of postoperative infection is increased only slightly.
• In this wound class, gross GI spillage or traumatic wounds place the patient at higher risk for infection.
• In this wound class, retained devitalized tissue or existing infection pose the greatest risk of infection.

4. A low-grade temperature present in the first 3 postoperative days is associated with the normal inflammatory response. Fever that persists may signify infection.

5. A clean, dry incision is at less risk for infection. Moisture can harbor microorganisms.

6. Aseptic technique prevents cross-contamination and transmission of bacterial infections to the surgical wound.

7. Educating the patient and family promotes their sense of control and minimizes anxiety and fear during preparation for discharge.

8. Sufficient intake of protein, calories, vitamins, and minerals is essential to promote tissue healing.

9. Rationales: _____
_____

NURSING DIAGNOSIS

Risk for postoperative urinary retention related to neuroendocrine response to stress, anesthesia, and recumbent position

Nursing priority

Prevent urine retention.

Patient outcome criterion

Within 1 day after surgery, the patient will void at least 200 ml of clear urine at a time.

Interventions

1. Assess for signs of urine retention. Include subjective complaints of urgency as well as objective signs, such as bladder distention, urine overflow, and marked discrepancy between the fluid intake amount and the time of the last voiding.

2. Initiate interventions to promote voiding as soon as the patient begins to sense bladder pressure.

3. Provide noninvasive measures to promote voiding, such as normal position for voiding, ambulation to the bathroom if possible, running water, relaxation, a warm bedpan if needed, pouring warm water over the perineum, or privacy.

4. Provide a supportive atmosphere: Use conscious positive suggestion; reassure the patient that voiding usually occurs eventually; don't threaten catheterization.

5. If the patient complains of bladder discomfort or hasn't voided within 8 hours after surgery, obtain an order for straight catheterization.

6. If the patient requires catheterization, drain the bladder of no more than 1,000 ml at a time. If urine output reaches 1,000 ml, clamp the catheter, wait 1 hour, then drain the rest of the urine from the bladder.

7. After catheterization, assess for dysuria, hematuria, pyuria, burning, and frequency and urgency of urination as well as for suprapubic discomfort. Assess and document the amount, appearance, odor, and clarity of urine. Report any signs of urinary infection.

8. Additional individualized interventions: _____

Rationales

1. The distended bladder can be palpated above the level of the symphysis pubis. Overflow incontinence occurs when intravesical pressure exceeds the restraining ability of the sphincter and enough urine flows out to decrease the intravesical pressure to a level at which the sphincter can control urine flow. A difference of several hundred milliliters between fluid intake and output, with the passage of several hours since the last voiding, implies retention.

2. Prompt treatment of potential voiding problems may reduce anxiety, which can further impair the ability to void.

3. These measures are designed to promote relaxation of the urinary sphincter and facilitate voiding. Successful use of noninvasive measures prevents unnecessary catheterization and related psychological strain and urethral trauma.

4. Conscious positive suggestion and reassurance promote relaxation and set up expectations for spontaneous voiding.

5. Straight catheterization poses less risk of infection than indwelling catheterization; an indwelling catheter can provide a pathway for bacteria to ascend into the bladder.

6. Draining more than 1,000 ml from the bladder releases pressure on the pelvic vessels. The sudden release of pressure allows subsequent pooling of blood in these vessels. Rapid withdrawal of this blood from the central circulating volume may cause shock.

7. Urine retention (stasis) and the introduction of a urethral catheter increase the risk for lower urinary tract infection.

8. Rationales: _____

_____

General plans of care

COLLABORATIVE PROBLEM

Risk for postoperative paralytic ileus, abdominal pain, or constipation related to immobility, surgical manipulation, anesthesia, and analgesia

Nursing priorities

• Detect paralytic ileus.
• Prevent constipation.

Patient outcome criteria

- Within 2 days after surgery, the patient will have normal bowel sounds.
- Within 4 days after surgery, the patient will:
  - have soft, formed bowel movements
  - not strain while defecating.
- Within 7 days after surgery, the patient will establish a regular bowel elimination pattern.

Interventions

1. Assess the abdomen twice daily for bowel sounds and distention. Assess for the presence of flatus or stool. Question the patient about abdominal fullness.

2. If paralytic ileus occurs, implement measures, as ordered, such as instructing the patient not to eat or drink anything, connecting a nasogastric (NG) tube to low intermittent suction, using a rectal tube to expel flatus, and administering I.V. fluids.

3. Implement comfort measures if paralytic ileus occurs: Provide frequent mouth care, position and tape the NG tube carefully, and administer analgesics.

4. Provide a diet appropriate to peristaltic activity. Make sure peristalsis has returned before progressing from nothing-by-mouth status to liberal fluid and solid food intake.

5. Encourage fluid intake of at least eight 8-oz (240-ml) glasses per day unless contraindicated (such as by heart failure). Provide fluids that the patient prefers.

6. Encourage frequent position changes and ambulation.

7. Provide privacy for the patient during defecation. Assist with ambulation to the bathroom if necessary.

8. Consult with the doctor concerning use of laxatives, suppositories, or enemas.

9. Additional individualized interventions: _____

Rationales

1. Bowel sounds will be hypoactive initially but should return to normal within the first 2 days after surgery. The presence of flatus or stool signals the return of peristalsis. Abdominal distention and absence of bowel sounds, flatus, and stool may indicate paralytic ileus.

2. These measures help prevent abdominal distention while promoting return of peristalsis. I.V. fluids maintain fluid and electrolyte balance while the patient has no oral intake.

3. Maintaining patient comfort is important for the prevention of further anxiety.

4. If peristalsis hasn't returned, feeding the patient will cause distention.

5. Sufficient fluid intake is required for proper stool consistency. Providing preferred fluids promotes hydration.

6. Activity promotes peristalsis.

7. Providing privacy eliminates possible embarrassment.

8. A laxative, suppository, or enema may be needed to promote bowel evacuation. These supplements should be used judiciously to avoid bowel dependence or possible damage to healing tissues.

9. Rationales: _____

COLLABORATIVE PROBLEM

Risk for malignant hyperthermia related to inherited skeletal muscle disorder, anesthetic agents, and abnormal calcium transport

Nursing priorities

- Detect malignant hyperthermia.
- Initiate treatment.

Patient outcome criteria

- Throughout the postoperative period, the patient will show no signs of malignant hyperthermia.
- By the time of discharge, the patient will be aware of risks for malignant hyperthermia.

Interventions

1. Assess the patient's susceptibility to malignant hyperthermia:

- personal and family history of malignant hyperthermia and response to anesthesia
- history of muscle abnormality: muscular hypertrophy, musculoskeletal problems (club foot, hernia, ptosis)
- young age, male.

2. Assess for signs and symptoms of malignant hyperthermia:
- ventricular arrhythmias (tachycardia, fibrillation)

- tachypnea

- hot, diaphoretic, mottled skin with or without cyanosis
- elevated temperature
- excessive muscle rigidity
- oliguria, anuria.

3. Monitor vital signs, arterial blood gases, electrolytes and ECG.

4. Alert anesthesiologist or nurse anesthetist to discontinue anesthesia (intraoperatively).

5. Administer dantrolene sodium (Dantrium), as ordered: initial I.V. dose is 2 to 3 mg/kg, followed by 1 mg/kg every 10 minutes up to 10 mg/kg.

6. Administer 100% oxygen.

7. Administer iced I.V. solutions or iced lavages of stomach, rectum, or bladder; employ hypothermia blanket.

8. Evaluate interventions; repeat regimen as indicated.

9. Before discharge, educate the patient and family about the future risk of malignant hyperthermia.

10. Additional individualized interventions: _____

Rationales

1. Malignant hyperthermia is an inherited skeletal muscle disorder causing a hypermetabolic state induced by anesthetic agents. Assessment identifies patients at risk for malignant hyperthermia, which can be fatal.
- A genetic predisposition exists for malignant hyperthermia.
- Musculoskeletal abnormalities may predispose the patient to malignant hyperthermia.
- The condition occurs in more children than adults and in more males than females.

2. Systematic observations aid in prompt detection of condition.
- Increased circulating catecholamines and hyperkalemia produce cardiac rhythm abnormalities.
- The respiratory rate increases to compensate for increased carbon dioxide production (respiratory acidosis).
- The body reacts to the hypermetabolic state by vasodilating and perspiring.
- Temperature increase reflects increased energy use.
- Anesthetic agents induce rigidity.
- Hypovolemia and decreased cardiac output cause decreased urine production.

3. Monitoring provides information about the extent of respiratory and metabolic acidosis and guides treatment of physiologic derangements.

4. Discontinuation of anesthesia removes a contributing factor.

5. Use of this skeletal muscle relaxant reduces muscular rigidity; this is the definitive pharmacologic treatment.

6. Oxygen administration provides increased oxygen to meet metabolic demands.

7. Cooling the body reduces the metabolic rate and lowers body temperature.

8. Hypermetabolic reaction can recur.

9. Malignant hyperthermia can recur.

10. Rationales: _____

General plans of care

COLLABORATIVE PROBLEM

Nausea or vomiting related to GI distention, rapid position changes, or cortical stimulation of the vomiting center or chemoreceptor trigger zone

Nursing priority

Prevent or relieve nausea or vomiting.

Patient outcome criteria

Within 1 hour of onset of nausea or vomiting, the patient will:
• verbalize relief of nausea
• be free from vomiting.

Interventions

1. Prevent GI overdistention: Maintain patency of the nasogastric tube; change the patient's diet only as tolerated.

2. Limit unpleasant sights, smells, and psychic stimuli, such as intense anxiety and pain.

3. Caution the patient to change position slowly.

4. As soon as possible, advance the patient from narcotics to other analgesics (as ordered), and then to nonpharmacologic pain-control measures.

5. Administer antiemetics, as ordered.

6. Additional individualized interventions: _____
_____

Rationales

1. Overdistention of the GI tract, particularly the duodenum, triggers the vomiting reflex.

2. These factors stimulate the chemoreceptor trigger zone in the medulla, which causes vomiting.

3. Rapid position changes also stimulate the trigger zone.

4. Medications, especially narcotics, may excite the chemoreceptor trigger zone.

5. Agents that depress the vomiting center or trigger zone responsiveness may be necessary when the measures described above are inappropriate or ineffective.

6. Rationales: _____
_____

DISCHARGE PLANNING

Discharge checklist
Before discharge, the patient should show evidence of:
❏ return to preoperative level of consciousness
❏ absence of fever
❏ absence of pulmonary and cardiovascular complications
❏ stable vital signs
❏ healing wound with no signs of infection
❏ hemoglobin level and white blood cell count within normal ranges
❏ I.V. lines discontinued for at least 24 hours
❏ ability to tolerate oral food intake
❏ ability to perform wound care independently
❏ ability to void and have bowel movements as before surgery
❏ ability to ambulate and perform activities of daily living as before surgery
❏ knowledge of activity restrictions
❏ ability to control pain using oral medications
❏ adequate home support, or referral to home care or nursing home if indicated by lack of home support system or by inability to perform self-care.

Teaching checklist
Document evidence that the patient and family demonstrate an understanding of:
❏ plan for resumption of normal activity
❏ wound care
❏ signs and symptoms of wound infection or other surgical complications

❑ all discharge medications' purpose, dosage, administration, and adverse effects requiring medical attention (postoperative patients may be discharged with oral analgesics)

❑ when and how to contact the health care provider

❑ date, time, and location of follow-up appointment with the surgeon

❑ community resources appropriate for surgical intervention performed such as a home health nurse.

Documentation checklist

Using outcome criteria as a guide, document:

❑ clinical status on admission

❑ significant changes in preoperative status (level of consciousness, emotional status, baseline physical data)

❑ preoperative teaching and its effectiveness

❑ preoperative checklist (includes documentation regarding preoperative consent, urinalysis, CBC, 12-lead ECG, chest X-ray, preoperative medication administration, surgical skin preparation, voiding on call from the operating room, and removal of nail polish, jewelry, prostheses, dentures, glasses, and hearing aids).

❑ clinical status on admission from the recovery room

❑ amount and character of wound drainage (on dressing and through drains)

❑ skin condition

❑ patency of tubes (I.V., nasogastric, indwelling urinary catheter, drains)

❑ pulmonary hygiene measures

❑ pain-relief measures

❑ activity tolerance

❑ nutritional intake

❑ elimination status (urinary and bowel)

❑ pertinent laboratory test findings

❑ patient and family teaching

❑ discharge planning.

ASSOCIATED PLANS OF CARE

Grieving
Impaired physical mobility
Ineffective individual coping
Knowledge deficit
Pain
Sensory-perceptual alteration

REFERENCES

Carpenito, L. *Nursing Diagnosis: Application to Clinical Practice,* 7th ed. Philadelphia: Lippincott-Raven Pubs., 1997.

Groah, L.K. *Perioperative Nursing,* 3rd ed. Stamford, Conn.: Appleton & Lange, 1996.

Lewis, S.M., et al. *Medical-Surgical Nursing: Assessment and Management of Clinical Problems,* 4th ed. St. Louis: Mosby–Year Book, Inc., 1996.

Meeker, M., and Rothrock, J. *Alexander's Care of the Patient in Surgery,* 11th ed. St. Louis: Mosby–Year Book, Inc., 1998.

Rothrock, J. *Perioperative Nursing Care Planning,* 2nd ed. St. Louis: Mosby–Year Book, Inc., 1996.

Sparks, S., and Taylor, C. *Nursing Diagnosis Reference Manual,* 4th ed. Springhouse, Pa.: Springhouse Corp., 1998.

Thompson, J., et al. *Mosby's Clinical Nursing,* 4th ed. St. Louis: Mosby–Year Book, Inc., 1997.

Winningham, M., and Preusser, B. *Critical Thinking in the Medical-Surgical Setting: A Case Study Approach.* St. Louis: Mosby–Year Book, Inc., 1996.

General plans of care

Part 3

Neurologic disorders

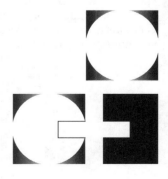

Alzheimer's disease

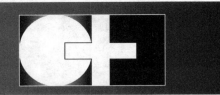

DRG information
DRG 012   Degenerative Nervous System Disorders.
               Mean LOS = 7.7 days
Additional DRG information: Patients are rarely admitted with only Alzheimer's disease (AD); usually, another disorder, such as pneumonia or dehydration, is the primary diagnosis. Because AD as a comorbidity would probably increase the other disorder's LOS and relative weight (depending on the primary diagnosis), a patient with AD is more likely to be assigned the DRG number of the primary diagnosis than DRG 012.

INTRODUCTION

Definition and time focus
AD is a chronic, irreversible neuronal degeneration of the central nervous system, leading to severe disorders of cognition in the absence of other neurologic manifestations. Senile plaques (conglomerations of protein) and neurofibrillary tangles (twisted nerve fibers) characterize the insidious, relentless progression of structural brain atrophy. This clinical plan focuses on the AD patient admitted at any stage of the disease.

Etiology and precipitating factors
Although the etiology is obscure, ongoing research suggests the following possible causes:
• neurochemical deficiency of the neurotransmitters acetylcholine and somatostatin (important for cognition and memory)
• neurometabolic disorder that diminishes cellular protein synthesis
• genetic and environmental factors, with autosomal-dominant transmission in certain families
• aluminum deposits in senile plaques and neurofibrillary tangles in the hippocampus of the brain, a cortical area necessary for memory
• slow viruses (those that invade the host but remain dormant for years before symptoms develop) whose effects sometimes resemble those of AD
• immune system dysfunctions.

FOCUSED ASSESSMENT GUIDELINES

Nursing history (functional health pattern findings)
Health perception–health management pattern
• Belief that memory loss results from normal aging
• Use of learned social skills and fabrication to disguise confusion and disorientation
• Family reports of patient's mental decline
Nutritional-metabolic pattern
• Anorexia (patient forgets to eat or does not recognize hunger signs)
• Weight loss
• Fatigue and malaise
• Dysphagia (in later stages)
Elimination pattern
• Constipation related to forgetfulness and disorientation
• Urinary and fecal incontinence in later stages
Activity-exercise pattern
• Limitation of activity to familiar environments as confusion and disorientation increase
• Growing inability to perform activities of daily living as patient loses ability to perform actions sequentially
• Deterioration in personal hygiene and appearance
• Incompetence in performing complex tasks, such as shopping, telephoning, and banking
• Personal safety jeopardized through wandering behavior or loss of locomotion
Sleep-rest pattern
• Nocturnal restlessness with insomnia
• Altered sleep-wake cycle
• Growing difficulty in awakening as the disease progresses
Cognitive-perceptual pattern
• Progressively impaired judgment
• Progressively impaired ability to orient self in the environment
• Loss of immediate, recent, and remote memory, including episodic (events) and semantic (knowledge) memory
• Incongruent, inconsistent, often depressed affect
• Progressively reduced conceptualization, attention, arousal, concentration, and abstract thinking
• Progressively impaired expressive language and increased receptive aphasia
• Repetitive actions or perseveration

Self-perception–self-concept pattern
• Attempt to sustain an internal center of control, dignity, and self-esteem
Role-relationship pattern
• Altered family dynamics resulting from role reversals and increased patient dysfunction
• Increased social withdrawal (isolationism)
Sexuality-reproductive pattern
• Rejection of intimate contact
Coping–stress tolerance pattern
• Defense mechanisms, such as rationalization, denial, and projection
• Apathy, depression, and helplessness
• Primary emotional lability, characterized by irritability, anger, fear, and agitation
• Symptoms of ego disintegration, including hallucinations, illusions, and suicidal ideation
Value-belief pattern
• Altered value system resulting from defective mental faculties

Physical findings
Neurologic
• Confusion
• Disorientation
• Memory loss
• Language disintegration
• Irritability
• Cognitive dysfunction
• Labile affect
• Clinical depression
Integumentary
• Poor skin turgor or other signs of dehydration
Musculoskeletal
• Decreased activity tolerance
• Lack of coordination
• Immobility
• Limited range of motion
Genitourinary
• Urine retention
• Urinary incontinence
Gastrointestinal
• Fecal incontinence

Diagnostic studies
Diagnostic tests are performed to rule out other diseases and allow the clinical diagnosis of AD, although postmortem brain biopsy is the only definitive diagnostic test.
• Hematologic measurements of neurotransmitters and neurotransmitter metabolites — low levels indicate a biochemical deficiency as the cause
• Complete blood count, Venereal Disease Research Laboratory test, blood chemistries, endocrine stud-

ies — performed for differential diagnosis of reversible cognitive impairment
• Vitamin B_{12} levels — low levels indicate a nutritional deficit
• Computed tomography scan — may indicate cortical atrophy and widening of the ventricles
• Lumbar puncture for cerebrospinal fluid examination — commonly shows abnormal protein levels
• Positron emission tomography — may reflect diminished brain metabolism
• Skull X-rays — may reflect cerebral atrophy
• Electroencephalography — may show decreased electrical activity contributing to dysfunction
• Magnetic resonance imaging — performed to rule out reversible cognitive impairment
• Language ability tests — performed for differential diagnosis
• Vision and hearing tests — establish sensory deficits (as opposed to cognitive impairment) as the cause of selected symptoms
• 12-lead electrocardiography — may indicate coronary insufficiency contributing to symptoms

Potential complications
• Total loss of mental faculties
• Pneumonia
• Injury

ALZHEIMER'S DISEASE

Major nursing diagnoses and collaborative problems	Key patient outcomes
Impaired cognitive function	Perform self-care as much as possible.
Nutritional deficit	Gain a predetermined number of pounds or maintain a stable weight.
Risk for injury	Avoid injury.
Constipation	Regularly eliminate soft, formed stools.
Risk for ineffective family coping	(The family is expected to) arrange a plan for care and mutual support.

COLLABORATIVE PROBLEM

Impaired cognitive function related to degenerative loss of cerebral tissue

Nursing priorities

• Provide a safe, structured environment.
• Promote an optimum level of functioning.
• Establish effective communication patterns.

Patient outcome criteria

Within 1 day of admission and then continuously, the patient will:
• remain free from injury
• perform self-care as much as possible
• communicate needs as clearly as possible
• wear some means of identification.

Interventions

1. Assess the patient's level of cognitive functioning, using a functional rating scale for symptoms of dementia or mini-mental status exam (see *Assessing Alzheimer's disease*). Prepare the patient for psychological testing.

2. Assign the patient to a room close to the nursing station for frequent observation.

3. Minimize hazards in the environment.

4. Maintain consistency in nursing routines.

Rationales

1. Information obtained from the patient and family provides a guide for planning care. Psychological testing will provide information necessary to structure a therapeutic regimen.

2. The patient may wander or require frequent attention.

3. The confusion and faulty judgment that result from AD make the patient more prone to injury.

4. Taking such measures as assigning the same nurse, serving meals on time, and scheduling rest periods provides the patient with structure in an unfamiliar environment.

Assessing Alzheimer's disease

Understanding how Alzheimer's disease progresses helps the nurse plan appropriate care and maximize the patient's functional ability. This chart summarizes the stages of disease progression.

Stage	Duration	Signs and symptoms	Nursing considerations
I	2 to 4 years	• "Fishing" for words • Forgetfulness progressing to inability to recall details of recent events • Irritability or apathy • Occasional episodes of getting lost • Periods of disorientation • Significantly impaired reasoning ability and judgment	• The patient typically can manage most daily activities and does not require institutionalization. • The patient senses a decrease in mental faculties and may use denial to cope with this. Do not force the patient to "face the facts."
II	2 to 12 years	• Reduced vision, hearing, and pain sensation • Hyperorality (chewing or tasting anything within reach) • Inability to recognize familiar things (may not recognize own mirror reflection) • Increased aphasia (language defect) • Increased appetite without weight gain • Perseveration (repeating the same word or action over and over) • Seizures • Social inappropriateness, such as poor table manners, personal hygiene, and grooming	• Assist the patient with hygiene and grooming to preserve self-esteem and dignity. • Avoid using puns or jokes because these will confuse the patient. • Call the patient by name, rather than "Honey," "Grandma," or another belittling term. • If the patient has trouble walking, accompany him on walks several times a day to prevent muscle contractures and other complications of immobility. • Maintain a consistent, calm environment to orient the patient. • Make sure the patient wanders only in safe areas. • Monitor the items the patient places in his mouth. • Maintain the patient on a toileting schedule to minimize incontinence. • Stay with the patient during meals to observe for swallowing problems and assist with table manners.
III	1 year	• Apraxia (inability to perform purposeful movements, even on command) • Bladder and bowel incontinence • Decreased appetite • Disappearance of perseveration and hyperorality • Generalized tonic-clonic seizures • Muteness • Unresponsiveness to verbal and physical stimuli	• Maintain a consistent routine. • Monitor the patient's skin for breakdown and pressure ulcers. • Monitor all body systems carefully for physiologic deterioration. • Perform passive range-of-motion exercises at least four times a day to prevent contractures, if the patient is bedridden.

From R. Charles, et al. "Alzheimer's Disease: Pathology, Progression, and Nursing Process," *Journal of Gerontological Nursing* 8(2):69-73, 1982. Adapted with permission of the publisher.

Neurologic disorders

5. Promote self-care within the scope of the patient's abilities; assist when necessary. Identify specific needs in the plan of care.

5. Allowing the patient to provide self-care preserves self-esteem. As the disease progresses, complete physical care — bathing, dressing, and toileting — becomes necessary. Identifying needs in the plan of care promotes appropriate care.

6. Establish and maintain a therapeutic relationship by dealing with the patient in a calm, reassuring, affirming, and nonthreatening manner.

6. Trust must be established to achieve any goal because of the patient's suspicions and increasing paranoia.

7. Capture and retain the patient's attention by giving simple, specific directions for accomplishing tasks; use eye contact and unobtrusive guidance.

7. The effects of memory loss and a reduced attention span can be minimized with clear directions and appropriate guidance.

8. Orient the patient to reality frequently and repetitively.

8. Although repetitive reorientation may not reduce disorientation, it may reduce the patient's anxiety.

9. Administer and document medications, as ordered.

9. Aricept (donepezil hydrochloride) for improving memory and bethanechol (Urecholine) for increasing neurotransmission may be used. Antianxiety drugs may be helpful. Other drugs may include ergoloid mesylates (Hydergine) or lecithin for cognition and memory; doxepin (Sinequan), nortriptyline (Pamelor), or amitryptyline (Elavil) as antidepressants; and temazepam (Restoril) or a similar drug for sleep maintenance.

10. Use aids to improve language skills and verbal repetition and pictures to improve recall.

10. Both methods may assist the patient with word recall.

11. Minimize communication barriers. Be aware that anxiety, cultural influences, spiritual beliefs, and language difficulties may contribute to paranoia and withdrawal.

11. Knowing and understanding the patient's cultural background and beliefs can further open communication.

12. Encourage social interaction with others by including the patient in unit activities when possible, allowing maximum flexibility in visiting hours, and providing occupational therapy referral.

12. Continued social interaction reinforces reality and contributes to a sense of self-worth and identity.

13. Prevent excessive stimulation and promote a regular sleep-wake pattern.

13. Moderate stimulation helps orient the patient, but excessive stimulation and sleep deprivation contribute to confusion.

14. Be attentive, and keep your verbal and nonverbal responses to the patient consistent.

14. Nurse-patient dialogue must reflect trust and understanding. Consistent verbal and nonverbal responses reduce cognitive dissonance.

15. When talking with the patient, encourage reminiscences.

15. Remembering past events helps the patient maintain self-identity. Distant memory may remain even when recent memory is impaired.

16. Prepare an identity card, a bracelet, or a name tag for the patient. Include name, address, phone number, medical problem, and other pertinent information.

16. Should the patient wander, identification information can help in the patient's prompt return.

17. Additional individualized interventions: _____

17. Rationales: _____

NURSING DIAGNOSIS

Nutritional deficit related to memory loss and inadequate food intake

Nursing priority

Stabilize and improve nutritional status.

Patient outcome criterion

By discharge, the patient will gain a predetermined number of pounds or maintain a stable weight.

Interventions

1. Assess present nutritional status: Weigh the patient and record customary dietary intake on admission. See the "Nutritional deficit" plan, page 80, and the "Total parenteral nutrition" plan, page 527, for more information on nutritional assessment.

2. Offer a balanced diet consisting of small meals at regular intervals and nutritious snacks between meals. Provide finger foods when possible.

3. Prepare the tray in advance — cut the meat, provide a spoon, open containers, and so forth — with appropriate portions of food arranged so that the patient may eat unassisted.

4. Provide time and privacy for meals.

5. Monitor and record daily weight and intake, including the amount and type of food. Adjust the dietary plan accordingly.

6. Provide dietary information to the home caregiver.

7. Additional individualized interventions: _____
_____

Rationales

1. Assessing the patient's nutritional status provides necessary information for determining actual deficits; an appropriate dietary regimen may then begin.

2. Regularly scheduled meals help maintain a structured environment. Small quantities may appeal to the patient and provide a sense of achievement when all the food is consumed. Finger foods are easier to handle than food that must be eaten with a utensil.

3. Coordination difficulties may develop, impairing use of utensils. Preparing food servings in advance decreases frustration and avoids the humiliation of being unable to provide self-care.

4. The patient who has difficulty chewing or swallowing will need more time to eat. Lack of coordination may result in socially unacceptable eating habits.

5. Evaluating weight and intake provides guidelines for modifying the dietary plan.

6. The patient will probably continue to need assistance in menu selection, cooking, and eating after discharge. The person shopping, cooking, and offering meals to the patient may need instruction in the patient's specific dietary needs.

7. Rationales: _____
_____

NURSING DIAGNOSIS

Risk for injury related to wandering behavior, aphasia, agnosia, or hyperorality

Nursing priority

Prevent injury while maximizing independence.

Patient outcome criteria

- Throughout the hospital stay, the patient will:
  - be appropriately dressed for the temperature
  - walk about only when attended
  - perform daily exercise to best of ability
  - avoid injury.
- By the time of the patient's discharge, the family will list five safety measures for the home environment.

Interventions

1. Consider putting a bell on the patient to alert caregivers to wandering.

Rationales

1. Wandering and restlessness characterize later stages of AD. If unattended, the patient may become lost, even in familiar surroundings.

2. Ensure that the patient is dressed appropriately for the temperature. Provide shoes that fit well.

2. The patient may not make appropriate choices about dress and may have a reduced ability to identify or verbalize discomfort. Loose shoes may be lost or contribute to injuries from falls.

3. Avoid using restraints.

3. Restraints increase the patient's agitation and paranoia and may contribute to injury.

4. Recommend specific safety measures to the family to prepare for home care, including:
• safely storing knives, medications, matches, firearms, and cleaning solutions and other toxic household chemicals
• using night-lights

• storing small objects safely

• securing door locks
• making sure objects remain in the same place

• explaining the patient's condition to neighbors.

4. An unprepared home environment may contribute to injuries.
• The patient may not recognize familiar objects (agnosia) and thus may inadvertently injure himself or others.
• Night-lights may decrease the risk of falling and help reorient the patient to the environment.
• AD patients may be prone to hyperorality (chewing or tasting anything within reach) and may put small objects in their mouths, swallowing or choking on them.
• Door locks may help prevent wandering.
• Consistency may help reorient the patient to the environment.
• If neighbors are aware of the patient's illness, they can alert the family if they see the patient wandering or engaging in unsafe behaviors.

5. Encourage a regular exercise program, as tolerated.

5. Regular exercise decreases restlessness and agitation, promotes muscle tone, and contributes to a sense of well-being. Overactivity, however, may contribute to fatigue and confusion.

6. Watch for nonverbal cues to injury, such as grimacing, rubbing, panting, or protecting an injured area, and note repetitive use of words or seemingly inappropriate statements. Alert the family to cues observed.

6. The patient may be unable to identify or express discomfort but may reveal illness or injury through nonverbal cues. Because aphasia may make expressions of discomfort convoluted, such words as *cold* or *hurt,* especially if repeated, may warrant investigation.

7. Additional individualized interventions: _____

7. Rationales: _____

Nursing diagnosis

Constipation related to memory loss about toileting behaviors and to inadequate diet

Nursing priority

Establish an effective elimination pattern.

Patient outcome criteria

Within 2 days of admission, the patient will:
• demonstrate knowledge of bathroom location
• regularly eliminate soft, formed stools.

Interventions

1. Identify the bathroom clearly—symbols or color codes may be helpful.

Rationales

1. An AD patient may develop constipation because of forgetting the location of the bathroom.

2. Prompt the patient, at regular intervals, to use the toilet. With an incontinent patient, use standard precautions.

3. Encourage a therapeutic diet with ample fluid and fiber intake during waking hours.

4. Observe the patient for nonverbal clues that signal the need for elimination.

5. Administer and document use of elimination aids (stool softener, laxative, or cathartic), as ordered.

6. Monitor and document the frequency of elimination.

7. Additional individualized interventions: _____
_____

2. When memory fails, the patient may neglect toileting. Reminders, with assistance at regular intervals, promote a regular elimination pattern and help prevent accidents.

3. Proper diet promotes effective elimination. Ample fluids and fiber help prevent constipation.

4. The patient may become restless, pick at clothing, or clutch the genitals but may be unable to verbalize the need to eliminate.

5. Such aids may help promote regular elimination.

6. Noting the frequency of elimination helps identify a regular bowel pattern and minimizes problems.

7. Rationales: _____
_____

NURSING DIAGNOSIS

Risk for ineffective family coping related to progressive mental deterioration of the patient with AD

Nursing priority

Aid in developing necessary role transitions while maintaining family integrity.

Patient outcome criteria

- Throughout the hospital stay, the family will be involved in teaching and providing care.
- By the time of the patient's discharge, the family will:
  - arrange a plan for care and mutual support
  - identify community support resources.

Interventions

1. Involve the family in all teaching. Use teaching as an opportunity to assess family roles, resources, and coping behaviors. See the "Ineffective family coping: Compromised" plan, page 63.

2. Offer support, understanding, and reassurance to the family. Support efforts to provide care for the patient in the home setting. Encourage family members to give each other "vacations" from providing care.

Rationales

1. Because AD patients require long-term care, the family must be taught how to cope effectively with this chronic, progressive disease. If the patient develops a childlike dependence after holding a strong provider role, others must assume new roles to maintain family stability. Assessment of family status provides a baseline for determining the best approach and needed interventions. The "Ineffective family coping: Compromised" plan contains additional information.

2. In many cases, caring for the AD patient is a frustrating and thankless task, involving endless repetition and, commonly, emotional confrontations that may leave family members drained. However, maintaining a stable home environment with familiar caregivers helps give the patient a sense of worth, reduces isolation, and may minimize disorientation. Frequent breaks from caregiving help increase family cohesiveness and prevent burnout.

Neurologic disorders

3. Involve a social worker or discharge planner in decisions regarding home care or nursing home placement. If appropriate, encourage family members to express their feelings about the decision to place the patient in a nursing home.

4. Provide information about community resources, such as home care, financial and legal assistance, and an Alzheimer's support group. Encourage use of all available resources.

5. Additional individualized interventions: _____
_____

3. Patient needs may become unmanageable at home. The social worker or discharge planner may offer special expertise in answering questions about long-term care. Family members may feel guilt, relief, anguish, or other conflicting emotions and will need support if this decision becomes necessary.

4. Community support may help lessen the family's burden and promote healthy adaptations to change. The AD patient is likely to appear in the emergency department when the family becomes overwhelmed. A social service referral may decrease such inappropriate use of resources and help avert family crises.

5. Rationales: _____
_____

Discharge planning

Discharge checklist
(See also discharge checklist for primary diagnosis if other than AD.) Before discharge, the patient shows evidence of:
❑ vital signs stable and within normal limits for this patient
❑ adequate nutritional intake
❑ regular bowel and bladder elimination
❑ adequate home support system or referral to home care or a nursing home if indicated.

Teaching checklist
Document evidence that the family demonstrates an understanding of:
❑ the diagnosis and disease process — for example, through literature from the Alzheimer's Association (70 East Lake Street, Suite 700, Chicago, IL 60601)
❑ plans for adequate supervision and behavior management
❑ recommended steps for minimizing environmental hazards
❑ instructions for promoting self-care independence
❑ recommended procedures for reorienting the patient to the home environment
❑ the need for an identification bracelet or other medical alert device
❑ the purpose, dosage, administration schedule, and adverse effects of prescribed medications
❑ techniques for continued improvement of language skills
❑ recommendations for meeting nutrition and elimination needs
❑ available community resources
❑ the need for restoring family equilibrium as roles change and patient dependence increases
❑ the probability of total patient regression
❑ how to contact the doctor.

Documentation checklist
Using outcome criteria as a guide, document:
❑ the patient's clinical status on admission, including level of cognitive function
❑ planned approach to maintain patient safety, security, and orientation
❑ laboratory data and diagnostic findings
❑ any change in the patient's behavioral response
❑ the patient's level of communication and social interaction
❑ the patient's dietary intake and elimination patterns
❑ patient and family teaching
❑ discharge planning.

Associated plans of care

Geriatric care
Grieving
Ineffective family coping: Compromised
Ineffective individual coping
Knowledge deficit

References

Costa, P.T. Jr., et al. "Recognition and Initial Assessment of Alzheimer's Disease and Related Dementias," *Clinical Practice Guidelines*, 19. Rockville, Md.: U.S. Department of Health and Human Services, Public Health Service, Agency for Health Care Policy and Research, 1996.

Crigger, N., and Forbes, W. "Assessing Neurologic Function in Older Patients," *AJN* 97(3):37-40, March 1997.

Handbook of Medical-Surgical Nursing, 2nd ed. Springhouse, Pa.: Springhouse Corp., 1998.

Hickey, J. *The Clinical Practice of Neurological and Neurosurgical Nursing*, 4th ed. Philadelphia: Lippincott-Raven Pubs., 1997.

Rakel, R. *Conn's Current Therapy*. Philadelphia: W.B. Saunders Co., 1997.

Stewart Amidei, C. "Horizons: Prevention of Alzheimer's Disease, Depression and Alzheimer's Disease," *Journal of Neuroscience Nursing* 28(2):128, April 1996.

Cerebrovascular accident

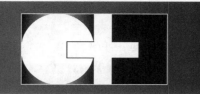

DRG information

DRG 014   Specific Cerebrovascular Disorders. Except
transient ischemic attack.
Mean LOS = 7.5 days
Principal diagnoses include:
- cerebral aneurysm
- aphasia
- nontraumatic intracerebral hemorrhage
- nontraumatic intracranial hemorrhage
- nontraumatic subarachnoid hemorrhage
- occlusion of cerebral arteries.

INTRODUCTION

Definition and time focus

A cerebrovascular accident (CVA), commonly called a
stroke or, more recently, a brain attack, can take the
form of any of several pathophysiologic events that disrupt cerebral circulation. The cells at the site of the resulting infarction then release chemicals that cause further damage and compromise blood flow, resulting in ischemia in the surrounding area. If the ischemic damage
continues, these cells also may die, worsening the patient's cognitive and functional deficits.

The most common causes of CVA include thrombosis,
embolism, and hemorrhage. Rarely, CVA may stem from
arterial spasm or compression of cerebral blood vessels
that results from tumor growth or another cause. The
consistent factor in all CVAs, regardless of the cause, is
brain injury resulting from disrupted blood circulation.

Deficits resulting from CVA may be temporary or permanent, depending on the portion of the brain and the
vessels involved, the extent of injury, the patient's preexisting physical and emotional health, and the presence of
other diseases or injuries.

This clinical plan focuses on the care of the noncritical
patient who is admitted to a medical-surgical unit for diagnosis and nonsurgical treatment of a CVA. Surgical interventions for CVA — such as carotid endarterectomy,
extracranial-intracranial bypass, and craniotomy — are
not discussed in this plan. For a sample clinical pathway,
see *Nonhemorrhagic stroke,* pages 128 to 130.

Etiology and precipitating factors

- Factors that cause occlusion of blood supply to cerebral tissue
  - Cerebral thrombosis, such as from atherosclerosis,
  inflammation from infection or other disease, mechanical constriction (for instance, from increased

intracranial pressure), prolonged vasoconstriction,
systemic hypotension, and hematologic disorders
that increase clotting tendencies
  - Cerebral embolism, such as from cardiac disease,
  plaques or clots from elsewhere in the circulatory
  system, substances (such as air, fat, or tumor parti -
  cles) that enter the bloodstream, and clotting disorders
- Factors that contribute to intracerebral bleeding
  - Hemorrhage, hypertension, ruptured aneurysm,
  trauma, ruptured arteriovenous malformations,
  bleeding from the growth of a tumor, bleeding associated with a disease (for example, leukemia, anemia, sickle cell disease, and hemophilia), anticoagulant therapy, and edema
- Factors causing cerebral ischemia
  - Arterial spasm, systemic hypoxemia, and compression of cerebral blood vessels
- Factors that increase an individual's risk of CVA
  - Hypertension, heart disease, smoking, diabetes, hypercholesterolemia, use of oral contraceptives, obesity, a family history of CVA, and congenital anomalies

FOCUSED ASSESSMENT GUIDELINES

Nursing history (functional health pattern findings)

Health perception–health management pattern
- Symptoms that may have developed over several days
(thrombosis), minutes to hours (hemorrhage), or just a
few minutes (embolus)
- Recent episodes of sudden weakness, vertigo, numbness or tingling in face or limbs, or speech or vision disturbances that resolved within 24 hours (transient ischemic attacks [TIAs]) or took longer than 24 hours to
resolve but left little or no deficit (reversible ischemic
neurologic deficits)
- Use of oral contraceptives
- Treatment for hypertension, heart disease, diabetes, or
other chronic condition
- Noncompliance with antihypertensive regimen or failure to see a doctor for many years
- History of smoking for many years

Nutritional-metabolic pattern
- Difficulty swallowing
- Nausea and vomiting (usually associated with hemorrhage)

Elimination pattern
- Urinary or fecal incontinence

Activity-exercise pattern
- Inability to move one side of body (hemiplegia)

(Text continues on page 130.)

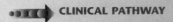

CLINICAL PATHWAY

Nonhemorrhagic stroke

DRG: 014 and 015
Estimated length of stay (LOS):
3 to 6 days

Plan	ED	Day 1
Laboratory studies	• Complete blood count (CBC) • Prothrombin time (PT)/partial thromboplastin time (PTT) • Blood chemistry studies	• PT/PTT every day if on anticoagulants • If lacunar infarct, sequential multiple analyzer with computer or Venereal Disease Research Laboratory test • Magnesium
Tests	• Computed tomography (CT) scan of brain • Chest X-ray • Electrocardiography • Telemetry, if indicated • Pulse oximetry	• Order CT scan for 48 hours after first CT scan if anterior, middle, or posterior cerebral artery stroke • Carotid duplex scan • Intensive care unit (ICU), if meets criteria, based on test results and assessment findings • Telemetry • 2-dimensional echocardiogram, if ordered • Magnetic resonance imaging (MRI) if lacunar or brain stem stroke suspected
Consultations		Consult if indicated: • Neurology • Dietitian • Social worker • Swallowing team • Rehabilitation: physical therapist (PT), occupational therapist (OT), speech therapist • Pastoral care • Psychiatric
Medications/I.V.	• I.V. • Aspirin	• Aspirin or anticoagulants • Stool softeners or laxatives • I.V. normal saline lock • Heparin S.C., I.V.
Treatments		
Nutrition		• Nothing by mouth until cleared by swallowing team or doctor • Diet consistent with diagnosis or condition
Elimination		• Assess normal pattern
Activity	• Head of bed > 20°	• Head of bed > 20° • High accident risk evaluation
Patient teaching		• Telemetry • ICU or critical care unit orientation • Diagnostic testing • Stroke teaching materials • Stroke educator consulted
Discharge planning		• Evaluate support systems and discharge needs

Day 2	Day 3
	• CBC • Blood chemistry studies
• Stop telemetry or discharge from ICU if stable	• CT scan/MRI repeat (48 hours after admission if anterior, middle, or posterior cerebral artery stroke)
• Rehabilitation unit • Functional independence measure score per rehabilitation	• Dietitian (if intake by mouth is < 75% daily caloric requirements), if no previous consult
• Diet recommendations followed • Calorie count if intake by mouth is < 75% daily caloric requirement	
	• Administer laxatives, if pattern is abnormal
• Appropriate bed positioning • Activities of daily living per PT or OT recommendation	• Progressive plan outlined by PT or OT

• Physical therapy education
• Occupational therapy education
• Speech therapy education (if needed)
For stroke patient, teaching materials include:
• Stroke effects
• "Why Am I So Emotional?" (American Heart Association [AHA] handout)
• "Why Am I So Depressed?" (AHA handout)
• Resource list
	• Diet
	• Swallowing team, if involved
	• Teaching materials (AHA handouts):
	  – "How Can I Reduce My Risk of Stroke?"
	  – "How Can I Reduce High Blood Pressure?"
	  – "Are There Complications from a Stroke?"
	• Smoking cessation information

• Complete assessment • Continue to evaluate for discharge needs	• Rehabilitation unit evaluation by PT, OT, speech therapist • Discharge to home if transient ischemic attack

(continued)

Neurologic disorders

Nonhemorrhagic stroke *(continued)*

Plan	Day 4	Day 5	Day 6	Goals met
Laboratory studies				• Laboratory values return to baseline
Tests				• No further progression of stroke
Consultations	• Dietitian (if intake by mouth is < 75% daily caloric requirements), if no previous consult			
Medications/ I.V.	• Discharge normal saline lock, I.V.			• Tolerating medications
Treatments				• Plan arranged for continued therapy in an appropriate setting
Nutrition	• Institute enteral feedings per dietitian • Determine that calorie and protein intake adequate	• Institute enteral feedings per dietitian • Determine that calorie and protein intake adequate	• Institute enteral feedings per dietitian • Determine that calorie and protein intake adequate	• Food and fluid intake meets caloric and protein needs
Elimination	• Administer laxatives, if pattern is abnormal	• Administer laxatives, if pattern is abnormal	• Administer laxatives, if pattern is abnormal	• Within normal limits
Activity	• Progressive plan has been outlined per PT/OT			• Plan safely addresses current functional status
Patient teaching	• Nutrition or drug instructions • Medications • AHA teaching handouts: – "Can I Live At Home After My Stroke?" – "What Is Stroke Rehabilitation?"	• Review teaching materials with patient and family		• Patient and family verbalize: – Medications (name, dosage, adverse effects, purpose, schedule, nutrient and drug interactions) – Signs and symptoms of complications – Appropriate diet
Discharge planning	• Discharge to home, rehabilitation unit, or extended care facility as appropriate for condition (lacunar infarct) • Home care intervention considered if outcome goals not met	• Discharge plan in place, referrals made	• Discharge to home, rehabilitation unit, or extended care facility as appropriate for condition (anterior, middle, or posterior cerebral artery stroke) • Make referrals if discharged to home and outcome goals not met	• Ensure follow-up plan is in place • Plan continued medical management, if discharged to rehabilitation unit

• Fear of falling
• Syncope
Cognitive-perceptual pattern
• Inability to understand explanations of what has happened or to respond to questions
• Dizziness, drowsiness, headache, burning or aching in extremities, and stiff neck

• Slowed thinking, clumsiness
Sleep-rest pattern
• Symptoms (most commonly from thrombosis) that develop during sleep or shortly after awakening
Self-perception–self-concept pattern
• Lack of awareness of affected side of body

Role-relationship pattern
• Emotional lability, behavioral changes, or altered speech or thinking abilities

Physical findings
Physical findings may or may not be present, depending on the site of the CVA.

General appearance
• Facial droop
• Lateralized weakness or flaccidity on side opposite brain lesion

Cardiovascular
• Hypertension
• Hypotension

Pulmonary
• Either increased or decreased respirations

Neurologic
• Seizures
• Altered level of consciousness
• Nuchal rigidity
• Memory impairment
• Confusion
• Retinal hemorrhage
• Hemianesthesia
• Hemianopia (visual field deficit in one or both eyes)
• Apraxia (inability to perform purposeful acts)
• Receptive aphasia (inability to understand words) or expressive aphasia (inability to say words)
• Agnosia (inability to recognize familiar objects)
• Disorientation
• Unequal pupil size
• Diplopia
• Disconjugate gaze
• Dysphagia
• Dysarthria (lack of muscle control to form words)
• Sensory deficits

Integumentary
• Flushing
• Pallor

Musculoskeletal
• Flaccidity
• Paralysis

Diagnostic studies
Initially, the need for specific diagnostic studies depends on whether the CVA stems from a hemorrhagic or a non-hemorrhagic cause (treatment is significantly different for each). Laboratory data may show no significant abnormalities unless other conditions are present.
• Complete blood count — performed to establish a baseline; may reveal blood loss if CVA was caused by significant hemorrhage
• Chemistry panel — performed to establish a baseline; assesses renal function and electrolyte levels (these may be significant in a patient requiring fluid restriction); rules out hypoglycemia and hyperglycemia as contributors to the altered mental state
• Prothrombin time/international normalized ratio (PT/INR) and partial thromboplastin time — performed to establish a baseline because the patient with a CVA caused by occlusion may need anticoagulants (INR expresses PT as a ratio to provide consistency for comparison from one laboratory to another)
• Urinalysis — rules out preexisting urinary tract infection (important because the patient is typically catheterized)
• Computed tomography (CT) scan of the head — differentiates infarction from hemorrhage and reveals extent of bleeding and brain compression (if present); may take several days for infarct to become visible
• Cerebral angiography — shows cerebral blood vessels and reveals site of bleeding or blockage
• Positron emission tomography scan — computer interpretation of gamma ray emissions provides information on cerebral blood flow, volume, and metabolism
• Brain scan — cerebral infarction indicated by areas of radioisotope uptake; may not become positive for up to 2 weeks after a CVA
• Electroencephalography (EEG) — reveals areas of abnormal brain activity and may help in diagnosing; however, a normal EEG does not rule out a pathologic condition
• Lumbar puncture — bloody cerebrospinal fluid may indicate intracerebral hemorrhage; used in fewer cases since CT scan became available
• Skull and cervical spine X-rays — rule out fractures, especially if the patient suffered a fall with the CVA
• Doppler ultrasonography — identifies abnormalities in blood flow in carotid, vertebral, basilar, and intracerebral arteries

Potential complications
• Brain stem failure and cardiopulmonary arrest
• Brain compression
• Brain infarction
• Brain abscess
• Encephalitis
• Pulmonary embolism
• Arrhythmias
• Heart failure
• Thrombophlebitis
• Pneumonia
• Dysfunctional limb contractures
• Pressure ulcers
• Malnutrition

Neurologic disorders

CLINICAL SNAPSHOT

CEREBROVASCULAR ACCIDENT

Major nursing diagnoses and collaborative problems	Key patient outcomes
Risk for ineffective airway clearance	Maintain a clear airway.
Risk for further cerebral injury	Show stable or improving neurologic signs.
Impaired physical mobility	Perform as much self-care as possible.
Risk for sensory-perceptual alteration	Demonstrate use of techniques to compensate for sensory loss.
Risk for impaired verbal communication	Establish some form of verbal or nonverbal communication.
Risk for knowledge deficit (CVA management)	Express understanding of the disease and the therapeutic regimen (patient and family).

NURSING DIAGNOSIS

Risk for ineffective airway clearance related to hemiplegic effects of a CVA

Nursing priorities
• Maintain a patent airway.
• Prevent pulmonary complications.

Patient outcome criteria

Throughout the hospital stay, the patient will:
• maintain a clear airway
• cough and perform deep-breathing exercises every 2 hours while awake
• have clear breath sounds or prompt identification and treatment of pulmonary problems
• take food and fluids (as ordered) without aspirating or choking.

Interventions

1. Position the patient with head turned to the side, supporting the trunk with pillows as needed. Elevate the head of the bed slightly. Never leave the patient supine while unattended. Provide a call button within easy reach of the unaffected arm, or provide alternative means of signaling for help, as needed.

2. If hemiplegia is present, position the patient on the affected side for shorter periods (less than 1 hour) than on the unaffected side (2 hours). Avoid positioning a patient's affected arm over the abdomen.

Rationales

1. Hemiplegia, impaired cough reflex, or dysphagia may render the patient unable to clear the airway. If left supine while unattended, the patient may aspirate; the supine position also increases the risk of airway obstruction from the tongue, especially if the patient is anesthetized. Providing the means to call for help is essential when the airway may become compromised.

2. Lying on the affected side may cause pooling of secretions, which are ineffectively cleared because of hemiplegia. The weight of an arm over the abdomen may further reduce the adequacy of thoracic expansion.

3. Encourage coughing (except in the patient with a hemorrhagic CVA) and deep breathing every 2 hours while the patient is awake. Set up equipment for oral suctioning, and suction accumulated secretions as necessary.

4. Assess breath sounds at least every 4 hours while the patient is awake. Also note the adequacy of respiratory effort, the rate and characteristics of respirations, and skin color. Investigate restlessness promptly, especially in the aphasic patient. Report any abnormalities.

5. Allow nothing by mouth until the patient's ability to swallow is evaluated. If the patient can swallow with minimum difficulty, assist with or observe the patient's eating, as needed. Place small bites of food in the unaffected side of the mouth. (Semisolid foods are usually handled better than thin liquids.)

6. Additional individualized interventions: _____

3. Accumulated secretions may obstruct the airway or predispose the patient to atelectasis or pneumonia. (Respiratory infection is one of the primary causes of death for CVA patients.) Coughing should be avoided in hemorrhagic CVA to prevent increasing intracranial pressure, which can cause further bleeding.

4. Many CVA patients have preexisting hypertension or heart disease, which may predispose them to heart failure. Abnormal breath sounds (crackles, gurgles) may be the first indicators of complications related to hypoventilation. Increased respiratory effort, tachypnea, ashen or cyanotic color, or restlessness may indicate hypoxemia. Early detection and reporting lead to prompt treatment.

5. Hemiplegia and associated dysphagia predispose the patient to aspiration. The patient may be better able to swallow if food is placed on the unaffected side. Small bites and thicker liquids decrease the risk of choking from aspiration.

6. Rationales: _____

COLLABORATIVE PROBLEM

Risk for further cerebral injury related to interrupted blood flow (embolus, thrombus, or hemorrhage)

Nursing priority

Improve cerebral tissue perfusion.

Patient outcome criteria

- Within 2 days of admission, the patient will:
  - show no further decrease in level of consciousness
  - show stable or improving neurologic signs.
- Throughout the hospital stay, the patient will:
  - maintain fluid balance
  - maintain electrolyte levels within normal limits.

Interventions

1. Assess neurologic status, checking level of consciousness, orientation, grip strength, leg strength, pupillary response, and vital signs every hour until neurologic status is stable; repeat assessment at least every 4 hours thereafter. Promptly report any abnormalities or changes, especially decreasing alertness, progressing weakness, restlessness, unequal pupil size, widening pulse pressure, flexor or extensor posturing, seizures, severe headache, vertigo, syncope, or epistaxis.

Rationales

1. When blood flow to and oxygenation of the brain is decreased, cerebral vasodilation and edema occur as the body attempts to compensate for the deficiency. Increasing cerebral edema causes increased intracranial pressure and may result in death if not treated promptly. Hemorrhage into enclosed intracranial spaces may also increase pressure. A decline in neurologic signs indicates progressive injury.

Neurologic disorders

2. Elevate the head of the bed slightly and provide supplemental oxygen as ordered.

3. Manage an occlusive CVA as follows:
• Administer anticoagulants, as ordered. Monitor appropriate laboratory findings (PT/INR or activated partial thromboplastin time [APTT]), and check current results before giving each dose. Observe carefully for (and advise the patient or family to report) melena, petechiae, epistaxis, hematuria, ecchymosis, oozing from wounds, or unusual bleeding. Observe for and report signs of intracranial bleeding (headache, irritability, weakness, decreased level of consciousness, or nuchal rigidity).

• Administer antiplatelet aggregation medications, as ordered. Observe for gastric irritation.

• Administer medications to control blood pressure, as ordered. Be alert for and immediately report signs of decreased cerebral perfusion. Check blood pressure at least every 4 hours while the patient is awake.

4. Manage a hemorrhagic CVA as follows:
• Maintain the patient on complete bed rest for the first 24 hours to 1 week, as ordered. Minimize stress and external stimulation as much as possible. Administer stool softeners or laxatives, as ordered.
• Administer medications to control blood pressure, as ordered. Be alert for signs of neurologic deterioration and immediately report any that occur.
• Monitor the patient to maintain optimal fluid status, observing fluid restrictions as ordered. Administer osmotic diuretics such as mannitol, as ordered. Monitor intake and output carefully.

2. Elevating the head of the bed helps minimize cerebral edema, which can contribute to increased ischemia. The brain uses 20% of the oxygen normally available to the body. When a CVA causes cerebral ischemia, supplemental oxygen may help prevent brain tissue death.

3. An occlusive CVA requires proper management:
• Use of anticoagulants, although still somewhat controversial, can inhibit stroke progression and possibly reduce the number of thromboembolic events. Heparin inactivates thrombin, thus preventing fibrin clots. Therapeutic APTT should be 1 to 1½ times the laboratory's normal value. Warfarin (Coumadin) interferes with vitamin K production, thus decreasing synthesis of several clotting factors. Therapeutic PT should be 1½ to 2½ times normal value. INR ranges vary depending on the reason for use. For all conditions that require anticoagulation therapy (except mechanical heart valve use or acute myocardial infarction), the recommended range is 2 to 3. Anticoagulants predispose the patient to systemic bleeding and may also cause intracranial bleeding.
• Drugs such as aspirin and ticlopidine (Ticlid) inhibit platelet aggregation and thus reduce the risk of embolus formation. Adverse effects include GI upset and bleeding, so these drugs may not be used if the patient has preexisting GI problems.
• Right after a CVA, the brain is in a hypermetabolic state and requires more blood flow to maintain perfusion, so blood pressure is allowed to run higher than normal. However, severe hypertension (systolic pressure greater than 200 mm Hg and diastolic pressure greater than 110 mm Hg) sustained over 30 to 60 minutes is treated because it may decrease perfusion to other organs and increase the risk of cerebral hemorrhage. Blood pressure should be brought down slowly because a sudden drop in cerebral blood flow may cause cerebral vasoconstriction, resulting in further ischemia.

4. A hemorrhagic CVA requires proper management:
• Minimizing activity and stimulation helps decrease the risk of further intracerebral hemorrhage. Stool softeners or laxatives prevent straining at stool, which can cause bleeding.
• Patients with hemorrhagic CVA commonly have significant vasospasm; a systolic blood pressure greater than 160 mm Hg may increase the risk of rebleeding.
• Fluid overload may cause fatal increases in intracranial pressure or recurrent hemorrhage. Osmotic diuretics reduce cerebral edema by drawing fluid into the intravascular space and stimulating diuresis. They also reduce the volume of circulating cerebrospinal fluid. Patients with other preexisting conditions, such as cardiac or renal disease, may not tolerate the temporary intravascular volume increase. Careful patient monitoring, including an accurate fluid intake and output record, helps prevent such complications.

5. Additional individualized interventions: _____ | **5.** Rationales: _____

NURSING DIAGNOSIS

Impaired physical mobility related to damage to motor cortex or motor pathways

Nursing priority

Minimize effects of immobility and prevent associated complications.

Patient outcome criteria

- Within 24 hours of admission, the patient will:
  - begin passive range-of-motion exercises
  - have clean and dry skin
  - have a patent urinary catheter or use a bedpan every 2 hours while awake with minimal incontinence.
- Throughout the hospital stay, the patient will:
  - maintain functional alignment
  - perform as much self-care as possible
  - maintain intact skin
  - maintain adequate bowel and bladder elimination, with no signs of infection
  - show no thromboembolic complications.

Interventions

1. Maintain functional alignment in positioning the patient at rest, using a footboard, handroll, or trochanter roll as necessary. Support the affected arm when the patient is out of bed.

2. Provide passive (and active, if appropriate) range-of-motion exercise to all extremities at least four times a day, beginning at admission. Increase activity levels as permitted and tolerated, depending on the cause of the CVA. Collaborate with the physical therapist to plan a rehabilitation schedule with the patient and family.

3. When permitted, encourage the patient to perform as much self-care as possible.

4. Provide antiembolism stockings, as ordered. Assess the patient for signs of thromboembolic complications. Report immediately any chest pain, shortness of breath, calf pain, or redness or swelling in an extremity.

Rationales

1. A functional position prevents contractures and deformities that can further complicate recovery and can help reduce intracranial pressure. The weight of an unsupported arm may cause shoulder dislocation, joint inflammation, or both.

2. Even passive exercise helps maintain muscle tone and establish new impulse pathways and neuron regeneration. Adjacent brain cells may take up the function of damaged cells, new nerve cell fibers may develop collaterally, or alternative nerve pathways may take over. Learning and repetition appear to be key factors in the development of new neuronal connections. Establishing a schedule helps the patient set goals, maintain a sense of control, and measure progress.

3. Independence in self-care helps maintain self-respect and may improve motivation to increase mobility.

4. Antiembolism stockings promote venous return, thus decreasing the risk of thrombus formation from immobility and venous stasis. The signs and symptoms listed may indicate pulmonary embolus or thrombophlebitis.

Neurologic disorders

5. Turn the patient from side to side at least every 2 hours. Keep bedding clean and dry. Massage bony prominences. Watch for fragile, thin, or excoriated skin, which may shear during turning. Provide a special mattress or foam or other padding. Report any red or broken skin areas immediately.

5. Impeccable skin care can prevent skin breakdown in the immobilized patient. Moisture promotes bacterial growth and increases skin friability. Turning and massage help prevent pressure sores from developing and promote circulation. An older patient is likely to have delicate skin, particularly if debilitated. If help did not arrive quickly after the CVA, the patient's skin may already be excoriated from the effects of urine, pressure, and dehydration. A special mattress or padding can help redistribute pressure. Prompt intervention can prevent serious skin problems that can interfere with recovery.

6. Maintain adequate elimination. If the patient is catheterized, begin bladder retraining as soon as possible, following an established protocol or medical order. If the patient is not catheterized, offer a bedpan every 2 hours. Report cloudiness, excessive sediment, or the presence of white blood cells in the patient's urine. Provide stool softeners and laxatives, as ordered, and monitor the frequency and characteristics of bowel movements. Reassure the patient that bowel and bladder control usually returns as rehabilitation progresses.

6. The interruption of neurosensory pathways that results from CVA may cause limited or altered sphincter control, either from actual brain damage or from CVA-related memory and inhibitory lapses. Incontinence and urinary stasis predispose the patient to infection. Bladder and bowel retraining reestablishes patterns and bolsters the patient's confidence in resuming activities as permitted. Reassurance that incontinence is usually temporary helps decrease anxiety, embarrassment, and a sense of helplessness.

7. Additional individualized interventions: _____

7. Rationales: _____

Nursing diagnosis

Risk for sensory-perceptual alteration related to cerebral injury

Nursing priority

Minimize the effects of deficits in perception and prevent related complications.

Patient outcome criteria

Throughout the hospital stay, the patient will:
• look at and touch the affected side of the body
• establish protective behavior for affected limbs
• demonstrate use of techniques to compensate for sensory loss.

Interventions

1. Use a calm and reassuring manner, eye contact, and touch to establish a relationship with the patient. Use the patient's preferred name, and approach the unaffected side.

2. Protect the patient from injury to the affected side. Give regular reminders to look at and touch the affected side.

Rationales

1. Sensory-perceptual and communication deficits may contribute to profound isolation for the patient who has suffered a CVA. Use of nonverbal communication establishes contact and helps decrease anxiety. The patient may be unable to see or feel on the affected side of the body.

2. Hemiplegia may be accompanied by full or partial hemianesthesia, making the patient unaware of actual or impending injury. Relearning awareness and acceptance of the affected side by using that side helps move the patient toward functional recovery.

3. If the patient has a visual field deficit, suggest frequent head-turning to widen the visual field. Make sure that food and other objects at the bedside are placed well within the patient's visual field.

4. Additional individualized interventions: _____

3. Visual field deficits may prevent the patient from observing the visual cues needed to prevent injury. Placing food and other objects in the patient's visual field helps prevent accidents and ensure adequate nutrition.

4. Rationales: _____

NURSING DIAGNOSIS

Risk for impaired verbal communication related to cerebral injury

Nursing priority

Establish effective means of communication.

Patient outcome criterion

Within 1 hour of admission, the conscious patient will establish some form of verbal or nonverbal communication.

Interventions

1. Assess communication ability. Explain to the patient that the CVA may have affected speech. Ask simple questions that evaluate the patient's ability to repeat words, interpret, follow directions, and express feelings. Allow ample time for responses.

2. Speak slowly and clearly, using short sentences; never shout. Use simple explanations and gestures. Always include the patient in conversation when others are present. Avoid answering for the patient. Never use baby talk. Provide an alternative means of communication (such as a word board or pencil and paper) if needed.

3. If significant speech deficits are present, arrange a referral to a speech therapist for more comprehensive evaluation and rehabilitation services.

4. Reassure the patient that functional recovery is possible with patience and consistent rehabilitation. Help the patient with repetition of verbal and physical exercises. Involve family members in the patient's exercises. If the patient uses inappropriate profanity, counsel the family.

5. Additional individualized interventions: _____

Rationales

1. Identifying speech problems (such as expressive or receptive aphasia) is the first step in planning rehabilitation. A patient with receptive aphasia may still be able to process information but is slower to interpret stimuli and form a response.

2. Rapid or complex explanations may cause neurosensory overload, adding to the patient's frustration. Hearing is usually not impaired, and shouting adds to the patient's distress over deficits. Answering for the patient, talking around the patient, and using baby talk are demeaning and contribute to the patient's sense of helplessness. Alternative means of communication may be needed while the patient relearns verbal skills.

3. A speech therapist can pinpoint and treat specific speech problems.

4. A patient with severe deficits may despair of resuming normal activities; maintaining hope is vital for the fullest recovery. Over time, the brain can develop new pathways for functions: Repetition aids this process. Family support helps maintain morale. Family members may be shocked by inappropriate profanity; advise them that this is typical in a patient whose speech has been affected by CVA.

5. Rationales: _____

Neurologic disorders

Nursing diagnosis

Risk for knowledge deficit (CVA management) related to lack of exposure to information on self-care

Nursing priority

Provide thorough patient and family teaching.

Patient outcome criteria

By the time of discharge, the patient or family will:
- express understanding of what has happened
- name risk factors associated with a potential recurrence of CVA
- list and discuss all medications for use at home
- list four signs of bleeding (if the patient is taking an anticoagulant)
- list signs of TIA and CVA
- demonstrate understanding of the activity regimen and perform activities
- use mobility aids appropriately, if needed
- name measures to protect the affected side
- verbalize understanding of the bowel and bladder control program
- express understanding of food and fluid intake recommendations
- tolerate frustration over speech deficits and use alternative measures to communicate
- understand the plan for ongoing rehabilitation
- express understanding of normal emotional responses.

Interventions

1. See the "Knowledge deficit" plan, page 72.

2. Explain to the family that some emotional lability is typically associated with cerebral injury but that such behavior usually decreases over time. Teach the family how to gently guide the patient back to appropriate emotional and physical responses. Encourage patience, affection, and the use of humor.

3. Maintain an attitude of acceptance and understanding. Do not exacerbate emotional outbursts by reacting personally to them. Encourage normal expression of feelings related to lost abilities.

4. Instruct the patient and family about all medications to be taken at home, including antihypertensive drugs, anticoagulants, and antiplatelet aggregation medication.

Rationales

1. This plan provides general information for use in patient and family teaching.

2. Family members may be confused and distressed by unexpected emotional outbursts, and they may be reassured to know that physiologic factors are at least partially responsible. The family may help the patient reestablish appropriate responses through supportive, gentle reminders. Family understanding and patience, with humor at appropriate moments, may defuse potentially volatile emotional outbursts.

3. A patient who has suffered a CVA typically exhibits excessive or inappropriate emotions as a result of brain injury. The profound alteration such deficits as aphasia cause in the patient's relationship with the environment can also cause widely varied emotional reactions, ranging from rage to grief; expression of such feelings is part of coping. The patient may be unable to control emotional responses, and strong reactions on the part of family members or caregivers may add to the patient's isolation and distress.

4. Understanding and complying with the drug regimen decreases the risk of a CVA recurring.

5. If the patient will be receiving anticoagulant therapy at home, provide thorough instructions about:

• the action, dosage, and schedule of the medication

• the need for frequent follow-up laboratory testing to determine dosage requirements
• signs of bleeding problems (melena, petechiae, easy bruising, hematuria, epistaxis) and the need to report them
• measures to control bleeding
• dietary considerations
• the need to avoid aspirin and other over-the-counter medications unless specifically approved by the doctor
• the need to avoid trauma

• the importance of wearing a medical alert tag and of notifying other health professionals (such as the dentist or optometrist) of anticoagulant therapy.

6. Teach the importance of lifestyle modifications to minimize the risk of CVA recurrence, including blood pressure control, weight control, cholesterol management, exercise, smoking cessation, diabetes control, diet modifications, and stress reduction.

7. Teach the patient and family to recognize and seek help for signs and symptoms associated with CVAs: vertigo, vision disturbances, sudden weakness or falls without loss of consciousness (drop attacks), paresthesia of the face or extremities, speech disturbances, lateralized temporary weakness, or sudden, severe, unexplained headache.

8. Teach the patient and family about rehabilitation plans, and arrange for home care follow-up or in-home assistance, as needed. Also teach the patient specific, individualized information on activities, safety measures, and proper positioning. Show how to use mobility aids (slings, braces, or walkers), and demonstrate airway maintenance and feeding techniques. Go over the patient's bowel and bladder control program. Reinforce the signs and symptoms of complications (decreasing neurologic status, infection, bleeding, or thromboembolic events). Make sure the patient and family understand food and fluid intake recommendations, skin care measures, communication techniques, and how to cope with emotional lability.

9. Discuss with the family the advisability of learning cardiopulmonary resuscitation techniques.

10. Additional individualized interventions: _____
_____

5. Because anticoagulant use may cause life-threatening bleeding, the patient and family must understand the regimen completely.
• Anticoagulants should be taken on a regular schedule in the prescribed dosage for maximum effectiveness.
• Tests determine the need for dosage adjustments.

• Excessive bleeding may indicate the need for a dosage adjustment, a therapeutic antidote, or both.

• Uncontrolled hemorrhage can be fatal.
• Vitamin K intake can affect dosage requirements.
• Some drugs can augment the effects of anticoagulants.

• Even minimal trauma may cause serious injury because of the effects of anticoagulants.
• Other health care providers must be aware of the patient's medication regimen so that they can adjust their care to prevent injury.

6. These lifestyle modifications may decrease the risk of a CVA recurring.

7. Recognizing the signs and symptoms of a CVA and quickly seeking medical help allows for medical interventions that can decrease the extent of brain tissue damage.

8. The rehabilitation level at discharge varies from patient to patient and may also depend on the availability of home care resources. Most CVA patients require some assistance at home after discharge, either from motivated and well-taught family members or from professional caregivers. Because of the impact of DRGs, a CVA patient may be discharged from the hospital early on in the rehabilitation process. Discharge planning should always address ongoing rehabilitation.

9. Many risk factors for CVA—such as hypertension and atherosclerosis—also are risk factors for myocardial infarction and cardiac arrest. Cardiac arrest also can cause further CVA from ischemia.

10. Rationales: _____
_____

Neurologic disorders

Discharge planning

Discharge checklist
Before discharge, the patient shows evidence of:
- absence of fever and pulmonary or cardiovascular complications
- stable vital signs
- absence of signs and symptoms indicating progression of neurologic deficit
- prothrombin level within acceptable parameters
- absence of skin breakdown and contractures
- ability to tolerate activity within expected parameters
- ability to transfer and ambulate
- ability to perform activities of daily living
- ability to compensate for neurologic deficit, such as paralysis, spasticity, or speech impairment
- ability to control bowel and bladder functions
- ability to tolerate nutritional intake
- physical and occupational therapy program with maximum benefit attained
- referral to home care if the patient is progressing toward maximum rehabilitation potential and home support system is adequate
- referral to a rehabilitation facility or nursing home for continued rehabilitation if the home support is inadequate or the patient needs continued rehabilitation outside the home
- referral form reflecting the patient's progress, potential, and goals and containing all other appropriate information necessary to provide continuity of care.

Teaching checklist
Document evidence that the patient and family demonstrate an understanding of:
- the injury or disease process and its implications
- the purpose, dosage, administration schedule, and adverse effects of all discharge medications (these may include anticoagulants, antiplatelet aggregation medications, and antihypertensives)
- the need for follow-up laboratory tests (if indicated)
- signs of cerebral impairment
- signs of infection
- signs of thromboembolic or other complications
- activity and positioning recommendations and mobility aids
- food and fluid intake recommendations
- the bowel and bladder control program
- risk factors
- safety measures
- use of medical alert tag
- the advisability of cardiopulmonary resuscitation classes for the family
- skin care
- communication measures
- verbal practice exercises

- expected emotional lability and coping methods
- community resources
- when and how to use the emergency medical system
- date, time, and location of follow-up appointment
- home care arrangements.

Documentation checklist
Using outcome criteria as a guide, document:
- clinical status on admission
- significant changes in status
- neurologic assessments
- pertinent laboratory and diagnostic test findings
- medication therapy
- activity and positioning
- food intake
- fluid intake and output
- bowel and bladder control measures
- communication measures
- patient and family teaching
- discharge planning.

Associated plans of care

Geriatric care
Grieving
Impaired physical mobility
Ineffective family coping: Compromised
Ineffective individual coping
Knowledge deficit
Nutritional deficit
Seizures
Thrombophlebitis

References

Adams, R.D., et al. *Principles of Neurology,* 6th ed. New York: McGraw-Hill Book Co., 1997.

McDowell, F. *Stroke: The First Hours. Emergency Evaluation and Treatment.* (Stroke Clinical Update and Consensus Statement). Englewood, Colo.: National Stroke Association, 1997.

National Stroke Association. *The Road Ahead: A Stroke Recovery Guide,* 3rd ed. Englewood, Colo.: National Stroke Association, 1995.

Severson, A.L., et al. "International Normalized Ratio in Anticoagulant Therapy: Understanding the Issues," *American Journal of Critical Care* 6(2):88-92, March 1997.

Craniotomy

DRG information

DRG 001   Craniotomy. Except for trauma. Age 17+.
Mean LOS = 11.1 days
Principal procedures include:
- biopsy of brain or cerebral meninges
- excision of brain or skull lesion
- clipping or repair of cerebral aneurysm
- insertion of ventricular shunt
- repair of arteriovenous fistula
- incision of brain or cerebral meninges
- incision or excision of intracranial vessels.

DRG 002   Craniotomy for Trauma. Age 17+.
Mean LOS = 1.6 days
Principal diagnoses include:
- concussion
- skull fracture
- hemorrhage (subarachnoid, subdural, or extradural) following injury
- cerebral laceration or contusion
- fracture of vertebral column with spinal cord injury.
Additional DRG information: These diagnoses must be treated surgically; see DRG 001 for examples of procedures.

DRG 003   Craniotomy. Ages 0 to 17.
Mean LOS = 2.7 days
Principal procedures for DRG 003: See principal procedures listed under DRG 001.

INTRODUCTION

Definition and time focus

Craniotomy, the most common neurosurgical procedure, is the surgical opening of the skull to provide access to the brain. It is performed to treat intracranial disease — for example, to remove tissue for biopsy or to remove a mass lesion (a substance that occupies the cranial cavity, compromising either the space or the integrity of the brain). The surgery involves making a series of small holes, called burr holes, in the cranium with a special drill, then cutting between the holes to allow removal of a flap of bone and scalp. At the end of the surgery, the flap is replaced and the muscle and scalp are realigned and sutured.

Although the surgical approach depends on the location of the lesion, surgery is performed in two general areas. In the supratentorial craniotomy, the cranium is incised above the tentorium (the fold of dura mater that separates the cerebral cortex from the cerebellum and

brain stem). This approach is used for lesions in the frontal, parietal, temporal, and occipital lobes of the cerebral hemispheres. The infratentorial approach, in which the cranium is incised below the tentorium, is used for lesions in the brain stem (midbrain, pons, and medulla) and cerebellum.

A craniotomy may be an emergency procedure for removal of a rapidly expanding lesion, such as an epidural hematoma or intracranial abscess, or an elective procedure to remove a slow-growing, space-occupying lesion such as a benign tumor. This clinical plan focuses on the immediate preoperative and postoperative care (in the critical care unit) of a patient undergoing an elective craniotomy.

Etiology and precipitating factors

- Tumor, abscess, aneurysm, chronic hematoma, cyst, or arteriovenous malformation
- Condition requiring repair of a cerebral injury

FOCUSED ASSESSMENT GUIDELINES

Nursing history (functional health pattern findings)

Health perception–health management pattern
- History of headache that is worse on arising in the morning and is aggravated by movement or straining at stool
- Personality changes
- Mental changes or mood swings
- Age (adults are at increased risk)
- Family or personal history of diabetes mellitus, intolerance to previous operative procedures, history of adrenocorticosteroid use, or signs and symptoms of endocrine dysfunction

Nutritional-metabolic pattern
- Vomiting

Activity-exercise pattern
- Recent hospitalization or bed rest
- Restricted physical activity because of motor or sensory deficits

Cognitive-perceptual pattern
- Changes in vision, hearing, touch, taste, or smell, depending on location and duration of lesion
- Language and memory problems (with chronic lesion)

Self-perception–self-concept pattern
- Negative self-image because of body disfigurement (if patient is undergoing radiation or chemotherapy for chronic lesion)

• Anger, embarrassment, or denial
Role-relationship pattern
• Altered role as spouse and breadwinner (depending on duration of lesion)
Sexuality-reproductive pattern
• Impaired sexual functioning (depending on location of lesion)
Coping–stress tolerance pattern
• Ineffective coping patterns
• Anticipatory grieving
Value-belief pattern
• Fear of the unknown and death brought on by the possible need for surgery, resulting in a delay in seeking medical attention
• Frustration with health care system if vague symptoms delayed diagnosis

Physical findings
Signs and symptoms depend on the lesion's site. The following are general findings that point to cerebral dysfunction.
Neurologic
• Decreased level of consciousness
• Mental changes, such as impaired memory, lack of initiative, or mood changes
• Visual deficits, such as decreased visual acuity, blurred vision, diplopia, or changes in extraocular eye movements
• Sensory deficits
• Motor deficits
• Seizures
• Papilledema
• Cranial nerve dysfunction
Gastrointestinal
• Vomiting

Diagnostic studies
• Complete blood count — decreased hemoglobin level may indicate anemia or blood dyscrasia as well as the need for blood transfusion before surgery to ensure adequate transport for oxygen in the blood; increased white blood cell (WBC) count may signal infection or an abscess, a contraindication for surgery (unless the abscess is in the brain)
• Blood urea nitrogen (BUN) level, serum creatinine — used to monitor renal function; increased values may indicate an impaired ability to cope with the sodium and water retention that results from the body's stress reaction to surgery
• Electrolyte analyses — used to monitor fluid status and detect hypokalemia and hyperkalemia; the patient may develop diabetes insipidus (DI) or syndrome of inappropriate antidiuretic hormone secretion (SIADH)
• Fasting blood glucose levels — used to detect diabetes mellitus, which would need to be controlled before and after surgery

• Typing and crossmatching — used to determine patient blood type and have blood products readily available in case the patient requires blood replacement from surgical loss
• Computed tomography (CT) scan — used to diagnose cerebral lesions, such as hematomas, tumors, cysts, hydrocephalus, cerebral atrophy, cerebral infarction, and cerebral edema; serial scanning may be done before and after surgery
• Cerebral angiography — used to diagnose cerebrovascular aneurysms, cerebral thrombosis, hematomas, tumors with increased vascularization, vascular plaques or spasm, arteriovenous malformations, cerebral fistulas, or cerebral edema
• Radionuclide imaging (brain scan) — used to diagnose intracranial masses, such as malignant or benign tumors, abscesses, cerebral infarctions, intracranial hemorrhage, arteriovenous malformations, or aneurysms; has been largely replaced by CT scans
• Magnetic resonance imaging — used to assess brain edema, hemorrhage, infarction, blood vessels, and tumors and to measure fluid flow
• Chest X-ray — can rule out congestion, pneumonia, atelectasis, or other pulmonary diseases that would compromise respiration
• Electrocardiography — can detect cardiac abnormalities such as arrhythmias that would be aggravated by the stress of a prolonged surgical procedure and drug therapy

Potential complications
• Increased intracranial pressure (ICP)
• Cerebral edema
• Shock (hemorrhagic or hypovolemic or from intracranial bleeding)
• Hematoma (subdural or epidural)
• Atelectasis
• Pneumonia
• Seizures
• Neurogenic pulmonary edema
• DI
• Meningitis
• Wound infection
• Neurologic deficits, such as decreased level of consciousness, motor weakness, or paralysis
• Loss of corneal, pharyngeal, or palatal reflexes
• Arrhythmias
• Thrombophlebitis
• Hyperthermia
• Postoperative hydrocephalus
• GI ulceration and bleeding
• Cranial nerve III damage (eye drop) and visual disturbances
• Personality changes
• Cerebrospinal fluid leakage

CLINICAL SNAPSHOT

CRANIOTOMY

Major nursing diagnoses and collaborative problems	Key patient outcomes
Preoperative knowledge deficit (impending craniotomy)	Verbalize understanding of upcoming surgery and its potential effects and complications.
Risk for cerebral ischemia	Demonstrate improved neurologic status.
Risk for infection	Have no signs or symptoms of wound or systemic infection or meningitis.
Risk for respiratory failure	Have a normal respiratory rate and pattern.
Risk for injury	Remain free from injury.
Risk for fluid volume excess or deficit	Have electrolyte levels, BUN level, hematocrit, and serum osmolality within normal limits.
Body-image disturbance	Verbalize feelings of self-worth.
Postoperative knowledge deficit (follow-up care)	Verbalize questions about follow-up care.

NURSING DIAGNOSIS

Preoperative knowledge deficit (impending craniotomy) related to lack of exposure to information

Nursing priority

Prepare the patient and family for the craniotomy.

Patient outcome criteria

Before surgery, the patient and family will:
• verbalize understanding of the upcoming surgery and its potential effects and complications
• describe their anxieties and how they are coping with them.

Interventions

1. Implement the measures in the "Knowledge deficit" plan, page 72, as appropriate.

2. Assess what the patient and family already know about the impending craniotomy and what they want to know. Consider the patient's educational level, level of consciousness, mental changes, and memory loss. As appropriate, ask the patient or family what they have learned from the doctor, other family members, or someone who has had a craniotomy.

Rationales

1. The "Knowledge deficit" plan contains detailed general information about teaching. This plan covers only specific information about craniotomy.

2. Level of consciousness, mental changes, and memory loss affect the patient's knowledge base. Although the doctor should have informed the patient and family about the procedure and potential complications, anxiety, memory loss, or limited comprehension may interfere with understanding and retention. Also, the patient and family may have limited or confusing information from various sources. Assessing the knowledge base allows the nurse to reinforce appropriate information, correct misconceptions, and fill in knowledge gaps.

Neurologic disorders

3. Describe the preoperative procedure, including neurologic assessment, weight measurement, the need for nothing by mouth after midnight, hair washing, and the possibility that long hair will be braided.

4. Explain that the patient's hair is cut and scalp shaved in the operating room. Explain the rationale and allow time for the patient to express any feelings. If the operating room personnel are willing to save the patient's hair, ask whether the patient wants it saved. Explain that, if desired, all hair can be shaved to promote uniform regrowth. If possible, have the family present during this explanation.

5. Discuss what the unit will be like and the effects of the craniotomy during the immediate postoperative period. Mention that headaches and altered consciousness may occur.

6. Encourage the patient and family to express fears and concerns about the impending surgery.

7. Additional individualized interventions: _____

3. Knowing what to expect usually decreases anxiety.

4. Hair is an important component of body image and self-concept. Having the hair cut may be extremely distressing to the patient. Knowing why it must be removed and that it may be saved may alleviate some of the distress and sense of loss. Allowing time for the patient to express feelings conveys sensitivity and validates the patient's emotions. Having the family present may provide the support necessary to cope with this situation and prepare them for how the patient will look after surgery.

5. Knowing in advance what the unit will be like may increase the patient's sense of security when awakening after surgery. Knowing that headaches and altered consciousness are common after the operation may help decrease the patient's and family's anxiety.

6. Fear of death, anxiety over other possible outcomes, and anticipatory grieving for the possible loss of body function interfere with learning. Providing an environment where the patient is comfortable discussing these feelings may improve learning and reduce preoperative and postoperative anxiety.

7. Rationales: _____

COLLABORATIVE PROBLEM

Risk for cerebral ischemia related to increased ICP

Nursing priorities
- Decrease ICP.
- Minimize fluctuations in cerebral perfusion pressure.

Patient outcome criteria
- Within 72 hours after surgery, the patient will:
  – have an ICP of 0 to 15 mm Hg and a cerebral perfusion pressure greater than 60 mm Hg
  – have a mean arterial pressure greater than 60 mm Hg
  – display no clinical signs of increased ICP or herniation.
- Within 1 week after surgery, the patient will demonstrate improved neurologic status.

Interventions

1. Implement the measures in the "Increased intracranial pressure" plan's "Risk for cerebral ischemia" collaborative problem, page 171.

2. Additional individualized interventions: _____

Rationales

1. Several factors can raise ICP to dangerous levels after a craniotomy, including surgical trauma, cerebral edema, blood pressure fluctuations, and nursing activities. The plan for "Increased intracranial pressure" covers this problem in detail.

2. Rationales: _____

Nursing diagnosis

Risk for infection related to surgery, invasive techniques, continuous intracranial monitoring, ventricular drains, or cerebrospinal fluid (CSF) leakage

Nursing priority

Prevent or promptly detect signs of infection.

Patient outcome criteria

- By 72 hours after surgery, the patient will:
  - have a normal temperature and WBC count
  - have no positive cultures.
- By the time of discharge, the patient will have no signs or symptoms of wound or systemic infection or meningitis.

Interventions

1. Implement the measures in the "Increased intracranial pressure" plan's "Risk for infection" nursing diagnosis, page 174.

2. Administer antibiotics as ordered, usually immediately before surgery begins.

3. Assess for respiratory infection:
- Auscultate lungs every 2 hours and as necessary for adventitious sounds.
- Assess sputum for color, consistency, amount, and odor; culture if necessary.
- Observe for temperature elevation and WBC elevation.

4. Observe the surgical wound daily for signs and symptoms of infection, such as redness, edema, suture stretch, pigskin appearance of the epidermis, tenderness, or drainage. Also observe for systemic signs, including fever, malaise, leukocytosis, or tachycardia.

Rationales

1. The "Increased intracranial pressure" plan provides general measures for prevention, assessment, and treatment of infection. This plan discusses additional care specific to the craniotomy patient.

2. Wound infection occurs in 0.7% to 5.7% of neurosurgical patients. Prophylactic antibiotic administration helps prevent infection by establishing the optimal tissue concentration of antibiotic before possible contamination. Antibiotic administration also may be repeated during a lengthy procedure. Antibiotics may be discontinued at the completion of surgery.

3. The overall pulmonary infection rate in the neurosurgery patient is 13% to 16%. Impaired mobility, characteristic of the surgical and postoperative periods, compromises the respiratory system by slowing the movement of secretions; this promotes atelectasis and produces generalized hypoxia. To decrease ICP, the patient's fluid balance may be maintained at a slightly lower level than normal. Dehydration makes the sputum thicker, increasing the risk of consolidation and pneumonia. Adventitious breath sounds, purulent or foul-smelling sputum, fever, and WBC elevation strongly suggest the development of pulmonary infection.

4. Scalp margin necrosis, wound dehiscence, CSF leakage, presence of a drain and monitoring device, possible scratching and manipulation by the patient, and environmental factors increase the risk of wound infection in the postcraniotomy patient. A stitch abscess may appear before a major wound infection. A true wound infection rarely occurs before the 2nd day after surgery and usually occurs within the first 2 weeks.

Neurologic disorders

5. Monitor the patient for signs and symptoms of meningitis, such as temperature elevation, chills, lethargy, severe headache, nausea and vomiting, nuchal rigidity, positive Kernig's sign or Brudzinski's sign, photophobia, irritability, decreased level of consciousness, or generalized seizures. Assist with CT scan and lumbar puncture if necessary.

5. Patients at risk for developing acute inflammation of the meninges of the brain or spinal cord include those with cranial or spinal wound infections, CSF fistulae following operative procedures on the dura mater, and subarachnoid bolts or ventricular drains. All of these are possible risk factors for the postcraniotomy patient. Abnormal lumbar puncture findings typically confirm the diagnosis. These findings include a positive culture, an elevated opening pressure of 200 to 700 mm H_2O, WBC count increased from 10 to 1,000 cells/µl, an increased protein count, decreased glucose and chloride levels and, in purulent bacterial meningitis, a tan or milky appearance of the fluid. A CT scan may be performed before the lumbar puncture to determine the risk of brain herniation from the sudden removal of CSF from the spinal canal.

6. Additional individualized interventions: _____

6. Rationales: _____

COLLABORATIVE PROBLEM

Risk for respiratory failure related to decreased level of consciousness, neurologic deficits, effects of anesthesia, immobility, altered respiratory patterns, and tenacious secretions associated with fluid loss and decreased fluid intake

Nursing priority

Maintain effective gas exchange.

Patient outcome criteria

- Within 24 hours after surgery, the patient will:
  - have an airway free from secretions
  - have arterial blood gas (ABG) levels within desired limits.
- By the time of discharge, the patient will:
  - have a normal respiratory rate and pattern
  - have normal ABG levels
  - have a clear chest X-ray.

Interventions

1. Implement the measures discussed in the "Increased intracranial pressure" plan's "Risk for respiratory failure" collaborative problem, page 176.

2. Additional individualized interventions: _____

Rationales

1. The neurosurgical patient requires meticulous respiratory assessment, support of oxygenation and ventilation, and pulmonary hygiene.

2. Rationales: _____

NURSING DIAGNOSIS

Risk for injury related to decreased level of consciousness, effect of anesthetics, seizures, or drug therapy

Nursing priority

Prevent injury.

Patient outcome criterion

Throughout the hospital stay, the patient will remain free from injury.

Interventions

1. Implement the measures discussed in the "Increased intracranial pressure" plan's "Risk for injury" nursing diagnosis, page 180.

2. Additional individualized interventions: _____
_____

Rationales

1. Although the risk factors for injury for the neurosurgical patient differ somewhat from those for the patient with increased ICP, the measures used to prevent them are the same.

2. Rationales: _____
_____

Nursing diagnosis

Risk for fluid volume excess related to physiologic stress response to surgery, steroid therapy, or SIADH

Nursing priority

Maintain fluid volume within prescribed limits.

Patient outcome criteria

By the time of discharge, the patient will:
• display electrolyte levels, BUN level, hematocrit, and serum osmolality within normal limits
• have a urine output within normal limits
• manifest hemodynamic values within normal limits.

Interventions

1. Implement the measures discussed in the "Increased intracranial pressure" plan's "Risk for fluid volume excess" nursing diagnosis, page 179.

2. Additional individualized interventions: _____
_____

Rationales

1. The "Increased intracranial pressure" plan discusses the potential for fluid volume excess in detail.

2. Rationales: _____
_____

Nursing diagnosis

Risk for fluid volume deficit related to diuretic therapy, fluid restriction, DI, hyperthermia, or GI suction

Nursing priority

Maintain fluid volume within prescribed limits.

Patient outcome criteria

By the time of discharge, the patient will:
• maintain a urine output within normal limits
• have electrolyte levels, hematocrit, BUN level, and serum osmolality within normal limits
• maintain hemodynamic values within normal limits.

Neurologic disorders

Interventions

1. Implement the measures discussed in the "Increased intracranial pressure" plan's "Risk for fluid volume deficit" nursing diagnosis, page 177.

2. Additional individualized interventions: _____

_____

Rationales

1. DI most commonly occurs after neurosurgery. The "Increased intracranial pressure" plan discusses this problem in detail.

2. Rationales: _____

_____

NURSING DIAGNOSIS

Body-image disturbance related to hair loss, possible disruption in sensory or motor function, or possible alteration in personality and thought processes

Nursing priorities

• Promote a healthy body image.
• Minimize damage to self-concept.

Patient outcome criteria

Within 5 to 7 days after surgery, the patient will:
• verbalize feelings of self-worth
• participate in self-care
• demonstrate an interest in personal appearance
• demonstrate an interest in occupational therapy, activities of daily living, and a potential rehabilitation program.

Interventions

1. Encourage the patient to express feelings, beliefs, and concerns about changes resulting from the diagnosis and craniotomy. Offer emotional support, as appropriate, based on knowledge of the diagnosis and the success of surgery.

2. Implement measures to minimize the patient's reaction to loss of hair and to the misshapen skull, if a bone flap was removed.
• Provide a surgical cap or scarf to wear; encourage usual grooming, makeup habits, and wearing a wig; reinforce that hair will regrow.

• Use therapeutic touch and visit frequently.

3. Provide appropriate stimuli:
• Place the patient in a room with a window, if possible.
• Provide a clock and calendar.
• Provide objects of interest to the patient such as photographs of loved ones.
• Play the radio, tapes, or television, if the patient wishes.
• Talk with the patient.
• Encourage the family to interact with the patient.

Rationales

1. The patient may have fears or misconceptions that can be clarified. Some residual effects of surgery are temporary. Recovery may be slow (months or years).

2. Specific interventions to minimize the body image changes may make the patient feel less self-conscious.

• These measures to improve appearance and help the patient become aware of the temporary nature of alterations in body image may encourage greater acceptance of the changes.
• Therapeutic touch and frequent visits convey acceptance, which may facilitate the patient's self-acceptance.

3. These measures provide stimulation and reality orientation. Talking with the patient and encouraging family interaction are particularly important because they reinforce a sense of human connection in the unfamiliar hospital environment.

4. Implement the measures in the "Impaired physical mobility" plan, page 50, as appropriate. Encourage participation in self-care, occupational therapy, activities of daily living, and ambulation, as permitted.

4. The measures in this plan prevent deformities and other complications resulting from the enforced immobility associated with major surgery. Maintaining motor function, muscle strength, and joint mobility are particularly important in preserving the patient's ability to benefit from later rehabilitation programs. Participation in activities fosters the patient's belief that independence can be reestablished.

5. Additional individualized interventions: _____

5. Rationales: _____

Nursing diagnosis

Postoperative knowledge deficit (follow-up care) related to lack of exposure to information

Nursing priority

Provide early teaching regarding rehabilitation and follow-up care.

Patient outcome criteria

By the time of discharge, the patient and family will:
• verbalize questions about follow-up care
• express satisfaction with the staff's willingness to answer questions
• begin identifying long-range learning needs.

Interventions

1. Implement measures in the "Knowledge deficit" plan, page 72, as appropriate. Wait to start formal teaching until the patient's condition stabilizes.

2. Provide informal teaching, as appropriate. Encourage questions, provide brief explanations about the current situation, and clarify misconceptions.

3. Identify and document long-range teaching needs as the patient or family raises questions or demonstrates a specific need. Upon the patient's discharge, communicate these needs to the receiving staff.

4. Provide information to the patient and family about community agencies and support groups, such as head injury support groups, vocational rehabilitation, and the American Cancer Society.

5. Additional individualized interventions: _____

Rationales

1. In the first days after surgery, the craniotomy patient usually is too ill for a structured teaching program, and the patient's and family's attention is directed toward more immediate needs. Formal teaching works best after the patient's condition has stabilized and the patient has been transferred to a better environment for learning.

2. Capitalizing on informal opportunities conveys a willingness to meet the patient's and family's immediate learning needs.

3. Planning for discharge teaching is most effective based on the specific needs of the patient and family. Documentation and colleague-to-colleague communication enhance continuity of care.

4. These organizations provide many forms of support for patients and families. In many cases, their credibility allows them to provide invaluable practical information on long-range education and rehabilitation. Knowing that others have coped with similar experiences may provide a sense of rapport and trust that encourages the learning necessary to adjust successfully to cranial surgery and possible residual deficits.

5. Rationales: _____

Neurologic disorders

DISCHARGE PLANNING

Discharge checklist

Before discharge, the patient shows evidence of:

❏ stable vital signs
❏ stable neurologic function
❏ ICP within normal limits
❏ healing incision
❏ headache controlled by oral analgesics
❏ absence of pulmonary, cardiovascular, or GI complications
❏ normal fluid and electrolyte balance
❏ absence of infection
❏ absence of fever.

Teaching checklist

Document evidence that the patient and family demonstrate an understanding of:

❏ the diagnosis and extent of surgery
❏ wound care
❏ the extent of neurologic deficits, if present
❏ the extent and demands of the rehabilitation process
❏ the need for continued family support
❏ date, time, and location of follow-up care
❏ purpose, dosages, and potential adverse effects of all discharge medications.

Documentation checklist

Using outcome criteria as a guide, document:

❏ clinical status on admission
❏ significant changes in status
❏ pertinent laboratory and diagnostic test findings
❏ fluid intake and output
❏ neurologic status
❏ neurologic deficits, if present
❏ GI bleeding, if any
❏ wound condition
❏ seizures, if any
❏ rehabilitation program needs
❏ patient and family teaching
❏ discharge planning.

ASSOCIATED PLANS OF CARE

Impaired physical mobility
Increased intracranial pressure
Ineffective family coping: Compromised
Ineffective individual coping
Knowledge deficit
Nutritional deficit
Pain
Seizures
Sensory-perceptual alteration
Surgery

REFERENCES

Clochesy, J.M., et al. *Critical Care Nursing*, 2nd ed. Philadelphia: W.B. Saunders Co., 1996.

Lewis, S.M., et al. *Medical-Surgical Nursing Assessment and Management of Clinical Problems*, 4th ed. New York: Mosby–Year Book, Inc., 1996.

Roberts, S.L. *Critical Care Nursing, Assessment and Intervention*. Stamford, Conn.: Appleton & Lange, 1996.

Ruppert, S.D., et al. *J.T. Dolan's Critical Care Nursing, Clinical Management Through the Nursing Process,* 2nd ed. Philadelphia: F.A. Davis Co., 1996.

Thompson, J.M., et al. *Mosby's Manual of Clinical Nursing,* 3rd ed. St. Louis: Mosby–Year Book, Inc., 1997.

Tilkian, S.M., et al. *Clinical and Nursing Implications of Laboratory Tests*, 5th ed. St. Louis: Mosby–Year Book, Inc., 1996.

Drug overdose

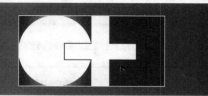

DRG information

DRG 449   Poisoning and Toxic Effects of Drugs
with Complication or Comorbidity
(CC); Age 17+.
Mean LOS = 4.5 days
Principal diagnoses include:
• poisoning by drugs of all varieties,
affecting multiple body systems
• toxic effects of alcohol.

DRG 450   Poisoning and Toxic Effects of Drugs
without CC; Age 17+.
Mean LOS = 2.3 days
Principal diagnoses include selected
principal diagnoses listed under DRG
449. The distinction is that DRG 450
excludes CC.

DRG 451   Poisoning and Toxic Effects of Drugs.
Ages 0 to 17.
Mean LOS = 2.1 days
Principal diagnoses include selected
principal diagnoses listed under DRG
449. The distinction is that DRG 451
excludes patients age 17+.

INTRODUCTION

Definition and time focus
The patient admitted after a drug overdose is a challenge. The patient may be comatose, withdrawn, agitated, somnolent, or otherwise unable to provide clear historical data. The type of drug involved may be unknown, or evidence may suggest the patient took more than one drug. If illegal substances are involved, family members may be reluctant to provide a full history because they fear possible criminal prosecution, even if assured of medical confidentiality.

Even when the patient or family clearly identifies a specific drug that was taken, the nurse must consider the potential interaction of the drug with other medications and the possibility that the patient took more than one drug. For the purposes of this plan, overdose is an intentional act in which the patient ingests, injects, sniffs, inhales, or otherwise self-administers a dose that proves to be toxic.

Using this definition, the plan omits discussion of overdoses from accidental poisoning, toxic reactions to prescribed medications taken at recommended dosages, and industrial or agricultural exposure to toxic substances. This plan focuses on the patient who is admit-ted to a hospital for treatment of an intentional overdose, commonly associated with a suicide gesture or attempt.

Etiology and precipitating factors
For each patient, different factors may cause the overdose event, but usually one or more of the following are involved:
• drug or alcohol abuse or addiction
• unhealthy coping patterns
• unusually stressful life event or circumstances
• despair, depression, anger, or the desire for revenge.

FOCUSED ASSESSMENT GUIDELINES

Nursing history (functional health pattern findings)
Health perception–health management pattern
• History of short- or long-term drug or alcohol abuse or addiction
• Intent to commit suicide
• Previous suicide attempt
Sleep-rest pattern
• History of insomnia or early morning awakening (associated with depression)
Cognitive-perceptual pattern
• Poor concentration or memory impairment
• Difficulty making decisions
Self-perception–self-concept pattern
• Helpless or hopeless self-perception (common)
• Self-deprecating statements
Role-relationship pattern
• Lack of significant other
• Recent conflict or breakup with significant other
• Recent or chronic job difficulties
• Recent death of a loved one
Coping–stress tolerance pattern
• Habitual use of unhealthy coping behavior such as drug abuse
Value-belief pattern
• Surprise or disbelief about the seriousness of overdose

Physical findings
Because physical findings vary widely with the drug taken, this section is omitted. See *Nurse's guide to common drug overdoses*, pages 152 and 153, or consult pharmacologic references for findings associated with specific drug overdoses.

(Text continues on page 154.)

Nurse's guide to common drug overdoses

Drug	Therapeutic effects	Signs and symptoms of overdose	Treatment	Complications
acetaminophen	Reduces fever and raises pain threshold; exact mechanisms unclear; metabolized in liver	• Anorexia • Nausea and vomiting • Diaphoresis • Right upper quadrant abdominal pain • Hypotension • Altered level of consciousness	• Drug level measured every 4 hours to guide treatment • Emesis or lavage • Cathartics • Acetylcysteine (Mucomyst) given orally, if more than 7.5 g ingested within 24 hours and serum level in toxic range 4 hours after ingestion	• Hepatic failure • Coagulation defects • Renal failure • Hepatic encephalopathy • Shock

alcohol (ethanol)	Central nervous system (CNS) depression, peripheral vasodilation	• Ataxia
		• Reduced comprehension
		• Vomiting
		• Respiratory depression
		• Hypotension
		• Seizures
		• Flushing
		• Coma
			• Emesis or lavage, if ingestion within 4 hours
			• I.V. fluids
			• Ventilatory support, especially in multiple drug overdose
			• Observation for withdrawal, including anxiety, tremors, diaphoresis, tachycardia, and hypertension (usually occurs 24 to 48 hours after last alcohol intake)
			• Sedation (if withdrawal symptoms are noted)
				• Respiratory depression
				• Aspiration
				• Hepatic failure
				• GI tract bleeding
				• With chronic abuse:
				  – Esophageal varices
				  – Portal hypertension
				  – Hepatic encephalopathy
				• Additive effects if taken with another CNS depressant

barbiturates	CNS depression	• Cardiopulmonary depression • Hypotension • Tachycardia • Sluggish pupil response • Nystagmus • Bullae • Hypothermia • Confusion • Ataxia • Coma	• Ventilatory support • Emesis or lavage (if ingested) • Activated charcoal • Cathartics • I.V. fluids • Observation for withdrawal, including tremors, vomiting, weakness, and hallucinations • Dialysis possible for large doses	• Arrhythmias • Respiratory arrest • Shock • Seizures • Pulmonary edema • Coma
benzodiazepines	CNS depression	• Lethargy • Hypotension • Tachycardia • Respiratory depression • Confusion • Ataxia • Coma	• Ventilatory support • Emesis or lavage (if ingested) • Activated charcoal • Cathartics • Flumazenil (Romazicon) given I.V. in repeated doses • I.V. fluids • Note: Hemodialysis and forced diuresis are *not* effective	• Taken alone, usually not fatal but when taken with other CNS depressants, additive effects can lead to respiratory depression, coma, and death

Nurse's guide to common drug overdoses *(continued)*

Drug	Therapeutic effects	Signs and symptoms of overdose	Treatment	Complications
cocaine	CNS stimulation, local anesthesia	• Hyperexcitability • Anxiety • Hypertension or hypotension • Fever • Tachypnea • Tachycardia • Confusion • Hallucinations • Dilated pupils • Diaphoresis • Seizures, coma	• Sedatives • Anticonvulsants • Cardiac monitoring • Emesis or lavage, if ingested • Activated charcoal, if ingested • Cathartic, if ingested • Fever control measures	• Myocardial infarction • Cerebral hemorrhage • Respiratory arrest • Status epilepticus • Cardiomyopathy • Rhabdomyolysis (rare)
opiates	CNS depression, analgesia, peripheral vasodilation	• Respiratory depression • Constricted pupils • Reduced level of consciousness • Hypothermia • Hypotension • Bradycardia	• Ventilatory support • Naloxone (Narcan) I.V. in repeated doses • Close monitoring, because respiratory depression may recur • Cardiac monitoring • Emesis or lavage, if ingested	• Respiratory arrest • Shock • Arrhythmias • Coma
salicylates	Analgesia	• Nausea and vomiting • Hyperthermia • Electrolyte imbalances • Acid-base imbalances (usually respiratory alkalosis and metabolic acidosis) • Hyperglycemia (in children, hypoglycemia) • Hyperpnea • Hyperventilation • Oliguria • Tinnitus • Confusion • Seizures • Petechiae	• Ventilatory support • Cardiac monitoring • I.V. fluids • Cooling measures • Correction of electrolyte and acid-base abnormalities • Emesis or lavage • Activated charcoal • Cathartics • Alkalinization of urine with sodium bicarbonate and potassium chloride (a urine pH between 7.5 and 8.5 promotes increased renal excretion)	• Respiratory failure • Arrhythmias or other life-threatening conditions caused by electrolyte or acid-base abnormalities • Renal tubular necrosis • GI bleeding • Hepatotoxicity • Pulmonary edema • Shock • Interference with normal clotting • Increased gastric motility
tricyclic antidepressants	Relieves symptoms of depression in patients with mood disorders	• Lethargy • Dry mouth • Dilated pupils • Confusion • Tremors • Urine retention • Tachycardia • Hypotension • Respiratory depression • Cardiac conduction delay • Hypothermia • Seizures • Coma	• Ventilatory support • Cardiac monitoring • Emesis or lavage • Activated charcoal • Cathartics • I.V. fluids • Sodium physostigmine 1 to 3 mg I.V., if large amount ingested • Cardiac pacing, if complete heart block • Anticonvulsants • Alkalinization with sodium bicarbonate • Temperature regulation measures • Note: Dialysis *not* effective	• Arrhythmias • Myocardial depression • Complete heart block • Heart failure • Shock • Paralytic ileus • Central and peripheral anticholinergic effects, myocardial depression

Neurologic disorders

Diagnostic studies

Appropriate laboratory tests vary widely, depending on the drug taken. The following are commonly performed for toxicity screening and evaluation.

• Serum electrolyte levels — may be abnormal; several drugs commonly seen in overdose cases, including salicylates and alcohol, may cause electrolyte abnormalities
• Arterial blood gas (ABG) values — essential for monitoring the adequacy of respiratory efforts; salicylates and other drugs cause acid-base abnormalities
• Liver enzymes — may reveal liver damage; many medications can cause liver damage at toxic levels, most notably acetaminophen and alcohol
• Blood alcohol level — an important screening test in any overdose because alcohol potentiates many drug effects, thus increasing central nervous system (CNS) depression
• Toxicology screening assay — checks for various substances, depending on the laboratory, but usually includes barbiturates, narcotics, amphetamines, salicylates, and acetaminophen
• Serum salicylate level — may reveal toxicity; time-elapsed nomograms are obtained in cases of acute overdose to assess toxicity level; because salicylates have a prolonged half-life, the sample should be ob-

tained at least 6 hours after ingestion; a level greater than 150 µg/ml is considered toxic
• Urine narcotic level — determines the presence and concentration of narcotics; most narcotics are excreted in urine within 48 hours of administration; toxic levels vary depending on the narcotic
• Serum barbiturate level — determines the concentration of barbiturates in the blood; salicylates may interfere with the test and alcohol ingestion may increase barbiturate levels; toxic levels vary depending on the barbiturate taken
• Serum antidepressant level — identifies and determines the concentration of antidepressant in the blood; toxic levels vary, depending on the antidepressant; for most tricyclic antidepressants, toxic level is greater than 1,000 ng/ml
• Abdominal X-rays — can reveal a mass of pills in the stomach
• Gastroscopy — may be performed to remove substances if X-rays reveal a coalesced mass of material that cannot be removed by lavage

Potential complications

See *Nurse's guide to common drug overdoses*, pages 152 and 153.

CLINICAL SNAPSHOT

DRUG OVERDOSE

Major nursing diagnoses and collaborative problems	Key patient outcomes
Ineffective airway clearance	Maintain a clear airway.
Risk for multiorgan dysfunction	Maintain vital organ function.
Hopelessness	Participate, as much as possible, in self-care and care planning.

NURSING DIAGNOSIS

Ineffective airway clearance related to reduced alertness, decreased or absent gag reflex, obstruction by tongue, vomiting, or lavage procedures

Nursing priority

Maintain a clear airway.

Patient outcome criteria

Throughout the hospital stay, the patient will:
• maintain a clear airway
• maintain a spontaneous respiratory rate of 12 to 24 breaths per minute or be placed on mechanical ventilation.

Interventions

1. Assess the patient's airway status continually by noting the adequacy of spontaneous respiratory efforts, chest excursion, breath sounds, gag reflex, skin color, and level of consciousness.

2. Place the patient in a side-lying position. Ensure that suction equipment is ready at the bedside.

3. If lavage is initiated, ensure airway protection by placing the patient in a head-down position; if the patient is sedated, assist with placement of a cuffed endotracheal tube.

4. If the patient's gag reflex is reduced or absent or if respirations are less than 12 or more than 24 per minute, shallow, or labored, anticipate and assist with endotracheal intubation and mechanical ventilation. See the "Mechanical ventilation" plan, page 283, for details.

5. Monitor ABG levels, as ordered. See Appendix B, Acid-Base Imbalances.

6. Additional individualized interventions: _____

Rationales

1. Initial and ongoing airway evaluation is essential in the patient who has taken a drug overdose because many medications cause CNS depression. If several medications were taken, their combined effects may further reduce the patient's ability to clear the airway.

2. The side-lying position makes drainage from the mouth easier and reduces the probability of aspiration. Suctioning may be needed if the patient vomits.

3. Aspiration of gastric contents may lead to aspiration pneumonitis, a complication associated with increased morbidity and mortality.

4. Toxic CNS effects may interfere with vital functions. Unless promptly corrected, respiratory impairment results in permanent damage to the brain and other organs.

5. Changes in ABG levels may provide early warning of impaired ventilatory status before clinical evidence is apparent. Also, toxic levels of many medications cause acid-base abnormalities; ABG studies serve as a guide for intervention.

6. Rationales: _____

COLLABORATIVE PROBLEM

Risk for multiorgan dysfunction related to systemic toxic drug effects

Nursing priorities
• Support and monitor vital organ functions.
• Identify and counteract drug effects.

Patient outcome criteria
• Within 1 hour of admission to the hospital, the patient will receive initial treatment for a specific drug overdose.
• Throughout the hospital stay, the patient will maintain vital organ functions.

Interventions

1. Collect as much information as possible about the overdose by questioning the patient, family, friends, and other caregivers. If possible, determine:
• what was taken
• how much was taken
• when the drug was taken
• how it was taken (for example, ingested or injected)
• whether there was also alcohol use
• if there are underlying health problems
• what other medications were taken
• what has been done for the patient so far.

Rationales

1. A thorough history may be difficult to obtain, but it provides vital clues for effective intervention and ongoing monitoring.

Neurologic disorders

2. Monitor vital signs, hemodynamic pressures, and electrocardiogram findings according to Appendix A, Monitoring Standards, or unit protocol.

3. Collaborate with the doctor and regional poison control center personnel in selecting and initiating measures to reverse or eliminate the drugs from the body (some measures may have already been implemented in the emergency department). Initiate one or more of the following, as appropriate:
• induced vomiting with ipecac syrup, 30 ml orally with 10 to 12 oz (300 to 350 ml) of fluids. Observe for onset of vomiting within 15 to 30 minutes. If no vomiting occurs, the dose may be repeated once. If the patient still does not vomit, consult the doctor and prepare for gastric lavage. Never administer ipecac if the patient has an absent gag reflex, signs of decreasing alertness, a history of seizures, or ingested corrosives. Consult with the poison control center before administering ipecac to a patient who has ingested a hydrocarbon or has taken an overdose of an antiemetic drug.

• gastric lavage, using a large-bore Ewald tube and normal saline solution or other ordered irrigant. Lavage with 100- to 200-ml fluid boluses and avoid overdistending the stomach. Lavage until return is clear, unless otherwise ordered, usually 1,000 to 1,500 ml total. Monitor inflow and outflow volumes and report discrepancies. Save aspirated fluid for analysis, as needed. Monitor serum electrolyte levels in conjunction with large-volume or prolonged lavage.

• dilution, usually with milk or water, unless the patient is obtunded.

• gut lavage, using a peristaltic pump to deliver warmed electrolyte solution to the stomach.
• activated charcoal, usually 25 to 50 g in a slurry, administered orally or via gastric tube after emesis or lavage is completed. Do not give charcoal at the same time as ipecac syrup.

• cathartics, as ordered, usually mixed with charcoal; cathartics ordered include magnesium sulfate and magnesium citrate.

2. At toxic levels, many drugs can interfere with the vasomotor center's control of cardiac function and blood vessel constriction. Baseline and ongoing assessment of these parameters provides early warning of cardiovascular dysfunction.

3. Since the institution of regional poison control centers, with their hot line consultative services, mortality from poisonings has fallen significantly. The poison control center provides expert advice on treating all types of drug overdoses.

• Ipecac syrup is thought to act both centrally and locally on the GI tract to stimulate vomiting. Fluids are given with ipecac because, without adequate gastric volume, esophageal injury may occur from forceful retching. Doses greater than 60 ml may have cardiotoxic effects. Ipecac administration is contraindicated if the patient's condition may result in aspiration. Also, vomiting of corrosives may cause or increase damage to esophageal and oropharyngeal mucosae. The treatment of hydrocarbon ingestion depends on the specific substance. Ipecac may not be effective if the patient has taken an overdose of antiemetic medication such as a phenothiazine.
• Gastric lavage is used when vomiting is contraindicated (for example, if the patient has a reduced or absent gag reflex). It effectively removes ingested substances from the stomach but is thought to be somewhat less effective than induced emesis. The choice of fluid is controversial and may depend on the drug ingested. Fluid boluses larger than 200 ml are thought to wash the toxin into the small bowel. A discrepancy between the amounts of instilled irrigant and returned fluid may indicate a need to reposition the patient to promote drainage or may indicate fluid reabsorption and the risk of fluid overload. The aspirate may be examined for diagnostic clues. Electrolyte imbalances and their cardiovascular sequelae may result from prolonged or large-volume lavage.
• Dilution is used primarily to treat ingestion of corrosives or other substances that preclude emesis. Distending the abdomen with fluid if the patient is not conscious may increase the risk of aspiration.
• This relatively new therapy may be used to aid clearance of certain herbicides from the bowel.
• Activated charcoal is an inert substance that adsorbs toxins. It should not be given at the same time as ipecac syrup because it will inactivate the ipecac and prevent emesis. Opinions vary on whether the charcoal should be removed after a given time or allowed to pass through the intestines.
• Saline cathartics stimulate peristaltic activity by drawing fluid into the bowel through osmosis, thus hastening drug excretion and reducing absorption from the gut.

• specific antidotes or antagonists, as ordered.

• other measures, as recommended by the doctor or poison control center, such as forced diuresis, peritoneal dialysis, hemodialysis, exchange transfusions, or gastroscopy.

4. Perform careful serial evaluations of level of consciousness, mental status, and gag and corneal reflex status every 1 to 2 hours during the first 24 hours or until the patient's condition stabilizes.

5. Monitor fluid intake and output and promptly report a dropping urine output (less than 60 ml/hour) to the doctor.

6. Assess and monitor initial or serial laboratory test findings, as ordered, for overdose substances.

7. Additional individualized interventions: _____

• A few drugs, notably narcotics and acetaminophen, are effectively treated with antidote-antagonist substances; however, because the patient may have taken more than one drug, close monitoring is still necessary.
• Forced diuresis may be used if the drug involved is excreted primarily through the urinary tract. Dialysis may help remove certain substances, but its effectiveness depends on the drug's pharmacologic properties and its distribution within body tissues. Exchange transfusions may be used for certain drugs if the dosage is massive and recent enough that tissue absorption has not yet taken place. Gastroscopy may be performed if abdominal X-rays reveal a coalesced mass of pills in the stomach.

4. Decreasing alertness and diminished or absent protective reflexes indicate CNS impairment and the likely need for airway management or ventilatory support. Serial evaluations allow early detection of subtle changes.

5. Because many medications are detoxified or excreted through the renal system, the possibility of renal failure from toxic effects must always be considered. Also, a dropping urine output is a clue to the early development of shock, another potential complication of drug toxicity

6. Specific initial and serial urine or serum studies provide information about the amount of drug taken and the rate of absorption, guiding treatment.

7. Rationales: _____

NURSING DIAGNOSIS

Hopelessness related to low self-esteem, emotional disorganization, or a sense of having inadequate resources to cope with life

Nursing priorities
• Promote a sense of hope.
• Foster self-esteem.

Patient outcome criteria

Before discharge from the unit, the patient will:
• discuss reasons for the overdose and identify precipitating factors
• participate as fully as possible in self-care and care planning
• begin to display healthy coping behaviors
• make contact with follow-up care providers.

Neurologic disorders

Interventions

1. Examine your attitudes toward suicide and drug abuse. Maintain a concerned but nonjudgmental attitude when providing care, avoiding all punishing behavior. If your feelings about suicide or drug abuse interfere with patient care, seek peer support or consult with a psychiatric liaison nurse.

2. Foster communication.

• Use touch, as appropriate.

• Use active listening skills.

• Note and acknowledge nonverbal cues (body posture and gestures, facial expression, tone of voice, and silences).
• Make eye contact.

3. Encourage the patient to participate in care-related decisions as soon as possible.

4. Arrange a referral to psychiatric resources (such as a psychiatric nurse specialist, psychiatrist, or other mental health professional). Place the patient on suicide precautions, if appropriate.

5. See the "Ineffective individual coping" plan, page 67, and the "Dying" plan, page 20.

6. Ensure appropriate follow-up care arrangements before discharge from the unit, including continuation of suicide precautions, if appropriate.

7. Additional individualized interventions: _____
_____

Rationales

1. Many health professionals have difficulty caring for a suicidal or self-abusive patient. Frustration and anger are common when the patient seems to be undermining the efforts of health care providers. Punishing attitudes, however, tend to further decrease the patient's already fragile self-esteem and reduce coping ability. The patient may interpret such behavior as "just one more sign I'm no good for anything," adding to self-directed anger and hopelessness. Peer or psychiatric liaison support can help professionals address and resolve issues raised by an abusive or noncompliant patient.

2. Commonly, the patient who has taken an overdose perceives a lack of personal resources or cannot communicate feelings because of emotional disorganization. Opening communication is the first step in identifying more positive responses to the problems that may have led to the overdose.
• Touch can convey profound messages of acceptance and caring and, for some patients, may be less threatening than verbal interaction as a way to initiate the therapeutic relationship.
• Active listening involves an attentive attitude, feedback, and rephrasing or reflection to help the patient clarify feelings and ideas. This reaffirms a sense of self-worth and the importance of feelings.
• Acknowledging nonverbal communication may help verify expressed feelings or open discussion of unexpressed feelings.
• Making eye contact in a nonthreatening manner expresses interest and the intent to communicate.

3. Considering the patient's stated wishes may, in many cases, be secondary to saving the patient's life. However, as the condition stabilizes, a return to participation in self-care helps bolster self-respect and reduces feelings of powerlessness.

4. Any patient admitted with an intentional overdose warrants psychiatric evaluation and counseling as part of the plan of treatment. Careful evaluation of suicide potential is essential. If suicidal ideation is present, suicide precautions are warranted.

5. The "Ineffective individual coping" plan contains interventions for patients struggling with emotional adjustments. The "Dying" plan addresses issues that may relate to the care of the patient who has attempted suicide.

6. The patient who has been severely depressed may try suicide again once physical energy has been restored and personal appearance seems improved. Careful follow-up, both on the unit to which the patient is transferred and after discharge from the hospital, is vital in helping the patient make the transition to everyday life.

7. Rationales: _____
_____

DISCHARGE PLANNING
Discharge checklist
Before discharge, the patient shows evidence of:
- [ ] spontaneous respirations and airway clearance
- [ ] stable vital signs for at least 12 hours
- [ ] completion of specific measures to remove or reverse drugs consumed
- [ ] drug levels (if applicable) declining since admission
- [ ] urine output greater than 60 ml/hour
- [ ] ABG values within normal limits
- [ ] initial psychiatric evaluation and follow-up arrangements made
- [ ] implementation of suicide precautions, if appropriate.

Teaching checklist
Document evidence that the patient and family demonstrate an understanding of:
- [ ] toxic effects of drugs and possible later complications
- [ ] the treatment measures undertaken
- [ ] the signs and symptoms of any potential complications
- [ ] healthy coping behaviors
- [ ] resources available for help.

Documentation checklist
Using outcome criteria as a guide, document:
- [ ] clinical status on admission
- [ ] significant changes in status
- [ ] pertinent laboratory and diagnostic test findings
- [ ] effectiveness of measures to promote elimination of drug or reversal of drug effects
- [ ] mental health measures
- [ ] suicide precautions, if used
- [ ] follow-up plans
- [ ] patient and family teaching
- [ ] discharge planning.

ASSOCIATED PLANS OF CARE
Acute renal failure
Dying
Grieving
Impaired physical mobility
Ineffective individual coping
Mechanical ventilation
Sensory-perceptual alteration

REFERENCES
Ayers, S.M., et al. *Textbook of Critical Care*, 3rd ed. Philadelphia: W.B. Saunders Co., 1995.
Clochesy, J.M., et al. *Critical Care Nursing*, 2nd ed. Philadelphia: W.B. Saunders Co., 1996.
Kitt, S., and Kaiser, J. *Emergency Nursing, A Physiologic and Clinical Perspective,* 2nd ed. Philadelphia: W.B. Saunders, Co., 1995.
Phipps, W.J., et al. *Medical-Surgical Nursing, Concepts and Clinical Practice,* 5th ed. St. Louis: Mosby–Year Book, Inc., 1995.
Thompson, J.M., et al. *Mosby's Clinical Nursing*, 4th ed. St. Louis: Mosby–Year Book, Inc., 1997.

Neurologic disorders

Guillain-Barré syndrome

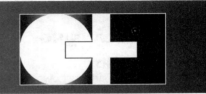

DRG information

DRG 018   Cranial and Peripheral Nerve Disorders
with Complication or Comorbidity (CC).
Mean LOS = 6.4 days
Principal diagnoses include:
- disorders of cranial or peripheral nerves
- mononeuritis of upper or lower limb
- neuritis or radiculitis of brachial or un-specified nerve
- various types of neuropathy (including Guillain-Barré syndrome)
- various types of polyneuropathy.

DRG 019   Cranial and Peripheral Nerve Disorders
without CC.
Mean LOS = 4.5 days
Principal diagnoses include select principal
diagnoses listed under DRG 018.

INTRODUCTION

Definition and time focus

Guillain-Barré syndrome, also known as acute idiopathic polyneuritis, Landry–Guillain-Barré–Strohl syndrome, and polyradiculoneuritis, is a demyelinating disorder affecting the peripheral nervous system. First described in 1859, it is diagnosed typically when the patient complains of sudden weakness or paralysis of the legs that progresses upward symmetrically. Its cause is unknown; however, the disorder may result from an autoimmune response in which sensitized lymphocytes infiltrate the peripheral nervous system and produce demyelination, edema, and inflammation. The destruction of the myelin sheath, which increases impulse transmission by allowing impulses to jump from node to node along the axon, results in slowed conduction or, if significant edema is present, complete blockage of impulse transmission.

Commonly, the disorder causes progressive loss of function over 2 to 3 weeks, at which time the patient may require ventilatory support because of respiratory paralysis. However, the symptoms are potentially reversible because the myelin sheath can regenerate; full recovery without residual deficits eventually occurs in 75% to 85% of cases. Complete recovery is slow and commonly takes 18 to 24 months from the onset of symptoms. This plan focuses on the patient who is admitted with a diagnosis of Guillain-Barré syndrome.

Etiology and precipitating factors

- Idiopathic origin
- Autoimmune factors (possible link)
- Immunizations (vaccinations for smallpox, tetanus, influenza, and measles have been implicated in the syndrome)
- Viral illnesses
- Immunosuppression (Hodgkin's disease and other lymphomas may increase risk)
- Previous surgery

FOCUSED ASSESSMENT GUIDELINES

Nursing history (functional health pattern findings)

Health perception–health management pattern
- Sudden, symmetric weakness of legs, increasing and moving upward over several days, and mild to moderate sensory changes, such as tingling and muscle pain
- Self-limiting, mild respiratory or GI illness 2 to 3 weeks before onset of symptoms
- Frequent paresthesia before onset of weakness, such as a "stocking-and-glove" numbness and tingling
- Difficulty speaking

Nutritional-metabolic pattern
- Dysphagia

Elimination pattern
- Retention of sphincter control; possible incontinence with autonomic nervous system (ANS) involvement

Activity-exercise pattern
- Leg weakness or paralysis that progresses upward to the trunk, arms, and head (common)
- Arms affected first (uncommon)
- Injuries from falling
- Shortness of breath
- Easy fatigability (uncommon)

Cognitive-perceptual pattern
- Pain, a tingling "pins and needles" sensation, or numbness in arms and legs
- Altered sense of position

Coping–stress tolerance pattern
- Extreme anxiety over progression of symptoms

Self-perception–self-concept pattern
- Feelings of helplessness
- Anxiety about his role and responsibilities

Physical findings
Cardiovascular
- Hypotension or, more commonly, hypertension (if ANS involved)
- Tachyarrhythmias or bradyarrhythmias (if ANS involved)

Pulmonary
- Diminished breath sounds
- Difficulty clearing secretions
- Shallow respirations
- Use of accessory muscles

Neurologic
- Diminished or absent deep tendon reflexes
- Symmetrical paralysis or paresis
- Loss of position and vibration sense
- Cranial nerve abnormalities, most commonly cranial nerve VII (facial); others, in order of frequency, include VI (abducens), III (oculomotor), XII (hypoglossal), V (trigeminal), and IX (glossopharyngeal); abnormalities can produce facial paralysis, dysphagia, ptosis, diplopia, deviated tongue, loss of gag and cough reflexes, and difficulty chewing, swallowing, or talking

Gastrointestinal or renal
- Occasional urine or fecal retention or incontinence (if ANS involved)

Musculoskeletal
- Ascending weakness or flaccid paralysis of arms and legs
- Tenderness on deep palpation of leg or arm muscles

Integumentary
- Warm, flushed skin
- Cold, clammy skin if ANS involved
- Occasional anhidrosis if ANS involved

Diagnostic studies
Diagnosis of Guillain-Barré syndrome is based primarily on clinical findings and progression of symptoms; although no specific diagnostic tests exist, studies may include the following:

- routine blood studies — may reveal no significant abnormalities
- lumbar puncture — reveals classic findings of albuminocytologic dissociation (elevated protein level of more than 45 mg/dl and a normal white blood cell count of 5 to 10/μl); serial punctures commonly are performed to monitor the disease course; cerebrospinal fluid protein level may be elevated until 1 to 2 weeks after onset of symptoms
- electromyography studies — reveal denervated areas; recordings show repetitive firing of single units, rather than normal sectional activity (may not appear until 2 weeks after onset of symptoms)
- nerve conduction velocity tests — reveal marked reduction in conduction speed
- pulmonary function studies — provide baseline data for evaluating degree of respiratory impairment; usually, decreased vital capacity (less than 20 ml/kg) is revealed

Potential complications
- Respiratory failure (occurs in about 25% of patients)
- Thrombophlebitis
- Pulmonary embolus
- Ileus
- Gastric dilation
- Atelectasis
- Pneumonia
- Skin breakdown
- Urinary tract stones and infection
- GI bleeding
- Septicemia
- Autonomic dysfunction and arrhythmias
- Muscle atrophy
- Ineffective coping
- Syndrome of inappropriate antidiuretic hormone secretion
- Nosocomial infection

Neurologic disorders

CLINICAL SNAPSHOT

GUILLAIN-BARRÉ SYNDROME

Major nursing diagnoses and collaborative problems	Key patient outcomes
Risk for respiratory failure	Maintain arterial blood gas (ABG) levels within normal limits.
Impaired physical mobility	Display no complications of impaired mobility, such as thromboembolism or pneumonia.
Risk for nutritional deficit	Eat without aspirating, if able to tolerate oral food.
Powerlessness	Participate in making choices about care.

COLLABORATIVE PROBLEM

Risk for respiratory failure related to weakness or paralysis of respiratory muscles

Nursing priority

Maintain adequate ventilatory status.

Patient outcome criteria

- On admission, the patient will have a clear airway.
- Within 4 hours of admission, the patient will have:
  - clear breath sounds
  - regular respirations
  - bilaterally equal chest excursion
  - partial pressure of oxygen (PO_2) greater than 70 mm Hg; partial pressure of carbon dioxide (PCO_2) of 35 to 45 mm Hg.

Interventions

1. Assess airway patency, breath sounds, respiratory rate and effort, ability to count slowly from 1 to 10, skin color, chest excursion, forced vital capacity (FVC) and maximum inspiratory force at least every 2 hours. Immediately report dyspnea, tachypnea, increasing restlessness, increasing use of diaphragmatic and accessory muscles, cyanosis, decreased breath sounds, shallow or irregular respirations, FVC of less than 15 ml/kg, a maximum inspiratory force of less than 20 cm H_2O, or reduced respiratory effort.

2. Encourage hourly coughing and deep breathing, and assist with pulmonary hygiene measures (postural drainage, percussion, and incentive spirometry). Monitor carefully for development of fever, crackles, or areas of consolidation.

3. Prepare to assist with endotracheal intubation or tracheotomy if FVC falls below 15 ml/kg, maximum expiratory force is less than 20 cm H_2O, the patient's speech becomes nasal, or the patient cannot clear secretions.

4. Use pulse oximetry to monitor oxygen saturation continuously or as needed. Obtain and monitor ABG values, as ordered. Report changes or abnormal findings promptly.

Rationales

1. Respiratory failure can occur subtly but rapidly in Guillain-Barré patients, and about 25% develop significant pulmonary problems. As muscular paralysis ascends, the phrenic nerve may become involved, affecting diaphragmatic excursion and impairing the patient's ability to maintain an adequate tidal volume and clear secretions from the airway.

2. Reduced ventilatory capacity and resultant stasis of secretions may lead to atelectasis or pneumonia. Pulmonary hygiene measures help promote airway clearance. Coughing may lead to microatelectasis from the associated increase in intrathoracic pressure if not followed by deep breathing to reexpand collapsed alveoli.

3. Because these findings indicate a high risk of respiratory failure, endotracheal intubation should take place before it occurs. Intubation can be indicated simply to protect or clear the airway, but it also allows the patient to receive positive-pressure mechanical ventilation quickly during the acute phase of the disorder.

4. Ventilatory support is indicated if the patient's PCO_2 increases 10 to 15 mm Hg or if the PO_2 decreases 10 to 15 mm Hg (or parameters established on admission) compared with normal ranges. ABG values help in the assessment of respiratory status. Pulse oximetry provides ongoing monitoring without invasive procedures.

5. Suction as necessary, hyperinflating and hyperoxygenating with 100% oxygen before and after suctioning. Observe for a vasovagal response during suctioning.

5. Careful suctioning can help avert mucus plugs or pulmonary infection from secretion stasis. Also, suctioning may be required because of facial or glossopharyngeal nerve involvement, which may cause drooling and impaired swallowing. Hyperinflation and hyperoxygenation are essential because lower oxygen levels are common with impaired respiratory effort, and suctioning further depletes the oxygen supply. ANS dysfunction in Guillain-Barré syndrome is linked to a vagal nerve (cranial nerve X) deficit. Hypoxia and vagal stimulation that can occur with suctioning can cause severe bradycardia or cardiac arrest. If oxygenation does not abolish the reflex, treat with I.V. atropine, as ordered.

6. Every 1 to 2 hours, monitor vital signs and neurologic status, including level of consciousness, muscle strength, and the ability to gag, cough, and swallow. Also monitor hemodynamic parameters and electrocardiography findings according to Appendix A, Monitoring Standards, or unit protocol. Assess for and immediately report the onset of sweating, flushing, altered vital signs, or arrhythmias. If life-threatening arrhythmias are present, institute appropriate pharmacologic treatment according to unit protocol.

6. Bradycardia, tachycardia, or blood pressure alterations may indicate hypoxemia or ANS involvement. Reduced cranial reflex responses, lethargy, or drowsiness may indicate increased carbon dioxide retention from respiratory insufficiency. Sweating, flushing, or arrhythmias may indicate ANS involvement. Vagus nerve involvement may be responsible for life-threatening arrhythmias.

7. When muscles of the upper arms or shoulders or changes in swallowing indicate reduced function, watch closely for respiratory changes.

7. These areas are commonly affected just before muscles used in respiration; dysfunction may herald impending respiratory problems.

8. If mechanical ventilation is required, maintain ventilator settings and monitor ABG levels. Teach the patient and family about ventilator use and alarm systems. Reassure the patient and family that mechanical ventilation is usually temporary and that independent breathing should return when the patient's condition improves. See the "Mechanical ventilation" plan, page 283.

8. Ventilator settings should correlate with current ABG levels and status. The patient and family may be extremely anxious over the use of and need for mechanical ventilation. Careful explanations may decrease fear and minimize the patient fighting against the effects of the ventilator. The "Mechanical ventilation" plan provides details regarding care of the patient on a ventilator.

9. Additional individualized interventions: _____
_____

9. Rationales: _____
_____

NURSING DIAGNOSIS

Impaired physical mobility related to slowed or absent conduction of motor nerve impulses, resulting in weakness or flaccid paralysis

Nursing priority

Prevent complications associated with immobility.

Neurologic disorders

Patient outcome criteria

- On admission and continuously, the patient will:
  - have intact skin
  - have normal eye lubrication or receive protective measures.
- Within 3 days of admission, the patient will:
  - have a bowel movement
  - receive regular active or passive range-of-motion exercise, as condition allows.
- As function returns, the patient will:
  - show no exacerbation of condition
  - suffer no accidental injuries.

Interventions

1. See the "Impaired physical mobility" plan, page 50, for detailed interventions regarding positioning, range-of-motion exercises, skin care, infection prevention and treatment, elimination aids, and promotion of circulation.

2. Caution the patient and family in handling arms and legs; they should be aware of the risks of pressure, temperature and, as function returns, overexertion and fatigue.

3. Administer corticosteroids or corticotropin, if ordered. Monitor closely for signs and symptoms of gastric irritation, edema, hypokalemia, hyperglycemia, or other adverse effects. Be aware that steroid use may mask signs and symptoms of underlying infection.

4. Prepare the patient for plasmapheresis, if ordered. For the patient undergoing plasmapheresis, monitor for complications: trauma or infection at the site of vascular access; hypovolemia; hypokalemia and hypocalcemia; and temporary circumoral and distal extremity paresthesia, muscle twitching, and nausea and vomiting related to the administration of citrated plasma.

5. Provide eye care, including use of artificial tears and eye protectors, as needed.

Rationales

1. The "Impaired physical mobility" plan contains interventions for preventing complications associated with prolonged immobility. The patient with Guillain-Barré syndrome is at increased risk for such immobility-related problems as infections, thromboembolic phenomena, joint contractures, muscle atrophy, skin breakdown, constipation or ileus, and urinary calculi. Preventive and therapeutic measures for these complications are essential in the care of the patient with Guillain-Barré syndrome. Frequent changes of position may also help reduce pain caused by the disease or immobility.

2. Reduced sensory capabilities associated with nerve dysfunction may cause the patient to be unaware of impending or actual injury. When function begins to return, the patient must resume activities slowly so that overexertion does not exacerbate symptoms.

3. Steroid use to reduce the inflammatory reaction that impairs mobility is controversial. Adverse reactions may outweigh potential benefits, so if such medication is ordered, monitor carefully. Corticotropin may shorten the syndrome's duration in some cases, but its use is still being investigated.

4. Plasmapheresis has been shown to have possible benefit in chronic relapsing or progressive Guillain-Barré syndrome. Although the reason for the benefit is unknown, the procedure may remove antimyelin antibodies that are linked to the development of the disorder, possibly shortening the disease course. However, neither this nor any other treatment has been proven to have direct therapeutic effects, so monitoring and support remain the primary interventions.

5. Trigeminal nerve impairment may cause the loss of corneal sensation. Facial nerve involvement commonly affects eyelid function.

6. Early in the hospital stay, provide assistance with physical activities and teach the patient to use splints and assistive devices, as needed. As soon as possible, encourage the patient to resume normal activities, beginning by assuming the upright position with the use of a tilt table or bed adjustment. Arrange a referral to a physical therapist, and supervise coordination of the activity program.

7. Additional individualized interventions: _____

6. Early activity and proper positioning prevent contractures and injuries from disuse. Gradually resuming an upright position helps regain vascular tone and diminishes the orthostatic hypotension that can result from the venous pooling associated with bed rest. Function may return asymmetrically, predisposing the patient to falls, back problems, or other injuries. A physical therapist can provide expert guidance in planning rehabilitation.

7. Rationales: _____

Nursing diagnosis

Risk for nutritional deficit related to dysphagia, depression, tracheostomy, or mechanical ventilation

Nursing priority

Provide adequate nutrition.

Patient outcome criteria

By the time of discharge, the patient will:
• be receiving optimal nutritional intake, as reflected by stable weight (plus or minus 2 or 3 lb [0.9 to 1.4 kg] per week)
• eat without aspirating, if able to tolerate oral food intake.

Interventions

1. See the "Nutritional deficit" plan, page 80.

2. Before the patient eats, assess the patient's gag reflex, ability to swallow, and motor and sensory function of upper extremities; note signs of facial paralysis.

3. If oral intake is tolerated, use techniques to help minimize choking and aspiration:
• elevate the patient's head and flex the neck while swallowing
• have suction equipment at hand and supervise the patient closely during meals
• provide semisolid foods; avoid liquids initially; allow the patient to make choices about diet when possible.

4. Administer enteral and parenteral feedings as ordered during the acute phase of illness. If enteral feedings are used, check for residual every 4 hours or before each feeding, and maintain the patient in a sitting position or with the head of the bed elevated during and for 1 hour after feeding.

5. Additional individualized interventions: _____

Rationales

1. The "Nutritional deficit" plan contains interventions for assessment and support of the patient with a potential nutritional deficit.

2. If the disease affects cranial nerves V (trigeminal), VII (facial), IX (glossopharyngeal), X (vagus), or XII (hypoglossal), the patient will have difficulty chewing and swallowing and will not have a gag reflex. Aspiration can occur easily if the patient attempts to eat or is fed orally.

3. Cranial nerve involvement may cause dysphagia; when the patient takes food by mouth before and after acute phase of illness, care is needed to avoid aspiration. Permitting choices, when possible, helps the patient maintain or regain a sense of self-control.

4. Adequate nutrition minimizes muscle wasting, maintains the body's defenses against infection, maintains skin integrity, and promotes healing. During the acute phase, dysphagia may be too severe to safely permit oral intake. Precautions must be taken with enteral feedings to prevent regurgitation and aspiration of feedings.

5. Rationales: _____

Neurologic disorders

Nursing diagnosis

Powerlessness related to rapidly progressing symptoms, altered communication, dependency on others for basic needs, and fear of death

Nursing priority

Maintain psychological equilibrium.

Patient outcome criteria

- Within 2 hours of admission, the patient will:
  - have an effective communication method
  - rate pain as less than 3 on a 0 to 10 pain rating scale.
- Within 24 hours of admission, the patient will:
  - participate in making choices about care
  - begin expressing feelings
  - display reduced anxiety and fear as evidenced by a relaxed expression.

Interventions

1. See the "Ineffective individual coping" plan, page 67.

2. Provide frequent, factual explanations about the condition, emphasizing the temporary, potentially reversible nature of the disorder. Prepare the patient and family for potential problems of the acute phase. Point out any small improvements in the patient's condition as they occur. Encourage family members to participate in care.

3. If the patient's ability to communicate is impaired, arrange for use of signals (eye blinks or motion-sensor call devices) or use a writing tablet or word board. Anticipate needs; be sensitive to nonverbal cues such as facial expression. Reassure the patient his needs will be met. Place a call button that is easy to push within the patient's reach.

4. Encourage the use of relaxation and stress-control techniques. Emphasize that proficient use of such techniques may benefit the patient even after the disorder has resolved. As appropriate assist and teach the patient about:
- progressive relaxation
- guided imagery
- "thought stopping" and positive affirmation
- meditation.

5. Whenever possible, encourage the patient to make choices regarding care and involve the family in care planning.

Rationales

1. The "Ineffective individual coping" plan provides interventions helpful in caring for the patient and family experiencing illness-related disorganization.

2. Depression and hopelessness are common emotional responses to the sudden losses caused by Guillain-Barré syndrome. Preparatory teaching may reduce panic as the acute phase progresses. Maintaining hope and providing encouragement throughout the extended course of the illness is an essential part of nursing care, especially because the patient usually remains alert and oriented despite functional deficits. Family participation in care provides tangible support for the patient.

3. Paralysis of the facial nerve (VII), paralysis of the extremities, and intubation alter the patient's ability to communicate. This inability to communicate can be terrifying. Providing the patient with some means of signaling helps reduce anxiety.

4. The patient who cannot do anything physically may still find comfort in psychological self-help. Learning and practicing such techniques helps the patient maintain control and a sense of active participation in recovery. Relaxation techniques have been shown to avoid many stress-related health problems.

5. The debilitating nature of Guillain-Barré syndrome promotes dependency and helplessness. Allowing some choices, even in small matters, increases the patient's sense of self-control and reduces powerlessness.

6. Encourage the patient and family to express their feelings. Cultivate an attitude of acceptance. If manipulative or dysfunctional behavior occurs, try to provide the patient with increased control and choices. Encourage family members to talk to the patient, even if the patient cannot respond. Refer the patient to a mental health professional, if appropriate.

6. The losses caused by Guillain-Barré syndrome and their long-term effects on the patient's life will cause normal reactions of anger, depression, grieving, and even paranoia. Acceptance of feelings aids in developing healthy coping behavior. Manipulative behavior can be an attempt to regain a sense of control. Although motor function is impaired, the patient can still hear and understand verbal communication. A mental health professional can provide long-term supportive therapy.

7. Provide appropriate referrals to social services staff or other agencies, as needed.

7. The sudden transition from healthy, working adult to hopeless, disabled patient is frightening enough, but the patient may have additional worries about income, child care, or other arrangements. Providing referrals promptly may lessen anxiety about such problems.

8. Provide pain-relief measures, as needed, with non-narcotic analgesics as ordered, supportive repositioning, and alternative pain-control techniques. See the "Pain" plan, page 88, for details.

8. Patients with Guillain-Barré syndrome may experience varying degrees of limb pain or uncomfortable paresthesia. Unrelieved pain decreases coping ability and adds to the patient's physiologic stress. The "Pain" plan contains interventions that apply to any patient in pain.

9. After the patient is physiologically stable, attempt to create a more normal environment; for instance, let the patient watch television and suggest to the family that they bring in flowers and personal items from home.

9. A normal environment reinforces improvement and decreases the depersonalizing effects of the hospital setting.

10. Additional individualized interventions: _____

10. Rationales: _____

_____

_____

Discharge planning

Discharge checklist
Before discharge, the patient shows evidence of:
- ❏ spontaneous respiration
- ❏ effective airway clearance
- ❏ FVC and maximum inspiratory force within normal limits
- ❏ stable vital signs within normal limits for the patient
- ❏ ABG measurements within normal limits
- ❏ effective communication ability.

Teaching checklist
Document evidence that the patient and family demonstrate an understanding of:
- ❏ the nature and progression of the syndrome and the expected prognosis
- ❏ signs and symptoms of possible exacerbation
- ❏ relaxation and stress-reduction measures
- ❏ activity programs and the use of assistive devices
- ❏ safety precautions
- ❏ name, dosage, purpose, and adverse effects of prescribed medications
- ❏ the need for periods of uninterrupted rest
- ❏ the need for adequate nutrition and fluids

- ❏ the need for exercise as tolerated
- ❏ the need for rehabilitation therapy.

Documentation checklist
Using outcome criteria as a guide, document:
- ❏ clinical status on admission
- ❏ significant changes in status
- ❏ pertinent laboratory and diagnostic test findings
- ❏ respiratory support measures
- ❏ nutritional status
- ❏ measures to prevent complications of immobility
- ❏ communication measures
- ❏ relaxation and stress-reduction teaching
- ❏ activity progression
- ❏ patient and family teaching
- ❏ discharge planning
- ❏ referral to a support group.

Associated plans of care
Dying
Grieving
Impaired physical mobility
Ineffective family coping: Compromised
Ineffective individual coping

Neurologic disorders

Knowledge deficit
Mechanical ventilation
Nutritional deficit
Pain
Sensory-perceptual alteration

REFERENCES

Hickey, J.V. *The Clinical Practice of Neurological and Neurosurgical Nursing*, 4th ed. Philadelphia: Lippincott-Raven Pubs., 1997.

Hund, E.F., et al. "Intensive Management and Treatment of Severe Guillain-Barré Syndrome," *Critical Care Medicine* 21(3):433-43, March 1993.

Lewis, S.M., et al. *Medical-Surgical Nursing Assessment and Management of Clinical Problems*, 4th ed. St Louis: Mosby–Year Book, Inc., 1996.

Roberts, S. L. *Critical Care Nursing: Assessment and Intervention*. Stamford, Conn.: Appleton & Lange, 1996.

Ruppert, S.D., et al. *Dolan's Critical Care Nursing, Clinical Management through the Nursing Process*, 2nd ed. Philadelphia: F.A. Davis Co., 1996.

Smeltzer, S.C., and Bare, B.G. *Brunner and Suddarth's Textbook of Medical-Surgical Nursing*, 8th ed. Philadelphia: Lippincott-Raven, Pubs., 1996.

Tilkian, S.M., et al. *Clinical and Nursing Implications of Laboratory Tests*, 5th ed. St. Louis: Mosby–Year Book, Inc., 1996.

Increased intracranial pressure

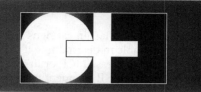

DRG information

Increased intracranial pressure (ICP) is a sign of an underlying problem and not a condition in and of itself in terms of coding guidelines. The DRG assigned for increased ICP depends entirely on the underlying cause that requires hospitalization, such as hemorrhage, hematoma, head trauma, abscess, or radiation. The length of stay depends entirely on the principal diagnosis.

INTRODUCTION

Definition and time focus

Increased ICP occurs when the components of the intracranial cavity — brain tissue, cerebral blood volume, and cerebrospinal fluid (CSF) — exceed the cavity's compensatory capacity. The volume of these three components usually remains relatively constant, with a normal ICP of 0 to 15 mm Hg.

Autoregulatory mechanisms in the brain compensate for volume changes of the contents, so an increase in one component is counteracted by a decrease in another. These mechanisms include displacement of CSF from the cranial cavity to the subarachnoid space surrounding the spinal cord (the primary compensatory mechanism), increased CSF reabsorption, and the reduction of cerebral blood volume by compression of the venous system, displacing venous blood from the intracranial cavity into the systemic circulation. Displacement of brain tissue without concurrent decompensation is extremely limited and occurs primarily with a slowly expanding mass, such as a tumor or chronic subdural hematoma.

When these autoregulatory mechanisms can no longer compensate for changes in the components of the intracranial cavity, increased ICP results. When ICP is sufficiently elevated to reduce cerebral perfusion pressure, irreversible brain damage may occur. This plan focuses on the critically ill patient with acutely increased ICP.

Etiology and precipitating factors

• Increased brain volume (caused by intracranial hemorrhage or hematoma, cerebral edema caused by surgical or head trauma, rapidly growing tumors, abscess, metabolic coma, radiation, chemotherapeutic agents, infarction, and anoxic events)

• Increased cerebral blood volume (from loss of autoregulation; hyperthermia; vasodilation caused by hypoxemia, hypercapnia, anesthetic agents, or narcotics; venous outflow obstruction caused by compression of the internal jugular veins or intrathoracic or intraabdominal pressure; fluctuations above a mean arterial pressure [MAP] of 160 mm Hg or below 60 mm Hg)
• Obstruction of CSF outflow (because of hematomas in the posterior fossa; brain shift and herniation; or impaired reabsorption from the subarachnoid space caused by inflammation of the meninges either by subarachnoid hemorrhage or infection, or obstruction of arachnoid villi by blood cells or bacteria)

FOCUSED ASSESSMENT GUIDELINES

Nursing history (functional health pattern findings)

Health perception–health management pattern

• Sudden change in level of consciousness, ranging from flattening of affect to coma; possible loss of consciousness for less than 24 hours
• History of head trauma resulting from a motor vehicle accident, fall, assault, gunshot or stab wound, or recreational accident; males between ages 15 and 24 are at an increased risk because of this group's higher incidence of head injury from motor vehicle accidents
• History of infection, particularly in middle ear, mastoid cells, or paranasal sinuses
• History of receiving anesthetics, narcotics, radiation, or chemotherapeutic drugs
• History of hypoxia from hypoventilation, apnea, chest trauma, pneumonia, or ventilation-perfusion abnormalities

Nutritional-metabolic pattern

• Vomiting (uncommon); if present, it is not preceded by nausea

Cognitive-perceptual pattern

• Headache (uncommon); if present, it is worse on arising in the morning; straining or movement may increase the pain.

Self-perception–self-concept pattern

• Anxiety or apprehension if the patient is alert enough to understand that something abnormal is happening

Physical findings

Many of the classic signs and symptoms of increased ICP now are considered indicators of brain shift and brain stem dysfunction. Clinical signs and symptoms alone are not reliable in determining if ICP is elevated, in detecting early increased ICP, or in determining the severity of increased ICP. Frequent neurologic assessment and ICP monitoring are the most reliable methods for detecting early deterioration.

Neurologic
Early findings
- Decreasing level of consciousness (most sensitive indicator of increased ICP), indicated by such signs as confusion, restlessness, or lethargy
- Pupillary abnormalities, with the pupil dilating gradually and becoming slightly ovoid and sluggish in the eye ipsilateral to the cause of the increased ICP
- Visual deficits, such as decreased visual acuity, blurred vision, diplopia, and changes in extraocular eye movements
- Motor weakness (monoparesis or hemiparesis) contralateral to the cause of increased ICP

Later findings
- Coma
- Pupillary abnormalities, including dilated and nonreactive (fixed) ipsilateral pupil; with herniation, pupils become bilaterally fixed and dilated
- Loss of deep tendon reflexes
- Hemiplegia and abnormal posturing (sometimes termed *decorticate* or *decerebrate posturing*), which may be unilateral or bilateral; as death approaches, the patient becomes bilaterally flaccid
- Babinski's positive sign
- Hyperthermia from hypothalamic injury
- Loss of brain stem reflexes, including corneal, oculocephalic (doll's eyes), and oculovestibular reflexes (the oculovestibular reflex is not as readily compromised as the oculocephalic and is a more sensitive indicator of any remaining brain stem function); gag, cough, and swallowing reflexes also are lost
- Papilledema (rarely); more common with chronically increased ICP

Cardiovascular
Later findings
- Cushing's reflex (compensatory mechanism to provide adequate cerebral perfusion pressure [CPP]) — rising systolic blood pressure, widening pulse pressure, and bradycardia (Cushing's triad); full, bounding pulse

Pulmonary
- Irregular respirations, commonly in patterns that relate to the level of brain dysfunction; Cheyne-Stokes respirations, central neurogenic hyperventilation, and ataxia are common in later stage of increased ICP; may be difficult to assess with the mechanically ventilated patient

Gastrointestinal
- Vomiting (uncommon); if present, not preceded by nausea

Diagnostic studies
Although no laboratory test for diagnosing increased ICP exists, tests may include the following:
- arterial blood gas (ABG) measurements — used to monitor the patient's acid-base balance and to detect hypoxemia and hypercapnia, which increase ICP
- complete blood count — may reveal elevated white blood cell (WBC) count, which may signify the beginning of an infection or abscess
- electrolyte panel — used to monitor the patient's fluid status and potassium and sodium levels; sodium is retained during stressful events and potassium is lost; sodium and potassium levels also are altered in diabetes insipidus (DI) and syndrome of inappropriate antidiuretic hormone secretion (SIADH), two abnormalities that may occur with increased ICP
- serum creatinine, blood urea nitrogen (BUN) levels — used to monitor renal function, particularly if osmotic diuretics are administered
- blood glucose test — used to monitor for hyperglycemia if dexamethasone (Decadron) therapy is used
- serum osmolality — used to monitor for hyperosmolality when mannitol therapy is used and aids in establishing a diagnosis of DI or SIADH
- urine specific gravity — may indicate DI if low or SIADH if high
- urine glucose and acetone levels — may reveal glucose in the urine, which may be an adverse reaction to dexamethasone therapy
- computed tomography (CT) scan — can differentiate among many conditions that cause increased ICP. It clearly outlines ventricles and shows size and position in relation to midline structures. CT scan is useful in diagnosing cerebral edema, hematomas caused by intracranial bleeding, abscesses, cerebral infarctions, and tumors. Serial scanning is useful in a deteriorating patient or one who does not improve as rapidly as expected. It may show intracranial hematomas in a patient whose initial CT scan was normal.
- skull X-rays — useful in detecting linear and depressed skull fractures; may demonstrate intracranial shifts. A high incidence of developing masses and intracranial hemorrhage occurs with linear fractures. Skull X-rays should be considered when the patient has an altered level of consciousness any time after injury, focal neurologic signs, or CSF discharge from the nose or ears.
- cerebral echoencephalography — may be used if a CT scan is not available. It is useful in detecting shifts of normally midline structures but is not reliable in detecting generalized cerebral edema that does not produce a midline shift.
- cerebral angiography — may be used if a CT scan is not available. It can reveal space-occupying lesions, such as subdural or epidural hematoma, and cerebral

edema. Because cerebral angiography is an invasive study, the CT scan is preferred.
• magnetic resonance imaging—gives clearer images of soft tissues than a CT scan and can detect brain edema, hemorrhage, infarction, and blood vessel disruptions more clearly. At this time, it has limited usefulness for a patient with increased ICP because it cannot be used on a patient whose care requires use of such metal devices as electrocardiogram electrodes, or a patient who is on mechanical ventilation.
• ICP monitoring—may reveal values of 15 to 40 mm Hg, indicating moderately elevated ICP, or 40 mm Hg or greater, indicating severely elevated ICP
• electrocardiography (ECG)—useful in assessing changes, such as the development of tall T waves in early increased ICP that become progressively flatter or inverted with an ICP greater than 45 mm Hg. ST-segment changes occur with transient changes in ICP and return to normal with the return of ICP to previous levels. Low levels of increased ICP produce abnormally shortened QT intervals; prolonged QT intervals occur with ICP greater 65 mm Hg.

Potential complications
• Brain herniation
• Permanent neurologic deficits
• Seizures
• Pneumonia
• Atelectasis
• GI ulceration and hemorrhage
• Infection
• DI
• SIADH
• Neurogenic pulmonary edema

CLINICAL SNAPSHOT

INCREASED INTRACRANIAL PRESSURE

Major nursing diagnoses and collaborative problems	Key patient outcomes
Risk for cerebral ischemia	Demonstrate improved neurologic function.
Risk for infection	Display no indications of infection.
Risk for increased cerebral metabolism	Maintain a normal temperature.
Risk for respiratory failure	Have a normal respiratory rate and pattern.
Risk for fluid volume deficit or excess	Maintain urine output, serum osmolality, electrolyte and BUN levels, and hematocrit within normal limits.
Risk for injury	Remain free from additional injury.

Neurologic disorders

COLLABORATIVE PROBLEM
Risk for cerebral ischemia related to fluctuations in arterial blood pressure, stressful events, nursing activities, hypoxemia, or hypercapnia

Nursing priority
Minimize fluctuations in cerebral perfusion pressure.

Patient outcome criteria
• Within 72 hours of admission, the patient will:
  – have an ICP of 0 to 15 mm Hg and a CPP greater than 60 mm Hg
  – have an MAP greater than 60 mm Hg
  – display no clinical signs of increased ICP and herniation.
• Within 1 week of admission, the patient will demonstrate improved neurologic status.

Interventions

1. Assess the patient's level of consciousness, behavior, motor and sensory function, pupillary reactions (size, position, and reactivity), and respiratory patterns every 1 to 2 hours and as necessary.

2. Monitor ICP (if an ICP monitoring device is in place) and MAP continually and compare readings to a desirable level. Document every hour or as changes occur. Calculate CPP as changes occur (see Appendix A, Monitoring Standards).

3. Maintain MAP at a level that will result in a CPP of 60 mm Hg or more.

• If pharmacologic support of blood pressure is needed, administer dopamine hydrochloride (Intropin) or other vasopressors, as ordered.
• If systemic hypertension is present, titrate fluid restriction, vasodilator administration, or other therapies according to CPP, as ordered.

4. Monitor ABG levels as ordered. Maintain ABG levels within prescribed parameters, typically partial pressure of arterial oxygen (PaO_2) greater than 80 mm Hg and partial pressure of arterial carbon dioxide ($PaCO_2$) between 28 and 32 mm Hg.

5. Use an ICP monitoring device to observe ICP levels, particularly during activities that are known to cause sustained increases in ICP, such as suctioning, moving the patient, emotional upsets, noxious stimuli, arousal from sleep, coughing, sneezing, or Valsalva's maneuver.

6. Instruct the alert patient to avoid the following activities: straining at stool, holding breath while moving or turning in bed, coughing, nose blowing, and extreme hip flexion (90 degrees or more).

Rationales

1. Changes in any of these parameters may indicate a deterioration in the patient's neurologic condition. The level of consciousness is the most sensitive and reliable indicator of increasing ICP. A change in respiratory patterns, also a sensitive indicator of increased ICP, is an early indicator of hypoxemia or hypercapnia, which also lead to increased ICP.

2. ICP indicates how well the three components of the intracranial cavity are balanced. CPP is the blood pressure gradient across the brain and is calculated as the difference between the incoming MAP and the opposing mean ICP (CPP = MAP–ICP). Alterations in either MAP or intracranial volume affect CPP and the integrity of brain tissue. A CPP of at least 60 mm Hg must be maintained to provide a minimally adequate blood supply to the brain. A CPP of less than 30 mm Hg results in cell death and is fatal.

3. Blood pressure must be maintained to ensure adequate CPP. Between a MAP of 60 and 160 mm Hg, the brain automatically regulates blood vessel diameter to maintain constant cerebral blood flow (CBF) and thus CPP. If the autoregulatory mechanism is lost, CBF and cerebral blood volume passively depend on the blood pressure and CPP so that hypotensive episodes provoke ischemia, whereas hypertensive bursts push fluid into the brain.
• An increase in systemic hypotension worsens cerebral ischemia and necrosis.

• Treating hypertension may be difficult because blood pressure already may be elevated as a compensatory mechanism for ischemia. Usually, blood pressure is lowered only after ICP is controlled. CPP is considered the best guide for gauging the effects of therapies to control systemic hypertension in a patient with increased ICP.

4. Hypoxemia (PaO_2 less than 60 mm Hg) and hypercapnia ($PaCO_2$ greater than 45 mm Hg) have a potent vasodilatory effect on cerebral vessels and increase CBF and ICP. Keeping the patient well-oxygenated and slightly hypocapnic helps limit CBF and therefore helps control ICP.

5. Clinical symptoms of increased ICP are not always present, even when a substantial increase in pressure occurs. By maintaining an awareness of activities that produce spikes in ICP and by monitoring ICP levels, you can modify or terminate these activities as ICP increases.

6. These activities increase intrathoracic and intra-abdominal pressure, which is transmitted to the jugular veins, impeding cerebral venous return and increasing ICP.

7. Instruct the alert patient to avoid pushing the feet against a footboard or the arms against the bed.

7. These activities produce isometric muscle contractions, which increase muscle tension without lengthening the muscle. These contractions elevate systemic blood pressure and result in increased ICP.

8. Administer pharmacologic agents, as ordered, for shivering and abnormal posturing, typically chlorpromazine hydrochloride (Thorazine) for shivering and pancuronium bromide (Pavulon) for severe abnormal posturing. Document administration and effects.

8. Shivering commonly occurs in response to hypothermia, which may be used to control ICP increase due to increased temperature. Shivering is a form of isometric contraction and thus can increase ICP. Abnormal posturing also produces muscle contractions, which elevate ICP.

9. Structure the environment to reduce unpleasant stimuli:
• Avoid unnecessary or unintended emotionally stimulating conversation (for example, about prognosis or condition).
• Provide a quiet room.
• Avoid jarring the patient's bed.
• Provide soft stimuli, such as a soft voice, soft music, and a gentle touch when necessary.
• Space painful nursing or medical procedures.
• When necessary to awaken the patient, use gentle touch and a soft voice.
• Avoid unnecessary disturbances.

9. Unpleasant or noxious stimuli can increase ICP. They also increase systemic blood pressure, which may increase ICP in the patient with poor or absent autoregulation.

10. Assess the patient's level of comfort and administer ordered medications as needed, documenting administration and effectiveness:
• analgesics when permitted for headache and pain
• antiemetics for nausea and vomiting
• stool softeners for constipation.

10. Pain, nausea, vomiting, and constipation are noxious stimuli that increase ICP. Vomiting also increases intra-abdominal and intrathoracic pressure, impeding venous return from the brain.

11. Use restraints only when absolutely necessary and as ordered.

11. Restraints may cause the patient to struggle. Both the stimulation and the resulting increased activity (producing increased heart rate and increased blood flow to the brain) elevate ICP.

12. Space activities when possible, especially routine care activities, such as baths, mouth care, and bed changes.

12. Closely spaced activities can have a cumulative effect, causing a greater and more prolonged elevation of increased ICP than a single activity.

13. Maintain venous drainage from the brain by proper alignment and positioning: keep the head and neck in a neutral position and the head of the bed elevated 30 to 60 degrees at all times, or as ordered.

13. Because the cerebral venous system has no valves, jugular vein compression causes increased pressure throughout the system, impeding drainage from the brain and increasing ICP. Placing the patient flat or in the Trendelenburg position prevents venous drainage as well; the Trendelenburg position actually increases blood flow to the brain. Elevating the head of the bed improves venous drainage.

14. Implement therapeutic measures, as ordered:

• corticosteroids, usually dexamethasone

14. Interventions help maintain ICP at a level consistent with optimal CPP.
• Although the value of corticosteroids in reducing ICP is controversial, clinicians usually consider them effective in reducing cerebral edema in some clinical problems such as tumors. Their exact mechanism of action is unknown.

• diuretics (see the "Risk for fluid volume excess" nursing diagnosis in this plan)

• Diuretics limit cerebral intracellular and extracellular swelling and CSF volume.

Neurologic disorders

• CSF drainage, via an intraventricular drain	• Draining CSF helps control erratic ICP increases and is most helpful when decreased CSF absorption is causing increased ICP.
• barbiturate coma, typically with pentobarbital (Nembutal) or thiopental (Pentothal), for severe, persistent, refractory increased ICP in adults.	• Barbiturate coma therapy is a controversial treatment that rapidly induces cerebral vasoconstriction and decreases cerebral metabolism and blood flow, thus lowering ICP, preserving ischemic cells, and preventing irreversible damage. Because barbiturate coma requires complete life support and extensive nursing supervision, it is used to manage uncontrolled intracranial hypertension unresponsive to conventional treatment. This therapy is used primarily in patients with head injuries, cerebral hemorrhage, encephalitis, and Reye's syndrome.
• neuromuscular blocking agents such as pancuronium.	• Because these drugs decrease the body's metabolism and control shivering and posturing, they help control ICP. A patient receiving one of these drugs needs complete life support and extensive monitoring.
15. When noninvasive therapeutic interventions do not control ICP, prepare the patient and family for surgical intervention (see the "Craniotomy" plan, page 141).	**15.** Surgical intervention may be necessary to control the cause such as intracranial hematoma or to gain time to prevent herniation while slower therapies reduce swelling — for instance, removing a bone flap to allow brain expansion.
16. Additional individualized interventions: _____	**16.** Rationales: _____

NURSING DIAGNOSIS

Risk for infection related to invasive techniques, immunosuppression, or surgical or other trauma

Nursing priorities

• Prevent infection.
• Monitor for signs and symptoms of infection.

Patient outcome criteria

• Within 48 to 72 hours of admission, the patient will:
  – have a normal body temperature
  – have a WBC count within normal limits.
• By the time of discharge, the patient will display no indicators of infection.

Interventions

1. Maintain strict sterile or aseptic technique as appropriate for catheterization, endotracheal tube care, and closed intracranial drainage system care.

2. Change dressings as ordered, using sterile technique. Change the dressing at the intracranial monitoring device site every 24 to 48 hours, or as ordered. Apply gentamicin (Garamycin) or other ointment around the insertion site only if ordered.

Rationales

1. Sepsis is the primary concern with any invasive equipment or procedure. Using the appropriate technique will help prevent infection.

2. Preventing infection and sepsis is crucial, particularly at sites with direct access to the brain. Cerebral infection increases the cerebral metabolic rate and CBF, thus increasing ICP. Practices regarding use of antibiotic ointment around the insertion site vary.

3. Maintain ICP monitoring devices as closed systems. Do not flush the system routinely. Instill antibiotic solutions (such as bacitracin or gentamicin) via the ICP monitoring line every 24 to 48 hours, followed by normal saline solution, only if ordered.

3. Maintaining a closed system may be critical in preventing infections in the CSF. Flushing an ICP monitoring line is not a routine procedure and is not considered a safe practice by many clinicians, so it should be performed only on specific orders. Prophylactic instillation of antibiotics may help control infection but is highly controversial.

4. Assess periodically for signs and symptoms of infection:
• redness, tenderness, or warmth around insertion sites or wounds (check daily)
• cloudy or foul-smelling drainage (check daily)
• fever (check every 4 hours)
• elevated WBC count (monitor as ordered)
• positive urine, sputum, blood, or wound cultures (monitor as ordered)
• infiltrates on chest X-ray (monitor as ordered).

4. Early detection of infection allows for prompt and appropriate intervention. An elevated WBC count may confirm an infection; however, the value may be elevated if the patient is on steroids.

5. Administer antibiotics, as ordered, typically if the patient has an ICP monitoring device or ventricular drainage system or if signs and symptoms of infection are present. Document your actions and monitor for effectiveness and adverse reactions.

5. Broad-spectrum antibiotics may be ordered prophylactically for direct access to the brain. Once infection has been documented, antibiotic choice depends on culture results.

6. Additional individualized interventions: _____

6. Rationales: _____

COLLABORATIVE PROBLEM

Risk for increased cerebral metabolism related to temperature elevations caused by infection and hypothalamic injury

Nursing priority

Maintain normal body temperature.

Patient outcome criterion

By the time of discharge, the patient will maintain a temperature within normal limits without the aid of a hypothermia blanket.

Interventions

1. Monitor and document temperature every 4 hours and as needed.

2. Administer antipyretics, as ordered, typically acetaminophen (Tylenol). Administer tepid sponge baths, as ordered.

Rationales

1. In the later stages of increased ICP, pressure on the hypothalamus may cause hypothalamic injury, disrupt normal thermoregulatory mechanisms, and cause extremely elevated temperatures. Because an elevated temperature increases systemic and cerebral blood flow and contributes to increased ICP, it should be controlled as soon as possible.

2. With infection, the temperature will rise because interleukin 1 (IL-1) may act as a pyrogen. Both IL-1 and the fever it triggers activate the body's defense mechanisms. These measures, along with antibiotic administration discussed earlier, may be sufficient to control an elevated temperature caused by infection.

Neurologic disorders

3. Apply a hypothermia blanket, as ordered, for an elevated temperature that does not respond to more conservative measures.

4. Take appropriate precautions when using the hypothermia blanket:
• Cover the hypothermia blanket with a sheet or bath blanket.

• Check the patient's rectal temperature every 30 minutes or use a rectal probe.

• Turn the blanket off when the rectal temperature slightly exceeds desired temperature, according to unit protocol.
• Control shivering by administering medication, as ordered, usually chlorpromazine hydrochloride (Thorazine).

5. Remove excess bed clothes, and allow for adequate ventilation in the patient's room.

6. Additional individualized interventions: _____
_____

3. Temperature elevation from hypothalamic injury and loss of autoregulatory control usually requires more aggressive intervention to return the temperature to normal levels.

4. Hypothermia has numerous physiologic effects that may result in injury.
• Direct contact between the patient's skin and the hypothermia blanket can cause skin damage similar to frostbite.
• The degree of hypothermia must be controlled carefully to prevent adverse reactions. A rectal thermometer or probe accurately measures body temperature.
• The patient's temperature will continue to drop and will return to normal gradually because the solution inside the blanket remains cold.
• Shivering is a form of isometric contraction that results in increased ICP.

5. Inadequate ventilation and excess bed clothes increase the time needed to reduce the patient's temperature to normal.

6. Rationales: _____

COLLABORATIVE PROBLEM

Risk for respiratory failure related to increased ICP, cerebral dysfunction, obstructed airway, absence of spontaneous respirations and gag or cough reflex, aspiration, atelectasis, ventilation-perfusion abnormalities, altered level of consciousness, or neurogenic pulmonary edema

Nursing priority

Maintain effective gas exchange.

Patient outcome criteria

• Within 24 hours of admission, the patient will:
 – have an airway free from secretions
 – have ABG levels within desired limits
 – have clear breath sounds in all lobes.
• By the time of discharge, the patient will:
 – have a normal respiratory rate and pattern
 – have normal ABG levels
 – have a clear chest X-ray.

Interventions

1. Assess and document the respiratory rate, depth, and pattern every 15 to 60 minutes. Notify the doctor of a rate less than 14 or greater than 24 breaths per minute, shallow respirations, or changes in the respiratory pattern. Assist with intubation if the patient cannot maintain an adequate airway, respiratory depth, and respiratory pattern

Rationales

1. Respiratory status is the result of a complex interplay of factors, including airway patency and medullary and pontine control mechanisms. The respiratory rate is a sensitive indicator of airway patency and increasing ICP; the respiratory pattern may correlate with the level of brain stem dysfunction. If the patient cannot maintain adequate gas exchange, intubation and mechanical ventilation may be necessary to avert cardiopulmonary arrest.

2. Auscultate for breath sounds every 2 hours and as needed to determine adequacy of aeration and the presence of adventitious sounds. Observe for restlessness and tachycardia. Assess for cyanosis around the mouth, in nail beds, and in earlobes.

2. Adventitious sounds may signal the need for intervention such as suctioning. Restlessness and tachycardia are key findings in early hypoxemia. Cyanosis, a late finding, indicates inadequate gas exchange.

3. Assess the color, amount, and consistency of respiratory secretions. Culture as needed.

3. Secretions may indicate infection or the need for hydration to help clear secretions.

4. Monitor ABG levels, as ordered. Maintain ABG levels within prescribed parameters, as described under the "Risk for cerebral ischemia" diagnosis in this plan. Obtain chest X-rays, as ordered. Correlate the findings with clinical observations.

4. Objective documentation of pulmonary status is an important adjunct to clinical observations.

5. Position the patient with the head of the bed elevated to the prescribed height and the patient's hips at the break in the bed.

5. Proper positioning allows for complete lung expansion.

6. Turn the patient every 2 hours, if ICP levels allow.

6. Dependent lung lobes cannot fully expand, thus compromising gas exchange. Turning allows for full expansion of all lobes and aids in preventing atelectasis and pneumonia, which interfere with gas exchange. However, turning may increase ICP levels, so the benefits of turning must outweigh the risks.

7. Suction as needed, hyperventilating with 100% oxygen before and after suctioning and limiting suctioning to no more than 10 seconds. Administer lidocaine (Xylocaine) through an endotracheal tube or I.V. line, as ordered. Monitor for seizures, depressed respirations, or cardiac arrhythmias. If given I.V., administer 2 minutes before suctioning; if given endotracheally, administer 5 minutes before suctioning.

7. Suctioning-induced hypoxemia contributes to increased ICP and compromised CPP. Suctioning can raise ICP up to 100 mm Hg. Used topically, lidocaine limits elevation of ICP in response to suctioning. When given as an I.V. bolus, lidocaine can sustain this effect over time. Lidocaine overdoses may cause seizures, respiratory arrest, or cardiac arrest.

8. Implement care related to mechanical ventilation, if used. See the "Mechanical ventilation" plan, page 283.

8. Carbon dioxide and oxygen levels are more precisely controlled when the patient is intubated and ventilated mechanically. The "Mechanical ventilation" plan contains detailed information about this intervention.

9. Additional individualized interventions: _____

9. Rationales: _____

NURSING DIAGNOSIS

Risk for fluid volume deficit related to diuretic therapy, fluid restriction, diabetes insipidus, hyperthermia, or GI suction

Nursing priority

Maintain fluid volume within prescribed limits.

Patient outcome criteria

By the time of discharge, the patient will:
• maintain a urine output within normal limits
• maintain electrolyte and BUN levels, hematocrit, and serum osmolality within normal limits
• maintain hemodynamic values within normal limits.

Neurologic disorders

Interventions

1. See Appendix C, Fluid and Electrolyte Imbalances.

2. Monitor and correlate fluid intake and output, both hourly and cumulatively. Measure and document urine specific gravity. Report the following:

• urine output greater than 200 ml/hour for 2 hours, with specific gravity 1.001 to 1.005

• urine output less than 30 ml/hour for 2 hours, with specific gravity greater than 1.030.

3. Monitor laboratory values, as ordered. Report the following:
• urine osmolality, usually less than 200 mOsm/kg
• serum osmolality, usually greater than 300 mOsm/kg
• serum sodium, usually greater than 145 mEq/L
• BUN levels and hematocrit usually elevated.

4. Monitor the ECG and hemodynamic pressures continually. Promptly report:
• the appearance of U waves, prolonged QT interval, depressed ST segment, and low T waves

• arrhythmias, particularly bradycardia and atrial arrhythmias, first-degree and second-degree heart block, and premature ventricular contractions (PVCs)
• low hemodynamic pressure and cardiac output.

5. Administer replacement therapy, as ordered, usually isotonic solution with potassium chloride added if serum potassium is low. Monitor the I.V. flow rate closely. Anticipate increased fluid requirements if hyperthermia or infection is present.

6. Administer exogenous ADH, such as vasopressin (Pitressin) or desmopressin (DDAVP).

Rationales

1. The Fluid and Electrolyte Imbalances appendix contains general information; this plan focuses on fluid and electrolyte problems specific to increased ICP.

2. Diuretic therapy, hyperthermia, restricted fluid intake, and DI may produce an overwhelming fluid deficit. Hourly and cumulative measurements allow prompt detection of any deficit.
• Urine output greater than 200 ml/hour usually indicates DI. In a patient with increased ICP, DI results from failure of the pituitary gland to secrete antidiuretic hormone (ADH) because of damage to the hypothalamus, the supraopticohypophyseal tract, or the posterior lobe of the pituitary gland. Such damage occurs most commonly after neurosurgery, but it can also occur secondary to vascular lesions or severe head injury. Because ADH is absent, the renal tubules fail to conserve water, resulting in the excretion of large volumes of dilute urine. The low specific gravity reflects the dilute urine. Urine output of this magnitude can rapidly create a fluid volume deficit.
• A urine output less than 30 ml/hour for 2 hours with a high specific gravity indicates that a fluid volume deficit already exists.

3. Laboratory values provide objective evidence of an imbalance. The low urine osmolality reflects diuresis; the elevated serum osmolality, serum sodium, and hematocrit reflect hemoconcentration.

4. Continual monitoring provides early warning of potentially fatal conditions.
• ECG signs reflect the decreased responsiveness of cardiac cells to stimuli — the result of hypokalemia secondary to renal potassium washout.
• Bradycardia, heart block, atrial arrhythmias, and PVCs reflect hypokalemia. Prompt treatment is necessary to prevent hypokalemic arrest.
• Low pressure reflects hypovolemia and decreased cardiac output indicates insufficient preload.

5. Isotonic solution is the replacement fluid of choice for lost body fluids. Close monitoring is needed to prevent fluid volume overload. Solutions with potassium should be carefully monitored because potassium is irritating to the vein and rapid potassium infusion can cause hyperkalemia, possibly leading to complete heart block, ventricular fibrillation, or ventricular standstill. Hyperthermia and infection accelerate fluid loss by increasing metabolic rate and increasing skin and respiratory fluid excretion.

6. DI occurs when circulating ADH is diminished or absent, resulting in massive free-water loss. A short-acting drug such as vasopressin or a long-acting drug such as desmopressin controls water loss.

7. Additional individualized interventions: _____

_____

7. Rationales: _____

_____

NURSING DIAGNOSIS

Risk for fluid volume excess related to stress, steroid therapy, or SIADH

Nursing priority

Maintain fluid volume within prescribed limits.

Patient outcome criteria

By the time of discharge, the patient will:
• display serum osmolality, electrolyte and BUN levels, and hematocrit within normal limits
• have a urine output within normal limits
• maintain hemodynamic values within normal limits.

Interventions

1. See Appendix C, Fluid and Electrolyte Imbalances.

2. Monitor and correlate fluid intake and output hourly. Report a urine output less than 30 ml/hour for 2 hours with a specific gravity greater than 1.030. Insert an indwelling urinary catheter, if necessary and as ordered.

3. Monitor urine and serum osmolality, serum electrolyte studies, hematocrit, and BUN levels daily or as ordered. Report the following:
• urine osmolality (usually high)
• serum osmolality (usually less than 280 mOsm/kg)
• serum sodium (usually less than 126 mEq/L)
• BUN levels and hematocrit (usually low).

4. Monitor the ECG and hemodynamic pressures continually. Report promptly:
• the appearance of U waves, prolonged QT interval, depressed ST segment, or low T waves
• arrhythmias, particularly bradycardia and atrial arrhythmias, first-degree and second-degree heart block, and PVCs

Rationales

1. The Fluid and Electrolyte Imbalances appendix contains general information on fluid and electrolyte problems. This plan focuses on problems specific to increased ICP.

2. Carefully monitoring fluid intake and urine output helps detect potential problems that increase ICP. Decreased urine output may reflect a fluid volume deficit or SIADH; high specific gravity reflects increased water reabsorption. SIADH is characterized by abnormally high levels or continuous secretion of ADH, resulting in water being continually reabsorbed from the renal tubules. Increased ADH secretion is caused by several factors related to increased ICP, including hyperthermia, hypotension, trauma, stress response, and administration of drugs, such as chlorpromazine, barbiturates, and acetaminophen. Sodium and water retention also are caused by corticosteroids and the stress response. Awareness of water retention may prevent further complications such as pulmonary edema.

3. High urine osmolality reflects water retention. Low serum osmolality, serum sodium, hematocrit, and BUN levels reflect hemodilution.

4. Constant monitoring provides early warning of impending problems.
• These ECG findings reflect dilutional hypokalemia.

• These rhythms are commonly caused by hypokalemia.

Neurologic disorders

• elevated hemodynamic pressures and decreased cardiac output.

5. Institute the following therapies, as ordered:

• fluid restriction

• diuretics, generally mannitol and furosemide (Lasix)

• potassium (if furosemide has been given).

6. Additional individualized interventions: _____

• Hemodynamic pressures indicate fluid overload, and decreased cardiac output results from the heart's inability to handle the excessive preload.

5. An increase in cerebral blood volume increases ICP, requiring therapy.
• Fluid restriction helps decrease extracellular fluid. Patients with increased ICP may be kept slightly dehydrated.
• Mannitol is an osmotic diuretic that moves water from the brain and CSF into plasma by an osmotic gradient, thus decreasing ICP. Furosemide, a loop diuretic, inhibits distal tubular reabsorption, promoting diuresis. Furosemide also appears to dehydrate injured cerebral tissue selectively, thus reducing cerebral edema and ICP.
• When furosemide is used, potassium is excreted along with fluid, so it may need replacement.

6. Rationales: _____

NURSING DIAGNOSIS

Risk for injury related to decreased level of consciousness, seizures, and drug therapy

Nursing priority

Maintain patient safety.

Patient outcome criterion

Throughout the hospital stay, the patient will remain free from new injury

Interventions

1. Observe the patient closely at all times. Keep side rails up at all times except during direct nursing care.

2. Assess for seizures. Implement seizure precautions, such as making sure that the bed has padded side rails and that airway and suction equipment is at the bedside. Administer and document antiseizure medication, as ordered, typically phenytoin (Dilantin) or phenobarbital.

3. Assess for gastric bleeding. Administer medications as ordered, usually an antacid, such as aluminum and magnesium hydroxide (Maalox), and such histamine$_2$ blockers as cimetidine (Tagamet), ranitidine (Zantac), or famotidine (Pepcid).

Rationales

1. Decreased level of consciousness is one of the earliest indications of increased ICP. The patient may not be aware of surroundings and possible dangers.

2. Seizures may be caused by the altered neuronal function associated with increased ICP. If the patient does have a seizure, padded side rails lessen the potential for such physical injuries as cuts, abrasions, and fractures. A patient may need help maintaining a patent airway or may need suctioning after a seizure.

3. Gastric irritation and GI bleeding are major adverse reactions to corticosteroid therapy. Also, gastric bleeding occurs with increased ICP, although the exact mechanism is unknown. Increased ICP hypothetically stimulates the vagal nuclei directly, resulting in hypersecretion of gastric acid and hyperacidity. A patient with increased ICP is usually placed on prophylactic antacid and histamine$_2$-blocker therapy to decrease the risk of bleeding.

4. Assess for an absent corneal reflex and apply artificial tears and eye patches, as needed.

4. During the later stages of increased ICP, brain stem dysfunction results in the loss of the corneal reflex. Artificial tears lubricate the eyes, and both the tears and patches prevent injury to the cornea.

5. Additional individualized interventions: _____

5. Rationales: _____

DISCHARGE PLANNING

Discharge checklist
Before discharge, the patient shows evidence of:
❒ stable ICP within normal limits
❒ stable vital signs
❒ absence of cardiopulmonary complications
❒ absence of GI bleeding
❒ normal fluid and electrolyte balance
❒ ABG levels within normal limits
❒ stable temperature
❒ stable neurologic function
❒ removal of ICP monitoring line.

Teaching checklist
Document evidence that the patient and family demonstrate an understanding of:
❒ the causes of increased ICP
❒ the extent of neurologic deficits, if present
❒ the need for continued family support
❒ the requirements for rehabilitation program, if known
❒ the date, time, and location of follow-up appointments
❒ the purpose, dosage, and potential adverse effects of all discharge medications.

Documentation checklist
Using outcome criteria as a guide, document:
❒ clinical status on admission
❒ significant changes in status
❒ pertinent laboratory and diagnostic test findings
❒ fluid intake and output
❒ neurologic status
❒ neurologic deficits, if present
❒ GI bleeding, if any
❒ seizures, if any
❒ patient and family teaching
❒ discharge planning.

ASSOCIATED PLANS OF CARE
Impaired physical mobility
Ineffective family coping: Compromised
Ineffective individual coping

Knowledge deficit
Nutritional deficit
Pain
Seizures
Sensory-perceptual alteration

REFERENCES

Chulay, M., et al. *AACN Handbook of Critical Care Nursing*. Stamford, Conn.: Appleton & Lange, 1997.

Clochesy, J.M., et al. *Critical Care Nursing*, 2nd ed. Philadelphia: W.B. Saunders Co., 1996.

Hartshorn, J.C., et al. *Introduction to Critical Care Nursing*, 2nd ed. W.B. Saunders Co., 1997.

Hickey, J.V. *The Clinical Practice of Neurological and Neurosurgical Nursing*, 4th ed. Philadelphia: Lippincott-Raven Pubs., 1997.

Lewis, S.M., et al. *Medical-Surgical Nursing Assessment and Management of Clinical Problems*, 4th ed. St. Louis: Mosby–Year Book, Inc., 1996.

Roberts, S.L. *Critical Care Nursing: Assessment and Intervention*. Stamford, Conn.: Appleton & Lange, 1996.

Ruppert, S.D., et al. *Dolan's Critical Care Nursing, Clinical Management through the Nursing Process*, 2nd ed. Philadelphia: F.A. Davis Co., 1996.

Smeltzer, S.C., and Bare, B.G. *Brunner and Suddarth's Textbook of Medical-Surgical Nursing*, 8th ed. Philadelphia: Lippincott-Raven Pubs., 1996.

Tilkian, S.M., et al. *Clinical and Nursing Implications of Laboratory Tests*, 5th ed. St. Louis: Mosby–Year Book, Inc., 1996.

Neurologic disorders

Laminectomy

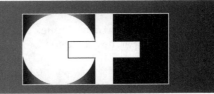

DRG information

DRG 499 Back and Neck Procedures except Spinal
Fusion with Complication or Comorbidity
(CC).
No mean LOS has been established yet.

DRG 500 Back and Neck Procedures except Spinal
Fusion without CC.
No mean LOS has been established yet.

INTRODUCTION

Definition and time focus

Laminectomy is a major spinal surgery in which one or
more vertebral laminae are removed to expose the
spinal cord and nearby structures. Most commonly, it is
performed to allow the removal of part or all of a disk
(nucleus pulposus) that has herniated and is pressing
on a spinal nerve root. Almost all herniated disks occur
in the lumbar spine, 90% to 95% occurring at the level
of L4 or L5 to S1.

A laminectomy also may be performed to relieve
spinal cord compression from a fracture, dislocation,
hematoma, or abscess and to allow for spinal nerve
surgery or the removal of a spinal cord tumor or vascular malformation. Less commonly, it may be performed
to treat intractable pain by sectioning posterior nerve
roots or interrupting spinothalamic tracts.

Lumbar laminectomy is more common than cervical
laminectomy. A posterior surgical approach is used
most commonly for lumbar laminectomy and an anteri-
or approach for cervical laminectomy.

If the spine is unstable, it may be fused at the same
time, typically using iliac crest bone fragments. Recovery takes longer with fusion because the bone graft
heals slowly.

This plan focuses on the patient undergoing lumbar
laminectomy for lumbar disk herniation that has not responded to conservative medical management. Spinal
fusion is not discussed.

Etiology and precipitating factors

For a herniated disk, causes include:
• disk degeneration
• trauma — for example, an accident, strain, or repeated
minor stresses
• poor body mechanics that cause low back strain
• congenital predisposition.

FOCUSED ASSESSMENT GUIDELINES

Nursing history (functional health pattern findings)

Health perception–health management pattern
• Pain in lumbosacral area accompanied by varying de-
grees of sensory and motor deficit
• Dull pain in the buttocks followed by unilateral or bi-
lateral leg pain that may extend to the foot, depending
on the level of disk herniation
• Numbness and tingling in the toes and feet
• Pain that usually increases with activities that cause
increased intraspinal pressure (such as sitting, sneezing,
coughing, straining, and lifting)
• Patient may have a natural deformity of the lumbar
spine
• Obesity
• History of chronic low back pain
• History of employment involving straining, lifting, or
twisting
• Sex and age (male patients between ages 20 and 45
are at increased risk)

Nutritional-metabolic pattern
• Dietary history consistent with obesity (high-calorie,
high-fat intake)

Activity-exercise pattern
• Altered mobility because of asymmetrical gait
• Lack of physical activity because of pain

Sleep-rest pattern
• Sleep disturbances related to chronic low back pain,
aggravated by sleeping on the stomach

Role-relationship pattern
• Greatest concern about the ability to return to work,
especially if work involves lifting

Physical findings

General appearance
• Anxious or pained facial expression

Cardiovascular
• Radiating pain elicited by jugular vein compression
with patient in a standing position (Naffziger's test)

Gastrointestinal
• Constipation (related to inactivity or pressure on
spinal nerve roots)

Genitourinary
• Urine retention (related to pressure on spinal nerve
roots)

Neurologic
• Increased pain in affected leg with straight-leg raising (positive Lasègue's sign)
• Sensory and motor deficit in affected leg and foot
• Pain with extension of knee when both hip and knee are at 90-degree flexion (positive Kernig's sign)
• Pain with deep palpation over the affected area
• Decreased or absent Achilles tendon and patellar reflexes
• Deformity of lumbar spine

Musculoskeletal
• Muscle spasms
• Muscle weakness or atrophy in the affected leg and foot
• Asymmetrical gait
• Decreased ability to bend forward
• Restricted lateral movement
• Leaning away from affected side during standing or ambulation
• Absence of normal lumbar lordosis and presence of lumbar scoliosis with reflex muscle spasms
• Tense posture

Diagnostic studies
• Cerebrospinal fluid (CSF) — protein level may be elevated 70 to 100 mg/dl
• Hemoglobin level and hematocrit — performed as a prerequisite for surgery and as a baseline for comparison with postoperative values to detect bleeding
• Computed tomography (CT) scan — may show disk protrusion or prolapse
• Spine X-ray — may show narrowed vertebral interspaces at the level of disk degeneration, with flattening of the lumbar curve
• Magnetic resonance imaging (MRI) — may reveal disk pressure on the spinal cord or nerve root
• Myelogram — may confirm a herniated disk and show the precise level of herniation
• Electromyogram — may indicate neural and muscle damage as well as the level and site of injury

Potential complications
• Unrelieved acute pain
• Muscle weakness and atrophy
• Paralysis
• Altered bowel or bladder function

CLINICAL SNAPSHOT

LAMINECTOMY

Major nursing diagnoses and collaborative problems	Key patient outcomes
Knowledge deficit (impending surgery)	Verbalize understanding of preoperative instructions.
Risk for sensory and motor deficits	Have circulatory, motor, and sensory function improve or return to prehospitalization level.
Risk for cerebrospinal fistula	Have no CSF drainage from incision.
Pain	Describe pain as within tolerable limits (typically less than 3 on a 0 to 10 pain rating scale).
Risk for paralytic ileus	Have normal bowel sounds.
Risk for hypovolemia	Have stable vital signs, typically with heart rate of 60 to 100 beats/minute; systolic blood pressure, 90 to 140 mm Hg; and diastolic blood pressure, 50 to 90 mm Hg.
Risk for urine retention	Show balanced fluid intake and output.
Risk for knowledge deficit (home care)	Verbalize understanding of recommended follow-up home care.

Neurologic disorders

NURSING DIAGNOSIS

Knowledge deficit (impending surgery) related to lack of exposure to information

Nursing priority

Prepare the patient to cope with the surgical experience.

Patient outcome criteria

By the day of surgery, the patient will:
• verbalize understanding of preoperative instruction
• correctly demonstrate logrolling, leg exercises, use of an incentive spirometer, and coughing and deep breathing.

Interventions

1. Provide specific preoperative teaching for the patient who will have a lumbar laminectomy. Also provide general preoperative teaching (see the "Surgery" plan, page 103, for details).

2. Explain what will happen postoperatively, including:
• frequent taking of vital signs and neurovascular observations of the extremities
• turning by logrolling during the first 48 hours
• positioning with pillows to maintain proper body alignment
• coughing and deep breathing with the back firmly against the mattress or with a pillow held against the chest for splinting purposes
• using a urinal or bedpan while the patient lies flat in bed
• wearing antiembolism stockings and performing ankle and foot exercises
• beginning progressive activity 24 to 48 hours after surgery, depending on the doctor's preference
• avoiding flexing, hyperextending, turning, or twisting the lumbar spine
• using the correct method for moving from the lying to the standing position (for example, maintaining spinal alignment and using arm and leg muscles to change position)
• exercising as ordered to strengthen arm, leg, and abdominal muscles
• using a trapeze as ordered by the doctor.

3. Demonstrate logrolling, leg exercises, incentive spirometry, coughing, and deep breathing, and have the patient practice these techniques before surgery.

Rationales

1. The patient having a laminectomy usually has undergone a long period or intermittent periods of conservative treatment. The surgery is preceded by chronic pain, a decrease in physical activity, and possible absence from work. The patient may view the surgery with relief but also with anxiety about the possible results. Information about the specific procedure will help to allay anxieties about having spinal surgery. The "Surgery" plan provides detailed information on general preoperative teaching.

2. The patient's understanding of the postoperative routine helps avoid complications, such as increased pressure on the operative site or twisting of the spinal column. Correct alignment of the body should be maintained in all positions to prevent trauma to the surgical site and to decrease discomfort. Other potential complications, such as pneumonia or atelectasis and thromboembolism, also may be prevented by proper postoperative care.

3. Practicing these techniques before surgery will help the patient perform them more effectively postoperatively, helping to prevent circulatory and respiratory complications.

4. Explain the sources of postoperative pain. Tell the patient that preoperative numbness or pain in the affected leg will remain for some time after the surgery because of nerve irritation and edema. Also explain that muscle spasms may occur.

5. Provide information about comfort measures, including:
• the importance of communication with the staff about the patient's pain (characteristics and tolerance) and anxiety
• the availability of analgesics

• giving injections in the least painful area

• positioning.

6. Additional individualized interventions: _____

4. This knowledge helps allay the patient's anxiety that the surgery might not be successful when numbness or tingling occurs or when weakness makes moving the extremities difficult. Muscle spasms that typically occur on the third or fourth postoperative day are accompanied by severe pain.

5. The patient should know that measures are available to promote postoperative comfort.
• Pain tolerance is individual, and the patient who is anxious about the potential for injury from movement may feel more discomfort.
• Medicating as needed and encouraging the patient to request medication before pain becomes severe can help maintain comfort.
• Intramuscular injections given in the unaffected buttock, or in the deltoid muscle if both buttocks are affected, cause the least pain.
• Proper body alignment increases patient comfort.

6. Rationales: _____

COLLABORATIVE PROBLEM

Risk for sensory and motor deficits related to the surgical procedure, edema, or hematoma at the operative site

Nursing priority

Prevent or minimize neurovascular impairment.

Patient outcome criteria

Within 48 hours after surgery, the patient will:
• have normal circulatory, motor, and sensory function in the lower extremities (the same as before hospitalization or improved)
• have no signs or symptoms of hematoma
• maintain correct body alignment.

Interventions

1. Document the lower extremities' neurovascular status every 2 hours or as needed for 24 to 48 hours: skin color and temperature, sensation and motion, edema, peripheral pulses, capillary refill time, ability to flex and extend the foot and toes, muscle strength, numbness or tingling in the extremities, and tone and strength in the quadriceps. Compare bilateral findings.

2. Assess pain in the lower extremities. Determine exact location and whether the pain is diminishing or worsening.

Rationales

1. Postoperative deficits may result from pressure on the spinal cord or spinal nerve roots caused by surgical trauma or hematoma. Early detection of altered function allows for prompt intervention.

2. Although preoperative numbness and pain in the lower back and affected leg will remain for some time after surgery, pain may increase from edema secondary to nerve compression. Early detection of nerve compression allows for prompt intervention.

Neurologic disorders

3. Assess for hematoma formation at the surgical site, looking for such indications as severe incision pain unrelieved by analgesics and decreased motor function and sensation in the involved area.

3. An untreated hematoma at the surgical site may cause such irreversible neurologic damage as paraplegia or bowel and bladder dysfunction.

4. If signs and symptoms of neurovascular damage occur, notify the doctor immediately.

4. Prompt intervention may help minimize neurovascular damage.

5. Implement measures to prevent neurovascular damage in the lower extremities:
• Maintain proper body alignment by logrolling (every 2 hours for the first 24 to 48 hours) and positioning with pillows.
• Use a firm mattress and a bed board.

5. These measures help reduce stress and pressure on the surgical site until healing occurs.

6. Maintain patency of the wound drainage system, if present.

6. Maintaining drainage decreases pressure on the surgical site. A hematoma may cause serious neurovascular complications.

7. Administer corticosteroids, if ordered, and document their use.

7. Corticosteroids decrease inflammation in the surgical area.

8. Implement measures to minimize neurovascular damage if initial signs and symptoms of impairment occur.
• Assess for and correct improper body alignment.
• If footdrop is present, initiate passive range-of-motion exercises every 1 to 2 hours while awake.
• Stabilize the foot with ancillary equipment, such as a footboard, sandbags, pillows, foam boots, or foot positioners.

8. These measures help prevent further damage from uneven or excessive pressure on the operative site. Permanent disability may be prevented by careful attention to the occurrence and prompt treatment of motor and sensory deficits.

9. Prepare the patient for surgical intervention if evacuation of a hematoma at the surgical site is indicated. See the "Surgery" plan, page 103.

9. Prompt evacuation of a hematoma may minimize damage. Adequate preparation of the patient for surgical intervention helps allay anxieties. The "Surgery" plan provides further details.

10. Additional individualized interventions: _____

10. Rationales: _____

COLLABORATIVE PROBLEM

Risk for cerebrospinal fistula associated with incomplete closure of the dura at the surgical site

Nursing priority

Detect any CSF leakage promptly.

Patient outcome criteria

Throughout the postoperative period, the patient will have:
• no CSF drainage from a lower back incision
• no signs or symptoms of meningitis.

Interventions

1. Observe the patient carefully every 2 to 4 hours for CSF drainage on the dressing: a clear halo or a watery pink ring around bloody or serosanguineous drainage.

2. Test the dressing with a reagent strip to check for glucose.

3. Determine if the patient has a headache.

4. Document any CSF drainage, and notify the doctor immediately if it occurs.

5. Implement measures to reduce stress on the surgical site. See the "Pain" nursing diagnosis later in this plan.

6. Change the dressing when it becomes damp, using strict aseptic technique. Assess for infection at the incision site.

7. Administer antibiotics, as ordered, and document their use.

8. Monitor temperature every 4 hours for 48 to 72 hours after surgery. Monitor the white blood cell (WBC) count daily, as ordered.

9. Assess for signs and symptoms of meningitis: headache, fever, chills, nuchal rigidity, photophobia, and positive Kernig's and Brudzinski's signs.

10. If a fistula occurs and does not heal spontaneously, prepare the patient for surgical closure. See the "Surgery" plan, page 103.

11. Additional individualized interventions: _____

Rationales

1. An abnormal opening between the subarachnoid space and the incision causes CSF to drain. Drainage on the dressing is an important sign of a fistula, usually a late postoperative complication occurring about a week after surgery. Early detection of CSF leakage allows for prompt intervention and treatment.

2. Glucose is a CSF component whose presence indicates a fistula; it is not normally present in serous wound drainage.

3. A headache is a common symptom associated with CSF loss.

4. Untreated CSF leakage may be fatal.

5. Decreasing stress on the surgical site promotes healing of the dura, which is incised during the surgical procedure. The "Pain" diagnosis contains specific details about stress reduction measures.

6. Microorganisms can pass through the fistula, multiply in the CSF, and infect the central nervous system. Changing a damp dressing immediately, using aseptic technique, helps prevent infection at the site and reduces the risk of meningitis.

7. Antibiotics help treat or prevent infection.

8. The temperature may be elevated to 102° F (38.9° C) for the first few postoperative days because of the body's normal response to tissue injury and inflammation. Temperature elevation from infection would normally be accompanied by an increased WBC count.

9. Meningitis is a common complication resulting from contamination of CSF. Undetected, it may be fatal within a short time.

10. Adequate preparation before surgical closure of the dura helps allay patient anxiety. The "Surgery" plan contains detailed information on preparation for surgery.

11. Rationales: _____

NURSING DIAGNOSIS

Pain related to immobility, muscle spasm, and paresthesia secondary to surgical trauma and postoperative edema

Nursing priority

Relieve discomfort or pain.

Neurologic disorders

Patient outcome criteria

- Within 1 day of surgery, the patient will:
  – describe pain as within tolerable limits (typically less than 3 on a 0 to 10 pain rating scale)
  – verbalize decreased pain, numbness, and tingling.
- Within 2 days of surgery, the patient will increase participation in activities (as allowed).
- Within 3 days of surgery, the patient will tolerate prescribed activity.
- By the time of discharge, the patient will use correct body mechanics and ambulate well.

Interventions

1. Refer to "Pain" plan on page 88.

2. Assess the patient for discomfort or pain — specifically, muscle spasm and pain in the lower back, abdomen, and thighs as well as pain, numbness, or tingling in the affected leg or legs — every 2 to 4 hours. Use a 0 to 10 pain rating scale.

3. Assess for associated signs and symptoms: rubbing of the lower back and hips, guarding of the affected extremity, and showing reluctance to move.

4. Administer muscle relaxants or anti-inflammatory agents, as ordered, and document their effects.

5. Administer analgesics judiciously, as ordered, and document their use. Assess for pain relief 30 minutes after giving medication and document findings.

6. To reduce the patient's discomfort, implement the following:
- Position the patient to maintain body alignment with the spine straight.
- Use a firm mattress or a bed board under the mattress.
- Avoid the prone position.
- Logroll for the first 48 hours after surgery to avoid twisting, flexing, or hyperextending the spine.
- Elevate the head of the bed with the patient's knees slightly flexed or positioned as ordered.
- Turn the patient every 2 hours.
- Use a bed cradle over areas of paresthesia.
- Place personal items and the call bell within the patient's reach.
- Teach the patient to avoid coughing, sneezing, or straining at stool.

Rationales

1. The "Pain" plan contains general information on pain. This plan presents additional information specific to laminectomy.

2. Preoperative numbness and pain in the lower back and affected leg will remain for some time after surgery. (Some patients experience pain and muscle spasm throughout the hospital stay). Postoperative pain and muscle spasms are usually caused by irritation of nerve roots and muscles from edema and surgical trauma. Muscle spasms tend to occur on the third or fourth postoperative day. Using a pain rating scale improves consistency of pain assessment.

3. The patient may not report pain, but nonverbal indicators may reveal its presence. Some patients are reluctant to request pain medication.

4. These drugs decrease pain and discomfort. Muscle relaxants (such as diazepam [Valium] or methocarbamol [Robaxin]) decrease muscle spasms; anti-inflammatory agents (such as dexamethasone [Decadron]) reduce edema and inflammation at the operative site.

5. Pain medication works best when given before the onset of severe pain. If accustomed to chronic back pain, the patient may wait until the pain is severe to request medication, when it may provide less relief.

6. These measures help alleviate discomfort by reducing stress and strain on the surgical site and by reducing pressure on the spinal nerve roots.

7. Maintain the patient on bed rest for 24 to 48 hours or as ordered.

8. Use a trapeze bar if prescribed.

9. When increased activity is ordered, instruct the patient about getting out of bed using arm and abdominal muscles; limiting initial activity to sitting in a straight-backed chair for short intervals or ambulating; and avoiding slumping or limping.

10. Consult with the doctor for antitussives, decongestants, laxatives, or stool softeners, as needed.

11. Additional individualized interventions: _____

7. Bed rest promotes healing.

8. A trapeze bar will assist the patient in moving.

9. Activity must be increased gradually and proper body alignment must be maintained at all times to prevent muscle spasm and spinal trauma. Although slumping and limping may be comfortable at first, they cause fatigue.

10. Use of these medications, as indicated, prevents pressure and associated stress on the surgical site.

11. Rationales: _____

COLLABORATIVE PROBLEM

Risk for paralytic ileus related to anesthesia, medications, retroperitoneal bleeding, or injury to the spinal nerve roots

Nursing priority

Prevent or promptly detect paralytic ileus.

Patient outcome criteria

- Within 2 days of surgery, the patient will:
  – have bowel sounds
  – expel flatus.
- By the time of discharge, the patient will have normal bowel sounds.

Interventions

1. Perform a complete abdominal assessment every 4 hours for at least the first 48 hours after surgery, then as needed. Auscultate for bowel sounds and inspect, palpate, and percuss for abdominal distention. Measure abdominal girth if distention is present.

2. Assess for associated signs and symptoms of ileus, such as nausea, vomiting, and increased back pain.

3. Document assessment findings and notify the doctor of abdominal distention or absent bowel sounds. See the "Surgery" plan, page 103, for further management.

4. Allow the patient to sit for bowel movements, condition permitting. Otherwise, logroll the patient onto a fracture bedpan.

5. Additional individualized interventions: _____

Rationales

1. Transient paralytic ileus is a common complication after laminectomy. Parasympathetic nervous system and sympathetic nervous system (SNS) innervation of the bowels originates in the lumbosacral spine. SNS stimulation contributes to loss of peristalsis and to decreased contraction of the internal sphincters, resulting in paralytic ileus. Normal bowel sounds (5 to 30 per minute) and a soft, tympanic, nondistended abdomen indicate normal bowel functioning.

2. If ileus is present, attempts to take fluids orally will cause nausea and vomiting. Back pain may worsen from increased pressure on the surgical site.

3. These signs may indicate ileus has developed. Immediate intervention is required. The "Surgery" plan provides further details.

4. The sitting position helps the patient to expel flatus and stool while maintaining correct spinal alignment.

5. Rationales: _____

Neurologic disorders

COLLABORATIVE PROBLEM

Risk for hypovolemia related to blood loss during surgery, vascular injury, hemorrhage at the incision site, or retroperitoneal hemorrhage

Nursing priority

Prevent or minimize bleeding.

Patient outcome criteria

- Within 4 hours of surgery, the patient will have no unusual bleeding or change in status.
- Within 24 hours of surgery, the patient will:
  - have stable vital signs (typically with heart rate 60 to 100 beats/minute, systolic blood pressure 90 to 140 mm Hg, and diastolic blood pressure 50 to 90 mm Hg)
  - show no signs of bleeding
  - have normal hemoglobin level and hematocrit.

Interventions

1. Implement standard postoperative care related to potential hypovolemia: monitor vital signs, clinical status, hemoglobin level and hematocrit, and surgical drainage. See the "Surgery" plan, page 103, for details.

2. Assess for flank pain, tenderness, and paresthesia every 2 to 4 hours for the first 72 hours, then every 8 hours. Compare findings with previous assessments.

3. Notify the doctor of any unusual bleeding or a change in status.

4. Additional individualized interventions: _____

Rationales

1. The "Surgery" plan contains detailed measures that apply to any postoperative patient. This plan provides additional measures specific to laminectomy.

2. These symptoms may indicate retroperitoneal hemorrhage.

3. Prompt intervention is essential to prevent shock.

4. Rationales: _____

NURSING DIAGNOSIS

Risk for urine retention related to supine positioning, pain, anxiety, anesthesia, decreased activity, or injury to the spinal nerve roots innervating the bladder

Nursing priority

Prevent or minimize urine retention.

Patient outcome criteria

- Within 3 hours of surgery, the patient will have:
  - adequate urine output
  - no complaints of urgency, fullness, or suprapubic discomfort
  - no suprapubic distention.
- Within 2 days of surgery, the patient will:
  - show balanced fluid intake and output
  - void sufficiently at normal intervals.

Interventions

1. Assess for signs and symptoms of urine retention, such as absence of voiding within 8 hours of surgery, frequent voiding of small amounts (50 ml or less), complaints of bladder fullness or urgency, and suprapubic distention.

2. Implement standard postoperative measures to monitor fluid intake and output, facilitate voiding, and provide catheterization. See the "Surgery" plan, page 103, for details.

3. Additional individualized interventions: _____

Rationales

1. Transient voiding problems caused by temporary loss of bladder tone from cord edema are common after lumbar laminectomy. Autonomic innervation of the bladder smooth muscle is from the thoracolumbar sympathetic outflow and the sacral parasympathetic outflow. The micturition center is located in the lumbosacral area.

2. These measures are the same for any postoperative patient and are explained further in the "Surgery" plan.

3. Rationales: _____

NURSING DIAGNOSIS

Risk for knowledge deficit (home care) related to lack of exposure to information

Nursing priority

Increase knowledge about home care.

Patient outcome criteria

By the time of discharge, the patient will:
• list signs and symptoms of complications to report to the doctor
• verbalize understanding of recommended follow-up home care
• list five ways to help prevent recurrent disk herniation.

Interventions

1. Tell the patient to report signs and symptoms to the doctor, including:
• any change in movement, sensation, color, pain, or temperature in the extremities
• increased pain at the incision site
• difficulty standing erect
• persistent or severe headache
• drainage from the incision site
• swelling or redness around the incision site or odor from site
• elevated temperature
• loss of bowel or bladder function.

Rationales

1. Knowing what to observe for and report will help minimize complications.

Neurologic disorders

2. Teach the patient about postsurgical restrictions and when to resume activities (at approximately 6 to 12 weeks postsurgery), including:
• restricting driving and riding in cars
• avoiding pulling, bending, stooping, pushing, lifting, twisting, or stair climbing
• logrolling into or out of bed
• avoiding tub bathing
• refraining from sexual activity
• standing or sitting for only short periods
• resting after activities
• avoiding heavy work for 6 to 12 weeks after surgery.

3. Provide information about comfort measures, including:
• lying with knees bent
• using stronger muscles, such as arm and leg muscles, to change positions
• shifting weight from one foot to the other when standing for long periods
• sitting with knees higher than hips
• using correct posture when sitting or standing
• sitting forward with knees crossed and with abdominal muscles tightened to flatten the back (if sitting for long periods)
• sleeping on one's side
• sleeping on one's back only if the knees are supported with a pillow
• using a heating pad as needed
• using prescribed muscle relaxants or analgesics
• avoiding fatigue and cold.

4. Provide information about recommended alterations in lifestyle to reduce back strain, such as:
• sleeping on a firm mattress or a bed board
• sitting on firm, straight-backed chairs
• using proper body mechanics (for example, bending at the knees, rather than at the waist, and carrying objects close to the body)
• maintaining correct posture
• wearing supportive shoes with moderate heels
• avoiding lifting heavy objects
• using thoracic and abdominal muscles when lifting objects
• using proper techniques for prescribed exercises
• scheduling adequate rest periods
• reducing or stopping any activity that causes or aggravates discomfort
• maintaining optimal weight using a prescribed, progressive exercise program, if necessary.

5. Additional individualized interventions: _____

2. Patients may hesitate to ask questions about home activities. Providing information before discharge about activities that place stress on the spinal column and incision site may prevent complications.

3. Muscle spasms and pain may persist for a time after surgery. Reducing pain, spasms, and stress on the lumbosacral spine will increase comfort.

4. Disk herniation can recur in the same area or at other levels of the lumbosacral spinal cord, particularly if degenerative changes are already present. Reducing back strain lessens the potential for disk herniation.

5. Rationales: _____

DISCHARGE PLANNING

Discharge checklist

Before discharge, the patient shows evidence of:
- ❏ stable vital signs
- ❏ absence of fever
- ❏ absence of signs and symptoms of infection
- ❏ absence of cardiovascular or pulmonary complications, such as atelectasis and thrombophlebitis
- ❏ WBC count, hematocrit, and hemoglobin level within normal parameters
- ❏ decreasing pain, muscle spasm, numbness, and tingling in lower extremities
- ❏ ability to control pain using oral medications
- ❏ absence of bowel or bladder dysfunction
- ❏ wound drainage within expected parameters
- ❏ ability to perform wound care independently or with minimal assistance, using appropriate technique
- ❏ ability to tolerate adequate nutritional intake
- ❏ knowledge of activity restrictions
- ❏ ability to perform activities of daily living and to transfer and ambulate independently or with minimal assistance
- ❏ completion of initial physical therapy assessment and instructions
- ❏ adequate home support system or referral to home care if indicated by inadequate home support system or inability to perform self-care.

Teaching checklist

Document evidence that the patient and family demonstrate an understanding of:
- ❏ the purpose, dosages, administration schedule, and adverse effects of all discharge medications (pain medications may be prescribed for continued pain and muscle spasm; laxatives may be prescribed to prevent constipation)
- ❏ infection prevention
- ❏ signs and symptoms of postoperative infection
- ❏ signs and symptoms of CSF drainage
- ❏ when and how to report signs and symptoms of complications
- ❏ recommended alterations in lifestyle to prevent recurrence of back problems
- ❏ comfort measures
- ❏ correct body mechanics
- ❏ use of pain-relief measures
- ❏ postsurgical activity restrictions
- ❏ date, time, and location of follow-up appointments
- ❏ how to contact the doctor
- ❏ adequate nutritional intake.

Documentation checklist

Using outcome criteria as a guide, document:
- ❏ clinical status on admission
- ❏ significant changes in status, especially motor or sensory deficits, headaches, and weakness
- ❏ results of myelography, spine X-ray, CT scan, electromyography, MRI, and hemoglobin and hematocrit testing
- ❏ episodes of muscle spasms, severe pain at incision site or in extremities
- ❏ pain-relief measures
- ❏ nutritional intake
- ❏ elimination habits
- ❏ preoperative teaching
- ❏ patient and family teaching
- ❏ discharge planning.

ASSOCIATED PLANS OF CARE

Impaired physical mobility
Ineffective individual coping
Knowledge deficit
Pain
Sensory-perceptual alteration
Surgery

REFERENCES

Cole, H.M., ed. "Diagnostic and Therapeutic Technology Assessment: Laminectomy and Microlaminectomy for Treatment of Lumbar Herniation," *JAMA* 264(11):1469-72, September 19, 1990.

Cyriax, J. *Textbook of Orthopaedic Medicine, Volume 1, Diagnosis of Soft Tissue Lesions,* 8th ed. Philadelphia: Bailliere Tindall, 1989.

Hickey, J.V. *The Clinical Practice of Neurological and Neurosurgical Nursing,* 4th ed. Philadelphia: Lippincott-Raven Pubs., 1997.

Jaffe, M.S. *Medical-Surgical Nursing Care Plans, Nursing Diagnoses and Interventions*, 3rd ed. Stamford, Conn.: Appleton & Lange, 1996.

LeMone, P., and Burke, K.M. *Medical-Surgical Nursing, Critical Thinking in Client Care*. Menlo Park, Calif.: Addison-Wesley-Longman Publishing Co., 1996.

Tilkian, S.M., et al. *Clinical and Nursing Implications of Laboratory Tests*, 5th ed. St. Louis: Mosby–Year Book, Inc., 1996.

Neurologic disorders

Multiple sclerosis

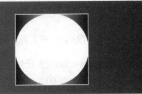

DRG information

DRG 013   Multiple Sclerosis and Cerebellar Ataxia.
         Mean LOS = 6.2 days

Additional DRG information: Patients with multiple sclerosis (MS) are most commonly admitted to an acute care setting for complications, such as pneumonia or bowel or bladder dysfunction. However, in the past 5 years, some neurologists have been admitting MS patients for trials of various I.V. medications used to counteract MS symptoms. Only in these rare circumstances would MS be the principal diagnosis. More commonly, an MS patient would be diagnosed with another illness, and the DRG would be one related to the principal diagnosis.

INTRODUCTION

Definition and time focus

MS is a relatively common, chronic, degenerative disease causing demyelinization of the central nervous system (CNS). Approximately 500,000 cases occur in the United States each year. The disease is characterized by recurrent inflammatory reactions and the formation of sclerotic plaques throughout the CNS, which interfere with normal impulse conduction and eventually cause irreversible neurologic deficits. Exacerbations and remissions are common, with some symptoms appearing only briefly or intermittently. The prognosis is variable: Approximately one-third of patients experience minimal disability and can continue most normal activities; the remaining two-thirds have moderate to severe limitations and are susceptible to complications associated with relative or absolute immobility. MS affects about five times more women than men and typically is diagnosed between ages 20 and 40. This clinical plan focuses on the patient admitted for diagnosis or management during an acute episode of MS.

Etiology and precipitating factors

Theories under study include:
• nutritional deficiencies
• excessive dietary animal fat
• heavy metal poisoning
• vascular disturbances
• acute viral infection
• viruses that invade the host early in life but remain dormant in the body for years before symptoms develop (results of slow-virus research studies bear some resemblance to the effects of MS)
• allergic or CNS hypersensitivity response to a common virus (90% of MS patients have high concentrations of measles antibodies in cerebrospinal fluid [CSF])
• immunologic disorder, particularly of cell-mediated immunity
• autoimmune response (immune cells are found in the demyelinated plaques)
• genetic and environmental predisposition
• stress, trauma, pregnancy, or fever (may induce first episode or exacerbation).

FOCUSED ASSESSMENT GUIDELINES

Nursing history (functional health pattern findings)

Health perception–health management pattern
• Onset generally between ages 20 and 40
• History of symptom-recovery cycles: mild, transient symptoms occurring in one body part, then subsiding, with the patient continuing to see self as healthy until symptoms appear on another body part
• Symptom-recovery cycles increasing in frequency and severity

Nutritional-metabolic pattern
• Difficulty chewing food
• Exhaustion from effort of eating
• Choking (dysphagia) episodes from poor muscle control

Elimination pattern
• Constipation, impaction, or incontinence (related to weakness or spasticity of anal sphincter)
• Urgency, frequency, or retention (from loss of bladder sphincter control)

Activity-exercise pattern
• Spasticity and weakness of limbs
• Weakness and fatigue with activity

Sleep-rest pattern
• Initially, reduction of symptoms with rest
• Later, spasticity that interrupts sleep

Cognitive-perceptual pattern
• Diplopia and eye pain
• Mentation disorders, such as impaired judgment and failure to comprehend or conceptualize

Self-perception–self-concept pattern
• Feelings of diminished self-worth as job performance becomes impaired (psychosocial disequilibrium)
• Emotional lability

Role-relationship pattern
• Increased dependence on others as disease progresses

Sexuality-reproductive pattern
• Occasional impotence in males
• Alterations in vaginal sensation in females

Coping–stress tolerance pattern
• Difficulty adjusting to the disease if diagnosed in early to middle adult life
• Effective coping mechanisms if in remission phase early in the disease
• Ineffective coping mechanisms if exacerbation cycles become more frequent and symptoms more disabling

Value-belief pattern
• Neglect of mild, transient symptoms (denial), only to seek medical attention later when recurring symptoms become more severe

Physical findings

Gastrointestinal
• Impaction or incontinence

Neurologic
• Charcot's triad (classic): nystagmus, intention tremors, and scanning (slow, monotonous, slurred) speech
• Loss of coordination
• Ataxia
• Paralysis
• Cranial nerve impairment
  – evidence of optic neuritis with visual field deficits
  – presence of blind spot
  – dysarthria
  – dysphagia
  – loss of facial muscle control
• Lhermitte's sign (sudden "shock wave" down the body on forward neck flexion)
• Hyperreflexic deep tendon reflexes
• Sensory loss, including paresthesia
• Decreased vibratory sensation
• Decreased or absent proprioception

Musculoskeletal
• Spasticity
• Reduced mobility
• Contractures (related to immobility)

Genitourinary
• Incontinence

Integumentary
• Reddened pressure points, skin breakdown (effects of immobility)

Diagnostic studies
• Electrophoresis—elevated oligoclonal banding of immunoglobulin G in 90% of patients (contributes evidence for differential diagnosis of MS)
• Hematology—gamma globulin levels abnormally high, reflecting increased immune system activity
• Evoked response potentials—delayed response after adequate stimulation of visual, auditory, or somatosensory mechanism suggests MS
• Computed tomography scan—may indicate lesion of CNS white matter, atrophy, or ventricular enlargement
• Lumbar puncture—increased protein and white blood cells in CSF
• Core hyperthermia—increasing body core temperature to 102° F (38.9° C) causes marginal conduction to become incomplete or blocked; use as a diagnostic procedure is controversial because results may resemble symptoms of other CNS diseases; besides being diagnostically inconclusive, the test presents some risk to the patient
• Magnetic resonance imaging—may identify discrete lesion

Potential complications
Those associated with immobility include:
• urinary tract infection
• respiratory tract infection
• phlebitis or other thromboembolic phenomena.

Neurologic disorders

CLINICAL SNAPSHOT

MULTIPLE SCLEROSIS

Major nursing diagnoses	Key patient outcomes
Impaired physical mobility	Show no evidence of skin breakdown or other effects of immobility.
Constipation and altered urinary elimination	Have satisfactory bowel and bladder elimination restored.
Risk for sexual dysfunction	Identify sexual concerns.
Self-esteem disturbance	Participate in care planning.
Risk for ineffective family coping	(The family will) participate in the patient's care.

NURSING DIAGNOSIS

Impaired physical mobility related to demyelinization

Nursing priorities

- Preserve maximum physical functioning.
- Protect from effects of immobility.

Patient outcome criteria

- Within 3 days of admission, the patient will:
  - recognize the need for rest
  - show no evidence of skin breakdown or other effects of immobility.
- Within 5 days of admission, the patient will:
  - verbalize the need for mobility assistance
  - list three safety measures
  - function at or above admission level.

Interventions

1. Provide rest and prevent fatigue.

2. Begin a physical therapy program, as ordered, including:
- active and passive range-of-motion exercises
- limb splints
- gait training
- use of leg weights and heavy shoes for balance during weight bearing
- swimming.

3. Administer medications, as ordered, to control pain and muscle spasm. Observe precautions and watch for adverse reactions, as follows:
- diazepam (Valium) — observe for increased fatigue, sedation, confusion, or depression
- dantrolene sodium (Dantrium) — monitor liver function studies (serum aspartate aminotransferase and serum alanine aminotransferase), as ordered, and observe for jaundice or other signs of liver damage as well as for drowsiness or increased weakness
- baclofen (Lioresal) — observe for increased fatigue, drowsiness, or dizziness.

4. Assess breath sounds at least every 8 hours. Report crackles, rhonchi, decreased breath sounds, or other abnormal findings promptly. Encourage incentive spirometer use, as ordered, or other pulmonary hygiene measures.

5. Teach the patient the need for and how to use specific mobility aids, such as a cane, a walker, crutches, or a wheelchair.

Rationales

1. Rest seems to alleviate symptoms; fatigue may worsen symptoms.

2. Exercising prevents joint contractures and improves muscle tone. Circulation improves with musculoskeletal activities. As exercise endurance increases, the patient gains a sense of achievement.

3. Medications (antidepressants, analgesics, and antispasmotics) relax the patient by relieving pain and spasm, promoting comfort, and permitting physical activity. Adverse reactions to these medications may make their use questionable in some MS patients. Reduced muscle tone may contribute to increased weakness and risk of injury.

4. Immobility contributes to stasis of lung secretions, predisposing the MS patient to infections and other complications related to inadequate chest excursion.

5. Teaching the patient the importance of mobility aids helps the patient adjust to using them. Although adjustment to them may be difficult, aids can prevent injury and offer the patient a sense of security while mobile.

6. Teach the patient safety measures to prevent injury related to sensory loss, including:
• using a thermometer to test water temperature
• wearing gloves in inclement weather
• wearing an eye patch to alleviate eye disturbances
• using kitchen utensils with insulated handles to prevent burns.

7. Frequently assess skin and bony prominences for pressure signs. Reposition the patient to alleviate pressure effects. Teach the patient and family how to assess skin and minimize pressure.

8. Minimize the cardiovascular effects of immobility by:
• using antiembolism stockings on the patient
• teaching leg exercises to increase venous return
• checking indices of peripheral circulation — pulses, color, temperature, sensation, mobility, and capillary refill time
• looking for signs of dependent edema.

9. Administer the following medications, as ordered, watching for adverse effects and providing appropriate patient teaching:
• corticotropin or corticosteroids — observe for hyperglycemia, excessive weight gain, and signs of bleeding, infection, or gastric distress. Caution the patient not to stop taking the medication abruptly without consulting the doctor.
• immunosuppressant drugs — caution the patient about the increased risk of infection, and review infection signs and symptoms and precautionary measures with the patient.

10. Use stress-reduction techniques, such as deep breathing, progressive relaxation, or visualization, when appropriate.

6. Impaired sensory perception may cause injury. Especially significant is the effect of temperature changes: Increased core temperature has the potential to accentuate MS symptoms by blocking impulse conduction.

7. Frequent assessment and treatment of pressure areas is necessary because immobility predisposes the patient to circulatory impairment and resultant skin breakdown. Frequent position changes redistribute pressure. Teaching the patient and family may avert postdischarge problems.

8. Immobility influences all systems. Increasing venous return may reduce venous stasis and the risk of thromboembolism. Identifying arterial insufficiency helps ensure peripheral oxygenation. Edema suggests decreased peripheral circulation and the need for prompt limb elevation.

9. Medication therapy varies widely, depending on patient status and doctor preference. Several medical therapies are under investigation.
• These drugs may reduce the length of exacerbations. Sudden withdrawal from corticosteroids may cause adrenal insufficiency.

• Immunosuppressants are still of questionable value for long-term MS therapy but may offer longer-lasting effects than corticosteroids.

10. Stress may induce an acute episode.

NURSING DIAGNOSIS

Constipation and altered urinary elimination related to demyelinization

Nursing priority

Maintain bowel and bladder function.

Patient outcome criteria

Within 5 days of admission, the patient will:
• comply with dietary recommendations
• have satisfactory bowel and bladder elimination restored
• list measures to maintain effective elimination.

Neurologic disorders

Interventions

1. Assess and record the patient's pattern of bowel and bladder function. Identify any dysfunctional pattern.

2. Evaluate dietary habits. Determine the need for high-fiber, high-bulk foods and foods low in saturated fat.

3. Increase and record fluid intake as appropriate.

4. Initiate a bowel or bladder program, as appropriate — for example, manual extraction, stimulation, Credé's maneuver, or an indwelling urinary catheter. Consult rehabilitation protocols for bowel or bladder retraining.

5. Administer laxatives, stool softeners, or propantheline bromide (Pro-Banthine), as ordered.

6. Prevent exposure to infection. If the patient develops a urinary tract infection, treat it vigorously, as ordered.

7. Teach the patient a bowel and bladder program for elimination management at home, suggesting the following guidelines:
• Establish regular voiding times.
• Use Credé's maneuver.
• Restrict fluids at night or before trips.
• Observe for signs of infection.
• Use suppositories, as ordered.
• Maintain adequate fluid and fiber intake.
• Monitor times and consistency of bowel movements.

8. Additional individualized interventions: _____

Rationales

1. MS may cause elimination problems from decreased peristalsis. Evaluating the patient's status helps identify elimination problems; for example, is the elimination problem constipation or retention?

2. A regulated diet high in fiber and bulk promotes normal peristalsis to move bowel contents through the alimentary canal. Foods low in saturated fat are thought to interrupt demyelinization.

3. Increased fluid intake promotes absorption and peristalsis.

4. Mechanical or manual assistance may be needed to overcome the effects of demyelinization on elimination. Protocols vary among institutions.

5. Medication may be required to adjust bowel absorption of metabolites and to reduce bowel spasticity problems.

6. The patient with MS is at increased risk for recurring infection, especially if urine retention is evident. (Urinary stasis is a precursor to urinary tract infection.)

7. In many cases, the patient can manage an effective elimination regimen at home, which can help reestablish a sense of independence and control.

8. Rationales: _____

NURSING DIAGNOSIS

Risk for sexual dysfunction related to fatigue, decreased sensation, muscle spasm, or urinary incontinence

Nursing priorities
• Promote healthy sexual identity.
• Teach ways to minimize the effects of disease on sexual functioning.

Patient outcome criteria
• During the admission interview, the patient will identify sexual concerns, if desired.
• Throughout the hospital stay, the patient will initiate affection, especially with partner.
• By the time of discharge, the patient will list three measures to minimize sexual dysfunction.

Interventions

1. Assess the effects of MS on the patient's sexual function. During the admission interview, ask the patient how the disease has affected sexual performance.

2. Encourage the patient and spouse or partner to share sexual concerns. Offer to be available as a resource, or refer the couple to another health professional.

3. Offer specific suggestions for identified problems, such as teaching the patient to:
• initiate sexual activity when energy levels are highest
• try different positions (for example, side-lying) if muscle spasm makes leg abduction difficult or if weakness limits activity
• empty the bladder before sexual activity and pad the bedding, as necessary, to protect against wetness
• try oral or manual stimulation if intercourse is difficult or unsatisfying.

4. Encourage expressions of affection between the patient and partner. If ongoing dysfunction has created anxiety about sexual encounters, suggest affectionate "play" sessions without intercourse as the goal.

5. Emphasize the importance of discussing birth control and family planning with a doctor.

Rationales

1. MS is extremely variable in its course and effects. The patient may be hesitant to broach the subject of sexuality. Gentle, matter-of-fact questioning during routine assessment provides the patient an opportunity to voice concerns.

2. Even couples who have no difficulty communicating in most areas may find it hard to verbalize feelings related to sexuality. Health professionals who are comfortable discussing sexual issues may be able to start and maintain a dialogue.

3. The patient needs concrete information on specific problems.
• Fatigue contributes to decreased libido.
• Muscle spasms commonly affect hip abductor and adductor muscles. Some positions require less energy expenditure.
• Urinary incontinence is more common during intercourse or masturbation.
• The MS patient may find intercourse less satisfying than before because decreased sensation makes orgasm more difficult to achieve.

4. Sexuality involves more than the act of coitus. Emphasis on playful, affectionate exchanges between partners helps reduce anxiety, promotes trust, and improves the patient's body image and self-esteem.

5. An intrauterine device may be contraindicated because decreased sensation may cause complications to go undetected. Birth control pills may exacerbate MS symptoms. The familial tendency to develop MS and lack of prenatal screening for the disease may be significant factors for the patient considering having a child because women of childbearing age are the primary victims of the disease.

Neurologic disorders

NURSING DIAGNOSIS

Self-esteem disturbance related to progressive, debilitating effects of disease

Nursing priority

Promote a healthy self-image and a realistic acceptance of limitations.

Patient outcome criteria

Throughout the hospital stay, the patient will:
• participate actively in care planning
• verbalize feelings related to losses
• participate in family activities as much as possible
• show interest in appearance and grooming
• initiate independent activities
• show an interest in others.

Interventions

1. Encourage the patient to participate in all decisions related to care planning. Discourage overdependent behaviors. Help the patient set goals and work toward them.

2. Promote the expression of feelings related to losses. Avoid overly cheerful responses but still maintain a positive outlook. See the "Grieving" plan, page 44, and the "Ineffective individual coping" plan, page 67.

3. Work with the family to promote maximum patient participation in familiar family roles and rituals or to identify new roles of value for the patient, such as humorist, correspondent, or arbitrator.

4. During care activities, encourage the patient to touch affected body parts, perform self-lifting activities as much as possible, and participate in grooming and wardrobe selection.

5. Provide recognition for goals achieved. Acknowledge evidence of inner strengths and growth as well as external achievements; for example, notice difficult emotional issues the patient has dealt with positively as well as activity goals achieved.

6. Additional individualized interventions: _____

Rationales

1. Active participation fosters a sense of control and increases self-esteem. The patient with MS experiences loss of control in many areas; encouraging responsibility for self-care helps maintain dignity and independence. Goal setting aids in maintaining hope.

2. The patient suffering from a chronic debilitating disease may see each hospital stay as a further step in disease progression and loss of control. Healthy grieving is a realistic response to multiple losses and a normal part of acceptance. Overly cheerful responses indicate a lack of understanding of the profound changes MS entails for the patient. Empathy and realistic optimism, in contrast, show respect for the patient. The general plans of care noted suggest other interventions that may be helpful for the patient with MS.

3. Disease progression and an increasing sense of helplessness are compounded by the inability to fulfill familiar family roles. Encouraging family recognition and support of these roles minimizes distress. Physical disability may nevertheless allow the patient to assume new roles within the family, thus helping the patient maintain a sense of self-worth.

4. Acceptance of altered body image and function is essential to a healthy self-concept. Touching one's body and becoming familiar with its limitations is the first step toward acceptance. Grooming promotes a positive self-concept.

5. Chronic progressive disease may narrow a patient's world view severely. Recognizing struggles and achievements decreases the sense of isolation. The patient can teach nurses much that may help them care for other patients. Acknowledging this gift may help provide a sense of meaning in difficult times and extend the patient's outlook toward others.

6. Rationales: _____

Nursing diagnosis

Risk for ineffective family coping related to progressive, debilitating effects of disease on family members and resultant alteration in role-related behavior patterns

Nursing priority

Maintain family integrity while promoting a healthy adjustment to necessary role changes.

Patient outcome criteria

By the time of the patient's discharge, family members will:
• appear healthy and well rested
• participate actively in the patient's care
• participate in home care planning.

Interventions

1. Assess the family system by observing family members' interaction with the patient, encouraging family participation in care activities, and talking with family members individually or as a group about changes brought about by the disease. See the "Ineffective family coping: Compromised" plan, page 63. Mention other resources for patients and families, such as the National Multiple Sclerosis Society, 733 Third Ave., New York, NY 10017, E-mail: info@nmss.org

2. Encourage family members to take turns in the caregiving role, as necessary.

3. Help the family understand and accept any mental changes that occur.

4. Promote healthy habits for family members: Urge adequate rest, proper dietary intake, exercise, and relaxation.

5. Help the family plan changes in the home environment to make care easier, such as making structural changes (ramps, rails), rearranging furnishings and supplies to allow easy access for the patient, and having special supplies for incontinence available. Help the family arrange for transportation and obtain help with caregiving by providing a social services referral.

6. Additional individualized interventions: _____

Rationales

1. Chronic diseases can have a devastating effect on families as well as affected individuals. As the primary support for most patients, families must be supported and considered in care planning. Open discussion among family members promotes mutual supportiveness and understanding. The "Ineffective family coping: Compromised" plan provides interventions especially helpful for families in or at risk for crisis. Knowing that others have coped with the same situation may create a sense of rapport and trust that facilitates the learning necessary to cope successfully with this disorder.

2. As the disease progresses, the patient becomes more dependent on others for care. Sharing care responsibilities helps prevent burnout, provides variety in care routines, and allows for mutual understanding.

3. From 40% to 60% of MS patients exhibit alterations in mental function, ranging from inattention and euphoria (early in the disease) to irritability, depression, disorientation, and loss of memory (later in the disease). Understanding that these symptoms are part of the disease and not intentional helps minimize distress for both the patient and family.

4. Adequate sleep, proper nutrition, exercise, and relaxation help family members remain strong, supportive, and capable of caring for the patient and each other. Guilt feelings may preclude meeting personal needs unless health care providers offer encouragement.

5. Without careful planning, the gradual progression of the disease may overwhelm the family with new demands. Social services can offer many resources for patient and family support at home through volunteer, charitable, church, or public institutions.

6. Rationales: _____

DISCHARGE PLANNING

Discharge checklist
Before discharge, the patient shows evidence of:
- ❏ stable vital signs
- ❏ absence of fever
- ❏ absence of pulmonary or cardiovascular complications
- ❏ ability to manage bowel and bladder functioning independently or with minimal assistance
- ❏ absence of signs and symptoms of urinary tract infection
- ❏ ability to transfer and ambulate at prehospitalization levels or with minimal assistance, using appropriate assistive devices as ordered
- ❏ ability to tolerate adequate nutritional intake
- ❏ control of muscle spasms and pain with oral medications
- ❏ adequate home support system or referral to home care or a nursing home if indicated by inadequate home support system or inability to perform self-care.

Neurologic disorders

Teaching checklist
Document evidence that the patient and family demonstrate an understanding of:
❏ the course and nature of MS
❏ the physical therapy program
❏ the purpose, dosage, administration schedule, and adverse effects of all discharge medications (usual discharge medications include corticosteroids, antispasmodics, and stool softeners)
❏ mobility aids
❏ safety instructions for protection from injury related to sensory deficits
❏ information regarding problems associated with immobility
❏ stress reduction techniques
❏ specific suggestions for sexual problems
❏ community resources
❏ recommended therapeutic diet, including selection of foods low in saturated fat
❏ bowel and bladder program
❏ the importance of avoiding exposure to infection
❏ the date, time, and location of follow-up appointments
❏ when to call the doctor
❏ how to contact the doctor.

Documentation checklist
Using outcome criteria as a guide, document:
❏ clinical status on admission
❏ significant changes in clinical status
❏ pertinent laboratory data and diagnostic findings
❏ physical therapy program and activity tolerance
❏ medication administration
❏ nutritional intake
❏ fluid intake and output
❏ bowel and bladder function
❏ patient and family teaching
❏ discharge planning.

ASSOCIATED PLANS OF CARE

Grieving
Ineffective family coping: Compromised
Ineffective individual coping

REFERENCES

Barnes, M.P. "Treating and Nursing Patients with Multiple Sclerosis," *Nursing Standard* 11(23):42-44, February 1997.
Fauci, A.S. *Harrison's Principles of Internal Medicine,* 14th ed. New York: McGraw-Hill Book Co., 1998.
Stuifbergen, A.K., and Rogers, S. "The Experience of Fatigue and Strategies of Self-Care Among Persons with Multiple Sclerosis," *Applied Nursing Research* 10(1):2-10, February 1997.
Swain, S.E. "Multiple Sclerosis: Primary Health Care Implications," *Nurse Practitioner* 21(7):40,43,47-50, July 1996.

Myasthenia gravis

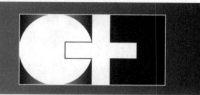

DRG information
DRG 012   Degenerative Nervous System Disorders.
          Mean LOS = 7.7 days

INTRODUCTION

Definition and time focus
Myasthenia gravis (MG) is a chronic debilitating disease resulting from defective transmission of nerve impulses at the neuromuscular junction. Characterized by remissions and exacerbations of progressive muscle weakness, MG is estimated to occur in 1 out of 10,000 to 50,000 persons and affects more women than men. Peak incidence occurs during the 20s and 30s. When full-blown, MG causes complete dependence.

   MG usually is treated pharmacologically. If symptoms persist despite medication, plasmapheresis may be used to remove autoantibodies. Thymectomy may be performed in patients with thymomas or thymic hyperplasia because these abnormal cells may trigger an autoimmune reaction; thymus gland removal decreases the response to new antigens. This clinical plan focuses on the patient admitted for initial diagnosis and pharmacologic treatment of MG.

Etiology and precipitating factors
• Autoimmune syndrome
• Antibodies to acetylcholine receptors, reducing the number of functional receptors on muscle cells
• Smoking
• Alcohol consumption
• Cold weather
• Prolonged exposure to sun
• Stress
• Menstruation
• Pregnancy
• Influenza

FOCUSED ASSESSMENT GUIDELINES

Nursing history (functional health pattern findings)
Health perception–health management pattern
• Vague symptoms in absence of objective findings
• Weak muscles, especially those involved in chewing, swallowing, and speaking
• Weakness of facial and extraocular muscles; diplopia
• Breathlessness (related to respiratory muscle weakness)

• Fatigue, with partial improvement of muscle strength with rest
• Weakness that is restricted to specific muscle groups or generalized; may be symmetrical or asymmetrical
• Increased weakness with repetitive use of the muscle group
Nutritional-metabolic pattern
• Difficulty in swallowing that worsens toward the end of meals
• Weight loss related to decreased nutritional intake
Elimination pattern
• Constipation
Activity-exercise pattern
• Increasing fatigue with delayed muscle strength recovery
• Sedentary lifestyle since the onset of symptoms
Self-perception–self-concept pattern
• Helplessness; inability to complete physical tasks
• Tiredness or depression
Sexuality-reproductive pattern
• Impotence
Coping–stress tolerance pattern
• Coping with symptoms by resting
• Ineffective coping mechanisms, such as frustration, denial, and anger
• Worsening of symptoms with stress
Value-belief pattern
• Delay in seeking medical attention because of vague and transient symptoms
• Belief that MG symptoms are manifestations of another autoimmune disease, such as lupus erythematosus, rheumatoid arthritis, or thyrotoxicosis

Physical findings
General appearance
• Expressionless face
• Fatigue
Pulmonary
• Dyspnea
• Limited chest excursion
• Possibly decreased tidal volume, vital capacity, and inspiratory force
Gastrointestinal
• Hypoactive bowel sounds (less common)
• Constipation (less common)
Neurologic
• Ptosis (worsened with upward gaze), squinting, and nystagmus
• Attempts to smile look snarl-like
• High-pitched, nasal voice

- Progressive weakening of voice during conversation
- Poorly articulated speech
- Normal sensory findings

Musculoskeletal
- Difficulty sitting upright, holding head up, and reaching above head
- Facial drooping
- Mouth hangs open
- Dysphasia
- Dysphagia

Diagnostic studies
- Acetylcholine receptor antibody titer — positive
- Arterial blood gas (ABG) levels — may reveal hypoxemia or hypercapnia related to ineffective ventilation
- White blood cell count — may reveal leukocytosis related to pulmonary infection
- Triiodothyronine and thyroxine — normal levels rule out thyroid disorder as cause of muscle weakness; however, abnormally high or low levels do not exclude MG

because a small percentage of MG patients also have thyroid abnormalities
- Magnesium — may be low because of protein-calorie malnutrition
- Edrophonium test — when 2 to 10 mg of edrophonium chloride (Tensilon) is administered I.V., marked improvement in muscle strength within 60 seconds confirms MG
- Electromyogram — shows rapid decreases in evoked muscle action potentials
- Computed tomography scan or chest X-ray — may reveal thymoma or thymic hyperplasia

Potential complications
- Airway obstruction
- Respiratory arrest
- Aspiration
- Myasthenic crisis
- Cholinergic crisis
- Corneal abrasion or ulceration

CLINICAL SNAPSHOT

MYASTHENIA GRAVIS

Major nursing diagnoses and collaborative problems	Key patient outcomes
Muscle weakness	Maintain muscle strength adequate to support ventilation.
Ineffective breathing pattern	Show clearing or absence of gurgles.
Ineffective airway clearance	Maintain a normal breathing pattern.
Activity intolerance	Perform activities of daily living without assistance.
Impaired verbal communication	Communicate needs.
Risk for aspiration	Not aspirate.
Nutritional deficit	Maintain a stable weight ±3 lb per week.
Ineffective management (individual) of therapeutic regimen	Verbalize intent to follow medication schedule exactly as prescribed.
Sexual dysfunction	Describe ways to improve sexual function.

COLLABORATIVE PROBLEM
Muscle weakness related to reduced number of acetylcholine receptors

Nursing priority
Promote optimal muscle strength.

Patient outcome criteria
• Within 12 hours of admission, the patient will show muscle strength adequate to support ventilation, as evidenced by a pH greater than 7.35 and a partial pressure of arterial carbon dioxide ($Paco_2$) less than 45 mm Hg.
• Within 2 days of admission, the patient will show improved muscle strength and the ability to turn in bed and assist with transfer to a chair.

Interventions

1. Administer anticholinesterase medication orally three or four times per day, 30 to 60 minutes before meals, as ordered. Give with milk. Watch for:
• therapeutic effect — increased muscle strength
• underdosage — continuation or worsening of myasthenic signs and symptoms (such as weakness, ptosis, dyspnea, and dysphagia)
• overdosage — cholinergic signs and symptoms (myasthenic signs and symptoms plus increased salivation, vomiting, diarrhea, fasciculation, and increased pulmonary secretions).

2. Keep emergency airway, suctioning, and ventilation equipment nearby. Monitor ABG measurements, as ordered.

3. Keep atropine sulfate nearby.

4. Periodically assess muscle strength by having the patient maintain a steady upward gaze and by having the patient drink through a straw.

5. Keep a daily log of periods of fatigue and times of increased and decreased muscle strength.

6. Contact the doctor if the patient says that more or less medication is needed.

7. Administer such medications as succinylcholine (Anectine) and pancuronium (Pavulon) with caution, as ordered.

Rationales

1. Anticholinesterases slow the breakdown of acetylcholine at the neuromuscular junction, promoting better impulse transmission to muscles and making chewing and swallowing during meals easier. Milk prevents gastric irritation. The margin between therapeutic effects, underdosage, and overdosage varies. Anticholinesterase need may fluctuate, depending on stresses (such as emotions or infection) and the effects of other therapies.
   Underdosage may induce myasthenic crisis, an abrupt exacerbation of motor weakness caused by inadequate impulse transmission at the neuromuscular junction. Overdosage may induce cholinergic crisis, an abrupt exacerbation of motor weakness caused by prolonged action of acetylcholine at the neuromuscular junction.
   Differentiating between underdosage and overdosage can be difficult because of their similar signs and symptoms. Parasympathetic effects help to identify overdosage but are not conclusive. The edrophonium test definitively distinguishes between underdosage and overdosage.

2. Anticholinesterase overdosage or underdosage leads to respiratory muscle weakness that might require artificial ventilation. ABG measurements provide objective evidence of the adequacy of ventilation.

3. Atropine sulfate is the antidote to anticholinesterase overdosage (cholinergic crisis).

4. MG commonly affects eye muscles the most dramatically. After 1 minute of upward gazing, the patient may exhibit progressive eyelid drooping. Drinking through a straw requires repetitive use of the facial and swallowing muscles, causing fatigue.

5. The log can help the doctor adjust the medication dosage and schedule.

6. The MG patient on long-term medication therapy typically can detect an overdose or underdose before clinical signs appear.

7. The MG patient is sensitive to the effects of curariform drugs, which produce symptoms similar to a further reduction in acetylcholine receptors.

Neurologic disorders

8. Observe for muscle weakness after the administration of aminoglycoside antibiotics or antiarrhythmic medications, especially quinidine (Quinora) and procainamide (Pronestyl).

9. Additional individualized interventions: _____

8. The MG patient is sensitive to the neuromuscular blocking effects of the aminoglycosides and class IA antiarrhythmics.

9. Rationales: _____

NURSING DIAGNOSIS

Ineffective breathing pattern related to muscle fatigue

Nursing priority

Promote adequate ventilation.

Patient outcome criteria

- Within 12 hours of admission, the patient will have:
  - no dyspnea
  - $Paco_2$ less than 50 mm Hg
  - an arterial partial pressure of oxygen (Pao_2) greater than 50 mm Hg
  - a respiratory rate less than 30 breaths per minute.
- Within 24 hours of admission, the patient will have:
  - a regular breathing pattern
  - a vital capacity greater than 15 ml/kg
  - a tidal volume greater than 5 ml/kg
  - an inspiratory force greater than -20 cm H_2O.

Interventions

1. Monitor and document respiratory rate and depth every 2 hours, and monitor ABG levels. Observe for changes.

2. Measure vital capacity, tidal volume, and inspiratory force before and 1 hour after administration of anticholinesterase medications. Alert the doctor if the patient's vital capacity falls below 10 ml/kg, if tidal volume falls below 5 ml/kg, or if inspiratory force falls below -20 cm H_2O or a pattern of decreasing values occurs.

3. Monitor and document the appearance of expectorated sputum.

4. Additional individualized interventions: _____

Rationales

1. Changes in rate and depth are clues to impending respiratory muscle failure; an increase in $Paco_2$ or a drop in Pao_2 indicates hypoventilation.

2. A therapeutic dose of anticholinesterase medication results in increased vital capacity, tidal volume, and inspiratory force. Both underdosage and overdosage result in muscle weakness, which is reflected as decreased vital capacity, tidal volume, and inspiratory force. Values that do not improve with I.V. administration of an anticholinesterase indicate the need for intubation and mechanical ventilation.

3. The ability to expectorate sputum indicates an effective breathing pattern.

4. Rationales: _____

NURSING DIAGNOSIS

Ineffective airway clearance related to decreased inspiratory force and increased secretion production

Nursing priority

Maintain a patent airway.

Patient outcome criteria
- Within 12 hours of admission, the patient will have PO_2 greater than 50 mm Hg.
- Within 5 days of admission, the patient will:
  - show clearing or absence of gurgles
  - expectorate any sputum produced.

Interventions

1. Demonstrate the cascade cough by having the patient take a deep breath, cough three or four times after the same inhalation, and repeat several times until the cough is productive.

2. Encourage the patient not to suppress coughs.

3. Perform chest physiotherapy (CPT) and suction every 2 to 4 hours, as needed. Evaluate breath sounds to judge efficacy.

4. Monitor and document ABG levels.

5. Additional individualized interventions: _____

Rationales

1. A deep breath followed by a single long, harsh cough is ineffective in airway clearance because it commonly causes bronchospasm. The cascade cough mimics the normal cough pattern, which moves sputum farther up the bronchial tree with each successive cough.

2. Because of pain or unpleasant sensations, the patient may try to stop the cough response.

3. CPT mechanically loosens secretions; suctioning helps remove them. Effective CPT clears secretions.

4. A drop in Pao_2 may signal inadequate ventilation resulting from airway obstruction.

5. Rationales: _____

NURSING DIAGNOSIS

Activity intolerance related to muscle fatigue

Nursing priority

Minimize fatigue and promote a tolerable level of activity.

Patient outcome criteria
- Within 2 days of admission, the patient will show little or no fatigue.
- Within 5 days of admission, the patient will be able to perform activities of daily living without assistance.

Interventions

1. Identify sources of excess energy consumption, such as frequent telephone conversations, reading, watching television, or chewing hard or tough food.

2. Space bathing, grooming, and other activities throughout the day to avoid fatigue.

3. Rearrange the environment to keep frequently used items close by.

4. Plan a rest period before each meal. Keep meals small.

5. Additional individualized interventions: _____

Rationales

1. Minimizing unnecessary actions helps conserve strength.

2. Muscles weaken rapidly when used repetitively. Several short rest periods may be more effective in restoring muscle strength than one longer rest period.

3. Keeping frequently used items within easy reach minimizes unnecessary muscle use.

4. The muscles used in chewing and swallowing weaken quickly.

5. Rationales: _____

Neurologic disorders

NURSING DIAGNOSIS

Impaired verbal communication related to fatigue of facial and respiratory muscles

Nursing priority

Establish effective communication.

Patient outcome criterion

Within 24 hours of admission, the patient will communicate needs.

Interventions

1. Avoid frequent or long conversations with the patient.

2. Provide alternative methods of communication, such as paper and pencil or a word board.

3. Additional individualized interventions: _____

Rationales

1. Facial and respiratory muscles are easily fatigued.

2. Alternative methods allow communication without using facial and respiratory muscles.

3. Rationales: _____

COLLABORATIVE PROBLEM

Risk for aspiration related to impaired swallowing

Nursing priority

Prevent aspiration.

Patient outcome criteria

• Throughout the hospital stay, the patient will not aspirate.
• By the time of the patient's discharge, the family will demonstrate airway clearance procedures.

Interventions

1. Plan mealtimes to coincide with peak anticholinesterase effects.

2. Ask the patient for a self-evaluation of swallowing ability, and order foods of appropriate consistency: liquid, pureed, soft, or regular. Give the patient nothing by mouth if swallowing is severely impaired.

3. Provide rest periods during meals.

4. Have suctioning equipment at the patient's bedside. Stay with the patient during meals.

5. Teach the patient and family what steps to take if choking or aspiration occurs, such as back blows, abdominal thrusts, and nasotracheal suctioning.

Rationales

1. Oral anticholinesterase medications achieve full effect within 60 minutes, with the duration of action ranging from 2 to 8 hours. The potential for aspiration increases when anticholinesterase levels are low.

2. Subjective evaluation of swallowing is usually accurate; it also allows the patient to take part in decision making and keep a sense of control.

3. Chewing and swallowing require repetitive use of the same muscle groups, causing fatigue.

4. Respiratory complications secondary to aspiration can lead to death.

5. Back blows and abdominal thrusts can loosen food obstructing the airway. Suctioning stimulates coughing and removes sputum and debris.

6. Additional individualized interventions: _____

6. Rationales: _____

Nursing diagnosis

Nutritional deficit related to decreased oral intake

Nursing priority

Maintain adequate oral nutrition.

Patient outcome criteria

• Within 2 days of admission, the patient will have $Paco_2$ levels within normal limits.
• Within 5 days of admission, the patient will maintain a stable weight ±3 lb per week.

Interventions

1. Refer to the "Nutritional deficit" plan, page 80.

2. Collaborate with the dietitian or nutritional support service to obtain a nutritional assessment on admission, including:
• height and weight
• midarm circumference measurement
• triceps skin-fold measurement
• arm muscle circumference calculation
• creatinine height index.

3. Provide a diet with the proper balance of protein, fat, carbohydrate, and calories.

4. Serve the main meal in the morning.

5. Provide liquids in a cup.

6. Have the patient sit erect during meals.

7. Record all food and nutritional supplements consumed. Evaluate protein, calorie, vitamin, and mineral intake.

8. Consult with a dietitian about nutritional supplements, tube feedings, and total parenteral nutrition, if indicated.

9. Additional individualized interventions: _____

Rationales

1. The "Nutritional deficit" plan covers the disorder in depth. This plan provides additional information pertinent to the MG patient.

2. These parameters indicate nutritional status, which affects muscle performance. Professionals with special nutritional expertise are best equipped to evaluate the patient's nutritional status.

3. A balanced diet meets nutritional needs while keeping the respiratory quotient (RQ) at a normal level (0.8). (RQ—the ratio of carbon dioxide [CO_2] produced to oxygen consumed during metabolism—indicates the patient's ability to increase ventilation to remove excess CO_2 produced by a large carbohydrate intake. If RQ is abnormal, the workload caused by increased CO_2 production may lead to respiratory failure.)

4. The muscles used for chewing are strongest in the morning.

5. Weak facial muscles make drinking with a straw difficult.

6. Sitting erect enhances the swallowing reflex.

7. A record of consumption provides the basis for dietary assessment; its evaluation forms the basis for further planning.

8. The dietitian's expertise helps meet the MG patient's special nutritional needs.

9. Rationales: _____

Neurologic disorders

NURSING DIAGNOSIS

Ineffective management of individual therapeutic regimen related to knowledge deficit and new medications

Nursing priority

Provide the knowledge needed for self-care.

Patient outcome criteria

- Within 5 days of admission, the patient will:
  - list signs and symptoms that should be reported to the doctor or nurse promptly
  - know how to order a medical alert tag
  - begin maintaining a medication-response log.
- By the time of discharge, the patient will:
  - list four factors that may lead to a crisis
  - verbalize intent to follow the medication schedule exactly as prescribed
  - verbalize ways to cope with decreased activity tolerance.

Interventions

1. Teach the patient and family about the disease and its implications. Find out what the doctor has stated, and reinforce that explanation. Clarify misconceptions. Stress the fluctuating nature of MG and the value of self-care.

2. Instruct about factors that may worsen the condition—stress, infection, smoking, alcohol, exposure to cold or heat, pregnancy, and medication overdosage or underdosage.

3. Teach the patient and family signs and symptoms of crises that may require notifying the doctor or nurse, including nausea, vomiting, diarrhea, abnormal sweating, increased salivation, irregular or slow heartbeat, muscle weakness, or severe abdominal pain.

4. Teach the patient about medications, particularly:
- the importance of following the schedule exactly if the patient must continue taking anticholinesterase on a fixed schedule after discharge
- the parameters within which the patient may adjust the dosage if following an on-demand anticholinesterase schedule
- signs of overdosage and underdosage
- the significance of alterations in GI function (such as nausea, cramping, diarrhea, or constipation)
- the need to check with the doctor before taking any other medications, including over-the-counter drugs.

5. Demonstrate how to keep a medication-response log.

Rationales

1. Because it is a chronic disease, MG requires a well-informed, motivated patient and family for best management. The doctor's initial explanation may not have been fully comprehended by the patient and family because of anxiety. Similar explanations from both the doctor and nurse improve comprehension and increase confidence.

2. The patient and family must be aware of risk factors in order to avoid them. Involving the patient in self-management may help restore a sense of control and provide reassurance that MG does not affect intellectual capability.

3. The signs and symptoms of myasthenic and cholinergic crises are similar. Both underdosage and overdosage of anticholinesterases can cause life-threatening respiratory insufficiency.

4. A knowledgeable, confident patient and family are crucial to successful management of MG. GI dysfunction may result from long-term anticholinesterase therapy or may signal anticholinesterase toxicity. If a doctor rules out the latter, the patient may be helped by small meals, altered fluid intake, antiemetics, or other interventions. Many medications, such as narcotics, sedatives, quinidine, and aminoglycoside antibiotics, interfere with neuromuscular transmission.

5. The medication-response log helps the doctor adjust medication dosages if needed.

6. Provide information about how to obtain a medical alert tag.

6. A medical alert tag provides information about the patient's name, diagnosis, current medication dosages, and the doctor's name and number in an emergency.

7. Teach ways to cope with decreased activity tolerance, including how to:
• conserve energy (for example, by using clothing that is easy to put on)
• space activities
• institute safety precautions (such as hand rails in the tub or by the commode).

7. Learning methods to cope with this chronic disease may reduce frustration, decrease exacerbations, and restore self-esteem.

8. Provide the following address: The Myasthenia Gravis Foundation, 53 West Jackson Boulevard, Suite 1352, Chicago, IL 60604.

8. The Myasthenia Gravis Foundation provides direct services to patients and families.

9. Additional individualized interventions: _____

9. Rationales: _____

Nursing diagnosis

Sexual dysfunction related to muscle weakness and fatigue

Nursing priority

Provide emotional support and the knowledge needed for alternative means of sexual expression.

Patient outcome criteria

By discharge, the patient will:
• verbalize concerns related to sexual function
• describe ways to improve sexual function.

Interventions

1. Using a direct, open approach, ask the patient what concerns he has about the effect of MG on sexuality.

2. Explain to the patient that MG does not affect sensation and the enjoyment of sex and has no effect on the ability to have children.

3. Explain to the patient that planning to have sex during periods of higher energy — early in the morning, when the medication is having its peak effect, and after rest periods — can improve the sexual experience.

4. Teach the patient what positions can help conserve energy and improve respiratory function — for instance, the supine position or sitting with back support.

5. Encourage open communication between the patient and the patient's partner or spouse about sexual performance.

6. Teach the patient about the effects of medications on sexuality; explain that immunosuppressants should be discontinued at least 4 months before conceiving.

Rationales

1. Such an approach can make the discussion of the effects of MG on sexual performance easier for the patient.

2. Information about those aspects of sexuality that MG does not affect can help dispel the patient's fears.

3. Teaching the patient to plan for times of higher energy can help increase sexual performance and enjoyment.

4. Using such positions should reduce fatigue and increase performance and enjoyment.

5. Open communication is essential for establishing and maintaining intimacy.

6. The patient needs to know that immunosuppressants can reduce spermatogenesis and cause amenorrhea.

Neurologic disorders

7. Tell the patient to discuss family planning with the doctor before beginning a family. The patient needs to know that:
• the pregnancy rate in MG patients is the same as it is in the general population
• MG remains stable in two-thirds of the patients during pregnancy, and one-third suffer exacerbations
• myasthenia crisis can occur at anytime during a pregnancy
• experience during previous pregnancies does not predict the course of a later pregnancy.

8. Additional individualized interventions: _____

7. Information about the effect of MG on pregnancy can help the patient make an informed decision about having children.

8. Rationales: _____

DISCHARGE PLANNING

Discharge checklist
Before discharge, the patient shows evidence of:
❏ normal ABG levels
❏ absence of fever
❏ absence of airway-compromising dysphagia for at least 48 hours
❏ ability to tolerate adequate nutritional intake
❏ absence of cardiovascular and pulmonary complications
❏ ability to tolerate at least minimal activity
❏ ability to perform activities of daily living independently or with minimal assistance
❏ ability to understand and maintain a medication response log
❏ adequate home support
❏ referral to home care or nursing home, if necessary. Because of the age-group and sex that MG usually strikes and the chronic nature of the illness, the health care provider must assess the patient's home situation, including problems associated with child care, finances, and the ability to cope with an altered lifestyle. In mid-stage and end-stage MG, patients typically need nursing home placement or around-the-clock home care assistance if they can afford it. Anticipate a social service referral for every MG patient.

Teaching checklist
Document evidence that the patient and family demonstrate an understanding of:
❏ the nature of the disease and its implications
❏ signs and symptoms of myasthenic and cholinergic crises
❏ activity recommendations and limitations
❏ airway clearance procedures
❏ the purpose, dosage, administration schedule, and adverse effects of all discharge medications (usual discharge medications include anticholinesterases)

❏ community resource and support groups
❏ how and where to obtain a medical alert tag
❏ when and how to contact the emergency medical system
❏ date, time, and location of follow-up appointments
❏ how to contact the doctor.

Documentation checklist
Using outcome criteria as a guide, document:
❏ clinical status on admission
❏ significant changes in status
❏ responses to medications
❏ periods of fatigue or increased weakness
❏ swallowing ability
❏ respiratory parameters before and after medication administration
❏ activity tolerance
❏ patient and family teaching
❏ discharge planning.

ASSOCIATED PLANS OF CARE

Grieving
Ineffective family coping: Compromised
Ineffective individual coping
Knowledge deficit
Total parenteral nutrition

REFERENCES

Hardy, E.M., et al. "Myasthenia Gravis: An Overview," *Orthopaedic Nursing* 13(6):37-42, November/December 1994.
Kernich, C.A., et al. "Myasthenia Gravis: Pathophysiology, Diagnosis, and Collaborative Care," *Journal of Neuroscience Nursing* 27(4):207-18, August 1995.
Kersten, L.D. *Comprehensive Respiratory Nursing*. Philadelphia: W.B. Saunders Co., 1989.
Maehling, J.S., ed. "Sexuality and the Myasthetic," in *The Myasthenia Gravis Manual for the Nurse*. Chicago: National Myasthenia Gravis Foundation, 1990.

Seizures

DRG information
DRG 024 Seizure and Headache with Complication or Comorbidity (CC); Age 17+.
Mean LOS = 5.8 days
Principal diagnoses include:
• cerebral arteritis
• convulsions or epilepsy (seizures)
• benign intracranial hypertension (increased intracranial pressure [ICP])
• reaction to spinal or lumbar puncture
• postconcussion syndrome.
DRG 025 Seizure and Headache without CC; Age 17+.
Mean LOS = 3.9 days
Principal diagnoses include selected principal diagnoses listed under DRG 024.
DRG 026 Seizure and Headache. Ages 0 to 17.
Mean LOS = 4.6 days
Principal diagnoses include selected principal diagnoses listed under DRG 024.

INTRODUCTION

Definition and time focus
A seizure represents uncontrolled, paroxysmal, abnormal electrical discharge in the central nervous system (CNS). The precise mechanism involved is not known, but a decreased neuronal firing threshold or excessive irritability is suspected.

Seizures are described as primary or secondary, depending on whether the cause can be identified. Primary (idiopathic) seizures appear without any identifiable cause, commonly arise in childhood, and may result from a congenital tendency. Secondary seizures are triggered by specific metabolic, structural, chemical, or physical abnormalities. Diagnostically, seizures are classified into two broad groups: partial and generalized. Partial seizures involve localized areas of brain irritability and are characterized by physical activity that corresponds to the affected area of the brain. Loss of consciousness may not occur. Generalized seizures involve both brain hemispheres and, usually, major bilateral muscle activity and loss of consciousness.

Seizures are commonly a sign of underlying abnormality, and any seizure, even in a patient with a preexisting seizure history, must be evaluated within the context of the patient's overall condition. In some patients, a single, brief seizure may be of minimal concern; in others, it may represent grave deterioration in the patient's neurologic status. Persistent or recurrent generalized seizures warrant immediate pharmacologic control and prompt identification and treatment of the underlying cause. Because seizures present such a wide range of physical manifestations, this plan focuses on the patient exhibiting generalized tonic-clonic seizures; you should, however, be knowledgeable about and alert for more subtle types of seizures as well.

Etiology and precipitating factors
• Metabolic conditions—hyperpyrexia, hypoxia, hypoglycemia, hyperglycemia, electrolyte imbalances, uremia, fluid overload
• Chemical or pharmacologic conditions—inadequate serum anticonvulsant levels, alcohol or drug overdose or toxicity, alcohol or drug withdrawal
• Infections—meningitis and encephalitis
• Structural or physical conditions—increased ICP, cerebral edema, cerebral or subdural hematoma, cerebral hemorrhage, eclampsia, malignant hypertension, tumor, congenital malformations
• Degenerative conditions—Alzheimer's disease, multiple sclerosis, systemic lupus erythematosus
• Reduced cardiac output—Stokes-Adams syncope, other arrhythmias
• Idiopathic origin

FOCUSED ASSESSMENT GUIDELINES

The patient exhibiting generalized seizures cannot always provide relevant historical information, so the nursing history (functional health patterns) section of this plan has been omitted. Instead, these guidelines for observing and documenting seizures can help in developing an accurate diagnosis and effective interventions.

Preictal phase
• Did an aura or warning precede seizure onset? What was the patient doing when the seizure began (or when the aura was noted)?

Tonic-clonic phases
• Did the patient give a shrill cry?
• Did the patient fall?
• What kind of movement was noted first?
• Where did it begin?
• Were other areas progressively involved? If so, in what pattern?
• If a tonic (rigid) phase occurred, how long did it last?

• If a clonic (jerking) phase occurred, how long did it last?
• How long did the entire seizure last?
• Did the patient lose bowel or bladder control?
• During the phases of the seizure, did the pupils react? Deviate?
• Did the patient lose consciousness? If so, when?

Postictal phase
• What was the patient's level of consciousness after the seizure?
• Did the patient exhibit amnesia, confusion, disorientation, or agitation when he regained consciousness?
• Did the patient have any motor, sensory, or perceptual deficits after the seizure?
• How long did the postictal phase last?

Physical findings
Physical findings vary widely, depending on the type of seizure activity, the area of brain tissue involved, and the phase of the seizure (see *Physical findings in seizures*). Keep in mind that the range of physical manifestations is almost limitless.

Diagnostic studies
Because a seizure represents a clinical sign, not a diagnosis, testing is usually needed to determine the seizure's cause. The following is a list of possible studies that may be ordered for this purpose.
• Serum glucose tests—can rule out hypoglycemia or hyperglycemia as a cause of seizure
• Serum phenytoin or serum phenobarbital levels—allows evaluation of adequacy of anticonvulsant dosage in the patient with a known seizure history
• Blood urea nitrogen, creatinine studies—allows evaluation of renal function because uremia may induce seizures
• Serum electrolytes—abnormal levels, particularly a calcium deficiency, may induce seizures
• Arterial blood gas values—may indicate hypoxia, which can induce seizures or result from prolonged seizures or associated respiratory depression
• Toxicology screening—may indicate drug ingestion as a cause of seizures
• Blood cultures—can rule out sepsis as a cause of seizures
• Computerized tomography scan—may identify cerebral abnormality, such as tumor, arteriovenous malformation, hemorrhage, or edema
• Lumbar puncture—may identify infection, indicated by bacteria, increased white blood cell count, and decreased glucose level in cerebrospinal fluid; increased pressure may indicate a space-occupying lesion, or bleeding may indicate hemorrhage
• Electroencephalography—may identify the lesion area. Increased electrical activity and spikes characterize generalized motor seizures. Repeated studies may be necessary to record actual seizure activity
• Magnetic resonance imaging—may reveal intracerebral abnormality
• Skull X-rays—may indicate fractures or areas of calcification
• Cerebral angiography—allows evaluation of cerebral circulatory status and identifies vascular abnormalities
• ICP monitoring—allows for identification of possible increased ICP as cause of seizure

Potential complications
• Status epilepticus
• Airway obstruction
• Respiratory arrest
• Aspiration pneumonia
• Hyperthermia
• Hypoglycemia
• Renal failure
• Cerebral ischemia

CLINICAL SNAPSHOT

SEIZURES

Major nursing diagnoses and collaborative problems	Key patient outcomes
Ineffective airway clearance	Maintain a clear airway.
Risk for status epilepticus	Maintain therapeutic drug levels.
Risk for injury	Experience no injury related to muscle contraction.
Knowledge deficit (seizure management)	Verbalize understanding of seizure management.

Physical findings in seizures

Body system	Tonic phase	Clonic phase	Postictal phase
Neurologic	• Shrill cry; then loss of consciousness • Pupils dilated and nonreactive	• Loss of consciousness • Pupils may or may not remain dilated and nonreactive • Excessive salivation	• Deep sleep; then confusion, disorientation, amnesia • Reactive pupils
Musculoskeletal	• Opisthotonos • Rigidity • Jaw clenching • Extension of extremities • Clenched fists	• Violent, bilateral, rhythmic jerking • Facial grimacing	• Flaccidity
Pulmonary	• Apnea	• Stertorous, irregular respirations	• Deep, regular respirations
Renal/Gastrointestinal		• Fecal incontinence • Urinary incontinence	
Integumentary	• Cyanosis	• Profuse diaphoresis • Flushing	
Cardiovascular	• Bradycardia	• Bradycardia or tachycardia • Hypertension	

NURSING DIAGNOSIS

Ineffective airway clearance related to loss of consciousness, apnea, excessive secretions, jaw clenching, or airway occlusion by tongue or foreign body

Nursing priorities

• Maintain patent airway.
• Promote adequate oxygenation.

Patient outcome criterion

Throughout the seizure, the patient will maintain a clear airway.

Interventions

1. If the patient reports seeing an aura or if a warning phase occurs, turn the patient to the side and use the chin lift or jaw thrust maneuver as needed to maintain an open airway. Never try to force the jaw open or insert an oral airway during the seizure.

Rationales

1. Turning the patient to the side promotes drainage of saliva from the mouth and reduces the risk of aspiration. Attempts to force the jaw open or insert objects during a seizure may cause damage to the teeth or injury to the caregiver. An apneic period of up to 60 seconds is usually followed by resumption of spontaneous respiration. If the airway becomes occluded during the tonic phase, significant hypoxia may ensue, so maintaining an open airway is essential.

Neurologic disorders

2. Suction the oropharynx, as needed. Provide supplemental oxygen via nasal cannula.

3. If seizures are persistent (unresponsive to drug therapy) or frequently recur, notify the doctor immediately and anticipate the need for endotracheal intubation and mechanical ventilation. See the "Mechanical ventilation" plan, page 283.

4. After the seizure, insert a nasogastric (NG) tube and connect it to low suction, as ordered. Do not attempt to insert an NG tube during an active seizure.

5. Additional individualized interventions: _____
_____

2. During the clonic and postictal phases, the patient who is not fully conscious is at risk for aspirating saliva that has accumulated during the tonic phase. Vomiting may also occur. Supplemental oxygen is indicated because seizures cause increased oxygen demands. Also, some degree of respiratory depression commonly follows generalized seizures. A cannula is preferred because a mask may hamper airway clearance if vomiting occurs.

3. Status epilepticus, in which seizure activity persists or recurs without the patient regaining consciousness, is a medical emergency. Irreversible brain damage may result from the prolonged apnea that occurs. Mechanical ventilation may be necessary to ensure adequate oxygenation while attempting to stop the seizures. The "Mechanical ventilation" plan contains detailed interventions for the care of the patient on a ventilator.

4. Emptying the stomach of gastric contents prevents accidental aspiration should vomiting occur. Attempting to insert an NG tube during an active seizure could stimulate a gag reflex and vomiting.

5. Rationales: _____
_____

COLLABORATIVE PROBLEM

Risk for status epilepticus related to inadequate pharmacologic control or misidentification of underlying cause

Nursing priorities

• Stop seizures.
• Treat underlying cause.

Patient outcome criteria

• Following onset of seizures, the patient will:
  – be recognized as being at risk for status epilepticus
  – receive appropriate anticonvulsants promptly
  – have underlying causes identified and treated.
• Throughout the hospital stay, the patient will:
  – maintain therapeutic drug levels
  – receive appropriate therapy for the underlying cause of seizures.

Interventions

1. Administer I.V. antiseizure medication, as ordered. Commonly ordered medications for acute seizures include the following:

Rationales

1. Prolonged seizures may result in respiratory depression or arrest, cardiovascular insufficiency, or cerebral edema. Antiseizure medications suppress the ectopic focus.

• diazepam (Valium), 5 to 10 mg, I.V.; may repeat every 10 to 15 minutes, not to exceed 30 mg in an hour. Observe the patient closely for respiratory depression. Monitor for drug interactions, especially if the patient is also taking phenothiazines, barbiturates, narcotics, or monoamine oxidase inhibitors.

• phenobarbital (Luminal) and other barbiturate anticonvulsants. The usual dose of phenobarbital ranges from 60 to 400 mg/day. Observe the patient closely for respiratory depression, especially if the patient also received diazepam. Monitor carefully for drug interactions, especially if the patient is taking phenothiazines, warfarin (Coumadin), digoxin (Lanoxin), or disulfiram (Antabuse).

• phenytoin (Dilantin; the usual loading dose is 10 to 15 mg/kg, followed by 100 mg every 6 to 8 hours. Administer phenytoin slowly in normal saline solution, giving no more than 50 mg/minute. Observe the patient's electrocardiogram (ECG) during phenytoin administration. Monitor closely for adverse reactions or indications of possible toxicity, such as anemia, elevated serum glucose levels, GI upset, and diplopia with nystagmus.
–Monitor therapeutic blood levels, as ordered.

–Monitor carefully for possible drug interactions. Drugs that may increase serum phenytoin levels include chloramphenicol (Chloromycetin)), isoniazid (Laniazid), salicylates, sulfonamides, cimetidine (Tagamet), warfarin, and benzodiazepines; acute alcohol ingestion also may increase serum phenytoin levels. Phenytoin may increase metabolism of warfarin and digitoxin (Cristodigin). Digitoxin, reserpine (Diupres), prednisone (Deltasone), phenobarbital, and chronic alcoholism may decrease phenytoin levels.

2. Consider possible underlying causes. Assist with identification and treatment. Underlying causes include:
• head trauma

• electrolyte imbalance

• hypoxia

• Diazepam is the initial drug of choice for generalized motor status epilepticus, although it is neither recommended nor sufficient for ongoing seizure control. It appears to act on the limbic system, thalamus, and hypothalamus to stop seizures. Respiratory depression is a common adverse reaction. The medications listed may potentiate the actions of diazepam and increase the risk of respiratory compromise.

• Like diazepam, phenobarbital depresses the CNS. Its precise action is unclear, but it appears to reduce cerebral oxygen consumption and may help decrease ICP. It also potentiates phenothiazines. Phenobarbital may decrease warfarin absorption and digoxin metabolism. Disulfiram may increase the likelihood of toxicity.

• Phenytoin appears to act on the motor cortex to stabilize the threshold against neuronal hyperexcitability, possibly by aiding the efflux of sodium from neurons. Phenytoin must be administered in saline solution because it precipitates in glucose-containing solutions. ECG monitoring is essential; giving phenytoin too rapidly may cause arrhythmias or cardiac arrest.

–Assessing serum phenytoin levels allows the determination of the optimal dosage and minimizes the risk of toxicity.
–Phenytoin reacts with many other medications so controlling seizures may involve balancing phenytoin with other drugs. Watch for adverse reactions and signs of toxicity or inadequate therapeutic effect.

2. In a patient without a history of seizures, treating the underlying cause is crucial to seizure control.
• Secondary seizures are caused most commonly by head trauma. If the patient was admitted after an acute traumatic event, this link may be obvious. However, seizures may occur months or even years after head injury, as scar tissue creates a focus for abnormal neuronal activity, so careful history taking is needed.
• Electrolyte imbalances may induce seizures by altering cell membrane permeability, thus interfering with normal neuronal electrical conduction.
• Sufficient oxygen is essential for maintaining the normal neuronal ionic gradient. Any condition that lowers the level of oxygen delivered to sensitive brain tissue may contribute to seizure activity.

Neurologic disorders

• hypoglycemia or hyperglycemia

• Cerebral neurons are extremely sensitive to decreased glucose levels because glucose is their primary substrate. A sudden drop in blood glucose seems more likely to cause neurologic problems than a gradual decline. Hyperglycemia may contribute to a hyperosmolar crenation of brain cells, with resultant irritability and altered conduction pathways. Also, seizure activity increases cerebral metabolic needs and depletes stores of glucose and energy.

• brain tumors

• Seizures are the major initial sign in as many as 18% of patients with undetected brain tumors. Tissue compression from tumor growth is usually the cause.

• infections

• Infections may contribute to seizures by leading to scarring (in response to inflammatory changes), cerebral edema (in acute infections), hyperpyrexia, abscesses, or autoimmune demyelinization (as in encephalomyelitis, for example).

• cerebral hemorrhage

• Localized ischemic damage to brain tissue may cause seizures.

• toxins.

• Toxins may cause seizures by interfering with the cell's metabolic processes, altering cell membrane function and integrity. Some hydrocarbons, lead, mercury, and arsenic may cause seizures in high concentrations. A hypersensitive patient may develop seizures in response to certain medications such as phenothiazines. Withdrawal from alcohol or barbiturates is a common cause of seizures because abrupt withdrawal from the CNS-depressant effects of either appears to increase neuronal irritability.

3. If seizures do not respond to drug therapy, anticipate possible preparation for neuromuscular blockade or general anesthesia, with mechanical ventilation.

3. Status epilepticus has a mortality of about 10% and causes one-third of all seizure-related deaths. As seizures persist, cerebral vasodilation occurs, perfusion pressure drops, and irreversible cell damage follows from nutritional depletion and neuronal exhaustion. Neuromuscular blockade stops motor activity but does not directly interrupt brain electrical activity. General anesthesia causes global depression of cerebral function, interrupting the cycle of hyperexcitability at its source.

4. Additional individualized interventions: _____

4. Rationales: _____

NURSING DIAGNOSIS
Risk for injury: Trauma or myoglobinuria related to excessive uncontrolled muscle activity

Nursing priority
Prevent injury.

Patient outcome criterion
During and after the seizure episode, the patient will experience no injury from muscle contractions.

Interventions

1. At the seizure's onset, ensure safe patient positioning. Place pillows or padding around the patient and raise and pad the side rails. Do not restrain the patient's arms and legs. Maintain the bed in low position.

2. During the seizure, stay with the patient. Maintain a patent airway and suction secretions as needed. Provide privacy, as possible.

3. After motor activity stops, place the patient in the side-lying position. Perform a neurologic evaluation, noting pupil size and reactivity, level of consciousness, responsiveness to stimuli, and respiratory status. Repeat the evaluation every 15 to 30 minutes until condition stabilizes. Inspect the oropharynx, tongue, and teeth for seizure-related injury.

4. Avoid excessive environmental stimulation during the postictal period.

5. If the seizure was prolonged, monitor urine for possible myoglobinuria, indicated by a red or cola color. Send urine specimen for myoglobin testing. Report findings to the doctor promptly.

6. Additional individualized interventions: _____

Rationales

1. Violent muscle contractions may cause injury without protective measures. Padded side rails help prevent injury if the patient strikes the rails during the seizure. Restraining arms and legs may result in fractures during the clonic phase.

2. The seizing patient is extremely vulnerable to injury because of uncontrollable muscle activity. After the seizure, the patient is commonly embarrassed and ashamed of the loss of control. Providing privacy helps protect the patient's dignity.

3. The side-lying position helps prevent aspiration. Careful monitoring of status during the postictal period is essential because respiratory depression is common. Violent seizure activity may result in mouth injury, and blood in the oropharynx and loose teeth may be aspirated.

4. Environmental stimulation (such as bright lights, abrupt movement, or loud, sudden noises) may reactivate neuronal irritability and stimulate further seizures.

5. Repeated, vigorous muscle contraction releases excess amounts of myoglobin into the bloodstream from muscle cell breakdown. If the quantity is sufficient, the accumulated myoglobin may occlude the kidneys and cause renal failure. Treatment involves flushing the renal system, using fluids and diuretics.

6. Rationales: _____

NURSING DIAGNOSIS

Knowledge deficit (seizure management) related to lack of exposure to information

Nursing priority

Instruct the patient and family on seizure management.

Patient outcome criteria

By the time of discharge, the patient and family will demonstrate and verbalize understanding of seizure management.

Interventions

1. Assess the patient's and family's current level of understanding. Refer to the "Knowledge deficit" plan, page 72.

2. Instruct the patient and family about the disorder and the need to adhere to a medical regimen.

Rationales

1. Determining the level of understanding allows the nurse to individualize learning to meet patient needs. The "Knowledge deficit" plan contains detailed information about this problem.

2. Understanding the disorder helps to increase compliance.

3. Instruct the patient and family about medications and causes of seizures.

4. Additional individualized interventions: _____

3. Teaching improves compliance. Failure to take medications is a common cause of recurrent seizures. Excessive stress, fatigue, and environmental factors may cause seizures in susceptible individuals.

4. Rationales: _____

DISCHARGE PLANNING

Discharge checklist
Before discharge, the patient shows evidence of:
- ❏ cause of seizures identified and treated
- ❏ seizures controlled
- ❏ respiratory status stable
- ❏ neurologic status stable.

Teaching checklist
Document evidence that the patient and family demonstrate an understanding of:
- ❏ the cause and implications of seizures
- ❏ treatments instituted
- ❏ signs of possible recurrence
- ❏ safety precautions.

Documentation checklist
Using outcome criteria as a guide, document:
- ❏ clinical status on admission
- ❏ significant changes in status
- ❏ pertinent diagnostic test findings
- ❏ seizure episodes
- ❏ safety precautions instituted
- ❏ pharmacologic interventions
- ❏ patient and family teaching
- ❏ discharge planning.

ASSOCIATED PLANS OF CARE

Craniotomy
Drug overdose
Hypoglycemia
Increased intracranial pressure
Mechanical ventilation
Multiple trauma
Sensory-perceptual alteration

REFERENCES

Ayers, S.M., et al. *Textbook of Critical Care*, 3rd ed. Philadelphia: W.B. Saunders Co., 1995.

Clochesy, J.M., et al. *Critical Care Nursing*, 2nd ed. Philadelphia: W.B. Saunders Co., 1996.

Hickey, J.V. *The Clinical Practice of Neurological and Neurosurgical Nursing*, 4th ed. Philadelphia: Lippincott-Raven Pubs., 1997.

Phipps, W.J., et al. *Medical-Surgical Nursing, Concepts and Clinical Practice*, 5th ed. St. Louis: Mosby–Year Book, Inc., 1995.

Thelan, L.A., et al. *Critical Care Nursing Diagnosis and Management*, 2nd ed. St. Louis: Mosby–Year Book, Inc., 1994.

Thompson, J.M., et al. *Mosby's Clinical Nursing*, 4th ed. St. Louis: Mosby–Year Book, Inc., 1997.

Part 4

Eye
disorders

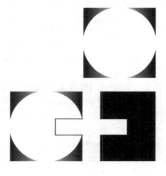

Glaucoma

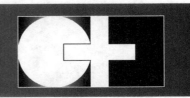

DRG information

DRG 038   Primary Iris Procedure.
Mean LOS = 2.6 days

DRG 045   Neurologic Eye Disorders (low tension glaucoma).
Mean LOS = 3.8 days

DRG 046   Other Disorders of the Eye with Complication or Comorbidity (CC) (associated with disorders of the lens or borderline glaucoma); Age 17+.
Mean LOS = 5.6 days

Additional DRG information: Patients with DRGs 038, 045, and 046 are rarely admitted to acute care facilities. DRG 038 patients are most commonly admitted to same-day surgery units or are treated as outpatients. This reduces the amount of time available for teaching and evaluation of the patient's ability to follow discharge instructions. Documentation must contain evidence of adequate home support to assist the patient after discharge. A referral to home care should always be considered. DRGs 045 and 046 are treated in the acute care setting if a CC necessitates admission.

INTRODUCTION

Definition and time focus

Glaucoma is the progressive loss of visual fields resulting from increased intraocular pressure, which damages the optic nerve. The increased intraocular pressure results from an imbalance between the formation and absorption of aqueous humor. Simple chronic glaucoma is characterized by a gradual loss of peripheral vision, eventually leading to total vision loss; the less common acute angle-closure glaucoma is usually characterized by a severe vision loss within a few hours of onset. This plan focuses on the patient admitted for definitive diagnosis and management of either type of glaucoma. Simple chronic glaucoma is sometimes referred to as open-angle or primary open-angle glaucoma. Acute angle-closure glaucoma is also known as acute (congestive) glaucoma, narrow-angle glaucoma, and angle-closure or primary angle-closure glaucoma.

Etiology and precipitating factors

• Simple chronic glaucoma (severe myopia; degenerative changes in the eye; swollen cataracts; ocular trauma, infection, tumor, inflammation, or hemorrhage; other factors that can narrow the trabecular meshwork openings and increase resistance to aqueous humor

drainage and raising intraocular pressure; and genetic predisposition)

• Acute angle-closure glaucoma (darkness; excitement, mydriatic medications, and other factors that can dilate the pupils and push the iris against the trabecular meshwork and thus block drainage of aqueous humor through the anterior-chamber angle and increase intraocular pressure)

FOCUSED ASSESSMENT GUIDELINES

Nursing history (functional health pattern findings)

Health perception–health management pattern

• Simple chronic glaucoma—slow onset, initially without symptoms; the patient then develops early symptoms, such as gradual loss of peripheral vision (tunnel vision), slightly blurred vision, persistent dull eye pain or tired feeling in the eye, or failure to detect color changes (particularly blue-green); later symptoms include blurred vision, halos around lights, morning headaches that disappear shortly after arising, or pain behind eyeballs

• Acute angle-closure glaucoma—the patient may report sudden onset of severe eye pain radiating to head, sudden blurred vision progressing to severe loss of vision within a few hours, decreased light perception, or colored haloes around lights; the eye may appear inflamed and watery and the pupil may be fixed and dilated; the patient may also experience nausea, vomiting, and abdominal discomfort

• History of frequent changes in eyeglass prescription after age 40 or of severe myopia

• Age, sex, race, preexisting condition—patient who is over age 40, female, black, or diabetic or who has a family history of glaucoma is at increased risk

Nutritional-metabolic pattern

• Acute angle-closure glaucoma—the patient may report nausea, vomiting, or abdominal pain

Activity-exercise pattern

• History of decreased ability to cope with activities of daily living (ADLs)

• Fatigue in performing ADLs

• Decreased time spent in leisure activities

• Self-care deficit such as inadequate grooming

• Alterations in mobility, such as bumping into people or objects and hesitancy in walking in unfamiliar environments

Sleep-rest pattern
• Difficulty adjusting to darkness
• Eye pain at night or in the early morning
Self-perception–self-concept pattern
• Concern about ability to be independent
Role-relationship pattern
• Decreased ability to maintain social, job, and family roles
• Increased isolation from other people
Value-belief pattern
• Delay in seeking medical attention because symptoms developed gradually
• Difficulty in comprehending or believing that lifelong treatment will be required

Physical findings
Gastrointestinal
With acute angle-closure glaucoma
• Vomiting
• Abdominal pain
Neurologic
• Increased intraocular pressure
• Cupping of optic disk
• Visual field losses with scotomas (blind spots)
• Optic disk degeneration
• Whiteness of optic nerve disk
• White or gray appearance of cornea
• Shallow anterior chamber
• With acute angle-closure glaucoma, the patient may also have a fixed and dilated pupil, corneal edema, hazy appearance of cornea, headache, and reddened eye
Musculoskeletal
• Pained or anxious facial expression
• Fatigue

• Hesitancy in walking

Diagnostic studies
• Ophthalmoscopy — shows a white optic disk with cupping and displaced and depressed large retinal vessels
• Tonometry — shows corneal indentation consistent with elevated intraocular pressure; values above 22 mm Hg indicate glaucoma, although individual norms vary
• Gonioscopy — shows characteristic changes over time, small defects progressing to larger visual field defects (the patient may have 20/20 central vision); optic disk becomes wider, deeper, and paler; impending angle closure may appear before rise in intraocular pressure
• Tonography — shows characteristic changes: a flat graphic tracing with increased intraocular pressure
• Visual field determination — shows characteristic loss of visual field as well as location, size, and density of scotomas
• Slit-lamp microscopy — shows characteristic changes, including a fixed and moderately dilated pupil, erythematous conjunctiva, and an edematous, cloudy cornea

Potential complications
• Total blindness
• Trauma or self-injury
• Nutritional deficits
• Failure to thrive
• Social isolation

CLINICAL SNAPSHOT

GLAUCOMA

Major nursing diagnoses and collaborative problems	Key patient outcomes
Risk for further vision loss	Show no signs or symptoms of increased intraocular pressure.
Eye pain	Verbalize the absence or relief of pain.
Risk for injury	Adjust to limitations on movement and activity.
Fear	Verbalize fears.
Knowledge deficit (surgery)	Verbalize understanding of surgery and postoperative care.

Eye disorders

COLLABORATIVE PROBLEM

Risk for further vision loss related to increases in intraocular pressure

Nursing priority

Prevent or minimize increases in intraocular pressure.

Patient outcome criteria

By the time of discharge, the patient will:
• show no signs or symptoms of increased intraocular pressure
• show no further decrease in vision
• list three signs of increased intraocular pressure
• list three techniques to minimize an intraocular pressure increase.

Interventions

1. Assess for the presence of or any increase in eye pain, pain around orbit, blurred vision, reddened eye, abdominal pain, nausea, vomiting, and neurologic changes, on admission and as needed.

2. Evaluate the visual fields on admission and as needed.

3. Assess the patient's use of medications before hospitalization by obtaining a comprehensive list of all current and past medications. Verify with the doctor the need to continue medications during the hospital stay.

4. Administer and document ocular medications, as ordered.

Rationales

1. A change from baseline assessment data may indicate increasing intraocular pressure affecting optic nerve function. With acute angle-closure glaucoma, this may indicate an emergency situation.

2. Progressive visual field losses indicate increasing intraocular pressure. Detection of subtle changes may require special equipment.

3. Certain medications can cause an acute episode; many preparations can produce increased intraocular pressure, including:
• steroids (all types)
• oral and nasal inhalants
• amphetamines
• nasal decongestants (oral or spray)
• nonprescription diet capsules or tablets
• anticholinergics
• antihistamines
• antidiarrheal agents
• some antidepressant drugs
• nonsteroidal anti-inflammatory drugs.

4. Consistent and timely use of medications will decrease intraocular pressure. Common medications used singly or in combination include:
• cholinergics (parasympathomimetics), such as pilocarpine hydrochloride (Pilocar) and carbachol (Carboptic), to promote aqueous outflow
• adrenergics (sympathomimetics) such as epinephrine (Epifrin, to decrease aqueous humor production and increase aqueous outflow
• carbonic anhydrase inhibitors such as oral acetazolamide (Diamox) and beta-adrenergic blockers such as timolol maleate (Timoptic) to reduce secretion of aqueous humor
• hyperosmotics such as mannitol (Osmitrol) used preoperatively to reduce intraocular pressure by reducing the volume of intraocular fluid.

5. Evaluate medications' effectiveness and observe for the presence of major adverse effects, including:
• cholinergics — headache, excessive salivation, diaphoresis, nausea, and vomiting
• adrenergics — headache, tachycardia, and tremors
• carbonic anhydrase inhibitors — paresthesia, anorexia, nausea, fatigue, and impotence
• beta-adrenergic blockers — bradycardia, hypotension, fatigue, and depression
• hyperosmotics — dehydration.

6. Assess for signs and symptoms of increased tolerance to ocular medications related to prolonged medical therapy: increased blurring of vision, increased headache, nausea, fixed and dilated pupil, increased blood pressure, allergic reaction, and asthmatic attack. Notify the doctor at once.

7. Minimize stressful events.

8. Use noninvasive techniques to reduce intraocular pressure.

9. Prepare the patient for diagnostic testing.

10. Additional individualized interventions: _____
_____

5. If signs or symptoms persist or increase, intraocular pressure is probably increasing, and the doctor needs to be notified. Adverse effects may compromise other body systems.

6. An increase in signs and symptoms may indicate that the prescribed medication is no longer effective and intraocular pressure is rising.

7. Stress — worry, fear, excitement, or anger — increases intraocular pressure. Anticipating and preventing stress reactions helps maintain intraocular pressure at a safe level.

8. Meditation, rest, a quiet environment, and a decrease in stimuli help decrease stress and, thus, intraocular pressure.

9. Some diagnostic tests such as tonometry involve application of direct pressure to the eyeball. These may be done repeatedly, at different times of the day, to assess intraocular pressure. Thorough explanations of tests may decrease the patient's anxiety and ensure compliance during the procedures.

10. Rationales: _____
_____

Nursing diagnosis

Eye pain related to progressive pressure on the optic nerve

Nursing priority

Minimize or relieve eye pain.

Patient outcome criteria

• Within 30 minutes of the occurrence of intraocular pain, the patient will verbalize the absence or relief of pain.
• By the time of discharge, the patient will:
  – practice selected noninvasive pain-relief measures
  – identify stressors that may increase pain.

Interventions

1. On admission, assess the patient for presence and degree of eye pain.

2. Monitor the patient every 2 hours while awake for the occurrence of, or an increase in, eye pain.

Rationales

1. Eye pain in the glaucoma patient indicates increased intraocular pressure.

2. Increased eye pain, or the occurrence of eye pain when not present previously, may indicate increasing intraocular pressure.

3. On admission, teach the patient to report any eye pain or change in symptoms.

3. Early intervention can prevent further damage to the optic disk.

4. Assess for associated signs and symptoms, such as blurred vision, nausea, vomiting, abdominal pain, or neurologic changes.

4. The patient may not report pain, but observation of associated signs or symptoms may lead to early intervention. Without early intervention, eye pain will eventually occur. These signs and symptoms may indicate increasing intraocular pressure or an episode of acute angle-closure glaucoma. Even if the patient does not report an increase in symptoms, be alert for hesitancy in walking, bumping into people or walls, or new bruises from hitting objects.

5. Administer eye medications, as ordered, and document your actions.

5. Eye medications are administered to permit better drainage of aqueous humor and to decrease the amount of humor produced. Consistent, accurate medication administration will reduce intraocular pressure and may prevent eye pain.

6. Administer analgesics judiciously, as ordered, and document their use. Assess pain relief 30 minutes after administering medication.

6. Continued pain can cause increased anxiety and stress, leading to increased intraocular pressure.

7. Use noninvasive pain-relief measures as well as medications. See the "Pain" plan, page 88, for details.

7. Alternative measures such as cold eye compresses may decrease painful eye spasms. Relaxation techniques and meditation as well as a quiet room with decreased stimuli may reduce the perception of pain.

8. Help the patient identify and modify causes of stress.

8. Stress may increase intraocular pressure. Knowledge and modification of individual stressors (worry, fear, anxiety, and anger) may decrease intraocular pressure and pain.

9. Explain unfamiliar procedures and new events.

9. The patient who is well prepared for new procedures and events experiences less stress.

10. Additional individualized interventions: _____

10. Rationales: _____

NURSING DIAGNOSIS

Risk for injury related to decreased visual field, medically induced blurred vision, use of eye patches, and hesitancy in walking

Nursing priority

Prevent patient injury.

Patient outcome criteria

By the time of discharge, the patient will:
• experience no falls or injuries
• list safety measures necessary to prevent injury
• adjust to limitations on movement and activity.

Interventions

1. Assess the patient's vision. Document blurred vision, the amount of peripheral vision, blindness, or patched eyes.

Rationales

1. Unable to see all or part of the environment as a result of tunnel or blurred vision, the patient may knock over, bump into, or fall over objects. Awareness of the patient's limitations helps determine what to teach about environmental hazards and if objects should be rearranged.

2. Assess for and document signs of decreasing vision each shift.

3. Orient the patient to the environment.

4. Ensure that items are placed within the patient's maximum field of vision.

5. Illuminate the room adequately, and provide a night-light.

6. Place the bed in a low position with the wheels locked.

7. Teach the patient that some medications may affect vision.

8. Encourage the patient to ask for assistance, as needed. Instruct the patient to avoid activities that may increase intraocular pressure, such as coughing, vomiting, bending at the waist, squeezing the eyes, and straining at stool.

9. Additional individualized interventions: _____

2. As the patient's visual acuity decreases, the potential for injury increases.

3. A thorough knowledge of surroundings, including the call system and available nursing assistance, decreases the possibility of falls or injury.

4. Placing objects within the patient's reach and sight will decrease the potential for self-injury and feelings of dependence. Thereafter, the environment should never be rearranged without first notifying the patient. Move unneeded objects out of the room so that the patient will not fall over them or bump into them.

5. When a patient has blurred or decreased vision, it is even more difficult to see in a dimly lit room. Appropriate lighting promotes safety and decreases the patient's risk of self-injury.

6. The patient's potential for injury is reduced if the bed is at an appropriate level at all times.

7. Knowing that vision may be further impaired after medication administration will alert the patient to the need for increased safety measures.

8. Calling for assistance may prevent falls and injuries, and instruction may keep the patient from engaging in activities that will increase intraocular pressure.

9. Rationales: _____

NURSING DIAGNOSIS

Fear related to previous vision loss, possible surgery, and possible total blindness

Nursing priority

Comfort and support the patient.

Patient outcome criteria

Within 2 days of admission, the patient will:
• verbalize fears
• exhibit calm, relaxed facial expressions, body movements, and behavior.

Interventions

1. Encourage expression of feelings.

Rationales

1. Expressing fear, anger, and helplessness may help the patient cope. Listening attentively, providing consistent care, reassuring the patient that support is available, and communicating sensitivity to the patient's problem encourages expression of feelings. Reinforcing that the patient's response is appropriate helps to develop the trust necessary for sharing of feelings.

Eye disorders

2. Provide a quiet environment.

2. The sudden onset of symptoms and the presence of pain, as in acute angle-closure glaucoma, may be very frightening. A quiet and distraction-free environment may reduce the patient's stress while enhancing the effect of prescribed medications. As intraocular pressure and symptoms subside, fear may decrease.

3. Explain the need for frequent administration of ocular medications, tonometry readings, and physical assessments.

3. Explaining each step of the therapy may reduce the patient's fear of the unknown and promote adjustment to the new routines.

4. Support the patient's preferred coping style.

4. Determining how the patient normally copes with fear and encouraging the use of those coping strategies while offering comfort and support may help reduce fear. Offering feedback about expressed feelings and supporting realistic perceptions may help the patient cope with the fear of blindness.

5. Explore the patient's strengths, and introduce resources to help the patient cope with the fear of blindness.

5. Focusing on strengths and capabilities may help the patient recognize the ability to cope with fear of the future regardless of outcome. Introducing the patient to a person coping successfully with glaucoma may also be helpful.

6. Observe for excessive stress levels resulting from fear.

6. The patient may feel stress to the point of incapacitation. Early intervention is needed to prevent this reaction because treatment requires the participation of a calm, relaxed patient.

7. Observe for evidence of a positive response to therapy.

7. Reduced fear and increased comfort indicate that the patient is responding in a positive manner and is coping effectively with fear.

8. Additional individualized interventions: _____

8. Rationales: _____

NURSING DIAGNOSIS

Knowledge deficit (surgery) related to lack of exposure to information

Nursing priority

Increase the patient's knowledge about the surgery.

Patient outcome criteria

- By the day of surgery, the patient will:
  - verbalize understanding of preoperative instructions
  - verbalize understanding of surgery and postoperative care
  - identify signs of postoperative complications and list ways to prevent them.
- By the time of discharge, the patient will have demonstrated the proper technique for administering eyedrops.

Interventions

1. Provide preoperative teaching for the patient who will have eye surgery. (See the "Surgery" plan, page 103, for details.) Assess the patient's level of knowledge regarding the disease, and incorporate relevant pathophysiology into the teaching, as needed, to correct any misconceptions.

2. Explain noninvasive procedures, such as laser iridotomy or laser trabeculoplasty, if appropriate.

3. Explain diathermy, cryothermy, or ultrasound therapy, as appropriate.

4. Provide instruction about the postoperative routine, precautions, and signs of complications. Explain the increased risk for injury related to the eye patch, possible poor vision in the other eye, and frustration from dependence on others and activity restrictions.

5. Administer medication as needed and encourage the patient to dim room lights and wear dark glasses.

6. Prevent infection by washing hands before administering eyedrops or changing a patch, keeping the tip of the eyedropper sterile, and checking regularly for drainage.

7. Additional individualized interventions: _____

Rationales

1. The patient is awake during eye surgery and must be cooperative. Information about the procedure and correction of misconceptions allays anxieties and helps ensure cooperation. Procedures include classic surgical (cutting) techniques, such as iridectomy (used for acute angle-closure glaucoma) and trabeculectomy (used for simple chronic glaucoma), and laser techniques (iridotomy and trabeculoplasty). Surgery is usually necessary with acute angle-closure glaucoma.

2. Knowing that these procedures involve less risk than surgery, are more cost-effective, and can be done in an outpatient setting may help ease the patient's fears. Intraocular pressure is checked after 2 hours and then in 24 hours. Discomfort is usually limited to headaches and blurred vision. Glaucoma medications are continued at least until the first checkup.

3. These techniques partially destroy cells of the ciliary body to reduce aqueous production and intraocular pressure. Explaining the purpose and desired result of the therapy will help reduce the patient's fears about further loss of vision. The patient is observed for several hours before discharge.

4. The patient's understanding of the postoperative routine will help avoid complications. Intraocular hemorrhage may be related to improper positioning or increased intraocular pressure. Intraocular pressure can be increased by sneezing, coughing, bending, vomiting, straining with bowel movement, or lifting heavy objects.

5. The eye will be sensitive to light after the eye patch is removed.

6. Eye infection may cause vision loss and negate the effects of surgery.

7. Rationales: _____

DISCHARGE PLANNING

Discharge checklist
Before discharge, the patient shows evidence of:
- ❏ stable intraocular pressure within acceptable limits, controlled by ocular medications or surgery
- ❏ healthy coping behaviors regarding vision loss and possibility of total blindness
- ❏ an understanding of glaucoma, glaucoma management, and signs and symptoms of increasing intraocular pressure
- ❏ an understanding of the pharmacologic regimen and the reasons for lifelong treatment.

Teaching checklist
Document evidence that the patient and family demonstrate an understanding of:
- ❏ the purpose, dosage, adverse effects, and administration schedule and technique for all discharge medications as well as which eye to medicate (usual discharge medications include adrenergics, cholinergics, carbonic anhydrase inhibitors, and beta-adrenergic blockers)
- ❏ infection prevention
- ❏ the need to avoid nonprescription medications
- ❏ the need to avoid medications that dilate the pupils

◻ signs and symptoms indicating increasing intraocular pressure, such as aching around the eye or any changes in vision
◻ the date, time, and location of follow-up appointments and the importance of lifelong medical supervision
◻ when and how to report any reappearance of symptoms or stressful events to the ophthalmologist
◻ safety precautions in taking eye medications, such as carrying medications when away from home, having a reserve bottle of eyedrops at home, and knowing which local pharmacies are open late in case of an emergency
◻ factors that increase the risk of injury
◻ the need to assess safety of home environment
◻ safety measures to use or the need for assistance when performing tasks that require clear vision
◻ circumstances that may increase intraocular pressure, such as emotional upsets, fatigue, constrictive clothing, heavy exertion, sneezing, coughing, bending, vomiting, straining at stool, lifting heavy objects, and sexual activity
◻ recommended activities and precautions, such as exercise in moderation, moderate reading and television watching, maintenance of regular bowel habits, and no driving for 2 hours after administration of ocular drugs
◻ transportation alternatives
◻ ways to mobilize support systems
◻ ways to adjust to social situations with vision loss and the need to follow medication routine
◻ the need for potassium supplement or high-potassium foods if acetazolamide is prescribed
◻ the need to alert health care providers about diagnosis and continued need for prescribed eyedrops
◻ the importance of wearing a medical alert tag indicating glaucoma diagnosis.

Documentation checklist
Using outcome criteria as a guide, document:
◻ clinical status on admission
◻ significant changes in status, especially regarding vision, headaches, and eye pain
◻ results of ophthalmoscopy, tonometry, gonioscopy, tonography, visual field determination, and slit-lamp microscopy
◻ episodes of eye pain or headache
◻ episodes of nausea, vomiting, or abdominal pain
◻ pain-relief measures
◻ serial tonometry results
◻ surgery or ocular medication management
◻ nutrition intake
◻ patient and family teaching
◻ discharge planning.

ASSOCIATED PLANS OF CARE
Grieving
Ineffective family coping: Compromised
Ineffective individual coping
Knowledge deficit
Pain
Sensory-perceptual alteration
Surgery

REFERENCES
Lewis, S.M., et al. *Medical-Surgical Nursing: Assessment and Management of Clinical Problems,* 4th ed. St. Louis: Mosby–Year Book, Inc., 1996.
Thompson, J.M., et al. *Mosby's Clinical Nursing,* 4th ed. St. Louis: Mosby–Year Book, Inc., 1997.
Tilkian, S.M., et al. *Clinical and Nursing Implications of Laboratory Tests,* 5th ed. St. Louis: Mosby–Year Book, Inc., 1996.
Wilson, B.A., et al. *Nursing Drug Guide.* Stamford, Conn.: Appleton & Lange, 1997.

Retinal detachment

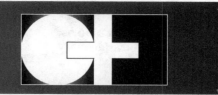

DRG information

DRG 036   Retinal Procedures.
                 Mean LOS = 1.6 days
DRG 046   Other Disorders of the Eye with Complica-
                 tion or Comorbidity (CC); Age 17+.
                 Mean LOS = 5.6 days
DRG 047   Other Disorders of the Eye without CC;
                 Age 17+
                 Mean LOS = 3.8 days
DRG 048   Other Disorders of the Eye. Ages 0 to 17.
                 Mean LOS = 2.9 days

Additional DRG information: If retinal detachment cannot or should not be repaired surgically, DRG 046, 047,
or 048 would be used. If surgery is attempted, DRG
036 would be used. Although the mean LOS for each
DRG is between 1.6 and 5.6 days, it would not be unusual for a patient with a retinal detachment to be discharged the day of or the day after the surgical procedure. Therefore, the patient's home support system
should be carefully analyzed and a referral to home care
should always be considered.

INTRODUCTION

Definition and time focus
Retinal detachment (RD) is the separation of the neural
retinal layer (rods and cones) from the pigment epithelium layer of the retina. RD most commonly results
from the entry of vitreous humor (a liquid) through a
hole or tear into the potential space between the layers.
Blindness can occur unless the separation is treated.
This clinical plan focuses on the patient admitted for
surgical treatment of RD.

Etiology and precipitating factors
• Myopic eye, causing thinness of the retina and vitreous degeneration
• Aphakic eye (absent lens), causing distortion of the
eye
• Degenerative systemic or eye disease (hypertension,
diabetic retinopathy, or tumors) that causes separation
or traction on the retina from holes, hemorrhage, or
anatomic distortion
• Trauma to the head or eye that causes tearing (rip-
ping) of the retina
• Strenuous physical exertion that causes separation
from increased pressure within the eye

FOCUSED ASSESSMENT GUIDELINES

Nursing history (functional health pattern findings)
Health perception–health management pattern
• Unilateral and blurred vision loss, described as being
like a veil or like a blind being drawn over the eye
• Flashing lights, usually lasting seconds
• Floating spots (floaters), typically red blood cells (RBCs)
• Diabetes mellitus, hypertension, or an eye condition
• Black eye or history of head trauma
• Age (those over age 40 are at higher risk)
Activity-exercise pattern
• Incident of heavy straining coinciding with onset of
vision changes
Cognitive-perceptual pattern
• Inability to recall or relate present condition to previ-
ous occurrence, such as a blow to head or eye
• Little or no pain
Self-perception–self-concept pattern
• Fears about the effects of vision loss on mobility and
work
Role-relationship pattern
• Concern about ability to take care of family
Value-belief pattern
• Disbelief over suddenness of vision loss

Physical findings
Cardiovascular
• Hypertension
Neurologic
• Sudden decrease in central and peripheral vision
Integumentary
• Bruising around eyes if RD was caused by trauma
Musculoskeletal
• Hesitancy and awkwardness during ambulation

Diagnostic studies
• Laboratory data—usually reflect no significant abnormalities
• Direct and indirect ophthalmoscopic measurements—show a bulging and hanging retina, curved
reddish tear, and floating RBCs
• Visual field and acuity examinations—show unilateral vision loss opposite the area of detachment
• Biomicroscopy—may indicate proliferation of cells
along retinal and vitreous surfaces (proliferative vitreo-
retinopathy)
• Ultrasonography—identifies areas of detachment

Potential complications
• Permanent loss of vision
• Extension of RD
• RD in other eye
• Retinal hemorrhage
• Infection (scleral, choroidal, or retinal)

• Intolerance to scleral circling or buckling devices (bands or implants that serve to indent the eye inward)
• Referred pain to face and head on affected side
• Exposure of sutures or implanted devices
• Endophthalmitis (inflammation of the inner eye)
• Vitreal fibroblastic growth
• Sympathetic ophthalmia in the other eye

CLINICAL SNAPSHOT

RETINAL DETACHMENT

Major nursing diagnoses and collaborative problems	Key patient outcomes
Sensory-perceptual alteration: Visual (preoperative)	Show no further loss of vision.
Sensory-perceptual alteration: Visual (postoperative)	Maintain activity and position limitations.
Eye pain	Rate pain level as less than 3 on a 0 to 10 pain rating scale.
Impaired physical mobility	Have no skin breakdown or other effects of immobility.
Risk for injury	Be free from injury.
Anxiety	Verbalize a realistic perception of the prognosis.
Diversional activity deficit	Verbalize satisfaction with diversional activity.

COLLABORATIVE PROBLEM

Sensory-perceptual alteration: Visual (preoperative) related to extension of detachment while awaiting surgery

Nursing priority

Prevent or minimize further vision loss during the preoperative period.

Patient outcome criteria

Throughout the preoperative period, the patient will:
• show no further vision loss
• maintain position and activity limitations.

Interventions

1. Evaluate and document visual acuity and visual fields on admission, every 2 hours, and as needed.

2. Restrict movement. Place the patient on continuous bed rest. Position the head with the affected area lowermost.

Rationales

1. Changes in visual acuity and visual fields may indicate worsening detachment. Sudden loss of central vision such as inability to read may indicate detachment in the macular area. An increase in blurring or the number of floaters may indicate hemorrhage.

2. Rest decreases the risk of further detachment. A dependent position helps reattachment by gravity.

3. Pad one or both eyes, as ordered, either continuously or intermittently.

4. Additional individualized interventions: _____
_____

3. Eye pads rest the eyes and prevent rapid eye movements, which may increase fluid accumulation between the retinal layers.

4. Rationales: _____
_____

COLLABORATIVE PROBLEM

Sensory-perceptual alteration: Visual (postoperative) related to extension of tear or nonapproximation of retinal layers, retinal hemorrhage, or eye infection

Nursing priority

Prevent complications that could cause further vision loss after surgery.

Patient outcome criteria

• Within the immediate postoperative period, the patient will:
  – show no further vision loss
  – have no nausea or vomiting
  – maintain position and activity limitations
  – remain free from complications, such as hemorrhage or infection.
• Within 3 days of surgery, the patient will be able to describe signs and symptoms of recurrent retinal detachment and what to do about them.

Interventions

1. Verify specific postoperative positioning restrictions with the doctor. Inform the patient about the restrictions. Place the patient on bed rest or limited activity for 1 to 2 days. Position the head with detached area lowermost, unless a gas bubble has been injected. Position the patient who has a gas bubble (injected into the eye cavity) so that the bubble will rise against the detachment and remain there (usually this requires a face-down position with the head turned to the side just enough for the patient to breathe); maintain the face-down position for several days while the patient is in bed, eating, using the commode, or ambulating.

2. Teach the patient to avoid quick, jerking head movements, such as hair combing, face washing, teeth brushing, head turning, shampooing, and coughing; rapid eye movements, such as those involved in reading or doing crafts; vomiting; and Valsalva's maneuver.

3. After eye pads are changed (within 1 to 2 days), instruct the patient to report any vision changes or other physical symptoms immediately.

4. Give antiemetics, as needed, for nausea.

5. Give antibiotics, as ordered, to prevent infection.

6. Monitor continually for such complications as retinal hemorrhage, evidenced by vision changes and the appearance of floaters.

Rationales

1. Rest decreases the risk of detachment while the area is healing. Maintaining the affected area in a dependent position aids approximation of the layers and development of adhesion scars. The gas bubble provides traction against the area and promotes adherence of the layers. The gas bubble is absorbed into the surrounding tissue in 5 to 10 days.

2. Jerking head movements, rapid eye movements, vomiting, Valsalva's maneuver, and other quickly executed activities increase intraocular pressure — and the risk of detachment.

3. Changes in visual fields or vision acuity may indicate detachment.

4. Vomiting increases intraocular pressure and can cause detachment.

5. Infection increases the risk of vision loss.

6. Complications such as hemorrhage can increase the risk of nonapproximation of retinal layers.

Eye disorders

7. Incorporate relevant teaching into all interventions.

8. Additional individualized interventions: _____

_____

7. A knowledgeable patient is more likely to comply with recommendations and to recognize complications.

8. Rationales: _____

_____

NURSING DIAGNOSIS

Eye pain related to postoperative inflammation

Nursing priority

Relieve eye pain.

Patient outcome criteria

Within 1 day of surgery, the patient will:
• rate pain level as less than 3 on a 0 to 10 pain rating scale
• have no swelling
• show a relaxed posture and facial expression.

Interventions

1. Assess the patient for pain immediately after surgery and every 2 hours thereafter using a 0 to 10 pain rating scale.

2. Administer analgesics, as ordered and needed. Document pain episodes and medication. Apply moist compresses, as ordered.

3. Keep the room dark and quiet immediately after surgery and as needed.

4. Avoid direct pressure to the eyeball.

5. Additional individualized interventions: _____

Rationales

1. Mild pain is expected after surgery; however, a sudden change in pain may indicate complications.

2. Pain increases intraocular pressure and the risk of detachment. Moist compresses reduce swelling and relieve pain.

3. Reduced light and noise may diminish the effects of photophobia caused by mydriatics and swelling.

4. External pressure may increase intraocular pressure, pain, and risk of detachment.

5. Rationales: _____

_____

NURSING DIAGNOSIS

Impaired physical mobility related to position and activity limitations

Nursing priority

Prevent complications related to immobility.

Patient outcome criteria

Within 3 days after surgery, the patient will:
• have no skin breakdown
• exhibit clear lungs
• show no further vision loss.

Interventions

1. See the "Surgery" plan, page 103.

2. Encourage isometric, deep-breathing, and range-of-motion exercises hourly while the patient is awake. Caution the patient to avoid coughing and Valsalva's maneuver.

3. Consult the doctor regarding activity progression. Maintain the head in the desired dependent position while the patient is ambulating, as ordered.

4. Instruct the patient about postdischarge activity:
• moderate, unhurried activities for the first few weeks, avoiding jerking the head or straining (such as by reading, bending the head below the waist, or driving)
• light activities after 3 weeks (such as light secretarial work)
• after 6 weeks, heavy work, sex, and exercise.

5. Additional individualized interventions: _____

Rationales

1. The "Surgery" plan contains general interventions related to postoperative immobility.

2. These activities will prevent venous stasis, skin breakdown, and atelectasis. Coughing and Valsalva's maneuver increase intraocular pressure.

3. Most patients are ambulatory by the 2nd day after surgery. Maintaining a dependent head position will aid in scar formation and adherence of retinal layers.

4. Abrupt or vigorous changes in position associated with activity increase the risk of detachment. Lowering the head below the waist or leaning over a bowl to shampoo hair increases intraocular pressure and jeopardizes reattachment. Gradual resumption allows activity increase to parallel healing.

5. Rationales: _____

NURSING DIAGNOSIS

Risk for injury related to vision loss or eye pads

Nursing priority

Prevent injuries.

Patient outcome criteria

• Within 2 hours after surgery, the patient will be reoriented to the environment.
• During the hospital stay, the patient will:
  – be free from injury
  – be able to perform activities of daily living (ADLs) with minimal assistance.

Interventions

1. Before surgery, after surgery, and as needed, orient the patient to the room, including the bathroom, call light, telephone, bed controls, and position of furniture.

2. Explain procedures as they are done.

3. Document vision limitations on the Kardex.

4. Additional individualized interventions: _____

Rationales

1. Knowledge of the location of furniture and equipment needed for ADLs will help prevent patient falls and injuries.

2. Concurrent explanations relieve the patient's anxiety and help the patient anticipate the nurse's touch.

3. A Kardex record will be available to other personnel and help provide continuity of care.

4. Rationales: _____

Eye disorders

NURSING DIAGNOSIS

Anxiety related to fear of blindness

Nursing priorities

- Reduce anxiety to a tolerable level.
- Provide realistic reassurance.

Patient outcome criteria

Within 3 days after surgery, the patient will:
- have a relaxed facial expression
- identify specific fears related to potential blindness
- verbalize a realistic perception of the prognosis.

Interventions

1. During caregiving, elicit and accept the patient's expressions of fear and anxiety. Help the patient identify and prioritize problems.

2. Offer realistic reassurance.

3. If the eye or eyes are patched, check the patient frequently, anticipate needs, speak when approaching the bedside, and use touch to offer reassurance.

4. Additional individualized interventions: _____

Rationales

1. Identifying the most significant components of the threat of blindness helps the patient regain control and initiate contingency planning.

2. Most retinal reattachments restore vision.

3. Inability to see increases the sense of helplessness, further contributing to anxiety. Speaking on approach alerts the patient. Because the patient cannot perceive the usual visual cues, touch may be especially meaningful.

4. Rationales: _____

NURSING DIAGNOSIS

Diversional activity deficit related to postoperative activity limitation

Nursing priority

Promote allowable activities.

Patient outcome criteria

Throughout the hospital stay, the patient will:
- verbalize satisfaction with diversional activity
- spend time daily visiting with friends and family, if available.

Interventions

1. Provide diversional activities that do not cause rapid eye movement or head jerking, such as radio, television, conversation, books, and visitors.

2. Additional individualized interventions: _____

Rationales

1. Such activities will not interfere with healing of the retinal tear and can relieve boredom and reduce isolation.

2. Rationales: _____

DISCHARGE PLANNING

Discharge checklist

Before discharge, the patient shows evidence of:
- ❒ absence of infection and pain
- ❒ ability to manage ADLs with minimal limitations
- ❒ ability to ambulate with minimal assistance
- ❒ stable vital signs and absence of pulmonary or cardiovascular complications
- ❒ expected amount of restored vision or ability to accept vision deficit
- ❒ ability to follow activity restrictions
- ❒ adequate home support system
- ❒ referral to home care if support system is inadequate or if further teaching is warranted
- ❒ knowledge of how to contact community resources that offer support to visually impaired persons.

Teaching checklist

Document evidence that the patient and family demonstrate an understanding of:
- ❒ extent of vision loss (if any) and expected time period needed for further return of vision
- ❒ the purpose, dosage, administration schedule, and adverse effects of all discharge medications as well as which eye to medicate (usual discharge medications include mydriatics)
- ❒ activity limitations
- ❒ the signs and symptoms of retinal detachment, such as changes in vision or seeing flashes of light
- ❒ the date, time, and location of follow-up appointments
- ❒ community resources for the visually impaired.

Documentation checklist

Using outcome criteria as a guide, document:
- ❒ clinical status on admission
- ❒ significant changes in status
- ❒ pertinent laboratory and diagnostic test findings
- ❒ vision changes
- ❒ pain-relief measures
- ❒ activity and position restrictions
- ❒ nutritional intake
- ❒ other therapies
- ❒ patient and family teaching
- ❒ discharge planning.

ASSOCIATED PLANS OF CARE

Grieving
Ineffective individual coping
Knowledge deficit
Pain
Surgery

REFERENCES

LeMone, P., and Burke, K.M. *Medical-Surgical Nursing: Critical Thinking in Client Care.* Menlo Park, Calif.: Addison-Wesley-Longman Publishing Co., 1996.

Lewis, S.M., et al. *Medical-Surgical Nursing: Assessment and Management of Clinical Problems.* St. Louis: Mosby–Year Book, Inc., 1996.

Monshizaden, R., and Haimovici, R. "Advances in Vitreoretinal Surgery: Macular Hole Repair and Perfluorocarbon Liquids," *Today's OR Nurse* 18(1):20-23, January-February 1996.

Eye disorders

Part 5

Respiratory disorders

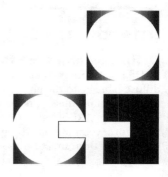

Adult respiratory distress syndrome

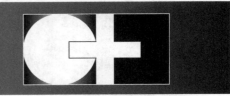

DRG information

DRG 099   Respiratory Signs and Symptoms with Complication or Comorbidity (CC).
Mean LOS = 3.5 days
Principal diagnoses include:
• adult respiratory distress syndrome (ARDS)
• dyspnea and other respiratory abnormalities
• hemoptysis
• cough.

DRG 100   Respiratory Signs and Symptoms without CC.
Mean LOS = 2.4 days
Principal diagnoses include selected principal diagnoses listed under DRG 099. The distinction is that DRG 100 excludes CC.

DRG 087   Pulmonary Edema and Respiratory Failure.
Mean LOS = 6.9 days
Principal diagnoses include:
• ARDS caused by trauma or after surgery
• respiratory failure
• pulmonary edema.

DRG 475   Respiratory System Diagnosis with Ventilator Support.
Mean LOS = 12.3 days
Principal diagnoses include:
• respiratory failure
• chronic obstructive pulmonary disease
• acute or chronic bronchitis
• pneumonia from various causes
• ARDS.

Additional DRG information: ARDS is rarely a principal diagnosis. It is usually a CC to other diseases, trauma, or surgery. Used as a secondary diagnosis, it can increase a particular DRG's weight because it qualifies as a CC. The above DRGs, however, are calculated with ARDS as a principal diagnosis.

INTRODUCTION

Definition and time focus

ARDS is a complex, poorly understood syndrome of diffuse damage to the alveolar-capillary membrane. The most common cause of respiratory failure in the critical care setting, ARDS may represent the ultimate manifestation of several unrelated physiologic insults that produce direct or indirect pulmonary injury. Key clinical features necessary for its diagnosis include a history consistent with ARDS, moderate to severe hypoxemia, bilateral diffuse infiltrates on chest X-ray, and exclusion of other causes of pulmonary congestion, specifically left-sided heart failure.

Known by many other names (such as noncardiogenic pulmonary edema, shock lung, and postpump lung), ARDS is characterized by interstitial and alveolar pulmonary edema resulting from increased permeability of the pulmonary microvasculature. Other key pathophysiologic features include a massive pulmonary shunt, decreased lung compliance, and increased alveolar dead space. On autopsy, lungs are heavy and wet, demonstrating congestive atelectasis, and marked by hyaline membrane formation and pulmonary fibrosis.

The chemical mediators involved in ARDS are complex and poorly understood. One theory is that in sepsis, bacteria stimulate granulocytes lodged in the lung. The resulting oxidative burst releases toxic metabolites (such as free radicals) and proteolytic enzymes, both of which can cause severe pulmonary injury. Other chemical mediators include histamine, serotonin, and prostaglandins. This plan focuses on the critically ill patient with a diagnosis of ARDS.

Etiology and precipitating factors

• Gram-negative sepsis, *Pneumocystis carinii* pneumonia, bacterial or viral pneumonia, or other infections
• Aspiration of gastric contents, fresh or salt water (near drowning), or other liquids
• Pulmonary contusion, nonthoracic trauma, burns, or other types of trauma
• Inhalation of smoke, toxic levels of oxygen, corrosive chemicals, or other toxins
• Shock
• Fat embolism, cardiopulmonary bypass, massive transfusions, disseminated intravascular coagulation, transfusion reaction, or other hematologic causes
• Drug overdose, particularly heroin, methadone (Dolophine), and propoxyphene (Darvon)

FOCUSED ASSESSMENT GUIDELINES

Nursing history (functional health pattern findings)

Health perception–health management pattern

• History of catastrophic pulmonary insult followed by a lag time of several hours to several days and then progressive dyspnea

Physical findings

General appearance

• Restlessness

Pulmonary

• Tachypnea
• Hyperventilation
• Progressive dyspnea
• Fine, diffuse crackles
• Increased peak inspiratory pressure (if on ventilator)

Neurologic

• Deteriorating level of consciousness

Integumentary

• Cyanosis

Diagnostic studies

No single diagnostic test exists for ARDS.
• Arterial blood gas (ABG) values — reveal moderate to severe hypoxemia (partial pressure of arterial oxygen [PaO_2] less than 50 mm Hg), even when the inspired oxygen concentration is greater than 60%, and hyper-capnia (partial pressure of arterial carbon dioxide [$PaCO_2$] greater than 50 mm Hg)
• Alveolar-arterial gradient — reveals increased gradient (greater than 15 mm Hg on room air or greater than 50 mm Hg on 100% oxygen)
• Shunt calculation — reveals pulmonary shunt in excess of 5%, typically 20% to 30%
• Bronchial fluid protein to serum protein ratio — greater than 0.5, indicating unusually high protein concentration in the bronchial fluid (implying that a damaged alveolar-capillary membrane is allowing proteins to leak through capillary walls)
• Chest X-ray — reveals bilaterally diffuse infiltrates
• Lung compliance — reduced below 50 ml/cm H_2O, typically 20 to 30 ml/cm H_2O
• Pulmonary artery wedge pressure — normal or only slightly elevated (less than 15 mm Hg), indicating that left-sided heart failure is not causing pulmonary congestion
• Functional residual capacity — reduced

Potential complications

• Respiratory arrest
• Respiratory failure
• Pulmonary fibrosis
• Disseminated intravascular coagulation
• Persistent pulmonary function abnormalities after recovery (such as mild restrictive disease, impaired gas transfer, or expiratory small-airway obstruction)

CLINICAL SNAPSHOT

ADULT RESPIRATORY DISTRESS SYNDROME

Major nursing diagnoses and collaborative problems	Key patient outcomes
Hypoxemia	Exhibit ABG levels within normal limits: typically, pH 7.35 to 7.45; PaO_2, 80 to 100 mm Hg; $PaCO_2$, 35 to 45 mm Hg; and HCO_3^-, 22 to 26 mEq/L.
Risk for injury: Complications	Maintain vital signs within normal limits: typically, heart rate, 60 to 100 beats/minute; systolic pressure, 90 to 140 mm Hg; and diastolic pressure, 50 to 90 mm Hg.
Risk for ineffective individual and family coping	Display effective coping skills.

COLLABORATIVE PROBLEM

Hypoxemia related to pulmonary shunt, interstitial edema, and alveolar edema

Nursing priorities
• Prevent further deterioration of lung function.
• Support the lung during healing.
• Maintain oxygenation.

Patient outcome criteria

Within 3 days of the initial insult and continuously thereafter, the patient will:
• display eupnea
• have a respiratory rate of 12 to 20 breaths/minute
• have clear breath sounds
• display a level of consciousness equal to or better than that on admission
• have normal chest X-rays
• maintain ABG values within normal limits: typically, pH, 7.35 to 7.45; Pa_{O_2}, 80 to 100 mm Hg; Pa_{CO_2}, 35 to 45 mm Hg; and HCO_3^-, 22 to 26 mEq/L
• have an arterial oxygen saturation (Sa_{O_2}) of 95% or better and a mixed venous oxygen saturation ($S\bar{v}_{O_2}$) of 60% to 80% if oximetry is used.

Interventions

1. Monitor for clinical signs and symptoms:

• initial insult period — persistent unexplained mild tachypnea, breathlessness, air hunger, and normal breath sounds

• latent period — persistent moderate tachypnea; increasing dyspnea; neck, chest, or abdominal muscle use; fatigue; restlessness; confusion; and crackles
• progressive pulmonary insufficiency — severe tachypnea and hyperventilation, progressive dyspnea, gurgles, and deteriorating level of consciousness

• terminal stage — depressed level of consciousness, arrhythmias, and profound shock leading to asystole.

2. Obtain chest X-rays daily, as ordered, and monitor serial findings. Be alert for reports indicating patchy infiltrates or "whiteout." Also note any other abnormal findings.

Rationales

1. Clinical signs and symptoms, when correlated with ABG values and chest X-ray results, indicate the syndrome's progression.
• The initial insult is followed by a variable lag period before signs and symptoms appear. About 60% of ARDS patients develop clinical indicators within 24 hours, 30% within 24 to 72 hours, and 10% after 72 hours. During the initial insult, signs and symptoms are mild and nonspecific. Tachypnea despite a normal Pa_{O_2}, the most characteristic finding, probably results from stimulation of juxtacapillary receptors in the alveolar interstitium.
• Signs and symptoms during the latent phase reflect borderline hypoxemia and interstitial edema.

• As the syndrome worsens, respiratory distress becomes marked. Increased dead space creates a need for high minute volumes while decreasing compliance creates a need for high inspiratory pressures. The continuing capillary leak produces frank alveolar edema, and the massive pulmonary shunt produces hypoxemia.
• In the terminal stage, hypoxemia refractory to therapy produces profound brain and heart dysfunction, terminating in cardiopulmonary arrest.

2. Chest X-rays are used to monitor the degree of edema and the development of complications. During the initial insult, the X-ray typically is normal. Patchy infiltrates appear during the latent period, worsen during pulmonary insufficiency, and culminate in a complete "whiteout" in the terminal stage.

3. Obtain ABG values at least every 4 hours, as ordered. Note degree of hypoxemia and any acid-base imbalance, typically:
• normal Pa_{O_2}, mild hypocapnia, and respiratory alkalosis during the insult period

• borderline hypoxemia during the latent period

• progressive hypoxemia, increasing hypercapnia, and worsening respiratory and metabolic acidosis as pulmonary insufficiency becomes more pronounced

• refractory hypoxemia, hypercapnia, and severe respiratory and metabolic acidosis during the terminal stage.

3. ABG values provide a way to assess and document gas exchange abnormalities.

• During the insult period, tachypnea maintains a normal Pa_{O_2}, but the accompanying carbon dioxide blow-off produces hypocapnia and respiratory alkalosis.
• Borderline hypoxemia reflects early impairment of gas diffusion.
• Hypercapnia develops later because carbon dioxide is much more diffusible than oxygen. Carbon dioxide retention produces respiratory acidosis. The worsening oxygen deprivation causes cells to switch from aerobic to anaerobic metabolism, resulting in lactic acidosis.
• Refractory hypoxemia results from a massive pulmonary shunt. Interstitial edema compresses alveoli and alveolar edema fills them with fluid. In both cases, the alveoli cannot oxygenate capillary blood flowing past them. The resulting perfusion without ventilation converts the alveolar-capillary units to shunt units. Without open alveoli, supplemental oxygen cannot reach capillary blood.

4. Continuously monitor gas exchange status, as ordered, by monitoring Sa_{O_2} with a pulse oximeter or $S\overline{v}_{O_2}$ with an $S\overline{v}_{O_2}$ catheter. Monitoring the end-tidal carbon dioxide ($ETCO_2$) level can also be helpful.

4. Conventional ABG sampling cannot provide a continuous indication of gas exchange and results are not immediately available. Continuous monitoring provides uninterrupted data, allowing early detection of impending deterioration and close monitoring of the effects of nursing interventions. It also permits assessment of the effects of multiple interventions that may have opposing effects on oxygenation and cardiac output — for instance, administration of dopamine (Intropin) and nitroprusside (Nitropress) to a patient on positive-pressure ventilation and positive end-expiratory pressure (PEEP). Pulse oximetry monitors oxygen supplied to tissues; $S\overline{v}_{O_2}$ monitoring indicates tissue oxygen consumption. $ETCO_2$ evaluates ventilation.

5. Prepare for endotracheal intubation if the respiratory rate exceeds 30 breaths/minute and the patient is elderly, chronically ill, or suffering from preexisting pulmonary disease; fatigued; or exhibiting an increasing Pa_{CO_2}.

5. Endotracheal intubation is usually necessary to protect the airway and allow for delivery of high levels of oxygen and PEEP. Advanced age, chronic illness, or preexisting pulmonary disease increases the likelihood the patient will be unable to tolerate the rapid respiratory rate. Fatigue and increasing Pa_{CO_2} indicate inadequate spontaneous ventilation.

6. Implement mechanical ventilation, as ordered. See the "Mechanical ventilation" plan, page 283.

6. The widespread pulmonary congestion impairs alveolar expansion. Surfactant production decreases, making alveoli even more difficult to expand. The high inspiratory pressures required to expand alveoli and the high minute volume needed to compensate for increased physiologic dead space increase the work of breathing so markedly that the patient cannot maintain spontaneous ventilation. Also, hypoxemia makes the patient prone to respiratory arrest. Mechanical ventilation conserves the patient's energy, prevents respiratory arrest, and allows time for the lung injury to heal.

7. Implement PEEP, as ordered, typically if an inspired oxygen concentration greater than 50% is needed for more than 24 hours or if Pa$_{O_2}$ falls below 50 mm Hg even though oxygen concentration exceeds 60%. Place the patient with severe ARDS in the prone position for 24 hours. Then alternate to supine position for 24 hours.

8. Monitor compliance, as described in the "Mechanical ventilation" plan, page 283.

9. Administer medications, as ordered. Document effectiveness and observe for adverse reactions.
• corticosteroids, typically methylprednisolone (Solu-Medrol)

• antibiotics

• sedatives

10. Additional individualized interventions: _____

7. PEEP, a mainstay in the treatment of ARDS, is believed to increase alveolar size and restore alveolar ventilation. It thus increases functional residual capacity, decreases shunting, improves ventilation-perfusion matching, and improves compliance. The prone position improves gas distribution to gravity-dependent areas of the lung.

8. Compliance objectively measures the ease of lung expansion. Decreasing compliance, implying increasing lung stiffness, indicates that ARDS is worsening. Interpreting compliance values is covered in the "Mechanical ventilation" plan.

9. Medications have limited effectiveness in ARDS but may be prescribed empirically.
• Corticosteroid administration in ARDS is controversial. Although anecdotal reports and limited clinical and animal studies suggest possible effectiveness in certain types of ARDS such as radiation pneumonitis, no randomized, controlled study in humans has demonstrated its effectiveness.
• Antibiotics are usually prescribed for suspected or documented infection. Although many doctors prescribe them prophylactically in ARDS, such use has not been proven effective.
• Morphine, diazepam, and other sedatives can help control struggling, thus improving oxygenation and decreasing the risk of barotrauma. The patient's level of sedation should be carefully monitored. If a paralytic agent such as pancuronium is used, the patient should also receive an amnesiac agent.

10. Rationales: _____

NURSING DIAGNOSIS

Risk for injury: Complications related to single or multiple organ failure

Nursing priority

Minimize the effects of related organ failure.

Patient outcome criteria

Within 24 hours of the initial insult and then continuously, the patient will:
• maintain vital signs within normal limits: typically, heart rate, 60 to 100 beats/minute; systolic blood pressure, 90 to 140 mm Hg; and diastolic blood pressure, 50 to 90 mm Hg
• display normal sinus rhythm
• produce an hourly urine output greater than 30 ml
• show no signs of infection.

Interventions

1. Maintain adequate cardiac output. Assist with pulmonary artery (PA) catheter insertion, if indicated. Monitor PA pressures, vital signs, electrocardiogram, and urine output according to Appendix A, Monitoring Standards.

2. Administer packed red blood cells, as ordered, to maintain the hemoglobin level between 12 and 15 g/dl.

3. Administer crystalloid or colloid I.V. fluids, as ordered. Monitor fluid administration closely.

4. If the patient has gastric distention, a decreased level of consciousness, or impaired airway protection reflexes, obtain an order to institute gastric drainage.

5. Provide nutritional support, as ordered. See the "Nutritional deficit" plan, page 80.

6. Maintain strict asepsis. Monitor for signs and symptoms of infection, and document and report them promptly to the doctor. Institute aggressive treatment measures, as ordered.

7. Observe for signs of single or multiple organ dysfunction syndrome, especially central nervous system failure, renal failure, and GI dysfunction.

8. Implement general supportive nursing measures to prevent the complications of immobility. See the "Impaired physical mobility" plan, page 50.

9. Additional individualized interventions: _____

Rationales

1. Arterial oxygen transport (the amount delivered to the tissues) depends on cardiac output and oxygen content. Close monitoring of hemodynamic values is essential: Enough fluid must be given to maintain cardiac output, but too much fluid worsens the pulmonary capillary leak. A PA catheter also helps differentiate cardiac from noncardiac pulmonary edema.

2. Oxygen content depends on the hemoglobin level, hemoglobin saturation, and PaO_2. This hemoglobin level maintains normal oxygen transport.

3. The choice of appropriate fluid in ARDS remains controversial. Crystalloids readily cross from the vascular to the interstitial space, potentially worsening edema. Colloids also cross the leaky capillary membrane, move into the interstitial space, and draw water to the space by osmosis, also worsening edema. Close monitoring minimizes the potential for developing shock and fluid overload, two risk factors for ARDS.

4. Aspiration of gastric contents is a risk factor for ARDS. Gastric drainage can prevent such aspiration.

5. The protracted period of mechanical ventilation necessary for most ARDS patients requires total parenteral nutrition to maintain pulmonary muscle strength and immunologic defense mechanisms.

6. A major infection in an ARDS patient can readily lead to death if the source of the infection cannot be identified. Once the source is identified, prompt, aggressive treatment can save the patient's life.

7. Failure or dysfunction of additional organ systems is linked with increased mortality in ARDS.

8. The patient on prolonged bed rest is at risk for many complications that worsen lung function, such as pneumonia, atelectasis, and pulmonary embolism. The "Impaired physical mobility" plan contains detailed interventions for these and other potential complications.

9. Rationales: _____

NURSING DIAGNOSIS

Risk for ineffective individual and family coping related to abrupt onset of life-threatening illness

Nursing priority

Maximize the patient's and family's coping skills.

Patient outcome criteria

The patient will indicate increased ability to cope, if able to communicate. The family will participate in establishing a family action plan to cope with the crisis.

Interventions

1. Implement the measures outlined in the "Ineffective family coping: Compromised" plan, page 63, and the "Ineffective individual coping" plan, page 67.

2. Allow the family to interact with the patient.

3. Encourage the patient and family to express their feelings about treatments, especially mechanical ventilation.

4. Provide another method of communication for the patient, such as eye blinks or paper and pencil.

5. Additional individualized interventions: _____
_____

Rationales

1. Whether ARDS occurs after a catastrophic incident such as trauma or complicates an already critical illness, its onset places the patient and family under severe stress. This stress is increased by the treatments the patient must undergo, particularly mechanical ventilation, which precludes oral communication at the time when the patient and family most need it. Using the measures detailed in the "Ineffective family coping: Compromised" and "Ineffective individual coping" plans not only makes the ordeal more bearable but also decreases anxiety-induced oxygen requirements.

2. Interaction with loved ones decreases the patient's sense of isolation and encourages a positive attitude toward treatment.

3. Becoming aware of feelings and expressing them clearly and appropriately are healthy coping behaviors.

4. Intubation prevents the patient from speaking. Providing another means of communicating increases the patient's sense of security and promotes safety.

5. Rationales: _____
_____

DISCHARGE PLANNING

Discharge checklist
Before discharge, the patient shows evidence of:
- [ ] stable vital signs within normal limits for the patient
- [ ] spontaneous respiratory rate of 12 to 24 breaths/minute
- [ ] patent airway without endotracheal intubation
- [ ] discontinuation of PA catheter.

Teaching checklist
Document evidence that the patient and family demonstrate an understanding of:
- [ ] definition and pathophysiology of ARDS
- [ ] probable cause
- [ ] prognosis
- [ ] rationale for mechanical ventilation, PEEP, and other therapies.

Documentation checklist
Using outcome criteria as a guide, document:
- [ ] clinical status on admission
- [ ] significant changes in status
- [ ] pertinent diagnostic test findings
- [ ] airway care
- [ ] tolerance of ventilator and PEEP
- [ ] response to medications
- [ ] fluid therapy
- [ ] nutritional support
- [ ] nursing care to combat effects of immobility
- [ ] psychological coping
- [ ] patient and family teaching
- [ ] discharge planning.

ASSOCIATED PLANS OF CARE

Disseminated intravascular coagulation
Grieving
Hypovolemic shock
Impaired physical mobility
Ineffective family coping: Compromised
Ineffective individual coping
Mechanical ventilation
Multiple trauma
Nutritional deficit
Sensory-perceptual alteration
Septic shock

REFERENCES

Chillcott, S, et al. "ECCO2R: An Experimental Approach to Treating ARDS," *Critical Care Nurse* 15(1):50-56, February 1995.

Delgado, E. "Pressure Controlled-Inverse Ratio Ventilation," *Critical Care Nurse Quarterly* 19(3):22-35, November 1996.

Kokkef, M.H., et al. "The Acute Respiratory Distress Syndrome," *New England Journal of Medicine* 332(1):27-37, January 1995.

Nerlich, S. "Critical Care Management of the Patient with ARDS, Part 1: Pathophysiology and Implications for Mechanical Ventilation," *Australian Critical Care* 10(2):49-54, June 1997.

Asthma

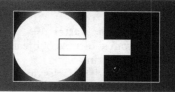

DRG information

DRG 087   Pulmonary Edema and Respiratory Failure.
Mean LOS = 6.9 days

DRG 088   Chronic Obstructive Pulmonary Disease.
Mean LOS = 6.1 days
Principal diagnoses include:
- asthma, chronic obstructive, with or without mention of status asthmaticus.

DRG 096   Bronchitis and Asthma with Complication or Comorbidity (CC); Age 17+.
Mean LOS = 5.5 days
Principal diagnoses include:
- bronchitis (acute and chronic)
- asthma.

DRG 097   Bronchitis and Asthma without CC; Ages 17+ to 69.
Mean LOS = 4.3 days

DRG 098   Bronchitis and Asthma; Ages 0 to 17.
Mean LOS = 4.3 days

DRG 475   Respiratory System Diagnosis with Ventilator Support.
Mean LOS = 12.3 days

INTRODUCTION

Definition and time focus

Asthma is characterized by widespread narrowing of the airways (bronchoconstriction), increased mucus production, mucosal inflammation and edema, and airflow obstruction. These effects result from an increased responsiveness and hyperreactivity of the tracheal and bronchial smooth muscle to various stimuli and are reversible, either spontaneously or as a result of therapy. Between asthma attacks, the individual may remain symptom-free. Attacks vary in severity, from mild obstruction to profound respiratory failure. *Status asthmaticus* is a nonspecific term used when usual medical treatment fails to relieve severe obstruction.

Asthma is divided into two types:
- extrinsic asthma — begins in childhood and usually disappears in the adult; positive family history; usually seasonal; multiple, well-defined allergies; positive response to allergy skin testing (indicates an antigen-antibody response)
- intrinsic asthma — seen in adults after age 30; may be more severe in nature and continuous; associated with a history of recurrent respiratory tract infections; multiple nonspecific conditions can provoke an attack; negative response to allergy skin testing.

The adult patient admitted to the acute-care setting usually has intrinsic asthma and is in acute respiratory distress. This plan focuses on the patient admitted after self-management or outpatient intervention has failed to stop an asthma attack.

Etiology and precipitating factors

- Acute episode may have numerous causes:
  - infection (viral or bacterial)
  - environmental exposure to a nonspecific allergen (such as secondhand smoke, dust, or cleaning compounds)
  - chronic sinusitis
  - weather changes (such as heat, cold, fog, or wind)
  - exercise
  - regurgitation
  - psychogenic factors
  - ingestion of aspirin (aspirin-sensitive individuals may also be sensitive to indomethacin [Indocin], mefenamic acid [Ponstel], or tartrazine [yellow dye found in many medications]).

FOCUSED ASSESSMENT GUIDELINES

Nursing history (functional health pattern findings)

Health perception–health management pattern
- Increasing shortness of breath, stated as "can't catch breath," "can't inhale," or "hyperventilating"
- Chest tightness
- Feeling of panic or suffocation (typically resists oxygen mask)
- Increased coughing, often dry and nonproductive, leading to shortness of breath
- Inability to move sputum out of lungs
- Attack in progress for some time before admission to acute-care setting
- Increasing fatigue and inability to handle the attack with usual measures
- Noncompliance with prescribed outpatient treatments
- Continual inhaler use (either prescription or nonprescription type) without benefit
- Identification of certain events or environmental factors as major contributors to the attack's development

Sleep-rest pattern
- Coughing that disturbs sleep

Nutritional-metabolic pattern
• Dehydration (from shortness of breath, mouth breathing, or reluctance to drink water)
• Lack of eating since the attack's onset because of preoccupation and shortness of breath; may complain of nausea, which may be related to medication use or abuse
• Weight gain (long-term corticosteroid users)

Activity-exercise pattern
• Ongoing exercise limitations because exercise can cause wheezing and shortness of breath
• Difficulty maintaining desired level of physical conditioning if exercise is limited

Cognitive-perceptual pattern
• Ability to describe complex strategies for self-management during an acute attack, but reported inability to put them into effect during an actual attack, when panic may overwhelm problem-solving skills and hypoxemia may impair thinking

Role-relationship pattern
• Avoidance of public events and activities because of embarrassment from severe dyspnea and cough
• Attack precipitated by laughing
• Attack precipitated by partner, family, or social group via such environmental irritants as cigarette smoke

Self-perception–self-concept pattern
• Changes in body image related to medication's cushingoid effects (if maintenance corticosteroid therapy is used)
• Discouragement with appearance and inability to prevent or alter physiologic changes

Coping–stress tolerance pattern
• Fluctuations in emotions, such as:
– denial of problem (may ignore potential irritants by refusing to give away a pet, stop smoking, or remove offending furniture; may refuse to learn medication routines and self-management strategies)
– anger (may blame others for causing attack; may describe asthma as a "kid's disease"; may not feel past health habits justify disease's extent)

Physical findings

Physical parameters, which vary with the attack's severity, are good indicators of treatment outcomes.

General appearance
• Anxiety
• Maintenance of upright position
• Fever (if infection is present)

Neurologic
• Initially, hyperalert, awake, and oriented; may become progressively less alert, although awake and oriented, as fatigue progresses
• Restlessness (from hypoxemia)
• Lethargy (from increased carbon dioxide levels)

Integumentary
• Color initially good; may be flushed; cyanosis a late, unreliable sign
• Diaphoresis
• Dry mucous membranes from rapid oral breathing and dehydration

Cardiovascular
• Sinus tachycardia (related to bronchodilating medications and stress response)
• Mild to moderate hypertension (related to medications and anxiety)
• Paradoxical pulse becoming more pronounced (greater than 15 mm Hg) as air trapping increases
• Potential arrhythmias

Respiratory
• Accessory neck muscles used during breathing; becomes more pronounced as obstruction worsens
• Respiratory rate less than 30 breaths/minute, increasing as attack worsens but possibly lessening with fatigue
• Prolonged exhalations
• Wheezing; may be audible from a distance (timing varies with severity: initially expiratory wheezing, then inspiratory-expiratory, finally no wheezing — "silent" chest indicates critical airflow limitation)
• Cough, possibly decreased sputum production (increased production a positive sign; can be yellow, thick, or crusted)
• Monosyllabic speech with worsening airflow limitation

Diagnostic studies

• Arterial blood gas (ABG) measurements — may be obtained only in severe or prolonged attack; hypoxemia always present; carbon dioxide level used to stage attack's progress
– Stage 1: decreased partial pressure of oxygen (Po_2) and partial pressure of carbon dioxide (Pco_2) levels (hyperventilation)
– Stage 2: decreased Po_2 level, normal Pco_2 level (increased fatigue)
– Stage 3: decreased Po_2 level (less than 50 mm Hg), increased Pco_2 level (critical hypoventilation and fatigue)
• Sputum specimens — Gram stain used to detect treatable organisms; eosinophil smear done if allergens are suspected as primary cause; culture and sensitivity testing difficult to obtain because mucus is initially thick, tenacious, and difficult to mobilize; casts and plugs are present when sputum is mobilized
• Complete blood count and differential — white blood cell (WBC) count increased with infection; eosinophil count increased with allergy
• Serum electrolyte levels — potassium level invariably decreased

• theophylline level — may be necessary in acute phase if the patient treated self extensively with nonprescription and prescription remedies; normal level is 10 to 20 mg/ml; an elevated level may indicate medication misuse; a decreased level may indicate noncompliance
• Chest X-ray — shows hyperinflation; air trapping decreases as airflow obstruction improves; between attacks, hyperinflation resolves; infiltrates are present if infection is a major cause
• Pulmonary function testing (PFT) — not usually performed during an acute attack; measures of airflow rate, peak expiratory flow rate (PEFR), and forced expiratory flow rate in 1 second (FEV_1) are less than 25% of predicted value in severe obstruction; full PFT demonstrates dramatic response to bronchodilators; metha-

choline or histamine challenge provokes increased airway resistance
• Allergen skin test — negative; positive skin test does not necessarily indicate that exposure will trigger a respiratory response

Potential complications
• Cardiopulmonary arrest
• Cardiac arrhythmias
• Rib fractures (from violent coughing)
• Pneumothorax
• Atelectasis
• Pneumonia
• Drug overdose related to noncompliance or knowledge deficit about medication use during an acute attack

---

CLINICAL SNAPSHOT

ASTHMA

Major nursing diagnosis and collaborative problem	Key patient outcomes
Risk for status asthmaticus or pulmonary arrest	Exhibit stable vital signs within the patient's normal limits: typically, heart rate, 60 to 100 beats/minute; systolic blood pressure, 90 to 140 mm Hg; and diastolic blood pressure, 50 to 90 mm Hg.
Knowledge deficit (self-care)	Describe personal plan of treatment for variations in peak flow.

COLLABORATIVE PROBLEM

Risk for status asthmaticus or pulmonary arrest related to airway obstruction, hypoxemia, and progressive fatigue

Nursing priorities
• Maintain effective airway clearance.
• Promote an efficient breathing pattern.

Patient outcome criteria
• Within 1 hour of beginning therapy, the patient will:
  – show an improved flow rate (FEV_1 and PEFR)
  – mobilize sputum
  – exhibit reduced anxiety while maintaining a normal level of consciousness
  – have reduced hypoxemia, with Pco_2 level at or below normal.
• Once stabilized, the patient will:
  – have improved breath sounds
  – decrease use of accessory muscles for breathing
  – exhibit stable vital signs within the patient's normal limits, typically heart rate 60 to 100 beats/minute, systolic blood pressure 90 to 140 mm Hg, and diastolic blood pressure 50 to 90 mm Hg
  – have improved ABG measurements.

Interventions

1. Administer oxygen via nasal cannula, 2 to 3 L/minute or more, as ordered.

2. Administer fluid therapy orally or I.V., as ordered. The usual fluid goal, eight to twelve 8-oz (240-ml) glasses every 24 hours, may vary with the patient's age and general status.

3. Monitor the patient's status continually until it stabilizes. Parameters to monitor include level of consciousness, skin color and moisture, speech pattern, use of accessory muscles for breathing, breath sounds, sputum production, respiratory rate, pulse, blood pressure, and paradoxical pulse. Obtain ABG measurements, as ordered, and expiratory flow rates. Once baselines are established, use a pulse oximeter to monitor oxygenation. Thoroughly document findings. Report changes that indicate deteriorating status.

4. Be especially alert for signs of a potentially fatal attack, and promptly report them to the doctor. Such signs include:
- previous severe asthma attacks
- FEV_1 of less than 500 cc or PEFR of less than 35% of predicted
- little or no response to bronchodilator therapy in 1 hour, as evidenced by flow rate measurements
- altered level of consciousness, gasping respirations, and no evidence of air movement on auscultation
- cyanosis
- PO_2 less than 50 mm Hg
- PCO_2 greater than 45 mm Hg
- paradoxical pulse (a drop in systolic pressure of more than 10 mm Hg on inspiration)
- electrocardiogram abnormality
- pneumothorax
- sweating
- use of accessory muscles.

5. Administer medications, as ordered. The medication regimen varies but typically includes:

- bronchodilators, such as beta-adrenergics and theophylline (Slo-Phyllin). Beta-adrenergics (such as epinephrine [Adrenalin], terbutaline [Brethaire], isoproterenol [Isuprel], and metaproterenol [Alupent]) are given subcutaneously, inhaled from a pressurized canister or nebulizer, or taken orally; observe for such adverse effects as nervousness or hypertension. Theophylline (methylxanthine) preparations such as aminophylline (Phyllocontin) are initially given I.V. and then orally; observe for and report arrhythmias, tachycardia, hypotension, vomiting, or other adverse effects.

Rationales

1. Hypoxemia is always present in an acute asthma attack because of ventilation-perfusion imbalance. Supplemental oxygen decreases the work of breathing and reduces the potential for cardiac dysfunction.

2. The patient is usually dehydrated on admission. Hydration promotes expectoration of thickened sputum and minimizes development of impacted mucus.

3. Parameters vary with the attack's severity, the patient's response to treatment, and patient fatigue. Because the patient is physiologically unstable during an attack, parameters may change rapidly.

4. One or more of these signs may indicate a potentially fatal attack. Prompt, aggressive therapy is needed to prevent pulmonary arrest.

5. Although some patients can control signs and symptoms with relaxation techniques, medication is usually necessary and is more effective when used before the attack becomes severe or prolonged.
- Cyclic adenosine monophosphate (cAMP) is a chemical mediator that controls bronchodilation. Beta-adrenergics and theophyllines stimulate production or prevent destruction of cAMP and thus produce bronchodilation. Effectiveness varies with blood level.

• corticosteroids. These are initially given I.V., then orally, and tapered off as soon as possible. Aerosolized corticosteroids, with or without oral agents, may be given to some patients.

6. Take steps to alleviate panic, ensure safety, and promote relaxation. Place the patient in an upright position with adequate support; promote exhalation of trapped air by instructing the patient to prolong exhalation and to exhale without force; maintain a calm, reassuring attitude; and reduce environmental stimulation, if possible.

7. Assess therapeutic medication levels daily, watching for associated electrolyte and glucose imbalances, as ordered. Report abnormal findings.

8. Initiate measures to mobilize sputum, such as postural drainage and percussion, suctioning (if necessary), and controlled coughing. Keep in mind that each of these measures can intensify hypoxemia. Use supplemental oxygen, temporarily increasing the liter flow if any respiratory distress is observed.

9. Monitor fluid balance, noting intake and output, weight, skin turgor, condition of mucous membranes, characteristics of sputum, presence or absence of edema, and urine specific gravity and hematocrit. Document and report abnormalities.

10. Do not administer narcotics or sedatives for anxiety.

11. Watch for indications that the patient needs intubation, including fatigue, further reduction in thoracic expansion, decreasing level of consciousness, an increase in Pco_2 level of more than 10 mm Hg above the resting level, severe hypoxemia, and decreasing breath sounds. Alert the doctor immediately if any of these appear.

12. Additional individualized interventions: _____

• I.V. and oral corticosteroids are believed to reduce inflammation, thereby reducing edema in bronchial mucosa. Aerosolized corticosteroids may provide beneficial effects with minimal adverse effects because they are delivered directly to the affected tissues.

6. The acutely asthmatic patient experiences extreme anxiety and panic and may try to lessen discomfort with counterproductive posturing and breathing patterns and with restless activity. Characteristically, the harder the patient attempts to breathe, the less productive the effort and the greater the amount of air trapped. Prolonged exhalation promotes a relaxed expiratory effort and reduces air trapping.

7. Establishing a therapeutic medication regimen requires monitoring of drug levels and electrolyte status as the patient is rehydrated and stabilized. Theophylline clearance may be impaired, or electrolyte or glucose levels may be altered, or both — especially in the patient who has cardiac or liver disease, is hypertensive, or uses other medications.

8. Once hydration is begun, the patient must mobilize the thick, crusty mucus rapidly to prevent bronchial plugging. The fatigued patient may need assistance.

9. During an asthma attack, profuse diaphoresis and tachypnea cause fluid loss. Because the patient is usually too dyspneic and panicked to take oral fluids, significant dehydration may quickly occur. I.V. fluid replacement must be tailored to each patient and monitored carefully; otherwise, aggressive hydration may lead to fluid overload in the patient with compromised cardiovascular status.

10. Anxiety in the asthmatic patient stems from hypoxemia; sedation would worsen the situation by depressing the respiratory drive and worsening hypoventilation.

11. When the work of breathing becomes overwhelming, exhaustion results. If intubation and mechanical ventilation are not started promptly, pulmonary arrest can occur.

12. Rationales: _____

NURSING DIAGNOSIS

Knowledge deficit (self-care) related to complexity of therapeutic regimen

Nursing priority

Improve the patient's ability to prevent or cope with breathing difficulties.

Patient outcome criteria

By the time of discharge, the patient will:
• demonstrate appropriate breathing techniques during activity-induced shortness of breath or coughing episodes
• describe assertive strategies for dealing with environmental irritants
• realistically describe body-image changes related to adverse effects of medications while continuing to comply with the medication regimen
• identify factors that may trigger attacks.

Interventions

1. After the acute episode resolves, help the patient identify triggers that may cause or contribute to attacks (see *Triggers of asthma attacks*) Such triggers may stem from the patient's diet, medications, emotional states, and specific environment.

2. Teach the patient how to use a peak flow meter (PFM) to assess his condition. Make sure the patient knows what to do when the PFM indicates a variation in flow, including when to use bronchodilators, anti-inflammatory agents, or antibiotics and when to contact the doctor, based on his specific plan of treatment.

3. After the acute episode resolves, discuss and demonstrate (through role-playing) assertive strategies the patient can use when confronted with an environmental irritant (such as secondhand smoke). Have the patient return the demonstration.

Rationales

1. Once the patient knows what can cause an attack, he can take steps to reduce or eliminate his exposure to these triggers.

2. Used for patients with limited expiratory flow rates, a PFM measures peak expiratory flow, an indicator of lung function. It can be used in the morning and at night when the patient is at an increased risk for attacks. If readings are abnormal, the patient needs to know how to follow his plan of treatment and when to contact the doctor, who may vary the dosage of the patient's medication or take other steps to prevent a major attack.

3. The patient will be more likely to implement an assertive, nonaggressive strategy for dealing with potentially hazardous situations if he has several alternative responses. The patient may not be aware of the right to request environmental changes or may not know how to make such requests.

Triggers of asthma attacks

The four categories below include examples of specific irritants that can cause or contribute to an asthma attack.

Allergic triggers	Chemical medication triggers	Irritant triggers	Physical triggers
• House dust and dust mites	• Alcohol	• Smog	• Sulfur dioxide (food additives)
• Feathers and animal dander	• Nose drops, sprays (Neo-Synephrine)	• Smoke	• Temperature and barometric pressure change
• Mold spores and mildew	• Aspirin	• Fumes (industrial, chemicals, household cleaners, paints, varnishes)	• Humidity
• Pollens	• Reserpine (Serpalan)	• Strong odors (perfumes, cooking odors)	• Winds
• Infections	• Guanethidine (Ismelin)	• Dusts (sawdust, chalk dust)	• Strenuous exercise
	• Propranolol (Inderal)	• Sprays (hair spray, insect spray)	• Menstruation, pregnancy, menopause, or other hormonal changes
	• Methyldopa (Aldomet)		
	• Methantheline (Banthine)		
	• Thioridazine (Mellaril)		

4. Teach the patient how to use a metered-dose inhaler. Discuss with the patient potential adverse effects the medications can cause, such as anxiety and tremor from bronchodilators or moon face, loss of muscle tissue, and a tendency to bruise from corticosteroids. Encourage expression of frustration about the effects on socialization that can result from these adverse effects.

5. Demonstrate strategies to be used during a coughing episode (for example, controlled cough technique or "huff" coughing) and for acute shortness of breath during an activity (for example, upright and forward posturing, with shoulder relaxation and prolonged exhalation). Coach the patient in using these strategies.

6. Demonstrate and have the patient practice relaxation and stress reduction exercises.

7. Teach the patient the symptoms of an attack — pain or tightness in the chest, shortness of breath, an itchy chin or throat, and a dry mouth. Review discharge and over-the-counter medications and bronchial hygiene measures, including the purpose, dosage schedule, and adverse effects of medications, particularly effects that require medical attention. Explain that the patient will be taking two basic types of asthma medications — one to prevent an attack, usually taken daily, and one to relieve the symptoms of an attack, taken as soon as symptoms occur.

8. Improve the patient's self-efficacy (a person's belief in his ability to produce or achieve goals). On a scale of 1 to 5 (1 = not at all; 5 = very much), have the patient rate his ability to:
• decrease asthma symptoms
• take medications appropriately
• use an asthma inhaler correctly
• avoid asthma attacks
• perform relaxation exercises.
Use teaching and return demonstration to improve the patient's confidence in his ability to perform these tasks.

9. Additional individualized interventions: _____

4. The patient needs to understand how to use a metered-dose inhaler to deliver asthma medications. Although adverse effects cannot be eliminated, compliance with the prescribed regimen may be improved if the patient is given a chance to express feelings about such effects.

5. Breathing strategies reduce forceful exhalation, which occurs during coughing or acute shortness of breath and results in increased airway obstruction. Using these strategies as soon as possible during an attack will lessen the anxiety that shortness of breath can cause.

6. These exercises may help reduce the frequency of attacks.

7. Teaching helps the patient follow the daily care principles needed to help prevent attacks and ensures that he knows what steps to take (including seeking emergency care) should an attack occur.

8. An improvement in self-efficacy correlates with an improvement in future success.

9. Rationales: _____

DISCHARGE PLANNING

Discharge checklist
Before discharge, the patient shows evidence of:
❑ WBC count within normal parameters
❑ oxygen and I.V. therapy discontinued for at least 24 hours
❑ stable vital signs
❑ ABG measurements within expected parameters
❑ absence of cardiovascular and pulmonary complications (such as arrhythmias or atelectasis)
❑ tolerance of and response to oral medication regimen
❑ absence of signs and symptoms of dehydration

❑ ability to tolerate adequate nutritional intake
❑ absence of acute shortness of breath on exertion
❑ ability to ambulate and perform activities of daily living at prehospitalization level
❑ adequate home support or referral to home care, if indicated by inadequate home support system or patient's inability to perform self-care.

Teaching checklist
Document evidence that the patient and family demonstrate an understanding of:
❑ factors that trigger an asthma attack (specific to the patient, if possible)

- ❏ how to assess home and work environments and how to modify them to counter potential irritants
- ❏ preventive measures for use when irritant exposure is unavoidable
- ❏ clinical indicators of an impending attack
- ❏ relaxation and breathing exercises to improve control during an attack
- ❏ purpose, dosage, administration schedule, and adverse effects requiring medical attention of all discharge medications (usual discharge medications include bronchodilators and corticosteroids)
- ❏ purpose and use of over-the-counter medications (bronchodilators, expectorants, cough suppressants, cold remedies, or sleep remedies) as well as precautions to take when using them
- ❏ bronchial hygiene measures, including indications, schedule, and use
- ❏ use and cleaning of respiratory therapy equipment such as metered dose inhaler, PFM, and nebulizers
- ❏ self-management plan, including decision-making strategies for mild attacks or early stages of an attack and an emergency plan for severe or progressing attacks
- ❏ hydration requirements
- ❏ controlled cough techniques
- ❏ exercise recommendations and limitations, if any
- ❏ measures to control shortness of breath when performing activities
- ❏ need for flu and pneumococcus vaccine
- ❏ date, time, and location of follow-up appointment
- ❏ how to contact the doctor.

Documentation checklist
Using outcome criteria as a guide, document:
- ❏ clinical status on admission
- ❏ significant changes in status
- ❏ pertinent laboratory and diagnostic test findings
- ❏ treatments, including patient responses
- ❏ respiratory status (each shift)
- ❏ oxygen therapy
- ❏ medications
- ❏ hydration status and fluid intake and output
- ❏ patient and family teaching
- ❏ discharge planning.

ASSOCIATED PLANS OF CARE

Ineffective individual coping
Knowledge deficit

REFERENCES

Barnes, P. "Current Therapies for Asthma: Promise and Limitations," *Chest* 111(2):17S-26S, February supplement 1997.

Janson-Bjerklie, S. "Status Asthmaticus," *AJN* 90(9):52-55, September 1990.

Keeley, D, and Rees, J. "New Guidelines on Asthma Management: Aim to Control Symptoms Rapidly with Higher Initial Doses of Steroid and Earlier Use of Beta Agonists," *British Medical Journal* 314(7077):315-16, February 1, 1997.

Matthews, P. "Using a Peak Flowmeter: Monitoring the Air Waves," *Nursing97* 27(6):57-59, June 1997.

McFadden, E., and Hejal, R. "Asthma," *Lancet* 345(8959):1215-50, May 1995.

Tobin, D., et al. "The Asthma Self-Efficacy Scale," *Annals of Allergy* 59(4):273-77, October 1987.

"Zafirlukast (Accolate): After 20 Years, a New Class of Asthma Drug," *AJN* 97(5): 54-55, May 1997.

Chronic obstructive pulmonary disease

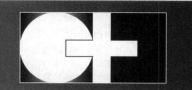

DRG information

DRG 079   Respiratory Infections and Inflammations with Complication or Comorbidity (CC); Age 17+.
Mean LOS = 9.3 days
Principal diagnoses include:
• complicated pneumonias (*Klebsiella, Staphylococcus,* gram-negative pneumonias, and the like)
• aspiration pneumonia

DRG 088   Chronic Obstructive Pulmonary Disease (COPD).
Mean LOS = 6.1 days
Principal diagnoses include:
• congenital bronchiectasis
• obstructive chronic bronchitis
• emphysema
• chronic respiratory conditions resulting from fumes or vapors.
This DRG is seen in many acute-care settings. Also, COPD patients commonly are readmitted within 15 days of previous hospitalization.

DRG 089   Simple Pneumonia and Pleurisy with CC; Age 17+.
Mean LOS = 7.1 days
Principal diagnoses include:
• bronchopneumonia
• influenza with pneumonia
• pneumonia with organism unspecified.

INTRODUCTION

Definition and time focus

COPD is a diagnostic category applied to patients whose primary respiratory difficulty involves exhalation. This plan focuses on two diseases, emphysema and chronic bronchitis. (Asthma, another disorder sometimes included in COPD, is covered in a separate plan.)

Emphysema is permanent, destruction of alveoli, resulting in dyspnea inappropriate for age and level of exertion. Chronic bronchitis (inflammation of the bronchi) is characterized by a chronic productive cough resulting from hyperplasia of mucus-producing cells and increased mucus production. Few patients have a "pure" disease process; most experience a combination of symptoms.

Common features of the stable state include:
• difficulty exhaling because of airway collapse, especially with increased effort (the harder the patient tries to exhale, the more difficult it becomes)
• air trapping with hyperinflation
• dyspnea
• history of smoking
• airway hypersensitivity to various stimuli
• difficulty clearing secretions.

Common features of an exacerbation include those of the stable state plus ventilation-perfusion imbalance resulting in:
• increased work of breathing
• increased myocardial work
• hypoxemia
• carbon dioxide retention.

This plan focuses on the COPD patient who is admitted to the acute care setting with an exacerbation of the disease and failure of prescribed therapies to control the symptoms.

Etiology and precipitating factors

Exacerbation is usually caused by a viral or bacterial infection; other common causes include exposure to environmental pollutants (secondhand smoke, dust, or cleaning compounds), exercise, and weather changes (heat, cold, fog, or wind)

FOCUSED ASSESSMENT GUIDELINES

Nursing history (functional health pattern findings)

Health perception–health management pattern
• Greater than normal shortness of breath, with inability to control symptoms with prescribed or nonprescribed therapies
• Increased fatigue and inability to cope with crisis
• Increasing anxiety and panic
• Increasing difficulty expectorating sputum

Nutritional-metabolic pattern
• Anorexia
• Inability to eat and digest without shortness of breath
• Nausea, possibly associated with medications
• Bloating, especially after eating foods known to cause flatulence
• Difficulty maintaining adequate fluid intake (at least eight 8-oz [240-ml] glasses per day)
• Symptoms of fluid and electrolyte disturbance, such as weakness, lethargy, confusion, weight changes, and muscle cramping

Activity-exercise pattern
• Shortness of breath with even minimal exertion or when performing activities of daily living
• Shortness of breath and panic controlled with breathing techniques

Sleep-rest pattern
• Sleep pattern disturbance
• Sleeping upright (usually in a reclining chair)
• Shortness of breath during the night, relieved by bronchial hygiene and expectoration of secretions
• Nervousness and trouble falling asleep
• Chronic fatigue and sleepiness during the day
• Nocturia (possibly related to medications)
• Morning headache

Cognitive-perceptual pattern
• Fluctuating compliance with therapeutic regimen (patient may perceive regimen as complex and difficult to understand and follow)

Role-relationship pattern
• Multiple role changes, resulting in depression, isolation, and increased dependence
• Difficulty verbalizing feelings because emotions intensify shortness of breath

Sexuality-reproductive pattern
• Complex interpersonal role changes with spouse or partner, with decreased desire for and frequency of sexual activity because of actual or potential shortness of breath

Coping–stress tolerance pattern
• Difficulty expressing either positive or negative emotions because of shortness of breath
• Fluctuating behavior (alternately passive, angry, abusive, or manipulative)

Value-belief pattern
• Ambivalence about resuscitative measures that may be necessary during hospital stay but may not ultimately improve the quality of life

Physical findings
General appearance
• Apprehension and anxiety; maintenance of upright, tense posture
• Tendency to panic easily if activity is requested
• Cachexia (emphysema); plethora (chronic bronchitis)

Cardiovascular
• Typically, rapid pulse because of medications; expected upper limit for medication-induced tachycardia is 120 beats/minute
• Atrial fibrillation or multifocal atrial tachycardia (common arrhythmias of COPD)
• Signs of cor pulmonale and right-sided heart failure (edema, jugular vein distention, or crackles)

Pulmonary
• Accentuated accessory neck muscles
• Barrel chest from hyperinflation
• Decreased breath sounds bilaterally
• Prolonged expiratory phase

• Productive cough: tapioca-like plugs (hallmark of emphysema) or copious amounts of sputum (hallmark of chronic bronchitis)
• Gurgles if secretions are copious; crackles if heart failure or pneumonia is present (crackles are not a common or expected finding in COPD)
• Chronic sinus drainage with accompanying sinus pain (may cause recurring infections)

Neurologic
• Anxiety
• Restlessness with hypoxemia
• Lethargy and sleepiness with increased partial pressure of carbon dioxide (Pco_2) levels

Integumentary
• Skin that discolors (mottling and cyanosis) easily during coughing spells, strenuous activity, or episodes of acute shortness of breath

Diagnostic studies
• Arterial blood gas (ABG) measurements—specific values vary with disease
  –Hypoxemia: most common; more pronounced with exercise; in stable state, partial pressure of oxygen (Po_2) level should be between 55 and 65 mm Hg because the patient may have a reduced respiratory drive when Po_2 level is greater than 65 mm Hg; in acute exacerbation, Po_2 level commonly falls below 55 mm Hg
  –Increased carbon dioxide level: in stable state, Pco_2 level should be maintained at 50 mm Hg or less; during exacerbation, Pco_2 level above 50 mm Hg is common
  –Acid-base imbalance: in stable state, body compensates for respiratory acidosis; during exacerbation, both respiratory and metabolic acidosis may be present
• Sputum specimens—if infection is suspected, Gram stain and culture and sensitivity tests are done to determine appropriate antibiotic
• Theophylline level—normal is 10 to 15 µg/ml (normal may be 5 to 12 µg/ml if the patient is using other drugs); may be elevated if the patient has adjusted theophylline dose
• Alpha$_1$-antitrypsin assay—uncommon; performed to determine alpha$_1$-antitrypsin deficiency in young patients with suspected emphysema
• Other tests—white blood cell count, hematocrit, and serum electrolyte levels are performed, according to suspected cause
• Chest X-ray—shows hyperinflation, with flattening of the diaphragm caused by air trapping in the chest, that may worsen during exacerbation; may also show infiltrates, depending on exacerbation's cause
• Pulmonary function test—usually not performed in acute exacerbation; common findings in stable state include:

– reduced expiratory flow rates, especially with effort; airway obstruction is more pronounced as the patient tries harder to exhale
– some response to bronchodilators in patients with chronic bronchitis; no response in patients with emphysema
– decreased diffusion capacity in patients with emphysema predominating

Potential complications
• Acute respiratory failure
• Cardiac arrhythmias
• Depressed brain function; permanent brain injury
• Other organ injury (such as kidney)
• Pneumonia
• Pneumothorax
• Cor pulmonale

CLINICAL SNAPSHOT

CHRONIC OBSTRUCTIVE PULMONARY DISEASE

Major nursing diagnoses and collaborative problems	Key patient outcomes
Risk for respiratory failure	Exhibit ABG levels within normal limits for the patient.
Ineffective breathing pattern	Display use of effective breathing techniques, especially when experiencing shortness of breath or during exercise.
Nutritional deficit	Eat meals without acute shortness of breath.
Activity intolerance	Demonstrate the method for gaining control of activity-related shortness of breath.
Sleep pattern disturbance	Report an improved sleep pattern.
Knowledge deficit	List four indicators of impending exacerbation.
Altered sexuality patterns	Describe ways to use therapies for maximum benefit in order to engage in sexual activity.

COLLABORATIVE PROBLEM

Risk for respiratory failure (Po_2 level less than 50 mm Hg, with or without Pco_2 level greater than 50 mm Hg) related to ventilation-perfusion imbalance

Nursing priorities

• Maintain adequate airway clearance.
• Reverse hypoxemia and carbon dioxide retention.
• Maintain optimum environment for adequate function of the patient's limited respiratory reserves.
• Resolve causative factors.

Patient outcome criteria

• Within 48 hours of admission, the patient will:
– exhibit a Po_2 level greater than 50 mm Hg, with or without supplemental oxygen
– exhibit a Pco_2 level within the patient's normal range, typically less than 50 mm Hg
– exhibit fewer and shorter periods of acute shortness of breath.
• By the time of discharge, the patient will:
– exhibit reduced evidence of infection or environmental irritation
– easily expectorate clear or white, thin sputum
– have lungs clear on auscultation, without gurgles or crackles.

(Text continues on page 261.)

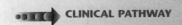 CLINICAL PATHWAY

Managing COPD or asthma

Patient problem	1-4 hours/Direct admission only	Day 1
Pulmonary Risk for altered pulmonary function	• Goal: Stable pulmonary function: respiratory rate 18 to 25 breaths/minute; effective airway clearance; no change in mental status or level of consciousness; use of diaphragmatic muscles for breathing; no restlessness or anxiety; antibiotics and theophylline I.V. given within 45 minutes of admission • Vital signs • Oxygen by nasal cannula or mask • Unit dose nebulizer with bronchodilator • Multidose inhaler • Antibiotic I.V. within 45 minutes of admission • Theophylline I.V. within 45 minutes of admission • Steroid I.V. within 45 minutes of admission • I.V. fluids/saline lock • Pharmacy to assess drug orders • Assess drug allergies and notify pharmacy	• Goal: Stable pulmonary function: respiratory rate 18-25 breaths/min; effective airway clearance; no change in mental status/LOC; use of diaphragmatic muscles for breathing; no restlessness or anxiety • Vital signs q 8 hr • Assess breath sounds q shift • O_2 — nasal/mask • Unit dose nebulizer with bronchodilator • Multidose inhaler • I.V. fluids
Tests High risk for anxiety related to tests, procedures, and hospitalization	• Goal: Laboratory work and tests completed within 45 minutes of admission: sputum culture and sensitivity (collect within 45 minutes of admission; document attempts; if unable, RT to induce); S7; complete blood count; chest X-ray; arterial blood gas values (collect within 45 minutes of admission); theophylline level; urinalysis; PBS (if indicated); electrocardiogram	• Goal: Labwork/tests within expected limits: assess sputum report for acceptability; notify doctor to re-order if unacceptable
Activity • Risk for activity intolerance • Risk for impaired mobility related to illness	• Assess for skin breakdown and document	• Goal: Tolerates activity progression: stable blood pressure and pulse and respiratory rates; performs self-care with assistance; feeds self • Assist with personal care daily • Active ROM q 2 hr • Initiate skin care protocol
Gastrointestinal • Risk for altered nutrition: Less than body requirements • Risk for altered bowel function	• Goal: Stable GI function: active bowel sounds; abdomen nondistended • GI assessment	• Goal: Stable GI function: active bowel sounds; abdomen nondistended; normal bowel pattern • GI assessment q 8 hr • Goal: Nutritional intake meets body requirements: dietary intake > 50% per meal; P.O. intake ≥ 2,000 ml/day • Assess intake P.O. (I&O q 8 hr) • Assess need for supplemental intake q 8 hr
Teaching • Knowledge deficit related to disease process, medication, and preventive measures		• Goal: Patient and family participate in identifying learning needs: They verbalize understanding of plan of care; demonstrate ability to follow instructions • Assess knowledge of disease process • Provide COPD and asthma patient booklets • Teach purse-lip breathing • Assess special needs
Discharge planning • Risk for self-care deficit • Risk for impaired home maintenance management	• Goal: Patient and family participate in identifying discharge needs: They verbalize needs; acknowledge discharge process • Notify case manager • Discharge planning assessment.	• Goal: Patient and family participate in identification of discharge needs: They verbalize needs; acknowledge discharge process • Discharge planning nurse to see if indicated
Psychosocial/spiritual • Risk for ineffective family coping • Risk for ineffective individual coping		• Goal: Patient and family demonstrate adequate coping: They verbalize fears and anxieties; demonstrate compliance with care; participate in care • Allow time to verbalize concerns • Pastoral care p.r.n. • Assess response to care/treatment • Assess support system

Day 2

- Goal: Stable pulmonary function:
respiratory rate 18-25 breaths/minute; effective airway clearance; no change in mental status/LOC; use of diaphragmatic muscles for breathing ; no restlessness or anxiety
- Vital signs q 8 hr
- Assess breath sounds q shift
- O_2 — nasal/mask
- Unit dose nebulizer with bronchodilator
- Multidose inhaler
- I.V. fluids
- Pharmacy for medication review

- Goal: Labwork/tests within expected limits:
theophylline level; CBC; survey 6 (repeat if abnormal previously); assess preliminary sputum results; pattern blood sugar (if indicated)

- Goal: Tolerates activity progression:
stable blood pressure and pulse and respiratory rates; performs self-care; tolerates chair 1 hour t.i.d.
- Out of bed in chair t.i.d.
- Up in chair with meals
- Skin care protocol

- Goal: Stable GI function:
active bowel sounds; abdomen nondistended; normal bowel pattern
- GI assessment q 8 hr
- Goal: Nutritional intake meets body requirements:
dietary intake > 50% per meal; P.O. intake ≥ 2,000 ml/day
- Assess P.O. intake
- Assess need for supplemental intake q 8 hr

- Goal: Identified learning needs met:
patient verbalizes understanding of plan of care; demonstrates ability to follow instructions; verbalizes special needs
- Provide smoking cessation information as appropriate
- Assess knowledge of disease process
- Encourage questions
- Teach progression of activity, pulmonary care and equipment needs

- Goal: Patient and family participate in identification of discharge needs:
they verbalize needs; acknowledge discharge process; participate in decision making
- Discharge planning nurse to see if indicated

- Goal: Demonstrates adequate coping:
patient verbalizes fears and anxieties; demonstrates compliance with care; participates in care
- Allow time to verbalize concerns
- Pastoral care p.r.n.
- Assess response to care and treatment
- Assess support system

Day 3

- Goal: Stable pulmonary function:
respiratory rate 18-25 breaths/minute; effective airway clearance; no change in mental status/LOC; use of diaphragmatic muscles for breathing; no restlessness or anxiety; vital signs within normal limits; SAO_2 ≥ 92%; breath sounds clear; weaning steroids
- Vital signs q 8 hr
- Assess breath sounds q shift
- O_2 — wean O_2
- Multidose inhaler
- Pulse oximetry (if on O_2). Call the doctor if < 90%
- Change to P.O. antibiotics
- Change I.V. to saline lock
- Assess need to change I.V. site

- Goal: Labwork/tests within normal limits:
theophylline level normal; CBC normal; survey 6 normal (if ordered); pattern blood sugar normal (if ordered)
- Pattern blood sugar (if indicated)

- Goal: Tolerates activity progression:
stable heart rate, blood pressure, and respiratory rate; performs self-care; tolerates ambulation t.i.d.
- Ambulate with assistance t.i.d.
- Up in chair with meals
- Skin care protocol

- Goal: Stable GI function:
active bowel sounds; abdomen nondistended; normal bowel pattern
- GI assessment q 8 hr
- Goal: Nutritional intake meets body requirements:
dietary intake > 50% per meal; P.O. intake ≥ 2,000 ml/day
- Assess P.O. intake
- Assess need for supplemental intake q 8 hr

- Goal: Identified learning needs met:
patient verbalizes understanding of progression of care; demonstrates ability to follow instructions; verbalizes special needs
- Assess knowledge of measures to prevent infection and symptoms to report to the doctor at home
- Teach progression of activity, pulmonary care, and equipment needs

- Goal: The patient and family participate in identifying discharge needs:
they verbalize needs; acknowledge discharge process; participate in decision making
- Assess and arrange for home health care and equipment needs
- Assess need for skilled nursing unit
- Assess need for pulmonary rehabilitation

- Goal: Demonstrates adequate coping:
patient verbalizes fears and anxieties; demonstrates compliance with care; participates in care
- Allow time to verbalize concerns
- Pastoral care p.r.n.
- Assess response to care and treatment
- Assess support system

Managing COPD or asthma *(continued)*

Patient problem	Day 4	Day 5
Pulmonary Risk for altered pulmonary function	• Goal: Stable pulmonary function: respiratory rate 18-25 breaths/minute; effective airway clearance; no change in mental status/LOC; use of diaphragmatic muscles for breathing; no restlessness or anxiety; normal vital signs; $Sao_2 \geq 92\%$; breath sounds clear; weaning steroids • Vital signs q 8 hr • Assess breath sounds q shift • Discontinue O_2 • Discontinue unit dose nebulizer • Multidose inhaler • Change to P.O. theophylline • Change to P.O. steroids • I.V. site care • Pharmacy to assess discharge medications	• Goal: Stable pulmonary function: respiratory rate 18-25 breaths/minute; effective airway clearance; no change in mental status/LOC; use of diaphragmatic muscles for breathing; no restlessness or anxiety; normal vital signs; $Sao_2 \geq 92\%$; breath sounds clear; weaning steroids • Assess vital signs q 8 hr • Assess breath sounds q shift • Multidose inhaler • Discontinue saline lock • Review pulmonary discharge instructions
Tests High risk for anxiety related to tests, procedures, and hospitalization	• Goal: Tolerates activity progression: stable heart rate, blood pressure, and respiratory rate; patient performs self-care; patient tolerates ambulation • Patient ambulates independently q.i.d. • Skin care protocol	• Pattern blood sugar (if indicated)
Activity • Risk for activity intolerance • Risk for impaired mobility related to illness	• Goal: Stable GI function: active bowel sounds; abdomen nondistended; normal bowel pattern • GI assessment q 8 hr	• Goal: Tolerates activity progression: stable heart rate, blood pressure, and respiratory rate; performs personal care; increased activity time; independent ambulation • Up at will • Skin care protocol
Gastrointestinal • Risk for altered nutrition: less than body requirements • Risk for altered bowel function	• Goal: Nutritional intake meets body requirements dietary intake > 50% per meal; P.O. intake $\geq$ 2,000 ml/day • Assess P.O. intake • Assess need for supplemental intake q 8 hr	• Goal: Stable G.I. function: active bowel sounds; abdomen nondistended; normal bowel pattern • GI assessment q 8 hr • Goal: Nutritional intake meets body requirements: dietary intake > 50% per meal; P.O. intake $\geq$ 2,000 ml/day • Assess P.O. intake • Assess need for supplemental intake q 8 hr
Teaching • Knowledge deficit related to disease process, medication, and preventive measures	• Goal: Identified learning needs met: patient verbalizes understanding of progression of care at home • Reinforce prior instructions p.r.n. • Discharge instructions: COPD booklet; asthma booklet; medications; pulmonary care; pursed-lip breathing	• Goal: Identified learning needs met: patient verbalizes understanding of progression of care at home • Reinforce prior instructions • Review discharge instructions: COPD booklet; asthma booklet; medications; pulmonary care; pursed-lip breathing
Discharge planning • Risk for self-care deficit • Risk for impaired home maintenance management	• Goal: Patient and family participate in identifying discharge needs: they verbalize needs; acknowledge D/C process; participate in decision making • Discharge plans completed	• Goal: Identified discharge needs met: patient and family describe home plan of care; demonstrate ability to manage home care • Review home plan of care • Review discharge medications and instructions
Psychosocial/spiritual • Risk for ineffective family coping • Risk for ineffective individual coping	• Goal: demonstrates adequate coping: patient verbalizes fears and anxieties; demonstrates compliance with care; participates in car. • Allow time to verbalize concern. • Pastoral care p.r.n. • Assess response to care and treatment • Assess support system	

Interventions

1. Obtain and report ABG measurements as needed to determine the patient's baseline, to monitor the appropriateness of therapy, and to determine the effect of an acute episode (if the patient becomes somnolent or increasingly restless or has a sudden personality change).

2. Administer oxygen as ordered, generally 2 L/minute during the day and 3 L/minute at night or during activity.

3. Administer pharmacologic agents and monitor therapeutic levels, as ordered.
• bronchodilators (often self-administered by patient using metered-dose inhalers)

• antibiotics
• corticosteroids

• expectorants

4. Perform bronchial hygiene measures, as ordered. Assess breath sounds before and after all treatments and at least every 4 hours when the patient is awake. Report and document the effectiveness of all of the following treatments that are used: aerosols, postural drainage and percussion, and suctioning (if the coughing mechanism is inadequate).

5. Maintain fluid intake at eight to twelve 8-oz (240-ml) glasses of water per day.

6. Monitor, document, and report signs of infection or further deterioration in respiratory status, such as an increase or decrease of sputum, changes in the sputum's color or consistency, fever, increased shortness of breath, and changes in breath sounds.

7. If possible, reduce or eliminate environmental irritants: Encourage the patient who smokes to quit, and do not use (or allow roommates or visitors to use) hair, deodorant, or room-freshening sprays or strong fragrances near the patient.

8. Additional individualized interventions: _____

Rationales

1. ABG evaluations are the only reliable way of assessing the patient's oxygenation and carbon dioxide status. No formula exists for determining the precise percentage of oxygen a patient needs because the appropriateness of the oxygen dosage can be evaluated only by serial ABG determinations.

2. The COPD patient may have an altered respiration-regulating mechanism. Instead of responding to an elevated carbon dioxide level (normal response), the COPD patient may respond only to a need for oxygen. Low percentages of oxygen are less likely to decrease the respiratory drive. Oxygen supply decreases at night (nocturnal desaturation) because of decreased intercostal muscle tone during sleep. Oxygen demand increases with activity.

3. Pharmacologic agents are ordered according to the severity of the disease.
• Three main classes of bronchodilators used in the treatment of COPD include anticholinergic agents (such as ipratropium bromide), beta agonists (such as albuterol), and methylxanthines (such as theophylline). The preferred route is by metered-dose inhaler. Proper use of the inhaler provides the maximum effective dosage; a spacer device or aerochamber can be used, especially for an elderly or very young patient, to ensure adequate dosing.
• Antibiotics are ordered for the specific organism.
• Corticosteroids (I.V. or oral) are believed to reduce inflammation.
• Expectorants may be used as an adjunct to fluid therapy.

4. Ventilation-perfusion abnormalities are the major reason for respiratory failure in the COPD patient. Bronchial hygiene measures open obstructed airways for more effective ventilation while conserving oxygen reserves.

5. Sputum viscosity is related to the patient's hydration status. Water is the most physiologically compatible expectorant.

6. Routine monitoring and accurate documentation allows early detection of subtle changes in the patient's condition that might signal illness progression.

7. Many environmental substances and sprays can cause airway irritation in the COPD patient (especially when the airways are already compromised) and exacerbate the condition.

8. Rationales: _____

NURSING DIAGNOSIS

Ineffective breathing pattern related to emotional stimulation, fatigue, or blunting of respiratory drive

Nursing priority

Maintain an effective breathing pattern.

Patient outcome criteria

• Immediately upon admission, after coaching by the nurse, the patient will use effective breathing techniques, especially when experiencing shortness of breath or during exercise.
• Within 24 hours, the patient will pace activities to coincide with periods of maximum bronchodilation and peak energy.

Interventions

1. Reduce the work of breathing and lessen depletion of oxygen reserves through teaching and by promoting relaxation as follows:
• Position the patient for comfort (upright may be best, with a pillow under the elbows and the patient leaning on the overbed table).
• Remind the patient to relax the shoulders and neck muscles.
• Instruct the patient to prolong exhalation.
• Sit with the patient and encourage rhythmic breathing.
• Use a calm, unhurried manner.

2. Teach and help the patient to perform breathing exercises and coordinate breathing with activity.

3. Pace all activities according to periods of maximum bronchodilation and peak energy. Encourage energy conservation.

4. Instruct the patient in breathing techniques to use when expressing feelings that may cause shortness of breath.

5. Avoid the use of sedatives or narcotics.

6. Additional individualized interventions: _____

Rationales

1. Inhalation normally requires muscle work and energy expenditure. Exhalation is ordinarily passive, not requiring extra energy and oxygen, but because the COPD patient in distress uses oxygen for both inhalation and exhalation, a large amount of oxygen from each inhalation is used to take and expel the next breath. Also, because shortness of breath causes anxiety, the patient tends to tighten muscle groups, thus using even more oxygen. Relaxation and easy, prolonged exhalation maximize lung expansion while minimizing energy and oxygen expenditures. Despite the value of breathing techniques, the COPD patient may forget them in a crisis and need the nurse's assistance to regain control.

2. Breath holding during exertion dramatically increases shortness of breath.

3. Pacing allows activity while conserving energy reserves.

4. Any expression of emotion, such as happiness, anger, or sadness, affects respiratory patterns and may increase shortness of breath.

5. These agents further depress the respiratory centers and may provoke respiratory arrest.

6. Rationales: _____

NURSING DIAGNOSIS

Nutritional deficit related to shortness of breath during and after meals and adverse reactions to medication

Nursing priorities

• Maintain adequate caloric and nutritional intake.
• Reduce deterrents to eating.
• Optimize environmental conditions to increase appetite.

Patient outcome criteria

• Within 48 hours of admission, the patient will take meals without episodes of acute shortness of breath.
• By the time of discharge, the patient will have a stable weight.

Interventions

1. Use supplemental oxygen during mealtimes, as ordered.

2. Perform bronchial hygiene measures before meals. Provide mouth care, and remove secretions from the eating area.

3. Provide frequent, small meals.

4. Monitor the patient's weight and nutritional intake.

5. Obtain a dietary consultation as soon as the patient can take foods or fluids, with special attention to needs for:
• high-protein, low-carbohydrate, high-fat supplements

• eliminating gas-producing foods from diet

• considering the patient's food preferences and conforming to any dietary restrictions such as limiting salt.

6. Additional individualized interventions: _____

Rationales

1. The act of eating requires oxygen. Supplemental oxygen during meals bolsters oxygen reserves.

2. Performing hygiene measures before meals ensures maximum bronchodilation and reduces activity-related ventilation-perfusion imbalances that may cause hypoxemia. The presence of sputum may decrease appetite.

3. Small meals require less oxygen for eating and digestion than large ones.

4. During periods of exacerbation, metabolic demands may increase, creating an increased demand for calories to maintain weight. A steady weight loss over weeks to months points to insufficient calories; a weight gain of 3 lbs or more within 4 days may indicate fluid retention.

5. Early dietary consultation can prevent complications from further debilitation.

• The COPD patient has an increased respiratory rate and increased work of breathing, resulting in greater metabolic demands. A diet with a low calorie-to-nitrogen ratio will meet metabolic demands without increasing carbon dioxide production (as occurs with a high-carbohydrate diet).
• Abdominal distention can cause diaphragmatic compression, increasing the sensation of shortness of breath.
• The patient is more likely to follow a nutritional plan that includes favorite, familiar foods. Necessary restrictions must be observed to promote optimal health.

6. Rationales: _____

NURSING DIAGNOSIS

Activity intolerance related to shortness of breath, avoidance of physical activity with resultant muscle weakness, deconditioning, depression, and (possibly) exercise-related hypoxemia

Nursing priority

Promote a gradual return to an optimal level of activity, with absent or controlled episodes of acute shortness of breath. (*Note:* Progress on this priority will depend on resolving the exacerbation and its causative factors.)

Patient outcome criteria

• Throughout the hospital stay, the patient will increase the ability to ambulate over longer times and distances without shortness of breath, pulse changes (rate or rhythm), blood pressure drop, or a color change.
• By the time of discharge, the patient will demonstrate the method for gaining control of activity-related shortness of breath.

Interventions

1. Assess the patient's ability to perform household chores, movements, work, family and social activities, volunteer work, and recreation. Help the patient identify barriers and develop alternative approaches to activities.

2. Instruct the patient in breathing techniques to use when performing activities of daily living (ADLs): slow and relaxed exhalation, avoidance of breath holding, and relaxation of accessory muscles. (For more information and pictures of these techniques for use during instruction, contact the local American Lung Association chapter.)

3. Administer oxygen during activity, as ordered.

4. Before recommending an activity level, assess for stable ABG measurements and level of fitness (the pulmonary function or respiratory therapy department can assist in determining an appropriate exercise level). Also assess for other factors that can contribute to inactivity (such as family relationships), concomitant diseases (such as arthritis), or environmental conditions.

5. Develop and implement a daily walking schedule, increasing time and distance as tolerated. Before beginning, teach the patient how to control shortness of breath. This includes telling the patient to stop, lean back, position his hips against a sturdy object or wall, and stand with his feet apart.

6. Before, during, and after walking, monitor the patient's response to exercise. Along with the time and distance walked, document the following: blood pressure (before and after), pulse rate and rhythm, patient's color, respiratory rate, and degree of shortness of breath.

7. Additional individualized interventions: _____

Rationales

1. An inability to cope psychologically with the disruptive effects of disease is significantly linked with increased mortality.

2. Breathing techniques make full exhalation easier, thereby promoting removal of stale air, increasing ventilatory efficiency, and permitting a wider range of physical activity.

3. Increased activity requires supplemental oxygen.

4. If undertaken prematurely, increased activity may worsen the patient's symptoms. The patient is unlikely to follow an activity prescription that does not take into account ABG measurements, level of fitness, and other deterrents to activity.

5. Implementing a walking schedule should start in the hospital, if possible, so that the patient can be observed and coached in appropriate breathing techniques. Gaining control over shortness of breath improves the patient's confidence in walking independently.

6. If a patient experiences desaturation or acidosis during the walk, these events will be reflected in vital sign changes. More sophisticated exercise testing may be needed to determine the extent of disability and the appropriate therapy.

7. Rationales: _____

NURSING DIAGNOSIS

Sleep pattern disturbance related to bronchodilators' stimulant effect, shortness of breath, depression, and anxiety

Nursing priority

Minimize sleep disruption.

Patient outcome criteria

By the time of discharge, the patient will:
• report less frequent episodes of nocturnal shortness of breath
• fall asleep easily at night
• sleep throughout the night, without early morning headache or excessive drowsiness during the day
• report an improved sleep pattern or more easily controlled episodes of nocturnal shortness of breath, or both.

Interventions

1. Identify the patient's normal sleep pattern as well as the abnormal pattern.

2. Consult with the doctor about adjusting medications to optimize bronchodilation with minimal stimulant effects.

3. Teach the patient how to perform bronchial hygiene before retiring and as needed for nocturnal dyspnea.

4. Administer oxygen therapy during the night, as ordered.

5. Monitor periods of sleeplessness, including degree of shortness of breath, pulse rate and rhythm, respiratory rate, and breath sounds. Observe which treatments seem to provide the most benefit.

6. Instruct the patient in relaxation techniques to be used at bedtime. (A COPD patient should not use sleeping medications unless the doctor specifically prescribes them.)

7. Additional individualized interventions: _____

Rationales

1. The patient may have misconceptions about normal and abnormal sleep patterns. Discussion may clarify factors contributing to sleep disturbance.

2. Bronchodilators vary in their stimulant properties. Stimulants may cause myocardial irritability, nervousness, and anxiety and may increase oxygen demand.

3. Nocturnal shortness of breath may be unavoidable so the patient needs to know how to deal with such an episode effectively.

4. PaO_2 levels normally decrease at night. Although most people can tolerate the decrease, the already hypoxemic COPD patient cannot because hypoxemia-induced pulmonary vasoconstriction can cause or exacerbate cor pulmonale.

5. Observing a sleeplessness episode and its resolution may provide clues for preventing or coping with future episodes.

6. Relaxation techniques can promote sleep and minimize oxygen demands. Sleeping medications may depress respirations in the already compromised patient.

7. Rationales: _____

NURSING DIAGNOSIS

Knowledge deficit (failure to recognize signs and symptoms indicating impending exacerbation) related to complexity of disorder

Nursing priority

Teach the patient to recognize an impending exacerbation and to seek appropriate treatment.

Patient outcome criteria

By the time of discharge, the patient will:
• list four indicators of an impending exacerbation
• correctly identify the rationale for notifying the doctor before adjusting the medication regimen.

Interventions

1. Teach the patient the signs and symptoms of an impending exacerbation, including:
• increased or decreased sputum production
• change in the color or character of sputum over a 24-hour period
• fever (based on baseline normal temperature)
• restlessness or inability to sleep for more than one night
• increased fatigue or sleepiness.

Rationales

1. Early detection and intervention increase the likelihood of successful reversal or control of the episode.

2. Emphasize the need to notify the doctor promptly if these symptoms occur rather than altering the medication regimen without the doctor's knowledge.

3. Caution the patient to avoid overmedication with prescription drugs or over-the-counter remedies.

4. Additional individualized interventions: _____
_____

2. Appropriate intervention requires medical judgment.

3. Overuse of some medications such as bronchodilators may actually increase oxygen demands. Over-the-counter remedies may contain substances such as ephedrine that increase or counteract the therapeutic effects of prescribed medication.

4. Rationales: _____
_____

NURSING DIAGNOSIS

Altered sexuality patterns related to shortness of breath, change in body image, deconditioning, change in relationship with spouse or partner, and adverse reactions to medications

Nursing priority

Help the patient and spouse (or partner) to discuss feelings and determine realistic expectations.

Patient outcome criterion

By the time of discharge, the patient will describe ways to use therapies for maximum benefit in order to engage in sexual activity.

Interventions

1. Establish rapport with the patient and spouse (or partner). Discuss their feelings concerning changes in sexual functioning.

2. Help the patient learn or arrange therapies (including medication schedule, oxygen level, bronchial hygiene, and energy conservation) to optimize sexual function, as desired.

3. Additional individualized interventions: _____
_____

Rationales

1. A sense of rapport makes discussion of this sensitive topic more comfortable. Discussion will help clarify the issues involved and the expectations held by the patient and spouse (or partner).

2. As with other activities, the patient must learn to arrange therapies to accomplish desired goals.

3. Rationales: _____
_____

DISCHARGE PLANNING

Discharge checklist

Before discharge, the patient shows evidence of:
❑ absence of fever and other signs of infection
❑ ABG levels within acceptable parameters
❑ absence of cardiovascular or pulmonary complications
❑ minimal shortness of breath
❑ breath sounds clear or normal for patient when not in exacerbated state
❑ ability to tolerate ambulation with minimal limitations, same as before exacerbation and hospitalization

❑ ability to perform ADLs independently (or with minimal assistance) at preexacerbation level
❑ ability to tolerate diet with minimal shortness of breath
❑ stabilized weight (within 5 lb [2.3 kg] of normal weight)
❑ adequate home support system or referral to home care if indicated because of inadequate home support, inability to perform ADLs at preexacerbation levels, or need for continued assistance with bronchial hygiene measures.

Keep in mind that the patient with COPD will not be "normal" when discharged. Therefore, discharge evaluation should relate to the patient's condition before the exacerbation. The most important thing to document is the absence of acute infection, but also note ABG levels on discharge. ABG levels must be within acceptable parameters because abnormal levels on discharge commonly cause readmission within a short time.

Teaching checklist
Document evidence that the patient and family demonstrate an understanding of:
❏ practical energy conservation and breathing techniques
❏ signs and symptoms of infection or exacerbation
❏ purpose, dosage, administration schedule, and adverse reactions requiring medical attention of all discharge medications (usual discharge medications include bronchodilators, corticosteroids, antibiotics, and expectorants)
❏ bronchial hygiene measures
❏ use, care, and cleaning of respiratory equipment
❏ need for drinking eight to twelve 8-oz glasses of water per day
❏ dietary restrictions
❏ twice-weekly weight monitoring
❏ importance of avoiding exposure to infections and need for flu vaccination
❏ importance of avoiding lung irritants, such as cold air, secondhand smoke, sprays, and dust
❏ exercise prescription
❏ referral to community agencies, as appropriate (such as Meals on Wheels, American Lung Association, Better Breathers Club, respiratory equipment company and name of representative, emergency response service, home care agency, and smoking-cessation group)
❏ date, time, and location of next appointment
❏ how to contact the doctor.

Documentation checklist
Using outcome criteria as a guide, document:
❏ clinical status on admission
❏ significant changes in status
❏ pertinent laboratory and diagnostic tests such as ABG levels
❏ episodes of shortness of breath, including physical assessment parameters during each episode, treatment administered, and treatment outcome
❏ respiratory status per shift, including breath sounds, character of cough, and character, color, and amount of sputum
❏ administration and outcome of therapies given
❏ nutritional intake
❏ fluid intake
❏ exercise ability and activity level

❏ patient and family teaching
❏ discharge planning.

ASSOCIATED PLANS OF CARE
Dying
Grieving
Ineffective individual coping
Knowledge deficit
Pneumonia

REFERENCES

Ball, P. "Epidemiology and Treatment of Chronic Bronchitis and its Exacerbations," *Chest* 108(2):Supplement, 43S-52S, August 1995.

Bone, R. "A Step-Care Approach to Managing COPD," *Journal of Respiratory Disease* 12(8):727-40, June-July 1995.

Friedman, M. "Changing Practices in COPD," *Chest* 107(5):Supplement, 194S-197S, May 1995.

Kong, G., et al. "Reducing Lengths of Stay for Patients Hospitalized with Exacerbation of COPD by Using a Practice Guideline," *Chest* 111(1):89, January 1997.

Kumar, A., et al. "Clinical and Personality Profiles and Survival in Patients with COPD," *Chest* 11(1):95, January 1997.

Leidy, N., and Haase, J. "Functional Performance in People with Chronic Obstructive Pulmonary Disease: A Qualitative Analysis," *Advances in Nursing Science* 18(3):77-90, March 1996.

Wilson, R. "Outcome Predictors in Bronchitis," *Chest* 108(2):Supplement, 53S-57S, August 1995.

Lung cancer

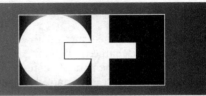

DRG information
DRG 075   Major Chest Procedures.
              Mean LOS = 11.2 days
DRG 076   Other Respiratory System O.R. Procedure
              with Complication or Comorbidity.
              Mean LOS = 12.5 days
DRG 082   Respiratory Neoplasms.
              Mean LOS = 7.9 days
DRG 410   Chemotherapy. Principal diagnosis: mainte-
              nance chemotherapy.
              Mean LOS = 3.4 days
DRG 409   Radiotherapy.
              Mean LOS = 6.7 days
DRG 412   History of Malignancy with Endoscopy.
              Mean LOS = 3.0 days

INTRODUCTION

Definition and time focus
Lung cancer is a condition of aberrant cellular growth causing morphologic tissue changes within the lung. It causes 13% of all cancer in men and 32% of all cancer-related deaths in men. It is responsible for 13% of all cancer in women and 25% of all cancer-related deaths in women.

    Tumors may be primary (original) or secondary (from distant metastasis). The most common types of primary lung cancer are squamous cell carcinoma (40% to 50% of cases), adenocarcinoma (25% of cases), small-cell anaplastic carcinoma (20% to 25% of cases), and large-cell anaplastic carcinoma (less than 15%).

    Surgical resection, lobectomy, or pneumonectomy may be performed alone or with radiation therapy, chemotherapy, or both to treat lung cancer. However, the 5-year survival rate for persons with this disease is below 13% regardless of the treatment used. This clinical plan focuses on the patient with primary lung cancer who is admitted to an acute care center for chemotherapy as an initial treatment.

Etiology and precipitating factors
• Cigarette smoking
• Exposure to carcinogens, such as asbestos, pollution, pitchblende, metals, radon, or chemicals
• Genetic predisposition

FOCUSED ASSESSMENT GUIDELINES

Nursing history (functional health pattern findings)
Health perception–health management pattern
• History of heavy smoking
• Dyspnea associated with activity or anxiety; degree of dyspnea may be disproportionate to overall clinical picture
• Chest pain aggravated by deep breathing (if pleura involved), cough (may be nocturnal), rust-streaked or purulent sputum, or hemoptysis
• Increased risk if older than age 45 or male
• Shoulder or arm pain if brachial plexus involved
• Hoarseness common with laryngeal involvement
• Easy bleeding from minor trauma as well as slowed clot formation (cancer inhibits factor VIII [antihemophilic factor] activity)
• Medical assistance sought only when cough, dyspnea, weakness, and weight loss caused patient to sense "something was wrong"
Nutrition-metabolic pattern
• Significant weight loss, anorexia, early satiety, changes in taste sensation, or reduced sensitivity to sweets
Elimination pattern
• Constipation along with abdominal discomfort or diarrhea
Activity-exercise pattern
• General fatigue and weakness
Sleep-rest pattern
• Sleep disturbed by cough
Self-perception–self-concept pattern
• Inability to carry out routine activities that may cause questioning of self-worth and a feeling of powerlessness
• Fear related to diagnosis, physical disabilities, and possible death
Role-relationship pattern
• Inability to assume family tasks and occupational role
• Feelings of loss related to changing roles and possible death
• Loss of a significant relationship before diagnosis
Sexuality-reproductive pattern
• Inability to be sexually active without experiencing dyspnea
Coping–stress tolerance pattern
• Feelings of depression or despondency

Value-belief pattern
• Feeling of personal control over circumstances (common in the patient with an above-average chance for successful remission)
• Equating of cancer with death (common in the patient with a below-average chance for successful remission)

Physical findings
Cardiovascular
• Rapid pulse rate if anemia is present
• Possible arrhythmias
• Edema of face or neck or distended neck veins if superior vena cava syndrome is present
Pulmonary
• Cough (may be nocturnal)
• Rust-streaked or purulent sputum
• Crackles, wheezes, and friction rub in affected lung
• Hoarseness if vocal cords are involved
• Finger clubbing
Neurologic
• Headache, mental confusion, and unsteady gait if central nervous system (CNS) is involved
• Diminished deep tendon reflexes
• Decreased mental alertness if anemia and hypoxemia are present
Musculoskeletal
• Pathologic fractures with metastasis

Diagnostic studies
• Carcinoembryonic antigen titer — high levels may be useful to monitor treatment responses; 50% of patients may have false-negative titers
• Arterial blood gas (ABG) measurements — may reveal hypoxemia
• Hemoglobin values — may be low from anemia
• Hematocrit — may be low from anemia
• Platelet count — may be low from bone marrow suppression
• White blood cell (WBC) count — may be low from bone marrow suppression
• Sputum collection for cytology — may be useful to determine cell type (according to continuum of classes from normal to malignant)
• Serum albumin level — hypoalbuminemia may indicate malnutrition
• Serum creatinine level — indicates altered renal function related to chemotherapy
• 24-hour urine creatinine test — nutritional index that indicates changes in lean body weight when compared with individual's height; also indicates altered renal function related to chemotherapy
• Chest X-ray — may reveal tumor position; usually does not show early tumor involvement
• Computed tomography scan — outlines tumor's size, shape, and position

• Bronchoscopy — useful in diagnosing centrally located lesions
• Mediastinoscopy — needle biopsy of nodes useful in diagnosis and tumor staging
• Radioisotopic scans — performed to assess for metastasis
• Scalene node biopsy — determines lymphatic involvement

Potential complications
From lung cancer
• Pleural effusion
• Pneumonitis
• Cardiac failure or arrhythmias
• Brachial plexus involvement
• Cushing's syndrome
• Hypercalcemia
• Syndrome of inappropriate antidiuretic hormone secretion
• Peripheral neuritis
• CNS degeneration
• Dermatomyositis
• Superior vena cava syndrome
• Paralysis of diaphragm
• Pathologic fractures
• Disseminated intravascular coagulation
From chemotherapy
• Bone marrow suppression
• Immunosuppression
• Renal tubular necrosis
• Liver toxicity
• Cardiotoxicity
• Pulmonary toxicity
• Neurotoxicity
• Sterility

CLINICAL SNAPSHOT

LUNG CANCER

Major nursing diagnoses and collaborative problems	Key patient outcomes
Hypoxemia	Exhibit less dyspnea while at rest
Risk for hemorrhage	Follow safety measures to prevent bleeding
Chronic pain	Express an increased sense of control over pain
Risk for infection	Display no signs of infection
Risk for sensory/perceptual alteration	Have no complaints of paresthesia
Nutritional deficit	Control any nausea or vomiting with antiemetics
Risk for constipation or diarrhea	Maintain regular bowel elimination
Risk for altered urinary elimination	Maintain urine output within normal limits
Activity intolerance	Perform activities of daily living (ADLs) with minimal assistance
Sleep pattern disturbance	Report 8 to 10 hours of sleep during a 24-hour period
Self-esteem disturbance	Verbalize measures to improve self-esteem
Altered sexuality patterns	Discuss the desire for sexual expression and intimacy, if desired

COLLABORATIVE PROBLEM

Hypoxemia related to aberrant cellular growth of lung tissue, bronchial obstruction, increased mucus production, or pleurisy

Nursing priority

Optimize oxygen availability to cells.

Patient outcome criteria

Throughout chemotherapy, the patient will:
• exhibit less dyspnea while at rest
• use pursed-lip breathing and relaxation techniques
• decrease smoking by at least one-half compared with preadmission rate
• demonstrate huff cough and cascade cough techniques on request.

Interventions

1. Initiate ABG measurements or continuous or intermittent pulse oximetry monitoring on admission, and monitor for changes in the partial pressure of oxygen (Po_2) daily or as the patient's clinical condition changes, as ordered.

Rationales

1. The Po_2 indicates the amount of pressure oxygen exerts against an artery. A decreased Po_2 reflects increased hypoxemia.

2. Administer humidified oxygen continuously, via mask or mechanical ventilator, as ordered and according to nursing judgment.

2. Oxygen administered at higher-than-room-air concentrations increases the oxyhemoglobin saturation of available red blood cells. An increase in hemoglobin saturation increases the amount of oxygen available for cellular metabolism if circulation is not impaired. The patient with lung cancer frequently needs high concentrations of oxygen that can be provided only by mask or mechanical ventilation. An oxygen humidifier decreases the drying effect of oxygen administration on the respiratory mucosa.

3. Elevate the head of the bed during dyspneic episodes.

3. Elevating the head of the bed aids respiratory movement by allowing gravity to displace abdominal organs downward, thus decreasing pressure on the diaphragm.

4. Evaluate and document breath sounds, respiratory rate, and chest movements every 8 hours or more frequently, based on the patient's condition. Observe for dyspnea: complaints of difficulty breathing, shortness of breath, flaring nostrils, and intercostal retractions on inspiration or bulging on expiration.

4. Dyspnea is a subjective finding that indicates hypoxemia. Abnormal findings common in the patient with a lung tumor include crackles, bronchial breath sounds, pleural friction rubs, and decreased breath sounds.

5. During dyspneic episodes, stay with the patient, explain all procedures, and support the patient and family. Do not increase the oxygen rate or concentration over the prescribed level; counsel the patient and family accordingly.

5. Dyspnea is commonly associated with anxiety and fear of impending death. Anxiety may be decreased if the patient feels in control and has confidence in caregivers. Increasing oxygen levels may remove the hypoxic stimulus for respiration in the patient with chronic obstructive pulmonary disease, cause carbon dioxide narcosis if a face mask is used, or cause oxygen toxicity.

6. Encourage the patient who smokes to stop or decrease smoking.

6. Smoking increases mucus production, irritates respiratory mucosa, and decreases oxyhemoglobin saturation.

7. Teach pursed-lip breathing and relaxation techniques.

7. Pursed-lip breathing increases end-expiratory pressure and helps prevent alveolar collapse. Controlled breathing and relaxation decrease the anxiety associated with dyspnea.

8. Teach huff cough or cascade cough.

8. Huff cough is accomplished as the patient takes a deep breath and, with mouth open, "huffs" several times. After repeating several times, the patient coughs. The cascade cough involves taking a deep breath and then coughing until the patient feels that no air is left in the lungs. These maneuvers maximize the coughing effort and help remove secretions while conserving energy.

9. Additional individualized interventions: _____

9. Rationales: _____

COLLABORATIVE PROBLEM

Risk for hemorrhage related to depression of platelet production by chemotherapy

Nursing priority

Prevent or minimize hemorrhage.

Patient outcome criteria

Throughout chemotherapy, the patient will:
• exhibit vital signs within normal limits: heart rate, 60 to 100 beats/minute; systolic blood pressure, 90 to 140 mm Hg; and diastolic blood pressure, 50 to 90 mm Hg
• have no evident bleeding
• follow safety measures to prevent bleeding.

Interventions

1. Caution the patient to report any bleeding immediately, including petechiae, ecchymoses, and oozing wounds.

2. Initiate and monitor serum platelet counts before, during, and after chemotherapy, as ordered.

3. Caution the patient to use a soft or sponge toothbrush for oral hygiene and to avoid spicy foods.

4. Teach the patient to monitor urine and stools for signs of bleeding and to report such signs at once.

5. Instruct the patient to use an electric razor for shaving or, if male, to grow a beard (unless alopecia is present).

6. Administer medications to suppress menses, as ordered. Make sure the patient does not use a vaginal douche.

7. Teach the patient to report any headaches, dizziness, or light-headedness immediately.

8. Avoid intramuscular injections. If they are unavoidable, apply pressure for at least 5 minutes after the injection. Do not take the patient's temperature rectally or allow the use of suppositories.

9. Avoid administering aspirin and medications that contain aspirin.

10. Apply ice packs to bleeding areas.

11. Administer stool softeners, as ordered.

12. Additional individualized interventions: _____

Rationales

1. Hemorrhage may occur rapidly. The patient may be able to assume some responsibility for observing for signs of bleeding. Petechiae, ecchymoses, and oozing wounds indicate clotting problems.

2. Chemotherapeutic agents suppress bone marrow and affect platelet production. A patient with a platelet count below 20,000/mm^3 is at high risk for spontaneous hemorrhage.

3. The oral mucosa may bleed if irritated from flossing or use of a hard toothbrush or a toothpick. Spicy foods also may irritate the oral mucosa.

4. Tea- or cola-colored urine or black, tarry, or blood-streaked stools indicate bleeding, which requires immediate attention.

5. An electric razor decreases the risk of lacerating the skin while shaving.

6. Prolonged menstrual bleeding may cause severe blood loss; douching may cause vaginal bleeding.

7. CNS bleeding may cause headaches, dizziness, or light-headedness. Dizziness and light-headedness also may indicate hypovolemia.

8. Decreased platelet counts prolong clotting time. Direct pressure for 5 minutes stops active bleeding in most patients. Objects inserted in the rectum may cause bleeding.

9. Aspirin decreases platelet aggregation and increases clotting time

10. Ice causes peripheral vasoconstriction, decreasing blood flow to the area and the risk of significant hemorrhage.

11. Soft stools decrease the risk of tearing the rectal mucosa and help minimize straining on defecation, which increases intracranial pressure and may lead to intracranial bleeding.

12. Rationales: _____

NURSING DIAGNOSIS

Chronic pain associated with involvement of peripheral lung structures, metastasis, or chemotherapy

Nursing priority

Relieve pain and promote comfort.

Patient outcome criteria

Throughout chemotherapy, the patient will:
• request pain-relief medication before pain peaks
• rate pain as less than 3 on a 0 to 10 pain rating scale
• express an increased sense of control over pain
• demonstrate the correct procedure for administering pain medication.

Interventions

1. Instruct the patient to report pain or discomfort immediately

2. Monitor the patient continually for signs or symptoms of pain or discomfort, such as facial grimaces, splinting of the chest (painful area), diaphoresis, or restlessness.

3. Involve the patient in pain-control strategies by using imagery and relaxation techniques. See the "Pain" plan, page 88, for details.

4. Administer pain medication, as needed, according to a set schedule or medical protocol and nursing judgment. Teach the patient or a family member how to administer pain medication after discharge.

5. Additional individualized interventions: _____

Rationales

1. Early intervention provides more effective pain relief than measures employed after the pain has peaked.

2. The patient may not report pain or discomfort. Careful observation may allow detection of nonverbal indications that the patient is in pain.

3. Cognitive measures may decrease pain perception. The "Pain" plan contains general interventions for pain.

4. Pain medication ordered for a terminally ill patient may be given more frequently and in larger doses than routinely recommended (the patient receiving pain medication over a prolonged period may develop an increased tolerance). A set schedule may improve ongoing pain control because analgesics are more effective if given before pain becomes severe. Self-administration or administration of medication by a family member enables the patient to control pain at home.

5. Rationales: _____

NURSING DIAGNOSIS

Risk for infection related to immunosuppression from chemotherapy and malnutrition

Nursing priority

Prevent infection.

Patient outcome criteria

• Within 1 day of admission, the patient will isolate self from infected family members or friends.
• Throughout chemotherapy, the patient will:
 – display no signs of infection
 – have normal temperature
 – present no growth from cultures.

Interventions

1. Observe strict medical and surgical asepsis during wound care, venipuncture, and any invasive procedures.

2. Monitor and record temperature every 8 hours. Report even slight temperature elevations.

3. Instruct the patient to avoid crowds and persons with infections. Do not place the patient in reverse isolation unless laminar airflow or another method is available.

4. Monitor WBC counts before, during, and after chemotherapy, as ordered.

5. Initiate routine cultures of stool, urine, sputum, nasopharynx, oropharynx, and skin, as ordered.

6. Instruct the female patient to use sanitary napkins instead of tampons.

7. Avoid using indwelling urinary catheters.

8. Additional individualized interventions: _____

Rationales

1. The immunosuppressed patient easily contracts infections because of diminished host defenses. Maintaining strict medical and surgical asepsis decreases the risk of exposing the patient to pathogenic organisms.

2. Elevated temperature is a sign of infection. The immunosuppressed patient may show slight or no temperature elevation even when extensive infection is present.

3. The risk of infection increases when a patient is exposed to individuals with contagious diseases. Reverse isolation is usually not effective unless laminar airflow is used because airborne organisms can still enter the patient's room.

4. Chemotherapy causes bone marrow depression, which may decrease the WBC count. Granulocyte counts below 1,000/µl increase the patient's risk of infection.

5. Cultures provide information about bacterial colony growth that may produce infection. Early information about possible causes of infection guides the doctor in prescribing appropriate antibiotic therapy.

6. Tampons may traumatize the vaginal mucosa and provide a favorable environment for pathogen growth.

7. Indwelling catheters may introduce pathogens into the bladder and increase the risk of urinary tract infections.

8. Rationales: _____

NURSING DIAGNOSIS

Risk for sensory-perceptual alteration related to peripheral neuropathies caused by chemotherapy

Nursing priority

Prevent or minimize sensory-perceptual deficits caused by chemotherapy.

Patient outcome criteria

Throughout chemotherapy, the patient will:
• have no complaints of paresthesia
• have normal deep tendon reflexes.

Interventions

1. Assess for, document, and report deficits in neurologic functioning, including paresthesia and abnormal deep tendon reflexes.

2. Discontinue or decrease the chemotherapy dosage, depending on the neuropathies' severity, as ordered.

Rationales

1. Chemotherapeutic agents such as vincristine (Oncovin) may cause peripheral neuropathies.

2. Discontinuation or dosage reduction of medications such as vinca alkaloids may reverse adverse neurologic effects and will prevent further neuropathies.

3. Explain that changes in sensation are related to chemotherapy, and allow the patient to express fears related to this situation.

4. Protect the area of decreased sensory perception from injury: Use a bath thermometer; assess the skin every 8 hours for signs of trauma; apply dressings to injured areas; use a night-light; and avoid clutter in areas of activity to prevent abrasions, contusions, or falls.

5. Additional individualized interventions: _____

3. Fear may be reduced when the patient confronts the situation.

4. Decreased perception at sensory nerve endings may reduce the patient's ability to judge temperature and pressure and may reduce pain sensation. Taking preventive measures reduces the potential for injury.

5. Rationales: _____

NURSING DIAGNOSIS

Nutritional deficit related to cachexia associated with tumor growth, anorexia, changes in taste sensation, or stomatitis

Nursing priorities
- Minimize weight loss.
- Promote return to optimum achievable body weight.

Patient outcome criteria
Throughout chemotherapy, the patient will:
- plan meals appropriately, with or without family assistance
- control any nausea or vomiting with antiemetics
- exhibit pink oral mucosa, with no lesions.

Interventions

1. Within 24 hours of admission, estimate the patient's required protein needs based on ideal body weight and serum total protein level.

2. With the patient and dietitian, develop a diet plan based on calculated dietary needs and the patient's food preferences.

3. Increase dietary protein levels by adding powdered milk to gravies, puddings, and milk products.

4. Provide small, frequent meals.

5. Document weight weekly.

Rationales

1. Caloric needs are altered by cancer-related cachexia. Serum total protein level reflects the status of visceral protein stores. Protein needs for a patient with cancer are calculated as 1 g/kg of ideal body weight (1 g of protein = 30 kcal).

2. Patient participation allows some feeling of control. Nutritional intake should increase if the patient's likes and dislikes are considered in planning meals.

3. Powdered milk increases protein content without increasing bulk.

4. Small, frequent meals increase total intake for the patient who experiences the early satiety common in cancer.

5. A weight record allows accurate assessment of changing nutritional needs. A patient with cancer commonly experiences significant weight loss.

6. Provide antiemetics, as ordered, before administering chemotherapeutic agents. To reduce nausea, provide diversionary activities during chemotherapy and encourage the patient to lick salt or a lemon slice or sip sweetened ice water.

6. The effects of chemotherapy on the CNS and gastric mucosa may induce vomiting. Granisetron (Kytril), ondansetron (Zofran), and prochlorperazine (Compazine) are effective antiemetics. Marijuana and tetrahydrocannabinol are being studied for control of nausea and vomiting. Nausea associated with chemotherapy may be psychogenic (it sometimes occurs before chemotherapy is administered); diversionary activities may distract the patient's attention and reduce nausea. The taste of lemon, salt, or sugar can relieve nausea in some patients.

7. Daily assess the oral mucosa for stomatitis and document findings.

7. Chemotherapeutic agents, such as methotrexate (Folex) and fluorouracil (Adrucil), affect cells that undergo rapid replication such as those in the GI system. Stomatitis interferes with the ability to eat.

8. Provide a mild mouthwash with viscous lidocaine (Xylocaine) before meals.

8. The local anesthetic action of lidocaine decreases oral discomfort during meals.

9. After meals, clean the patient's mouth with ½ tsp of sodium bicarbonate and ½ tsp salt mixed with 8 oz (240 ml) tap water. Follow with a 1:5 solution of hydrogen peroxide and water. Rinse with the sodium bicarbonate and salt solution. Do not use the hydrogen peroxide solution if bleeding occurs in the mouth, and do not use lemon-glycerin swabs.

9. Rinsing and cleaning with a sodium bicarbonate and salt solution followed by water and hydrogen peroxide reduces the bacterial count in the mouth and decreases the risk of infection. Using hydrogen peroxide in the presence of bleeding may disrupt clot formation. Lemon-glycerin swabs can dry the mouth, causing further discomfort.

10. Lubricate the patient's lips with petroleum jelly.

10. Lubrication with petroleum jelly reduces lip drying and cracking.

11. Assess oral mucosa daily for signs of lesions from opportunistic infections such as *Candida*.

11. *Candida* is an opportunistic organism that may cause infection in an immunosuppressed patient.

12. Instruct the patient to swish and swallow with yogurt or buttermilk three times a day.

12. Yogurt and buttermilk restore to the GI tract the natural flora destroyed by chemotherapeutic agents. Growth of opportunistic organisms is decreased if normal flora is maintained.

13. Administer oral nystatin (Mycostatin), as ordered.

13. Oral nystatin is effective against candidal infections.

14. Additional individualized interventions: _____

14. Rationales: _____

Nursing diagnosis

Risk for constipation or diarrhea related to chemotherapy

Nursing priority

Maintain normal bowel elimination.

Patient outcome criteria

Throughout chemotherapy, the patient will:
• maintain regular bowel elimination
• have soft stools.

Interventions

1. Assess and document the patient's bowel elimination pattern on admission. Reassess the patient's bowel elimination pattern before chemotherapy.

2. Administer antidiarrheal medication such as diphenoxylate hydrochloride (Lomotil), as ordered.

3. Assess for signs of paralytic ileus (such as diminished or absent bowel sounds and abdominal discomfort) every 8 hours. If present, report them to the doctor immediately.

4. Prevent constipation by increasing dietary fiber, providing warm fluids, and promoting the optimal amount of exercise. Do not check for fecal impaction if thrombocytopenia is present.

5. Administer stool softeners, as ordered.

6. Additional individualized interventions: _____
_____

Rationales

1. Chemotherapeutic agents may cause constipation or diarrhea. Information about the patient's previous bowel elimination pattern provides a baseline for evaluating bowel elimination during the hospital stay.

2. Diphenoxylate anticholinergic activity slows gastric motility, effectively controlling diarrhea.

3. Paralytic ileus is a medical emergency that may be caused by chemotherapeutic agents.

4. Bran, raw vegetables, fruits, and whole grain breads provide dietary fiber and promote bowel elimination. Liquids increase peristalsis. Exercise causes abdominal muscle contraction and promotes bowel elimination. Checking for fecal impaction may cause the thrombocytopenic patient to bleed.

5. Stool softeners promote bowel elimination by increasing the water content of stools and easing their passage.

6. Rationales: _____
_____

NURSING DIAGNOSIS

Risk for altered urinary elimination related to possible development of renal toxicity or hemorrhagic cystitis from chemotherapy

Nursing priority

Maintain normal urinary elimination pattern.

Patient outcome criteria

Throughout chemotherapy, the patient will:
• maintain urine output within normal limits
• have amber-colored urine
• feel no pain on urination.

Interventions

1. Assess and document the patient's urinary elimination pattern on admission.

2. Force fluids and administer allopurinol (Lopurin) before administering chemotherapeutic agents, as ordered.

Rationales

1. Accurate assessment directs appropriate care planning.

2. Cyclophosphamide (Cytoxan) may cause hemorrhagic cystitis. Methotrexate may cause renal toxicity. Increasing fluid intake increases the glomerular filtration rate and reduces the risk of potentially toxic renal effects from chemotherapy. Allopurinol decreases uric acid calculi formation from chemotherapy by inhibiting uric acid synthesis.

3. Alkalinize the patient's urine before and during chemotherapy to prevent uric acid calculi formation.

3. Chemotherapy may cause uric acid calculi formation because acidic urine increases uric acid excretion. Fruits (such as oranges, tomatoes, and grapefruit), vegetables, and milk increase urine alkalinity and decrease uric acid calculi formation.

4. Monitor serum creatinine and 24-hour urine creatinine, as ordered, before chemotherapy.

4. Serum creatinine and 24-hour urine creatinine studies provide information about renal function. Normally functioning kidneys should clear creatinine.

5. Additional individualized interventions: _____

5. Rationales: _____

NURSING DIAGNOSIS

Activity intolerance related to weakness from cachexia, altered protein metabolism, muscle wasting, or hypoxia

Nursing priority

Optimize activity level without inducing dyspnea.

Patient outcome criteria

Within 1 week of admission, the patient will:
* manage activities with less dyspnea than on admission
* perform ADLs with minimal assistance.

Interventions

1. Immediately on admission, determine what activities the patient can tolerate without dyspnea.

Rationales

1. Dyspnea occurs as energy requirements exceed oxygen availability. Determining what activities the patient can tolerate without dyspnea guides activity recommendations.

2. Instruct the patient to organize activities into manageable units.

2. Activities performed without fatigue promote comfort and decrease dyspnea.

3. Teach proper body mechanics to decrease the energy expenditure associated with ADLs: Explain the need to slide objects rather than carry them, work close to the body, sit when possible, use gravity, and avoid unnecessary bending or reaching.

3. The use of proper body mechanics reduces energy expenditure.

4. Additional individualized interventions: _____

4. Rationales: _____

NURSING DIAGNOSIS

Sleep pattern disturbance related to nocturnal cough

Nursing priority

Optimize sleep patterns.

Patient outcome criterion

Within 3 days of admission, the patient will report 8 to 10 hours of sleep within a 24-hour period, including 4 hours of uninterrupted sleep.

Interventions

1. Assess and document sleep patterns on admission. Discuss sleep patterns before the diagnosis was made.

2. Provide quick, efficient assistance with respiratory hygiene when coughing disrupts sleep.

3. Instruct the patient to sleep with his head elevated.

4. Exercise caution in administering sedatives and hypnotics.

5. Administer cough suppressants, as ordered.

6. Additional individualized interventions: _____

Rationales

1. Sleep pattern goals should be based on the patient's perception of normal sleep patterns. Sleep disruption, commonly caused by the psychological distress of the diagnosis, robs the patient of energy needed to cope with the illness.

2. Sleep disturbance is minimized if care is provided quickly and efficiently.

3. Head elevation while sleeping eases the work of breathing by decreasing pressure on the diaphragm.

4. Sedatives and hypnotics may blunt respiratory drive and worsen hypoxia.

5. Cough suppressants may lessen sleep disruption.

6. Rationales: _____

NURSING DIAGNOSIS

Self-esteem disturbance related to weight loss, cough, sputum production, hair loss, or role changes

Nursing priority

Promote a positive self-concept.

Patient outcome criteria

Throughout chemotherapy, the patient will:
• wear well-fitting clothes
• express the desire to wear a wig, a hat, or scarf or verbalize acceptance of baldness
• verbalize measures to improve self-esteem
• initiate interaction with friends, family, and health care providers.

Interventions

1. Approach the patient with an accepting attitude.

2. Assess and document the patient's self-concept and attitudes and responses to role changes.

3. Encourage the patient and family to share feelings.

4. Discuss methods to accentuate the patient's positive features and minimize weight loss through changes in hairstyle and clothing.

5. Encourage the use of a portable disposal unit for discarding tissues and sputum.

6. Encourage frequent contact, in person or by telephone, with loved ones.

Rationales

1. An individual needs to experience acceptance from others to develop a positive self-concept.

2. Accurate assessment of the patient's self-concept promotes appropriate care planning.

3. Expression of feelings promotes honest, open relationships.

4. Clothing that fits well without accentuating weight loss improves general feelings of well-being. A well-groomed appearance improves self-concept.

5. Knowing how to dispose of unsightly tissues and sputum improves the patient's feelings of control and increases self-esteem.

6. Contact with others minimizes isolation and improves self-concept.

7. Discuss probable hair loss before chemotherapy starts (keep in mind that hair loss may affect all parts of the body, not just the scalp). With the patient's permission, cut hair before loss occurs. Natural hair may be used to fashion a wig, or the patient can be fitted for a wig before hair loss. The patient may want to wear a hat or scarf instead of a wig.

8. Remind the patient that hair loss is not permanent and that hair regrows after chemotherapy ends. Be sure to mention that new hair may be different in color and texture.

9. Explain to the patient about scalp tourniquets and scalp hypothermia treatments that may diminish hair loss. Inform the patient that these procedures are time-consuming and may be unsuccessful.

10. Additional individualized interventions: _____

7. Knowledge about hair loss will decrease the anxiety associated with it. Hair loss is more manageable when hair is short. A wig, hat, or scarf helps minimize the impact of hair loss on body image and self-esteem.

8. Hair regrowth usually begins within a few days to a few weeks after the end of chemotherapy.

9. Scalp tourniquets and scalp hypothermia treatments diminish the contact of chemotherapeutic agents with hair follicles and may decrease hair loss. The patient should be allowed to make an informed choice.

10. Rationales: _____

NURSING DIAGNOSIS

Altered sexuality patterns related to dyspnea and possible sterility

Nursing priorities

• Promote acceptance of optimal expressions of sexuality.
• Promote long-range plans for childbearing, if desired.

Patient outcome criteria

Throughout chemotherapy, the patient and spouse or partner will:
• discuss the desire for sexual expression and intimacy, if desired
• request time for privacy, if desired.

Interventions

1. During initial assessment, discuss any changes in patterns of sexual expression that have resulted from the diagnosis and treatments.

2. Help the patient and spouse or partner discuss their desires for sexual expression and intimacy. Help them differentiate between the two needs and stress the importance of love and affection in maintaining a sense of closeness with each other.

3. Discuss options for sexual expression within the patient's physical limitations. For example, if intercourse is fatiguing or impossible for physical reasons and if the couple is receptive, suggest alternative forms of sexual and sensual expression that appeal to all senses, such as massage with scented oils, listening to music, sharing foods with various tastes and textures, and reading romantic literature.

Rationales

1. Open discussion helps the patient to develop realistic goals and expectations related to sexual expression.

2. Honest, caring communication between partners about their sexual needs promotes adjustment to cancer's impact on sexuality. Differentiating the desire for sexual activity from the desire for emotional closeness may allow the couple to focus on the strengths in their relationship, rather than on a loss of a specific sexual activity.

3. Sexual expression is closely tied to self-esteem, and the patient and spouse or partner may find that their self-esteem suffers when they can no longer participate in intercourse. Knowledge of alternative methods of sexual and sensual gratification can restore sexual intimacy and increase self-esteem when intercourse is no longer an option.

4. Encourage the use of supplemental oxygen during intercourse.

5. Provide privacy for the patient and spouse or partner to maintain intimacy through such activities as private discussions and affectionate cuddling, if desired.

6. Explain that reduced sexual responsiveness may result from fatigue or chemotherapy.

7. Explain that chemotherapy may cause sterility. If appropriate, discuss sperm banking before chemotherapy. Inform the patient that childbearing plans should be postponed for at least 18 months after chemotherapy ends.

8. Additional individualized interventions: _____
_____

4. Exercise increases oxygen demands.

5. Intimacy is encouraged when individuals can share uninterrupted time.

6. Knowing the reasons for reduced sexual responsiveness decreases anxiety about sexuality.

7. Chemotherapy may affect gonadal function and diminish sperm and ovum production. Sperm may be saved in sperm banks for future fertilization. Drug-induced changes in sperm and ova should reverse by 18 months after the end of chemotherapy. Although the prognosis for these patients may be poor, discussion of future plans may help maintain hope.

8. Rationales: _____
_____

DISCHARGE PLANNING

Discharge checklist
Before discharge, the patient shows evidence of:
❏ absence of fever and pulmonary or cardiovascular complications
❏ stable vital signs
❏ absence of infection
❏ nausea or vomiting and diarrhea controlled by oral medications
❏ adequate hydration
❏ normal renal function
❏ adequate nutritional and fluid intake
❏ ability to control pain using oral and subcutaneous medication
❏ absence of bowel complications
❏ coughing controlled by medication
❏ minimal use of oxygen to assist breathing
❏ ability to demonstrate or explain proper oxygen administration technique, including how to acquire oxygen for home use
❏ ability to tolerate ADLs and ambulation with minimal difficulty
❏ adequate home support system or, if appropriate, referral to hospice, home care, or both
❏ knowledge of community support programs.

Teaching checklist
Document evidence that the patient and family demonstrate an understanding of:
❏ diagnosis
❏ effects of chemotherapy
❏ prevention, detection, and management of bleeding
❏ use of supplemental oxygen
❏ smoking cessation
❏ breathing exercises

❏ purpose, dosage, administration schedule, and adverse effects requiring medical attention of all discharge medications; usual discharge medications include analgesics, antiemetics, and stool softeners or antidiarrheals, as appropriate
❏ pain-relief measures
❏ signs of and methods to prevent infection
❏ signs of neurologic changes
❏ dietary modifications
❏ measures to control nausea and vomiting
❏ measures to promote normal renal function
❏ measures to decrease dyspnea
❏ measures to minimize effects of changing body image
❏ plans for sexual expression
❏ date, time, and location of follow-up appointments
❏ how to contact the doctor
❏ when and how to seek emergency medical care
❏ community resources.

Documentation checklist
Using outcome criteria as a guide, document:
❏ clinical status on admission
❏ significant changes in status
❏ pertinent laboratory and diagnostic test findings
❏ response to chemotherapy
❏ episodes of dyspnea
❏ oxygen therapy
❏ bleeding episodes
❏ nutritional status
❏ bowel elimination
❏ urinary elimination
❏ activity tolerance
❏ sleep patterns
❏ patient and family teaching
❏ discharge planning.

Associated plans of care

Dying
Grieving
Ineffective family coping: Compromised
Ineffective individual coping
Knowledge deficit
Pain

References

Groenwald, S.L., et al., eds. *Comprehensive Cancer Nursing Review,* 4th ed. Sudbury, Mass.: Jones & Bartlett Pubs., Inc., 1998.

McCorkle, R., et al., eds. *Cancer Nursing: A Comprehensive Textbook,* 2nd ed. Philadelphia: W.B. Saunders Co., 1996.

Murphy, G.P., et al. *Textbook of Clinical Oncology,* 2nd ed. Atlanta: American Cancer Society, Inc., 1995.

Parker, S.L., et al. "Cancer Statistics, 1997" *CA: A Cancer Journal for Clinicians* 47(1):5-27, January-February 1997.

Sarna, L., and McCorkle, R., "Burden of Care and Lung Cancer" *Cancer Practice* 4(5):245-51, September-October 1996.

Mechanical ventilation

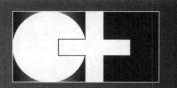

DRG information

DRG 475   Respiratory System Diagnosis with Ventilator Support.
Mean LOS = 9.7 days
Principal diagnoses include:
• respiratory failure
• chronic obstructive pulmonary disease (COPD)
• acute or chronic bronchitis
• pneumonia from various causes
• adult respiratory distress syndrome (ARDS)
• mechanical respiratory assistance.

Additional DRG information: A patient must have a principal respiratory system diagnosis to receive DRG 475. An intubated patient with Guillain-Barré syndrome complicated by respiratory failure will not be assigned DRG 475. Likewise, a patient with a principal diagnosis of heart failure will not be assigned DRG 475, even if that patient is intubated.

INTRODUCTION

Definition and time focus

Mechanical ventilation (providing gas volumes sufficient to maintain alveolar ventilation) commonly is required for patients with significant breathing abnormalities that may lead to apnea or respiratory failure. This plan focuses on the patient receiving positive-pressure ventilation, the most common type of mechanical ventilation in critical care.

Etiology and precipitating factors

• Central respiratory depression, such as from drug overdose, head trauma, cerebrovascular accident, anesthesia, or cardiac arrest
• Airway diseases, such as asthma and bronchitis
• Parenchymal diseases, such as ARDS, pulmonary edema, pneumonia, and emphysema
• Neuromuscular disorders, such as myasthenia gravis and Guillain-Barré syndrome
• Chest wall injury, such as pneumothorax, flail chest, and major thoracic surgery

FOCUSED ASSESSMENT GUIDELINES

Nursing history (functional health pattern findings)

Health perception–health management pattern
• Sudden or progressive onset of abnormal ventilatory patterns or airway obstruction
• Severe dyspnea or air hunger (if patient is able to speak)
• History of motor vehicle accident, assault, or other head, chest, or orthopedic trauma
• Treatment for long-standing chronic respiratory disease
• Recent major surgical procedure involving the thorax or upper abdomen
• History of drug or alcohol abuse
• History of cardiac disease

Physical findings

Pulmonary
• Labored breathing
• Shallow breathing
• Agonal breathing or other abnormal breathing pattern
• Tachypnea
• Intercostal retractions
• Nasal flaring
• Accessory muscle use
• Decreased or absent breath sounds
• Crackles, gurgles, or wheezes
• Increased secretions

Neurologic
• Restlessness
• Confusion
• Agitation
• Somnolence
• Unconsciousness

Cardiovascular
• Tachycardia (early), bradycardia (late)
• Arrhythmias
• Hypertension or hypotension

Integumentary
• Diaphoresis
• Cyanosis (central or peripheral)

Diagnostic studies

• Arterial blood gas (ABG) levels — reveal hypercapnia (partial pressure of arterial carbon dioxide [$Paco_2$] greater than 50 mm Hg) in a patient who previously had normal levels (or greater than 10 mm Hg increase

above usual value in a COPD patient). ABG levels also reveal hypoxemia with a partial pressure of arterial oxygen (PaO_2) less than 50 mm Hg on supplemental oxygen
• Alveolar-arterial (A-a) gradient — may be greater than 300 mm Hg on 100% oxygen
• Shunt — may be greater than 30%
• Minute ventilation (spontaneous) — may be less than 5 L/minute, indicating insufficient ventilation to remove carbon dioxide adequately, or greater than 10 L/minute, indicating excessive work of breathing
• Vital capacity (VC) — may be less than 15 ml/kg body weight, indicating poor ventilatory reserve

• Maximum inspiratory force (MIF) — may be less than 20 cm H_2O, indicating weak respiratory drive or respiratory musculature
• Dead space: tidal volume (V_D:V_T) ratio — may be greater than 0.6, indicating excessive wasted ventilation

Potential complications
• Tension pneumothorax
• GI hemorrhage
• Shock
• Pneumonia
• Ventilator malfunction
• Airway obstruction
• Long-term ventilator dependency

CLINICAL SNAPSHOT

MECHANICAL VENTILATION

Major nursing diagnoses and collaborative problems	Key patient outcomes
Ineffective alveolar ventilation	Maintain ABG levels within expected limits for the underlying disorder.
Risk for hypoxemia	Maintain partial pressure of oxygen and oxygen (O_2) saturation within expected limits.
Ineffective airway clearance	Maintain a patent airway.
Risk for injury: Complications	Remain free from pulmonary infection and other complications.
Fear	Be able to communicate needs, if conscious.
Risk for ineffective weaning	Maintain a spontaneous respiratory rate of 12 to 24 breaths/minute.

COLLABORATIVE PROBLEM

Ineffective alveolar ventilation related to failure to maintain prescribed ventilator settings

Nursing priority

Maintain settings as ordered.

Patient outcome criteria

Upon institution of mechanical ventilation and continuously thereafter, the patient will:
• have bilaterally equal chest excursion and breath sounds
• manifest compliance values within usual limits for the underlying disorder
• maintain ABG levels within expected limits for the underlying disorder.

Interventions

1. Confirm orders for mechanical ventilation, particularly:
- ventilator type

- inspiratory mode

– control

– assist-control

– synchronized intermittent mandatory ventilation (SIMV)

Rationales

1. Mechanical ventilation may be achieved with many combinations of modes and settings.
- The type of ventilator is determined by how the machine controls inspiration. In the acute care setting, ventilators that can deliver a prescribed volume are indicated; these are volume-cycled ventilators. Other types include time-cycled and pressure-cycled ventilators, both of which can have variable tidal volumes (V_T) and are used only for special situations.

Advances in technology and an increased need for equipment have resulted in a proliferation of different ventilators. The ventilator selected depends on the patient's ventilation requirements, type of monitoring desired, and weaning options.
- Inspiratory modes determine the type and degree of control over inspiration.
– The control mode provides complete ventilatory support by delivering a set number of breaths per minute, regardless of the patient's inspiratory efforts. The least-used mode, it is appropriate only for an apneic or paralyzed patient (such as a patient with central nervous system dysfunction or drug-induced paralysis), or in chest trauma where negative inspiratory pressure would be harmful (such as in flail chest). Keep in mind that this mode prevents the patient from taking *any* additional breaths.
– Assist-control, the most common mode, is suitable for almost all initial ventilator setups. This mode ensures delivery of a preset minimum number of breaths per minute but allows the patient to initiate the breath and to breathe more rapidly if desired. If the patient initiates a breath, the machine delivers the desired volume; if the patient does not breathe, the machine supplies the breath. Because the ventilator delivers a preset volume even on patient-initiated breaths, it lessens the work of breathing while improving alveolar ventilation.
– SIMV, once used only for the difficult-to-wean patient, is now considered a standard ventilatory mode for full or partial ventilatory support. The machine delivers a preset number of mandatory breaths. In between, the patient can breathe spontaneously through the ventilator circuit. The ventilator senses each breath and synchronizes the mandatory breaths in such a way as not to "stack" breaths on top of each other. Because these spontaneous breaths depend on the negative pressure the patient can generate, their V_T may vary significantly from the ventilator V_T. SIMV has several advantages; it maintains lower mean airway pressures (reducing the risk of barotrauma—lung damage from excessive pressure—and depression of cardiac output), reduces the risk of hyperventilation, helps maintain respiratory muscle strength, provides ventilatory support at rapid respiratory rates, and assures more even ventilation throughout the lung.

– pressure support

– pressure control

• expiratory maneuvers

– positive end-expiratory pressure (PEEP)

– continuous positive airway pressure (CPAP)

2. Collaborate with the respiratory therapist to monitor prescribed settings when settings are changed, when arterial blood is drawn for ABG measurements, or when pulse oximetry or capnography is used.

• respiratory rate: Count the machine rate and the patient's rate for 1 minute each and compare. Check controls for proper settings.

• tidal volume: Compare delivered V_T with desired V_T, typically 10 to 15 ml/kg. On newer models, read inspired V_T from the digital readout. On models with no readout, measure exhaled V_T with a Wright respirometer.

– Pressure support uses small amounts of pressure at the end of inspiration to increase V_T in a spontaneously breathing patient. Similar to intermittent positive-pressure breathing machines, pressure support can be used in combination with SIMV or as a weaning mode for a patient with inadequate spontaneous volumes.

– Pressure control uses peak pressure to limit the inspiratory cycle, although V_T will vary. Close monitoring is essential.

• Expiratory maneuvers determine the degree of resistance to expiration.

– PEEP is used commonly with positive-pressure ventilation of the patient with alveolar collapse (from loss of surfactant, early small-airway closure, or atelectasis) or alveolar filling (as in pulmonary edema and ARDS). In such a patient, nonfunctioning alveoli, unable to oxygenate blood flowing through pulmonary capillaries, produce an abnormal pulmonary shunt and hypoxemia refractory to oxygen therapy. PEEP is thought to help keep alveoli from collapsing and to recruit nonfunctioning alveoli. It also increases functional residual capacity (FRC) and allows gas diffusion to take place throughout the respiratory cycle. Because PEEP improves ventilation-perfusion matching, oxygenation improves. PEEP permits lowering of inspired oxygen concentration, helpful in preventing lung damage from excessive oxygen exposure. However, care needs to be taken to prevent trauma from higher pressures.

– Similar to PEEP, CPAP is used for a spontaneously breathing patient. It maintains positive airway pressure throughout the respiratory cycle. Its benefits are similar to those of PEEP. It can be applied through a ventilator during spontaneous respiration or via a special device, such as nasal CPAP, for a nonintubated patient.

2. Depending on the unit protocol, either the nurse or the respiratory therapist may be responsible for checking the ventilator. If the respiratory therapist checks, the nurse should confirm that ventilator settings are as ordered when first assuming responsibility for the patient. The nurse and the respiratory therapist must collaborate closely to provide the best patient care. Checking at the times indicated ensures that prescribed settings are accurate.

• With all ventilatory modes, the ventilator may not actually deliver the number of breaths set. Also, with assist-control or SIMV, the patient can breathe above the set rate.

• V_T is the amount of air inspired. Measuring exhaled V_T indicates the volume actually received. Decreasing V_T may indicate a machine, cuff, or bronchopulmonary leak.

• minute ventilation (MV): If the patient is on assist-control or SIMV, compare actual and desired MV. If the patient is on SIMV, also compare total and non-SIMV MV.

• MV, the product of the respiratory rate and the V_T, determines alveolar ventilation. MV is related inversely to $Paco_2$: As MV increases, $Paco_2$ decreases, and vice versa. Decreased MV is associated with carbon dioxide retention and respiratory acidosis, whereas increased MV is associated with carbon dioxide blow-off and respiratory alkalosis.

Comparing actual and desired MV indicates how well the machine meets the patient's ventilatory needs. Comparing total and non-SIMV MV indicates what amount the patient's spontaneous breaths are contributing to total MV; monitoring this amount can help the doctor or respiratory therapist evaluate the patient's readiness for weaning.

• inspiratory flow rate

• This rate is the speed of airflow per unit of time. Slower flow rates are preferred because they result in better gas flow characteristics: less turbulence, lower mean airway pressure, and better gas distribution within the lungs. It may be necessary to increase the flow rate so that the patient has time to exhale before the next breath is triggered or gas may be trapped in the lungs; this is called autoPEEP. Newer models contain demand valves so the patient can receive the flow needed.

• inspiratory-expiratory (I:E) ratio (typically 1:2 or greater)

• Expiration should be longer than inspiration to avoid air trapping. In some situations, reversing the I:E ratio may help improve oxygenation. Inspiration is then controlled by inspiratory flow, and expiratory time is controlled by respiratory rate.

• airway pressure (normally 20 to 40 cm H_2O and relatively constant): Monitor both peak inspiratory pressure and inspiratory plateau pressure, noting sudden changes in airway pressures or a trend of increasing pressures.

• Peak inspiratory pressure is the pressure at peak inspiration. It reflects the maximum pressure needed to overcome resistance to flow and to lung and chest wall expansion. Increased peak inspiratory pressure implies increased airway resistance, such as from secretions or bronchospasm. Plateau pressure is the pressure at end-inspiration. It reflects the pressure necessary to hold the airways open and deliver the volume of gas. Increased plateau pressure implies stiffness of lung tissue, pneumothorax, or a decrease in chest wall mobility.

• pressure limit

• This setting limits the amount of pressure that the machine can exert when delivering volume in order to prevent barotrauma. Once this level is reached, inspiration stops even if the desired V_T has not been delivered. The pressure limit may be reached occasionally if the patient is coughing or has excessive airway secretions or if the ventilator tubing is kinked. Consistently reaching the pressure limit suggests decreased compliance or a pneumothorax.

• sensitivity (typically 2 cm H_2O below zero or PEEP level)

• The sensitivity knob controls the amount of negative inspiratory pressure the patient must generate in order to trigger an inspiration.

• sigh

• A sigh is a periodic deep breath delivered by the ventilator. Thought to prevent atelectasis, sighing is not commonly used. Instead, the patient is ventilated with large V_Ts to prevent atelectasis.

• alarms and monitors

• Alarms need to be set for high airway pressure (usually the same as the pressure limit), low airway pressure (disconnect alarm), high and low volumes (to detect leaks), and high and low fraction of inspired oxygen (FIO_2). Many other parameters can be monitored and alarms set. Newer ventilators employ microprocessors that can simultaneously and continuously monitor almost all parameters related to the ventilator.

3. In collaboration with the respiratory therapist, monitor compliance every 8 hours:

3. Compliance measures the resistance to expansion. It is determined by the amount of change in volume that results from a given change in pressure (volume in milliliters divided by pressure in centimeters of water pressure equals compliance [in ml/cm H_2O]). Decreased lung compliance signifies that the lungs require more pressure to ventilate; they are stiffer than usual, as in ARDS. Increased compliance, rarely a clinical problem, indicates the lungs are easier to ventilate than usual. For example, in emphysema, where elasticity is lost, lung compliance increases, although airway obstruction still may render the patient difficult to ventilate.

• Monitor static compliance (V_T divided by end-inspiratory [plateau] pressure) or dynamic compliance (V_T divided by peak inspiratory pressure). If PEEP is used, subtract PEEP value from pressure before dividing.

• Static compliance indicates compliance when the lungs are at rest, whereas dynamic compliance indicates compliance when airflow is occurring. Static compliance values reflect lung compliance; dynamic compliance values also reflect airway resistance.

• Compare the patient's values with normal values (static: 100 ml/cm H_2O; dynamic: 50 ml/cm H_2O). Monitor compliance curves or note trend of values.

• Comparing static and dynamic values can help identify the source of difficulty in ventilating a patient. For example, a near-normal static compliance with a low dynamic compliance suggests the problem is increased airway resistance, whereas both low static and low dynamic compliance suggest the problem is the lung itself, as occurs with ARDS. Compliance curves—serial plotting of pressure changes compared to volume changes—indicate trends graphically and may allow determination of the best combination of pressure and volume for a patient.

4. Evaluate pulmonary status at least every 2 hours. Note particularly the symmetry of chest excursion, bilateral breath sounds, and any adventitious sounds.

4. These factors provide data about adequacy of airflow throughout the pulmonary tree and about secretions or obstructions to flow.

5. Additional individualized interventions: _____

5. Rationales: _____

COLLABORATIVE PROBLEM

Risk for hypoxemia related to insufficient oxygen delivery or inadequate PEEP level

Nursing priority

Maintain optimal oxygenation.

Patient outcome criteria

Within 24 hours of onset of mechanical ventilation and then continuously, the patient will:
• maintain a PaO_2 and O_2 saturation within expected limits
• display no signs or symptoms of oxygen toxicity.

Interventions

1. Compare delivered oxygen percentage with the desired percentage, typically 100% initially and thereafter adjusted according to PaO_2. With newer models, read the delivered oxygen percentage from the digital display of the built-in oxygen analyzer. With older models, use a handheld oxygen analyzer. Initially, use pulse oximetry, if desired, to titrate the FIO_2. Confirm the pulse oximetry readings with ABG oxygenation values.

2. Be aware if the FIO_2 is greater than 50%.

• In conjunction with the doctor, consider the risk of oxygen toxicity in relation to the need for oxygen therapy. If possible, implement ways to reduce the oxygen dose, as ordered.
• If it is not possible to reduce the oxygen dosage, observe the patient for sharp, pleuritic chest pain (typically after about 6 hours on 100% oxygen), decreased VC and decreased compliance (typically after 18 hours), and signs and symptoms of ARDS (typically after 24 to 48 hours). Document your observations and promptly notify the doctor if any of these signs or symptoms occur.

3. Monitor PEEP, typically ordered if the patient cannot maintain a PaO_2 greater than 60 mm Hg on less than 50% oxygen.
• Visually monitor the PEEP level (usually 5 to 15 cm H_2O) on the PEEP gauge or inspiratory pressure gauge (instead of dropping to zero at the end of expiration, the needle drops to the PEEP level).
• Assist the respiratory therapist with titration of PEEP by correlating the PEEP level with inspired oxygen percentage, the resulting PaO_2 level, and hemodynamic values. Apply PEEP in increments of 3 to 5 cm H_2O to reach a maintenance level of 5 to 15 cm H_2O, as ordered.

4. Additional individualized interventions: _____

Rationales

1. The machine may not deliver the set oxygen percentage. The oxygen analyzer evaluates the accuracy of oxygen delivery. Too low a percentage promotes hypoxemia, whereas too high a percentage promotes oxygen toxicity (see the "Risk for injury" collaborative problem, page 291).

2. Prolonged exposure to high alveolar oxygen tension promotes oxygen toxicity. Although an FIO_2 greater than 60% does not cause clinically significant parenchymal abnormalities in normal lungs, an FIO_2 greater than 50% may cause serious lung dysfunction in previously damaged or susceptible lung tissue.
• Lowering the oxygen dose, as can be achieved through PEEP, helps decrease the risk of toxicity. However, the need to treat hypoxemia takes precedence over the potential danger of oxygen toxicity.
• Signs and symptoms of oxygen toxicity reflect the progression from the initial phase of tracheobronchitis through the exudative phase of alveolar-capillary membrane damage. If unchecked, the syndrome progresses to a proliferative stage that results in pulmonary fibrosis. To assess for chest pain in an intubated patient, look for indications of pain such as grimacing and analyze pain characteristics by asking the patient questions that can be answered with a "yes" or "no" signal.

3. By increasing FRC and recruiting shunt units, PEEP improves oxygen transport and allows use of a lower inspired oxygen concentration.
• Visual monitoring confirms that the prescribed PEEP level is being maintained.

• The optimal PEEP level for a given patient depends on several factors, including shunt reduction, lung compliance, and cardiac output. The desired goal is maintenance of an adequate PaO_2 level on less than 50% oxygen. PEEP levels above 15 cm H_2O are associated with increased barotrauma and depressed cardiac output.

4. Rationales: _____

NURSING DIAGNOSIS

Ineffective airway clearance related to presence of endotracheal tube, increased secretions, and the underlying disease

---

Nursing priority

Maintain airway patency.

Patient outcome criteria

Continuously during mechanical ventilation, the patient will:
• maintain a patent airway
• have clear breath sounds bilaterally, as underlying condition allows.

Interventions

1. Provide artificial airway care according to unit protocol or as ordered, including the following:
• Support the ventilator tubing so it does not press on the edge of the patient's nose or mouth.

• Measure cuff pressures at least every 8 hours. Optimally, maintain cuff pressure at less than 20 mm Hg with a minimal leak.

2. Monitor endotracheal tube position. When oral or nasal endotracheal tube position is confirmed after intubation, mark the tube and trim excess. Check tube placement frequently by noting the relationship between the mark and the patient's lip or nostril. Also assess breath sounds every 1 to 2 hours.

3. Keep a manual self-inflating bag and mask connected to 100% oxygen at the bedside. If accidental extubation occurs, open the airway and ventilate with the bag and mask. Summon medical assistance.

4. Change the patient's position every 1 to 2 hours, including prone position. Provide chest physiotherapy as indicated.

5. Suction when needed, as indicated by dyspnea, coughing, gurgles, appearance of visible secretions in the tube, or a high-pressure alarm. Follow these guidelines for suctioning:
• Use a self-inflating bag to hyperoxygenate the patient with 100% oxygen before, during, and after suctioning. For suctioning, use a catheter with a diameter less than 50% of endotracheal tube diameter. Suction for no more than 15 seconds. Always reset the oxygen to its previous level after hyperoxygenation. Alternatively, use an in-line suction catheter to suction the trachea without disconnecting the patient from the ventilator. Hyperoxygenate the patient before, during, and after suctioning, and return the ventilator to its previous setting.

Rationales

1. Meticulous airway care can prevent many potential complications associated with endotracheal intubation.
• Maintaining proper alignment prevents accidental extubation, tube advancement, or nasotracheal or orotracheal erosion.
• Monitoring cuff pressures permits early detection of pressures high enough to cause tracheal ischemia and necrosis.

2. An endotracheal tube can migrate downward and rest against the carina, obstructing airflow and causing the patient to cough and fight the ventilator, or enter one of the bronchi (usually the right mainstem bronchi), preventing ventilation of the opposite lung. It also can migrate upward, increasing the risk of unintended extubation. Checking tube position and assessing breath sounds allows for detection of tube movement and repositioning as needed. Trimming oral tubes decreases mechanical dead space.

3. The bag and mask allow for emergency ventilation in the event of accidental extubation or mechanical failure. Reintubation must be performed by someone skilled in the technique.

4. Position changes help drain secretions and promote ventilation of all lung areas. Placing the patient in a prone position may optimize ventilation and oxygenation in acute hypoxemia. Chest physiotherapy promotes secretion drainage.

5. Intubation prevents an effective cough reflex and subsequent airway clearance. Frequent suctioning decreases the risks of suction-induced hypoxemia, arrhythmias, bronchospasm, and loss of PEEP.
• Suctioning causes arterial oxygen desaturation, the degree of which depends on the presuctioning PaO_2 level, catheter size in relation to endotracheal tube size, duration of suctioning, and other factors. Following the recommended guidelines helps minimize hypoxemia. Resetting the oxygen level minimizes the risk of oxygen toxicity.

• If the patient is on PEEP, use a manual self-inflating bag with a PEEP valve or a closed suctioning system when suctioning.

• A bag with a PEEP valve minimizes loss of PEEP support. A closed suctioning system maintains the ventilator connection, including PEEP, and may minimize hypoxemia. However, if suction flow is greater than the volume delivered by the ventilator, alveolar collapse may occur, producing arterial desaturation.

• Apply suction only while withdrawing the catheter.
• Monitor blood pressure, heart rate, and electrocardiogram (ECG) pattern during suctioning. If adverse reactions, such as bradycardia, hypotension, or arrhythmias occur, immediately remove the suctioning catheter and ventilate the patient with 100% oxygen.
• While suctioning, observe for paroxysmal coughing without deep breaths; remove the catheter if it occurs.

• This technique minimizes trauma to the endothelium.
• Bradycardia, hypotension, and arrhythmias may result from stimulation of vagal fibers at the carina, hyperinflation, or hypoxemia.

• Paroxysmal coughing mimics the effects of a sustained Valsalva's maneuver at pressures high enough to cause bradycardia and hypotension. Removing the catheter reduces airway obstruction.

• If the patient reacts adversely to traditional suctioning, consult with the doctor about administering an anticholinergic agent such as atropine or an anesthetic such as lidocaine (Xylocaine) before suctioning.

• An anticholinergic agent will prevent bradycardia caused by vagal stimulation. Lidocaine decreases coughing and, in a patient with increased intracranial pressure (ICP), helps prevent further pressure increases.

6. Additional individualized interventions: _____

6. Rationales: _____

COLLABORATIVE PROBLEM

Risk for injury: Complications related to patient deterioration, mechanical breakdown, increased intrathoracic pressure, or bypassed defense mechanisms

Nursing priorities
• Prevent complications when possible.
• Respond appropriately if complications occur.

Patient outcome criteria
Throughout the period of mechanical ventilation, the patient will:
• maintain vital signs within acceptable limits: typically, heart rate, 60 to 100 beats/minute; systolic blood pressure, 90 to 140 mm Hg; and diastolic blood pressure, 50 to 90 mm Hg
• maintain a cardiac index of 2.5 to 4.0 L/minute/m^2
• remain free from pulmonary infection and other complications.

Interventions

Abrupt respiratory distress
1. Keep ventilator alarms turned on at all times.

Rationales

1. The patient's life depends on this therapy, and alarms can warn of potentially fatal problems. Turning the alarms off places the patient at risk for unobserved disconnection, cardiac arrest, or other catastrophe.

2. Be familiar with troubleshooting techniques before they are needed.

2. Troubleshooting techniques are complex and vary among ventilators. Learning troubleshooting techniques in advance reduces anxiety and improves the likelihood of prompt, successful resolution of a problem.

3. Continually observe whether the patient is breathing in synchrony with the ventilator. If the patient develops sudden respiratory distress or the ventilator fails abruptly, take the following steps:

• Immediately disconnect the ventilator, open the airway if necessary, and ventilate the patient using a manual self-inflating bag and 100% oxygen.

• Once ventilation is established, reevaluate the patient. If the distress has cleared, check the ventilator settings. Obtain ABG levels or evaluate oximetry readings.

• If the distress continues, perform a rapid cardiopulmonary assessment, suction the airway if indicated, or obtain medical assistance.
• Evaluate for signs of tension pneumothorax, such as a sudden unexplained increase in inspiratory pressure, shock, decreased or absent breath sounds on the affected side, tracheal deviation away from the affected side, air hunger, or intense anxiety. If any of these signs are present, anticipate immediate chest X-ray, needle thoracentesis, or chest tube insertion.
• If the problem's source cannot be identified and you suspect patient panic, hand-ventilate at a rate faster than the patient's, gradually slow down to the ventilator rate, and then reconnect the ventilator, coaching the patient in a calm, reassuring tone to breathe with the ventilator. Sedate as needed.

• If the problem persists, implement changes in ventilator settings, sedate the patient (usually with morphine sulfate), or paralyze the patient (for example, with diprovan or pancuronium bromide [Pavulon]), as ordered. If paralysis is prescribed, be sure that sedation with an amnesic agent, such as diazepam (Valium) or midazolam (Versed), also is prescribed. Carefully monitor the level of sedation.

3. Breathing out of synchrony (sometimes called "fighting the ventilator" or "breathing out of phase with the ventilator") markedly increases intrathoracic pressure; failure of mechanical ventilation places the patient's life in jeopardy.
• Determining whether the cause of the respiratory distress is patient- or ventilator-related is crucial. Patient-related problems (such as airway obstruction or tension pneumothorax) require immediate intervention, while distress from ventilator malfunction can be relieved by ventilating the patient manually until the exact cause can be evaluated. Manual ventilation provides a quick way to distinguish between the two categories, supplies adequate emergency ventilation, and allows rapid detection of increased airway resistance or decreased compliance.
• If the respiratory distress has cleared, the ventilator is at fault. ABG levels or oximetry readings may reveal hypoxemia or hypercapnia, possible indicators of inadequate mechanical ventilation. The ventilator may need to be replaced or adjusted to meet the patient's needs.
• Your assessment may reveal the cause of the distress, such as airway obstruction or tension pneumothorax.

• Positive pressure ventilation increases the risk of barotrauma. Tension pneumothorax, a life-threatening emergency, may result from such factors as rupture of lung blebs, friable tissue, suture disruption, or central line insertion. Immediate chest decompression is needed to prevent cardiopulmonary arrest from mediastinal shift.
• The patient may panic about the need for mechanical ventilation or the sensations associated with it. Hyperventilation may worsen the panic. Adjusting the ventilatory rate as described helps the patient gain control over hyperventilation. Conveying calmness while coaching the patient in specific maneuvers helps build a sense of trust and provides reassurance that the situation is under control. Sedation lessens the patient's awareness of mechanical ventilation.
• Persistent struggling may indicate the need for ventilator adjustments or pharmacologic support. Morphine reduces anxiety and respiratory drive. Because of its short half-life, diprovan is very effective. Pancuronium bromide induces apnea, eliminating the problem of "fighting" the ventilator, but does not blunt consciousness. Because paralysis can be terrifying for the fully conscious patient, sedation with an amnesic agent is indicated.

4. Monitor the patient on PEEP closely for barotrauma, decreased cardiac output, water retention, and, if the patient has an ICP monitor, increased ICP.

5. Additional individualized interventions: _____

Decreased cardiac output
1. Monitor the patient for signs and symptoms of decreased cardiac output, such as hypotension, tachycardia, deteriorating mental status, and arrhythmias. Report findings promptly to the doctor. Administer I.V. fluid or vasopressors, as ordered.

2. Read pulmonary artery (PA) and wedge pressures at the end of expiration.

3. If the patient is on PEEP, consult the doctor about the specific technique for reading wedge pressures. In general, leave the patient on the ventilator, and do not make any adjustments in response to the readings; instead, watch for trends over time.

4. Additional individualized interventions: _____

Pulmonary infection
1. Monitor the humidifier's water level and temperature, usually set at body temperature.

4. Because PEEP is superimposed on intrathoracic pressure already increased from mechanical ventilation, it further increases the risks of barotrauma and cardiovascular deterioration. The mechanism by which PEEP alters fluid imbalance is unclear, but it may be mediated by antidiuretic hormone, baroreceptors, renin production, or stimulation of the sympathetic nervous system. PEEP may increase pressure in the superior vena cava, impeding cerebral venous drainage and raising ICP.

5. Rationales: _____

1. Increased intrathoracic pressure associated with mechanical ventilation diminishes venous return and may cause a right-to-left shift of the interventricular septum, impinging on left ventricular filling. Reducing the work required for breathing and administering oxygen, sedatives, or other therapies such as vasodilators can cause abrupt, significant decreases in the level of sympathetic tone supporting blood pressure. Most patients placed on mechanical ventilation develop hypotension, but it usually responds well to fluid and vasopressor support.

2. PA waveforms reflect fluctuations in intrathoracic pressure. Positive pressure ventilation causes the waveforms to rise during inspiration and drop during expiration. Reading pressures at the end of expiration minimizes the effects of respiratory variation.

3. Controversy exists over the extent to which PEEP affects wedge pressures. Usually, wedge pressures obtained on the ventilator are similar to those obtained with the ventilator disconnected (probably because poorly compliant lungs do not transmit airway pressures well to the heart and pulmonary capillary bed), so the benefit of maintaining PEEP argues in favor of reading pressures on the ventilator. If there is a discrepancy, the doctor may wish to confirm by X-ray that the catheter tip lies in the basal third of the lung, where pulmonary vascular pressures may be least affected by alveolar pressure. A recently developed volumetric right-sided heart catheter, which measures blood volume rather than pressure, may eliminate this problem.

4. Rationales: _____

1. Artificial airways bypass the upper-airway mechanisms for warming, humidifying, and purifying inspired air. Humidification is added to the ventilator to prevent mucosal dehydration and thickened secretions. The temperature is controlled to prevent loss of body heat or tracheal burns.

2. Drain condensed fluid in the ventilator tubing.

2. This condensation, from humidified air passed through the ventilator, must be discarded because it increases expiratory pressure and resistance in the ventilatory circuit. It also could be aspirated.

3. Maintain aseptic technique, good oral care, and careful positioning, and observe for signs and symptoms of pulmonary infection, such as fever, purulent secretions, or elevated white blood cell count.

3. Artificial airways provide a direct access for contaminants to enter the lungs. Aseptic technique, good oral care, and careful positioning help prevent nosocomial infections.

4. If signs and symptoms of infection are present, consult with the doctor.

4. Pulmonary infections are a major contributor to mortality from mechanical ventilation. Because they usually occur in debilitated patients and are caused by virulent pathogens, pulmonary infections require prompt, aggressive therapy.

5. Additional individualized interventions: _____

5. Rationales: _____

Gastrointestinal bleeding
1. Insert a nasogastric (NG) tube, as ordered.

1. NG intubation helps prevent gastric dilatation and reduces the risk of aspiration.

2. Administer antacids, ranitidine (Zantac), or cimetidine (Tagamet), as ordered, spacing doses. Implement additional measures from the "Gastrointestinal hemorrhage" plan, page 505, as appropriate.

2. GI hemorrhage may result from the development of a stress ulcer, a complication of prolonged mechanical ventilation. Although their exact cause is not well understood, stress ulcers are thought to result from excess gastric acid secretion and decreased gastric mucosal resistance. Antacids neutralize gastric acid; cimetidine and ranitidine decrease gastric acid secretion. Antacids should not be given concurrently with cimetidine because they may impair its absorption. The "Gastrointestinal hemorrhage" plan contains detailed interventions for ulcer-related bleeding.

3. Additional individualized interventions: _____

3. Rationales: _____

Fluid retention
1. Monitor for signs and symptoms of fluid retention. If present, consult with the doctor about treatment.

1. Fluid retention may result from the humidifier's interference with insensible water loss via the lungs, decreased lymphatic flow, or altered secretion of ADH.

2. Additional individualized interventions: _____

2. Rationales: _____

Tracheal trauma
1. Monitor cuff pressure and the position of the endotracheal tube. Maintain cuff pressure well below diastolic blood pressure; a safe cuff pressure ranges from 15 to 20 mm Hg.

1. An endotracheal tube can damage vocal cords and tracheal mucosa, resulting in scarring and stenosis. Maintaining cuff pressure below diastolic blood pressure permits mucosal perfusion.

2. With the doctor, consider tracheostomy for long-term ventilation.

2. To prevent a range of upper airway problems, including sinusitis and tracheal stenosis, an endotracheal tube should be replaced with a tracheostomy tube, which is better tolerated for long-term ventilation.

3. Additional individualized interventions: _____

3. Rationales: _____

Nursing diagnosis

Fear related to inability to speak and dependence on a machine for life support

Nursing priority

Promote acceptance of mechanical ventilation.

Patient outcome criteria

Within 2 hours of being placed on mechanical ventilation and then continuously, the patient will:
• be able to communicate needs, if conscious
• appear relaxed.

Interventions

1. Implement the general measures in the "Ineffective individual coping" plan, page 67, as appropriate.

2. Establish a communication method, such as eye blinks, magic slate, or paper and pencil. Be sure the call light is always within the patient's reach.

3. Reduce the patient's need for communication by anticipating needs, providing consistency in staffing and routines, using frequent eye contact, and reassuring the patient that monitoring is constant. Emphasize that a nurse is available immediately if needed.

4. Explain the reason for mechanical ventilation. Briefly orient the patient and family to the ventilator's features, if appropriate, stressing features (such as alarms) that may be important to them. Encourage questions. Stress the temporary nature of ventilation, if applicable.

5. Additional individualized interventions: _____

Rationales

1. Mechanical ventilation is an extremely stressful experience for most patients. The "Ineffective individual coping" plan contains comprehensive information on ways to decrease the stress of critical illness and promote positive coping.

2. Intubation prevents use of the vocal cords. Needing to communicate and being unable to do so is extremely stressful. Providing alternative methods increases security and promotes patient safety.

3. Although alternative communication methods do work, they are cumbersome and fatiguing. Reducing the need for communication helps reduce the patient's fatigue and frustration, and reassurance helps reduce fear.

4. Mechanical ventilation commonly is instituted under crisis conditions, when explanation and emotional preparation may not have been possible. Even if the patient and family were prepared, stress may have caused them to block or selectively filter information. Briefly reviewing the procedure and encouraging questions may relieve unstated anxiety about the device.

5. Rationales: _____

Collaborative problem

Risk for ineffective weaning related to lack of physiologic or psychological readiness

Nursing priority

Promote a smooth transition to spontaneous ventilation.

Patient outcome criteria

During weaning and continuously thereafter, the patient will:
• maintain a clear airway
• maintain a spontaneous respiratory rate of 12 to 24 breaths/minute
• manifest ABG levels within normal limits
• display pulmonary function measurements within normal limits
• display normal sinus rhythm with no ectopic beats, or a benign variant such as sinus arrhythmia or a normal sinus rhythm with fewer than four premature ventricular contractions/minute
• remain alert and oriented.

Interventions

1. Anticipate weaning when the patient meets these criteria: improvement in respiratory status (as evidenced by an A-a gradient less than 300 mm Hg on 100% oxygen, shunt less than 20%, V_D: V_T less than 0.6, respiratory rate less than 24 breaths/minute, and MV 5 to 10 L), stable hemodynamic status, and adequate muscle strength (as evidenced by VC greater than 10 to 15 ml/kg and MIF greater than –20 cm H_2O).

2. Make sure the patient is rested, well nourished, oriented, able to follow commands, and not receiving any respiratory depressants.

3. Explain weaning to the patient and family. Mention that the patient may feel short of breath initially. Stress that the patient will be attended closely during the trial of spontaneous breathing and that if it is not successful, it will be tried again later.

4. Obtain baseline vital signs, ABG levels, and pulmonary function measurements. Suction the airway.

5. Implement the weaning method ordered: CPAP, SIMV, T-piece, or pressure support.

6. Monitor the blood pressure, heart rate, pulse oximeter oxygen saturation, ECG rhythm, respiratory rate, ease of breathing, level of consciousness, and level of fatigue constantly for the first 20 to 30 minutes and every 5 minutes thereafter until weaning is complete.

Rationales

1. Many factors affect the success of weaning attempts. Premature attempts to wean impose unnecessary physiologic stress on the patient, jeopardizing recovery. Meeting the listed criteria increases the likelihood that weaning will be accomplished with few or no setbacks.

2. Reestablishing spontaneous ventilation is physically demanding, and the patient must have enough energy reserves to succeed. The ability to take a deep breath and cough on command helps prevent atelectasis and airway obstruction. A strong respiratory drive is crucial to resume spontaneous breathing.

3. Weaning is stressful psychologically. Thorough emotional preparation promotes a sense of security. Preparing the patient for the possibility of trying again later may reduce the sense of failure if the weaning attempt is unsuccessful.

4. These measurements provide a basis for comparison to evaluate the appropriateness of weaning. Suctioning the airway reduces the risk of aspiration because secretions may have accumulated above the cuff.

5. CPAP or pressure support may make weaning easier for the patient on PEEP by maintaining some positive pressure during the trial of spontaneous breathing. SIMV supplies periodic mandatory deep breaths; the rate can be decreased by two breaths at a time until the patient's breathing is completely spontaneous. A T-piece provides supplemental oxygen during weaning. Pressure support can increase V_T in a patient too weak to wean on a T-piece alone.

6. Frequent monitoring provides ongoing indications of the success or failure of the weaning attempt.

7. In collaboration with the doctor, terminate weaning if adverse reactions occur, such as a heart rate increase greater than 20 beats/minute, systolic blood pressure increase greater than 20 mm Hg, arterial oxygen saturation less than 90%, respiratory rate less than 8 or greater than 24 breaths/minute, ventricular arrhythmias, labored or erratic breathing, fatigue, or panic.

7. Attempts to persist in weaning an unstable patient may cause cardiorespiratory arrest from hypoxia or arrhythmias.

8. If weaning continues, measure the V_T, MV, and ABG values in 20 to 30 minutes. Compare with desired values for the patient, determined in collaboration with the doctor, typically V_T 300 to 700 ml, MV 5 to 10 L, pH 7.35 to 7.45, Pao_2 greater than 70 mm Hg, and $Paco_2$ 35 to 45 mm Hg.

8. Values at this point help determine the appropriateness of continuing weaning.

9. If physiologic parameters indicate weaning is feasible but the patient resists, consider the possibility of psychological dependence on the ventilator. Consult with the doctor, pulmonary nurse specialist, or psychiatric nurse clinician, as appropriate.

9. Psychological dependence is a common problem after prolonged mechanical ventilation. Possible causes for dependency include fear of dying, depression from chronic illness, and secondary gains from the illness role. Consulting with other professionals may help to uncover causes and allow the formulation of appropriate interventions to resolve underlying fears or conflicts.

10. Assist with extubation, when ordered. Confirm that someone qualified to reintubate is present.

10. The same criteria used to evaluate readiness for weaning are used to determine readiness for extubation. A patient ventilated for short periods (24 to 48 hours) usually is ready for extubation after a 30-minute trial of spontaneous breathing, whereas those ventilated for longer periods may require days to weeks of gradual weaning. Availability of immediate reintubation is critical because postextubation airway obstruction can be sudden and fatal.

11. Additional individualized interventions: _____

11. Rationales: _____

DISCHARGE PLANNING

Discharge checklist
Before discharge, the patient shows evidence of:
☐ respiratory status (after extubation) stable for more than 12 hours
☐ absence of significant arrhythmias (without I.V. antiarrhythmic drugs) for more than 12 hours
☐ level of consciousness stable for more than 12 hours
☐ vital signs within normal limits.

Teaching checklist
Document evidence that the patient and family demonstrate an understanding of:
☐ reason for mechanical ventilation
☐ communication measures
☐ alarms
☐ weaning.

Documentation checklist
Using outcome criteria as a guide, document:
☐ clinical status on admission
☐ significant changes in status
☐ pertinent diagnostic test findings
☐ ventilator and patient checks
☐ ventilator alarm status
☐ airway care
☐ measures to prevent or detect and treat complications
☐ communication measures
☐ emotional support
☐ sedative or paralyzing pharmacologic agents, if used
☐ weaning
☐ patient and family teaching
☐ discharge planning.

ASSOCIATED PLANS OF CARE

Adult respiratory distress syndrome
Impaired physical mobility
Ineffective individual coping
Nutritional deficit
Sensory-perceptual alteration

REFERENCES

Batrientos-Bega, R., et al. "Prolonged Sedation of Critically Ill Patients with Midazolam or Propofol: Impact on Weaning and Costs," *Critical Care Medicine* 25(1):33-40, January 1997.

Burns, S.M. "Understanding, Applying and Evaluating Pressure Modes of Ventilation," *AACN Clinical Issues in Critical Care Nursing* 7(4):495-507, November 1996.

Burns, S.M., et al. "Weaning from Long-Term Mechanical Ventilation," *American Journal of Critical Care* 4(1):4-22, January 1995.

Chang, V.M. "Protocol for Prevention of Complications of Endotracheal Intubation," *Critical Care Nurse* 15(5):19-27, October 1995.

Macintyre, N.R. "Respiratory Facts in Weaning from Mechanical Ventilatory Support," *Respiratory Care* 40(3):244-48, March 1995.

Thorens, J.B., et al. "Influence of the Quality of Nursing on the Duration of Weaning from Mechanical Ventilation in Patients with Chronic Obstructive Pulmonary Disease," *Critical Care Medicine* 23(110):1807-15, November 1995.

Pbneumonia

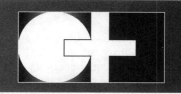

DRG information

DRG 079   Respiratory Infections and Inflammations with Complication or Comorbidity (CC); Age 17+.
Mean LOS = 9.3 days

DRG 080   Respiratory Infections and Inflammations without CC; Age 17+.
Mean LOS = 6.6 days

DRG 081   Respiratory Infections and Inflammations; Ages 0 to 17.
Mean LOS = 7.8 days

DRG 089   Simple Pneumonia with CC; Age 17+.
Mean LOS = 7.1 days

DRG 090   Simple Pneumonia without CC; Age 17+.
Mean LOS = 5.1 days

DRG 091   Simple Pneumonia; Ages 0 to 17.
Mean LOS = 4.5 days

Additional DRG information: Identifying the pneumonia's cause can increase the potential DRG (for example, staphylococcal pneumonia or aspiration pneumonia would place a patient into DRGs 079 to 081, rather than 089 to 091).

INTRODUCTION

Definition and time focus

Respiratory infections account for a significant number of hospitalizations each year, particularly among the very old and the very young—the two groups most susceptible to serious respiratory illness. Respiratory infections include bacterial pneumonias (most commonly caused by pneumococci), viral pneumonias (most commonly caused by influenza and other viral diseases), tuberculosis, lung abscesses, fungal infections, bronchitis from various causes, and pulmonary empyema resulting from another disorder.

Pneumonia is the second most common nosocomial infection in the United States and is linked with substantial morbidity and a mortality rate estimated at 30% to 70%. It is especially dangerous in the elderly and those with severe underlying diseases (such as cardiopulmonary disease).

Since the advent of antibiotic therapy, patients are hospitalized for treatment less commonly today than in the past. Although many patients still need hospitalization, a patient may receive treatment at home if he prefers and can drink fluids and take medications by mouth, has a willing and capable caregiver, and has no severe underlying medical conditions.

This plan focuses on the patient with pneumonia who is admitted to the medical-surgical setting for diagnosis and treatment. Similar nursing interventions apply to most patients with respiratory infections of other types.

Etiology and precipitating factors

For community-acquired disease

• Particularly virulent organism or high level of exposure in otherwise healthy person
• Chronic obstructive pulmonary disease, alcoholism, influenza, pulmonary neoplasms, heart failure, altered consciousness, or swallowing disorders in older person
• Viruses, pneumococci, or *Mycoplasma pneumoniae*

For nosocomial disease

• Presence in medical-surgical units and intensive care units
• Intubation, mechanical ventilation, recumbent position, increased risk for aspiration, incompetent lower esophageal sphincter, which allows gastric contents to flow back up
• Patient's age, severity of underlying disorder, primary diagnosis, and response to therapy
• Gram-negative bacteria, which colonize the oropharynx in hospitalized patients (the stress that typically occurs in hospitalized patients is believed to alter saliva composition, changing the resident flora in the mouth and thus increasing the risk of pneumonia if sufficient numbers of these organisms are aspirated into the lungs)

FOCUSED ASSESSMENT GUIDELINES

The manifestations of pneumonia vary considerably, depending on the degree of inflammation, the disease stage, and the pathogenic organism involved.

Nursing history (functional health pattern findings)

Health perception–health management pattern

• Fatigue, malaise, and respiratory signs and symptoms, such as cough, pleurisy (chest pain with inspiration), and sputum production
• Recent upper respiratory infection or sinus disease if disease is community-acquired; self-treatment common—patient may have used outdated antibiotics

(prescribed for a previous illness), over-the-counter medications, or both
• History of smoking, alcohol abuse, or multiple stressors contributing to overall fatigue
• Multiple risk factors (with nosocomial disease), such as activity restriction, depressed inspiratory effort, depressed cough reflex, and use of respiratory equipment or an artificial airway; patient may not have been admitted for a primary respiratory disorder

Nutritional-metabolic pattern
• Anorexia during illness; poor nutrition before onset of respiratory illness

Activity-exercise pattern
• Limited activity because of fatigue and shortness of breath

Sleep-rest pattern
• Fatigue with inability to "catch up" on needed rest
• Sleep disturbance if cough is present

Cognitive-perceptual pattern
• Community-acquired disease: questioning of why illness occurred despite good physical condition; failure to relate subtle increase in stress to present illness; possible delay in seeking medical attention because illness seemed like "just a little cold"
• Nosocomial disease: failure to understand connection between primary reason for hospitalization and present illness

Physical findings
General appearance
• Fever — low grade or with shaking chills, depending on pathogenic organism (if possible, compare with patient's normal temperature because low-grade fever may actually represent a significant elevation such as in an older patient)

Pulmonary
• Crackles
• Decreased breath sounds over area of infection
• Increased respiratory rate
• Shallow, labored breathing (may not report shortness of breath)
• Possible abnormal bronchial breath sounds heard on auscultation over area of consolidation
• Fremitus — normal or increased
• Possible cough
• Possible sputum production and rhinorrhea — character, color, and odor of secretions depend on pathogenic organism (generally, viral organisms produce clear secretions, whereas bacterial organisms produce discolored and purulent secretions)

Gastrointestinal
• Possible vomiting

Integumentary
• Warm, moist skin
• Possible cyanosis, pallor, or flushing

Lymphoreticular system
• Possible cervical lymphadenopathy or tenderness in salivary glands

Musculoskeletal
• Weakness

Diagnostic studies
• Arterial blood gas (ABG) measurements — may show hypoxemia; possible hypocapnia related to increased minute volume in response to hypoxemia
• Sputum specimen (Gram stain or culture and sensitivity testing or both) — performed to identify causative organisms; may be difficult to differentiate between colonization by an organism that is not the primary cause of infection and the pathogenic organism; even isolation of a specific pathogen does not necessarily prove pneumonia's cause
• Transtracheal aspiration — may be performed in an attempt to obtain a sputum specimen free from saliva or mouth flora; an increased number of polymorphonuclear cells with few squamous cells indicates an acceptable specimen
• Blood culture — may match organism in sputum, increasing likelihood that organism is causative pathogen
• Bronchoscopy — may be performed to obtain a sputum specimen, identify the problem, or clear the airways
• Chest X-ray — shows pulmonary infiltrates in affected areas from the inflammatory process (occasionally clear); may show pleural effusion
• Thoracentesis — done to identify organism if significant pleural fluid is present on chest X-ray and sputum specimen is unobtainable
• Pulmonary function tests — forced vital capacity decreased
• White blood cell (WBC) count — may be elevated but does not contribute directly to diagnosis

Potential complications
• Severe hypoxemia
• Adult respiratory distress syndrome (ARDS)
• Empyema
• Sepsis
• Lung abscess
• Pulmonary embolism
• Pneumothorax
• Pericarditis
• Meningitis

CLINICAL SNAPSHOT

PNEUMONIA

Major nursing diagnoses and collaborative problems	Key patient outcomes
Risk for nosocomial infection	Remain free from nosocomial infections.
Risk for hypoxemia	Maintain partial pressure of arterial oxygen (Pao_2) levels with normal limits on room air, typically 80 to 100 mm Hg.
Pain	Rate pain as less than 3 on a 0 to 10 pain rating scale.
Knowledge deficit (home care and preventive measures)	Demonstrate effective pulmonary hygiene measures for home use.

NURSING DIAGNOSIS

Risk for nosocomial infection related to stress and other risk factors

Nursing priority

Prevent nosocomial infection, if possible.

Patient outcome criteria

Throughout the hospital stay, the patient is expected to remain free from nosocomial infections.

Interventions

1. Wash hands between patients.

2. Elevate the head of the patient's bed.

3. Consult the doctor about administering sucralfate in place of antacids to prevent stress-induced GI bleeding.

4. Additional individualized interventions: _____

Rationales

1. Oropharyngeal secretions on unwashed hands increase the risk of cross-contamination.

2. An elevated head helps prevent the reflux of oropharyngeal secretions and endotracheal tube condensate.

3. Antacids alkalinize the stomach; when aspirated, the high pH fosters overgrowth of gram-negative organisms.

4. Rationales: _____

COLLABORATIVE PROBLEM

Risk for hypoxemia related to inflammatory response to pathogen and inadequate airway and alveolar clearance

Nursing priority

Optimize oxygenation and airway and alveolar clearance.

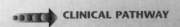 CLINICAL PATHWAY

Managing pneumonia

Level of care	Day 1 (admission)	Day 2
Assessments	• Breath sounds q 4 hr and as needed (p.r.n.) • Respiratory effort — prevent fatigue • Intake and output (I&O) • Skin care needs • Sputum • Daily weight • Immunization status for Pneumovax, flu shot, diphtheria/tetanus	• Breath sounds • Respiratory effort • I&O • Skin care needs • Weight
Diagnostic testing	• AA Chem • Complete blood count (CBC) • Sputum culture and sensitivity, Gram stain • Blood culture × 2 • Sputum for AFB smear/culture • Cold agglutinins • Urinalysis • Electrocardiogram if indicated • Arterial blood gases (ABGs) • Chest X-ray	• CBC • ABGs
Treatments	• Oxygen (O_2)	• O_2 • Discontinue O_2 per criteria
Activity	• Active and passive range of motion • Bedrest with bedside commode • Head of bed elevated • Turn, cough, and deep breathe q 2 hr	• Rest times postactivity • Chair b.i.d.
Consultations	• Social Services p.r.n. • Respiratory care assessment	• Social Services p.r.n. • Dietary p.r.n.
Medications/I.V.	• I.V. fluids • Antibiotics • Antipyretics • Home medications	• I.V. fluids • Antibiotics • Antipyretics • Home medications
Nutrition	• Regular diet • Encourage fluids	• Regular diet • Encourage fluids
Psychosocial, emotional, spiritual needs	• Chaplain p.r.n.	• Chaplain p.r.n.
Patient and family education	• Orient patient to unit • Call nurse if the patient is dyspneic • Call for assistance to bedside commode • Institute isolation technique if appropriate • Follow proper hand-washing guidelines • Diet, medications, activity, safety	• Cough technique • Fluid intake • Disease process, symptoms, and therapy prescribed (printed materials)
Discharge planning	• Initial assessment • Advanced directives review • Review pathway	• Facilitate team conference • Home O_2 if indicated • Assess need for follow-up care
Expected outcomes	• Antibiotics initiated within 4 hr of order • Fluid intake > 2,000 ml/24 hr • Resting quietly	• Temperature decreasing • Tolerates P.O. intake of 1,500 ml/24 hr • Tolerates activity • 50% diet consumed

Day 3	Day 4	Day 5
• Breath sounds • Respiratory effort • I&O • Weight	• Breath sounds • I&O • Weight	• Breath sounds • I&O • Weight
• ABGs	• CBC • Chest X-ray	
• O_2 • Discontinue O_2 per criteria • Immunize as indicated		
• Ambulate in room at will • Chair t.i.d.	• Ambulate at will • Chair q.i.d.	• Activity at will • Chair q.i.d.
• Social Services p.r.n. • Dietary p.r.n. • Home infusion p.r.n.	• Social Services p.r.n. • Dietary p.r.n.	
• I.V. → intermittent infusion device • P.O. antibiotics if possible • Home medications	• Home medications • P.O. antibiotics or arrange for outpatient I.V. antibiotics	• I.V. discontinued • P.O. antibiotics • Home medications
• Regular diet • Encourage fluids	• Regular diet • Encourage fluids	• Regular diet • Encourage fluids
• Chaplain p.r.n.	• Chaplain p.r.n.	• Chaplain p.r.n.
• Medications: dosage, frequency, precautions, potential adverse effects • Importance of taking all of the prescribed antibiotic • Signs and symptoms of pneumonia and importance of reporting to doctor • Risks for recurring respiratory infections • Home care instructions	Same as Day 3	Same as Day 3
Same as Day 2	Same as Day 2	Same as Day 2
• Temperature decreasing • Dyspnea decreasing • O_2 discontinued • ADLs with minimal assistance • 75% diet consumed • Effective cough	• Chest X-ray without progression • WBC ↓ by 50% • Temperature decreasing • Breath sounds without progression	• Rx reviewed • Room air • Temperature < 100.5° F • Breath sounds without progression • Home support system in place • Discharged

Patient outcome criteria

Within 2 days of admission, the patient will:
• maintain Pa_{O_2} levels within normal limits on room air, typically 80 to 100 mm Hg
• easily expectorate less purulent sputum
• exhibit decreased crackles
• perform pulmonary hygiene measures hourly while awake
• exhibit increased vigor and ability to perform self-care measures
• have no fever
• take oral fluids to recommended level
• have adequate dietary intake.

Interventions

1. Administer oxygen therapy, as ordered. Document therapy on initiation and once per shift.

2. Maintain oxygen therapy during activities such as ambulation to the bathroom. Note activity tolerance, observing for increased fatigue, tachypnea, cyanosis, tachycardia, and other signs of impaired oxygenation.

3. Administer and document antibiotic therapy, as ordered. Monitor the results of indicated blood level studies. Monitor and document the antibiotic's adverse effects.

4. Evaluate the patient's progress, and document the following parameters once per shift and as needed: level of consciousness, sputum character and color, presence or absence of cough, temperature, pulse, respiratory rate, skin color, breath sounds, and activity tolerance.

5. Collect sputum specimens in the recommended manner. Maintain a sterile collection cup. When the patient expectorates lower respiratory tract secretions, send the specimen to the laboratory immediately to prevent overgrowth of normal oral flora. If necessary, ask the respiratory therapy department to perform a sputum induction to collect an adequate specimen.

Rationales

1. Until the airway and alveoli are clear, supplemental oxygen is necessary to reduce the system's need to maintain high minute volumes. Although high minute volumes help compensate for hypoxemia, they may contribute to respiratory fatigue and, ultimately, respiratory failure. Usual administration ranges from 1 to 6 L/minute by nasal cannula.

2. Increased activity levels increase oxygen demands and further tax the already compromised system.

3. Specific treatments vary, depending on when the pneumonia developed, prior antibiotic therapy, and the specific flora that exists on the unit; the antibiotic of choice depends on the pathogen identified. Optimum antibiotic blood levels, necessary to achieve desired results, vary among individuals. Some adverse effects require changes in medication levels or therapy to prevent immediate or long-term complications.

4. Changes in level of consciousness, such as increased restlessness or lethargy, can indicate deterioration and impending respiratory failure. Other parameters should improve if antibiotic and airway clearance therapy is effective.

5. Appropriate antibiotic therapy depends on accurate pathogen identification.

6. Perform noninvasive measures to promote airway clearance:
• If the patient is able to cooperate, have him breathe deeply and cough each hour and use an incentive spirometer, as ordered.
• If the patient is unable to cooperate, perform artificial sighing and coughing each hour, using a manual resuscitation bag.
• Perform postural drainage and percussion with vibration every 4 hours or as ordered.

7. Perform nasotracheal suctioning if the patient cannot cough effectively. Suction as needed, as indicated by gurgles heard over the major airways. Consider the use of a nasal trumpet for frequent nasal suctioning. Follow standard precautions, including wearing eye protection and gloves.

8. Use increased levels of supplemental oxygen before and during airway clearance procedures.

9. Encourage the patient to increase fluid intake to at least eight 8-oz (240-ml) glasses per day.

10. Encourage small, frequent, high-protein, high-calorie meals. If the patient cannot eat, begin total parenteral nutrition, as ordered.

11. Monitor ABG levels, as ordered and as needed, if dyspnea increases or respiratory effort is inadequate. Report abnormalities immediately, and prepare the patient for possible ventilatory support.

12. Additional individualized interventions: _____

6. Noninvasive clearance measures move purulent, infectious secretions from the alveoli up toward the major airways, where they can be expectorated or suctioned.

7. Nasotracheal suctioning is effective only if secretions are within reach of the suction catheter, typically above the carina (at the level of the angle of Louis). Because nasotracheal suctioning can damage the tracheal mucosa, it should be performed only if secretions are within reach. Although a nasal trumpet can also cause some damage, it can reduce trauma in a patient who must undergo frequent nasal suctioning. Following standard precautions reduces exposure to infectious organisms.

8. Measures used to clear the airways may intensify hypoxemia while they are being performed, especially if the patient has concomitant cardiovascular disease. Supplemental oxygen can be maintained via nasal prongs during nasotracheal suctioning.

9. Sputum's viscosity is related to the patient's overall hydration status. Fever contributes to dehydration. Adequate fluid intake promotes thinner secretions that can be expectorated more easily, decreasing the risk of hypoxemia related to sputum plugs in airway.

10. Protein and calorie malnutrition may contribute to impaired humoral and cell-mediated host defenses. Malnutrition also weakens the patient, contributing to a less vigorous respiratory effort.

11. Indications of severe hypoxemia and developing ARDS include a dropping partial pressure of oxygen level despite a stable or increasing level of supplemental oxygen.

12. Rationales: _____

NURSING DIAGNOSIS

Pain related to fever and pleuritic irritation

Nursing priority

Minimize discomfort while promoting adequate oxygenation.

Patient outcome criteria

Within 24 hours of admission, the patient will:
• demonstrate splinting technique while performing pulmonary hygiene measures (if stable)
• rate pain using oral medications as less than 3 on a 0 to 10 pain rating scale
• demonstrate adequate chest expansion during inspiration.

Interventions

1. See the "Pain" plan, page 88.

2. Administer antipyretics, analgesics, or both, as ordered and as needed. Use caution in administering sedatives or narcotics, if ordered. Document response.

3. Teach the patient to splint the chest wall with hands or pillows, as needed, while coughing, deep breathing, or performing other pulmonary hygiene measures.

4. Apply a heating pad or hot packs to areas of chest wall discomfort, as ordered.

5. Additional individualized interventions: _____

Rationales

1. The "Pain" plan contains general interventions for the care of the patient in pain. This plan contains additional measures specific to pneumonia.

2. Pleuritic pain and discomfort from fever may be so severe that the patient inhibits thoracic expansion to minimize pain, increasing the likelihood of atelectasis, hypoventilation, inadequate airway clearance, and hypoxemia. Sedatives or narcotics may cause respiratory depression.

3. Splinting may help reduce unnecessary chest wall movement, which contributes to pain. Supporting painful areas helps promote fuller chest expansion.

4. Heat reduces inflammation and promotes muscle relaxation.

5. Rationales: _____

NURSING DIAGNOSIS

Knowledge deficit (home care and preventive measures) related to lack of exposure to information

Nursing priority

Teach home care and preventive measures.

Patient outcome criteria

By the time of discharge, the patient will:
• demonstrate effective pulmonary hygiene measures for home use
• list three preventive measures
• list three symptoms indicating possible recurrence.

Interventions

1. Emphasize the importance of an ongoing pulmonary hygiene regimen. Teach the patient and family techniques for home use, based on the patient's condition and capabilities at discharge.

2. Teach the importance of rest during convalescence at home.

Rationales

1. Deep-breathing exercises should be continued at home for at least 4 to 6 weeks to help reduce atelectasis and promote healing. Ongoing pulmonary hygiene measures may be indicated for the patient with a coexisting condition such as emphysema that is associated with a higher incidence of recurrence.

2. Respiratory infections place significant stresses on the body. Overexertion may further tax compromised defenses. Rest promotes healing.

3. Teach the patient to:
• avoid respiratory irritants
• avoid crowds and persons with known infections
• be aware of the mode of transmission of infection (usually airborne) and to keep in mind that saliva and sputum contain increased concentrations of pathogens
• get an influenza vaccination, once he is stable, if the doctor recommends it.

4. Teach the patient and family the importance of promptly reporting signs and symptoms that may indicate recurrence: headache, fever, dyspnea, chest pain, and other signs and symptoms of a cold or the flu.

5. Additional individualized interventions: _____

_____

3. Persons recovering from respiratory infections tend to be susceptible to other infections and are also at increased risk for recurrence after healing. Preventive measures may help the patient avoid further illness.

4. Early and appropriate treatment of respiratory infections results in shorter periods of illness. In older patients and other high-risk groups, a delay in reporting symptoms is associated with higher mortality rate.

5. Rationales: _____

_____

DISCHARGE PLANNING

Discharge checklist
Before discharge, the patient shows evidence of:
❏ absence of pulmonary or cardiovascular complications (dullness on auscultation may still be present)
❏ normal ABG levels and WBC count
❏ absence of fever for at least 24 hours
❏ clearing pleural effusion on chest X-ray
❏ decreasing sputum production
❏ no need for supplemental oxygen for 48 hours
❏ I.V. antibiotics discontinued for at least 24 hours
❏ ability to tolerate adequate dietary and fluid intake
❏ ability to control pain using oral medications
❏ ability to ambulate and perform activities of daily living at the same level as before hospitalization
❏ adequate home support system or referral to home care or a nursing home.

Teaching checklist
Document evidence that the patient and family demonstrate an understanding of:
❏ purpose, dosage, administration schedule, and adverse effects requiring medical intervention of all discharge medications
❏ recommended dietary plan and need for ongoing fluid intake
❏ realistic plan for rest and activity
❏ care and use of oxygen equipment
❏ pulmonary hygiene measures
❏ preventive measures to avoid recurrence
❏ signs and symptoms requiring medical intervention
❏ date, time, and location of follow-up appointments
❏ how to contact the doctor.

Documentation checklist
Using outcome criteria as a guide, document:
❏ clinical status on admission

❏ significant changes in status
❏ pertinent diagnostic findings
❏ ABG test results
❏ pain-relief measures
❏ nutrition and fluid intake
❏ oxygen therapy
❏ airway clearance measures and results
❏ patient and family teaching
❏ discharge planning.

ASSOCIATED PLANS OF CARE

Acquired immunodeficiency syndrome
Chronic obstructive pulmonary disease
Geriatric care
Ineffective individual coping
Knowledge deficit
Pain

REFERENCES

Agency for Health Care Policy and Research website: http://www.ahcpr.gov/
Craven, D. "Prevention of Hospital-Acquired Pneumonia: Measuring Effect in Ounces, Pounds and Tons," *Annals of Internal Medicine*122(3):229-31, February 1, 1995.
Crowe, H. "Nosocomial Pneumonia: Problems and Progress," *Heart and Lung* 25(4): 418–21, September 1996.
"New Guidelines Are Out for Nosocomial Pneumonia," *The Brown University Long-Term Care Quality Advisor* 9(9):2, 1997.
"New Prediction Method Could Cut Hospital Admissions and Costs for Pneumonia Patients," *PR Newswire* 21(121), 1997.
Nishioka, S., et al. "Nosocomial Pneumonia and Mortality." *JAMA* 276(4):866-69, July 1996.
Tablan, O., et al. "Guidelines for the Prevention of Nosocomial Pneumonia." *Infection Control Hospital Epidemiology*, 15(9):587–627, September 1994.
"What's New for Clinicians: Pneumonia. New Prediction Model Proves Promising," *AHCPR* Pub. No. 97-R031, January 1997.
"What's New for Consumers: Pneumonia. More Patients May Be Treated at Home," *AHCPR* Pub. No. 97-R003, January 1997.

Pulmonary embolism

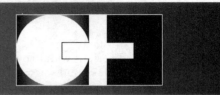

DRG information

DRG 07   Other Respiratory System or Procedure with Complication or Comorbidity.
Mean LOS = 12.5 days
Procedures include:
Vena Cava Filter Insertion.

INTRODUCTION

Definition and time focus

A pulmonary embolus (PE) is debris deposited in a branch of the pulmonary artery that partially or completely obstructs blood flow. Venous thromboemboli are the most common cause of obstruction, accounting for approximately 95% of all cases; most arise from deep venous thrombosis (DVT) in the lower extremities. Other types of PE include air, fat, and amniotic fluid emboli, septic emboli, and bone fragments.

The severity of the associated signs and symptoms depends on the size of the embolus and amount of lung affected by the altered perfusion. Emboli range in size from small to massive. Small emboli usually lodge in the peripheral pulmonary arterial bed and may cause cardiopulmonary compromise. A massive PE that obstructs more than 50% of the pulmonary artery circulation leads to severe cardiopulmonary compromise. The location and size of the embolus or emboli may vary; for instance, a single embolus may block the pulmonary artery bifurcation (a saddle embolus), or small emboli may be scattered throughout pulmonary tissue, causing anywhere from no symptoms to significant symptoms depending on the amount of tissue affected. If the embolus is not a venous thromboembolus, other systems may be compromised (for example, fat emboli may cause opthalmic complications, result in acute renal failure, or compromise perfusion to distal extremities).

This plan covers all phases of care, from the initial diagnosis in the medical-surgical setting, through the critical care phase, to readying the client for discharge.

Etiology and precipitating factors

• Venous stasis, such as from DVT, immobility, burns, varicose veins, heart failure, atrial fibrillation, right ventricular infarction, or myocardial infarction (diminished or absent ventricular motion)
• Injury of the vascular endothelium, such as from venipuncture of the legs, surgery (especially of the abdomen, pelvis, or hip), I.V. drug abuse, or trauma (particularly long-bone fractures or myocardial injury)
• Hypercoagulability, such as from sepsis, dehydration, oral contraceptive use, blood dyscrasias, pregnancy, or recent childbirth

FOCUSED ASSESSMENT GUIDELINES

Nursing history (functional health pattern findings)

Health perception–health management pattern
• Sudden shortness of breath (most common symptom)
Cognitive-perceptual pattern
• A sense of impending doom
• Chest pain that worsens with inspiration
• Headache
Coping–stress tolerance pattern
• Apprehension or fear
• Anxiety

Physical findings

More than half of all patients who have DVT have no signs or symptoms. If they do, signs and symptoms may include the following.
General appearance
• Restlessness
• Acute distress
Neurologic
• Altered (decreased) level of consciousness
• Confusion
• Hallucinations
• Euphoria
Cardiovascular
• Tachycardia (in 60% to 75% of patients)
• Arrhythmias (commonly atrial)
• Murmur
• Hypotension
• Low-grade fever (with massive PE)
• Accentuated heart sound (P_2)
• Neck vein distention
• S_3 gallop (rare)
Integumentary
• Pallor
• Cyanosis
• Diaphoresis (with massive PE)
• Petechiae of face, neck, and chest (especially with fat embolism)
Renal
• Oliguria
• Altered electrolyte, creatinine, and blood urea nitrogen levels

Pulmonary
- Tachypnea
- Localized crackles
- Wheezes
- Decreased breath sounds
- Pleural friction rub
- Cough (may be associated with pulmonary injury)
- Unexplained hemoptysis (may be associated with pulmonary injury)

Musculoskeletal
- Swelling (variation in calf size)
- Pain
- Warmth
- Erythema

Diagnostic studies
Laboratory data are used to rule out other conditions or provide general confirming evidence.
- Ventilation-perfusion lung scan — typically performed in two stages; stage 1, perfusion, uses radioisotope-tagged albumin to identify perfusion defects in pulmonary vasculature; stage 2, ventilation, is performed if stage 1 is inconclusive and requires the patient to breathe radioactive gas in a closed system while lung fields are scanned with a special camera
- Pulmonary angiography — considered the standard test for detecting and confirming PE; it uses multiple films to reveal constant intraluminal filling defects and a sharp cutoff in vessels greater than 2.5 mm in diameter; this procedure can cause pulmonary vascular compromise
- Arterial blood gas (ABG) levels — may reveal partial pressure of arterial oxygen less than 60 mm Hg, partial pressure of arterial carbon dioxide ($Paco_2$) less than 35 mm Hg, and an increased alveolar-arterial gradient
- 12-lead electrocardiogram (ECG) — used to rule out myocardial infarction; in PE, it shows ST-segment depression, right axis deviation, right bundle-branch block, peaked P waves, and Q waves in lead III.
- Chest X-ray — may be normal or may reveal:
  - elevated diaphragm on affected side
  - enlarged pulmonary arteries
  - sudden cutoff of a pulmonary shadow
  - cardiac enlargement with prominent right atrial border
  - right ventricular dilation
  - dilated superior vena cava or hump-shaped shadow on the affected side, if pulmonary infarction is present
- Noninvasive vasculature ultrasonography — supports the diagnosis of PE if thrombosis is present

Potential complications
- Recurrent embolism
- Right-sided heart failure
- Shock (cardiogenic or distributive)
- Arrhythmias
- Hypoxemia
- Pulmonary hemorrhage
- Pulmonary infarction
- Cardiopulmonary arrest

CLINICAL SNAPSHOT

PULMONARY EMBOLISM

Major nursing diagnoses and collaborative problems	Key patient outcomes
Risk for injury	Maintain stable vital signs: heart rate, 60 to 100 beats/minute; systolic blood pressure, 90 to 140 mm Hg; and diastolic blood pressure, 50 to 90 mm Hg.
Hypoxemia	Maintain normal ABG levels: pH, 7.35 to 7.45; partial pressure of arterial carbon dioxide ($Paco_2$), 35 to 45 mm Hg; HCO_3^-, 22 to 26 mEq/L.
Risk for cardiogenic shock	Maintain normal hemodynamic values: pulmonary artery (PA) systolic pressure, 20 to 30 mm Hg; PA diastolic pressure, 10 to 15 mm Hg; and PA wedge pressure, 4 to 12 mm Hg.
Risk for complications	Experience minimal, if any, bleeding.
Knowledge deficit (identification of recurrent emboli and anticoagulant therapy)	Describe safety considerations while on anticoagulant therapy.
Risk for ineffective individual and family coping	Display effective coping methods.

NURSING DIAGNOSIS

Risk for injury related to presence of risk factors

Nursing priority

Provide early recognition of PE signs and symptoms in high-risk patients.

Patient outcome criteria

Within 24 hours of admission, the patient will:
• maintain normal vital signs: typically, heart rate, 60 to 100 beats/minute; systolic blood pressure, 90 to 140 mm Hg; and diastolic blood pressure, 50 to 90 mm Hg
• be alert and oriented
• have lungs clear to auscultation
• have no complaints of leg or chest pain
• maintain oxygen saturation greater than 90%
• remain free from respiratory distress.

Interventions

1. Identify patient at risk for vascular injury, venous stasis, or hypercoagulability.

2. Perform a thorough physical assessment of the patient on admission, and review the patient's initial laboratory and diagnostic information.

3. Assess the patient for changes every 2 hours and p.r.n.

4. Take steps to help prevent thromboemboli: Use antiembolism stockings or sequential compression devices, perform passive range-of-motion exercises or have the patient perform active exercises, ensure adequate fluid intake, and avoid the high Fowler position, knee gatching, and leg massages.

5. Help the patient mobilize as soon as possible.

6. If the patient's condition starts to deteriorate, collaborate with the appropriate health care professionals.

7. Additional individualized interventions: _____

Rationales

1. Early identification of patients at risk allows for close monitoring for initial indications of PE.

2. A thorough physical assessment and initial laboratory and diagnostic information establish a baseline that can be used to gauge changes in the patient's condition.

3. Regular assessment allows the detection of initial, subtle changes, such as restlessness, a feeling of apprehension, or a slight drop in oxygen saturation.

4. These measures help maintain peripheral venous blood flow by preventing stasis, hypercoagulability, and clot dislodgment and by minimizing clot formation.

5. Early mobilization helps stimulate peripheral venous blood flow, minimizing clot formation.

6. A team of health care professionals can provide the interventions necessary to prevent complications.

7. Rationales: _____

COLLABORATIVE PROBLEM

Hypoxemia related to ventilation-perfusion mismatch

Nursing priority

Maintain adequate spontaneous ventilation.

Patient outcome criteria

Within 48 hours of onset, the patient will:
• have ABG levels returning to the patient's normal range: typically, pH, 7.35 to 7.45; $Paco_2$, 35 to 45 mm Hg; HCO_3^-, 22 to 26 mEq/L; Po_2, 80 to 100 mm Hg; Sao_2, greater than 90%
• have clear bilateral breath sounds
• display no dyspnea
• no longer require mechanical ventilation.

Interventions	Rationales
1. Assess pulmonary status at least every hour. Note the presence of: • tachypnea and dyspnea	**1.** Serial assessments indicate the disorder's severity and the effectiveness of interventions. • Tachypnea, a cardinal sign, is a compensatory measure to increase oxygenation and is attributed to stimulation of intrapulmonary receptors in the alveolar-capillary wall. Dyspnea results from apprehension or the sudden increase in alveolar dead space from alveoli that are ventilated but not perfused. Ventilation without perfusion impairs gas exchange.
• wheezing	• Wheezing results from pneumoconstriction following hypocapnia and platelet degranulation. Local hypocapnia constricts bronchial smooth muscle, increasing airway resistance and redirecting ventilation to better perfused areas; the resulting reduction in wasted ventilation is a protective mechanism. The thromboembolus consists of fibrin, red blood cells, and platelets; platelet degranulation releases substances that provoke bronchoconstriction and vasoconstriction.
• decreased or absent breath sounds	• Normally, surfactant reduces surface tension as alveoli deflate, preventing alveolar collapse and lessening the work necessary to reinflate alveoli. Decreased surfactant production leads to atelectasis, as evidenced by decreased or absent breath sounds.
• crackles and gurgles	• Normally, surfactant also minimizes leakage of capillary fluid into alveoli by controlling alveolar surface tension. Decreased surfactant increases surface tension and allows fluid leakage, resulting in interstitial edema, as evidenced by crackles and gurgles.
• mentation changes, such as restlessness, changes in level of consciousness, or irritability.	• Mentation changes reflect cerebral hypoxia.
2. Monitor ABG levels or pulse oximeter readings (Sao_2) or both, as ordered.	**2.** ABG levels and pulse oximeter readings provide objective evidence of the degree of hypoxemia, which is useful in evaluating the severity of the PE and the effectiveness of interventions.
3. Administer supplemental oxygen, as ordered.	**3.** Supplemental oxygen prevents the immediate consequences of hypoxemia, which may include arrhythmias, cerebral ischemia, and myocardial infarction.
4. Elevate the head of the bed 30 to 45 degrees. Use pillows to support the patient in a comfortable position.	**4.** This position promotes respiratory excursion and reduces the cardiopulmonary workload.
5. Maintain strict bed rest. Assist the patient with bathing, eating, and other activities that increase dyspnea.	**5.** Rest conserves energy needed for breathing.

6. Implement a program of vigorous pulmonary hygiene, including deep-breathing exercises, coughing, incentive spirometry, and frequent repositioning. Suction as necessary.

7. Assist with intubation and mechanical ventilation with positive end-expiratory pressure (PEEP), as needed. Refer to the "Mechanical ventilation" plan, page 283, for guidelines.

8. Additional individualized interventions: _____

6. Adequate alveolar ventilation can reduce elevated $Paco_2$ levels. Restoring effective aeration may prevent the onset of pneumonia from retention of secretions in the atelectatic area.

7. If the above measures fail to control hypoxemia, intubation and mechanical ventilation with PEEP may reopen collapsed alveoli. The "Mechanical ventilation" plan details the care involved in this therapy.

8. Rationales: _____

COLLABORATIVE PROBLEM

Risk for cardiogenic shock related to pulmonary hypertension and right-sided heart failure

Nursing priority

Maintain adequate cardiac output.

Patient outcome criteria

- Within 48 hours of symptom onset, the patient will have:
  - stable vital signs: typically, heart rate, 60 to 100 beats/minute; systolic blood pressure, 90 to 140 mm Hg; and diastolic blood pressure, 50 to 90 mm Hg
  - cardiac rhythm within normal limits
  - hemodynamic parameters within normal limits: typically, PA systolic, 20 to 30 mm Hg; PA diastolic, 10 to 15 mm Hg; PAWP, 4 to 12 mm Hg; and cardiac output, 4 to 6 L/minute
  - warm and dry skin
  - urine output greater than 60 ml/hour.
- Within 72 hours of symptom onset, the patient will:
  - have the pulmonary artery catheter removed
  - have no complications from pulmonary artery catheter monitoring.

Interventions

1. Institute constant ECG monitoring if it is not already taking place. Observe for arrhythmias, particularly paroxysmal atrial tachycardia (PAT) or right bundle-branch block.

2. Maintain I.V. line patency and administer fluids, as ordered.

3. Assist with pulmonary artery (PA) catheter insertion, as ordered. Monitor pulmonary artery pressure and pulmonary artery wedge pressure (PAWP), as ordered, typically every hour until the patient is stable and then every 2 to 4 hours.

4. Monitor for signs and symptoms of right-sided heart failure, such as neck vein distention and elevated central venous pressure readings. If any are present, notify the doctor.

Rationales

1. The right ventricle may decompensate in response to the sudden elevation in pulmonary pressure. PAT or other atrial arrhythmias reflect atrial stretching from volume overload, whereas bundle-branch block probably reflects right ventricular strain. Other arrhythmias may result from cardiac ischemia or hypoxemia; cardiopulmonary arrest may occur in massive embolism.

2. Although the PE patient is not volume depleted, I.V. access is critical for medication administration.

3. A PA catheter provides objective data useful in assessing hemodynamic function of the left and right sides of the heart.

4. Mechanical obstruction from the embolus and release of vasoconstrictors, described above, elevate pulmonary vascular resistance. The increased resistance to right ventricular ejection may cause right-sided heart failure.

5. Monitor for signs and symptoms of cardiogenic shock, such as severe hypotension and elevated PAWP. If present, notify the doctor and implement measures in the "Cardiogenic shock" plan, page 392, as appropriate.

6. If above measures are ineffective or the PE is life-threatening, prepare the patient for emergency surgery, if ordered.

7. Additional individualized interventions: _____

---

5. Major obstruction to ventricular ejection produces cardiogenic shock. The "Cardiogenic shock" plan presents detailed assessment and interventions for this complication.

6. Pulmonary embolectomy may be a life-saving operation.

7. Rationales: _____

COLLABORATIVE PROBLEM

Risk for complications related to thrombolytic or anticoagulant therapy

Nursing priority

Prevent or minimize complications.

Patient outcome criteria

Throughout the hospital stay, the patient will:
• experience minimal, if any, bleeding
• display no signs of recurrent emboli.

Interventions

1. Administer a continuous low-dose heparin infusion, as ordered or following protocol. Monitor the activated partial thromboplastin time (APTT) or international normalized ratio (INR) daily or following protocol. Maintain values within the therapeutic range (APTT is normally twice the control value and INR is normally 2.0 to 3.0). If APTT exceeds 100 seconds, the infusion is generally stopped for a period of time. For anticoagulant overdosing, administer protamine sulfate, as ordered.

2. Administer streptokinase (Streptase) or urokinase (Abbokinase), according to unit protocol, as ordered. Protocols vary but generally include:
• contraindications, such as recent surgery or cerebrovascular accident, active bleeding, and severe hypertension
• administration via a PA catheter or systemic infusion
• a loading dose followed by constant infusion for several hours
• maintaining thrombin time at two to five times normal
• monitoring for bleeding episodes.

Rationales

1. Heparin is a potent anticoagulant that inactivates thrombin and blocks further clot formation. It also inhibits platelet degranulation around the thrombus and limits the release of vasoconstrictors. Subtherapeutic values place the patient at continued risk for recurrent emboli; values beyond the therapeutic range place the patient at risk for bleeding episodes. Protamine sulfate counteracts the effects of heparin.

2. Streptokinase or urokinase therapy may be ordered for the unstable patient with massive embolism. These thrombolytic agents dissolve already formed clots, decreasing symptoms. Streptokinase, the enzyme from beta-hemolytic streptococci, converts plasminogen to plasmin, producing fibrinolysis and resulting in decreased blood viscosity, improved microcirculation, and improved oxygen delivery. Urokinase also converts plasminogen to plasmin, degrading fibrin clots, fibrinogen, and other plasma proteins. Unit protocols vary regarding details of administration.

3. Start a second vascular access site for collection of blood samples for laboratory tests. Maintain the site with normal saline flushes. Minimize the risk of bleeding by avoiding intramuscular injections when possible and collaborating with the doctor or clinical pharmacist to limit interactions between anticoagulants, thrombolytic agents, and other medications. Monitor for both apparent and occult bleeding, such as by observing for hematomas and by guaiac-testing gastric contents and stool.

4. If emboli recur despite the above measures, prepare the patient for surgery, as ordered.

5. Teach the patient and family about the prescribed anticoagulant therapy, clot formation, and safety considerations.

6. Additional individualized interventions: _____

3. Anticoagulation and thrombolytic therapies increase the risk of bleeding. The second access site allows the collection of blood samples without increasing the risk of bleeding from multiple venipunctures. Early detection of bleeding permits dosage adjustment before massive hemorrhage occurs.

4. Vena cava ligation or insertion of a vena cava umbrella can trap recurrent emboli, which fibrinolysis can then dissolve.

5. Such information will help prevent clotting and bleeding complications.

6. Rationales: _____

NURSING DIAGNOSIS

Knowledge deficit (identification of recurrent emboli and anticoagulant therapy) related to complex disorder and therapy

Nursing priority

Teach the patient how to prevent complications.

Patient outcome criteria

By the time of discharge, the patient and family will:
• describe the action, dosage, frequency, and adverse effects of the prescribed anticoagulant
• describe activities that can cause or prevent clot formation
• describe safety considerations while the patient is on anticoagulant therapy.

Interventions

1. Teach the patient and family what activities can trigger clot formation and what steps they can take to prevent clot formation; make sure the patient can describe the safety considerations he should follow while on anticoagulant therapy. These include using an electric razor, wearing shoes, taking safety precautions when using potentially dangerous mechanical equipment, preventing cuts, and avoiding trauma to extremities.

2. Make sure the patient and family can describe the dosage, frequency, actions, and adverse effects of the prescribed anticoagulant. Give the patient information about follow-up laboratory testing to monitor anticoagulant therapy.

3. Additional individualized interventions: _____

Rationales

1. The patient and family need to understand what activities are safe and how to prevent clots from forming.

2. The patient and family need to understand how the patient should take discharge medications, what adverse effects to look for, and when to report for follow-up testing (usually at least three times a week initially and then as directed).

3. Rationales: _____

NURSING DIAGNOSIS

Risk for ineffective individual and family coping related to potentially life-threatening situation

Nursing priority

Provide emotional support to the patient and family.

Patient outcome criteria

• By the time of discharge, the patient and family will verbalize increased ability to cope and participate in establishing a family action plan to cope with crisis.
• Should the patient die, the family will meet the outcome criteria identified in the "Dying" plan (such as making contact with support persons).

Interventions

1. Implement measures in the "Ineffective individual coping" plan, page 67, and "Ineffective family coping: Compromised" plan, page 63, as appropriate. If death is imminent, implement measures in the "Dying" plan, page 20, as appropriate.

2. Additional individualized interventions: _____
_____

Rationales

1. Pulmonary embolism is a major psychological threat, evidenced by the classic finding of a sense of impending doom. The "Ineffective individual coping" and "Ineffective family coping: Compromised" plans contain measures to help the patient and family deal with the emotional aftermath of a PE. If therapeutic measures are ineffective and the patient's condition continues to deteriorate, measures in the "Dying" plan may help the patient and family cope with approaching death.

2. Rationales: _____
_____

DISCHARGE PLANNING

Discharge checklist

Before discharge, the patient shows evidence of:
❏ stable blood pressure, pulse, and respiratory rate
❏ ABGs within normal limits for patient

Teaching checklist

Document evidence that the patient and family demonstrate an understanding of:
❏ underlying reasons for clot development
❏ rationale for therapy
❏ measures to prevent recurrence.

Documentation checklist

Using outcome criteria as a guide, document:
❏ clinical status on admission
❏ significant changes in status
❏ pertinent diagnostic test findings
❏ oxygen therapy
❏ heparin therapy
❏ thrombolytic therapy
❏ patient and family teaching
❏ discharge planning.

ASSOCIATED PLANS OF CARE

Cardiogenic shock
Dying
Ineffective individual coping
Ineffective family coping: Compromised
Pain

REFERENCES

Kinney, M.R., et al. *AACN's Clinical Reference for Critical Care Nursing,* 3rd ed. St. Louis: Mosby–Year Book, Inc., 1993.
Majoros, K., and Moccia, J. "Pulmonary Embolism," *Nursing96* 26(4):26-32, April 1996.
Thompson, J.M., et al. *Mosby's Clinical Nursing,* 4th ed. St. Louis: Mosby–Year Book, Inc., 1997.

Thoracotomy

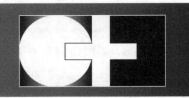

DRG information

DRG 075   Major Chest Procedures.
Mean LOS = 11.2 days
Principal procedures include:
- exploratory thoracotomy
- biopsy of diaphragm, pericardium, thymus, bronchus, or lung
- surgical collapse of lung
- incision of lung, bronchus, or thoracic vessels
- reopening of recent thoracotomy site
- pleurectomy or repair of pleura
- repair of diaphragmatic hernia, abdominal or thoracic approach.

Additional DRG information: Thoracotomy as an operative approach for other procedures may or may not be classified under DRG 075, depending on the definitive procedure accomplished.

INTRODUCTION

Definition and time focus

A thoracotomy is an incision into the chest wall (thorax); its location depends on the surgery's purpose. A posterolateral or anterolateral approach (through the ribs) is common with general thoracic surgery, whereas a median sternotomy (through the sternum) is commonly used for cardiothoracic surgery. The ribs or sternal halves are spread to gain access to the pleural cavities or the mediastinum. Common thoracotomy procedures on the lungs include exploratory thoracotomy, pneumonectomy (removal of a lung), lobectomy (removal of a lobe), segmental resection (removal of one or several lung segments), wedge resection (removal of part of a lung segment), decortication (removal of scarred, fibrous tissue over the pleura), and thoracoplasty (removal of ribs). Thoracotomies are also used to perform esophageal, diaphragmatic, aortic, or open-heart procedures. Used in patients who have accessible peripheral lesions, the recently developed video or endoscopic thoracotomy involves inserting a fiberoptic camera and instruments through small, inch-sized chest incisions to remove lesions. A full thoracotomy is a major surgical procedure that requires careful preoperative and postoperative patient management and may require mechanical ventilation and closed chest drainage. This plan focuses on preoperative care, postoperative stabilization, and initial recovery of the thoracotomy patient.

Etiology and precipitating factors

- Pulmonary conditions, such as cancer, benign tumors, tuberculosis, abscesses or infection, bronchiectasis, blebs or bullae caused by emphysema, or empyema
- Cardiac conditions, such as arteriosclerotic coronary arteries, valvular disease, mural wall defects, aortic aneurysm, cardiomyopathy, or congenital heart disease
- Hiatal hernias or esophageal problems
- Chest trauma involving one or more of the vital chest structures (lungs, heart, aorta, trachea, esophagus, or superior or inferior vena cava)

FOCUSED ASSESSMENT GUIDELINES

Nursing history (functional health pattern findings)

Health perception–health management pattern
- Shortness of breath or labored breathing on exertion
- Bloody or excessive sputum
- Tiredness and less tolerance for exercise than usual
- Swelling of feet and ankles
- Family history of heart disease or lung conditions such as asthma
- High-risk cardiac and respiratory health patterns, such as sedentary lifestyle, overeating, lack of exercise, stress, smoking, or exposure to respiratory toxins
- Major traumatic accident with a blow to the chest

Nutritional-metabolic pattern
- Loss of appetite (respiratory or cardiac problem)
- Weight gain (cardiac problem)
- Weight loss (respiratory problem)

Activity-exercise pattern
- Difficulty in breathing at rest and during exercise
- Weakness and fatigue

Cognitive-perceptual pattern
- Fear about serious nature of illness and impending major surgery
- Periods of dizziness

Self-perception–self-concept pattern
- Fear of disfigurement and scarring

Role-relationship pattern
- Fear of inability to return to work after surgical procedure
- High-risk job that subjects patient to excessive stress or exposure to respiratory toxins

Sexuality-reproductive pattern
- Fatigue and inability to sustain sexual activity

Physical findings

Physical findings may vary depending on the nature of the condition requiring the thoracotomy.

General appearance
• Cardiac condition: possibly typical signs and symptoms of angina, acute myocardial infarction, or heart failure. See the "Angina" plan on page 367, "Acute MI" plans on pages 338 and 355, or the "Heart failure" plan on page 420 for the general appearance of a patient with these problems.
• Pulmonary condition: possibly respiratory distress or general debilitation, depending on whether the condition is rapidly progressing or more chronic
• Chest trauma: possibly respiratory and cardiac distress and obvious crushing or penetrating injuries to the chest

Cardiovascular
• Arrhythmias
• Classic angina (substernal pain radiating to the left shoulder and arm that is relieved by nitroglycerin or rest)
• Unstable angina (substernal and radiating pain that is not relieved by nitroglycerin or rest and that is more serious, prolonged, and unpredictable)
• Noncardiac chest pain
• Hypotension
• Tachycardia

Pulmonary
• Dyspnea
• Shortness of breath
• Tachypnea
• Use of accessory muscles
• Gurgles, wheezes, crackles
• Chest trauma: possible open sucking wound, flail chest, paradoxical asymmetrical chest movements, or orthopnea

Gastrointestinal
• Hiatal hernia or esophageal problem: may have regurgitation, heartburn 30 to 60 minutes after meals, substernal pain, dysphagia, or feelings of fullness
• Cardiac problem: may have nausea and vomiting

Integumentary
• Cyanosis
• Pallor
• Chest trauma: abrasions or open wounds

Diagnostic studies

Because of the various conditions for which thoracotomy may be performed, no typical laboratory data exist. This section instead presents monitoring tests.
• Arterial blood gas (ABG) levels — monitor oxygenation, ventilation, and acid-base status
• Cardiac enzymes, creatine kinase, lactic acid dehydrogenase — may reveal cardiac tissue damage

• Complete blood count — monitors red blood cell count, white blood cell (WBC) count, and platelet count. Altered hemoglobin level and hematocrit reflect any potential blood loss and the blood's oxygen-carrying ability. An elevated WBC count and an elevated sedimentation rate may reflect an inflammatory response.
• Serum creatinine, blood urea nitrogen levels — monitor the adequacy of renal function
• Serum electrolyte panel — monitors fluid, electrolyte, and acid-base status
• Urinalysis — monitors renal status, including renal secretion and concentration abilities
• Sputum assessment — monitors for infection
• Blood coagulation studies — monitor clotting
• *For all conditions:*
  – Chest X-ray: may reveal abnormalities of the chest structures and heart and lung tissues
  – Electrocardiogram: may reveal changes associated with ischemia
  – Fluoroscopy: may reveal mobility abnormalities of the intrathoracic structures
  – Magnetic resonance imaging: may reveal abnormalities of the thoracic structures and organs
• *For cardiac or pulmonary conditions:*
  – Computed tomography: may reveal abnormalities of the lung, such as tumors, calcium deposits, or cavities, and abnormalities of the heart such as enlargement
  – Biopsy: may aid in definitive diagnosis of lung or heart problems
  – Gallium scan: may reveal inflammation or tumors of the heart or lungs
• *For pulmonary conditions:*
  – Ventilation-perfusion pulmonary scan: may reveal areas of nonventilation and nonperfusion
  – Pulmonary function tests: monitor static and dynamic lung volumes and capacities
  – Bronchoscopy: may reveal abnormalities of the pulmonary tree
  – Sonogram of the lung: may reveal collections of fluid and may be used postoperatively to locate the best site for thoracentesis
  – Thoracentesis: may reveal abnormal fluid or tissue specimens
  – Bronchograms: may reveal abnormal airway structures or a tumor
• *For cardiac conditions:*
  – Cardiac radionuclide imaging: may reveal areas of cardiac ischemia and necrosis
  – Echocardiography: may reveal structural and motion abnormalities of the heart
  – Cardiac catheterization: may reveal abnormalities of the coronary arteries (during left-sided heart catheterization) or pulmonary artery vasculature (during right-sided heart catheterization)

- *For esophageal conditions:*
  - Barium swallow, esophagoscopy, motility studies: may reveal esophageal abnormalities

Potential complications
- Cardiac arrhythmias
- Atelectasis
- Pleural effusion
- Pericardial effusion

- Tension pneumothorax
- Hemothorax
- Infection
- Pulmonary edema
- Pulmonary embolism
- Hemorrhage
- Cardiac arrest
- Shock
- Cardiac tamponade

CLINICAL SNAPSHOT

THORACOTOMY

Major nursing diagnoses and collaborative problems	Key patient outcomes
Knowledge deficit (preoperative and postoperative thoracotomy care)	Verbalize or demonstrate understanding of preoperative and postoperative thoracotomy care.
Hypoxemia	Maintain normal ABG and oximetry levels: typically, pH, 7.35 to 7.45; partial pressure of arterial carbon dioxide ($Paco_2$), 35 to 45 mm Hg; HCO_3^-, 22 to 26 mEq/L; partial pressure of arterial oxygen (Pao_2), 80 to 100 mm Hg; and arterial oxygen saturation (Sao_2), greater than 90.
Risk for respiratory distress	Have a normal respiratory status.
Risk for injury: Complications	Display no signs of complications.
Risk for infection	Have a clean, dry, and healing wound.

NURSING DIAGNOSIS

Knowledge deficit (preoperative and postoperative thoracotomy care) related to unfamiliarity with procedure

Nursing priority

Prepare the patient and family preoperatively for surgery and postoperative care.

Patient outcome criteria

Within 2 hours after preoperative teaching, the patient, on request, will:
- explain the purpose and goal of thoracotomy and describe the general procedure and specific points covered during teaching
- verbalize or demonstrate understanding of preoperative and postoperative thoracotomy care.

Interventions

1. Refer to the "Knowledge deficit" plan, page 72.

Rationales

1. The "Knowledge deficit" plan contains general assessments and interventions for teaching and learning. This plan provides information specific to thoracotomy.

2. Provide information about the surgery. Document teaching and the patient's and family's response. Include the following points:
- purpose, goal, and general procedure

- type of incision

- usual scar

- preoperative medication

- anesthesia

- expected location for recovery in the immediate postoperative period
- I.V. and other lines

- oxygen therapy

- chest tubes and drainage system

- nasogastric (NG) tube

- indwelling urinary catheter.

3. Describe endotracheal intubation and mechanical ventilation, if appropriate. See the "Mechanical ventilation" plan, page 283. Document teaching and patient response.

4. Explain thoracotomy's general effects on the lungs and describe reexpansion methods. Coach the patient on deep breathing, coughing, and using an incentive spirometer, if ordered. Describe measurement of vital capacity and maximum inspiratory pressures. Observe return demonstrations. Document teaching and patient response.

2. Preoperative teaching may allay fears and anxiety about the unknown and help the patient cooperate with care and summon energy for healing.
- A general understanding of the purpose and goal of a thoracotomy and what the procedure will be like will help orient the patient to upcoming nursing and medical care.
- Knowing what the incision will look like beforehand helps reduce the patient's anxiety.
- Knowing that the incision will heal to a thin, white line helps reduce the patient's fear of major disfigurement.
- Knowing that preoperative sedation is available helps reduce the patient's anxiety.
- Teaching about the methods and effects of anesthesia helps prepare the patient for possible adverse reactions after surgery.
- Telling the patient where recovery will take place helps reduce postoperative disorientation.
- A postoperative thoracotomy patient may have peripheral I.V., central I.V., and monitoring lines. The necessary tubing and equipment could be frightening without preoperative preparation.
- All thoracotomy patients require oxygen therapy after surgery because of the atelectasis and hypoxemia produced by opening the chest and by anesthesia. The specific type of oxygen therapy depends on the surgery. Preoperative explanation about the oxygen therapy to be used may increase postoperative cooperation, particularly with the patient who will be intubated and placed on mechanical ventilation.
- Explaining the need for chest tubes and a drainage system to help reexpand the lungs and hasten recovery may allay anxiety about the invasive nature of these tubes.
- Explaining that an NG tube reduces abdominal discomfort until the GI tract resumes function may increase patient tolerance.
- Explaining the need to closely monitor fluid intake and output, including urine, after surgery may reduce anxiety about the catheter.

3. Explaining intubation and mechanical ventilation, including the temporary loss of speech, may allay anxiety about this treatment. The "Mechanical ventilation" plan includes detailed information about caring for a mechanically ventilated patient.

4. Explaining the effect that opening the chest wall has on the lungs and describing reexpansion methods provide an incentive for active patient involvement. The patient's postoperative efforts to reexpand the lungs, remove secretions, and participate in respiratory function measurements may be more successful if practiced preoperatively, when the patient is under less stress and is free from pain.

5. Discuss methods to relieve postoperative pain, including using pain medication and splinting the incision with a pillow during deep breathing and coughing. Document teaching and patient response.

6. Describe and document the expected level of postoperative activity, including turning from side to side, as allowed, every 2 hours on the day of surgery; sitting in a semi-Fowler's position and sitting on the side of the bed with legs dangling on the first day after surgery; getting into a chair with assistance on the first or second day after surgery; and ambulating in the room and hallway on the second or third day after surgery. Emphasize the importance of activity despite postoperative discomfort.

7. Explain and demonstrate the use of antiembolism stockings. Document teaching.

8. Additional individualized interventions: _____

5. Most patients describe thoracotomy pain as severe. The patient may be reassured to learn that pain relief is an important part of therapy. Explanations about the timely use of pain medication and pillow splinting may increase the patient's willingness to initiate and perform coughing and deep-breathing exercises.

6. A thoracotomy patient is likely to resist activity because of pain, fatigue, and weakness. Knowledge of expected activity and its importance provides a foundation on which the nurse can build when implementing the activity schedule.

7. Antiembolism stockings aid venous return and help prevent thrombus formation in the lower extremities.

8. Rationales: _____

COLLABORATIVE PROBLEM

Hypoxemia related to hypoventilation from anesthesia, pain, and analgesic medications as well as arrhythmias, atelectasis, and thickened secretions

Nursing priority

Optimize ventilation and oxygenation.

Patient outcome criteria

- Within 4 hours after surgery, the patient will:
  - perform deep breathing and coughing
  - use the incentive spirometer
  - request pain medication when needed.
- Within 8 hours after surgery, the patient will:
  - manifest normal vital signs: typically, heart rate, 60 to 100 beats/minute; systolic blood pressure, 90 to 140 mm Hg; and diastolic blood pressure, 50 to 90 mm Hg
  - display usual level of consciousness; minimally diminished breath sounds and chest movements
  - maintain trachea in normal position
  - have pink mucous membranes
  - have minimal dullness to percussion over operative side, except for pneumonectomy
  - be free from subcutaneous emphysema and premature ventricular contractions (PVCs) or other arrhythmias
  - turn every 2 hours with assistance.
- Within 2 days after surgery, the patient will:
  - use a spirometer two to three times an hour while awake
  - display minimal or absent crackles, gurgles, or wheezes
  - maintain normal ABG levels and oximetry levels: typically, pH, 7.35 to 7.45; $Paco_2$, 35 to 45 mm Hg; HCO_3^-, 22 to 26 mEq/L; Pao_2, 80 to 100 mm Hg; Sao_2, greater than 90%
  - display minimal pain and sit up in a chair.
- Within 3 days after surgery, the patient will:
  - have nearly equal bilateral breath sounds, chest expansion, and resonance to percussion, as appropriate for type of surgery
  - begin to ambulate.

Interventions

1. After surgery, assess the following every 15 minutes until stable, every 30 minutes for 2 hours, then every 1 to 2 hours and as needed. Document and notify the doctor of abnormal findings:

• respiratory rate, depth, and pattern; pulse rate; and blood pressure
• level of consciousness

• bilateral breath sounds and bilateral chest movements

• accessory muscle use
• tracheal position

• color of mucous membranes, circumoral skin, and earlobes

2. Assess percussion notes and vocal fremitus as well as the amount, color, and consistency of sputum every 1 to 2 hours and as needed.

3. Palpate the chest wall every 1 to 2 hours and as needed. Note the presence of tenderness, pain, or subcutaneous emphysema.

4. Monitor cardiac rhythm constantly. Note and report to the doctor atrial fibrillation, PVCs, or other cardiac arrhythmias. Refer to Appendix A, Monitoring Standards.

5. Monitor ABG levels every shift and as needed for suspected changes in respiratory status, as ordered. Notify the doctor and document results.

6. Monitor and document arterial oxygen levels using pulse oximetry twice a shift and as needed, as ordered.

7. Provide humidified oxygen for the first 1 to 2 days and as needed for respiratory distress. Document its use.

Rationales

1. The patient usually returns from surgery with a pulmonary artery catheter, arterial line, peripheral I.V. lines, and pleural or mediastinal chest tubes or both. Frequent assessments of the cardiopulmonary system may reveal problems and permit timely interventions.
• Hypoxemia is reflected in vital sign changes.

• Decreased oxygen delivery to the brain is reflected in changes in level of consciousness and mentation.
• After thoracotomy, sounds and chest movements may be diminished over the operative area. These findings usually lessen and then disappear as recovery progresses. Adventitious sounds or persistence or further diminishing or chest sounds and movements may reflect fluid accumulation, atelectasis, or other respiratory problems.
• Use of accessory muscles may reflect dyspnea.
• Tracheal deviation from midline may indicate increased intrathoracic pressure on the side opposite the deviation or lung collapse on the same side as the deviation.
• Cyanotic mucous membranes, circumoral skin, and earlobes may indicate hypoxemia.

2. Dullness to percussion and decreased vocal fremitus are common after surgery and reflect consolidation from atelectatic areas. Resonance to percussion and normal vocal fremitus should return gradually as recovery progresses, except in pneumonectomy. Sputum characteristics may reflect hydration status, bleeding or infection, or pulmonary edema.

3. Areas of increasing tenderness or pain imply infection or another complication. Subcutaneous emphysema may occur when an air leak increases intrapleural pressure and eventually results in air spreading throughout the surrounding tissues. Subcutaneous emphysema is usually self-limiting and reabsorbs in several days; however, it may indicate a need for increased pleural suction pressures.

4. Cardiac arrhythmias, including atrial fibrillation and PVCs, are common after a thoracotomy, particularly after open-heart surgery. Monitoring Standards includes specific assessments and interventions for arrhythmias.

5. ABG levels reflect general oxygenation levels. Low PaO_2 levels may indicate a need for increased oxygen therapy and more vigorous pulmonary hygiene.

6. Oximetry monitors arterial oxygen levels without needle sticks.

7. Oxygen therapy may be required until the lungs are fully reexpanded and the breathing pattern and airway clearance are more effective.

8. Medicate with analgesics for pain every 1 to 4 hours and as needed, as ordered. Monitor respiratory status to prevent respiratory depression. Document findings. Refer to the "Pain" plan, page 88, for further details.

8. Pain relief promotes effective deep breathing and coughing. Respiratory depressants such as morphine sulfate must be used cautiously to prevent inadequate ventilation, which would be counterproductive to deep breathing and coughing. The "Pain" plan contains general assessments and interventions for pain.

9. Show the patient how to support the incision with the hands or a small, hard pillow as needed during deep breathing and coughing efforts. Encourage deep breathing and coughing two to three times every hour while awake.

9. Support over the incision may decrease pain during deep breathing and coughing. Regular deep breathing and coughing promotes reexpansion of the lungs, mobilizes secretions, and prevents atelectasis.

10. Promote and document incentive spirometer use, as ordered, several times an hour while the patient is awake.

10. Spirometers encourage deep inspiratory efforts, which are more effective in reexpanding alveoli than forceful expiratory efforts.

11. Provide adequate hydration. Document fluid intake.

11. Adequate hydration promotes liquid, easily removed lung secretions. Other means of humidification, such as intermittent positive-pressure breathing, may be undesirable because of the danger of a pneumothorax.

12. Provide an overhead trapeze bar or hand pulls attached to the end of the bed frame to assist the patient to the upright position for deep breathing and coughing efforts.

12. An upright position promotes lung expansion by gravity. These devices provide better mobility than does pushing against the bed.

13. Implement and document a progressive activity program, as allowed, typically:
• turning from side to side every 2 hours on the day of surgery, and sitting in a semi-Fowler's position and on the side of the bed with legs dangling on the first postoperative day

13. Progressive activity is important to restore optimal cardiopulmonary function.
• Frequent position changes reexpand the lungs and prevent atelectasis and pooling of secretions. A patient who has had a pneumonectomy can be turned slightly toward the operative side or onto the back. Turning toward the nonoperative side could collapse the remaining lung, drain secretions into that lung, or cause a dangerous mediastinal shift. Semi-Fowler's position may aid reexpansion of the lungs by gravity; leg dangling allows the neurovascular reflexes to adjust to the upright position.

• getting into a chair with assistance on the first or second postoperative day and ambulating in the room and hallway on the second or third postoperative day.

• Early chair sitting and ambulation may prevent thrombus formation in the lower extremities and aid adjustment to the upright position.

14. Additional individualized interventions: _____

14. Rationales: _____

Collaborative problem

Risk for respiratory distress related to pneumothorax, hemothorax, or mediastinal shift secondary to malfunction or removal of chest drainage system

Nursing priorities
• Maintain patency of chest drainage system.
• Observe for complications after chest tube removal.

Patient outcome criteria

- On admission and continuously, the patient will have a properly functioning chest drainage system.
- Within 3 to 4 days after surgery, the patient will:
  - have fully expanded lungs
  - be free from air and fluid in the pleural space
  - have chest tubes removed.
- Within 1 week after surgery, the patient will:
  - display no dyspnea
  - have normal respiratory status.

Interventions

1. Maintain an intact water-seal drainage system, if used. In the event of disconnection or a broken chamber, reattach the tube or submerge it in water while the patient exhales. If reattachment is not possible or water is unavailable, leave the chest tube open to air until a new system can be attached. Notify the doctor and document occurrence. Arrange for a chest X-ray.

2. Inspect the chest tube insertion site every 2 hours and as needed for the presence of:
- intact occlusive dressings

- blood or drainage on the dressing

- proper position of the chest tubes within the chest and attachment to the chest wall.

3. Observe the drainage tubing and connectors every 1 to 2 hours for proper connection and taping of connectors. Coil the tubing to prevent dependent loops.

4. Milk and strip the tubing every 1 to 2 hours and as needed, as ordered, during the first postoperative day. Document these actions.

5. Assess the drainage receptacle every 1 to 2 hours and as needed for secure attachment to the drainage tubing. If bottle drainage is used, maintain the end of the tube in the water-seal chamber ³/₄″ (2 cm) below the water level.

Rationales

1. Although most thoracotomy patients have chest tubes, chest tubes are not usually used after pneumonectomy because serous fluid collection promotes the development of fibrotic tissue in the empty space. If the patient does have a chest tube, disconnection may allow air to enter the pleural space and cause a pneumothorax. Exhalation during reattachment may force excess air from the pleural space. Leaving the tube open to air creates the potential for a small open pneumothorax but may be less harmful than clamping the tube and possibly causing a tension pneumothorax, especially in a patient with an air leak. A chest X-ray may be necessary to assess respiratory status.

2. Frequent inspection may reveal problems and allow for timely interventions.
- Occlusive dressings are used to prevent air from entering the pleural space around the chest tube insertion site and to prevent accidental dislodgment of the tubes.
- Blood or drainage on the dressing may indicate recent bleeding or infection.
- Dislodgment of the tubes can create a dangerous increase of air or drainage within the pleural space, which could cause the lung to collapse.

3. The closed drainage system must be sealed to prevent air from entering the pleural space. Taped connectors are less likely to disconnect or develop air leaks. Improperly looped tubing may inhibit gravity flow of drainage.

4. This procedure assists drainage by creating negative pressure and preventing clotting and plugging of the tubes.

5. Securely attaching the drainage tubing to the drainage receptacle and placing the end of the water-seal tube below the water level prevent air from entering the drainage system and the pleural space.

6. Observe for and document tidalling (fluctuation of water level during respirations) in the submerged water-seal tube every 2 hours. To do this, turn off the suction or pinch the suction tubing temporarily.

6. Tidalling indicates a functioning, airtight system between the pleura and the drainage receptacle. During spontaneous ventilation, inspiration creates negative pressure in the pleura and the drainage system, which pulls the water level upward in the tubing. The level moves downward on expiration. Fluctuations are the reverse for a patient on mechanical ventilation: the positive pressure applied during inspiration pushes the water level downward, whereas termination of the positive pressure on expiration allows the water level to move upward. Absence of tidalling may indicate a blocked chest tube or complete lung expansion.

7. Observe the water-seal chamber for intermittent bubbling during respiration every 2 hours and as needed. Document the amount of bubbling and where in the respiratory cycle it occurs.

7. Intermittent bubbling represents drainage of air from within the pleural spaces. Bubbling occurs normally during expiration with spontaneous ventilation or during inspiration with mechanical ventilation.

8. If continuous bubbling occurs in the water-seal chamber, briefly clamp consecutive parts of the system, beginning at the chest wall, until the bubbling stops. If the bubbling stops when the clamp is proximal to the chest wall, notify the doctor. If the bubbling stops when the clamp is distal to the chest wall, replace the system beyond that point.

8. Continuous bubbling indicates an air leak within the patient or the drainage system. Clamping as described helps isolate the leak. Bubbling that stops when the clamp is proximal to the chest wall indicates an air leak within the patient, which requires medical evaluation. Bubbling that stops when the clamp is distal to the chest wall indicates a leak in the drainage system, which requires replacement of the system.

9. Maintain and document the ordered amount of suction, if used. With Emerson suction, check the pressure set on the dial and the pressure registering on the gauge. With a multiple-chamber system (such as Pleur-evac), check the water level in the suction control chamber to ensure that it equals the ordered amount of negative pressure.

9. Negative pressure may be required to remove secretions and air from the intrapleural space. Inadequate negative pressure may prevent drainage and reexpansion of the lungs, whereas excessive pressure may damage pleural tissue.

10. Monitor the amount, color, and consistency of chest tube drainage every 30 minutes for 2 hours, every hour for 6 hours, and then every 2 hours and as needed. Notify the doctor if large amounts of drainage occur (more than 200 ml/hour for 3 hours). Document findings.

10. Large amounts of drainage may indicate bleeding and require immediate intervention to prevent shock. Absence of drainage, particularly in the immediate postoperative period, may indicate a plugged chest tube, which could cause a dangerous increase in intrapleural pressure. Chest tubes commonly drain up to 500 ml in the first 8 hours, decreasing to zero drainage 3 to 4 days after surgery as the pleurae realign and the lungs reexpand.

11. Assist with removal of chest tubes 3 to 4 days after surgery.
• Before removal, look for an absence of chest tube drainage, tidalling with respirations, and the return of breath sounds in the affected area.
• Medicate with an analgesic before removal, as ordered.
• Place the patient in a high Fowler's position. Have the patient take a deep breath and cough vigorously. At maximum inspiration, assist in removing the tube and tightening the purse-string skin suture.

• Apply a sterile occlusive dressing.

11. Chest tubes are removed when the lungs have reexpanded.
• These signs indicate lung reexpansion.

• An analgesic helps decrease pain during removal.
• A high Fowler's position, deep breathing, and vigorous coughing may prevent the development of a pneumothorax during tube removal and suture tightening by providing maximum lung expansion and positive intrapleural pressure.
• A sterile occlusive dressing may prevent infection and air leaks into the pleural space.

• After chest tube removal, assess the patient for signs and symptoms of respiratory distress, including dyspnea, pain, absent breath sounds, uneven chest movement, dull percussion sounds, cardiac arrhythmias, or anxiety.

12. If necessary, assist the doctor with reinsertion of the chest tubes or thoracentesis. Document the procedure.

13. Additional individualized interventions: _____

• Rarely, the patient may develop such complications as pneumothorax, hemothorax, or mediastinal shift, which may compromise the respiratory and cardiac systems. Careful assessment allows early identification and intervention.

12. Rarely, the patient may accumulate fluid or air and may require reinsertion of chest tubes or thoracentesis.

13. Rationales: _____

NURSING DIAGNOSIS

Risk for injury: Complications related to surgical procedure, such as hemorrhage, pneumothorax, pleural effusion, atelectasis, pulmonary edema, or pulmonary embolism

Nursing priority

Monitor for and promptly report signs and symptoms of complications.

Patient outcome criterion

By 3 to 7 days after surgery, the patient will display no signs of complications, such as hemorrhage, cardiac arrhythmias, hemothorax, cardiac tamponade, pneumothorax, pleural effusion, atelectasis, subcutaneous emphysema, bronchopleural fistula, or mediastinal shift.

Interventions

1. See the "Surgery" plan, page 103.

2. Monitor for signs and symptoms of hemorrhage. If present, alert the doctor immediately and document. Observe for:
• tachycardia, hypotension, low hemodynamic measurements, and excessive chest drainage
• decreasing or absent breath sounds, increasing dullness to percussion, or decreased or absent fremitus
• decreased heart sounds, paradoxical pulse greater than 10 mm Hg on inspiration, or high central venous pressure.

3. Monitor for signs of pneumothorax, including tachypnea, dyspnea, decreased or absent breath sounds, absent vocal fremitus, and hyperresonance. Notify the doctor and document their occurrence.

4. Monitor for signs of pleural effusion, including decreased or absent breath sounds, decreased vocal fremitus, increased dullness, and tachypnea. Notify the doctor and document their occurrence.

5. Monitor for signs of increasing atelectasis, including fever, tachypnea, tachycardia, increasing dullness, increased vocal fremitus, and bronchial or bronchovesicular breath sounds in the lung periphery. Notify the doctor and document their occurrence.

Rationales

1. The "Surgery" plan covers general postoperative problems and interventions. This plan focuses on thoracotomy.

2. Hemorrhage may result from surgical trauma, inadequate hemostasis, or other factors. It always requires immediate medical evaluation and intervention.
• These signs may indicate hemorrhage and require a return to surgery to ligate bleeding vessels.
• These signs may reflect a hemothorax. Thoracentesis or reinsertion of chest tubes may be necessary.
• These signs may indicate cardiac tamponade, which requires immediate pericardiocentesis.

3. A pneumothorax prevents reexpansion of the lungs and may require reinserting chest tubes.

4. A pleural effusion may compress the lungs, causing hypoxemia. Chest tube reinsertion may be necessary to remove the fluid and reexpand the lungs. Failure to remove the fluid may result in empyema.

5. Atelectasis (collapsed alveoli), commonly caused by poor bronchial hygiene, produces hypoxemia reflected in tachypnea and tachycardia. Dullness, increased fremitus, and abnormal breath sounds all result from consolidation.

6. Monitor for signs and symptoms of pulmonary edema, including tachypnea; tachycardia; dyspnea; shortness of breath; cough; crackles; wheezing; pink, frothy sputum; and anxiety. Notify the doctor and document their occurrence.

7. Continuously monitor a pneumonectomy patient for the following complications:
• hemorrhage — If a patient has a sudden, large hemoptysis, place the patient in high Fowler's position, turned toward the operative side; summon immediate medical assistance.

• bronchopleural fistula — Observe for hemoptysis, an extensive air leak, subcutaneous emphysema, or fever.

• subcutaneous emphysema — Observe for swelling, puffiness, or crepitation of the skin.

• excessive mediastinal shift — Observe for excessive deviation of the trachea at the sternal notch, hypotension, tachycardia, weak peripheral pulses, and other signs of decreased cardiac output.

8. Monitor for signs and symptoms of pulmonary embolism, including chest pain, dyspnea, fever, hemoptysis, changes in vital signs, and increased central venous pressure. Notify the doctor and document. Refer to the "Pulmonary embolism" plan, page 308, for further information.

9. Additional individualized interventions: _____

6. Pulmonary edema is a life-threatening condition that requires immediate intervention, such as use of diuretics, inotropic agents, rotating tourniquets, and positive-pressure breathing. A patient with other problems, particularly cardiac problems, may be at high risk for this complication.

7. A pneumonectomy, the most traumatic form of thoracotomy, has a high incidence of complications.
• Hemorrhage may result from inadequate surgical hemostasis, development of a bronchopleural fistula, or other factors. Placing the patient in high Fowler's position toward the operative side may prevent drainage into the remaining lung.
• A bronchopleural fistula may develop after surgery, most commonly during the first week, causing bleeding, air leaks, or infection. Depending on the size and location of the fistula, it may require surgery (to close the bronchial stump) and antibiotics.
• A bronchial stump leak may cause a large amount of subcutaneous emphysema. An air leak usually resolves over 3 days to a week but may require surgery.
• After lung removal, the mediastinum is not supported on one side and may shift. The residual pleural space should fill after surgery by a combination of mediastinal shift, diaphragm elevation, coagulation of serous drainage, and development of fibrotic tissue. If mediastinal shift is excessive, decreased cardiac output may occur, requiring mediastinal stabilization by fluid or air injection or thoracentesis.

8. Pulmonary embolism, a serious complication, may result from deep vein thrombosis and cause varying signs and symptoms depending on the size of the embolus. Prompt medical treatment is required to prevent further pulmonary tissue damage. The "Pulmonary embolism" plan covers this disorder in detail.

9. Rationales: _____

NURSING DIAGNOSIS

Risk for infection related to surgical incision and endotracheal intubation

Nursing priority

Prevent infection.

Patient outcome criteria

• Within 3 days after surgery, the patient will:
– have a clean, dry, and healing wound
– display normal vital signs: heart rate, 60 to 100 beats/minute; systolic blood pressure, 90 to 140 mm Hg; and diastolic blood pressure, 50 to 90 mm Hg
– display a normal WBC count and sedimentation rate.
• By the time of discharge, the patient will have clear breath sounds, normal fremitus, and normal resonance to percussion, as appropriate to type of surgery.

Interventions

1. Monitor for and document signs of pneumonia, including fever, tachypnea, bronchial or bronchovesicular breath sounds in the periphery, increased vocal fremitus, increased dullness, and dyspnea. Notify the doctor if any of these signs occur.

2. Assess for signs and symptoms of wound infection every 2 to 4 hours and as needed. When the incision can be seen directly, observe for redness and swelling. Monitor for elevated WBC count or sedimentation rate, as ordered.

3. Monitor culture and sensitivity test results for wound drainage, as ordered.

4. Reinforce or change dressings as needed, using aseptic technique.

5. Additional individualized interventions: _____

Rationales

1. Invasive chest surgery and endotracheal intubation place the patient at high risk for pneumonia. Treatment may require aggressive pulmonary hygiene, antibiotics, and positive-pressure breathing treatments.

2. Regular assessments may provide early warning of infection. Occlusive dressings may remain over the incision sites for 1 to 3 days, making direct observation of the sites difficult.

3. Culture and sensitivity tests help identify the infective organism and the most effective antibiotic treatment.

4. The dressing is usually reinforced, not changed, during the first 1 to 2 days after surgery to prevent exposure to microorganisms.

5. Rationales: _____

DISCHARGE PLANNING

Discharge checklist

Before discharge, the patient shows evidence of:
❏ stable vital signs and monitoring parameters
❏ clear breath sounds, bilateral lung expansion, and bilateral resonance to percussion, as appropriate
❏ absence of major complications
❏ healing surgical incision.

Teaching checklist

Document evidence that the patient and family demonstrate an understanding of:
❏ surgical procedure, including expected postoperative course
❏ deep breathing, coughing, and spirometer use
❏ comfort measures
❏ ROM and other exercises
❏ purpose and mechanism of chest drainage system.

Documentation checklist

Using outcome criteria as a guide, document:
❏ clinical status on admission
❏ significant changes in status
❏ pertinent diagnostic test findings
❏ chest drainage (amount, consistency, and color)
❏ functioning of chest drainage equipment
❏ complications such as subcutaneous emphysema
❏ deep breathing, coughing, and spirometer efforts
❏ oxygen therapy
❏ pain and effects of medication

❏ activity levels and range-of-motion and other exercises
❏ patient and family teaching discharge planning.

ASSOCIATED PLANS OF CARE

Mechanical ventilation
Pain
Pulmonary embolism

REFERENCES

Davidson, J.E., and Colt, H.G. "Advanced Technology. Thoracoscopy: Nursing Implications for Optimal Patient Outcomes," *Dimensions of Critical Care* 16(1):20-28, January 1997.
Lewis, S.M., et al. *Medical-Surgical Nursing: Assessment and Management of Clinical Problems*, 4th ed. St. Louis: Mosby–Year Book, Inc., 1997.

Part 6

Cardiovascular disorders

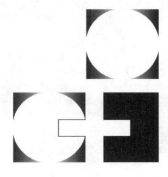

Abdominal aortic aneurysm repair

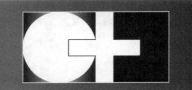

DRG information

DRG 110   Major Cardiovascular Procedures with Complication or Comorbidity (CC).
Mean LOS = 10.9 days

DRG 111   Major Cardiovascular Procedures without CC.
Mean LOS = 6.76 days
Principal diagnoses include abdominal aortic aneurysm (ruptured, nonruptured, or dissecting).

INTRODUCTION

Definition and time focus

The arterial wall consists of three tissue layers: the intima, the media, and the adventitia. In abdominal aneurysm, degeneration of the media causes the aorta to dilate, usually distal to the renal arteries. The vessel wall progressively weakens, increasing the risk of life-threatening rupture. In traditional abdominal aortic aneurysm repair, the diseased portion of the artery (aneurysm) is surgically replaced with a synthetic polyester (Dacron) graft. The graft may be tubular and straight or bifurcated (split into two branches), depending on the segment involved. Although cardiopulmonary bypass is not performed, the aorta is cross-clamped to prevent forward flow of blood during repair. The graft is then placed in the lumen of the aneurysm so that the outer layers of the arterial wall will close over and protect the graft.

One more recent technique to repair an aneurysm is endovascular stenting. In this procedure, a large catheter is inserted through a femoral incision to place expandable synthetic polytetrafluoroethylene balloon stents into the lumen of the aneurysm. The stents may also be used with Dacron grafts. The Dacron graft is sutured to hold the stent in place. Instead of the aneurysm being resected, blood flow is diverted from the aneurysm through the lumen of the stent; the aneurysm tissue eventually adheres to the outer wall of the stent. Another technique under investigation in some medical centers involves endoscopic aneurysm repair. The technique is similar to traditional aneurysm repair but is performed using endoscopic equipment and techniques. Both endovascular stenting and endoscopic techniques require shorter hospital stays, and patients typically can ambulate within 24 hours of surgery.

The abdominal aortic aneurysm patient typically spends 24 to 48 hours in the intensive care unit (ICU). Most patients are elderly and have one or more comorbidities, such as cardiovascular disease, diabetes, renal failure, and pulmonary disease. This plan focuses on preoperative care as well as the management of potential multisystem complications during the initial recovery period in the ICU and the medical-surgical unit.

Etiology and precipitating factors

The most common cause of aneurysm is atherosclerosis. Risk factors for atherosclerosis include:
- cigarette smoking
- hypercholesterolemia
- hypertension
- diabetes mellitus
- obesity
- hypertriglyceridemia
- sedentary lifestyle
- stress
- family history of cardiovascular disease.
  Other causes of aneurysm include:
- congenital disorders such as Marfan syndrome
- bacterial or fungal infections that invade the vessel wall (mycotic aneurysm)
- syphilitic aortitis
- blunt or sharp trauma
- chronic aortitis, related to Takayasu's arteritis or rheumatic spondylitis

FOCUSED ASSESSMENT GUIDELINES

Nursing history (functional health pattern findings)

Health perception–health management pattern
- Abdominal or back discomfort
- Feeling of heartbeat in the abdomen
- History of exercise intolerance
- Family history of atherosclerosis
- Cardiac and respiratory risk factors, such as cigarette smoking; high-fat, high-cholesterol diet; or sedentary lifestyle

Activity-exercise pattern
- Intermittent claudication or pain at rest
- Shortness of breath if a heavy smoker

Sexuality-reproductive pattern
- Impotence

Cognitive-perceptual pattern
- Fear about impending surgery

Physical findings
Cardiovascular
- Hypertension
- Arrhythmias
- Diminished peripheral pulses, claudication or pain at rest, trophic changes (if associated with atherosclerosis)
- Palpable abdominal mass above or at the umbilicus, extending toward the epigastrium
- Carotid, femoral, or abdominal aortic bruits

Integumentary
Integumentary changes are associated with atherosclerotic changes or distal embolization, including:
- cyanosis of lower extremities
- dependent rubor, with pallor on elevation
- thickened toenails
- decreased hair growth on lower extremities
- coolness of lower extremities

Diagnostic studies
- Arterial blood gas (ABG) levels — monitor oxygenation, ventilation, and acid-base status
- Complete blood count — monitors red blood cell, white blood cell (WBC), and platelet counts. Altered hemoglobin levels and hematocrit reflect any blood loss and the oxygen-carrying ability of the blood. An elevated WBC count reflects an inflammatory response.
- Serum electrolyte panel — monitors fluid, electrolyte, and acid-base status
- Serum creatinine and blood urea nitrogen (BUN) levels — monitor renal function
- Blood coagulation studies — monitor clotting

- Urinalysis — monitors renal status, including secretion and concentration
- Blood typing and cross-matching — necessary for blood replacement
- Electrocardiography (ECG) — may reveal cardiac changes associated with ischemia
- Chest X-ray — may reveal abnormalities of the chest, heart, and lungs
- Abdominal X-ray — may reveal calcium in the aneurysm wall
- Abdominal ultrasound — may reveal the aneurysm's size
- Abdominal computed tomography scan — may reveal a leaking aneurysm
- Aortic arteriogram — may show aberrant renal arteries, mesenteric artery patency, and iliac artery involvement
- Magnetic resonance angiography — form of magnetic resonance imaging that may give information on blood flow within the aneurysm

Potential complications
- Myocardial infarction
- Hemorrhage
- Microembolization
- Respiratory failure
- Lower limb ischemia
- Renal failure
- Bowel ischemia
- Spinal cord ischemia
- Infection
- Impotence

CLINICAL SNAPSHOT

ABDOMINAL AORTIC ANEURYSM REPAIR

Major nursing diagnoses and collaborative problems	Key patient outcomes
Knowledge deficit (preoperative and postoperative care)	Verbalize understanding of perioperative routines.
Risk for cardiac decompensation	Maintain stable vital signs: typically, heart rate, 60 to 100 beats/minute; systolic blood pressure, 90 to 140 mm Hg; and diastolic blood pressure, 50 to 90 mm Hg.
Risk for hypercapnia, hypoxemia, or both	Maintain ABGs within normal limits: typically, pH, 7.35 to 7.45; partial pressure of arterial carbon dioxide ($PaCO_2$), 35 to 45 mm Hg; HCO_3^-, 22 to 26 mEq/L; partial pressure of arterial oxygen (PaO_2), 80 to 100 mm Hg; arterial oxygen saturation (SaO_2), greater than 90%.
Risk for bleeding	Remain free from signs and symptoms of bleeding.
Risk for injury: Complications	Have any complication immediately detected, reported, and treated, as appropriate.
Pain	Rate pain with oral medication as less than 3 on a 0 to 10 pain rating scale.

Cardiovascular disorders

Nursing diagnosis

Knowledge deficit (preoperative and postoperative care) related to unfamiliarity with aortic surgery

Nursing priority

Prepare the patient and family for the impending surgery.

Patient outcome criteria

Within 2 hours after preoperative teaching, the patient, on request, will:
• verbalize understanding of perioperative routines
• demonstrate the ability to cough, breathe deeply, and use an incentive spirometer, if applicable, and to splint the incision.

Interventions

1. See the "Knowledge deficit" plan, page 72.

2. See the "Surgery" plan, page 103.

3. Describe endotracheal intubation and mechanical ventilation. Refer to the "Mechanical ventilation" plan, page 283.

4. Explain to the patient and family the need for close monitoring after surgery and the expected length of stay in the ICU, usually 24 to 48 hours.

5. Explain the need for frequent vascular checks to assess graft patency and peripheral vascular status.

6. Go over activities that may prevent graft kinking or compression and postoperative edema in the lower extremities: reclining while sitting in a chair, avoiding leg crossing or dangling the legs over the bedside, elevating the foot of the bed, and keeping the head of the bed at an angle of less than 45 degrees. The reverse Trendelenburg position may benefit a patient who has pulmonary complications.

7. Additional individualized interventions: _____

Rationales

1. The "Knowledge deficit" plan provides general patient teaching information. This plan focuses specifically on abdominal aortic aneurysm repair.

2. The "Surgery" plan describes what to teach the patient about perioperative routines.

3. The patient undergoing abdominal aortic aneurysm repair may require intubation and mechanical ventilation for the first 8 hours after surgery. Intubation time may be shorter with endoscopic or endovascular repair. Explaining mechanical ventilation and weaning may allay the patient's anxiety. The "Mechanical ventilation" plan provides detailed information about teaching a mechanically ventilated patient.

4. Explaining the expected postoperative course may minimize the patient's and family's anxiety. The length of time spent in the ICU varies among institutions.

5. Peripheral pulses are checked hourly for the first 24 hours. Assessing capillary refill time and the appearance of skin on the feet can lead to early detection of microembolization. A Doppler ultrasound stethoscope may also be used. Knowing that frequent assessment is normal may allay the patient's fears that the surgery failed.

6. Reclining positions may prevent pressure on the graft site and kinking of an aortobifemoral graft in the groin. Preventing leg crossing or dangling the legs over the bedside and elevating the foot of the bed may prevent or decrease lower extremity edema.

7. Rationales: _____

COLLABORATIVE PROBLEM

Risk for cardiac decompensation related to changes in intravascular volume, third space fluid shift, and increased systemic vascular resistance

Nursing priority

Promptly detect changes in cardiac status.

Patient outcome criteria

Within the first 24 hours after surgery, the patient will:
• maintain stable vital signs, typically heart rate 60 to 100 beats/minute, systolic blood pressure 90 to 140 mm Hg, and diastolic blood pressure 50 to 90 mm Hg
• be free from cardiac complications
• maintain graft patency.

Interventions

1. After surgery, monitor the patient's vital signs according to unit protocol and nursing judgment (typically every 15 minutes until stable, then every hour for the first 12 hours, then every 2 hours until discharge to the medical-surgical unit, then every 4 hours until discharge from the hospital).

2. Monitor hemodynamic parameters (central venous pressure [CVP], pulmonary artery wedge pressure [PAWP], cardiac output, and cardiac index) according to ICU protocol or doctor's orders until the pulmonary artery catheter is removed.

3. Continuously monitor heart rate and ECG for arrhythmias, particularly atrial fibrillation, and ST-segment elevation until the patient is discharged to the medical-surgical unit. Document and report abnormalities to the doctor. Obtain a 12-lead ECG if ST-segment elevation or chest pain develops.

4. Monitor effectiveness of antihypertensive or vasopressor medications, if prescribed.

5. Monitor for fluid and electrolyte imbalances. See Appendix C, Fluid and Electrolyte Imbalances.

6. Additional individualized interventions: _____

Rationales

1. Cardiac decompensation is the major complication that leads to morbidity following aortic surgery.

2. The patient usually returns from surgery with an arterial line, peripheral I.V. lines, and an indwelling urinary catheter. The patient may also have a pulmonary artery catheter. Hemodynamic monitoring provides an accurate evaluation of myocardial sensitivity and guides drug and fluid therapy to prevent cardiac complications.

3. Frequent cardiopulmonary assessments may reveal problems and allow for timely interventions. (Thromboembolism from atrial fibrillation may interfere with vital arterial blood flow.)

4. Hypertension and hypotension affect graft patency.

5. The Fluid and Electrolyte Imbalances appendix addresses assessment parameters and interventions.

6. Rationales: _____

COLLABORATIVE PROBLEM

Risk for hypercapnia, hypoxemia, or both related to endotracheal intubation, physiologic changes associated with aging, effects of general anesthesia, and presence of an abdominal incision

Nursing priority

Optimize ventilation and oxygenation.

Cardiovascular disorders

Patient outcome criteria

- Within 4 hours after surgery, the patient will:
  - exhibit bilaterally clear breath sounds
  - have minimal endotracheal secretions
  - maintain ABG levels within normal limits: typically, pH, 7.35 to 7.45; $Paco_2$, 35 to 45 mm Hg; HCO_3^-, 22 to 26 mEq/L; Po_2, 80 to 100 mm Hg; Sao_2, greater than 90%
  - maintain oxygen saturation greater than or equal to 95%.
- Within 4 hours of extubation, the patient will:
  - perform incentive spirometry without difficulty
  - have bilaterally clear anterior and posterior breath sounds
  - maintain oxygen saturation greater than or equal to 95%.

Interventions

1. Assess the patient's vital signs on admission to the ICU and every hour for 24 hours, then every 2 hours until the patient is returned to the medical-surgical unit, then every 4 hours. Note respiratory effort and the amount and character of sputum. Provide routine suctioning according to unit protocol while the patient is intubated. Document and report abnormalities.

2. See the "Mechanical ventilation" plan, page 283.

3. Once the patient is extubated, provide supplemental oxygen, as ordered. Have the patient turn, cough, and deep breathe with an incentive spirometer every 2 hours. Monitor oxygen saturation through pulse oximetry, ABG levels, or both, as ordered. See the "Mechanical ventilation" plan for details on pulse oximetry.

4. Administer analgesics for pain, as ordered. Monitor for signs and symptoms of respiratory depression. See the "Pain" plan, page 88.

5. Additional individualized interventions: _____

Rationales

1. Patients undergoing abdominal aortic aneurysm repair may be intubated overnight after surgery. Elevated temperature may indicate atelectasis. Respiratory effort may be minimal immediately after surgery. Suctioning promotes airway clearance.

2. The "Mechanical ventilation" plan provides specific information on assessments and interventions for the intubated patient.

3. Supplemental oxygen may be ordered to promote adequate tissue oxygenation. Position changes, deep breathing, and coughing exercises clear the airway and prevent atelectasis.

4. Pain medications may be necessary to increase the force of coughing. However, some narcotic analgesics exacerbate respiratory depression, particularly in the older patient. The "Pain" plan provides detailed information on assessing and managing this problem.

5. Rationales: _____

COLLABORATIVE PROBLEM

Risk for bleeding related to extensive retroperitoneal dissection and vascular anastomosis

Nursing priority

Promptly detect signs and symptoms of bleeding.

Patient outcome criteria

Within 24 hours after surgery, the patient will:
- remain free from signs and symptoms of bleeding
- have a dry, intact dressing
- maintain stable vital signs: typically, heart rate, 60 to 100 beats/minute; systolic blood pressure, 90 to 140 mm Hg; and diastolic blood pressure, 50 to 90 mm Hg.

Interventions

1. Monitor and document intake and output and vital signs every hour for 24 hours; monitor and document CVP, PAWP, and laboratory values according to protocol or doctor's orders. Measure abdominal girth every 2 hours for 12 hours, then once every shift. Be alert for decreased urine output, tachycardia, hypotension, decreased CVP or PAWP, decreased hematocrit, increased girth, and back pain. Document and report abnormalities.

2. Assess the dressings when the patient is admitted to the unit and every hour for 8 hours, then every 4 hours. Be alert for an expanding pulsatile groin mass.

3. Monitor and document the amount and character of nasogastric (NG) tube drainage every 2 hours for 12 hours, then every 8 hours.

4. Additional individualized interventions: _____

_____

Rationales

1. These signs may indicate intra-abdominal bleeding.

2. Frequent assessment allows for prompt detection of hemorrhage. An expanding pulsatile groin mass may indicate hemorrhage at the distal anastomosis of a bifurcated graft.

3. Bloody NG tube drainage may indicate intra-abdominal bleeding.

4. Rationales: _____

NURSING DIAGNOSIS

Risk for injury: Complications related to surgical procedure and atherosclerosis

Nursing priority

Promptly detect complications.

Patient outcome criteria

- Within 24 to 48 hours after surgery, the patient will:
  - have adequate perfusion to the upper and lower extremities, kidneys, bowel, and spinal cord, as evidenced by palpable 3+ pulses, urine output 60 ml/hour or more, normal-appearing bowel movements, spontaneous movement of extremities, and warm, dry skin
  - have any complications immediately detected, reported, and treated, as appropriate.
- Before discharge, the patient will:
  - have clean, dry, and intact incision lines
  - be afebrile, with a WBC count within normal limits.

Interventions

1. Monitor for decreased peripheral tissue perfusion: check peripheral pulses (both upper and lower extremities) immediately upon admission and every hour for the first 12 hours, then every 4 hours until discharge. Document the location and character of the pulse using this scale:
0 = absent
1 = detectable by Doppler ultrasound stethoscope only
2 = weakly palpable
3 = strong.
 Document evidence of capillary refill and signs of cyanosis and mottling. Notify the doctor of any changes.

Rationales

1. A decrease in peripheral tissue perfusion in the legs may result from graft thrombosis or distal embolization of atherosclerotic plaque. An arterial line may cause distal embolization as well as arterial dissection, arteriovenous fistula, false aneurysm, and hematoma formation. Accurate assessment of perfusion is crucial in the early postoperative period to detect early thrombosis formation and prevent limb loss.

Cardiovascular disorders

2. Monitor for acute renal failure. Record hourly urine output until the indwelling urinary catheter is removed. Monitor BUN and creatinine levels, as ordered. Be alert for a urine output of less than 30 ml/hour for 2 consecutive hours and elevated BUN and creatinine levels, and notify the doctor if they occur.

3. Monitor for signs and symptoms of bowel ischemia, including diarrhea (may be positive for occult bleeding), abdominal tenderness, fever, prolonged ileus, sepsis, shock, leukocytosis, and metabolic acidosis.

4. Monitor for signs and symptoms of spinal cord or cerebral ischemia. Monitor sensory and motor function of the lower extremities as well as temperature, color, and pulses every hour for the first 24 hours. Assess the patient's level of consciousness and orientation every hour for 12 hours, then every 4 hours.

5. Monitor for intra-abdominal graft infection by noting temperature elevations, leukocytosis, or prolonged ileus.

6. Monitor for local wound infection by inspecting incision lines for erythema and edema, and observe the amount, color, and odor of any drainage every 4 hours and as needed until discharge. Document and notify doctor of any changes.

7. Additional individualized interventions: _____
_____

2. Renal failure may result from atheromatous embolization to the renal arteries or prolonged cross-clamping of the aorta. A low urine output associated with elevated serum creatinine and BUN levels may indicate renal failure. (Creatinine clearance may be a better indicator of renal failure in the older patient.)

3. Approximately 2% of patients undergoing abdominal aortic aneurysm repair develop mesenteric artery ischemia, with a 50% mortality rate. This complication is related to low flow states, thrombosis, embolization, and fibrillatory cardiac disease. Signs and symptoms are most likely to occur in the first 48 hours after surgery.

4. The incidence of spinal cord ischemia after abdominal aortic aneurysm repair is quite low but warrants monitoring. Interruption of the arterial supply to the spinal cord may result from hypotension or embolus to the artery, causing lower extremity paraplegia. A decreased level of consciousness or change in mental status may indicate cerebral ischemia.

5. Unexplained fevers, leukocytosis, or prolonged ileus may indicate graft infection (a late complication).

6. Regular assessment may provide early warning of local wound infection.

7. Rationales: _____
_____

Nursing diagnosis

Pain related to surgical tissue trauma or ischemia

Nursing priority

Relieve pain.

Patient outcome criteria

Within 1 hour of complaint of pain, the patient will:
• rate pain (with oral medication) as less than 3 on a 0 to 10 pain rating scale
• appear relaxed.

Interventions

1. Assess patency and stability of the epidural catheter, if used. Monitor effectiveness of epidural analgesia and watch for adverse reactions.

2. See the "Pain" plan, page 88.

3. Additional individualized interventions: _____

Rationales

1. Epidural analgesia may be used to manage pain after abdominal aortic aneurysm repair.

2. The "Pain" plan specifically addresses pain assessment and management.

3. Rationales: _____

DISCHARGE PLANNING

Discharge checklist

Before discharge, the patient shows evidence of:
- ❏ stable vital signs
- ❏ normal body temperature
- ❏ absence of pulmonary and cardiovascular complications
- ❏ ability to tolerate oral intake
- ❏ ability to void and defecate same as before surgery
- ❏ healing wound free from signs of infection
- ❏ ability to ambulate according to progressive activity plan
- ❏ pain controlled with oral medication
- ❏ knowledge of activity and position restrictions
- ❏ adequate home support or referral to home health care or skilled care facility if indicated by lack of home support or by self-care limitations.

Teaching checklist

Document evidence that the patient and family demonstrate an understanding of:
- ❏ progressive activity and ambulation plan
- ❏ incision care
- ❏ signs and symptoms of wound infection and graft thrombosis
- ❏ purpose, dosage, administration, and adverse effects of all discharge medications
- ❏ risk factors for atherosclerosis and how to reduce them
- ❏ available community resources
- ❏ date, time, and location of follow-up appointments.

Documentation checklist

Using outcome criteria as a guide, document:
- ❏ clinical status on admission
- ❏ significant changes in status
- ❏ pertinent diagnostic test findings
- ❏ presence or absence of peripheral pulses
- ❏ pain-relief measures
- ❏ wound site appearance and amount, color, and consistency of any drainage
- ❏ activity tolerance and the patient's response to progressive ambulation
- ❏ patient and family teaching
- ❏ discharge planning.

ASSOCIATED PLANS OF CARE

Knowledge deficit
Mechanical ventilation
Pain
Surgery

REFERENCES

Black, J.M., and Matassarin-Jacobs, E. *Medical-Surgical Nursing: Clinical Management for Continuity of Care*, 5th ed. Philadelphia: W.B. Saunders Co., 1997.

Fellows, E. "Abdominal Aortic Aneurysm: Warning Flags to Watch for," *AJN* 95(5):26-35, May 1995.

Mialhe, C., et al. "Endovascular Treatment of Infrarenal Abdominal Aneurysms by the Stentor System: Preliminary Results of 29 Cases," *Journal of Vascular Surgery* 26(2):199-209, August 1997.

Sabiston, D.C., and Lyerly, H.K. *Textbook of Surgery: The Biological Basis of Modern Surgical Practice*. Philadelphia: W.B. Saunders Co., 1997.

Sandler, R. "Clinical Snapshot: Abdominal Aortic Aneurysm," *AJN* 95(1):38-39, January 1995.

Yuan, J.G., et al. "Endovascular Grafts for Noninfected Aortoiliac Anastamotic Aneurysms," *Journal of Vascular Surgery* 26(2):210-21, August 1997.

Cardiovascular disorders

Acute MI: Critical care unit

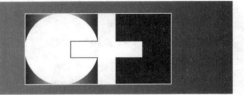

DRG information

DRG 121   Circulatory Disorders with Acute Myocardial Infarction (AMI) and Major Complications, Discharged Alive.
Mean LOS = 7.8 days

DRG 122   Circulatory Disorders with AMI, without Major Complications, Discharged Alive.
Mean LOS = 5.3 days

DRG 123   Circulatory Disorders with AMI, Expired.
Mean LOS = 4.7 days

Additional DRG information: In order for any of these three DRGs to apply:
• principal diagnosis must be a Circulatory Disorder (including AMI)
• AMI must be being treated during the initial episode of care.

DRG 121 is established when AMI and major complications are present. These major complications include:
• heart failure
• acute renal failure
• cardiogenic shock
• atrial or ventricular fibrillation or flutter
• ventricular tachycardia
• cerebrovascular accident
• pneumonia
• atelectasis
• respiratory failure
• pressure ulcer.

DRG 123 is established when the patient expires, regardless of major complications.

INTRODUCTION

Definition and time focus
AMI is the death of myocardial tissue, usually resulting from coronary artery occlusion or spasm. It may present as subendocardial infarction, involving the inner myocardial layer, or transmural infarction, involving the full thickness of the myocardium. Mortality depends on the extent and location of the infarct, the patient's preexisting health status, and the speed and effectiveness of therapy.

This plan focuses on the critically ill patient admitted for diagnosis and management during an attack of severe crushing chest pain, the classic presentation in AMI.

Etiology and precipitating factors
• Coronary artery disease, coronary artery spasm, hypotension, hypoxemia, severe bradycardia or tachycardia (especially with poor cardiac reserve), or other factors decreasing myocardial oxygen supply
• Exercise, emotional stress, exposure to extreme heat or cold, eating, tachycardia, or other factors increasing myocardial oxygen demand

FOCUSED ASSESSMENT GUIDELINES

Nursing history (functional health pattern findings)
Health perception–health management pattern
• Sudden onset of severe chest pain — heavy, tight, crushing, or constricting quality; usually retrosternal; usually radiates to the left arm but may radiate to the right arm, back, epigastrium, jaw, or neck; lasts longer than 30 minutes; unrelieved by rest or nitroglycerin; however, AMI is painless in some instances
• Treatment for angina, atherosclerosis, hyperlipidemia, hypertension, heart failure, arrhythmias, cerebrovascular accident, peripheral vascular disease, or diabetes mellitus
• History of previous AMI, cardiac surgery, or oral contraceptive use
• Coronary artery disease risk factors, such as obesity or cigarette smoking
• Other high-risk categories (such as male over age 40 or postmenopausal female)

Nutritional-metabolic pattern
• Indigestion, nausea, or vomiting
• Diet high in calories, fat, and salt (common)

Elimination pattern
• Feeling of fullness or bowel movement coinciding with onset of chest pain

Activity-exercise pattern
• Shortness of breath
• Sporadic exercise or sedentary lifestyle (common)

Sleep-rest pattern
• Sleep disturbances

Cognitive-perceptual pattern
• History of recurrent chest pain

Self-perception–self-concept pattern
• Great concern about ability to return to work as soon as possible

Role-relationship pattern
• Description of self as someone upon whom others depend

• Family history of death from AMI (especially before age 50)

Coping–stress tolerance pattern
• Anxiety, tension, type A personality (aggressive, competitive, impatient)
• Fear of death or of the unknown

Value-belief pattern
• Delayed pursuit of medical attention or expressed disbelief over condition (denial)

Physical findings

Cardiovascular
• Hypotension or hypertension
• Tachycardia or, uncommonly, bradycardia
• Other arrhythmias
• S_3 or S_4 heart sounds
• Slowed capillary refill time (in shock)

Pulmonary
• Crackles (if heart failure present)

Gastrointestinal
• Vomiting
• Abdominal distention

Neurologic
• Restlessness
• Irritability
• Confusion

Integumentary
• Diaphoresis
• Cool, clammy skin
• Variable skin color (may be normal, pale, ashen, or cyanotic)

Musculoskeletal
• Pained or anxious facial expression
• Tense posture

Diagnostic studies
Initial laboratory data may reflect no significant abnormalities; subsequent tests may reveal the following:
• cardiac isoenzymes — show characteristic trends, particularly elevated creatine kinase MB (CK-MB) and "flipped" lactate dehydrogenase (LD) pattern (LD_1 greater than LD_2)
• positive troponin I or increased myoglobin levels or both
• arterial blood gas (ABG) levels — may reveal hypoxemia and acid-base abnormalities
• electrolyte panel — used to rule out disturbances affecting cardiac conduction and contractility (such as hypokalemia, hyperkalemia, hypocalcemia, hypercalcemia, or hypomagnesemia)
• white blood cell count and sedimentation rate — usually rise on second day because of inflammatory response
• blood urea nitrogen levels and creatinine clearance — may rise, indicating diminished renal perfusion

• serum cholesterol and triglyceride levels — may be elevated, indicating increased risk of atherosclerosis
• serum drug levels — may indicate subtherapeutic or toxic levels of antiarrhythmic agents such as digitalis glycosides
• 12-lead electrocardiography (ECG) — with transmural infarction, elevated ST segment and upright T waves in hyperacute phase, progressing to deeply inverted T waves and pathologic Q waves in leads overlooking the infarcted area; with subendocardial infarction, depressed ST segment and inverted T waves
• chest X-ray — may show cardiac enlargement produced by heart failure
• myocardial imaging (radionuclide) studies — demonstrate areas of poor or absent perfusion, wall motion abnormalities, and reduced ejection fraction
• echocardiography — may illustrate structural or functional cardiac abnormalities

Potential complications
• Arrhythmias
• Sudden death
• Cardiogenic shock
• Heart failure
• Pulmonary edema
• Papillary muscle dysfunction or rupture
• Ventricular rupture
• Pericarditis
• Pulmonary embolism
• Ventricular aneurysm
• Cardiac tamponade

Cardiovascular disorders

CLINICAL SNAPSHOT

ACUTE M.I.:
CRITICAL CARE UNIT

Major nursing diagnoses and collaborative problems	Key patient outcomes
Risk for cardiogenic shock	Maintain vital signs within normal limits: typically, heart rate 60 to 100 beats/minute; systolic blood pressure, 90 to 140 mm Hg; diastolic blood pressure, 50 to 90 mm Hg.
Hypoxemia	Maintain arterial partial pressure of oxygen (PaO_2) greater than 80 mm Hg. Maintain oxygen saturation on pulse oximetry greater than 90%.
Chest pain	Rate pain as 0 on a 0 to 10 pain rating scale, with oral medications.
Risk for ineffective individual coping	Verbalize feelings appropriate to initial stage of coping.
Risk for constipation	Resume a regular bowel elimination pattern.
Risk for injury: Complications	Show no signs of complications.
Knowledge deficit (diagnostic procedures, therapeutic interventions, and long-range implications)	Begin to identify long-range learning needs.

COLLABORATIVE PROBLEM

Risk for cardiogenic shock related to arrhythmias, impaired contractility, or thrombosis

Nursing priority

Optimize cardiac output and cellular perfusion.

Patient outcome criteria

- Within 24 hours of admission, the patient will:
  - maintain vital signs within normal limits: typically, heart rate, 60 to 100 beats/minute; systolic blood pressure, 90 to 140 mm Hg; and diastolic blood pressure, 50 to 90 mm Hg
  - show normal skin color
  - have a capillary refill time less than 3 seconds.
- Within 3 days of admission, the patient will experience no life-threatening arrhythmias.

Interventions

1. Institute and document continuous ECG monitoring on admission, with alarms on at all times. Preferably, monitor lead MCL_1 or MCL_6. See the "Risk for injury" nursing diagnosis in this plan for details about specific arrhythmias.

2. Record and analyze rhythm strips following unit protocol and as needed for significant variations. Mount strips in chart.

3. Obtain serial 12-lead ECGs on admission, daily for 3 days, and as needed for chest pain.

Rationales

1. Arrhythmias are the primary cause of death in the first 24 hours after infarction. MCL_1 and MCL_6 best differentiate supraventricular aberration from ventricular ectopy.

2. Systematic analysis may warn of impending problems with impulse initiation or conduction.

3. The ECG obtained on admission provides a baseline for infarct localization. Serial ECGs monitor changes.

4. Every hour or as needed, evaluate and document level of consciousness, pulse, blood pressure, heart sounds, breath sounds, urine output, skin color and temperature, and capillary refill time.

4. Level of consciousness is a sensitive indicator of cerebral ischemia. Pulse rate may indicate fluid deficit, pulse rhythm may indicate ectopic beats, and pulse volume may indicate fluid deficit or overload. A systolic blood pressure reading more than 20 mm Hg below the patient's normal value or a systolic blood pressure of 80 mm Hg or less indicates shock. Abnormal heart sounds indicate various problems: S_3 or S_4 indicate heart failure, murmurs indicate incompetent or stenotic valves, and pericardial friction rub indicates pericarditis. Abnormal breath sounds (particularly crackles that do not clear with coughing) suggest heart failure. A urine output of less than 60 ml/hour suggests decreased renal perfusion. Pale, cyanotic, mottled, or cool skin indicates decreased peripheral perfusion, as does a capillary refill time greater than 3 seconds.

5. Establish and maintain a patent I.V. line on admission. Document cumulative fluid intake and output hourly.

5. An I.V. line is necessary for emergency fluid and drug administration. The usual order is for dextrose 5% in water at a keep-vein-open rate. If the patient does not need fluid, a heparin or saline lock may be ordered instead. Intake and output records provide clues to developing fluid imbalances.

6. Administer aspirin, as ordered.

6. Commonly used to decrease platelet aggregation, aspirin may be used along with thrombolytic therapy.

7. Administer heparin, warfarin sodium (Coumadin), or both, as ordered.

7. Heparin commonly is ordered prophylactically to minimize the risk of thromboembolism from arrhythmias or immobility. It also may be used to limit extension of a thrombus that produced an AMI. Warfarin provides long-term anticoagulation.

8. Prepare the patient for aggressive treatment measures, as ordered, which may include:

• thrombolytic therapy with streptokinase (Kabikinase), alteplase (Activase), anistreplase (Eminase), or urokinase (Abbokinase)
• emergency coronary arteriography

• percutaneous transluminal coronary angioplasty (PTCA)

• coronary artery bypass surgery.

8. Infarctions that are impending, in progress, or complicated may require immediate aggressive interventions.
• Thrombolytic therapy may be administered to lyse fresh clots, thus relieving the occlusion and reestablishing perfusion to the damaged area.
• Coronary arteriography normally is not performed during AMI because of the risk of furthering the infarct. It is necessary before angioplasty or emergency bypass surgery, however, to locate the site of occlusion precisely.
• PTCA may increase coronary artery blood flow by compressing occluding lesions and dilating the vessel lumen. The resulting increase in luminal cross-sectional area improves blood flow to ischemic tissue.
• Emergency surgery may be necessary to bypass life-threatening lesions.

9. Additional individualized interventions: _____

9. Rationales: _____

Cardiovascular disorders

(Text continues on page 345.)

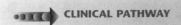 CLINICAL PATHWAY

Acute MI

Plan	Day 1 (CCU)	Day 2
Assessments	• History and physical exam • Nursing admission assessment • Review of systems assessment q shift and p.r.n	• 24-hr summary, physical exam • Review of systems assessment q shift and p.r.n.
Consults	• Social work if indicated	
Laboratory studies, diagnostics, and procedures	• Total CK and isoforms q 8h until peak, PTT (and with heparin changes), urinalysis • ECG • Echocardiogram (day 1 or 2)	• Total CK and isoforms if not baseline, PTT (if heparin and with changes), Chem 7, CBC • ECG • Echocardiogram (day 1 or 2)
Interventions	• Continuous ECG monitoring • Noninvasive blood pressure monitoring • Continuous oximetry • Rhythm strip q shift and p.r.n. • Vital signs per routine • I&O per routine • Chest pain protocol • Guaiac stools • Lytic therapy care per standard • I.V. site care • Immobility complication prevention	• Continuous ECG monitoring • Noninvasive blood pressure monitoring • Continuous oximetry • Rhythm strip q shift and p.r.n. • Vital signs per routine • I&O per routine • Chest pain protocol • Guaiac stools • I.V. site care • Immobility complication prevention
Medications and I.V.	• As indicated: heparin drip, nitroglycerin, aspirin, beta blocker, analgesics, stool softener, antiemetic, sedative • Oxygen (O_2)	• As indicated: heparin drip, nitroglycerin, aspirin, beta blocker, analgesics, stool softener, antiemetic, sedative • Discontinue O_2 if indicated
Diet	• Low-salt, low-fat diet, house or ADA	• Continued ordered diet
Activity	• Bed rest with commode • Assist with ADLs	• Have patient get out of bed and to a chair • Assist with ADLs
Teaching		• Cardiac teaching: critical pathway, CCU handbook, pain scale per protocol
Discharge, planning, and follow-up		• Begin discharge teaching
Key indicators	• Chest pain? Y_ N_ • Chest pain protocol effective in resolving chest pain? Y_ N_ • Sao_2 >90% Y_ N_ • Does patient have symptomatic arrhythmia? Y_ N_ • Is patient hemodynamically stable? Y_ N_	• Does the patient have chest pain? Y_ N_ • Was the chest pain protocol effective in resolving chest pain? Y_ N_ • Sao_2 >90% without O_2? Y_ N_ • Does patient have symptomatic arrhythmia? Y_ N_ • Is patient hemodynamically stable? Y_ N_ • Is patient out of bed for 1hr t.i.d.? Y_ N_

Day 3	Day 4	Day 5
• 24-hr summary, physical exam • Review of systems assessment q shift and p.r.n.	• 24-hr summary, physical exam • Review of systems assessment q shift and p.r.n.	• 24-hr summary, physical exam • Review of systems assessment q shift and p.r.n.
• Cardiac rehab	• Dietary	
• Total CK/ISOs if not baseline, PTT (if on heparin and with changes) • Schedule stress test	• Total CK/ISO's if not baseline, PTT (if on heparin and with changes) • Stress test • Schedule cardiac catheter if indicated	• Total CK/ISOs if not baseline, PTT (if on heparin and with changes) • Diagnostic cardiac catheter • Schedule PTCA/intervention if indicated
• Continuous ECG monitoring • Noninvasive blood pressure monitoring • Rhythm strip q shift and p.r.n. • Vital signs per routine • I&O per routine • Chest pain protocol • Guaiac stools • I.V. site care • Immobility complication prevention	• Continuous ECG monitoring (if stress test is negative, discontinue monitoring) • Rhythm strip q shift and p.r.n. • Vital signs per routine • Chest pain protocol • Guaiac stools • I.V. site care (if stress test is negative, discontinue I.V. access) • Immobility complication prevention	• Continuous ECG monitoring • Rhythm strip q shift & p.r.n. • Vital signs per routine • Chest pain protocol • Guaiac stools • I.V. site care • Immobility complication prevention
• As indicated: heparin drip, nitroglycerin, aspirin, beta blocker, analgesics, stool softener, antiemetic, sedative	• As indicated: heparin drip, nitroglycerin, aspirin, beta blocker, analgesics, stool softener, sedative	• As indicated: heparin drip, nitroglycerin, aspirin, beta blocker, analgesics, stool softener, sedative
• Continue ordered diet N.P.O. after midnight for stress test	• Continue ordered diet N.P.O. after midnight for stress test	• Continue ordered diet. • Resume diet after stress test.
• Have the patient ambulate with assistance. • Assist with ADLs.	• Have patient ambulate with assistance • Assist with ADLs	• Have patient ambulate independently. • Assist with ADLs.
• Provide teaching for a cardiac patient • Differentiate CCU and telemetry • Provide stress test instructions	• Provide cardiac teaching. • If stress test is negative, review discharge medications and instructions.	• Provide cardiac teaching. • If stress test is negative, review discharge medications and instructions
• Discharge teaching • Request transfer bed for day 4	• Discharge teaching	• Discharge teaching • If stress test is negative, discharge patient.
• Is the patient weaned off NTG? Y_ N_ • Have arrhythmias ceased without antiarrhythmics? Y_ N_ • Does the patient ambulate in room? Y_ N_ • Can the patient perform ADLs with moderate assistance? Y_ N_	• Can the patient ambulate in room? Y_ N_ • Can the patient perform ADLs with minimal assistance? Y_ N_ • Transfer to stepdown unit? Y_ N_ • Can the patient ambulate in hallway with assistance? Y_ N_	• Can patient perform ADLs independently? Y_ N_ • Can patient ambulate in hallway independently? Y_ N_ • Did patient comply with post catheter/intervention instructions and activity restrictions? Y_ N_ • Is site free of signs and symptoms of hematoma, hemorrhage, and infection? Y_ N_ • Are distal pulses present in affected extremity? Y_ N_ • Urine output >600ml per shift? Y_ N_ • Post intervention only: –Does patient have chest pain? Y_ N_ (on a scale of 0-10) –Was chest pain protocol effective in resolving chest pain? Y_ N_

Cardiovascular disorders

Acute MI *(continued)*

Plan	Day 6	Day 7
Assessments	• 24-hr summary, physical exam • Review of systems assessment q shift and p.r.n.	• 24-hr summary, physical exam • Review of systems assessment q shift and p.r.n.
Consults		
Laboratory studies, diagnostics, and procedures	• Total CK and isoforms if not baseline, PTT (if on heparin and with changes) • PTCA or interventional treatment	• PTT, hemoglobin, hematocrit, CK, BUN, creatinine
Interventions	• Continuous ECG monitoring • Rhythm strip q shift and p.r.n. • Vital signs per routine • Chest pain protocol • Guaiac stools • I.V. site care • Immobility complication prevention	• Continuous ECG monitoring • Rhythm strip q shift and p.r.n. • Vital signs per routine • Chest pain protocol • Guaiac stools • I.V. site care • Immobility complication prevention
Medications and I.V.	• As indicated: heparin drip, nitroglycerin, aspirin, beta blocker, analgesics, stool softener, sedative	• As indicated: heparin drip, nitroglycerin, aspirin, beta blocker, analgesics, stool softener, sedative
Diet	• Continue ordered diet	• Discontinue I.V. access.
Activity	• Have patient ambulate independently. • Assist with ADLs.	• Continue ordered diet.
Teaching	• Cardiac teaching per protocol.	• Have patient engage in activity per intervention standard. • Assist with ADLs.
Discharge, planning, and follow-up	• Discharge teaching	• Review discharge medications and instructions.
Key indicators	• Can patient perform ADLs independently? Y_ N_ • Can patient ambulate in hallway independently? Y_ N_ • Did patient comply with post catheter/intervention instructions and activity restrictions? Y_ N_ • Is site free of signs and symptoms of hematoma, hemorrhage, infection? Y_ N_ • Are distal pulses present in affected extremity? Y_ N_ • Urine output >600ml per shift? Y_ N_ • Post intervention only: –Does the patient have chest pain? Y_ N_ (on a scale of 0-10) –Was chest pain protocol effective in resolving chest pain? Y_ N_ –Is patient without significant ECG changes after procedure? Y_ N_ –Was bleeding noted from puncture sites or other source? Y_ N_ Note source _____	• Is patient hemodynamically stable per standards? Y_ N_ • Is patient free of chest pain, heart failure, ischemia, or significant arrhythmia? Y_ N_ • Can patient perform ADLs? Y_ N_ • Can patient demonstrate knowledge of discharge instructions? Y_ N_

COLLABORATIVE PROBLEM

Hypoxemia related to ventilation-perfusion imbalance

Nursing priorities

- Optimize myocardial oxygen demand-supply ratio.
- Minimize the risk of further infarction.

Patient outcome criteria

Within 24 hours of admission, the patient will:
- show no dyspnea
- maintain Pao_2 greater than 80 mm Hg
- maintain arterial oxygen saturation (Sao_2) greater than 90% on pulse oximetry
- display normal sinus rhythm or controlled arrhythmias
- have normal skin color
- rest comfortably.

Interventions

1. Observe for signs of hypoxemia, such as tachycardia, restlessness, irritability, or tachypnea. Monitor Sao_2 by pulse oximetry and ABG values, as ordered.

2. Administer and document oxygen therapy on admission, according to medical protocol and nursing judgment — typically 3 to 5 L/minute by nasal cannula for the first 24 to 48 hours.

3. If blood pressure is stable within normal limits, place the patient in semi-Fowler's position.

4. During the period of acute instability, place the patient on bed rest or chair rest. Once stabilized, increase activity as tolerated. See the "Activity intolerance" nursing diagnosis, page 399, in the "Cardiogenic shock" plan.

5. Provide adequate rest periods. Set priorities for care and group procedures. Refer to the "Sensory-perceptual alteration" plan, page 96, for further suggestions.

6. Additional individualized interventions: _____

Rationales

1. Cellular hypoxia commonly results from impaired coronary artery perfusion, decreased systemic perfusion, and respiratory depressant effects of analgesics and sedatives. Sao_2 and ABG values provide objective evidence of the degree of hypoxemia. Prompt treatment minimizes ischemic damage.

2. Supplemental oxygen will elevate arterial oxygen content and may relieve myocardial ischemia.

3. The semi-upright position facilitates breathing.

4. Rest reduces myocardial oxygen demands. Controlling oxygen demands helps limit infarct extension. Gradual resumption of activity helps promote a sense of well-being. The "Activity intolerance" nursing diagnosis contains detailed information on assessing activity tolerance and promoting safe resumption of physical activity.

5. Sleep deprivation, common in the critical care setting, can lead to increased irritability, confusion, increased sensitivity to pain, and other problems. The "Sensory/perceptual alteration" plan provides detailed interventions and rationales related to sleep deprivation.

6. Rationales: _____

COLLABORATIVE PROBLEM

Chest pain related to myocardial ischemia

Nursing priority

Relieve chest pain.

Cardiovascular disorders

Patient outcome criteria

Within 1 to 2 hours of admission, the patient will:
• rate pain as 0 on a 0 to 10 pain rating scale
• display no associated signs and symptoms of pain
• assume a relaxed posture
• have a relaxed facial expression.

Interventions

1. On admission, teach the patient to report immediately any unusual chest sensation, such as chest pain, tightness, heaviness, or burning.

2. Monitor continually for indications of chest pain, such as complaints of discomfort, sternal rubbing, tense posture, emotional withdrawal, facial grimacing, shortness of breath, diaphoresis, or restlessness.

3. Document pain episodes: Analyze pain characteristics (including value on pain rating scale), record a monitor rhythm strip, and obtain a 12-lead ECG.

4. Administer medication promptly at the onset of pain and document its use, according to medical protocol or orders. Administer oxygen when pain occurs. Evaluate and document blood pressure, pulse, and respirations before and after administration. Assess pain relief after 30 minutes.

5. During the initial period of cardiovascular instability, titrate I.V. morphine, typically in 2- to 5-mg doses (if ordered), according to the level of pain and vital signs. Withhold morphine and contact the doctor if the respiratory rate is less than 12 breaths/minute or the systolic blood pressure is less than 90 mm Hg (for a previously normotensive patient), or more than 20 mm Hg below the baseline value (for a previously hypertensive patient).

6. Remain with the patient until pain is relieved.

7. Position the patient comfortably. Use noninvasive pain-relief measures and medications, as appropriate. See the "Pain" plan, page 88, for details.

8. Additional individualized interventions: _____

Rationales

1. Symptoms other than obvious pain may indicate ischemia. Awareness of more subtle symptoms suggesting ischemia promotes early intervention.

2. The patient may not report pain, but astute observation may detect associated signs and symptoms and allow for early intervention. Shortness of breath and diaphoresis may result from sympathetic stimulation; restlessness may reflect cerebral ischemia.

3. Careful analysis of characteristics allows for differential diagnosis of pain. The rhythm strip can document new arrhythmias and the 12-lead ECG can document infarct extension.

4. Pain medication is more effective when given before severe pain develops. Pain may stimulate the sympathetic nervous system and increase myocardial workload. Supplemental oxygen may relieve pain and plays a role in reducing infarct size. Vital sign measurements before medication administration provide objective indicators of the degree of physiologic stress imposed by pain; those taken afterward indicate relief of such stress.

5. Administering narcotics I.V. relieves pain more rapidly and reliably than by the intramuscular (I.M.) route because poorly perfused muscles absorb medication erratically. I.M. injections also elevate CK levels, obscuring their diagnostic value. Morphine is the drug of choice for pain associated with AMI because it is a potent analgesic and causes peripheral vasodilation (lessening venous return and myocardial workload) and euphoria. The vital sign parameters listed indicate respiratory depression and excessive vasodilation, both possible adverse reactions to morphine.

6. The presence of a competent, confident caregiver may reassure the patient, relieving anxiety and thus lessening sympathetic stimulation.

7. Comfortable positioning and noninvasive pain-relief measures, such as rhythmic breathing, distraction, and relaxation, may reduce the perception of pain and promote endorphin release. The "Pain" plan discusses numerous alternative pain-relief strategies.

8. Rationales: _____

NURSING DIAGNOSIS

Risk for ineffective individual coping related to fear of death, anxiety, denial, or depression

Nursing priority

Promote healthy coping.

Patient outcome criteria

• Within 24 hours, the patient will display feelings appropriate to initial stage of coping.
• Within 72 hours, the patient will display the first signs of effective coping.

Interventions

1. Implement measures in the "Ineffective individual coping" plan, page 67, as appropriate.

2. Administer tranquilizers, as ordered, typically a benzodiazepine, such as diazepam (Valium), lorazepam (Ativan), or alprazolam (Xanax).

3. Additional individualized interventions: _____

Rationales

1. AMI is a major threat to psychological equilibrium and may provoke various protective responses. The "Ineffective individual coping" plan contains comprehensive information on evaluating and promoting healthy responses.

2. Minor tranquilizers may be used to keep anxiety at a tolerable level and avoid the harmful physiologic effects of anxiety-triggered catecholamine release.

3. Rationales: _____

NURSING DIAGNOSIS

Risk for constipation related to diet, bed rest, immobility, or medications

Nursing priority

Prevent or minimize constipation.

Patient outcome criteria

Within 3 days, the patient will:
• resume a regular bowel elimination pattern
• experience no straining during defecation
• have soft stool.

Interventions

1. Encourage the patient to follow the prescribed diet, which is usually low in calories, salt, and fat. Limit intake of caffeine. Document intake, likes, and dislikes.

2. Supply a bedside commode when the patient's condition allows.

3. Administer stool softeners and laxatives judiciously, as ordered, and document their use. Use alternatives and supplements to stool softeners and laxatives, such as increased dietary fiber and prune juice. Encourage increased fluid intake, if appropriate to medical status.

Rationales

1. Dietary prescriptions vary with the patient's needs. Caffeine is avoided because it is a cardiac stimulant. The patient is more likely to adhere to a diet plan that respects personal food preferences.

2. A bedside commode requires less energy to use than a bedpan, so constipation can be relieved with less myocardial oxygen demand.

3. Straining to defecate produces Valsalva's maneuver, which can cause bradycardia and decrease cardiac output. Rebound tachycardia and myocardial ischemia may follow. Dependence on laxatives diminishes the urge for spontaneous defecation.

Cardiovascular disorders

4. Provide privacy, a room deodorizer, and television or radio noise while the patient is defecating.

5. Additional individualized interventions: _____
_____

4. Without such measures, the patient may resist the urge to defecate because of embarrassment over expulsive sounds and odors.

5. Rationales: _____
_____

NURSING DIAGNOSIS

Risk for injury: Complications related to myocardial ischemia, injury, necrosis, inflammation, or arrhythmias

Nursing priority

Prevent or minimize complications.

Patient outcome criteria

• Within 24 hours of admission, the patient will:
  – display normal sinus rhythm or a controlled arrhythmia with a ventricular rate of 60 to 100 beats/minute
  – manifest strong, bilaterally equal peripheral pulses
  – show no signs of complications.
• Within 3 days of admission, the patient will:
  – have hemodynamic values within expected limits: typically, pulmonary artery (PA) systolic, 20 to 30 mm Hg; PA diastolic, 10 to 15 mm Hg; pulmonary artery wedge pressure (PAWP), 4 to 12 mm Hg; and cardiac output, 4 to 6 L/minute
  – have clear breath sounds
  – have clear heart sounds with decreasing or no S_3 or S_4, rub, or new murmurs
  – experience no further chest pain
  – show decreasing or no neck vein distention.

Interventions

1. Monitor constantly for general complications of AMI:

Arrhythmias
• Observe constantly for ventricular arrhythmias: ventricular premature beats, accelerated ventricular rhythm, ventricular tachycardia, and ventricular fibrillation.

• Observe constantly for supraventricular arrhythmias: premature atrial or junctional beats; atrial tachycardia, flutter, or fibrillation; or supraventricular tachycardia.

Rationales

1. Several complications can impair recovery from AMI. Many occur with any type of infarct and are associated less with the infarct's location than with the extent of myocardial damage and degree of the underlying coronary artery disease. Other complications have a pathophysiologic correlation with a specific type of infarct.

• Ventricular arrhythmias are the most common complication of AMI. In the first few hours after infarction, they probably result from an ischemia-induced reentry mechanism, whereas later arrhythmias probably result from increased automaticity.
• Supraventricular arrhythmias may result from ischemia, heart failure, catecholamine stimulation, and other factors. Although less serious than ventricular arrhythmias, they may contribute to an unstable physiologic status or to thromboembolism. Tachycardias increase myocardial oxygen demand, reduce left ventricular filling time, and reduce coronary artery perfusion time. The loss of atrial "kick" (normally coordinated atrial contraction) also may reduce cardiac output.

• Administer and document antiarrhythmic agents, as ordered. Monitor effectiveness and adverse effects. Typical agents include:
– Class IA agents, such as procainamide (Pronestyl), quinidine (Duraquin), and disopyramide (Norpace)

– Class IB agents, such as lidocaine (Xylocaine), ordered prophylactically or as needed for warning ventricular premature beats (more than 6 per minute, sequential, multifocal, or close to the preceding T wave), ventricular tachycardia, or ventricular fibrillation

– Class II agents, such as propranolol (Inderal), meto prolol (Lopressor), and atenolol (Tenormin)

– Class III agents, such as bretylium tosylate (Bretylol) and amiodarone (Cordarone)|

– Class IV agents, such as verapamil (Calan), nifedipine (Procardia), and diltiazem (Cardizem)

• Implement and document emergency measures as needed, based on medical protocol and nursing judgment.

Heart failure and cardiogenic shock
• Implement measures in the "Cardiogenic shock" and "Heart failure" plans, pages 392 and 420, respectively.

Infarct extension
• Monitor for new, increased, or persistent chest pain. Obtain a 12-lead ECG reading and administer oxygen and pain medication, as ordered. Notify the doctor about the pain and any new indicators of infarction on the ECG reading.

Pericarditis
• Observe for pericardial chest pain, typically stabbing, localized pain that worsens on deep inspiration and with movement. Also monitor for fever, tachycardia, and pericardial friction rub.
• If you observe signs and symptoms of pericarditis, notify the doctor. Administer anti-inflammatory agents, as ordered, typically aspirin, corticosteroids, or non-steroidal anti-inflammatory agents.
• Monitor for indicators of pericardial effusion: weak peripheral pulses, paradoxical pulse greater than 10 mm Hg, or a decreased level of consciousness. If present, notify the doctor promptly.

• Arrhythmias may impair cardiac output or progress to cardiac arrest. Antiarrhythmic agents are classified according to their electrophysiologic properties.
– Class IA drugs, used for both atrial and ventricular arrhythmias (particularly reentrant ones), decrease automaticity, conduction, and repolarization.
– Class IB agents, used to prevent and treat ventricular arrhythmias, inhibit ventricular automaticity. Lidocaine also increases the threshold for fibrillation. Prophylactic lidocaine may be ordered because of AMI's high incidence of ventricular fibrillation, which commonly occurs without warning.
– Class II agents, beta-adrenergic blockers, are used to control supraventricular arrhythmias. Their complex mechanisms include suppressing sinus node automaticity and decreasing atrioventricular (AV) conduction.
– Bretylium suppresses reentrant ventricular arrhythmias and elevates the threshold for ventricular fibrillation. Amiodarone increases the refractory period and is useful in life-threatening ventricular tachyarrhythmias.
– Class IV drugs, calcium channel blockers, inhibit sinoatrial (SA) and AV automaticity and prolong AV conduction. They are particularly useful in treating supraventricular tachycardias.
• Protocols usually allow for emergency treatment of warning and lethal arrhythmias (ventricular premature beats, tachycardia, fibrillation, asystole; symptomatic sinus bradycardia; and Mobitz II second- and third-degree AV blocks).

• Varying degrees of myocardial failure, such as heart failure or cardiogenic shock, are common during the first week after the infarction. Several factors place the AMI patient at risk for myocardial failure, including myocardial ischemia, hypoxemia, acidosis, hypotension, and paradoxical movement of the injured myocardial wall.

• Infarct extension may result from progressive ischemia of the myocardium secondary to swelling of damaged cells and inflammatory responses that compress surrounding tissue. Other factors that may cause extension of the infarct include hypoxemia and microemboli.

• Pericardial sac inflammation is a relatively benign complication. Focal pericarditis usually develops within 5 days; generalized pericarditis (Dressler's syndrome) typically develops within 14 days.
• Anti-inflammatory agents reduce inflammation, relieving signs and symptoms and reducing the risk of pericardial effusion.

• In pericardial effusion, fluid leaks across the walls of inflamed cells. The degree of leakage may vary from mild to major. Left untreated, an effusion may produce a cardiac tamponade large enough to induce cardiac arrest.

Cardiovascular disorders

• Monitor for indicators of cardiac tamponade, including Beck's triad (elevated central venous pressure [CVP], profound hypotension, and distant heart sounds), neck vein distention, tachycardia, decreased pulse pressure, paradoxical pulse, and pericardial friction rub. If you observe these signs, summon immediate medical assistance and prepare for emergency pericardial aspiration.

Ventricular aneurysm
• Observe for indications of a possible ventricular aneurysm, which include signs and symptoms of heart failure, thromboembolism, and persistent ectopy. Alert the doctor and prepare the patient for surgery, as ordered.

Rupture
• Monitor for signs and symptoms of papillary muscle rupture — sudden shock, a loud holosystolic murmur radiating from the apex to the left axilla, and signs of severe left-sided heart failure. If these signs and symptoms occur, call for immediate medical assistance. Assist with treatment of cardiogenic shock or prepare the patient for surgery, as ordered.

• Observe for signs and symptoms of potential septal rupture — severe chest pain, severe heart failure, a loud holosystolic murmur at the apex and lower left sternal border, or sudden cardiac death. If they occur, initiate cardiopulmonary resuscitation (CPR), if necessary, and call for immediate medical assistance. Implement measures to treat cardiogenic shock or prepare the patient for surgery, as ordered.
• Be alert for signs and symptoms of a possible impending myocardial rupture, especially in a patient with a transmural infarction who is on anticoagulant therapy — persistent chest pain without ECG changes, persistent hypertension after the infarction, M-shaped QRS complexes, or pericardial blood or fluid detected by an echocardiogram. Notify the doctor of such signs and symptoms immediately. Assist with emergency pericardiocentesis and treatment of cardiogenic shock, as ordered.

2. Monitor constantly for complications of particular types of AMI:

• Cardiac tamponade is a medical emergency. Because it impinges on ventricular expansion, it severely limits ventricular filling and therefore cardiac output. Immediate removal of the pericardial fluid permits ventricular filling and prevents cardiac arrest.

• Ventricular aneurysm is thought to occur in about 10% of AMI patients. Dilation most commonly occurs in the anterolateral area, although it may also occur in the posterior or septal walls or the apical area. The systolic outward bulging of the area weakened by the infarction decreases stroke volume. In addition, clots may occur in the dilated area and embolize to other organs. Aneurysmectomy removes the bulging, weakened area and prevents potentially fatal myocardial rupture.

• Papillary muscle rupture results from necrosis of the muscles that anchor the chordae tendineae of the mitral valve. It occurs most commonly with inferior infarction involving the posterior papillary muscle, although the anterior papillary muscle may be damaged with an anteroseptal infarct. The resulting acute mitral insufficiency may severely limit cardiac output. Definitive treatment is mitral valve replacement.
• Septal rupture, a rare but life-threatening emergency, results from necrosis of the interventricular septum. It may occur in inferior or anteroseptal infarcts and is most likely if significant disease is present in both the right and left anterior descending coronary arteries. CPR and measures to combat cardiogenic shock may keep the patient alive until the ventricular septal defect can be repaired surgically.
• A devastating complication, rupture of the free ventricular wall occurs most commonly in the anterior or lateral walls. It may occur anywhere from 3 days to 3 weeks after the infarction during the healing stage when leukocytic removal of myocardial debris thins the myocardial wall. Hypertension, anticoagulation, and full-thickness infarction increase the risk of rupture. The resulting massive cardiac tamponade leads to death. The invariable mortality from rupture emphasizes the urgency of action when any signs and symptoms of impending rupture are detected.

2. Certain complications correlate with a particular type of infarct because they stem from a common pathophysiologic cause.

Anterior, anteroseptal, or anterolateral infarct
• Monitor for signs or symptoms of potential bundle-branch block. Constantly monitor QRS complex width and the pattern of deflections in V_1 and V_6 (or MCL_1 and MCL_6). On serial ECGs, note axis deviation.

• Document and alert the doctor to the presence of any of the following:
– Right bundle-branch block (RBBB): QRS greater than 0.12 seconds, RSR′ pattern in V_1

– Left bundle-branch block (LBBB): QRS greater than 0.12 second, absent Q wave, and large monophasic R wave in V_6

– Left anterior hemiblock or left posterior hemiblock

• Observe closely for development of Mobitz II second-degree AV block or complete heart block, particularly if RBBB with left anterior hemiblock or left posterior hemiblock is present. Prepare for prophylactic pacemaker insertion, as ordered.

Inferior infarct
• Monitor for sinus bradycardia and AV block, particularly first-degree AV block and Mobitz I second-degree AV block.

• Because the left anterior descending coronary artery nourishes the ventricular septum, where the bundle branches are located, an anterior infarct may produce septal ischemia or necrosis with resulting bundle-branch block. Bundle-branch block widens the QRS complex beyond the normal limit because it disrupts the usual sequence or speed of depolarization. Because V_1 (MCL_1) is oriented to the right ventricle and V_6 (MCL_6) to the left, the pattern of deflections in these leads best indicates the timing and sequence of bundle-branch conduction.
• Untreated, certain blocks increase risk of mortality from AMI.
– RBBB produces delayed right ventricular stimulation, prolonging the QRS duration. It also alters the usual sequence of deflections, in which septal depolarization is followed by simultaneous depolarization of both ventricles. Instead, RBBB produces a small positive wave of septal depolarization, a large negative wave of left ventricular depolarization, and a large positive wave of right ventricular depolarization.
– LBBB disrupts the depolarization pattern to a greater extent than RBBB. It causes loss of the normal septal Q waves in leads oriented to the left ventricle and allows the right ventricle to depolarize before the left ventricle.
– Hemiblocks are blocks of one fascicle of the left bundle branch. Left anterior hemiblock is more common than left posterior hemiblock because the anterior fascicle is thinner and has a more vulnerable blood supply. Left anterior hemiblock is considered relatively benign, whereas left posterior hemiblock is more serious because it implies extensive infarction.
• Progression to a more advanced blockage is possible at any time. RBBB with hemiblock indicates a blockage of two of the three fascicles responsible for ventricular conduction, leaving the patient dependent on a single fascicle. Mobitz II block is an ominous sign because it indicates intermittent blockage of all three fascicles, implies extensive myocardial necrosis, and commonly heralds complete heart block. Prophylactic pacemaker insertion prevents ventricular asystole if complete heart block occurs.

• Although these rhythms may occur with any type of infarct from excess vagal stimulation, they are most common in inferior infarction. An inferior infarct typically results from occlusion of the right coronary artery, which nourishes the SA node in about 90% of the population and the AV node in about 55%. Ischemia of the SA node produces sinus arrhythmias; AV nodal ischemia above the bundle of His produces progressive slowing of impulse conduction through the AV node. Such ischemia usually is transient and responds promptly to administration of atropine.

Cardiovascular disorders

– Correlate rhythm with clinical status, noting the presence of hypotension, altered level of consciousness, chest pain, or increased ventricular premature beats.
– If the patient is symptomatic, administer atropine, as ordered and according to unit protocol. Notify the doctor and document the episode.
• Observe for indicators of right ventricular infarction, such as:

– neck vein distention, positive hepatojugular reflux, positive Kussmaul's sign (increased neck vein distention on inspiration), or elevated CVP or right atrial pressure with normal or mildly elevated PAWP.
– widely split S_2, right ventricular S_3 or S_4 heart sounds (audible at the third to fourth intercostal space at the left sternal border), or tricuspid insufficiency murmur

– bradycardia, AV blocks, and hypotension.

• If the patient is dehydrated on admission, be especially alert for the above signs after I.V. hydration.

• When recording 12-lead ECGs on a patient with suspected inferior or posterior infarction, routinely record right ventricular leads such as V_{4R}.

• If indicators of right ventricular infarction are present, alert the doctor. Obtain a chest X-ray and other noninvasive diagnostic studies, as ordered.

• If right ventricular infarction is confirmed, collaborate with the doctor to modify therapy.

– These signs indicate the arrhythmia is decreasing cardiac output.

– Atropine blocks vagal stimulation, thereby increasing SA node impulse formation and AV node conduction.

• Right ventricular infarction may occur with inferior or posterior left ventricular infarction because all these areas are perfused by the right coronary artery. Right ventricular infarction occurs in about 30% of inferior AMIs.
– These signs reflect the increased venous pressure that results from impaired right ventricular compliance and inability to pump blood effectively.

– The wide S_2 split reflects delayed pulmonary valve closure, the result of prolonged right ventricular ejection caused by the increased right ventricular volume and pressure. The S_3 or S_4 sound indicates decreased right ventricular compliance, and the tricuspid insufficiency murmur reflects a functional valvular insufficiency secondary to right ventricular dilation.
– Bradycardia probably reflects SA nodal ischemia, AV blocks indicate AV nodal ischemia, and hypotension results from impaired right ventricular stroke volume.
• Because the AMI patient may be dehydrated from nausea, vomiting, and diaphoresis, signs of right ventricular infarction may appear only after rehydration.
• The routine 12-lead ECG is not helpful in detecting right ventricular infarction, although it will reveal signs of concomitant inferior or posterior infarction. Right ventricular leads typically reveal Q waves, ST-segment elevation, and T-wave inversion with acute right ventricular infarction.
• A chest X-ray and other diagnostic studies provide objective evidence of right ventricular infarction. With right ventricular infarction alone, the chest X-ray typically is clear. An echocardiogram helps differentiate right ventricular infarction from cardiac tamponade, whereas radionuclide studies identify areas of infarction or decreased right ventricular ejection fraction. Diagnostic studies also help differentiate hypotension resulting primarily from right ventricular dysfunction from that resulting from left ventricular dysfunction—an important distinction because the therapy for each is quite different.
• Although the treatment of right ventricular infarction differs from that for left ventricular infarction, the goal is the same: to improve left ventricular filling pressure and thereby optimize cardiac output.

–Avoid diuretics. Administer fluid boluses, as ordered, typically to maintain right atrial pressure at 20 to 25 mm Hg and PAWP at 15 to 18 mm Hg.

–Administer inotropes and vasodilators judiciously, as ordered.

• Monitor hemodynamic parameters and clinical indicators of the effectiveness of therapy closely.

3. Additional individualized interventions: _____

–Because strong right ventricular contraction is absent with right ventricular infarction, blood flow from the right to the left side of the heart becomes passive and dependent on preload. Diuretics lower preload. Fluid is administered, rather than limited as in left ventricular infarction, to improve preload-dependent right ventricular systolic ejection, thereby increasing left ventricular filling pressure and cardiac output.
–Inotropes may increase right ventricular contractility. Vasodilators may be used to decrease pulmonary vascular resistance; the resulting right ventricular afterload reduction may improve left ventricular filling; the simultaneous left ventricular afterload reduction may improve left ventricular systolic emptying.
• The association of right ventricular infarction with left ventricular infarction can be confusing to interpret and a challenge to manage. The treatment of right ventricular infarction described above must take into consideration the therapy for left ventricular infarction. Continual surveillance is necessary to make sure that therapies are modified as necessary to achieve optimal cardiac output.

3. Rationales: _____

NURSING DIAGNOSIS

Knowledge deficit (diagnostic procedures, therapeutic interventions, and long-range implications for lifestyle changes) related to complex diagnosis and therapeutic regimen

Nursing priority

Educate the patient and family about health status, as appropriate.

Patient outcome criteria

Within 48 hours of admission, the patient and family will:
• provide feedback indicating an adequate knowledge base for immediate needs (for example, by asking appropriate questions and by respecting dietary restrictions)
• begin to identify long-range learning needs.

Interventions

1. Implement measures in the "Knowledge deficit" plan, page 72, as appropriate.

2. Defer a formal rehabilitation and education program until the period of physiologic instability has passed. In the meantime:

• Establish rapport. Use eye contact, reflective listening, and nonverbal communication. Emphasize and display consistency as much as possible.

Rationales

1. The "Knowledge deficit" plan contains detailed information helpful in assessing and meeting learning needs for all patients. This plan focuses on information specific to AMI.

2. Implementing a major teaching program during this period is inappropriate because physiologic recovery is a higher priority. Nevertheless, capitalizing on unexpected teaching opportunities provides a way to assess learning needs and meet immediate concerns.
• Excessive anxiety interferes with learning. Establishing rapport through consistent, caring contact helps promote trust and relaxation, which can help the patient and family retain new information.

Cardiovascular disorders

• Assess immediate learning needs, encourage questions, and provide brief explanations, correcting any misconceptions; repeat as necessary.

• As appropriate, provide brief information about the pathophysiology of AMI, risk factor reduction, medications, dietary recommendations, activity restrictions, rehabilitation programs, community agencies, and support groups. Consult the "Acute MI: Telemetry unit" plan, page 355.
• Note and document long-range learning needs. Upon transfer to the telemetry unit, communicate these needs to the new unit's staff.

3. Additional individualized interventions: _____
_____

• AMI usually raises major questions for the patient and family about health and lifestyle. Responding to expressed needs displays sensitivity to the patient and family. Brief, repeated explanations may be necessary because high anxiety levels or medication effects may cause the patient to screen out information unintentionally.
• Careful selection of initial teaching content helps prevent information overload. The "Acute MI: Telemetry unit" plan contains comprehensive information on long-range learning needs and rehabilitation programs, usually addressed after the patient has become physiologically stable.
• Documentation and communication of long-range learning needs allow continuity of care and personalization of ongoing educational efforts.

3. Rationales: _____
_____

DISCHARGE PLANNING

Discharge checklist
Before discharge, the patient shows evidence of:
❏ stable blood pressure within normal limits without I.V. inotrope or vasodilator support
❏ stable cardiac rhythm with arrhythmias (if any) controlled by oral, sublingual, or transdermal medications or by permanent pacemaker
❏ spontaneous ventilation.

Teaching checklist
Document evidence that the patient and family demonstrate an understanding of:
❏ extent of infarction
❏ activity restrictions
❏ recommended dietary modifications
❏ smoking-cessation program as needed
❏ common emotional changes
❏ community resources for lifestyle modification support and cardiac rehabilitation.

Documentation checklist
Using outcome criteria as a guide, document:
❏ clinical status on admission
❏ significant changes in status
❏ pertinent diagnostic test findings
❏ chest pain
❏ pain-relief measures
❏ rhythm strip analyses
❏ use of emergency protocols
❏ hemodynamic trends and other data
❏ I.V. line patency
❏ oxygen therapy
❏ other therapies
❏ nutritional intake

❏ patient and family teaching
❏ discharge planning.

ASSOCIATED PLANS OF CARE

Acute MI: Telemetry unit
Cardiogenic shock
Grieving
Heart failure
Impaired physical mobility
Ineffective family coping: Compromised
Ineffective individual coping
Knowledge deficit
Pain

REFERENCES

Black, J., and Matassarin-Jacobs, E., eds. *Medical-Surgical Nursing: Clinical Management for Continuity of Care,* 5th ed. Philadelphia: W.B. Saunders Co., 1997.

Clochesy, J., et al. *Critical Care Nursing,* 2nd ed. Philadelphia: W.B. Saunders Co., 1996.

Kinney, M., and Packa, D., eds. *Andreoli's Comprehensive Cardiac Care,* 8th ed. St. Louis: Mosby–Year Book, Inc., 1996.

Luckmann, J., ed. *Manual of Nursing Care.* Philadelphia: W.B. Saunders Co., 1997.

Riegel, B., et al. "Nursing Care of Patients with Acute Myocardial Infarction: Results of a National Survey," *Critical Care Nurse* 17(5):23-33, October 1997.

U.S. Department of Health and Human Services. "Heart Failure: Evaluation and Care of Patients with Left-Ventricular Systolic Dysfunction," *AHCPR Publication No. 94-0612.* Rockville, Md., 1994.

U.S. Department of Health and Human Services. "Unstable Angina: Diagnosis and Management," *AHCPR Publication No. 94-0602.* Rockville, Md., 1994.

Acute MI: Telemetry unit

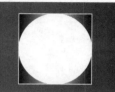

DRG information
(see "Acute MI: Critical care unit ," page 338)

DRG 121 Circulatory Disorders with Acute Myocardial Infarction (AMI) and Major Complications; Discharged Alive.
Mean LOS = 7.8 days

DRG 122 Circulatory Disorders with AMI without Major Complications; Discharged Alive.
Mean LOS = 5.3 days

INTRODUCTION

Definition and time focus
AMI is necrosis (death) of the myocardium resulting from an interrupted or diminished supply of oxygenated blood from the coronary arteries. This plan focuses on the patient who has passed through the critical stage of AMI and is ready to begin recovery. For information about problems seen in the critical care phase, see the "Acute MI: Critical care unit" plan.

Etiology and precipitating factors
The underlying disease is usually atherosclerosis that results in coronary occlusion or thrombosis, although severe coronary spasm may also be a cause. Contributing factors include:
• increased myocardial oxygen demand, such as from physical exertion, emotional stress, heavy meals, tachycardia, hyperthyroidism, hypertension, valvular insufficiency, and pregnancy
• decreased myocardial oxygen supply, such as from vasoconstriction, smoking, air pollution, anemia, bradycardia, hypotension, and sleep.

FOCUSED ASSESSMENT GUIDELINES

Nursing history (functional health pattern findings)
Health perception–health management pattern
• History of chest pain or previous infarction
• Treatment for hypertension, diabetes mellitus, heart failure, arrhythmias, hyperthyroidism, or anemia
• Cardiac risk factors, such as smoking, obesity, hyperlipidemia, high-stress occupation, sedentary lifestyle, or positive family history
• Increased risk for white males over age 40
• Postmenopausal females at increased risk

• Noncompliance with treatment program (diet, exercise, and medication)
Nutritional-metabolic pattern
• Diet usually high in calories, fat, and salt
Elimination pattern
• Constipation
Activity-exercise pattern
• Lack of energy for personal care and activities
• Sedentary lifestyle, lack of regular exercise, and lack of leisure activities
Sleep-rest pattern
• Difficulty sleeping because of unfamiliar surroundings, noise, or anxiety
• Need for frequent rest periods
Cognitive-perceptual pattern
• Recurring chest pain
Self-perception–self-concept pattern
• Realization of vulnerability and mortality
Role-relationship pattern
• Concern over inability to continue in usual family roles
• Concern for family's ability to manage
• Concern about ability to return to work
• Financial concerns
Sexuality-reproductive pattern
• Concern about decreased libido and resumption of sexual activities
Coping–stress tolerance pattern
• Type A personality (aggressive, ambitious, competitive, work-oriented, time-driven, impatient, and hostile)
• Anxious, expressing fear of sudden death, loss of employment, and loss of independence
• Depressed over losses
• Denial of seriousness of illness
Value-belief pattern
• Need for spiritual counseling

Physical findings
Cardiovascular
• Normal sinus rhythm or controlled arrhythmias
• S_3 or S_4 (less common)
• Hypotension (related to medications)
Pulmonary
• Shortness of breath
• Crackles (less common)
• Tachypnea secondary to pain or anxiety

Musculoskeletal
• Weakness
• Fatigability

Diagnostic studies
• Cardiac enzymes — after an infarct, elevated creatine kinase levels should return to normal within 3 to 4 days, lactate dehydrogenase levels (LD) within 7 to 10 days; sustained levels or levels that go up again indicate further cell death (expanding or recurrent infarction)
• Electrolyte levels — should be within normal limits; however, hypokalemia is common because of diuretic therapy
• Cholesterol and triglyceride levels — may be elevated
• Blood urea nitrogen and creatinine levels — should be within normal ranges; however, they may be elevated if blood supply to kidneys is diminished
• Serum drug levels — should be within therapeutic range
• White blood cell count — should return to normal 5 to 7 days after infarct
• Erythrocyte sedimentation rate — may remain elevated for several weeks
• Chest X-ray — may show cardiomegaly; if heart failure is present, may show lung congestion, pleural effusion, and pulmonary edema
• Telemetry — may show arrhythmias
• 12-lead electrocardiogram (ECG) — abnormal ST-segment elevation, signifying ischemia, and depressed or inverted T wave, indicating injury (may be present for days to weeks or longer); abnormal Q waves, signifying necrosis (may remain indefinitely)
• Echocardiography — may show valvular dysfunction, mural thrombi, dilated chambers, abnormal or decreased wall motion, and decreased cardiac output
• Exercise stress test — submaximal tests, used to measure exercise capacity and to help set activity and exercise guidelines, may show intolerance, as evidenced by arrhythmias, chest pain, shortness of breath, claudication, ST-segment changes, and blood pressure changes
• Thallium scan — used to detect location and extent of infarction and scarring; when performed during exercise, scan can reveal ischemic areas that are adequately perfused at rest

Potential complications
• Pulmonary edema
• Thromboembolism
• Ventricular aneurysm
• Extension of the infarction
• Recurrent myocardial infarction
• Arrhythmias
• Angina
• Heart failure
• Valvular dysfunction
• Pericarditis, Dressler's syndrome
• Shoulder-hand syndrome

CLINICAL SNAPSHOT

Acute M.I.: Telemetry unit

Major nursing diagnoses	Key patient outcomes
Activity intolerance	Maintain vital signs within normal limits: typically, heart rate, 60 to 100 beats/minute; systolic blood pressure, 90 to 140 mm Hg; and diastolic blood pressure, 50 to 90 mm Hg.
Risk for ineffective individual coping	Exhibit less anxiety, denial, or depression.
Altered sexuality pattern	List three recommendations for minimizing myocardial stress during sexual activity.
Knowledge deficit (risk factors and lifestyle modifications)	Express a willingness to adhere to prescribed therapy.

Nursing diagnosis

Activity intolerance related to myocardial ischemia, decreased contractility, or arrhythmias

Nursing priorities
• Minimize the risk of further infarction.
• Implement safe measures to increase activity or exercise tolerance.

Patient outcome criteria

By the time of discharge, the patient will:
• maintain vital signs within normal limits: typically, heart rate, 60 to 100 beats/minute; systolic blood pressure, 90 to 140 mm Hg; and diastolic blood pressure, 50 to 90 mm Hg
• perform self-care activities independently
• ambulate independently
• comply with the recommended activity and exercise program.

Interventions

1. Using telemetry, continuously monitor heart rate, rhythm, and conduction, as ordered. Document according to hospital protocol and as needed, noting pain and shortness of breath.

2. Promote physical comfort and rest.

3. Prohibit smoking and intake of stimulants, such as coffee, tea, and other beverages that contain caffeine.

4. Encourage the patient to perform activities of daily living (ADLs) and diversionary activities, as permitted and tolerated. Allow the patient to make as many decisions as possible.

5. Implement the prescribed activity or exercise program according to unit protocol, starting with low-energy activities, such as range-of-motion (ROM) exercises and progressing to full self-care. Encourage regular rest periods.

6. Assess and document intolerance to activity or exercise, as evidenced by:
• a pulse rate greater than 110 beats/minute or increased more than 20 beats/minute over baseline
• a pulse rate that does not return to baseline within 5 minutes
• new arrhythmias or a change in preexisting arrhythmias
• a blood pressure decrease during activity
• chest pain, diaphoresis, or dyspnea
• dizziness, increased weakness or fatigue, or syncope
• ST-segment elevation (if monitored).
   Monitor vital signs before and after activity or exercise and every 5 to 15 minutes during each session, depending on the patient's tolerance.

Rationales

1. A myocardial infarction may produce arrhythmias by promoting reentry and increased automaticity. Early detection allows for prompt treatment and prevention of life-threatening arrhythmias. Activity or exercise may cause new arrhythmias or a change in preexisting arrhythmias, which can result in decreased cardiac output.

2. Rest reduces myocardial oxygen needs and allows the heart to heal. Physical comfort reduces anxiety as well as oxygen demand. Controlling the extent of myocardial ischemia limits the infarction's size.

3. Stimulants increase the heart rate, thus increasing oxygen demands. Smoking decreases oxygen availability because hemoglobin molecules have a greater affinity for carbon monoxide (present in smoke) than for oxygen.

4. Participation in ADLs and diversionary activities increases the patient's sense of well-being and decreases anxiety. Making decisions about care activities and their timing, when possible, increases the patient's sense of control.

5. Progressive activity increases the heart's strength and collateral circulation. Starting with low-energy activities avoids creating an oxygen demand that exceeds supply. Alternating activity or exercise with rest periods prevents fatigue. Early ROM exercises decrease the risk of thromboembolism and other harmful effects of bed rest.

6. Exercise places increased demands on the heart that it may not be able to meet. AMI decreases contractility. Cardiac output may be reduced, resulting in decreased blood pressure and tissue perfusion. The heart rate may increase as a compensatory mechanism to maintain cardiac output. The absence or presence of symptoms helps determine when the activity or exercise program should be increased or stopped.

Cardiovascular disorders

7. Stress the importance of avoiding Valsalva's maneuver and isometric exercises.

7. Valsalva's maneuver may lead to bradycardia and a corresponding decrease in cardiac output and tissue perfusion. Isometric exercises cause a greater increase in blood pressure and heart rate than isotonic exercises do because sustained muscle tension impedes blood flow. The resultant increase in afterload increases myocardial work and myocardial oxygen demand.

8. Provide supplemental oxygen as ordered.

8. The healing myocardium requires a constant supply of oxygen. Supplemental oxygen increases arterial oxygen tension and may increase activity tolerance.

9. Administer vasodilators, as ordered, and monitor the patient's response. Also monitor for adverse effects, particularly hypotension.

9. Vasodilators dilate coronary arteries and peripheral blood vessels, thus increasing myocardial oxygen supply while decreasing demand.

10. Teach the patient to monitor pulse rate before and after activity or exercise.

10. Pulse rate best reflects the cardiac workload during activity or exercise.

11. Stress the importance of complying with the activity or exercise program and with rest requirements.

11. Regular periods of activity improve myocardial healing. Fatigue should be avoided because fatigued muscles require increased oxygen.

12. Encourage family members to support the patient's activity or exercise program.

12. Support from family members as well as health care professionals can motivate the patient to increase activity and exercise based on the therapeutic plan and individual tolerance.

13. Additional individualized interventions: _____

13. Rationales: _____

NURSING DIAGNOSIS

Risk for ineffective individual coping related to anxiety, denial, or depression

Nursing priority

Encourage healthy coping.

Patient outcome criteria

Within 3 days of admission to the intermediate care unit, the patient will:
• appear less anxious by exhibiting a calm expression, relaxed posture, dry palms, steady voice and hands, no tremors, and a normal heart rate. The patient will also sleep easily, have no morning insomnia, and be able to recall explanations and make reasonable decisions.
• confront denial (if present), and express concern about the AMI by discussing problems, gradually showing other signs of grief (such as crying, anxiety, or anger), taking responsibility for cooperating with the health plan, and allowing others to take over business affairs
• exhibit less depression (if present), participate in self-care, show a return of appetite, sleep restfully, discuss problems openly, talk about feelings without uncontrollable crying, express interest in learning about lifestyle modifications, make appropriate decisions, and express an intention to use available resources.

Interventions

1. Encourage the patient to express his feelings.

Rationales

1. The patient may perceive reactions as bizarre or otherwise inappropriate and may need "permission" to express them.

2. Anticipate feelings of denial, shock, anger, anxiety, and depression.

3. Explain the grieving process to the patient and family.

4. Evaluate the meaning of the patient's altered body image and role responsibilities.

5. Assess daily for indicators of anxiety, such as apprehensive expression, tense posture, continuous talking, difficulty remembering explanations, sweaty palms, tachycardia, shaky voice, tremulousness, disturbed sleep, and indecision. Take steps to relieve the patient's anxiety:
• Introduce yourself and other caregivers to the patient and family.

• Assign a primary care nurse, and limit the number of other nurses caring for the patient.
• Care for the patient calmly and confidently.

• Explain the purpose and routine nature of frequent assessments.
• Repeat explanations as necessary.

• Orient the patient to the unit.

• Administer minor tranquilizers, as ordered, using nursing judgment. Document their use.

• Help the patient explore ways to resolve unfinished business.

6. Assess daily for indicators of denial, such as refusal to discuss the AMI, minimal acceptance of its significance, apparent lack of concern about status, verbal acknowledgment that the AMI has occurred while ignoring diet and activity restrictions, and ongoing attempts to continue usual activities. Take steps to help resolve denial:
• Evaluate the impact of denial on the patient's health.

• If the patient verbalizes denial, listen nonjudgmentally.

2. These are normal responses to loss. They may become exaggerated in the face of overwhelming, life-threatening experiences and intense psychological threats.

3. The patient and family may be bewildered and alarmed about their emotional responses.

4. Responses vary because of the unique meaning of loss to each person.

5. Systematic assessment and comparison with previous findings increase the likelihood that coping problems will be detected early. Anxiety may result from fear of the unknown, unfamiliar surroundings, unfinished business, or other causes.

• Introductions reduce the depersonalizing effects of the hospital environment and lay the foundation for establishing rapport and trust.
• Continuity of caregivers promotes trust.

• Calm, confident behavior provides nonverbal reassurance of the caregiver's competence.
• Explaining that frequent assessment is normal dispels fears that the patient's condition is deteriorating.
• Anxiety interferes with memory; repetition enhances learning.
• Orientation increases the predictability of experiences, reducing the need for vigilance (wary watchfulness) and defining the patient's role in care.
• Minor tranquilizers may help calm the patient during periods of physiologic instability but can interfere with psychological adjustment by creating an air of unreality and by disturbing rapid-eye-movement (REM) sleep. A benzodiazepine, such as diazepam (Valium), lorazepam (Ativan), or alprazolam (Xanax), is usually given.
• The patient may feel compelled to keep appointments, conduct business, and so forth, and may need assistance in determining realistic ways to handle such situations. The patient may also need such reassurances as "It's okay to let go" and "People will understand that your health needs come first now."

6. Early detection allows prompt resolution of denial. Denial may be associated with the patient's current grieving process or previous coping pattern.

• Some denial is normal and may be a healthy initial response to an overwhelming situation. Denial that promotes self-destructive behavior, however, requires intervention.
• Confronting denial and forcing the patient to "face facts" prematurely may cause distraught behavior.

• If denial is demonstrated through acting-out behavior, document it, express concern, and promote greater patient control over the environment. Involve the patient in solving the problem, compromising and modifying restrictive aspects of care, and allow choices where appropriate.
• Be alert for topics the patient consistently fails to raise or refuses to discuss when prompted.
• Encourage the patient to focus on remaining abilities.

• Encourage the resumption of full self-care, as physical abilities allow.
• Consult psychiatric resources for further assistance, if needed.

7. Assess the patient daily for indicators of depression. For instance, the patient may express an excessive concern about the condition of his heart; focus on past physical accomplishments; express negative feelings about his body; express feelings of sadness, helplessness, or hopelessness; have a lack of appetite; experience insomnia or excessive sleeping; have psychosomatic complaints (such as headache, neck ache, backache, or stomachache); feel apathetic; have frequent crying episodes (or express a desire to cry); and maintain poor personal hygiene.
• Assess for and document specific psychological, spiritual, and pathophysiologic causes of depression as well as the depressive effects of medications.
• Assess and document the patient's sleep pattern. Promote restful sleep by grouping procedures, minimizing external stimuli, and providing relaxation measures at bedtime.
• Encourage the patient to express feelings and cry, as appropriate.

• Assist with realistic problem solving.

• When the patient expresses pessimistic thoughts, point out hopeful aspects of the situation.

• Encourage physical activity, as appropriate, and document the patient's responses.

• Help the patient identify and implement enjoyable diversions.

• Share information with the patient about his status, as appropriate. Emphasize even small signs of progress.

• These interventions promote a greater sense of control for the patient and are more likely to promote behavioral changes than are confrontation and threats.

• The patient may avoid topics that produce anxiety.

• The patient may be preoccupied with or panicked about perceived losses and may need encouragement to focus on strengths.
• Enforced dependence contributes to low self-esteem.

• A psychiatric clinical specialist, psychiatrist, or social worker can provide additional insight and guidelines for further intervention.

7. Accurate interpretation of cues helps the nurse intervene appropriately. Depression is most likely to result from body-image changes and altered role performance.

• Treatment of depression is most effective when it focuses on specific causes and patient concerns.

• Depression may contribute to sleep disturbances (especially feeling less than fully rested on awakening). Depression also can result from lack of REM sleep.

• Sharing feelings can help the patient identify causes of depression. Because crying is discouraged in American society, the patient may need permission and active encouragement to release pent-up tears.
• The patient who has mental "tunnel vision" may need help identifying and evaluating options.
• Depression may be self-perpetuating. Focusing on hopeful, positive factors may encourage the patient to break the cycle of depressive thoughts.
• Depression is immobilizing, and lack of activity reinforces depression. Physical activity usually elevates mood.
• Boredom may encourage an unhealthy preoccupation with illness. Pleasurable diversions include reading, doing crossword puzzles, listening to music, participating in arts and crafts (which involve the patient directly), and watching television (a passive activity).
• A depressed person tends to focus on negative thoughts. Emphasizing even small gains may help the patient recognize signs of recovery.

NURSING DIAGNOSIS

Altered sexuality pattern related to physical limitations secondary to cardiac ischemia and medications

Nursing priority

Provide information to the patient and spouse (or partner) regarding resumption of sexual activity.

Patient outcome criteria

Within 4 days of admission, the patient will:
• verbalize understanding of sexual activity's effects on cardiovascular function
• list three recommendations for minimizing myocardial stress during sexual activity.

Interventions

1. Obtain a sexual history, including incidence of chest pain during or after foreplay and intercourse.

2. Encourage the patient and spouse or partner to express fears and anxieties. Provide time for joint and individual discussion.

3. Be aware of personal feelings about sexuality; if you feel unable to counsel the couple effectively, make an appropriate referral.

4. Provide printed material about AMI and resumption of sexual activities.

5. Inform the patient that some medications can cause impotence or decrease libido. Encourage discussion with the doctor if such problems occur.

6. Discuss ways to decrease the effects of sexual activity on the cardiovascular system — for instance, through the use of medications.

7. Emphasize that sexual activity should be avoided after large meals or alcohol intake, in extreme temperatures, and under conditions of fatigue or increased stress.

Rationales

1. The history provides baseline information and identifies previous sexual problems.

2. Expressing fears and anxieties may help identify important issues and allow an opportunity to correct misconceptions.

3. Lack of awareness of personal feelings may inhibit sensitivity to sexual concerns. The caregiver's discomfort may keep the couple from expressing their concerns.

4. Accurate information may allay fears and anxieties and dispel misconceptions. Providing printed material will avoid misinterpretation and may increase the likelihood that sexual activity will resume.

5. Awareness of possible pharmacologic causes of sexual dysfunction helps decrease the patient's anxiety. Some commonly used medications with these adverse effects include antihypertensives (such as methyldopa [Aldomet], reserpine [Serpalan], guanethidine [Ismelin], and clonidine [Catapres]); diuretics (such as spironolactone [Aldactone] and hydrochlorothiazide [Esidrix]); and beta blockers (such as propranolol [Inderal] and nadolol [Corgard]).

6. Nitroglycerin or another vasodilator may be prescribed before intercourse to reduce the heart's workload.

7. Digestion of a large meal requires increased visceral blood flow and increases cardiac workload. In low doses, alcohol increases heart rate and cardiac output; in higher doses, alcohol causes myocardial depression and corresponding decreases in heart rate and cardiac output. Stress causes catecholamine release, increasing cardiac workload and oxygen demand.

Cardiovascular disorders

8. As ordered, evaluate activity tolerance by means of low-level treadmill exercise testing or two-flight stair climbing, followed by a resting ECG.

8. These tests provide specific information that can be used in counseling and as a guide for resuming sexual activity. The myocardial oxygen requirement for two-flight stair climbing is similar to that required for sexual activity. Walking on a treadmill at 3 to 4 miles/hour without ECG changes or excessive increases in blood pressure and heart rate indicates that the patient is more than able to meet the cardiac work requirements of sexual activity.

9. Teach symptoms that should be reported to the doctor if they occur during foreplay or intercourse, particularly increased heart rate and respirations persisting 10 minutes after activity, extreme fatigue the day after sexual activity, and chest pain during intercourse.

9. These symptoms indicate that the activity is too strenuous and that the increased myocardial oxygen demand is not being met.

10. Additional individualized interventions: _____

10. Rationales: _____

NURSING DIAGNOSIS

Knowledge deficit (risk factors and lifestyle modifications) related to newly diagnosed, complex disease and to unfamiliar therapy

Nursing priority

Assist in identifying cardiac risk factors and ways to modify lifestyle.

Patient outcome criteria

By the time of discharge, the patient will:
• verbalize knowledge of preventive health measures
• express a willingness to adhere to prescribed therapy
• list personal risk factors
• explain the rationale for dietary modifications
• identify specific ways to reduce salt and fat intake
• have begun a smoking-cessation program, if appropriate
• identify two personal stressors and ways to cope with them
• verbalize understanding of the medication regimen.

Interventions

1. To increase understanding of the disease:

• Describe the basic anatomy and physiology of the heart, how atherosclerosis develops, and the pathophysiology of chest pain and AMI.
• Discuss the symptoms of angina and go over what to do if they occur. Instruct the patient to call the doctor if chest pain is unrelieved by nitroglycerin (see *Medication therapy after myocardial infarction* for guidelines).
• Instruct the patient about medication therapy (see *Medication therapy after myocardial infarction*).

Rationales

1. The patient who understands the disease is more likely to implement therapeutic recommendations.
• Comprehension of AMI's pathophysiology provides a basis for understanding therapy.

• The prepared patient is more likely to react appropriately when angina occurs.

• Accurate information dispels misconceptions, reduces anxiety, and increases patient compliance.

Medication therapy after myocardial infarction

Drug	Action	Administration	Patient teaching	Possible adverse reactions
Vasodilator (such as nitroglycerin or long-acting nitrates)	Primarily dilates peripheral blood vessels, reducing myocardial workload	Can be given by mouth before meals. Sublingual: 1 tablet every 5 minutes up to a maximum of three tablets; if no relief, call doctor. Dermal: patch or cream	Take prophylactically before activities, as prescribed, or at onset of chest pain. Take sitting or lying down to prevent orthostatic hypotension. If no relief after three tablets, do not drive self to hospital: Call an ambulance. Record number of tablets taken. Check expiration date. Carry nitroglycerin at all times. Wear medical alert bracelet. Avoid alcohol, which has additive vasodilating effects. Replace tablets at 4 months. If ointment or patch is prescribed, follow guidelines for correct application, skin care, site rotation, and frequency of change.	Transient headache, flushing, faintness, dizziness, or hypotension
Beta blocker (such as propranolol [Inderal], metoprolol [Lopressor], or atenolol [Tenormin])	Blocks beta-adrenergic receptors to decrease blood pressure, heart rate, and contractility; also decreases automaticity to slow sinus rate, suppress ectopic beats, and improve myocardial oxygenation	Initially given I.V., then by mouth	Monitor pulse rate and blood pressure; report rate under 60 beats/minute and irregular or changed pulse rate. Do not stop drug abruptly—may cause chest pain or myocardial infarction.	Bradycardia, hypotension, dizziness, nausea, vomiting, diarrhea, bronchoconstriction, or impotence
Calcium channel blocker (such as verapamil [Calan], nifedipine [Procardia], diltiazem [Cardizem])	Blocks transport of calcium across cell membrane, resulting in vasodilation and decreased contractility; verapamil also increases refractory period of atrioventricular node and decreases sinoatrial node rate	By mouth, 1 hour before meals or 2 hours after meals	Monitor pulse rate and blood pressure; report pulse rate under 50 beats/minute.	Orthostatic hypotension, bradycardia, headache, dizziness, syncope, nausea, edema, or constipation
Aspirin	Antiplatelet action; decreases aggregation	By mouth daily, or every other day, usually with food	Report ongoing GI upset or burning, dark tarlike stool, or easy bruising or bleeding; avoid aspirin and over-the-counter aspirin-containing products	GI upset and irritation; GI bleeding; increased bruising

Cardiovascular disorders

2. To increase compliance with necessary dietary modifications:
• Explain the rationale for a diet low in calories (if the patient is obese), saturated fats, and salt.

• Take a dietary history, and help the patient identify eating patterns.
• Have the dietitian help the patient plan a diet low in calories, fat, and salt that fits the patient's lifestyle, culture, and socioeconomic status.
• Discuss the role of exercise in reducing weight, blood pressure, and serum lipid levels.
• Stress the need for the entire family to follow the modified diet.

• Give information about antilipemic medications (if prescribed), including action, dosage, scheduling, and adverse effects.
• Provide a list of weight-reduction programs, if appropriate.
• Give printed diet information for home use.

3. To stress the importance of hypertension management:

• Explain the risks of high blood pressure.

• Discuss medication therapy, including action, dosage, scheduling, and adverse effects, such as electrolyte imbalances, sexual dysfunction, orthostatic hypotension, lethargy, headache, flushing, nausea, vomiting, and palpitations.

• Describe ways to reduce salt intake, based on the diet history.

• Emphasize the need for follow-up visits.

2. Obesity, hypertension, and hyperlipidemia greatly increase the risk of coronary heart disease (CHD).
• Reducing weight and salt intake helps decrease blood pressure. Reducing saturated fat intake decreases blood lipid levels and increases the level of high-density lipoproteins (HDLs), which protect against atherosclerosis. Explanations improve patient compliance.
• The dietary history provides baseline information and identifies patterns that need to be changed.
• The patient is more apt to adhere to a prescribed diet if it is acceptable and affordable.

• Exercise decreases blood pressure, weight, triglyceride levels, and anxiety. It also increases HDL levels.
• Obesity, hypertension, and hyperlipidemia have familial tendencies. Compliance is more likely if the patient can share family meals.
• Antilipemics inhibit lipid synthesis. Information about medications will help the patient assume responsibility for self-care.
• Programs can provide motivation and increase compliance.
• Giving the patient printed material will avoid misinterpretation and increase compliance.

3. Hypertension is a significant predictor of CHD: The risk of heart disease increases in direct proportion to increases in systolic and diastolic blood pressure.
• Hypertension increases afterload and makes the heart increase its rate and force of contraction over a period of time. Left ventricular hypertrophy occurs, resulting in an increase in cardiac workload and oxygen demand. Also, a structural change in the coronary arteries accelerates atherosclerosis.
• Noncompliance is a common problem with antihypertensive medication therapy. Lack of symptoms makes it difficult to convince the patient that he has a serious health problem requiring lifelong treatment and follow-up care; adverse effects may further increase noncompliance. The patient should know that the doctor can change medications or dosage if adverse effects occur.
• Reduced salt intake decreases fluid volume and myocardial workload. Although the relationship between salt intake and hypertension is not well understood, a reduced intake in susceptible people is known to decrease blood pressure. Excessive salt intake causes fluid retention, which increases blood volume and peripheral vascular resistance and can lead to elevated blood pressure. Reducing salt intake also enhances the effectiveness of most antihypertensives.
• Follow-up visits provide opportunities to monitor blood pressure, evaluate the patient's response to medication and other forms of treatment, and detect early signs of complications.

• Provide printed information about antihypertensive medications.
• Stress the importance of contacting the doctor promptly if any of these signs or symptoms occur: chest pain, dizziness, headache, blurred vision, edema, nausea, vomiting, nose bleeds, or shortness of breath.

4. To stress the importance of smoking cessation:

• Explain the rationale for quitting.

• Discuss the benefits of not smoking.

• Help the patient identify needs currently met by smoking and explore substitutes.

• Discuss with the patient's spouse, partner, or family the need to assist and support the patient's efforts to stop smoking.
• Provide a list of community smoking-cessation programs.

5. To promote stress reduction:
• Discuss stress and its effect on the cardiovascular system.

• Help the patient identify stressors and learn health-promoting behaviors.

• Identify the characteristics of type A behavior, and review their relationship to AMI.
• Teach stress-reduction techniques, such as progressive relaxation, guided imagery, and aerobic exercise within recommended guidelines. Refer the patient to an outpatient stress-reduction program, as needed, and to a cardiac rehabilitation program, where available.

6. Additional individualized interventions: _____

• Giving the patient printed material helps prevent misinterpretation and increases compliance.
• These symptoms, which indicate increased hypertension, cardiac failure, or both, require therapeutic intervention.

4. Smoking increases the risk of premature heart disease three to six times; smoking cessation markedly decreases that risk.
• Smoking causes vasoconstriction, alters coagulation, and increases carbon monoxide levels and platelet aggregation. Also, nicotine (a stimulant) increases heart rate and the occurrence of arrhythmias.
• Knowledge of these benefits may make smoking cessation during the hospital stay a positive experience. The many benefits include improved senses of smell and taste, improved lung function, increased longevity, monetary savings, and the appreciation of nonsmokers.
• Smoking satisfies complex needs. For a smoking-cessation program to be successful, it must address those needs and ideally meet then with less harmful substitutes.
• Support from others provides motivation and encouragement to stop smoking.

• These programs offer support, motivation, and methods.

5. Stress is an important risk factor for AMI recurrence.
• Tension and psychological stress cause sympathetic stimulation, increasing blood pressure, pulse rate, and cardiac workload.
• The patient needs to learn health-promoting behaviors to reduce stress and improve health. The program should include specific and regular times for recreation and relaxation.
• A correlation exists between type A behavior patterns and the prevalence of CHD.
• Decreasing stress reduces myocardial oxygen demands and increases the patient's feeling of well-being.

6. Rationales: _____

DISCHARGE PLANNING

Discharge checklist
Before discharge, the patient shows evidence of:
❏ absence of chest pain
❏ tolerance of activity without signs of orthostatic hypotension, dyspnea, pain, or shortness of breath
❏ angina controlled by medication

❏ oxygen therapy discontinued for at least 48 hours before discharge
❏ ECG within expected parameters
❏ arrhythmias (if present) controlled by oral medication
❏ I.V. lines discontinued for at least 48 hours before discharge
❏ ability to tolerate ambulation and perform ADLs

Cardiovascular disorders

❏ vital signs within expected parameters for at least 48 hours before discharge
❏ absence of fever and of pulmonary or cardiovascular complications
❏ blood chemistry levels and laboratory values within expected parameters
❏ ability to tolerate diet and any diet restrictions
❏ normal elimination pattern
❏ referral to an outpatient cardiac rehabilitation program (if applicable).

Teaching checklist
Document evidence that the patient and family demonstrate an understanding of:
❏ the disease and its implications
❏ how to measure radial pulse rate accurately
❏ purpose, dosage, administration schedule, and adverse effects requiring medical attention of all discharge medications (usual discharge medications include nitrates, beta blockers, antiarrhythmics, calcium antagonists, antihypertensives, and inotropes)
❏ need for risk-factor modification
❏ prescribed diet
❏ prescribed activity or exercise program
❏ need for regularly scheduled rest periods
❏ signs and symptoms to report to health care providers
❏ need for follow-up care
❏ when to resume sexual activity
❏ availability of community resources
❏ how to contact the doctor.

Documentation checklist
Using outcome criteria as a guide, document:
❏ status on admission
❏ significant changes in status
❏ pertinent laboratory and diagnostic test findings
❏ telemetry monitoring
❏ chest pain
❏ interventions for pain relief
❏ dietary intake
❏ medical therapies, including medications
❏ emotional status
❏ activity tolerance
❏ patient and family teaching
❏ discharge planning.

ASSOCIATED PLANS OF CARE
Dying
Geriatric care
Grieving
Ineffective family coping: Compromised
Ineffective individual coping
Knowledge deficit
Pain

REFERENCES
Black, J., and Matassarin-Jacobs, E., eds. *Medical-Surgical Nursing-Clinical Management for Continuity of Care,* 5th ed. Philadelphia: W.B. Saunders Co., 1997.
Clochesy, J., et al. *Critical Care Nursing,* 2nd ed. Philadelphia: W.B. Saunders Co., 1996.
Kinney, M., and Packa, D., eds. *Andreoli's Comprehensive Cardiac Care,* 8th ed. St. Louis: Mosby–Year Book, Inc., 1996.
Luckmann, J., ed. *Manual of Nursing Care.* Philadelphia: W.B. Saunders Co., 1997.
U.S. Department of Health and Human Services. "Heart Failure: Evaluation and Care of Patients with Left-Ventricular Systolic Dysfunction," *AHCPR Publication No. 94-0612.* Rockville, Md., 1994.
U.S. Department of Health and Human Services. "Unstable Angina: Diagnosis and Management," *AHCPR Publication No. 94-0602.* Rockville, Md., 1994.

Angina pectoris

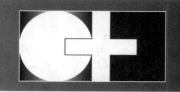

DRG information
DRG 132   Atherosclerosis with Complication or Co-
            morbidity.
            Mean LOS = 3.6
DRG 140   Angina Pectoris.
            Mean LOS = 3.5 days
            Principal diagnoses include:
            • angina pectoris
            • intermediate coronary syndrome
            • acute heart ischemia without acute myo-
              cardial infarction (AMI).

    Additional DRG information: When the underlying cause of angina pectoris is known (for example, arteriosclerotic disease of native coronary arteries or bypassed coronary vessels), arteriosclerosis should be the principal diagnosis.

INTRODUCTION

Definition and time focus
Angina pectoris is transient insufficient coronary blood flow caused by obstruction, constriction, or spasm of the coronary arteries. Angina is characterized by brief episodes of substernal or retrosternal chest pain, commonly felt beneath the middle and upper third of the sternum. Angina pain commonly radiates to the left shoulder, left arm, neck, jaw, or upper abdomen. The cells within the heart muscle do not die in angina as they do in AMI because the ischemia is transient.

    Angina may be classified as stable or unstable (also known as preinfarction or crescendo) angina. The patient also may experience nocturnal angina, which occurs while sleeping, or angina decubitus, which occurs only when the patient is supine, disappearing when the patient stands. Variant (Prinzmetal's) angina occurs at rest, usually during the same time each day, and may be caused by coronary artery spasm. These categories differ according to cause, precipitating factors, descriptions of pain, and electrocardiography (ECG) findings. This plan focuses on the patient admitted for diagnosis and medical management during an initial acute attack.

Etiology and precipitating factors
Classic angina
• Any condition that decreases oxygen delivery by the coronary arteries, increases the cardiac workload, or increases myocardial need for oxygen, such as atherosclerosis, severe aortic stenosis, mitral stenosis or regurgitation, hypotension, hyperthyroidism, marked anemia, ventricular arrhythmias, early menopause, oral contraceptive use, or hypertension
• Classic coronary artery disease risk factors, such as physical or emotional stress, physical inactivity, obesity, smoking, increased serum cholesterol level (above 200 mg/dl),or diabetes mellitus
• Genetic factors, such as hypertension or type II familial hyperlipoproteinemia
Prinzmetal's angina
• Coronary artery spasm

FOCUSED ASSESSMENT GUIDELINES

Nursing history (functional health pattern findings)
Health perception–health management pattern
• Sudden onset of substernal chest pain, pressure, or both; not sharply localized — pain may radiate to arms, shoulders, neck, jaw, upper abdomen; untreated and usually lasts 2 to 5 minutes but not more than 30 minutes
• Pain described as "pressure," "tightness," "aching," or "squeezing"; rest or nitroglycerin provides relief
• Recent emotional stress, heavy exercise, a large meal, or exposure to cold (classic angina)
• Cyclical pain in absence of precipitating factors (Prinzmetal's angina)
• Treatment for hypertension, hyperlipidemia, or diabetes mellitus
• Left ventricular hypertrophy
• Obesity or cigarette smoking
• History of chronic stress, type A behavior, or sedentary lifestyle
• Increased risk among white males over age 40, white females over age 50, or black males or females under age 45 with hypertension
Nutritional-metabolic pattern
• Nausea or indigestion
• Feeling of fullness
• Diet high in calories, cholesterol, saturated fat, and caffeine
• Pain episode after large, heavy meal

Activity-exercise pattern
• Shortness of breath during chest pain episode
• Sedentary lifestyle with only sporadic exercise reported by patient (when stable)
• Transient chest pain episodes during increased activity, alleviated by rest

Sleep-rest pattern
• Sleep disturbance such as chest pain during dreams or when lying flat

Cognitive-perceptual pattern
• Feeling of impending doom during chest pain

Self-perception–self-concept pattern
• Difficulty believing something is physically wrong during pain-free intervals

Role-relationship pattern
• Family history of coronary artery disease
• Perception of responsibility for others
• Involvement in multiple high-stress roles, such as business executive, president of community group, and parent of teenager
• Concern that hospitalization will prevent resumption of occupation and lifestyle

Sexuality-reproductive pattern
• History of oral contraceptive use
• Previous chest pain episodes during sexual activity
• Concern over resuming normal sexual relations

Coping–stress tolerance pattern
• Type A personality traits are typical, such as overreaction to stress, exaggerated sense of urgency, excessive aggressiveness, and competitiveness
• Involvement in high-stress occupation
• Delay in seeking medical attention because chest pain subsided with rest (denial)

Value-belief pattern
• Compulsive striving for achievement

Physical findings
Cardiovascular
• Increased heart rate
• Elevated blood pressure at onset of pain
• Arrhythmias
• S_3 and S_4 gallop
• Transient jugular venous pressure elevations

Pulmonary
• Shortness of breath during chest pain episode
• Abnormal breath sounds, particularly crackles

Neurologic
• Anxiety
• Restlessness

Integumentary
• Cool, clammy skin
• Diaphoresis

Musculoskeletal
• Pained facial expression
• Clenched fists
• Tense, rigid posture

Diagnostic studies
• Cardiac enzyme and isoenzyme levels—no elevations, or minor elevations without pattern characteristic of AMI
• Complete blood count—may show decreased hemoglobin level, hematocrit, and red blood cell level, suggesting anemia-induced angina
• Serum cholesterol, lipid profile—may be elevated, indicating increased risk for coronary artery disease
• Serum electrolyte levels—used to determine imbalances, particularly in potassium levels, that can cause arrhythmias
• Serum drug levels — may indicate toxic or subtherapeutic levels of cardiotonics or antiarrhythmics
• 12-lead ECG—resting ECG usually normal in angina, with ischemic changes during chest pain: Classic angina causes T-wave inversion and ST-segment depression; Prinzmetal's angina causes ST-segment elevation
• Treadmill or exercise test—may reveal chest pain and ECG signs of ischemia on exertion, especially ST-segment and T-wave changes, ventricular arrhythmias, and downsloping or horizontal ST-segment depression
• Myocardial perfusion studies—may show ischemic areas of the myocardium (imaged with thallium 201) as "cold spots"
• Echocardiogram—may illustrate structural problems, such as valvular disease or stenosis
• Cardiac catheterization and angiography—used to visualize blockage and to demonstrate coronary artery patency and ability to adequately perfuse myocardium

Potential complications
• Sudden death
• AMI
• Intractable, unstable, or crescendo angina
• Arrhythmias, especially ventricular arrhythmias
• Decreased ventricular function

CLINICAL SNAPSHOT

ANGINA PECTORIS

Major nursing diagnoses and collaborative problems	Key patient outcomes
Chest pain	Rate chest pain as 0 on a 0 to 10 pain rating scale.
Risk for arrhythmias or AMI	Maintain a normal sinus rhythm on ECG or have arrhythmia controlled by medications.
Activity intolerance	Increase activity according to activity prescription.
Risk for ineffective management of therapeutic regimen (individual)	Indicate specific plans for appropriate lifestyle modifications.
Knowledge deficit (cardiac catheterization, PTCA, or surgery)	Verbalize knowledge of cardiac catheterization, PTCA, or surgery.

NURSING DIAGNOSIS

Chest pain related to myocardial ischemia

Nursing priority

Identify and relieve chest pain.

Patient outcome criteria

- Within 30 minutes of chest pain onset, the patient will:
  - rate pain as 0 on a 0 to 10 pain rating scale
  - display relaxed facial expression and body posture
  - display normal depth and rate of respirations
  - show no restlessness, grimacing, or other signs and symptoms of pain.
- Within 1 hour of chest pain onset, the patient will:
  - display vital signs within normal limits: typically, heart rate, 60 to 100 beats/minute; systolic blood pressure, 90 to 140 mm Hg; and diastolic blood pressure, 50 to 90 mm Hg
  - increase participation in appropriate activities
  - show no life-threatening arrhythmias.

Interventions

1. Assess and document chest pain episodes according to the following criteria: location, duration, quality (on a scale of 0 to 10), causative factors, aggravating factors, alleviating factors, and associated signs and symptoms.

2. Assess the patient for nonverbal signs of chest pain: restlessness; clenched fists; rubbing of the chest, arms, or neck; chest clutching; and facial flushing or grimacing.

Rationales

1. Many conditions can produce chest pain. The nurse must carefully assess the chest pain to differentiate angina from pain related to other causes, such as pleuritic, gastric, or musculoskeletal disorders.

2. Each patient differs in the ways he expresses pain and in the meaning pain has for him. Denial of cardiac symptoms is common initially. An increase or change in the degree or intensity of pain may indicate increasing myocardial ischemia.

3. Obtain a 12-lead ECG immediately during acute chest pain.

3. Resting ECGs are usually normal in myocardial ischemia. Ischemic changes may be noted only during periods of actual chest pain.

4. Administer sublingual nitroglycerin promptly at the onset of pain, as ordered. (The typical protocol is one 0.4-mg tablet every 5 minutes to a maximum of three tablets.) Assess pain relief after 15 to 20 minutes. Evaluate and document blood pressure, pulse rate, respirations, and pain before and after medication administration. If the pain is unrelieved after 15 to 20 minutes (or after three tablets), notify the doctor immediately.

4. Nitrates decrease myocardial oxygen demands by causing vasodilation, which reduces preload and afterload and thus decreases cardiac workload and oxygen consumption. Pain unrelieved by nitroglycerin suggests extended ischemia or myocardial cell death.

5. Implement measures to improve myocardial oxygenation: Institute oxygen therapy, place the patient on bed rest in semi-Fowler's to high-Fowler's position with the shoulders pulled slightly back if possible, and minimize environmental noise and distractions.

5. These measures reduce the heart's oxygen demand and help alleviate chest pain and ensuing anxiety. Chest and head elevation eases lung ventilation. Sitting with the shoulders pulled slightly back allows unrestricted movement of the diaphragm. Decreasing anxiety reduces circulating catecholamine levels, thus decreasing blood pressure and myocardial oxygen consumption.

6. Stay with the patient during chest pain episodes.

6. The presence of a competent caregiver may decrease anxiety and promote patient comfort. It also allows for immediate intervention if problems occur.

7. Monitor and document the therapeutic effects of beta blockers (such as propranolol [Inderal], metoprolol [Lopressor], and nadolol [Corgard]), calcium channel blockers (such as verapamil [Calan] and nifedipine [Procardia]), vasodilators (such as hydralazine [Apresoline] and prazosin [Minipress]), and platelet aggregation inhibitors (such as aspirin, dipyridamole [Persantine], ticlopidine [Ticlid], and sulfinpyrazone [Anturane]). Monitor for bradycardia, hypotension, arrhythmias, signs and symptoms of heart failure, constipation, and exacerbation of ischemic symptoms from medication therapies.

7. Beta blockers block the myocardial response to sympathetic stimulation, thus decreasing oxygen demand and preventing or relieving anginal pain. Beta blockers also decrease heart rate, blood pressure, and myocardial contractility. Calcium channel blockers dilate the coronary arteries, thus decreasing coronary artery spasm and improving myocardial perfusion. Vasodilators that act on the arterial system may lessen the hypertensive response to exertion, which may prevent anginal attacks. Platelet aggregation inhibitors prevent platelet clumping, thus decreasing ischemia from platelet obstruction and decreasing the risk of occlusion of the coronary artery by platelet thrombi.

8. Establish and maintain I.V. access.

8. I.V. access is necessary for possible emergency medication administration or until the differential diagnosis is completed. The usual order is for a saline (or intermittent infusion) lock or dextrose 5% in water to keep the vein open.

9. Additional individualized interventions: _____
_____

9. Rationales: _____
_____

COLLABORATIVE PROBLEM
Risk for arrhythmias or AMI related to myocardial hypoxia and ischemia

Nursing priorities
• Optimize cardiac oxygenation and perfusion.
• Decrease myocardial oxygen demands.

Patient outcome criteria

• Within 30 minutes of chest pain onset, the patient will have stable vital signs: typically, heart rate, 60 to 100 beats/minute; systolic blood pressure, 90 to 140 mm Hg; and diastolic blood pressure, 50 to 90 mm Hg.
• Within 24 hours of admission, the patient will:
 – display a heart rate of 60 to 100 beats/minute
 – maintain a normal sinus rhythm on ECG or have arrhythmias controlled with medications
 – have no syncope, palpitations, or skipped beats
 – have no pulse deficit.
• Within 3 days of admission, the patient will:
 – have no elevation of cardiac enzymes
 – have a resting ECG negative for ST-segment elevation and Q waves
 – have normal blood pressure, pulse, and respirations
 – display clear lungs
 – maintain normal urine output.

Interventions

1. Monitor, report, and document signs and symptoms of arrhythmias, such as irregular apical pulse, pulse deficit, pulse rate below 60 beats/minute or above 100 beats/minute, syncope, dizziness, palpitations, chest "fluttering," or abnormal configurations on rhythm strips or 12-lead ECGs.

2. Administer antiarrhythmic medications, as ordered, noting and documenting their effectiveness and adverse effects.

3. Decrease myocardial oxygen demands by restricting activity (based on the arrhythmia's severity), maintaining oxygen therapy, and providing a calm, supportive environment.

4. Monitor, report, and document signs and symptoms of inadequate tissue perfusion, such as decreasing blood pressure; cool, clammy skin; cyanosis; diminished peripheral pulses; decreased urine output; increased restlessness and agitation; and respiratory distress.

5. Monitor and report signs and symptoms of developing myocardial infarction, such as chest pain lasting longer than 30 minutes and unrelieved by a short-acting nitrate, elevation of creatine kinase isoenzymes, ST-segment elevation, and pathologic Q wave on a 12-lead ECG.

6. Additional individualized interventions: _____

Rationales

1. Ventricular irritability secondary to myocardial ischemia can lead to life-threatening ventricular arrhythmias. Prompt arrhythmia identification is essential for stabilizing the patient's cardiovascular condition.

2. Common antiarrhythmic medications include lidocaine (Xylocaine), procainamide (Pronestyl), quinidine (Cardioquin), bretylium (Bretylol), and atropine. Lidocaine is the medication of choice for dangerous premature ventricular contractions (more than six per minute, sequential, multifocal, or early diastolic), which are common with myocardial hypoxia and ischemia.

3. Activities that increase myocardial oxygen demands may trigger arrhythmias by promoting increased automaticity and impeding electrical conduction through the myocardium.

4. Arrhythmias may lead to decreased cardiac output, resulting in inadequate tissue perfusion. Prompt recognition can help minimize damage and complications.

5. When myocardial ischemia is severe or prolonged, irreversible injury (tissue necrosis) occurs. Chest pain that does not respond to nitroglycerin within 30 minutes strongly suggests AMI.

6. Rationales: _____

Cardiovascular disorders

NURSING DIAGNOSIS

Activity intolerance related to development of chest pain on exertion

Nursing priority

Promote gradual activity restoration, balancing myocardial oxygen supply and demand.

Patient outcome criteria

- Within 24 hours of admission, the patient will:
  - adhere to activity restrictions
  - avoid Valsalva's maneuver.
- Within 48 hours of admission, the patient will:
  - increase activity according to activity prescription
  - have normal bowel elimination without straining.

Interventions

1. Instruct the patient to stop immediately any activity that causes chest pain. If chest pain occurs, maintain the patient in Fowler's position, and administer oxygen therapy, as ordered.

2. Instruct the patient to avoid Valsalva's maneuver by not straining at bowel movements and avoiding heavy lifting.

3. Document activity tolerance, and instruct the patient to increase activity gradually; monitor his pulse rate before and after activity; stop activity when he feels chest pain, fatigue, or marked tachycardia; and pace activities to avoid sudden demands on the heart.

4. Promote physical rest and emotional comfort.

5. Additional individualized interventions: _____
_____

Rationales

1. Pain may be relieved when the patient stops the physical activity that preceded its onset. Changing from a supine to a sitting position decreases central blood volume because blood pools in the extremities, reducing the heart's oxygen demand. Fowler's position allows maximum lung expansion; oxygen therapy decreases the heart's workload.

2. Valsalva's maneuver induces parasympathetic stimulation, which can cause bradycardia and decrease cardiac output, leading to increased ischemia.

3. Physical activity increases myocardial oxygen demand and can cause chest pain. An activity prescription is determined for each patient to maintain cardiovascular stability and prevent fatigue.

4. Fear and anxiety increase sympathetic nervous system responses, increasing myocardial oxygen demand. Relaxation increases the patient's ability to cooperate and participate in therapeutic activities.

5. Rationales: _____
_____

NURSING DIAGNOSIS

Risk for ineffective management of therapeutic regimen (individual) related to complexity of cardiovascular risk factors

Nursing priority

Minimize the development of complications from modifiable risk factors.

Patient outcome criteria

Within 3 days of admission, the patient will:
• verbalize knowledge of diet, lifestyle, and health-habit modifications
• eliminate smoking
• indicate specific plans for appropriate lifestyle modifications.

Interventions

1. Teach the patient about factors that may cause anginal attacks after discharge, such as strenuous exercise, changes in sexual habits or partners, exposure to extreme cold, strong emotions, stress, and smoking. Teach ways to decrease the risk of chest pain, such as using sublingual nitroglycerin prophylactically; monitoring pulse rate before and after activity; and stopping activity if chest pain, dyspnea, or palpitations ensue. Use the patient's experience as a basis for teaching. Document the patient's response to teaching.

2. Instruct the patient to maintain a diet low in saturated fat and cholesterol and to achieve ideal body weight. Document current height and weight.

3. Provide six light meals per day rather than three heavy ones.

4. Tell the patient to avoid foods and beverages high in caffeine.

5. Discourage cigarette smoking.

6. Instruct the patient in stress-reduction techniques.

7. Start the patient on a cardiovascular fitness regimen when approved by the doctor.

8. Additional individualized interventions: _____

Rationale

1. Teaching the patient ways to avoid anginal attacks will decrease anxiety and may increase participation in self-care. Controlling risk factors may minimize the disease's progress and lessen its impact on the patient's lifestyle. Relating teaching to the patient's experience capitalizes on the principle that adults learn better when material is relevant to their needs and integrated with prior experience.

2. Exacerbation of coronary artery disease may be related to increased dietary intake of cholesterol, which contributes to increased plaque formation and narrowing of coronary arteries. Obesity elevates blood pressure and places a greater demand on the heart.

3. Although subject to debate, large meals are believed to require an increased blood supply to the GI tract for digestion, increasing myocardial work. An anginal attack may be caused by a large, heavy meal. Small meals prevent epigastric fullness or indigestion that might be mistaken for anginal pain. In addition, small meals place less demand on myocardial oxygen consumption during digestion, reducing the risk of angina.

4. Coffee, tea, chocolate, and colas contain varying amounts of caffeine, a myocardial stimulant that increases myocardial oxygen consumption.

5. Nicotine causes vasoconstriction, is a cardiac stimulant, and reduces oxygen availability.

6. Unresolved anxiety and a stressful lifestyle increase myocardial oxygen demands, so they are risk factors for cardiovascular disease. By decreasing stress levels, the patient may decrease circulating catecholamine levels and thus decrease blood pressure and overall myocardial oxygen consumption.

7. Supervised exercise enhances cardiovascular fitness while minimizing the chance of another cardiac event.

8. Rationales: _____

Cardiovascular disorders

NURSING DIAGNOSIS

Knowledge deficit (cardiac catheterization, PTCA, or surgery) related to unfamiliarity with diagnostic or therapeutic procedures

Nursing priority

Teach the patient about upcoming procedures.

Patient outcome criteria

Before cardiac catheterization, PTCA, or surgery, the patient will, on request, verbalize knowledge of the procedure, risks and benefits, preprocedure and postprocedure care, possible complications, and postprocedure activity restrictions.

Interventions

1. See the "Knowledge deficit" plan, page 72.

2. Explain hospital protocol for cardiac catheterization to the patient and family. Include procedural steps, risks and benefits, preprocedure and postprocedure care, possible complications, and postprocedure activity restrictions.

3. Based on the results of cardiac catheterization, the patient may require percutaneous transluminal coronary angioplasty (also know as balloon angioplasty), coronary artery bypass graft surgery (CABG), or one of the more recently developed procedures, such as laser angioplasty, atherectomy, or intracoronary stenting. Assess the patient's level of anxiety, fear, and understanding of the planned procedure. Begin patient teaching as soon as appropriate and clarify any misconceptions.

Rationales

1. The "Knowledge deficit" plan provides helpful interventions for patient teaching. This plan contains additional specific information for the patient undergoing an invasive diagnostic or corrective procedure.

2. Currently, the most accurate way to determine the extent of coronary artery disease is through cardiac catheterization. A special catheter is inserted through a distal vein or artery (usually the femoral) and advanced into the right or left chambers of the heart. During angiography, radiopaque contrast dye is injected through the catheter to trace coronary artery blood flow. Teaching the patient about the procedure will decrease anxiety and enhance cooperation.

3. When the coronary arteries are significantly blocked, when the patient develops intractable angina, or when medical management no longer controls anginal attacks, the doctor usually recommends further interventions. Balloon angioplasty is an invasive, nonsurgical procedure in which a balloon-equipped catheter is passed under fluoroscopy into a partially blocked coronary artery. When the balloon is inflated, it stretches the artery, opening the lumen and relieving the blockage. Laser angioplasty uses either argon or neodymium-yttrium-aluminum garnet radiation to vaporize atherosclerotic plaque in the coronary artery. Atherectomy uses a catheter with a rotating cutting blade to scrape off and remove the atherosclerotic plaque and reopen the blocked coronary artery. In intracoronary stenting, a mesh tube is inserted into the artery to hold it open. CABG is indicated for the patient who either does not respond to balloon angioplasty or has more significant blockage. CABG uses a saphenous or mammary vein graft to bypass one or more blocked coronary arteries. The patient will be more receptive to teaching about the procedure if anxieties and fears are addressed first. Adequate preparation helps ensure cooperation.

4. For the patient undergoing CABG, see the "Cardiac surgery" plan, page 376.

5. For the patient undergoing PTCA, see the "Percutaneous transluminal coronary angioplasty" plan, page 441.

6. Additional individualized interventions: _____

_____

4. This plan specifies nursing care for the patient undergoing cardiac surgery.

5. This plan contains detailed information on this procedure.

6. Rationales: _____

_____

DISCHARGE PLANNING

Discharge checklist

Before discharge, the patient shows evidence of:
- ❏ absence of chest pain, or angina controlled by oral or sublingual medications
- ❏ stable vital signs for at least 48 hours
- ❏ absence of fever and pulmonary or cardiovascular complications
- ❏ ability to perform activities of daily living and ambulate without chest pain
- ❏ blood chemistry studies within expected parameters
- ❏ normal sinus rhythm or arrhythmias controlled with drugs
- ❏ ability to tolerate activity at prescribed levels
- ❏ ability to tolerate diet and dietary restrictions
- ❏ normal voiding and bowel movements
- ❏ ability to list activities that may cause angina
- ❏ referral to outpatient cardiac programs (if applicable).

Teaching checklist

Document evidence that the patient and family demonstrate an understanding of:
- ❏ angina's pathophysiology and implications
- ❏ recommended modifications of risk factors (smoking, stress, obesity, lack of exercise, diet high in fat and cholesterol)
- ❏ prescribed dietary modifications
- ❏ resumption of daily activities
- ❏ purpose, dosage, administration schedule, adverse effects, and toxic effects of all discharge medications
- ❏ common emotional adjustments
- ❏ community resources for lifestyle and risk-factor modification, such as stress- and weight-reduction groups, cardiac-exercise programs, and smoking-cessation programs
- ❏ signs and symptoms indicating need for medical attention, such as chest pain unrelieved by three nitroglycerin tablets within 20 minutes, new pattern of anginal attacks, palpitations or skipped beats, syncope, dyspnea, or diaphoresis
- ❏ date, time, and location of follow-up appointments
- ❏ how to contact the doctor.

Documentation checklist

Using outcome criteria as a guide, document:
- ❏ clinical status on admission
- ❏ significant changes in status
- ❏ chest pain episodes — precipitating, aggravating, and alleviating factors
- ❏ pertinent laboratory and diagnostic test results
- ❏ pain-relief measures
- ❏ oxygen therapy
- ❏ I.V. therapy
- ❏ use of protocols
- ❏ nutritional intake
- ❏ response to medications
- ❏ emotional response to illness; coping skills
- ❏ activity tolerance
- ❏ patient and family teaching
- ❏ discharge planning.

ASSOCIATED PLANS OF CARE

Acute MI: Critical care unit
Acute MI: Telemetry unit
Cardiac surgery
Ineffective individual coping
Knowledge deficit
Pain
Percutaneous transluminal coronary angioplasty

REFERENCES

Braunwald, E., ed. *Heart Disease, Vol. 2,* 5th ed. Philadelphia: W.B. Saunders Co., 1997.

Clochesy, J., et al. *Critical Care Nursing,* 2nd ed. Philadelphia: W.B. Saunders Co., 1996.

Gardner, E., et al. "Intracoronary Stent Update: Focus on Patient Education," *Critical Care Nurse* 16(2):65-75, April 1996.

Hayes, D. "Understanding Coronary Atherectomy," *AJN* 96(12):38-45, December 1996.

Kinney, M., et al. *Comprehensive Cardiac Care,* 8th ed. St. Louis: Mosby–Year Book, Inc., 1996.

Lazzara, D., and Sellergen, C. "Chest Pain Emergencies," *Nursing 96* 26(11):42-51, November 1996.

O'Donnell, L. "Complications of MI," *AJN* 96(9):25-31, September 1996.

Polaski, A., and Tatro, S. *Luckmann's Core Principles of Medical-Surgical Nursing.* Philadelphia: W.B. Saunders Co., 1996.

Smeltzer, S., and Bare, B. *Brunner and Suddarth's Textbook of Medical Surgical Nursing,* 8th ed. Philadelphia: Lippincott-Raven Pubs., 1996.

Woods, S., et al. *Cardiac Nursing,* 3rd ed. Philadelphia: Lippincott-Raven Pubs., 1995.

Cardiac surgery

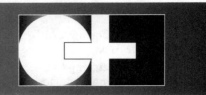

DRG information

Cardiac surgery may be classified under several DRGs, depending on the principal operating room procedure and whether cardiac catheterization was performed.

DRG 104   Cardiac Valve Procedure with Pump and with Cardiac Catheterization.
Mean LOS = 14.6 days
Principal operating room procedures include:
- open-heart mitral, aortic, pulmonary, or tricuspid valvuloplasty without replacement
- replacement of mitral, aortic, pulmonary, or tricuspid valve with biologic or mechanical prosthesis
- implantation or replacement of automatic cardioverter defibrillator, total system.

DRG 105   Cardiac Valve Procedure with Pump and without Cardiac Catheterization.
Mean LOS = 11.0 days

DRG 106   Coronary Bypass with Cardiac Catheterization.
Mean LOS = 11.7 days
Principal operating room procedures include aortocoronary bypass of one or more coronary arteries.

DRG 107   Coronary Bypass without Cardiac Catheterization.
Mean LOS = 8.8 days

DRG 108   Other Cardiothoracic or Vascular Procedures with Pump.
Mean LOS = 12.6 days
Principal operating room procedures include:
- open-chest coronary angioplasty to remove artery obstruction, with pump
- biopsy of pericardium
- cardiotomy
- excision of aneurysm or other heart lesion
- open-chest cardiac massage
- procedures on structures adjacent to heart valves
- pericardiotomy
- pericardiectomy
- repair of atrial or ventricular septa with tissue graft or prosthetic device
- total repair of certain congenital cardiac anomalies
- closed cardiac valvotomy.

Additional DRG information: Hundreds of additional vascular operating room procedures also are classified under DRG 108. The above list details only coronary procedures. Other cardiac surgical procedures not addressed in the following plan (such as permanent pacemaker insertion) have still other DRG numbers.

INTRODUCTION

Definition and time focus

Cardiac surgery can correct many structural and physiologic problems. During surgery, the surgical team stops the heart and collapses the lungs; cardiopulmonary bypass (CPB) maintains systemic perfusion and gas exchange during this time. CPB causes some predictable physiologic and hemodynamic changes during the early postoperative period; more recently developed, minimally invasive techniques may not require the use of CPB. Nursing care during this period focuses on assessing for anticipated changes, maintaining organ function, preventing complications, and providing emotional support to the patient and family. This clinical plan focuses on the patient in the critical care unit during the first 12 to 24 hours after coronary artery bypass graft (CABG) or valve repair or replacement. It assumes that a cardiovascular nurse specialist or a similarly qualified person provided preoperative teaching and that a formal postoperative teaching and rehabilitation program has been planned. (For teaching guidelines on cardiovascular health promotion, risk factor modification, and rehabilitation, see Kinney et al., 1996.)

Etiology and precipitating factors

- Severe coronary artery disease of one or more vessels, particularly the left anterior descending coronary artery
- Acute myocardial infarction (AMI), especially if complicated by cardiogenic shock, infarct extension, uncontrollable failure, papillary muscle rupture, or septal rupture
- Unstable or crescendo angina pectoris
- Previous bypass grafting with recurrent angina or angiographic evidence of graft closure
- Ventricular aneurysm
- Valvular stenosis or insufficiency with hemodynamic compromise

Focused assessment guidelines

Nursing history (functional health pattern findings)

Health perception–health management pattern
• History of acute or chronic coronary artery disease or valvular dysfunction
• Existence of a condition refractory to less invasive therapies such as medication. *Note:* Remaining health pattern findings are those of the underlying disease; refer to "Acute MI: Critical care unit," page 338, "Acute MI: Telemetry unit," page 355, "Heart failure," page 420, and "Cardiogenic shock," page 392, for examples.

Physical findings
Because the preoperative physical findings are those of the underlying disorder, they are not repeated here; instead, this section presents typical postoperative findings.

General appearance
• Increase of 2 to 18 lb (1 to 8 kg) above preoperative weight

Cardiovascular
• Blood pressure variable
• Arrhythmias
• Heart sounds variable; may have early flow murmur or audible clicking after valve replacement
• Chest tube drainage variable
• Peripheral pulses usually equal bilaterally
• Slow capillary refill

Pulmonary
• Variable rate and depth, depending on ventilator settings
• Breath sounds usually diminished in left base
• Crackles or gurgles
• Persistent atelectasis

Neurologic
• Level of consciousness variable (patient usually can be awakened)
• Confusion
• Disorientation

Integumentary
• Cool skin
• Dry skin
• Pallor
• Generalized edema
• Serosanguineous oozing from incisions

Gastrointestinal
• Absent bowel sounds
• Nasogastric tube drainage variable
• Pain may be increased or paralytic ileus prolonged with use of abdominal arterial bypass conduits (gastroepiploic or inferior epigastric arteries)

Renal
• Polyuria

Diagnostic studies
The following tests are performed before surgery for baseline data. Common early postoperative findings include:
• hemoglobin level and hematocrit — decreased because of hemodilution; hematocrit is usually about 25% or lower
• coagulation panel — may reveal prolonged prothrombin time/international normalized ratio (PT/INR) and activated partial thromboplastin time (APTT), reflecting intraoperative heparinization, and decreased platelet level, reflecting history of antiplatelet medication (aspirin, dipyridamole [Persantine]), and platelet destruction by CPB equipment, especially roller and filtration unit
• serum glucose level — elevated from stress-induced glycogenolysis and decreased insulin production
• serum electrolyte levels — vary, depending on preoperative status, replacement during surgery, fluid shifts, and other factors
• cardiac isoenzymes — may be elevated if AMI is present (slight elevation normal after surgery)
• 12-lead electrocardiography (ECG), resting and stress — findings vary, depending on preexisting disorders (such as AMI), acid-base status, electrolyte status, or medications
• chest X-ray — reveals cardiac size, mediastinal position, and pulmonary status; postoperatively, it confirms endotracheal tube, chest tube, central venous pressure line, and pulmonary artery (PA) catheter placement
• preoperative cardiac catheterization and coronary arteriography — reveal critical coronary artery occlusion, poor or normal left ventricular function, or hemodynamically significant valve stenosis or insufficiency (manifested by elevated left ventricular end-diastolic and pulmonary pressures, cardiac index (CI) less than 2.5 L/minute/m^2, tight valve areas, increased valvular gradients, occlusive lesions, or shunts)
• echocardiography — compares preoperative and postoperative function (especially for valve repairs)

Potential complications
• Cardiogenic shock
• Hypovolemic shock
• AMI
• Heart failure
• Endocarditis
• Graft occlusion
• Thromboembolism
• Atelectasis
• Cerebrovascular accident
• Hemorrhage
• Renal failure

Cardiovascular disorders

Cardiac surgery

Major nursing diagnoses and collaborative problems	Key patient outcomes
Risk for low cardiac output syndrome	Maintain cardiac output and other hemodynamic values within desired limits: typically, cardiac output, 4 to 6 L/minute; PA systolic, 20 to 30 mm Hg; PA diastolic, 10 to 15 mm Hg; and pulmonary artery wedge pressure (PAWP), 4 to 12 mm Hg.
Risk for endocarditis or other infection	Display no signs or symptoms of endocarditis.
Interstitial edema	Return to preoperative weight.
Hypovolemia	Experience no signs or symptoms of excessive bleeding.
Risk for hypoxemia	Maintain arterial blood gas (ABG) levels within normal limits: typically, pH, 7.35 to 7.45; partial pressure of arterial carbon dioxide ($Paco_2$), 35 to 45 mm Hg; HCO_3^-, 22 to 26 mEq/L; partial pressure of arterial oxygen (Pao_2), 80 to 100 mm Hg; arterial oxygen saturation (Sao_2), greater than 90%.
Risk for sensory-perceptual alteration	Display a level of mentation within the patient's normal limits.
Knowledge deficit (postoperative care)	Verbalize questions and concerns (patient and family).

Collaborative problem

Risk for low cardiac output syndrome related to hypothermia, excessive vasoconstriction, myocardial depression, arrhythmias, cardiac tamponade, or graft occlusion

Nursing priority

Maintain optimal cardiac output.

Patient outcome criteria

Within 24 hours after surgery, the patient will:
• have a mean arterial pressure (MAP) of 70 to 90 mm Hg
• have a regular supraventricular rhythm with a ventricular rate of 60 to 100 beats/minute (normal sinus rhythm is ideal)
• have peripheral pulses bilaterally equal and full
• have warm, dry arms and legs
• have a temperature of 98.6° to 101° F (37° to 38.3° C)
• display no signs of cardiac tamponade
• maintain right atrial pressure (RAP), pulmonary artery diastolic pressure (PADP), pulmonary artery systolic pressure (PASP), and PAWP within desired limits: typically, RAP, 2 to 6 mm Hg; PASP, 20 to 30 mm Hg; PADP, 10 to 15 mm Hg; and PAWP, 4 to 12 mm Hg.

Interventions

1. Monitor blood pressure continuously with an arterial catheter. Maintain MAP within desired limits; determine limits in consultation with the surgeon. In general, report a systolic blood pressure less than 80 mm Hg or greater than 150 mm Hg, a diastolic blood pressure greater than 100 mm Hg, or a MAP less than 60 mm Hg or greater than 90 mm Hg. Report any value abnormal for the patient.

2. Measure cardiac output (CO), as ordered, typically every hour until normal and then every 2 hours. If not using a computerized monitoring system, calculate CI by dividing CO by body surface area (obtain body surface area value from a chart or nomogram); calculate SVR by subtracting RAP from MAP and dividing the result by CO. Follow the trend of CI and SVR values, comparing them with normal ranges and previous values.

3. Monitor PADP continuously until stable. Monitor RAP, PASP, and PAWP, as ordered, typically every hour until stable. Compare with preoperative values and desired limits; determine limits in consultation with the surgeon.

4. Provide constant ECG monitoring. Observe for indicators of possible myocardial damage (such as ST-segment deviation, T-wave inversion, or pathologic Q waves) and for preexisting arrhythmias, new ventricular arrhythmias, and arrhythmias associated with the specific surgical procedure (see *Arrhythmias associated with cardiac surgery,* page 383). If present, assess for underlying causes, treat according to standing orders (usually with medications or temporary pacing), and document their occurrence.

5. Monitor for indicators of myocardial ischemia caused by graft occlusion: ECG changes, angina pectoris (must be differentiated from sternal incision pain), or cardiac enzymes (creatine kinase-MB [CK-MB]) elevated above expected postoperative level (consult surgeon for acceptable level). Expect slight elevations 4 to 7 hours after CABG and higher elevations after valve replacement or repair than after CABG. Immediately report an elevation greater than 50 U/L or any other significant changes.

Rationales

1. Low cardiac output syndrome, a potential postoperative problem, may result from preexisting abnormalities or the stress of surgery. Arterial monitoring provides the most direct and accurate blood pressure measurements. Because perfusion is directly related to blood pressure, maintaining optimal MAP ensures adequate organ perfusion. Hypothermia, used during surgery to lower metabolic demand and protect organs from ischemia, induces vasoconstriction, which increases systemic vascular resistance (SVR) and the risk of hypertension. Stress triggers the release of catecholamines, antidiuretic hormone (ADH), and aldosterone, which also may produce hypertension. Persistent hypertension can cause leaking or rupture of suture lines. The causes of hypotension are discussed later in this plan.

2. CO may drop in the postoperative period because of decreased preload from a fluid volume deficit (discussed below), increased afterload from elevated SVR, or impaired contractility (discussed below). Any of these factors may cause the already stressed heart to fail. CO measurements and CI calculations provide objective data on the adequacy of output, and SVR values show the degree of resistance to ventricular ejection. Increased afterload and hypertension both increase myocardial workload. SVR values typically are elevated in the early postoperative period. SVR and blood pressure values should return to normal gradually as rewarming occurs.

3. PADP is a useful indirect indicator of left ventricular performance. RAP reflects central venous pressure; PASP, the force of right ventricular ejection; and PAWP, left ventricular function. These values provide objective data for assessing the patient's fluid volume, cardiovascular function, and pulmonary status.

4. Constant monitoring provides early warning of possible myocardial damage or arrhythmias. Underlying causes may include pain, anxiety, hypokalemia, preexisting conditions (such as chronic atrial fibrillation), hypoxemia, and volume depletion. Arrhythmias usually respond to standard protocols such as lidocaine (Xylocaine) administration for premature ventricular beats. In many patients, pacing wires are inserted during surgery and brought out through the chest wall. If necessary, they can be connected to a pacemaker to provide a stable rhythm until cardiac irritability or the underlying cause resolves.

5. Early graft occlusion results from thrombus formation caused by poor runoff, graft injury, or faulty anastomosis. Late graft closure is related to subintimal thickening of the graft. The normal stress of surgery causes a slight CK-MB elevation a few hours after CABG. An elevation greater than 50 U/L after 18 to 30 hours may indicate a perioperative AMI. Higher CK-MB levels are normal after valve surgery because of greater tissue trauma. (*Text continues on page 383.*)

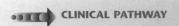

Managing CABG without catheterization

Level of care	Preop	Day of surgery
Intermediate progression toward discharge	• Open heart preop workup complete • Informed consent complete • Patient/family state expected LOS and postop activities via clinical path (CP)	• Patient extubated w/adequate oxygenation • Patient hemodynamically stable • Patient verbalizes pain relief on I.V. meds • Patient/family state path expectations for DOS
Consults	• Cardiac surgery • Cardiology • Anesthesia	
Tests and diagnostic studies	• CBC with differential and platelet count, Chem 7, PT • 12-lead ECG • Blood bank per protocol	• On admission: –12-lead ECG (hold if 100% paced); portable CXR – CPK with ISO, CBC/plt, Chem panel, ABG • PRN labs: Coag panel for chest tube bleeding, additional Hct and K+ (per protocol) • Repeat ABG: on CPAP, post-extubation per protocol
Medications, I.V.s, blood work	• Discontinue Coumadin 3 days prior to admission • Discontinue aspirin 5 days prior to admission • Preop meds per attending MD	• Analgesics (I.V.) as ordered • Antibiotics as ordered • Titrate vasoactive meds as ordered • K+ replacement per protocol • Aspirin as ordered • Volume replacement per protocol; discontinue after extubation • Autotransfuse MCT drainage per protocol
Treatments and interventions	• Betadine shower • Preop weight and height on chart • Shave/prep	• Monitor VS/hemody q 30 min × 2 → q 1 hr • Systemic rewarming to 36° C • Pacemaker as ordered • Chest tube @ –20 cm, Foley to gravity • I&O q 1 hr • Wean FIO_2 to 40% using SaO_2, $S\bar{v}O_2$, and $ETCO_2$; initiate early extubation protocol if criteria met • Post extubation: –Titrate O_2 via FM/NC; keep SaO_2 >92% –ICS q 1 hr when awake
Activity and mobility	• Ad lib	• Once hemodynamically stable: –Turn q 2 hr and elevate HOB 30° • Post extubation: –Dangle at side of bed
Nutrition	• N.P.O. after midnight	• N.P.O.: ice chips postextubation
Patient and family education	• Review preop teaching video/booklet • Review CABG Recovery Path w/patient family • Ask if patient has or wants information about advance directives	• Reorient patient upon reawakening • Instruct patient about: –CPAP/extubation and ICS procedures –Request pain meds p.r.n. • Instruct family/significant others about: –ICU routines, patient care updates
Case management and discharge planning	• Identify support systems and home situation	• Review clinical path expectations with patient/family

Postop day 1	Postop day 2	Postop day 3
• Patient extubated w/adequate oxygen on nasal O₂; is hemodynamically stable w/o I.V. meds; tolerates ambulation to chair b.i.d.; responds to p.r.n. diuretic therapy; obtains pain relief on oral medication; states CP expectations for POD1	• Oxygenation WNL for patient on RA • Cardiac rhythm/BP WNL for patient • Patient tolerates ambulation in room/hall b.i.d.; verbalizes pain relief on oral medication; tolerates oral intake without causing nausea/vomiting; states CP expectations for POD2	• Oxygenation WNL for patient • Cardiac rhythm/BP WNL for patient • Patient tolerates ambulation in hall >5 min t.i.d.; verbalizes pain relief on oral medication; tolerates oral intake without nausea/vomiting; states CP expectations for POD3
• Cardiac Rehabilitation	• Cardiac Rehabilitation	• Case management (PRN for DC planning needs)
• a.m.: – Chem panel, CBC/platelets, CPK w/ISO – 12-lead ECG – portable CXR	• Electrolytes, CBC	• K+ p.r.n. for continued diuresis
• Analgesics: start oral meds; I.V. for breakthru pain • Discontinue vasoactive meds as tolerated • Diuresis/K+ replacement p.r.n. wt > preop • Enteric aspirin P.O., multivitamin, stool softener daily • Restart needed preop meds • Start heparin lock prior to D/C central line	• Analgesics: Offer meds q 3-4hrs • Diuresis/K+ p.r.n. for wt > preop • Multivitamin daily • Enteric aspirin daily • Stool softener daily • Preop meds as needed • Peripheral heparin lock	• Analgesics: Offer meds q 3-4 hr • Diuresis/K+ p.r.n. for wt > preop • Multivitamin daily • Enteric aspirin daily • Stool softener daily • Preop meds as needed • Peripheral heparin lock
• Discontinue CVP/PA/A line per protocol • Monitor VS q 1-2 hr → q 4 hr posttransfer • Weight in a.m. • I&O q 1 hr → qs after transfer • Change dressings per protocol • TED hose to lower extremities • Discontinue NG tube and Foley (unless diuresing) • O₂ via NC/RA to maintain Sao₂ >92% • ICS q 1 hr when awake • Cap pacer wires if unused • Discontinue chest tube per protocol	• Monitor VS q 4 hr • Weight in a.m. • I&O q shift • Discontinue dressings if not oozing • TED stockings • Discontinue O₂ if Sao₂ >92% on RA • ICS q 1-2 hr when awake • Cap pacer wires if unused • Discontinue remaining Foley or chest tube	• Monitor VS q 4 hr • Weight in a.m. • I&O q shift • Incisions open to air; wash daily • TED stockings • Discontinue O₂ if Sao₂ >92% on RA • Encourage independent ICS use • Discontinue pacer wires if unused • Discontinue telemetry if no arrhythmias
• Nursing: – Out of bed for meals with left extremity elevated – Bath/grooming at bedside and BRP w/assist	• Out of bed t.i.d. for meals with left extremity elevated • Bath/grooming with assist • Bathroom privileges with assist • Assist to ambulate b.i.d., distance as tolerated	• Out of bed t.i.d. for meals with left extremity elevated • Bath/grooming unassisted • Bathroom privileges unassisted • Ambulate t.i.d. >5 min, distance as tolerated • assess for needed assistance
• Clear liquid, advance as tolerated	• LSF as tolerated (diabetic diet p.r.n.)	• LSF (diabetic diet p.r.n.)
• ICU: – Prepare patient/family for transfer – Reinforce pulmonary care – Provide patient care updates • Telemetry: – Introduce patient education materials – Begin cardiac rehab instruction	• Reinforce pulmonary care • Provide patient care progress updates • Review patient education booklets and videotapes • Cardiac rehab	• Reinforce pulmonary care • Provide patient care progress updates • Review patient education booklets and videotapes • Cardiac rehab
• Review clinical path expectations with patient/family	• Review clinical path expectations with patient and family • Assess home care situation and available resources	• Review clinical path expectations with patient and family • Notify case manager if home care or placement anticipated

Cardiovascular disorders

Managing CABG without catheterization *(continued)*

Level of care	Postop day 4	Postop day 5
Intermediate progression toward discharge	• Cardiac & respiratory status stable off telemetry • Patient tolerates ambulation in hall >5 min q.i.d. • Patient verbalizes pain relief on oral medication • Dietary intake and elimination normal for patient • Patient/family finalize plans for discharge per CP	• Cardiac & respiratory status stable • Independent with activity and ADLs • Scripts for home meds including pain Rx written • Dietary intake and elimination normal for patient • Patient/family education for home care completed
Consults	• Case management (p.r.n. for discharge planning needs)	• Outpatient cardiac rehab • SNF/Visiting Nurses p.r.n.
Tests and diagnostic studies	• PA and lateral chest X-ray prior to discharge • PRN for abnormal pulmonary exam	
Medications, I.V.s, blood work	• Doctor to write pain med prescription • Multivitamin daily • Enteric aspirin daily • Stool softener daily • Doctor to write discharge prescriptions • Discontinue heparin lock if off telemetry/I.V. med	• Home with discharge meds and instructions, continue after discharge: –multivitamin daily –enteric aspirin daily –stool softener as needed • Discontinue heparin lock
Treatments and interventions	• Monitor VS q8hrs • Weight in a.m. • Discontinue I&O • Incisions open to air; wash daily • TED stockings • Discontinue O_2 if Sao_2 >92% on RA • Encourage independent ICS use • Discontinue remaining pacer wires • Discontinue remaining telemetry	• VS q shift prior to discharge • Weight in a.m. • Discontinue chest tube sutures and cover sites w/steri-strips; TED stockings on • Continue ICS use at home
Activity and mobility	• OOB tid (minimum of 4 hrs/day) • Independent self-are • Independent ambulation at slow pace q.i.d.: increase distance as tolerated • Up/Down stairs w/assist	• Home transport arranged • Walk 5-10 min, 4-5 × day unassisted • Up/down stairs • Independent with ADLs
Nutrition	• LSF (diabetic diet p.r.n.)	• LSF (diabetic diet p.r.n.)
Patient and family education	• Continue rehab education and begin home instructions • Review appropriate diet with patient and family, including meal preparer at home	• Home care instructions given and reviewed with patient and family • Teaching booklet sent home w/patient • Home exercise plan reviewed • Discharge meds reviewed w/patient and family
Case management and discharge planning	• Finalize plans for discharge with patient/family per CP • Consult case manager if home care or placement pending	• Discharge orders written in a.m. • Outpatient follow-up with doctors' offices scheduled

Arrhythmias associated with cardiac surgery

Certain cardiac procedures place the patient at risk for arrhythmias related to the underlying pathophysiology of the disorder or to the procedure itself.

Surgery	Possible ECG changes	Significance
Coronary artery bypass grafting	• ST-segment (ischemic) changes	• Related to myocardial ischemia, residual air in the coronary arteries, or an occluded graft
	• Ventricular ectopy	• Related to surgical manipulation, ischemia, or hypoxemia
	• New Q waves	• Indicate perioperative myocardial infarction
	• Atrial fibrillation	• Related to surgical manipulation of the atrium
Aortic valve replacement	• ST-segment (ischemic) changes	• Related to embolization of valve debris (such as calcium or tissue)
	• Left bundle-branch block	• Related to left ventricular hypertrophy
Mitral valve repair or replacement	• Atrial fibrillation	• Related to preoperative left atrial enlargement
	• ST-segment (ischemic) changes	• Related to embolization of valve debris
	• Heart block	• Usually associated with valve disease
Tricuspid valve repair or replacement	• Heart block	• Related to surgical manipulation of the bundle of His

Cardiovascular disorders

6. Monitor level of consciousness; apical pulse rate; skin color, warmth, and temperature; peripheral pulse rates; and urine output every 15 minutes to 1 hour until normal and stable. Report abnormalities to the surgeon promptly.

7. Monitor core body temperature continuously (via bladder or rectal probe or PA catheter) or every hour (with a rectal thermometer) until normal and then every 4 hours.

8. If body temperature is low, cover the patient with warmed blankets until it returns to normal. As the temperature rises, monitor for signs of fluid volume deficit. If the temperature rises above 101° F (38.3° C), assess for underlying causes; administer antipyretics such as acetaminophen (Tylenol), as ordered; and use a hypothermia blanket, as ordered, for high fever. Do not give the patient aspirin.

6. These parameters indicate the adequacy of central and peripheral perfusion. Abnormalities may signal the development of several complications and warrant medical evaluation.

7. The patient's body temperature is usually low after surgery from induced hypothermia and heat loss from the open chest. The temperature then typically rises somewhat above normal (because of the inflammatory response after surgery) and gradually returns to normal in approximately 3 days or less.

8. Gradual rewarming gives the heart time to adjust to the expanded vascular bed as vasoconstriction lessens. As body temperature rises, vasodilation may unmask a previously hidden fluid volume deficit. Temperatures above 101° F suggest a cause other than the normal inflammatory response, such as dehydration or sepsis. Because fever increases cardiac workload, reducing the patient's body temperature will reduce the stress on his heart. Aspirin usually is avoided because it decreases platelet aggregation and may contribute to bleeding.

9. Administer vasodilators, such as sodium nitroprusside (Nipride), as ordered. Refer to the "Heart failure" plan, page 420, for details regarding administration. Correlate vasodilator administration with body temperature and rewarming.

9. Vasodilators control dilation of the vascular bed and reduce hypertension. Because afterload reduction lessens resistance to ventricular ejection, it also lessens myocardial workload. The "Heart failure" plan covers vasodilator administration. Vasodilators, fever, and rewarming all cause vasodilation, so their combined effects must be taken into account to avoid excessive vascular bed expansion.

10. Administer positive inotropic agents, as ordered, typically dopamine (Intropin) or dobutamine (Dobutrex). Refer to the "Heart failure" plan, page 420, for details on administration.

10. Mild, transient depression of contractility is common because of hypothermia and myocardial edema. Dopamine improves contractility through its beta$_1$-adrenergic effects but may cause tachycardia and arrhythmias. Dobutamine also increases contractility but is less likely to cause tachycardia and arrhythmias. An inotrope may be used for the first 12 to 24 hours in an uncomplicated recovery; in cases of preoperative myocardial depression or intraoperative infarction, it may be used for a longer period. The "Heart failure" plan covers administration of inotropic agents.

11. Monitor for indicators of cardiac tamponade, even when mediastinal chest tubes are draining freely. Observe for rapid hypotension, marked central venous pressure elevation, neck vein distention, muffled heart sounds, paradoxical pulse, or decreased QRS voltage on ECG; also observe for a sudden decrease in chest tube drainage.

11. Cardiac tamponade results when blood or fluid accumulates in the pericardium. Clotted chest tubes can produce tamponade; however, patent tubes do not necessarily reduce the risk of tamponade because fluid can accumulate in areas not drained by the tubes. Tamponade can rapidly interfere with ventricular filling and CO.

12. If tamponade with cardiac decompensation occurs, immediately notify the doctor. Assemble supplies and equipment for open chest massage and maintain fluid replacement.

12. Cardiac decompensation is a medical emergency. Opening the chest allows evacuation of blood or fluid while cardiac massage perfuses the brain and other vital organs.

13. Additional individualized interventions: _____

13. Rationales: _____

COLLABORATIVE PROBLEM

Risk for endocarditis or other infection related to perioperative contamination

Nursing priorities
• Promote wound healing.
• Prevent nosocomial infection.

Patient outcome criterion

After surgery, the patient will display no signs or symptoms of endocarditis or any other infection.

Interventions

1. Identify conditions that place the patient at risk for endocarditis or another infection: previous endocarditis; valvular heart disease; rheumatic heart disease; Marfan syndrome; congenital heart disease; presence of foreign bodies, such as a pacemaker or prosthetic valves or grafts; or presence of invasive lines or a urinary catheter.

Rationales

1. These conditions increase the risk of endocarditis and other infections.

2. Administer prophylactic antibiotics, as ordered.

3. Use strict aseptic technique during wound care and dressing changes.

4. Assess for signs and symptoms of endocarditis or another infection: elevated temperature; elevated white blood cell count; red, tender, or draining incision; changes in urine color, odor, clarity, or amount; malaise, weakness, diaphoresis, or easy fatigability; new murmur after valve surgery; or positive wound, blood, or urine cultures.

5. If signs and symptoms of endocarditis or another infection develop, notify the doctor promptly. Obtain wound cultures and administer antibiotics as ordered. See the "Surgery" plan, page 103, for further details.

6. Additional individualized interventions: _____
_____

2. Antibiotics are routinely administered for 24 hours after surgery (until invasive lines are removed).

3. Aseptic technique prevents cross-contamination and transmission of bacteria to incision sites.

4. These are common findings for endocarditis or another infection.

5. Because of the high mortality rate associated with postoperative endocarditis and other infections, prompt, aggressive treatment is indicated. Cultures help to identify specific sites of infection, and antibiotics fight the organism involved. The "Surgery" plan contains general information on infection control.

6. Rationales: _____
_____

COLLABORATIVE PROBLEM

Interstitial edema related to hemodilution, excessive fluid replacement, and stress adaptation syndrome

Nursing priority

Restore normal fluid volume.

Patient outcome criterion

Within 24 hours after surgery, the patient will have a 24-hour fluid output greater than intake.

Interventions

1. Expect signs and symptoms of interstitial fluid overload; monitor degree of overload and speed of resolution:

• Monitor generalized edema and tissue turgor.

• Monitor the patient's weight daily. Compare with preoperative and previous day's values.

• Monitor for neck vein distention and S_3 heart sounds; if present, notify the doctor.

Rationales

1. During CPB, hemodilution is achieved with I.V. crystalloid solution. Because hemodilution decreases blood viscosity and peripheral vascular resistance, it minimizes microcirculatory sludging, thus protecting organs from ischemia during surgery.
• Hemodilution lowers plasma oncotic pressure, which allows fluid to shift from the vascular to interstitial spaces, producing generalized edema.
• Weight gain from hemodilution may approach 18 lb (8 kg). Daily weight comparisons provide objective evidence of the degree of fluid retention and the speed with which fluid is mobilized and excreted after surgery.
• Although most of the excess fluid is in the interstitial space, central blood volume may increase. These findings may reflect such an increase or may result from cardiac dysfunction (described below) and require medical evaluation.

Cardiovascular disorders

2. Administer I.V. solutions, as ordered. Unless the patient is hypovolemic, limit fluid intake from all sources to 100 ml/hour or less.

2. Early hypovolemia is common, and I.V. fluids may be needed initially to compensate for interstitial fluid shifts, to increase plasma volume, and to optimize preload. Hemodilution during bypass pushes fluids to the interstitial space; however, this fluid shifts back into the vascular space between the second and fifth postoperative day. This, in addition to the large number of I.V. lines, can cause fluid overload unless total intake is monitored.

3. Monitor intake and output measurements, usually hourly on the first postoperative day and then every 8 hours.

3. The stress reaction triggered by surgery causes the release of ADH, the secretion of aldosterone, and sympathetic stimulation of the kidneys, all of which result in fluid retention. Monitoring intake and output records provides objective data on which to gauge fluid retention and base therapeutic decisions.

4. Administer I.V. diuretics, such as furosemide (Lasix), if ordered.

4. Aggressive diuresis may be used to eliminate excess interstitial fluid.

5. Monitor for signs and symptoms of electrolyte imbalance, particularly hypokalemia. See Appendix C, Fluid and Electrolyte Imbalances, for details. If hypokalemia is present:
• observe for arrhythmias
• add potassium to I.V. fluids, as ordered
• monitor serum levels closely, typically every 4 hours in the first 24 hours
• monitor for hyperkalemia.

5. Hypokalemia is common after surgery. It may result from preoperative diuretic administration, hemodilution, or postoperative diuresis. Supplemental I.V. potassium usually is necessary. Close monitoring of serum potassium level is essential to guide replacement and to avoid hyperkalemia from potassium administration and potassium release from hemolyzed blood cells.

6. Additional individualized interventions: _____

6. Rationales: _____

COLLABORATIVE PROBLEM

Hypovolemia related to bleeding or diuresis

Nursing priority

Maintain normal fluid volume.

Patient outcome criteria

• Within 3 hours after surgery, the patient will have chest tube drainage of less than 200 ml/hour and declining.
• Within 4 hours after surgery, the patient will have a urine output greater than 0.5 ml/kg/hour.
• Within 24 hours after surgery, the patient will:
  – display minimal drainage from incisions
  – have vital signs within normal limits: typically, heart rate, 60 to 100 beats/minute; systolic blood pressure, 90 to 140 mm Hg; and diastolic blood pressure, 50 to 90 mm Hg
  – show hemoglobin levels, hematocrit, PT/INR, APTT, and platelet levels returning to normal
  – experience no signs or symptoms of excessive bleeding.

Interventions

1. Monitor PT/INR, APTT, and platelet counts, as ordered. Consult the surgeon about reportable values, particularly prolonged PT/INR, prolonged APTT, low platelet level, or other coagulation deficiencies. Note any use of aprotinin during surgery, and monitor activated clotting time

2. Monitor hemoglobin levels and hematocrit. Consult the surgeon about reportable values, particularly declining ones. Have blood and blood products available.

3. Measure and document chest tube drainage. If drainage is constant or increasing, bright red, or exceeds 200 ml/hour, notify the surgeon. Also assess dressings for signs of drainage.

4. Maintain autotransfusion system, if used.

5. Observe for other signs of bleeding, such as excessive oozing from incisions, petechiae, and ecchymoses. If hemoglobin levels, hematocrit, or coagulation values are abnormal, test urine, feces, and vomitus for occult blood.

6. Monitor vital signs for tachycardia or hypotension.

7. Administer protamine sulfate, platelet concentrate, fresh frozen plasma, or red blood cells, as ordered.

Rationales

1. Blood loss has multiple causes during and after surgery. During surgery, some blood loss is inevitable, and heparin is used to prevent clotting in the extracorporeal circuit. This anticoagulation is reversed with protamine sulfate, but inadequate reversal may result in bleeding. Heparin rebound also may occur from the release of heparin stored in the tissues. The CPB equipment, especially the roller pump and filtration unit, damages platelets. Finally, the patient may have a history of antiplatelet medication use. All of these factors may alter normal coagulation, so abnormal values are expected after surgery. Aprotinin is used to reduce bleeding during surgery by decreasing clotting time, as measured by activated clotting time. Reportable values vary among surgeons.

2. Hemoglobin levels and hematocrit are low after surgery as a result of hemodilution. As postoperative diuresis occurs, the values should return to normal. Failure to do so implies continued bleeding. Usually, the patient will be transfused when the hematocrit drops below 25%.

3. Postoperative bleeding includes oozing of incisions, suture disruption, and chest tube drainage. Excessive or bloody drainage warrants surgical exploration.

4. Conserving the patient's blood avoids allergic reactions and the risks associated with blood from a blood bank.

5. Although laboratory tests provide valuable objective data of bleeding tendencies, they are no substitute for astute clinical assessment. Signs of frank or occult bleeding may be the first indication of abnormal coagulation.

6. Vital sign changes are usually nonspecific, relatively late indicators of bleeding; however, tachycardia is a compensatory response to hypovolemia, and hypotension can reflect significant blood loss or cardiac depression.

7. Protamine sulfate treats anticoagulation from inadequate heparin reversal. Platelet concentrate restores missing platelets, and fresh frozen plasma replaces platelets, clotting factors, and volume. Red blood cells provide hemoglobin.

Cardiovascular disorders

8. Monitor for urine output greater than 1 L/hour for the first 4 hours or increasing output thereafter. Also observe for urine output less than 0.5 ml/kg/hour. Monitor specific gravity every 2 hours for the first 24 hours. Report abnormal urine output and specific gravity values. Monitor serum glucose levels, as ordered. Correlate glucose values with urine output.

9. Additional individualized interventions: _____

_____

8. Mannitol, commonly administered during surgery to maintain CO, produces osmotic diuresis. Diuretics may also be administered after surgery to eliminate retained fluid. Urine output may be as much as 1 L/hour for the first 4 hours. Oliguria with high specific gravity may indicate hypovolemia, whereas oliguria with low specific gravity may indicate renal damage. Hyperglycemia results from stress-induced glycogenolysis and decreased insulin production, producing osmotic diuresis. Correlating glucose levels with urine output may identify hyperglycemia as the cause of excessive diuresis.

9. Rationales: _____

_____

COLLABORATIVE PROBLEM

Risk for hypoxemia related to alveolar collapse, increased pulmonary shunt, increased secretions, capillary leak, or pain

Nursing priority

Maintain oxygenation and ventilation.

Patient outcome criteria

Within 24 hours after surgery, the patient will:
• have a spontaneous respiratory rate of 12 to 24 breaths/minute
• maintain ABG levels within normal limits: typically, pH, 7.35 to 7.45; $Paco_2$, 35 to 45 mm Hg; HCO_3^-, 22 to 26 mEq/L; Po_2, 80 to 100 mm Hg; Sao_2, greater than 90%.

Interventions

1. Monitor pulmonary status and provide conscientious postoperative care to prevent pulmonary complications. Refer to the "Surgery" plan, page 103.

2. Monitor mixed venous oxygen saturation ($S\overline{v}o_2$) through a fiber-optic PA catheter to assess oxygen supply-demand balance.

Rationales

1. Many factors place the patient undergoing cardiac surgery at risk for impaired gas exchange. Lung collapse during CPB results in atelectasis, and reduced surfactant production makes the lungs more difficult to expand after surgery. Hemodilution promotes interstitial fluid accumulation. CPB also activates complement and kinin systems, creating a capillary leak syndrome. Microcirculatory clotting increases pulmonary shunt. Anesthesia irritates the airways, increasing production of secretions, and depressed ciliary action impairs secretion removal. After surgery, lingering anesthetic effects and narcotics cause respiratory depression, and pain and splinting reduce lung expansion. As a result, close observation of pulmonary status and aggressive pulmonary hygiene are important after surgery. The "Surgery" plan details the nursing measures used to achieve these goals.

2. Fiber-optic oximetry allows continuous monitoring of oxygen balance.

3. Monitor Sao_2 with pulse oximetry.

4. Provide care according to the "Mechanical ventilation" plan, page 283.

5. Additional individualized interventions: _____

3. Monitoring Sao_2 alerts the clinician to potential hypoxemia.

4. The patient undergoing cardiac surgery usually is mechanically ventilated for several hours after surgery to reexpand collapsed alveoli and decrease cardiopulmonary workload. The "Mechanical ventilation" plan details appropriate nursing care.

5. Rationales: _____

NURSING DIAGNOSIS

Risk for sensory-perceptual alteration related to sensory overload or deprivation from unit environment, anesthesia, cerebral ischemia or infarction, or prolonged CPB

Nursing priority

Optimize sensory-perceptual processing.

Patient outcome criterion

Within 48 hours, the patient will be awake, alert, and oriented, if so preoperatively.

Interventions

1. Implement measures in the "Sensory-perceptual alteration" plan, page 96, as appropriate.

2. For the first 12 to 24 hours postoperatively, assess for indicators of sensory-perceptual alteration every 4 hours while the patient is awake or more frequently if the patient is disoriented. If present, reassure the patient and family that these alterations are usually transient, continue implementing the measures in the "Sensory-perceptual alteration" plan, and arrange for early transfer to a telemetry unit, if the patient's condition allows.

3. Assess for indicators of cerebral ischemia or infarction: change in mental status or level of consciousness (compare with preoperative status), motor weakness, hemiparesis, change in pupil size, or slurred speech.

4. Additional individualized interventions: _____

Rationales

1. The "Sensory-perceptual alteration" plan describes interventions to reduce or eliminate sensory/perceptual dysfunction in any acutely ill patient.

2. Sensory-perceptual alteration may result from many factors in the critical care setting, including anxiety, sensory deprivation or overload, and sleep disruption; personality also plays a role. In addition, prolonged CPB, decreased CO, hypotension, and vasoactive medications can contribute to disorientation. It usually resolves by the time the patient is transferred from the unit. Measures in the "Sensory-perceptual alteration" plan are helpful, as is early transfer to a less hectic environment.

3. Cerebrovascular accident is one of the most serious complications of open-heart surgery. It is more common in older patients, who are more likely to have atherosclerotic disease of the aorta or carotid and vertebral arteries. Possible causes include carotid disease and emboli from the heart (thrombi, calcium fragments from diseased valves, or air remaining in the cardiac chambers).

4. Rationales: _____

Cardiovascular disorders

NURSING DIAGNOSIS

Knowledge deficit (postoperative care) related to complex, unfamiliar therapeutic regimen

Nursing priority

Educate the patient and family about the early postoperative period, as needed.

Patient outcome criterion

Throughout the unit stay, the patient (after extubation) and family will verbalize questions and concerns.

Interventions

1. Refer to the "Knowledge deficit" plan, page 72.

2. Ascertain whether preoperative teaching was provided. If the patient and family did receive preoperative teaching, reinforce explanations, as necessary. If emergency surgery was performed, provide explanations as the opportunity arises.

3. Encourage questions.

4. Begin discharge planning. Evaluate needs for discharge teaching. Explain to the family that detailed discharge education will be done after discharge to the telemetry unit. Document and communicate needs to staff members on the new unit when the patient is transferred.

5. Tailor education to the nature of the patient's surgery. For CABG, teach about risk factors; lifestyle modifications related to diet, exercise, and stress; and antiplatelet medication regimen (aspirin and dipyridamole). For valve repair or replacement, teach about signs and symptoms of infection, antibiotic prophylaxis before invasive procedures, anticoagulation medication (in patients with mechanical valves or history of chronic atrial fibrillation), signs and symptoms of valve failure, and signs and symptoms of thromboembolism.

6. Additional individualized interventions: _____
_____

Rationales

1. The "Knowledge deficit" plan contains general information on assessing and meeting learning needs.

2. Before elective cardiac surgery, the patient and family usually receive extensive teaching. However, anxiety may limit retention of information and, for the patient, pain and medications affecting consciousness further limit recall. In emergency cardiac surgery, preoperative preparation is minimal, so teaching should be done as the opportunity arises.

3. Questions provide an opportunity for dealing with initial concerns, clarifying misconceptions, and eliminating knowledge gaps.

4. Discharge planning is most effective when awareness of its importance pervades all phases of the hospital stay. Detailed discharge education is most appropriate after the patient is physiologically stable. Early identification of needs sets the stage for later teaching; documentation and communication enhance continuity of care.

5. An adult is more likely to learn information specific to personal needs. Coronary artery disease is progressive; knowledge of risk factors and potential lifestyle changes may retard disease progression. Antiplatelet medications decrease risk of thrombus formation and may maintain graft patency. The success of valve repair or replacement depends on both patient-related and prosthetic valve-related factors.

6. Rationales: _____
_____

DISCHARGE PLANNING

Discharge checklist

Upon the patient's discharge, documentation shows evidence of:

- ❏ blood pressure within normal limits for 12 hours without I.V. drugs
- ❏ normal sinus rhythm or acceptable variant for 12 hours without I.V. antiarrhythmic drugs
- ❏ CI, SVR, and other hemodynamic values within desired limits
- ❏ removal of PA catheter, arterial line, chest tubes, and indwelling urinary catheter
- ❏ spontaneous ventilation within normal limits for at least 12 hours
- ❏ ABG, hemoglobin, and electrolyte levels; hematocrit; and coagulation panel within normal limits.

Teaching checklist

Document evidence that the patient and family demonstrate an understanding of:

- ❏ signs and symptoms of prosthetic valve malfunction, if appropriate
- ❏ need for follow-up laboratory studies (PT/INR if taking anticoagulants)
- ❏ signs and symptoms of endocarditis
- ❏ surgical procedure
- ❏ anticipated postoperative course
- ❏ rationale for interventions
- ❏ common emotional reactions
- ❏ medications (warfarin [Coumadin], antiplatelet therapy)
- ❏ discharge planning.

Documentation checklist

Using outcome criteria as a guide, document:

- ❏ clinical status on admission
- ❏ significant changes in status
- ❏ pertinent diagnostic test findings
- ❏ CI, SVR, and other hemodynamic parameters
- ❏ diuretic, inotropic, or vasodilator administration
- ❏ routine postoperative care
- ❏ emotional response
- ❏ fluid and electrolyte status
- ❏ pulmonary care
- ❏ complications, if any, and related interventions
- ❏ patient and family teaching
- ❏ discharge planning.

ASSOCIATED PLANS OF CARE

Cardiogenic shock
Heart failure
Grieving
Hypovolemic shock
Impaired physical mobility
Ineffective coping
Knowledge deficit
Mechanical ventilation
Pain
Sensory-perceptual alteration
Surgery

REFERENCES

Berne, R., and Levy, M. *Cardiovascular Physiology*, 7th ed. St. Louis: Mosby–Year Book, Inc., 1996.

Ginsberg, R.J., et al. *The 1997 Year Book of Thoracic and Cardiovascular Surgery*. St. Louis: Mosby–Year Book, Inc.,1997.

Kinney, M., et al. *Comprehensive Cardiac Care*, 8th ed. St. Louis: Mosby–Year Book, Inc., 1996.

Ott, R.A., et al. *Managed Care and the Cardiac Patient*. St. Louis: Mosby–Year Book, Inc., 1995.

Piwnica, A., and Westaby, S. *Surgery for Acquired Aortic Valve Disease*. St. Louis: Mosby–Year Book, Inc., 1996.

Seifert, P.C. "Advances in Myocardial Protection," *Journal of Cardiovascular Nursing* (in press).

Seifert, P.C. *Cardiac Surgery*. St. Louis: Mosby–Year Book, Inc., 1994.

Seifert, P. "Cardiac Surgery," in *Alexander's Care of the Patient in Surgery*, 11th ed. Edited by Meeker, M., and Rothrock, J. St. Louis: Mosby–Year Book, Inc. (in press).

Cardiovascular disorders

Cardiogenic shock

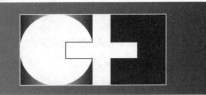

DRG information
DRG 121   Circulatory Disorders with Acute Myocardial Infarction and Major Complications, Discharged Alive.
           Mean LOS = 7.8 days
DRG 123   Circulatory Disorders with Acute Myocardial Infarction, Expired.
           Mean LOS = 4.7 days
DRG 127   Heart Failure and Shock.
           Mean LOS = 6.2 days

Acute Myocardial Infarction (AMI) takes precedence in DRG grouping, so a patient in cardiogenic shock will usually fall into DRG 121 or 123. Should the cardiogenic shock patient receive operating room treatment, that procedure (such as percutaneous transluminal coronary angioplasty, coronary artery bypass graft, or pacemaker insertion) would determine the DRG.

INTRODUCTION

Definition and time focus
Cardiogenic shock occurs when the heart fails to produce a cardiac output (CO) sufficient to meet metabolic demands, producing hypotension, vasoconstriction, and peripheral hypoperfusion. A major problem in critical care, cardiogenic shock usually results from a loss of 40% or more of functional myocardium, although it may be due to heart failure from any cause. Signs and symptoms result from the backup of fluid behind the failing ventricle (backward failure) or from decreased stroke volume (forward failure). When CO is significantly decreased and physiologic compensatory mechanisms are ineffective, cardiogenic shock results. Because cardiogenic shock is associated with an 80% mortality rate, this plan focuses on the patient with acute heart failure and the interventions necessary to prevent or decrease the complications of cardiogenic shock.

Etiology and precipitating factors
• Increased preload, such as in severe valvular stenosis or insufficiency, ruptured interventricular septum, papillary muscle rupture, or rupture of chordae tendineae
• Decreased myocardial contractility, such as in massive AMI, cardiomyopathy, ventricular aneurysm, myocarditis, or cardiac tamponade
• Increased afterload, such as in systemic hypertension, pulmonary hypertension, or massive pulmonary embolism

• Severely abnormal heart rate, such as in severe tachycardia, bradycardia, or conduction disturbances

FOCUSED ASSESSMENT GUIDELINES

Nursing history (functional health pattern findings)
Health perception–health management pattern
• Fatigue, weakness, or shortness of breath
• Failure to comply with low-salt diet or medication regimen, if under treatment for chronic heart failure
Nutritional-metabolic pattern
• Anorexia, nausea, or vomiting
Activity-exercise pattern
• Dyspnea on exertion or at rest
• Palpitations
• Dizziness or fainting (syncope)
Sleep-rest pattern
• Insomnia, paroxysmal nocturnal dyspnea, or nocturia
• Use of several pillows to elevate head (orthopnea)
Coping–stress tolerance pattern
• Marked anxiety, apprehension, or sense of impending doom

Physical findings
Cardiovascular
• Hypotension
• Tachycardia or other arrhythmias
• S_3 or S_4 heart sounds or both
• Weak or irregular pulses
• Decreased pulse pressure
Pulmonary
• Crackles, usually bibasilar
• Air hunger
• Hyperventilation
Gastrointestinal
• Decreased bowel sounds
Integumentary
• Cyanosis
• Diaphoresis
• Pallor
Renal
• Oliguria

Diagnostic studies
• Arterial blood gas (ABG) analysis — may reveal respiratory alkalosis (early stage) or hypoxemia and respiratory acidosis (late stage)

• Serum digitalis glycoside level — may reveal subtherapeutic range
• 12-lead electrocardiography (ECG) — reveals sinus tachycardia, frequent premature ventricular contractions, atrial fibrillation, or other arrhythmias
• Pulmonary artery pressures — reveal elevated pulmonary artery diastolic pressure and pulmonary artery wedge pressure (PAWP)
• Chest X-ray — reveals pulmonary infiltrates or cardiac enlargement

• Complete blood count — may reveal dilutional changes
• Gated blood pool imaging — may reveal reduced ejection fraction
• Echocardiography — may reveal chamber enlargement, ventricular dyskinesia, or valvular abnormalities

Potential complications
• Cardiac arrest
• Pulmonary edema
• Fluid and electrolyte imbalance

CLINICAL SNAPSHOT

CARDIOGENIC SHOCK

Major nursing diagnoses and collaborative problems	Key patient outcomes
Risk for hypoxemia	Display ABGs within acceptable range for individual.
Inadequate cardiac output	Manifest cardiac index greater than 2.2 L/minute/m² and PAWP less than 18 mm Hg.
Activity intolerance	Show no activity intolerance during self-care activities.

Cardiovascular disorders

COLLABORATIVE PROBLEM

Risk for hypoxemia related to pulmonary congestion, decreased systemic perfusion, or both

Nursing priority

Maintain optimal gas exchange.

Patient outcome criteria

Within 3 days, the patient will:
• show no signs or symptoms of hypoxemia
• have ABG levels within acceptable range for individual
• display a level of consciousness (LOC) similar to or better than that before admission
• be free from restlessness, irritability, confusion, and somnolence
• have a PAWP within normal limits
• have lungs essentially clear to auscultation
• have an acceptable chest X-ray.

Interventions

1. Monitor pulmonary status as needed, typically every 15 minutes until stable and then every 2 hours. Observe for:

• crackles, gurgles, wheezes, dyspnea, orthopnea, shallow respirations, accessory muscle use, cough, or S_3 or S_4 heart sounds

• tachypnea, cyanosis, restlessness, irritability, confusion, somnolence, or slow or irregular respirations

• elevated PAWP.

2. Monitor ABG values as ordered, typically every 4 hours until stable or as needed. Obtain chest X-rays, as ordered.

3. If pulmonary congestion is present, place the patient in semi- or high-Fowler's position.

4. Administer supplemental oxygen, as ordered, typically by nasal cannula at 6 L/minute.

5. Monitor peripheral oxygen saturation (SpO_2) continuously by pulse oximetry.

Rationales

1. Baseline and ongoing monitoring of pulmonary status provides data to guide priorities and interventions.

• Left ventricular end-diastolic pressure (LVEDP) most directly determines the strength of left ventricular contraction and the resulting adequacy of stroke volume. As the heart fails, decreased ventricular compliance raises LVEDP beyond the optimal stretch of myocardial fibers and, according to the Frank-Starling mechanism, optimal contractility. The elevated LVEDP is transferred to the pulmonary capillary bed and increases hydrostatic pressure in pulmonary capillaries, producing pulmonary congestion (backward failure). Elevated pulmonary capillary hydrostatic pressure causes fluid to shift across capillary walls into the interstitium and eventually into the alveoli. Crackles may result when pulmonary interstitial fluids compress the alveoli or when fluid accumulates in them. Gurgles and wheezes indicate fluid accumulation in the large airways. Interstitial edema produces dyspnea, shallow respirations, and accessory muscle use, while alveolar edema produces orthopnea and cough. S_3 and S_4 heart sounds reflect decreased ventricular compliance or volume overload.

• Fluid-filled alveoli cannot oxygenate the capillary blood flowing past them, producing a pulmonary shunt and hypoxemia. Tachypnea is an early compensatory mechanism for hypoxemia, while cyanosis is a late sign. Decreased CO (forward failure) produces cerebral ischemia, resulting in an altered LOC. Ischemia of medullary and pontine respiratory centers causes altered breathing patterns.

• PAWP correlates with the degree of pulmonary congestion. Usually, a PAWP of 18 to 20 mm Hg correlates with the onset of congestion, 20 to 25 mm Hg with moderate congestion, 25 to 30 mm Hg with severe congestion, and more than 30 mm Hg with pulmonary edema.

2. ABG values provide evidence of hypoxemia and accompanying respiratory and metabolic acidosis, while chest X-rays provide evidence of pulmonary fluid infiltration.

3. Elevating the head of the bed improves diaphragmatic excursion, facilitating ventilation.

4. Supplemental oxygen helps saturate hemoglobin, raising arterial oxygen content and improving oxygen transport. A cannula is less likely to produce the feelings of suffocation that an air-hungry patient experiences with a mask.

5. Continuous pulse oximetry is a safe, noninvasive method for early detection of hypoxemia. SpO_2 reflects arterial oxygen saturation (SaO_2). SpO_2 trends provide important information about the effects of therapy on SaO_2.

6. Suction as needed.

7. Assist with insertion of a pulmonary artery (PA) catheter, as ordered. A fiberoptic PA catheter for continuous venous oxygen saturation ($S\bar{v}o_2$) monitoring may be indicated.

8. Monitor PA pressure every hour, PAWP every 2 hours, and cardiac index (CI) every 4 hours, or as indicated by patient status and institutional standards (CI equals CO divided by body surface area, determined from a DuBois nomogram). Note both individual values and trends.

9. Determine the presence and severity of heart failure according to PAWP and CI. (See *Classification of heart failure by hemodynamic subsets,* page 396.)

10. Anticipate medical therapy. Administer therapy as ordered.

• For patients with no signs of failure (Subset I), observe for its development.

• For patients with pulmonary congestion only (Subset II), administer medication, as ordered.

• If blood pressure is normal, administer diuretics, typically furosemide (Lasix) or bumetanide (Bumex). Document effectiveness and monitor for adverse effects, especially excessive diuresis or electrolyte imbalances (particularly hypokalemia).

• If blood pressure is elevated, administer vasodilators, typically:

6. In heart failure, the lungs may produce sputum so rapidly that the patient cannot clear it spontaneously. Prompt suctioning not only improves gas exchange but also lessens the patient's anxiety.

7. The multiple therapies used in cardiogenic shock can affect the determinants of CO. Interpreting these effects based on clinical signs alone can be confusing. A PA catheter allows objective CO measurement and PAWP monitoring. PAWP monitoring is particularly important because it provides the most direct bedside indication of left ventricular function. In mitral valve or pulmonary disease, however, PAWP does not necessarily reflect left ventricular performance. $S\bar{v}o_2$ monitoring continuously reflects CO and helps determine if the body's oxygen supply can meet tissue oxygen demand. Evaluation of tissue oxygenation provides early identification of hemodynamic changes and immediate evaluation of therapeutic interventions.

8. Objective measurements of PAWP and PA diastolic pressure provide a means of evaluating left ventricular filling pressure, while CI indicates adequacy of CO. CI takes the patient's size into consideration, so it provides a more precise indication of the adequacy of CO than does CO alone. Isolated values provide immediate data, while trends indicate whether cardiogenic shock is resolving or worsening over time.

9. Classification by hemodynamic status is used to distinguish disease patterns and plan therapy.

10. Anticipation of therapy allows systematic planning and adequate patient preparation. Goals and therapeutic measures follow logically from the characteristics of each subset.
• Patients in Subset I have acceptable PAWP and CI. However, because critically ill patients decompensate rapidly, continuing observation is warranted.
• Patients in Subset II have an elevated PAWP and good CI. Drug therapy is designed to decrease circulating blood volume, thereby relieving pulmonary congestion.
• Diuretics reduce preload rapidly and effectively, improving ventricular compliance. Because diuretics block renal fluid reabsorption and increase renal tubular flow, potassium excretion increases. Excessive diuresis and hypokalemia are exaggerations of diuretics' therapeutic effects.
• When blood pressure is high enough to cause pulmonary congestion and reduce oxygenation, the patient's condition is too serious to wait for the action of diuretics. By expanding the vascular bed, vasodilators allow the vessels to accommodate the same amount of fluid in a larger area, thus lowering pressure. Vasodilation also lowers preload, which improves left ventricular performance.

Cardiovascular disorders

–venodilators, such as nitroglycerin or morphine. Observe for and report adverse effects, especially hypotension and, with morphine, respiratory depression.

–arteriolar dilators, such as sodium nitroprusside (Nipride). Monitor for and report adverse effects, especially hypotension, signs of hypoxemia, and thiocyanate and cyanide toxicity.

11. If administering morphine sulfate, observe for and report hypotension, nausea, and vomiting. Titrate doses to achieve desired effects without causing respiratory depression.

–Nitroglycerin produces significant venodilation and relatively little arteriolar dilation. Used primarily for its venodilating properties, nitroglycerin decreases preload and pulmonary congestion. It also redistributes myocardial blood flow, causing greater dilation of large vessels than of small ones, thus increasing flow to ischemic areas. As myocardial perfusion improves, more efficient contraction increases CO. Morphine, the drug of choice in pulmonary edema, also induces vasodilation. The resulting reductions in preload, afterload, and myocardial work all improve CO. Morphine also induces euphoria, particularly helpful in lessening the severe anxiety present with pulmonary edema.

–Although sodium nitroprusside dilates both arteriolar and venous beds, it is used primarily for its arteriolar effects. Because sodium nitroprusside reduces afterload, systolic emptying is improved and myocardial work decreases. As a result, it produces a greater increase in CO than nitroglycerin. Hypotension results from excessive dosage. Hypoxemia may result from reversal of pulmonary vasoconstriction, a compensatory mechanism that shunts blood to better-aerated alveoli. Thiocyanate and cyanide toxicity may develop from accumulation of toxic metabolites with long-term use, high dosage, or impaired liver or renal perfusion.

11. Morphine decreases pain, anxiety, catecholamine stimulation, and tachypnea, lessening the work of breathing. In a patient with respiratory center depression, however, it causes further depression and may trigger respiratory arrest. Titrating doses minimizes the risk of adverse effects. Morphine sulfate decreases the brain's oxygen requirement by nearly 50%, thereby decreasing the arterial blood flow needed to oxygenate the brain. Antiemetics may be administered with morphine sulfate to control nausea and vomiting.

Classification of heart failure by hemodynamic subsets

Subset	Classification
• Subset I: pulmonary artery wedge pressure (PAWP) 18 mm Hg and cardiac index (CI) 2.2 L/minute/m² (no failure)	• A PAWP of 18 mm Hg is the level above which signs of pulmonary congestion appear and a CI of 2.2 L/minute/m² is the level below which signs of peripheral hypoperfusion appear. Increased PAWP and depressed CI are the "final common pathways" for almost all signs of heart failure. In Subset I, a relatively normal PAWP and CI indicate the absence of heart failure.
• Subset II: PAWP greater than 18 mm Hg and CI greater than 2.2 L/minute/m² (pulmonary congestion)	• In Subset II, PAWP is elevated, but CI is relatively normal. Clinically, the patient shows signs of pulmonary congestion.
• Subset III: PAWP less than 18 mm Hg and CI less than 2.2 L/minute/m² (peripheral hypoperfusion)	• In Subset III, PAWP is relatively normal, but CI is depressed. Clinically, the patient shows signs of peripheral hypoperfusion.
• Subset IV: PAWP greater than 18 mm Hg and CI less than 2.2 L/minute/m² (pulmonary congestion and peripheral hypoperfusion)	• In Subset IV, PAWP is elevated and CI is depressed. Clinically, the patient presents with both pulmonary congestion and peripheral hypoperfusion.

12. Alert the doctor immediately if the patient develops crackles in bilateral peripheral lung fields, severe dyspnea, pink frothy sputum, or marked neck vein distention or describes a sense of impending doom.

12. These findings indicate pulmonary edema, a life-threatening condition. Immediate medical intervention is crucial.

13. Additional individualized interventions: _____

13. Rationales: _____

COLLABORATIVE PROBLEM

Inadequate CO related to heart rate abnormalities or diminished contractility

Nursing priority

Maintain adequate CO.

Patient outcome criteria

Within 3 days, the patient will have:
• blood pressure within acceptable limits
• heart rate within normal limits, ideally 60 to 80 beats/minute
• CI greater than 2.2 L/minute/m² and PAWP less than 18 mm Hg
• strong, bilaterally equal peripheral pulses.

Interventions

1. Observe for signs and symptoms of decreased CO, such as:

• arterial hypotension, tachycardia, narrowed pulse pressure, weak peripheral pulses

• restlessness, irritability, confusion, somnolence

• weakness and fatigue

• cool, mottled, or cyanotic skin

• decreased urine output.

Rationales

1. Cardiogenic shock is considered a form of heart failure because of several interrelated mechanisms. Decreased contractility makes the heart unable to move blood efficiently. The resulting distention causes ventricular fibers to exceed optimal stretch according to the Frank-Starling curve, so the ejection fraction falls and systemic perfusion suffers. Failure of the left ventricle affects all body systems.
• Systemic vascular resistance (SVR) increases initially in an attempt to maintain mean arterial pressure. Pulse pressure narrows because the decreased CO lowers systolic pressure, while the increased SVR elevates diastolic pressure. Tachycardia, although a compensatory response to decreased CO, may actually impair it further by limiting ventricular filling time.
• Changes in LOC or mentation reflect cerebral hypoxemia or ischemia.
• Weakness and fatigue result from diminished skeletal muscle perfusion, excessive work of breathing, and sleep disturbances.
• Skin changes reflect shunting away from skeletal muscles as the body attempts to preserve perfusion of core organs.
• Decreased urine output reflects diminished renal perfusion resulting from decreased circulating blood volume and intense sympathetic vasoconstriction of afferent arterioles.

Cardiovascular disorders

2. Monitor the ECG continuously. Document and report significant findings (see Appendix A, Monitoring Standards, for details).

3. For patients with hypoperfusion only (Subset III), provide the following care, as ordered:
• If heart rate is elevated, administer fluids. Document effectiveness and observe for adverse effects, especially fluid overload.

• If heart rate is depressed, assist with pacemaker insertion. Document effectiveness and observe for pacemaker malfunction.

4. For patients with pulmonary congestion and peripheral hypoperfusion (Subset IV), administer medications, as ordered.
• If blood pressure is depressed, administer positive inotropes, typically:

– digitalis glycoside preparations. Observe for and report signs of toxicity, including GI distress, bradycardia, atrioventricular block, premature beats, and atrial tachycardia with block.
– dopamine hydrochloride (Intropin). Observe for and report hypotension, tachyarrhythmias, ectopic beats, vasoconstriction with high doses, and I.V. fluid infiltration.

– dobutamine hydrochloride (Dobutrex). Monitor for and report adverse effects, especially tachycardia and arrhythmias.

– combined inotrope and vasodilator therapy, such as dopamine and sodium nitroprusside or amrinone (Inocor). With dopamine and sodium nitroprusside, monitor for and report adverse reactions, especially chest pain or increased ventricular arrhythmias. With amrinone, observe for and report adverse reactions, including arrhythmias, hypotension, and GI distress.

• If blood pressure is normal, administer vasodilators. See the "Risk for hypoxemia" collaborative problem above for details.

2. Because CO depends on the heart rate and stroke volume, arrhythmias can affect CO significantly; a dramatic drop in CO can cause cardiac arrest. Continuous monitoring allows for prompt treatment of arrhythmias.

3. Measures for patients in Subset III are designed to increase CO, thereby increasing peripheral perfusion.
• Tachycardia is a primary compensatory response to hypovolemia. Administering fluid increases preload and thus increases CO. The resulting increase in circulating blood volume restores peripheral perfusion and relieves tachycardia because as stroke volume increases, heart rate returns to normal.
• Because heart rate is a primary determinant of CO, bradycardia with hypoperfusion indicates a need to restore the normal heart rate. Pacemaker insertion provides an immediate way to increase the heart rate while the underlying problem such as heart block is identified and resolved.

4. Patients in Subset IV have an elevated PAWP and depressed CI, so the treatment goals are to lower PAWP and improve CI.
• Elevated PAWP, depressed CI, and depressed blood pressure strongly suggest depressed myocardial contractility. Positive inotropic agents increase myocardial contractility, thus improving CI and lowering PAWP as fluid is moved more efficiently through the heart.
– Digitalis glycosides improve contractility, but they also slow heart rate and cardiac conduction. They also may provoke various arrhythmias by increasing automaticity.
– Dopamine has complex dose-related pharmacologic actions. In heart failure, midrange doses of dopamine (2 to 10 mcg/kg/minute) increase renal perfusion via dopaminergic effects, and increase heart rate and contractility via beta$_1$-adrenergic stimulating effects.
– Dobutamine, primarily a direct beta$_1$ stimulator, is a potent inotropic agent that exerts less effect on heart rate than dopamine. As such, it significantly improves contractility with less tendency to cause arrhythmias than dopamine.
– Two synergistic drugs improve CO better and more safely than either agent used alone. For example, dopamine and sodium nitroprusside in combination reduce preload, augment contractility, and reduce afterload better than if used singly. However, both agents may decrease myocardial oxygen supply. Amrinone has both inotropic and vasodilating properties that lessen pulmonary congestion and improve CO. It is used commonly for short-term management of heart failure patients unresponsive to other therapies.
• Patients with congestion, hypoperfusion, and normal blood pressure may benefit from afterload reduction achieved through vasodilation.

5. For patients in Subsets III and IV who do not respond to fluid and drug therapy, assist with intra-aortic balloon pump (IABP) counter pulsation, as ordered. Monitor augmentation as necessary, every 15 minutes until stable and then every hour. Document the effectiveness of counterpulsation, and observe for complications and IABP malfunction.

6. Additional individualized interventions: _____

5. IABP counterpulsation increases coronary artery perfusion, contractility, and vital organ perfusion and reduces afterload and myocardial oxygen demand. Balloon inflation during diastole displaces blood from the aorta, augmenting coronary artery and peripheral perfusion by increasing the diastolic pressure. Balloon deflation at the end of diastole decreases pressure in the ascending aorta, thus reducing LVEDP and workload.

6. Rationales: _____

NURSING DIAGNOSIS

Activity intolerance related to hypoxemia, weakness, or diminished cardiovascular reserve

Nursing priority

Promote rest.

Patient outcome criterion

By the time of discharge, the patient will show no signs or symptoms of activity intolerance during self-care activities.

Interventions

1. Assess for signs and symptoms of activity intolerance, such as heart rate increase greater than 25%, blood pressure increase greater than 25%, any heart rate or blood pressure decrease, chest pain, arrhythmias, decreased LOC, or complaints of weakness or fatigue.

2. Place the patient on complete bed rest. Assist with activity, as needed. Implement measures in the "Impaired physical mobility" plan, page 50, as appropriate.

3. Pace nursing care to promote rest. If possible, allow at least 90 minutes of uninterrupted sleep at a time.

4. When the patient's condition stabilizes, increase activity gradually, as ordered.

• Maintain supplemental oxygen.

• Monitor the patient's response to increased activity. Slow or discontinue activity progression if the patient shows any signs of intolerance.

5. Additional individualized interventions: _____

Rationales

1. A dysfunctional myocardium may be unable to adjust stroke volume and oxygen during exertion. The unmet oxygen needs may cause tachycardia and myocardial or cerebral ischemia. Anaerobic metabolism resulting from impaired skeletal muscle perfusion results in weakness or fatigue.

2. Bed rest decreases myocardial workload. Assisting with activity conserves cardiovascular and energy reserves. The "Impaired physical mobility" plan contains measures to counteract the complications of immobility.

3. The numerous medical and nursing measures necessary to treat heart failure and cardiogenic shock may interrupt rest and exhaust the patient. The average sleep cycle lasts 90 minutes. Providing at least this much uninterrupted rest at a time allows the patient to progress through both rapid eye movement (REM) sleep, which helps restore psychological equilibrium, and non-REM sleep, which helps restore physiologic well-being.

4. A gradual activity increase allows neurovascular compensatory mechanisms to adjust to increased demands.
• Supplemental oxygen helps meet increased tissue oxygen demands during exercise.
• Close monitoring allows the nurse to match exercise level with energy resources.

5. Rationales: _____

Discharge planning

Discharge checklist
Before discharge, the patient shows evidence of:
- ❏ blood pressure within 30 mm Hg of normal value for at least 12 hours without I.V. vasodilators
- ❏ no significant arrhythmias for at least 12 hours without I.V. antiarrhythmic agents
- ❏ stable hemodynamic status for at least 12 hours without IABP counterpulsation
- ❏ absence of arterial and PA line
- ❏ stable respiratory status for at least 12 hours without mechanical ventilation.

Teaching checklist
Document evidence that the patient and family demonstrate understanding of:
- ❏ cause and implications of cardiogenic shock
- ❏ purpose of medications
- ❏ rationales for other therapeutic interventions
- ❏ need for continued treatment of underlying cause, including lifestyle modifications if appropriate.

Documentation checklist
Using outcome criteria as a guide, document:
- ❏ clinical status on admission
- ❏ significant changes in status
- ❏ pertinent laboratory and diagnostic test findings
- ❏ hemodynamic measurements
- ❏ oxygen therapy
- ❏ response to cardiac assist devices, such as a pacemaker or IABP
- ❏ fluid therapy or restrictions
- ❏ response to inotropics, vasodilators, or other drugs
- ❏ dietary modifications
- ❏ activity restrictions
- ❏ patient and family teaching
- ❏ discharge planning.

Associated plans of care

Acute MI: Critical care unit
Hypovolemic shock
Impaired physical mobility
Knowledge deficit

References

Barry, W.L., et al. "Cardiogenic Shock: Therapy and Prevention," *Clinical Cardiology* 21(2):72-80, February 1998.

Forrester, J., et al. "Medical Therapy of Acute MI by Applications of Hemodynamic Subsets," *New England Journal of Medicine* 295(23):1356-62, December 1976.

Goldberg, I.F. "Pathogenesis and Management of Cardiogenic Shock and Postoperative Shock," *Chest: The Cardiopulmonary Journal* 102(5):Supplement 2: 589s-632s, November 1992.

McGhie, A.I., and Goldstein, R.A. "Pathogenesis and Management of Acute Heart Failure and Cardiogenic Shock: Role of Inotropic Therapy," *Chest: The Cardiopulmonary Journal* 102(5): Supplement 2: 626s-32s, November 1992.

O'Donnell, L. "Complications of MI beyond the Acute Stage," *AJN* 96(9):Nurse Practitioner Extra Ed: 24-32, September 1996.

O'Neal, P.V. "How to Spot Early Signs of Cardiogenic Shock," *AJN* 94(5):L36-41, May 1994.

Shinn, A.E., and Joseph, D. "Concepts of Intraaortic Balloon Counterpulsation," *Journal of Cardiovascular Nursing* 8(2):45-60, January 1994.

Urban, N. "Integrating the Hemodynamic Profile with Clinical Assessment," *AACN Clinical Issues in Critical Care Nursing* 4(1):161-79, February 1993.

Carotid endarterectomy

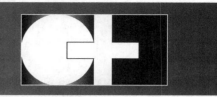

DRG information
DRG 005   Extracranial Vascular Procedures.
Mean LOS = 4.4 days
Includes Carotid Endarterectomy with synthetic or tissue patch graft.

INTRODUCTION

Definition and time focus
Carotid endarterectomy is the surgical removal of atherosclerotic plaque from the inner lining of the carotid artery to widen the vessel lumen. Endarterectomy increases cerebral blood flow and reduces the risk of cerebrovascular accident (CVA).

The surgical incision is made along the anterior sternocleidomastoid muscle to expose the carotid bifurcation, the most common site of plaque formation. The diseased artery is dissected away from surrounding tissue and nerves and clamped above and below the obstruction. Once the plaque is removed, the artery is sutured or closed with a vein or synthetic polyester (Dacron) patch graft.

Carotid endarterectomy is generally viewed as preventive surgery and is best performed before the patient shows significant neurologic loss. The patient may have had transient ischemic attacks (TIAs) or a CVA with minimal reversible ischemic neurologic deficits (RINDs). Symptoms usually occur when the artery is 70% occluded.

This plan focuses on the immediate postoperative care of a patient undergoing elective carotid endarterectomy for an atherosclerotic lesion of an internal carotid artery.

Etiology and precipitating factors
Atherosclerosis is the underlying cause in 90% of extracranial carotid disease, resulting in partial or complete occlusion. Indicators for surgery include:
• TIAs or RINDs with arteriographic evidence of an atherosclerotic carotid lesion. TIAs and RINDs usually affect the face and extremities (on the side opposite the involved cerebral hemisphere) as a result of temporarily insufficient blood supply to focal brain areas. TIAs resolve in 24 hours or less with no residual deficits, while RINDs last from 24 hours to a week.
• CVA from a carotid lesion with severe stenosis of the internal carotid artery and a good recovery (mild or no residual neurologic deficits) at least 5 weeks after the CVA. A CVA is characterized by hemiplegia and sensory loss on the side of the body opposite the involved hemisphere and visual-field defects on the same side as the involved hemisphere.
• asymptomatic carotid bruits with severe stenosis of one internal carotid artery and total occlusion of the opposite carotid artery, bilateral stenosis, a markedly ulcerated plaque, or stenosis in the artery to the dominant hemisphere
• recurrence of stenosis after endarterectomy.

FOCUSED ASSESSMENT GUIDELINES

Nursing history (functional health pattern findings)
Health perception–health management pattern
• History of TIAs, RINDs, or completed CVA
• Treatment of hypertension or diabetes mellitus
• History of atherosclerosis elsewhere, such as coronary artery disease (angina) or peripheral arterial occlusive disease (intermittent claudication)
• History of acute myocardial infarction (AMI)
• Risk factors, such as smoking, obesity, and sedentary lifestyle; high stress levels; high serum cholesterol, lipoprotein, and triglyceride levels; vasospasms of cerebral arteries; clotting abnormalities; polycythemia; or substance abuse
• Increased risk, if a black male
• At increased risk if over age 45; if over age 65, risk increases further
• Noncompliance with antihypertensive regimen; may not have sought medical attention for many years
Nutritional-metabolic pattern
• Diet high in calories, fat, cholesterol, and salt
• Transient or ongoing difficulty swallowing
Elimination pattern
• Transient or ongoing bowel or bladder incontinence
Activity-exercise pattern
• Sedentary lifestyle and lack of regular exercise (with history of TIAs, RINDs, or CVA) because of transient visual deficits (blurred vision, diplopia, blindness in one eye, or tunnel vision), motor deficits (contralateral weakness or paralysis in arm, hand, or leg), or vertigo (less common); may have minimal residual deficits that interfere with activity and exercise
• Fear of falling because of previous TIAs, RINDs, or CVA
Cognitive-perceptual pattern
• Dizziness

• Slowed mentation or clumsiness associated with prior TIAs or CVA

Sleep-rest pattern
• History of TIAs or CVA as a result of thrombosis, symptoms may have developed during sleep or shortly after awakening

Self-perception–self-concept pattern
• Altered self-concept, particularly if residual neurologic deficits are present

Role-relationship pattern
• Fear of inability to perform usual roles because of residual neurologic deficits or fear that TIA or CVA will occur during role performance

Physical findings

Clinical manifestations will vary depending on the extent of the disease at the bifurcation and the adequacy of collateral blood supply to the affected area. The patient may remain asymptomatic if there is sufficient collateral blood supply.

General appearance
• Some residual facial drooping from CVA

Neurologic
• Transient motor and sensory deficits, such as numbness, weakness, or paralysis of the face, hand, arm, or leg on the side opposite the lesion (contralateral); less commonly, gait disturbance (ataxia)
• Visual deficits, such as transient scotoma (area of poor vision surrounded by normal vision), tunnel vision, diplopia, blurred vision, or amaurosis fugax (transient blindness in one eye, lasting 10 minutes or less) on same side as affected carotid artery
• Speech difficulties, such as transient motor or expressive aphasia if the dominant hemisphere is involved

Cardiovascular
• Hypertension
• Carotid bruit localized to site of carotid bifurcation: characteristically loud, harsh, high-pitched systolic murmur that extends into diastole, associated with a decreased carotid pulse (no bruit is heard in about 20% of patients with significant obstruction of internal carotid artery)
• Decreased facial and superficial temporal pulses on side of lesion

Musculoskeletal
• Minimal residual weakness on side opposite lesion

Diagnostic studies

Screening tests are recommended before arteriography. Commonly used noninvasive tests include:
• oculoplethysmography — reveals significant disruption of blood flow to the ophthalmic artery, an important branch of the internal carotid artery, when carotid stenosis is present

• B-mode ultrasonography — reveals restricted blood flow when carotid stenosis is present
• carotid Doppler ultrasound — differentiates thrombotic from ulcerative plaques in the stenosed carotid artery
• Doppler imaging — detects abnormal carotid blood flow and ulcerative plaques within carotid arteries; highly accurate
• carotid phonoangiography — identifies origin of bruits and estimates severity of stenosis
• computed tomography scan — reveals ischemia and hemorrhage and identifies other causes of signs (such as tumors, hematomas, or cerebral aneurysms); discovery of a cerebral infarction may alter timing of surgery and indicate need for an intraluminal shunt during surgery; serves as baseline in event of perioperative neurologic deficit

Commonly used invasive tests include:
• digital subtraction angiography (DSA) — provides anatomic detail of the aortic arch, subclavian and vertebral arteries, and extracranial carotid arteries; identifies moderate to severe carotid artery stenosis; may be used in place of standard angiography for the asymptomatic patient in whom noninvasive tests demonstrate a significant stenosis; if DSA appears normal in symptomatic patients, standard angiography should be performed because minor stenoses and small ulcerations may be overlooked
• cerebral arteriography — identifies exact location and extent of atherosclerotic lesions; indicated if noninvasive screening reveals severe obstruction with harsh, bilateral bruits or progressive atherosclerosis elsewhere (recommended for all patients being considered for surgery)
• blood urea nitrogen and creatinine levels — monitor renal function before and after angiography or DSA because dyes used in these tests may affect renal function
• hemoglobin level and hematocrit — provide baseline for comparison with postoperative values to detect bleeding
• coagulation panel — may be increased if the patient takes antiplatelet medications such as aspirin; before surgery, provides a baseline for comparison with postoperative values to detect clotting abnormalities
• electrolyte panel — provides a baseline for comparison with postoperative values because electrolyte imbalances may occur after surgery (existing electrolyte imbalances are corrected before surgery)
• arterial blood gases (ABGs) — provide a baseline for comparison because hypoxemia is a major concern after surgery
• electrocardiography (ECG), treadmill exercise test, myocardial perfusion scans, and coronary angiography — screen for cardiac disease

Potential complications
• Blood pressure lability (hypertension most common, hypotension less common)
• AMI
• Cerebral ischemia or CVA
• Cranial nerve injury
• Airway obstruction secondary to hemorrhage and hematoma formation

• Acute respiratory insufficiency
• Hyperperfusion syndromes (rare), such as ipsilateral vascular type headaches, seizures, or intracerebral hemorrhage
• Increased ICP secondary to cerebral hemorrhage
• Rarely, vocal cord paralysis
• Infection

CLINICAL SNAPSHOT

CAROTID ENDARTERECTOMY

Major collaborative problems	Key patient outcomes
Blood pressure lability	Maintain stable blood pressure within desired limits.
Risk for cerebral ischemia	Exhibit signs of adequate cerebral blood flow.
Risk for cranial nerve injury	Manifest no signs or symptoms of cranial nerve injury.
Risk for acute myocardial infarction	Have an ECG with no evidence of infarction.
Risk for hypoxemia	Have ABG values within normal limits.

Cardiovascular disorders

COLLABORATIVE PROBLEM

Blood pressure lability related to carotid sinus dysfunction, hypovolemia secondary to intraoperative or postoperative bleeding or fluid imbalance, AMI, or hypoxia

Nursing priority

Maintain blood pressure within prescribed limits.

Patient outcome criteria

Within 24 hours after surgery, the patient will:
• maintain stable systolic or diastolic blood pressure or mean arterial pressure (MAP) within desired limits without antihypertensive or vasopressor drugs: typically, heart rate, 60 to 100 beats/minute; systolic blood pressure, 90 to 140 mm Hg; and diastolic blood pressure, 50 to 90 mm Hg
• exhibit fluid balance, as evidenced by approximately equal intake and output, blood pressure within desired limits, and pulmonary artery pressures within normal limits
• have ABGs within normal limits: pH, 7.35 to 7.45; Pco_2, 35 to 45 mm Hg; and HCO_3^-, 23 to 28 mEq/L
• exhibit little or no bleeding from the surgical site.

Interventions

1. Assess blood pressure every 15 minutes for the first hour, then every hour or as needed for the first 24 hours after surgery. Ideally, use an arterial line for the first 24 hours or until the blood pressure stabilizes. If medication is needed to control blood pressure, assess blood pressure every 15 to 30 minutes, and as needed.

2. Implement measures to control hypertension:
• Administer antihypertensive medications such as sodium nitroprusside (Nipride) to maintain a systolic blood pressure at no more than 120 to 150 mm Hg, diastolic blood pressure at 70 to 90 mm Hg, or MAP at 86 to 110 mm Hg, or as ordered. Notify the doctor immediately if the medication cannot maintain blood pressure within this range.
• Administer pain medication as ordered.
• Provide a quiet, restful environment.
• Maintain activity restrictions as ordered, usually bed rest for the first 24 hours.
• Maintain fluid restrictions as ordered.

3. Implement measures to control hypotension:

• Assess fluid intake and output every hour or as needed for the first 24 hours. If a pulmonary artery catheter is in place, assess cardiac output (CO), pulmonary artery wedge pressure, and central venous pressure every hour or as needed for the first 24 hours.
• If hypotension results from fluid loss, replace fluids as ordered.
• Assess for evidence of AMI (ECG changes, elevated creatine kinase [CK] and CK_2-MB isoenzymes, elevated troponin level and chest pain); if hypotension is caused by AMI, see the "Acute MI: Critical care unit" plan, page 338, for further interventions.
• Administer vasopressors, such as dopamine (Intropin) or dobutamine (Dobutrex), to maintain blood pressure within the limits specified above, as ordered.

• Administer pain medications judiciously.

• Monitor the incision and drainage system for bleeding and drainage.

Rationales

1. Baroreceptors at the carotid bifurcation normally control blood pressure. Surgical manipulation of these baroreceptors may impair carotid sinus reflexes, causing blood pressure instability. Additionally, hypovolemia and hypoxia contribute to fluctuating blood pressure. If uncontrolled, extreme hypertension or hypotension can cause a CVA. Blood pressure is most accurately measured with an arterial line.

2. Surgical trauma may render the carotid sinus insensitive to increasing blood pressure, resulting in hypertension. Because surgery increases blood supply to the cerebrum, capillaries are more prone to rupture when hypertension occurs, causing intracerebral bleeding and cerebral infarction. As blood pressure exceeds the limits of cerebral autoregulation (MAP of 60 to 160 mm Hg), increased pressure forces more blood into the cerebrum, leading to increased ICP and cerebral ischemia (see the "Increased intracranial pressure" plan, page 169). Research shows that stimuli (particularly noxious stimuli), hypervolemia, pain, and stress increase blood pressure. Hypertension may also cause the graft site to rupture.

3. Hypotension is less common after surgery than hypertension. The carotid sinus may be hypersensitive after surgery if the removed plaque had been dampening pressure signals. Frequent checks of the indicated parameters alert the nurse to hypotension and help differentiate between two common causes, hypovolemia and AMI.
• Frequent assessment provides early warning of developing problems.

• Fluid volume replacement increases CO, thus increasing blood pressure and cerebral perfusion.
• Hypotension may result from fluid deficit or myocardial dysfunction.

• Hypotension, whether caused by hypovolemia or decreased contractility with an AMI, results in decreased cerebral perfusion, decreased oxygenation, and cerebral ischemia and possible infarction. Short-acting drugs, such as dopamine or dobutamine, increase cardiac contractility, thus increasing CO and blood pressure.
• Pain medications keep the patient comfortable while maintaining blood pressure within desired limits.
• Excessive bleeding or drainage indicates the need for prompt intervention to prevent hypovolemia.

4. Maintain oxygenation as ordered, usually 2 to 5 L by nasal cannula after extubation. Assess oxygenation levels by continuous pulse oximetry or ABG levels, as needed.

4. Hypoxemia contributes to blood pressure fluctuations because the heart rate increases to supply additional oxygen to vital organs, thus increasing CO and blood pressure. Conversely, if the carotid body has been damaged, there may be a loss of the normal circulatory response to hypoxia. Because hypoxia causes the cerebral arteries to dilate, blood flow to the cerebrum increases, potentially increasing ICP and causing ischemia.

5. Additional individualized interventions: _____

5. Rationales: _____

COLLABORATIVE PROBLEM

Risk for cerebral ischemia related to multiple factors

Nursing priority

Prevent or minimize cerebral ischemia.

Patient outcome criteria

Within 24 hours after surgery, the patient will:
• exhibit signs of adequate cerebral blood flow as evidenced by alertness and orientation, intact motor and sensory function, and normal pupil reactions
• maintain stable vital signs: typically, heart rate, 60 to 100 beats/minute; systolic blood pressure, 90 to 140 mm Hg; and diastolic blood pressure, 50 to 90 mm Hg
• have hemoglobin levels, hematocrit values, and bleeding times within prescribed limits
• exhibit little or no bleeding.

Interventions

1. Assess level of consciousness (LOC), orientation, pupillary reaction, and motor and sensory function hourly or as needed for the first 24 hours. Document and report immediately decreased level of consciousness (LOC); change in orientation; pupillary changes, such as unequal pupils, a sluggish or absent pupillary reaction to light, or pupil deviated from midline position; motor and sensory deficits such as paresthesia, motor weakness, or contralateral hemiparesis; and slurred speech or seizures. When the patient is fully recovered from anesthesia, report any visual disturbances (such as blurred or dimmed vision, diplopia, or ipsilateral change in visual field) or headache.

2. Assess blood pressure, pulse, and respiratory rate hourly or as needed for the first 24 hours after surgery. Report increased or decreased pulse rate, marked fluctuations in blood pressure, and changes in respiratory rate and pattern (refer to the "Risk for hypoxemia" and "Blood pressure lability" problems in this plan).

3. Assess for patency of the internal carotid artery by lightly palpating the superficial temporal and facial arteries hourly, or by monitoring vital signs. Document and report any change from the baseline assessment.

Rationales

1. Cerebral ischemia or infarction is a major concern after endarterectomy. It may result from carotid artery clamping during surgery or vasospasm from clamping and manipulating cerebral vessels, hypovolemia secondary to blood loss, cerebral vessel compression from hematoma or edema, cerebral embolization from manipulation of the arteries, marked fluctuations in blood pressure, or thrombosis at the endarterectomy site. Depending on the extent of ischemia, signs vary from mild ischemia to CVA. Assessing frequently for signs of decreased cerebral perfusion reduces the risk of permanent damage, as appropriate action can be taken immediately.

2. Such changes as increased pulse and respiratory rates and decreased blood pressure may indicate hypovolemia caused by fluid deficit or bleeding. Hypovolemia leading to decreased CO, hypertension, and hypoxia increases the risk of cerebral ischemia. Bradycardia contributes to decreased CO and may be caused by vagal nerve stimulation.

3. Strong palpable pulses indicate good flow through the carotid artery and are a useful adjunct to other assessments.

4. Assess for signs of bleeding: increased neck circumference, bright red blood on the dressing, deviated trachea and respiratory distress (see the "Risk for hypoxemia" problem in this plan), or increased drainage in the collection system, if used. Monitor vital signs. Document and immediately report any changes from baseline. Assess hemoglobin levels, hematocrit values, and bleeding times, as ordered, and report changes that indicate bleeding, such as decreasing hemoglobin level and hematocrit and increasing bleeding times.

5. If bleeding is present, prepare the patient for corrective procedures, such as noninvasive or invasive testing, surgery to correct a suture line bleed, or arteriotomy and thrombectomy to remove a thrombus. Consult the "Surgery" plan, page 103, for details.

6. Implement measures to promote adequate cerebral blood flow, as ordered:
• Detect and treat hypovolemia.
• Maintain drain patency by keeping tubing free from kinks and emptying the collection device as necessary.
• Change or reinforce the dressing as necessary.
• Apply an ice pack at the incision line, as ordered.
• Support the patient's head and neck during position changes and maintain alignment.
• Position on the unoperated side.
• Avoid flexion of the neck.
• Administer corticosteroids, if ordered, and monitor for therapeutic and nontherapeutic effects.
• Control hypertension with antihypertensive medications such as sodium nitroprusside.
• Control hypotension with fluid replacement or vasopressors, such as dopamine or dobutamine.
• Maintain activity restrictions.

7. Implement measures to minimize injury, if signs and symptoms of cerebral ischemia occur:
• Continue the measures above to promote cerebral blood flow.
• Assess and report progression of sign and symptoms.

• Maintain the patient on bed rest with the head of the bed flat, unless contraindicated. The head of the bed may be elevated 30 degrees, or as ordered, when vital signs are stable.
• Initiate seizure precautions.
• Provide emotional support to the patient and family.

8. Additional individualized interventions: _____
_____

4. The patient undergoing carotid endarterectomy usually receives aspirin before surgery, sometimes up until the time of surgery, as well as heparin during surgery. Immediate detection of increased bleeding is therefore a high priority because decreased circulating blood volume increases the potential for cerebral ischemia. In addition to compromising cerebral blood flow, hematomas may cause tracheal compression, obstructing the airway. The patient may require further surgery to detect the cause of bleeding.

5. Prompt detection and correction of the cause of cerebral ischemia may minimize damage. Adequate patient preparation for testing or surgery helps allay anxieties. The "Surgery" plan provides detailed information for this problem.

6. These measures promote cerebral circulation, help prevent hematoma formation, or reduce edema and stress at the suture line, reducing the risk of bleeding.

7. Minimizing injury reduces the risk of permanent neurologic damage.
• Promoting cerebral blood flow reduces the risk of further injury.
• The progression of signs and symptoms alerts the nurse to the need for more aggressive intervention. Continued deterioration, bleeding, hematoma formation, or increased ICP may require further surgery.
• The supine position improves blood flow to the brain, while elevation of the head of the bed decreases edema in the operative site.

• Cerebral ischemia may trigger seizures.
• Keeping the family informed about what is happening may help to reduce anxiety and secure their cooperation in the patient's care.

8. Rationales: _____
_____

COLLABORATIVE PROBLEM

Risk for cranial nerve injury (particularly cranial nerves III, VII, IX, X, XI, XII) related to surgical trauma or blood accumulation and edema in the surgical area

Nursing priority

Detect and minimize neurologic impairment.

Patient outcome criteria

- Within 24 hours after surgery, the patient will manifest no signs and symptoms of cranial nerve damage.
- If damage has occurred, within 72 hours after surgery the patient will:
  - experience beginning resolution of cranial nerve damage as evidenced by a gradual improvement in facial muscle tone, movements and sensation, ability to chew and swallow, speech, and shoulder movements
  - begin therapy for more severe cranial nerve damage, such as speech therapy or physical therapy.

Interventions

1. Assess cranial nerve function hourly for the first 24 hours after surgery or as needed. Check for the following:

- full extraocular movements (EOMs)

- ability to smile and clench teeth symmetrically; general facial symmetry present
- swallows easily, uvula in the midline position, gag reflex intact, speaks clearly with normal tones, symmetrical movements of vocal chords and soft palate
- shoulders symmetrical; able to rotate head to side and shrug shoulders against resistance (may be contraindicated for the first 24 hours because both maneuvers exert pressure on the operative site)
- tongue midline, able to protrude tongue in the midline position and move it laterally with normal movements; able to speak, eat, and swallow without difficulty
- facial sensation, particularly in the earlobe and over the mastoid process.

2. Compare cranial nerve assessment to preoperative or recovery room baseline. Immediately report the following: incomplete EOMs, ipsilateral facial drooping (loss of nasolabial fold, drooping of corner of mouth or lower eyelid), difficulty swallowing, absent or diminished gag reflex, hoarse speech, early voice fatigue, unilateral shoulder sag, difficulty raising arm on affected side to horizontal position or raising shoulder against resistance, ipsilateral tongue deviation, dysphagia, tongue biting while eating, or loss of facial sensation.

Rationales

1. The cranial nerves lie close to the endarterectomy site. Clamping of or trauma to the nerves during surgery can impair their normal function. Nerves also may be severed accidentally during dissection to access the carotid artery.
- Normal EOMs indicate that the oculomotor nerve (cranial nerve III) is intact.
- These findings demonstrate normal facial nerve (cranial nerve VII) function.
- These findings demonstrate normal glossopharyngeal (cranial nerve IX) and vagus nerve (cranial nerve X) function (these two nerves are tested together).
- These movements indicate normal spinal accessory nerve (cranial nerve XI) function.

- These capacities demonstrate hypoglossal nerve (cranial nerve XII) function.

- These sensations show normal greater auricular nerve function.

2. An awareness of preexisting deficits facilitates prompt detection of cranial nerve damage. Dysfunction may be caused by stretching of the nerves during retraction, pressure from blood accumulation, or edema in the surrounding tissues. Prompt detection of cranial nerve damage facilitates appropriate interventions to minimize complications and injury to the patient.

Cardiovascular disorders

3. Implement measures to reduce edema or accumulation of fluid in the surgical area:
• Elevate the head of the bed as prescribed.
• Maintain patency of surgical drains, if present.
• Keep the head and neck in the midline position when the patient is supine. Support the patient's head and neck when turning.
• Keep the head and neck in correct alignment with pillows or rolls when the patient is turned to the side. Position on the unoperated side.
• Apply an ice pack at the incision line, as ordered.
• Monitor for therapeutic and nontherapeutic effects of corticosteroids, if administered.

4. If nerve damage occurs, particularly to the facial, hypoglossal, vagus, or glossopharyngeal nerves, implement measures to prevent injury to the patient:
• Keep suctioning equipment at the bedside and perform oral, pharyngeal, or tracheal suctioning as needed.

• Withhold oral fluids and food until the gag reflex returns.
• Assess the patient's ability to chew and swallow before offering fluids or food.
• Place the patient in high Fowler's position, unless contraindicated, during and after oral intake.
• Instill isotonic eyedrops or tape the eyelids shut if the patient's blink reflex is decreased or absent.

5. If the vagus or glossopharyngeal nerve is damaged (as shown by hoarseness, difficulty speaking clearly, or asymmetrical movement of vocal cords), implement measures to facilitate communication: Maintain a quiet environment; establish a means of communication with the eyes (for blinking for yes and no); provide pencil and paper, magic slate, flash cards, or pictures; pay close attention when the patient communicates.

6. If nerve damage occurs, provide emotional support to the patient and family by listening and providing information as appropriate.

7. Initiate appropriate referrals for follow-up care when cranial nerve damage persists.

8. Additional individualized interventions: _____
_____

3. Reducing edema and fluid accumulation in the surgical area minimizes pressure on the cranial nerves, reducing the potential for dysfunction. Corticosteroids are used to reduce edema.

4. Compensating for nerve deficits reduces the risk of injury.

• Suctioning excess secretions reduces the risk of aspiration and subsequent aspiration pneumonia. This is particularly important for the endarterectomy patient, who should avoid hypoxemia (see the "Risk for hypoxemia" problem in this plan).
• Withholding fluids and food when the gag reflex is absent prevents aspiration.
• Assessing ability to chew and swallow helps the nurse gauge the risk of aspiration.
• Placing the patient in this position facilitates swallowing and decreases the risk of aspiration.
• Artificial tears and taping help prevent corneal irritation and permanent eye damage.

5. The inability to communicate effectively can be stressful, if not terrifying. Providing the patient with a means of communication or signaling helps reduce anxiety.

6. The effects of cranial nerve damage can be frightening for both the patient and family. Providing the opportunity to express concerns and giving appropriate information can relieve anxiety and stress.

7. Nerve damage is usually not permanent, but the symptoms may take months to resolve. Working with such health care team members as the speech pathologist, physical therapist, or dietitian facilitates recovery and should begin as soon as the deficits are discovered.

8. Rationales: _____
_____

COLLABORATIVE PROBLEM

Risk for AMI related to atherosclerosis and trauma of surgery

Nursing priority

Promptly detect and treat AMI.

Patient outcome criterion

Within 24 hours after surgery, the patient will exhibit stable cardiac status as evidenced by vital signs within normal limits and an ECG with no evidence of further infarction.

Interventions

1. Assess for chest pain (see the "Acute MI: Critical care unit" plan, page 338). Also evaluate laboratory and diagnostic tests specific to cardiac function: 12-lead ECG, arrhythmia monitoring, CK, and CK isoenzymes and troponin. Document and report immediately ECG changes consistent with AMI, elevated CK, CK_2-MB, and troponin 1 levels, elevated ST segment, and premature ventricular contractions during continuous monitoring. Compare to baseline values.

2. Assess blood pressure, pulse rate, respiratory rate, central venous pressure (CVP), and urine output hourly, or as ordered. If a pulmonary artery (PA) catheter is used, assess wedge pressure every 2 hours and CO or cardiac index (CI) every 4 hours, or as ordered. Correlate abnormal findings with laboratory and diagnostic test results.

3. Administer nitroglycerin, as ordered, until preoperative cardiac medications can be resumed.

4. Implement the measures in the "Acute MI: Critical care unit" plan for the patient with AMI.

5. Additional individualized interventions: _____

Rationales

1. Because generalized atherosclerosis is common in patients undergoing endarterectomy, coronary artery disease (CAD) is usually present. AMI is the leading cause of death after endarterectomy. Continuous cardiac monitoring after surgery may detect ischemia and arrhythmias. Early detection of ischemia or an AMI facilitates prompt treatment and may help prevent cardiovascular complications.

2. Decreased blood pressure, CO, and CI, along with increased pulse and respiratory rates, wedge pressure, and CVP help to differentiate a myocardial infraction from other postoperative complications. Laboratory and diagnostic test results also help rule out other complications. Urine output is one of the best indicators of CO, particularly if a PA catheter is not in place.

3. Nitroglycerin may be ordered for the patient with known CAD to increase blood flow and decrease cardiac workload by vasodilation.

4. The "Acute MI: Critical care unit" plan provides detailed information about the care of the patient with an AMI.

5. Rationales: _____

COLLABORATIVE PROBLEM

Risk for hypoxemia related to airway obstruction from tracheal compression or aspiration

Nursing priorities

• Minimize or prevent airway obstruction and aspiration.
• Maintain oxygenation.

Cardiovascular disorders

Patient outcome criteria

Within 24 hours after surgery, the patient will:
• have a patent airway as evidenced by normal respiratory rate and effort, normal breath sounds, and appropriate LOC
• have ABG values within normal limits: typically, pH, 7.35 to 7.45; P_{CO_2}, 35 to 45 mm Hg; and HCO_3^-, 23 to 28 mEq/L
• produce minimal drainage from the incision
• display trachea in the midline position.

Interventions

1. Assess airway patency every 15 minutes for the first hour after surgery and then hourly, as needed, for 24 hours. Assess respiratory rate and effort, respiratory pattern, chest excursion, position of trachea, breath sounds, level of consciousness, and color. Document and report immediately increased respiratory rate, accessory muscle use, unequal chest excursion, altered LOC (such as lethargy, restlessness, or confusion), pale to cyanotic color, shortness of breath, tracheal deviation, stridor, wheezing, or labored respirations.

2. Assess oxygenation levels by continuous pulse oximetry or ABG levels, as needed. Also monitor ABG levels to ensure that pH and partial pressure of arterial carbon dioxide stay within normal limits. Document and report oxygen saturation below 95%, or as ordered, and ABG values outside the prescribed limits.

3. If airway obstruction occurs, prepare to assist with endotracheal (ET) intubation, tracheostomy, or drainage of an incisional hematoma. Anticipate intubation even if signs of hypoxemia have not yet developed. A tracheostomy tray should be available at the bedside or in the critical care unit.

4. Assess for bleeding and hematoma formation:

• Assess neck size closely every 15 minutes for the first hour, then hourly, as needed, for the first 24 hours after surgery. To maintain accuracy, mark the point at which the circumference is measured on the dressing. Observe for blood on the dressing. Document and immediately report excessive bleeding or a sudden increase in the neck's circumference.
• Check for bleeding behind the neck of the supine patient. If a bulky neck dressing makes inspection difficult, use the quality of respirations and ability to swallow as guidelines.

Rationales

1. Maintaining a patent airway is essential. The most common cause of acute postoperative airway obstruction is compression of the trachea by a hematoma or edema at the surgical site. Tracheal deviation and signs of hypoxemia, including altered LOC, labored respirations, and wheezing or stridor, are key assessment findings for the obstructed airway.

2. Pulse oximetry provides ongoing noninvasive monitoring of arterial oxygen saturation. ABG values provide objective documentation of acid-base status and are a helpful adjunct to observations of respiratory status. Acidosis, hypoxemia, or hypercapnia may increase cerebral edema.

3. Although usually done in the operating room, emergency drainage of a life-threatening hematoma in the neck may be performed at the patient's bedside. Drainage may be necessary before an ET tube can be inserted. The postoperative carotid endarterectomy patient must avoid hypoxemia because sufficient damage to the carotid body impairs ventilatory and circulatory responses to hypoxia. Therefore, the patient may be intubated before hypoxemia develops. If the doctor is unable to intubate, a tracheostomy may be performed.

4. Bleeding can lead to hypovolemia, while hematoma formation may compress the airway.
• Neck size increases with a developing hematoma. Closely observing neck size, ensuring consistency in measurements, and monitoring for bleeding promotes early detection of hypoxia.

• Blood may pool, promoting hematoma formation posterior to the incision.

• Monitor hemoglobin levels and hematocrit as ordered, and report any decreases.
• If a drain is present, maintain patency, and note the amount of drainage. Document and report excessive drainage.

5. Evaluate the patient's ability to swallow.

6. Assess for an intact gag reflex, ability to swallow and speak clearly with normal tones, and symmetrical movements of the vocal cords and soft palate.

7. Keep suctioning equipment at the bedside for oral, pharyngeal, or ET suctioning as needed.

8. Implement measures to increase gas exchange and prevent hypoxemia:
• Elevate the head of the bed as ordered, as soon as vital signs are stable.
• Encourage deep breathing every 2 hours. Remind the patient to yawn and sigh periodically. Provide frequent position changes after vital signs have stabilized, minimizing stress on the operative site by supporting the head and maintaining proper alignment when turning and positioning the patient. Suction secretions as necessary.
• Discourage the patient from coughing during the first 24 hours after surgery.

• Evaluate respiratory rate and effort before administering analgesics or sedation.
• Maintain supplemental oxygen as ordered.

9. Additional individualized interventions: _____

• Decreasing hemoglobin levels and hematocrit may indicate slow bleeding.
• Excessive bleeding through a drain may lead to hypovolemia and hypotension.

5. Edema that exerts pressure on the trachea and esophagus makes swallowing difficult and increases the risk of airway obstruction.

6. Damage to the laryngeal branches of the vagus nerve prevents closure of the glottis, which can lead to aspiration and subsequent aspiration pneumonia. Pneumonia may cause hypoxia, a potentially dangerous condition after carotid endarterectomy.

7. Prompt suctioning can prevent aspiration.

8. Facilitating gas exchange helps prevent hypoxemia and the complications associated with it.
• An upright position facilitates diaphragmatic excursion.
• These measures lessen postoperative atelectasis.

• Coughing during the first 24 hours can exert excessive pressure on the incision and may cause it to rupture.
• Analgesics and sedatives can depress the respiratory center, promoting hypoxemia.
• Supplemental oxygen increases blood oxygen content.

9. Rationales: _____

DISCHARGE PLANNING

Discharge checklist
Before discharge, the patient shows evidence of:
❑ patent airway
❑ stable blood pressure within normal limits without I.V. inotrope or vasodilator support
❑ ABG measurements within normal limits
❑ no bleeding from incision
❑ stable neurologic function
❑ absence of cardiovascular, respiratory, or neurologic complications
❑ normal fluid and electrolyte balance
❑ absence of infection
❑ absence or control of seizures
❑ absence of headaches.

Teaching checklist
Document evidence that the patient and family demonstrate an understanding of:
❑ extent of surgery
❑ extent of neurologic deficits, if any
❑ rehabilitation, if needed
❑ risk factors for atherosclerosis
❑ need for lifestyle modifications
❑ recommended dietary modifications
❑ lifestyle modification programs, such as stress management, cardiovascular fitness, weight loss, smoking-cessation, and alcohol rehabilitation programs, as needed
❑ community resources for lifestyle modification support
❑ all discharge medications' purpose, dosage, schedule, and adverse effects
❑ signs and symptoms to report to health care provider.

Documentation checklist

Using outcome criteria as a guide, document:

❏ clinical status on admission
❏ significant changes in status, especially regarding motor, sensory, or visual deficits, or episodes of hypertension or hypotension
❏ wound condition
❏ pertinent laboratory and diagnostic test findings
❏ episodes of headaches or seizures
❏ respiratory support measures
❏ pain-relief measures
❏ nutritional status
❏ preoperative teaching
❏ patient and family teaching
❏ rehabilitation needs
❏ discharge planning.

ASSOCIATED PLANS OF CARE

Acute MI: Critical care unit
Cerebrovascular accident
Geriatric care
Impaired physical mobility
Increased intracranial pressure
Ineffective individual coping
Knowledge deficit
Mechanical ventilation
Pain
Sensory or perceptual alteration
Surgery

REFERENCES

Black, J.M., and Matassarin-Jacobs, E. *Medical-Surgical Nursing, Clinical Management for Continuity of Care*, 5th ed. Philadelphia: W.B. Saunders Co., 1997.

Fahey, V., ed. *Vascular Nursing*, 2nd ed. Philadelphia: W.B. Saunders Co., 1994.

Frattini, W.H. "AANA Journal Course: Update for Nurse Anesthetists — Carotid Endarterectomy: Anesthetic Implications," *Journal of the American Association of Nurse Anesthetists* 64(2):175-83, April 1996.

Lemone, P., and Burke, K.M. *Medical-Surgical Nursing, Critical Thinking in Client Care*. Menlo Park, Calif.: Addison-Wesley-Longman, 1996.

Smeltzer, S.C., and Bare, B.G. *Brunner and Suddarth's Textbook of Medical-Surgical Nursing*, 8th ed. Philadelphia: Lippincott-Raven Pubs., 1996.

Femoral popliteal bypass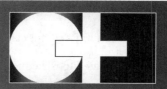

DRG information
DRG 478   Other Vascular Procedures with Complica-
tion or Comorbidities (CC).
Mean LOS = 8.3 days
DRG 479   Other Vascular Procedures without CC.
Mean LOS = 4.6 days

INTRODUCTION

Definition and time focus
Femoral popliteal bypass is one of several surgical revascularization techniques used to relieve symptoms of acute or chronic ischemia of the lower extremities. Femoral popliteal bypass involves using an autologous graft (usually the saphenous vein) or synthetic graft (polytetrafluoroethylene or Dacron) to route arterial blood from the femoral artery around a blocked popliteal artery, thus reestablishing blood flow in the tibial arteries. If revascularization fails, amputation is the treatment of last resort.

Femoral popliteal bypass may be the primary treatment or an adjunct to other revascularization techniques, such as angioplasty or intravascular stent placement. These newer, less invasive approaches to revascularization are associated with problems characteristic of any evolving technology, such as unsuitable design, insufficient technical guidance, and operator inexperience. These new techniques also carry a higher reported incidence of rapid thrombus formation, vessel perforation, vessel dissection, and rapid reocclusion of the manipulated vessel.

This plan focuses on postoperative care for the patient undergoing femoral popliteal bypass surgery.

Etiology and precipitating factors
Acute occlusion (Note: Acute occlusion is usually treated with anticoagulants, antiplatelet agents, vasodilators, embolectomy, or plasty repairs. Femoral popliteal bypass may be used when these approaches fail or the vessel is destroyed.)
• traumatic transection or occlusion
• disorders associated with embolus formation, such as endocarditis, aneurysms of the left ventricle or aorta, and atrial fibrillation
• collagen diseases and vasospastic disorders, such as thromboangiitis obliterans (Buerger's disease)
• diagnostic procedures such as angiography

Chronic occlusion (Note: Chronic occlusion may present with signs and symptoms of long-term ischemia or with evidence of acute limb-threatening ischemia. A stenosis of 60% or greater will produce significant symptoms. The typical blockage ranges in length from 1½" to 9½" [4 cm to 24 cm].)
• atherosclerosis, especially in a person over age 60 with a coexisting vascular disorder
• aneurysm of the popliteal artery
• chronic infection
• restenosis of previous grafts

FOCUSED ASSESSMENT GUIDELINES

Nursing history (functional health pattern findings)
Nutritional-metabolic pattern
• Obesity
• Type 1 or type 2 diabetes mellitus
• Adherence to a low-salt, low-cholesterol diet to control cardiovascular disease
• Severe nutritional deficit related to multisystem vascular insufficiency or advanced age
Elimination pattern
• Sudden onset of severe abdominal distress if ischemia is associated with multiple emboli and infarction of mesenteric vessels
• Symptoms of acute renal failure if ischemia is associated with multiple emboli and infarction of the renal or arcuate arteries
• Symptoms of chronic renal failure associated with hypertension and diabetes
• Neurosensory impairment of bowel function (constipation or diarrhea) associated with long-term diabetes
• Constipation associated with decreased physical activity
• Inability to perform activities of daily living (ADLs)
Activity-exercise pattern
• Sedentary lifestyle typical before onset of symptoms
• Limited mobility related to the onset of ischemic muscle pain with physical activity typically reported
• Leg muscle weakness associated with ischemic changes
• Sports- or work-related injury (dislocation of the knee)
• Fractures resulting from muscle weakness and sensory loss
• Inability to perform ADLs

• Unilateral or bilateral intermittent claudication

Sleep-rest pattern
• Sleep disturbance related to ischemic pain occurring at rest

Cognitive-perceptual pattern
• Low self-esteem as a result of inability to exercise or perform usual activities
• Depression
• History of cerebrovascular accident (CVA) with residual neurologic damage

Role-relationship pattern
• Diminished social interaction related to inability to maintain usual activities
• History of chronic alcohol abuse
• Diminished cognitive abilities associated with previous CVA

Sexuality-reproductive pattern
• Decreased libido if diabetic
• Impotence, if diabetic male
• Developing symptoms after menopause, if female
• Atrophy of secondary sex characteristics, if age 60 or older
• Oral contraceptive use or the recent birth of a child (uncommon)

Coping–stress tolerance pattern
• History of cigarette smoking
• History of chronic alcohol abuse

Physical findings
Cardiovascular
• Hypertension
• Decreased or absent peripheral pulses
• Bruits over abdominal aorta, femoral artery, or popliteal artery
• Increased capillary refill time
• Dependent rubor or cyanosis
• Atrial fibrillation
• Ventricular, aortic, or popliteal aneurysm

Renal
• Chronic renal failure
• Acute renal failure

Pulmonary
• Symptoms of heart failure or chronic obstructive pulmonary disease

Gastrointestinal
• Diarrhea or constipation
• Paralytic ileus

Neurologic
• Decreased sensory perception (heat, cold, pressure, vibration, and pain) in affected extremities
• Decreased proprioception in affected extremities
• Altered cognitive function

Integumentary
• Thinning
• Hair loss

• Paresthesia
• Ulcerations that fail to heal
• Skin cool or cold to touch
• Gangrene

Musculoskeletal
• Weakness
• Atrophy

Diagnostic studies
• Multiplane (retrograde femoral or translumbar) arteriography — visualizes abdominal aorta and vessels in the lower extremities
• Ultrasound Doppler and duplex waveform analyses — demonstrate direction and velocity of arterial flow
• 99mTc-hexametazime-labeled leukocyte imaging — radioactive scan, localizes infection in grafts from previous bypass procedures
• Ankle-brachial index (ABI) — noninvasive hemodynamic study, estimates the degree of arterial occlusion (a normal ABI is 1.0; single vessel occlusion, 0.5 to 1.0; multiple vessel occlusion, below 0.5)
• Toe-ankle index — noninvasive hemodynamic study, estimates degree of occlusion (normal toe-ankle index is above 0.65)
• Stress tests — estimate the degree of disease based on development of claudication
• Serum cholesterol — may be elevated if arterial occlusion is related to systemic vascular disease
• Serum triglycerides — may be elevated if symptoms are related to systemic vascular disease
• Blood glucose — may be elevated because diabetes mellitus is commonly associated with peripheral vascular disease
• Blood urea nitrogen — may be elevated if hypertension has affected renal function
• Liver function tests — may be altered in the patient with a history of alcohol abuse

Potential complications
• Hematoma formation
• Infection
• Emboli or thrombi
• Gangrene
• Skin ulcers

CLINICAL SNAPSHOT

FEMORAL POPLITEAL BYPASS

Major nursing diagnoses and collaborative problems	Key patient outcomes
Arterial insufficiency	Have bilaterally equal peripheral pulses.
Impaired skin integrity	Display no signs of infection.
Impaired physical mobility	Comply with activity restrictions.
Pain	Report pain, if any, (controlled by oral medications) as less than 3 on a 0 to 10 pain rating scale.

COLLABORATIVE PROBLEM

Arterial insufficiency related to arterial graft occlusion, reperfusion injury, or coexisting microangiopathy associated with diabetes or microemboli

Nursing priority

Maintain arterial flow.

Patient outcome criteria

Within 24 hours after surgery and then continuously, the patient will have:
• no ischemic pain
• bilaterally equal peripheral pulses.

Interventions

1. Assess and document appearance of surgical site. Include type of dressing, extent of drainage, and any drainage devices (such as a Hemovac).

2. Note the contours of the surgical site and compare with the opposite side. Observe for masses, ecchymoses, and skin changes. Monitor hemoglobin levels and hematocrit.

3. Measure calf circumference hourly for the first 24 hours, then as condition warrants. Observe for increased capillary refill time; diminished or absent pulses; mild pain beginning in the feet and lateral to the tibia, progressing to pain unrelieved by narcotics; decreased range of motion and ABI; or cold, cyanotic skin. Document findings.

Rationales

1. Baseline assessment permits later comparison of data. A surgical drain may be in place to remove lymph or blood. Drainage should be minimal and bright red initially, becoming serous within 24 hours.

2. Disruption of graft anastomosis, hemorrhage of soft tissues, or drainage from severed lymph vessels can produce enough fluid to occlude the graft. Fluid collection causes the skin at the site to become taut, with a dimpled appearance. A mass will be palpable. Surgical fluid removal is necessary if graft occlusion is imminent. Ecchymoses indicate arterial bleeding and possible disruption of the anastamosis. Decreased hemoglobin levels and hematocrit may indicate bleeding also.

3. These signs and symptoms suggest anterior compartment syndrome caused by tissue edema and hemorrhage. Emergency fasciotomy may be necessary to relieve signs and symptoms.

4. Position the leg to avoid hyperextension and undue pressure on the graft site.

5. Observe for symptoms of fluid volume deficit or hypotension. Document findings.

6. Administer ordered drugs and monitor for adverse reactions. If the antiplatelet medication will be continued after discharge, teach the patient about administration and possible adverse effects.

7. Observe for signs and symptoms of reperfusion injury (same as for severe hypoxia—cyanosis, coldness, and pain—with pulses still present). Maintain adequate hydration. If cyanosis, coldness, or pain occurs, check for presence of peripheral pulses using a Doppler waveform analysis. Notify the doctor of findings promptly and administer treatment as ordered, typically mannitol.

8. Additional individualized interventions: _____
_____

4. Hyperextension of the knee or pressure from body weight can retard venous flow, increasing tissue edema. Pressure also can diminish arterial flow through the graft. The resulting thrombosis calls for an emergency embolectomy.

5. The patient is at greatest risk for shunt occlusion immediately after surgery. Factors which decrease blood pressure could cause shunt collapse.

6. Antiplatelet drugs, such as dipyridamole (Persantine), ticlopidine hydrochloride (Ticlid) and aspirin, and anticoagulant drugs, such as heparin and warfarin (Coumadin), usually are ordered. Urokinase (Abbokinase) or streptokinase (Kabikinase) may be used to reverse shunt occlusion. The patient is usually continued on antiplatelet therapy after discharge.

7. In reperfusion injury, reperfused tissues typically demonstrate initial improvement, only to undergo severe hypoxic changes within 2 hours after surgery. Reperfused cells produce high levels of free oxygen radicals, which injure cells. Adequate hydration lessens the risk of reperfusion injury. The presence of peripheral pulses differentiates arterial reocclusion (in which pulses are absent) from reperfusion injury. Mannitol helps control reperfusion injury by acting as a free-radical scavenger.

8. Rationales: _____
_____

NURSING DIAGNOSIS

Impaired skin integrity related to surgical incision and possible preexisting stasis ulcers

Nursing priorities
• Promote wound healing.
• Prevent infection.

Patient outcome criteria

By the time of discharge, the patient will:
• demonstrate evidence of wound healing by primary intention
• display no symptoms of infection.

Interventions

1. Maintain strict aseptic technique in caring for the surgical wound, drains, and stasis ulcers of the feet and legs.

2. Do not administer injections on the affected side.

Rationales

1. The arterial graft lies close to the skin surface. As a result, infection at the surgical site can extend quickly to the shunt. In addition, lymph channels are severed during surgery, so debris from infected stasis ulcers drains into the surgical site, fostering infection at the graft.

2. Edema, tissue swelling, and the severing of lymph channels all slow circulation on the affected side, resulting in unpredictable drug absorption.

3. Assess for signs and symptoms of infection: fever, chills, malaise, increased pain at the surgical site, signs of arterial insufficiency distal to the site, incisional edema, drainage, and redness. Instruct the patient to observe for signs and symptoms of infection daily for 90 days after surgery.

4. Administer antibiotics and observe for adverse reactions.

5. Reposition the patient and perform skin care every 2 hours. Consider using a specialty bed or mattress for the patient with a chronic mobility problem, such as a multisystem disorder, obesity, or advanced age. Document your actions.

6. Monitor and document fluid and food intake.

7. Additional individualized interventions: _____

3. Tissue hypoxia before surgery increases the risk of infection. Infection with shunt occlusion can occur as late as 90 days after surgery.

4. Antibiotics are prescribed routinely because the risk of infection with subsequent shunt loss is high.

5. The skin, particularly on bony prominences, is prone to breakdown. Ulcers may already be present.

6. Adequate hydration and nutrition are necessary for wound healing and prevention of skin breakdown.

7. Rationales: _____

NURSING DIAGNOSIS

Impaired physical mobility related to surgery and preexisting disability

Nursing priority

Help the patient return to highest level of self-care and mobility possible.

Patient outcome criteria

By the time of discharge, the patient will:
• demonstrate no complications associated with immobility
• demonstrate improved mobility
• verbalize an understanding of the prescribed treatment regimen
• comply with activity restrictions.

Interventions

1. Before surgery, instruct the patient about positioning the affected extremity: avoiding hyperextension of the knee, leg-crossing, any position that puts pressure on the popliteal space, sitting for more than 20 minutes, or wearing clothing that restricts arterial flow.

2. After surgery, maintain the patient on bed rest as ordered, usually for 24 to 48 hours. Position the affected joint as ordered.

3. Encourage active range-of-motion (ROM) exercises of all unaffected joints 3 to 4 times daily or, if the patient is unable, perform passive ROM exercises.

4. Collaborate with the health care team to design an appropriate rehabilitation program. Instruct the patient accordingly.

Rationales

1. Preoperative teaching helps the patient avoid positions that could cause shunt occlusion.

2. Bed rest is usually maintained until shunt patency is ensured. Positioning depends on the type of surgery.

3. Exercise maintains joint flexibility and prevents postoperative complications associated with bed rest.

4. Extensive reconditioning may be necessary for the patient with long-term hypoxic injury to muscles and nerves or a history of myocardial infarction or CVA. Patient compliance with the rehabilitation regimen depends on an understanding of the prescribed treatment.

Cardiovascular disorders

5. Additional individualized interventions: _____

_____

5. Rationales: _____

_____

NURSING DIAGNOSIS

Pain related to the surgical incision

Nursing priority

Control pain.

Patient outcome criterion

Upon discharge, the patient will report pain (controlled with oral medication) as less than 3 on a 0 to 10 pain rating scale.

Interventions

1. See the "Pain" plan, page 88.

2. Identify and document the source and degree of pain, using 0 to 10 pain rating scale. Instruct the patient to report unrelieved pain.

3. Elevate the affected extremity.

4. Administer pain medication, as necessary, and observe for adverse reactions.

5. Additional individualized interventions: _____

_____

Rationales

1. General interventions for pain control are detailed in the "Pain" plan.

2. Prolonged or increasing pain could indicate hematoma or seroma formation at the surgical site. Unrelieved pain distal to the surgical site indicates anterior compartment syndrome, described under the "Arterial insufficiency" collaborative problem above, or shunt occlusion.

3. Moderate elevation, so as to not impair arterial flow, helps decrease tissue edema and swelling associated with surgical trauma.

4. Narcotic analgesics are used judiciously in the early postoperative period.

5. Rationales: _____

_____

DISCHARGE PLANNING

Discharge checklist

Before discharge, the patient shows evidence of:
❏ wound healing
❏ vital signs within limits for age and coexisting disorders
❏ absence of infection
❏ shunt patency
❏ absence of or minimal reports of pain
❏ restored arterial flow.

Teaching checklist

Document evidence that the patient and family demonstrate an understanding of:
❏ medication regimen
❏ proper positioning

❏ desirable lifestyle changes such as smoking cessation
❏ rehabilitation regimen
❏ dates and times of follow-up care
❏ symptoms of infection
❏ symptoms of arterial insufficiency
❏ symptoms requiring medical intervention.

Documentation checklist

Using outcome criteria as a guide, document:
❏ clinical status on admission
❏ significant changes in the preoperative state
❏ completion of preoperative checklist
❏ preoperative teaching
❏ clinical status on admission from postanesthesia unit
❏ amount and character of drainage from wounds or drains
❏ tube patency

❏ pain-relief measures
❏ activity tolerance
❏ nutritional intake
❏ elimination status
❏ pertinent laboratory finding
❏ patient and family teaching
❏ discharge planning
❏ clinical status upon discharge.

ASSOCIATED PLANS OF CARE

Amputation
Pain
Surgery

REFERENCES

Katzung, B., ed. *Basic and Clinical Pharmacology*, 7th ed. Stamford, Conn.: Appleton & Lange, 1998.
Handbook of Signs and Symptoms. Springhouse, Pa.: Springhouse Corp., 1998.
Noble, J., ed. *Textbook of Primary Care Medicine,* 2nd ed. St. Louis: Mosby–Year Book, Inc., 1996.
Stabo, J., ed. *The Principles and Practices of Medicine*. Stamford, Conn.: Appleton & Lange, 1996.

Cardiovascular disorders

Heart failure

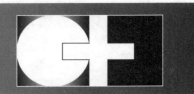

DRG information

DRG 127   Heart Failure and Shock.
Mean LOS = 6.2 days

DRG 127 is one of the most prevalent DRG's in the United States; however, heart failure frequently accompanies other diagnoses, particularly other cardiovascular diagnoses. In these instances, heart failure is not likely to be the principal diagnosis. Shock, likewise, is usually preceded by an underlying cause (such as sepsis, myocardial infraction, or trauma), which would generate the DRG.

INTRODUCTION

Definition and time focus

Heart failure is the end result of several disease states in which cardiac output (CO) fails to meet the body's metabolic demands, resulting in pulmonary and systemic congestion. Inadequate CO stimulates the sympathetic nervous system, resulting in increased heart rate, myocardial contractility, vasoconstriction, and salt and water retention. Cardiac and peripheral oxygen demands also increase. If the underlying problem cannot be corrected, these compensatory mechanisms lead to progressive fluid retention and further deterioration of cardiac efficiency. This plan focuses on the care of the patient admitted for treatment of an acute exacerbation of chronic heart failure or treatment of heart failure resulting from an acute event (such as acute myocardial infarction [AMI]).

Etiology and precipitating factors

• Conditions that reduce myocardial contractility, such as cardiomyopathies, ischemic cardiac disease, ventricular aneurysms, or constrictive pericarditis
• Conditions that increase fluid volume and lead to circulatory overload (increased preload), such as too-rapid infusion of I.V. fluids, increased sodium intake, or inadequate diuretic therapy
• Conditions that alter cardiac rhythm, such as severe bradycardia in the presence of decreased contractility, or tachycardia severe enough to decrease cardiac filling time and diminish CO
• Conditions that increase resistance to blood flow out of the heart (increased afterload), such as arteriosclerotic heart disease, hypertensive heart disease, or pulmonary hypertension
• Conditions that interfere with blood flow through the heart, such as valvular insufficiency or stenosis

• Conditions that increase oxygen demands beyond the heart's capabilities, such as hyperthyroidism, fever, pregnancy, or anemia

FOCUSED ASSESSMENT GUIDELINES

Nursing history (functional health pattern findings)

Health perception–health management pattern
• Long-term treatment for heart failure or a precipitating disease such as hypertensive heart disease
• No experience with signs and symptoms if episode occurs in response to an acute event such as an AMI
• Noncompliance with prescribed diet, medications, or activity restrictions
• Peripheral edema or fatigue (common)

Nutritional-metabolic pattern
• Anorexia (common); occasionally, reports nausea or vomiting from congested peripheral circulation or from medication adverse effects
• Weight loss and cachexia from decreased caloric intake and poor nutrient absorption

Elimination pattern
• Altered urinary patterns (from diuretic treatment or decreased renal blood flow)
• Constipation (from edema of the GI tract)

Activity-exercise pattern
• Inability to participate in exercise or leisure activities (common)
• Difficulty participating in everyday activities because of fatigue or shortness of breath

Sleep-rest pattern
• Disturbed sleep patterns from dyspnea and nocturia (common)
• Use of 2 or 3 pillows during sleep because of orthopnea (common)
• Paroxysmal nocturnal dyspnea

Cognitive-perceptual pattern
• Failure to understand problem and treatment protocols (if heart failure is an acute event)
• Headaches, confusion, or memory impairment

Self-perception–self-concept pattern
• Body-image disturbances related to edema and decreased activity level

Role-relationship pattern
• Difficulty fulfilling role responsibilities because of fatigue, weakness, or decreased activity tolerance (common)

Sexuality-reproductive pattern
• Decreased libido and impotence or orgasmic dysfunction related to fatigue or medications

Coping–stress tolerance pattern
• Anxiety related to shortness of breath
• Anxiety related to chronic illness
• Grief over loss of former level of health and loss of former roles and function
• Anticipation of premature death

Physical findings

Cardiovascular
• Tachycardia
• S_3 heart sound
• S_4 heart sound with summation gallop (with tachycardia)
• Atrial and ventricular arrhythmias
• Jugular vein distention
• Systolic murmur (in advanced heart failure)
• Decreased peripheral pulses

Pulmonary
• Dyspnea
• Crackles
• Nonproductive cough
• Progressive bilateral diminishing of breath sounds, beginning at bases

Neurologic
• Increased irritability
• Impaired memory
• Confusion (rare)

Gastrointestinal
• Abdominal distention
• Vomiting
• Tenderness over liver
• Liver enlargement

Renal
• Decreased urine output

Integumentary
• Dependent edema, such as in feet and sacrum
• Cyanosis
• Clubbing of fingers (in chronic failure)

Musculoskeletal
• Weakness and easy fatigability
• Muscle wasting (rare)

Diagnostic studies

• Serum electrolyte levels—electrolyte imbalances may occur from fluid shifts, diuretic therapy, or response of organ systems to decreased oxygen and increased congestion
–hyponatremia: volume overload causes dilutional hyponatremia; sodium restriction and diuretics may also lead to low serum sodium level
–hypokalemia: most common diuretics cause potassium loss

–hyperkalemia: can occur with oliguria or anuria, or excess potassium replacement
• Arterial blood gas measurements
–lowered Po_2 related to pulmonary congestion
–elevated Pco_2 (respiratory acidosis) may be from pulmonary edema or hypoventilation
• Prothrombin time/international normalized ratio (PT/INR), activated partial thromboplastin time (APTT)—obtained to determine baseline before beginning anticoagulant therapy or to evaluate clotting status during anticoagulant therapy
• Blood urea nitrogen (BUN) and creatinine levels—elevated, reflecting decreased renal function
• Bilirubin, aspartate aminotransferase, lactic dehydrogenase levels—elevated, indicating decreased liver function
• Urinalysis—reveals proteinuria and elevated specific gravity
• Chest X-ray—may reveal enlarged cardiac silhouette (common), distended pulmonary veins from redistribution of pulmonary blood flow, and interstitial and alveolar edema (common)
• Electrocardiogram—nonspecific diagnostically, but useful in identifying rhythm disturbances, conduction defects, axis deviations, and hypertrophy
• Echocardiography—can identify valvular abnormalities, chamber enlargement, abnormal wall motion, hypertrophy, pericardial effusions, and mural thrombi
• Multigated blood pool imaging scan—demonstrates decreased ejection fraction and abnormal wall motion

Potential complications
• Cardiogenic shock
• Pulmonary edema
• AMI
• Arrhythmias
• Thrombolytic complications
• Renal failure
• Liver failure

Cardiovascular disorders

CLINICAL SNAPSHOT

HEART FAILURE

Major nursing diagnoses and collaborative problems	Key patient outcomes
Decreased CO	Display signs of a normal CO.
Fluid volume excess	Have fluid intake and output in approximate balance.
Activity intolerance	Perform activities of daily living (ADLs) independently.
Nutritional deficit	Meet daily calorie requirement.
Knowledge deficit (lifestyle modifications)	Give name, purpose, dosage, schedule, and possible adverse effects for all discharge medications.
Risk for ineffective individual management of therapeutic regimen	Identify areas of potential ineffective management.

COLLABORATIVE PROBLEM

Decreased CO related to decreased contractility, altered heart rhythm, fluid volume overload, or increased afterload

Nursing priority

Maintain optimum CO.

Patient outcome criteria

By the time of discharge, the patient will:
• exhibit heart rate under 100 beats/minute
• exhibit optimal CO, as manifested by capillary refill time of less than 3 seconds, minimal or absent peripheral edema, normal peripheral pulses, and warm, dry skin
• have no S_3 heart sound
• have stable cardiac rhythm with any life-threatening arrhythmias under control
• have lungs clear to auscultation
• perform ADLs without incapacitating dyspnea
• have mental status within normal limits.

Interventions

1. Monitor and document heart rate and rhythm, heart sounds, blood pressure, pulse pressure, and the presence or absence of peripheral pulses. Compare to the baseline assessment. Report abnormalities to the doctor, particularly tachycardia, a new S_3 heart sound or systolic murmur, hypotension, decreased pulse pressure or pulse loss, or increased arrhythmias.

Rationales

1. One of the earliest signs of worsening heart failure is increased heart rate. A new S_3 heart sound or a systolic murmur may reflect increased fluid volume, leading to increased cardiac congestion and failure. Hypotension can reflect decreased CO from impaired myocardial contractility or overdiuresis. Diminished pulse pressure or peripheral pulse loss can indicate a decrease in CO. Increased arrhythmias can reflect an increased number of premature atrial or ventricular contractions — signs of increasing failure or medication toxicity.

2. Administer cardiac medications, as ordered, and document the patient's response. Observe for therapeutic and adverse effects:

• angiotensin converting enzyme (ACE) inhibitors such as captopril (Capoten) and enalapril (Vasotec) and angiotensin II receptor antagonists such as losartan — monitor for hypotension, hyperkalemia, and cough.

• inotropic agents (digitalis derivatives) — monitor for anorexia, pulse rate less than or above 100 beats/ minute, irregular heart rate, nausea, vomiting, and visual disturbances. Withhold the dose and contact the doctor if any of these signs or symptoms occur.

• diuretics such as hydrochlorothiazide (Esidrix) and furosemide (Lasix) — monitor for hypovolemia and hypokalemia. (See Appendix C, Fluid and Electrolyte Imbalances, for details.)
• nitrates such as isosorbide dinitrate (Isordil) — monitor for signs of hypovolemia.

• afterload reducers (vasodilators) such as hydralazine (Apresoline) — monitor for hypotension.

3. Observe for signs and symptoms of hypoxemia, such as confusion, restlessness, dyspnea, arrhythmias, tachycardia, and cyanosis. Ensure adequate oxygenation with proper positioning (semi-Fowler's or upright) and supplemental oxygen, as ordered.

4. Ensure adequate rest by monitoring the noise level, limiting visitors, grouping diagnostic tests (such as by ordering multiple blood tests on one blood sample, when possible), and spacing therapeutic interventions.

5. Monitor fluid status:

• Obtain accurate daily weights.

2. Pharmacotherapeutic agents may relieve heart failure by altering preload, contractility, or afterload — major determinants of CO. However, many of these agents have narrow therapeutic ranges or adverse effects that can worsen the underlying disease.
• The renin-angiotensin-aldosterone system is activated by low CO and decreased renal blood flow. Stimulation of the system results in the production of angiotensin II (a vasoconstrictor) and contributes to sympathetic nervous system stimulation and aldosterone production. The physiologic result of these substances is increased renal sodium retention and fluid retention. ACE inhibitors are the foundation of medical treatment for heart failure and relieve symptoms, improve exercise capacity, and reduce mortality.
• Inotropic agents increase contractility but also can increase myocardial oxygen consumption and cardiac workload, increasing heart failure. Digitalis glycosides, one of the most common medications used, have a narrow therapeutic range. (Therapeutic range via immunoassay is 0.5 to 2.0 ng/ml.) Early toxic adverse effects include anorexia; later, severe bradyarrhythmias, tachyarrhythmias, and irregular cardiac rhythms can compromise CO. Digitalis toxicity is more common in patients with compromised renal function and in the elderly.
• Diuretics decrease preload but can cause true hypovolemia from excessive fluid loss, or hypokalemia from potassium loss.

• Nitrates cause venodilation, reducing preload but also increasing the risk for relative hypovolemia from redistribution of blood volume to the periphery.
• Afterload reducers lower resistance to ventricular ejection but may lower blood pressure enough to compromise organ perfusion.

3. Prompt detection of hypoxemia allows timely intervention. The semi-Fowler position prevents abdominal organs from pressing on the diaphragm and interfering with its movement. An upright position permits a severely dyspneic patient to use accessory muscles for breathing; it also redistributes blood to dependent areas, decreasing blood return to the heart and reducing preload in a patient with volume overload. A patient who has difficulty maintaining an arterial oxygen level above 60 mm Hg may benefit from supplemental oxygen.

4. Rest reduces myocardial oxygen consumption.

5. Fluid volume may be increased from the heart's inability to maintain adequate flow and pressure through the kidneys.
• Rapid weight gain (1 to 2 lb [0.5 to 1 kg] a day) indicates fluid retention and the need for increased diuresis.

• Maintain an accurate intake and output record.

• Assess the lungs for crackles, decreased sounds, and a change from vesicular to bronchial breath sounds.

• Assess for dependent edema and increasing dyspnea.

• Assess for signs of dehydration.

6. Assess for increasing confusion.

7. Decrease the patient's fear and anxiety by providing information and by eliciting concerns and responding to them. See the "Ineffective individual coping" plan, page 67, for details.

8. Additional individualized interventions: _____

• Accurate intake and output records can warn of early fluid excess.
• Crackles, decreased sounds, and bronchial breath sounds indicate fluid in the lungs and signal increasing left-sided heart failure.
• Dependent edema and dyspnea are signs of increasing right-sided and left-sided heart failure respectively.
• Fluid volume may be decreased from excessive diuresis.

6. When CO is decreased, cerebral perfusion suffers, producing confusion.

7. Fear and anxiety activate the sympathetic nervous system and increase heart rate, myocardial contractility, and vasoconstriction. All these factors increase myocardial oxygen consumption. The "Ineffective individual coping" plan contains general interventions to reduce anxiety.

8. Rationales: _____

NURSING DIAGNOSIS

Fluid volume excess related to decreased myocardial contractility, decreased renal perfusion, and increased sodium and water retention

Nursing priority

Optimize and monitor volume status and electrolyte balance.

Patient outcome criteria

By the time of discharge, the patient will:
• have fluid intake and output in approximate balance
• exhibit sodium, potassium, creatinine, and BUN levels within expected parameters.

Interventions

1. See Appendix C, Fluid and Electrolyte Imbalances.

2. Monitor hourly fluid intake and output and 24-hour fluid balance. Weigh the patient daily.

3. Administer I.V. solutions, as ordered. Avoid saline solutions.

Rationales

1. The Fluid and Electrolyte Imbalances appendix describes the causes, signs and symptoms, laboratory findings, and treatments of these disorders.

2. Intake and output monitoring provides an objective method of tracking fluid gains or losses, while 24-hour summaries indicate net fluid balance. Daily weight measurements are a rough measure of fluid status; a weight change of 2.2 lb (1 kg) corresponds with a 1-L change in fluid balance.

3. The type and amount of I.V. fluid ordered depends upon the patient's current condition and the cause of heart failure. Saline solutions can cause water retention.

4. If the patient is placed on fluid restriction:
• explain the rationale to the patient and family

• establish a fluid intake schedule, teach the patient how to record oral fluids, and use microdrip tubing or an infusion pump to control I.V. intake.

5. Monitor creatinine and BUN levels and report increasing values.

6. Monitor sodium and potassium levels. Report abnormal values and signs of imbalances.

7. Additional individualized interventions: _____

4. Fluid restriction helps limit excessive preload.
• The patient and family are more likely to comply with fluid restriction if they understand the reasons behind it. Thirst is a powerful need and restricting fluids may cause the patient to feel deprived or punished. Explaining the rationale may help the patient view the situation positively.
• Regular fluid intake, consistent measurements, and use of microdrip tubing or infusion devices help ensure maintenance of fluid restrictions.

5. Creatinine and BUN levels reflect decreased renal perfusion from worsening heart failure. The BUN level rises disproportionately; the BUN-creatinine level ratio can increase from the normal of 10:1 to as high as 40:1.

6. Hyponatremia can cause decreased blood pressure, confusion, headache, and seizures; hypokalemia, weakness, fatigue, ileus, and ventricular fibrillation; and hyperkalemia, bradycardia, and ventricular asystole.

7. Rationales: _____

NURSING DIAGNOSIS

Activity intolerance related to bed rest and decreased CO

Nursing priorities
• Prevent complications of bed rest.
• Increase activity level without exceeding cardiac energy reserves.

Patient outcome criteria
By the time of discharge, the patient will:
• exhibit no evidence of thrombophlebitis or pulmonary embolism
• maintain a normal bowel pattern
• perform ADLs (feeding, bathing, and dressing) independently, with no significant change in heart rate or blood pressure
• walk in hall with no significant change in heart rate and blood pressure and no complaints of chest pain or profound fatigue.

Interventions

1. Determine cardiac stability by evaluating blood pressure, heart rhythm and rate, and indicators of oxygenation, such as level of consciousness (LOC) and skin color.

Rationales

1. Activity increases myocardial contractility, heart rate, blood pressure, and myocardial oxygen consumption. If CO is already compromised (as in tachycardia or severe arrhythmias), activity will reduce it further.

Cardiovascular disorders

2. When the patient is stable, institute a graduated activity program according to unit protocol. Begin with regular position changes and range-of-motion (ROM) exercises during bed rest. Then, as tolerated, progress to active ROM exercises, chair sitting, and ambulation.

3. Evaluate patient tolerance to new activities. Monitor blood pressure and pulse; respiratory rate, pattern, and depth; LOC and coordination; and patient reports of energy and strength. Discontinue activity, and resume it later at a slower pace, if any of the following occur:
• pulse rate greater than 30 beats/minute above resting level (or greater than 15 beats/minute if taking beta blockers)
• systolic blood pressure 15 mm Hg or more below resting level
• diastolic blood pressure 10 mm Hg or more above resting level
• new or increased pulse irregularity
• dyspnea, slowed respiratory rate, or shallow respirations
• decreased LOC or loss of coordination
• chest or leg pain
• fatigue disproportionate to activity level
• profound weakness.

4. Alternate activity with rest periods.

5. Administer anticoagulants, as ordered. Monitor appropriate coagulation studies and report results that exceed set limits.

6. Teach the patient how to avoid Valsalva's maneuver (forced expiration against a closed glottis), such as by exhaling when changing position and increasing fiber intake to promote bowel elimination.

7. Additional individualized interventions: _____

2. Bed rest has many detrimental effects, including cardiac deconditioning, increased risk of atelectasis and pneumonia, and skin breakdown. It also promotes venous stasis, further increasing the risk of thromboembolism from depressed myocardial contractility and atrial fibrillation—an arrhythmia common in heart failure because of atrial distention. Position changes and exercises that involve a change in muscle length (such as active or passive limb flexion) improve peripheral circulation and reduce the risks associated with immobility.

3. A too-rapid activity increase can exacerbate heart failure, myocardial ischemia, or peripheral vascular insufficiency. It also may cause hypotension, syncope, or cardiovascular collapse. At the least, activity goals that exceed the patient's capabilities may cause a psychological setback.

4. Bed rest and inactivity cause cardiac and muscle deconditioning. Initially, even short periods of activity can induce symptoms of cardiac compromise. Regular rest prevents depletion of cardiac reserves.

5. Heparin inactivates thrombin, preventing fibrin clot formation. Warfarin sodium (Coumadin) interferes with vitamin K production, decreasing synthesis of several clotting factors. The therapeutic APTT should be 2 to 2½ times normal; the therapeutic PT, 1½ to 2½ times normal. The therapeutic level of INR depends on why the patient is taking warfarin and other risk factors. For prevention of deep vein thrombosis, the therapeutic range of INR is 2.0 to 3.0.

6. Valsalva's maneuver increases intrathoracic pressure and decreases blood return to the heart. When the breath is released, venous return increases by reflex. Valsalva's maneuver has been associated with syncope and premature ventricular contractions.

7. Rationales: _____

NURSING DIAGNOSIS

Nutritional deficit related to decreased appetite and unpalatability of low-sodium diet

Nursing priority

Ensure adequate intake of nutrients needed for healing and increased energy requirements.

Patient outcome criterion

By the time of discharge, the patient will meet daily calorie requirements.

Interventions

1. Consult the "Nutritional deficit" care plan on page 80. Keep a daily record to monitor calorie intake. Consult with the dietitian to identify the patient's calorie needs.

2. Assess the patient's food preferences, and honor them when appropriate.

3. Additional individualized interventions: _____

Rationales

1. The "Nutritional deficit" care plan contains detailed information on assessing and meeting a patient's nutritional needs. Calorie needs vary with the patient's illness stage, activity level, and weight.

2. A low-sodium diet reduces cardiac preload by decreasing water retention. Unfortunately, low-sodium diets may be unpalatable to the patient accustomed to seasoned foods. The patient may be more compliant if food preferences are considered whenever possible.

3. Rationales: _____

NURSING DIAGNOSIS

Knowledge deficit (lifestyle modifications) related to complex disease process and treatment

Nursing priority

Prepare the patient to implement necessary lifestyle modifications to prevent recurrent episodes of heart failure, if possible.

Patient outcome criteria

By the time of discharge, the patient will:
• state intent to follow dietary recommendations
• demonstrate correct method for measuring pulse rate
• list five signs or symptoms of activity intolerance, on request
• give name, purpose, dosage, schedule, and possible adverse effects for all discharge medications
• verbalize understanding of when to seek emergency medical care
• have made first appointment for follow-up care
• verbalize understanding of daily weight measurement and weight gain requiring notification of the doctor.

Interventions

1. Once the patient is stable, institute a structured teaching plan only as the condition allows. See the "Knowledge deficit" plan, page 72, for details.

Rationales

1. The acutely ill patient usually is unable to tolerate sustained teaching. Planned teaching is more efficient and effective than haphazard instruction. The "Knowledge deficit" plan describes assessing readiness to learn and selecting teaching methods.

Cardiovascular disorders

2. Briefly explain the pathophysiology of heart failure. Relate the explanation to the patient's signs and symptoms.

3. Emphasize the patient's role in controlling the disease and the importance of medical follow-up.

4. With the dietitian, instruct the patient and family about the prescribed diet, usually one low in sodium, fat, cholesterol, and (if the patient is overweight) calories. Explain the rationale for such dietary restrictions as reducing sodium intake. Provide a list of high-sodium foods and suggest alternatives to salt, such as lemon juice and herbs. Recommend low-sodium cookbooks. Stress the importance of family support in making the necessary lifestyle changes.

5. Explain the rationale for activity restrictions. Provide specific information about recommended activities. Teach the patient to monitor activity tolerance by measuring pulse rate before and after activity and by watching for symptoms of over exertion. (See the "Activity intolerance" nursing diagnosis in this plan for details.)

6. Teach about discharge medications—typically inotropes, diuretics, vasodilators, or anticoagulants. Provide information sheets, and review the medications' purpose, dosage, schedule, adverse effects, and toxic effects. Stress the importance of taking doses on time. Suggest labeling a pillbox with days and times for doses.

7. Emphasize the importance of self-monitoring for signs and symptoms of increasing heart failure, such as ankle or leg swelling, breathlessness, tachycardia, and new or increased pulse irregularity. Teach the patient about the importance of measuring his weight daily on the same scale at the same time of day. Instruct the patient to contact the doctor based on specified weight parameters, such as when a 2-lb (1 kg) or greater weight gain occurs in 1 day or when a 4-lb (2 kg) weight gain occurs over 1 week.

8. Discuss with the patient and family an emergency plan, if needed, including:
• a medical alert bracelet
• circumstances that warrant emergency medical care, such as severe chest pain, marked difficulty breathing, and cessation of breathing
• access to emergency care
• cardiopulmonary resuscitation classes for the family.

2. Although extensive teaching should be deferred until the patient is stable, a brief explanation may help the patient understand the rationales for therapy. An adult learns best when the information relates directly to personal experience. Relevant information is helpful, but excessive detail can overwhelm and confuse.

3. Heart failure commonly becomes chronic or recurrent. The patient's active participation in implementing and monitoring treatment can be instrumental in limiting the disease's progression.

4. Many of the therapies for chronic or recurrent heart failure involve lifestyle modifications, such as a low-sodium diet, that may affect other family members. Other changes may involve habits the patient finds pleasurable, such as smoking. In either case, family support can smooth the transition to a more healthful lifestyle. Successful management of heart failure requires lifelong lifestyle modifications; changing eating habits is one of the most difficult. Understanding the reason for restrictions may help motivate the patient to establish and maintain the prescribed diet.

5. Vague instructions to "take it easy" leave the patient confused and may impair adjustment to an altered lifestyle, thus creating a "cardiac cripple." Providing information specific to the patient's condition lessens uncertainty and facilitates adjustment to recommended activity levels.

6. Successful heart failure management typically involves a long-term, complex drug regimen. Information about those medications better equips the patient and family to manage therapy at home. Understanding the drugs' purpose may increase the patient's motivation to take them; understanding dosage may increase accuracy. A properly labeled pillbox may decrease confusion and improve compliance.

7. An alert, informed patient and family are the first line of defense against recurrence or aggravation of heart failure. Knowing what to observe for and what measures to take increases the likelihood that the patient will receive prompt treatment. Early detection of increasing heart failure allows prompt adjustment of the therapeutic regimen. The patient is best able to identify subtle physiologic changes.

8. The patient with heart failure is at increased risk for other cardiovascular complications, such as AMI or cardiac arrest. Planning increases the likelihood of prompt, appropriate action in an emergency.

9. Review the plan for follow-up care — the doctor's name and telephone number and the date, time, and location of the next appointment.

10. Additional individualized interventions: _____

9. Management of heart failure requires consistent follow-up care.

10. Rationales: _____

NURSING DIAGNOSIS

Risk for ineffective individual management of therapeutic regimen related to complexity of therapeutic regimen, health beliefs, or negative relationship with caregivers

Nursing priority

Maximize likelihood of effective management.

Patient outcome criteria

Within 2 days of admission, the patient will:
• identify areas of potential ineffective management
• identify reasons for potential ineffective management
• verbalize willingness and ability to follow modified therapeutic plan, when possible.

Interventions

1. Observe for indicators of ineffective management, such as exacerbation of signs and symptoms, development of complications, failure to keep follow-up appointments, reports of behavior contrary to health recommendations, failure to seek health care when indicated, despairing remarks about health status, or belligerent exchanges with caregivers.

2. Evaluate the extent and result of ineffective management.

3. Differentiate possible causes of ineffective management, such as knowledge deficit, lack of family support, memory deficits, adverse effects of treatment, transportation difficulties, denial, poor self-esteem, or self-destructive behavior. Consult the "Ineffective individual coping" plan, page 67, and the "Knowledge deficit" plan, page 72, for possible interventions. Take appropriate steps, such as providing information or making necessary referrals, as indicated.

4. Initiate discussion of the situation with the patient and family, involving a psychiatric clinician or other health care team members as needed.

5. Express concern for the patient as a person.

Rationales

1. Ineffective management can have serious repercussions. Early identification of a problem increases the likelihood of its successful resolution.

2. If ineffective management is limited to areas of minor consequence in the overall plan of care, no further action may be necessary.

3. Identifying problems accurately increases the likelihood of appropriate intervention and resolution.

4. Open discussion can help reveal the reasons for ineffective management. The patient, family, and health care team members all can contribute insights and observations helpful in reevaluating the plan of care.

5. Expression of human caring and warmth may help break a cycle of negativity, if present, and free emotional energy for improved self-care. Nurturing behavior also may help establish rapport and trust.

Cardiovascular disorders

6. Emphasize the seriousness of heart failure and the importance of self-care. Use the patient's situation to explain how ineffective management affects health, and emphasize the positive outcomes of effective management.

7. Discuss the following with the patient:
• life priorities
• perception of prognosis
• feelings about the illness's length
• complexity of treatment
• degree of confidence in caregivers
• health care beliefs.

8. Consider the patient's cultural and spiritual heritage.

9. Ask the patient about satisfaction with caregivers. Also, examine caregivers' attitudes: if nontherapeutic, either help establish more positive attitudes or assign other caregivers to the patient.

10. Validate conclusions about reasons for behavior with the patient and loved ones.

11. Collaborate with other caregivers to reevaluate the goals and implementation of care. Consider possible modifications.

12. Search for alternative solutions. Ask what the patient wants or is willing to do to bring about agreement to the plan of care.

13. Use creative negotiation strategies to set goals with the patient. Consider changing the agreement's scope, shortening its length, or making trade-offs.

14. If the patient makes an informed choice not to follow the recommendations, and if negotiation is not possible:
• avoid punitive responses, and accept the decision

• keep open the option for treatment

• respect the patient's readiness to die.

15. Additional individualized interventions: _____

6. Failure to accept an illness's seriousness can be linked to ineffective management. Discussion that incorporates the patient's experiences is most effective in making points "come alive."

7. Apparent deliberate ineffective management may actually reflect preoccupation with more pressing needs, such as food and shelter. The patient's perception of expected outcomes may be overly pessimistic. Prolonged illness, complex treatment, lack of confidence in caregivers, and health care beliefs that differ from caregivers' beliefs increase the likelihood of ineffective management.

8. The patient is less likely to accept treatment that clashes with cultural or spiritual beliefs.

9. The patient's level of dissatisfaction with caregivers influences management of therapeutic regimen. A caregiver's negative attitude that results from frustration may be changed through expression and peer support. A negative attitude that results from burnout or personality clashes, however, may be best handled by removing the caregiver from the situation.

10. Obtaining feedback about the accuracy of conclusions helps avoid erroneous assumptions and inappropriate interventions.

11. Insisting on a plan to which the patient objects may create a power struggle between patient and caregivers. Flexibility and adaptability are more likely to achieve the desired ends.

12. Focusing on what the patient wants or is willing to do interrupts negativism and recasts the situation in a positive light. Such refocusing may free energy for creative problem solving and increase the patient's sense of control.

13. If full agreement is not possible, partial or temporary agreement may be. The patient may be willing to trade compliance in one area (such as medications) for greater freedom in another (such as food intake).

14. Patients have the right of self-determination.

• Exhibiting rejecting or other punitive behavior is disrespectful and may provoke the patient to terminate contact with health care resources.
• As the patient's condition changes, resistance may soften.
• Every person has the right to die with dignity. The patient's decision to refuse care may be a rational choice to live out the remaining period of life in a meaningful way.

15. Rationales: _____

DISCHARGE PLANNING

Discharge checklist
Before discharge, the patient shows evidence of:
❑ stable vital signs
❑ absence of fever and pulmonary or cardiovascular complications
❑ ability to tolerate adequate nutritional intake
❑ stable cardiac rhythm with arrhythmias controlled
❑ shortness of breath no worse than usual
❑ peripheral edema within acceptable limits or no worse than usual
❑ ABG measurements within acceptable parameters
❑ clear lung fields shown on chest X-ray within 48 hours of discharge
❑ absence of supplemental oxygen for at least 48 hours before discharge
❑ absence of signs and symptoms of dehydration
❑ mental status within normal limits
❑ laboratory values within expected parameters
❑ absence of urinary or bowel dysfunction
❑ ability to perform ADLs and ambulate same as before admission
❑ adequate home support system, or referral to home care if indicated by inadequate home support or inability to perform ADLs
❑ referral to community heart failure support group.

Teaching checklist
Document evidence that the patient and family demonstrate an understanding of:
❑ cause and implications of heart failure
❑ signs and symptoms of increasing heart failure
❑ all discharge medications' purpose, dosage, administration schedule, and adverse effects requiring medical attention (usual discharge medications include inotropes, diuretics, vasodilators, or anticoagulants)
❑ need for lifestyle modifications
❑ dietary restrictions
❑ activity restrictions
❑ plan for follow-up care
❑ plan for emergency care
❑ how to contact the doctor.

Documentation checklist
Using outcome criteria as a guide, document:
❑ clinical status on admission
❑ significant changes in clinical status
❑ pertinent laboratory and diagnostic findings
❑ intake and output
❑ nutritional intake
❑ response to activity progression
❑ response to illness and hospitalization
❑ family's response to illness
❑ patient and family teaching
❑ discharge planning.

ASSOCIATED PLANS OF CARE
Acute MI: Critical care unit
Acute MI: Telemetry unit
Chronic renal failure
Dying
Grieving
Ineffective individual coping
Knowledge deficit
Nutritional deficit

REFERENCES

Beattie, S., and Pike, C. "Left Ventricular Diastolic Dysfunction: Case Report," *Critical Care Nurse,* (16)2:37-50, April 1996.

Gibbar-Clements, T., et al. "PT and APTT: Seeing Beyond the Numbers," *Nursing97* 27(7):49-51, July 1997.

Kinney, M.R., et al. *AACN's Clinical Reference for Critical Care Nursing,* 4th ed. St. Louis: Mosby–Year Book, Inc., 1998.

Konstam M., et al. *Heart Failure: Management of Patients with Left-Ventricular Systolic Dysfunction, Clinical Practice Guideline No. 11.* AHCPR Publication No. 94-0612. Rockville, Md.: Agency for Health Care Policy and Research, Public Health Service, U.S. Department of Health and Human Services, June 1994.

Schwabaurer, N.J. "Retarding Progression of Heart Failure: Nursing Actions," *Dimensions of Critical Care Nursing* 15(6):307-17, November 1996.

Stanley, M. "Current Trends in the Management of an Old Enemy: Congestive Heart Failure in the Elderly," *AACN Clinical Issues* 8(4):616-26, November 1997.

Waterer, C.H., et al. "Dilated Cardiomyopathy: Strategies for Improving Survival," *The Journal of Critical Illness,* (9)3:231-43, 1994.

Cardiovascular disorders

Hypovolemic shock

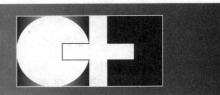

DRG information
DRG 127   Heart Failure and Shock.
Mean LOS = 6.2 days
Note: Hypovolemic shock is more likely to be coded by its cause than by DRG 127 because the principal diagnosis or procedure determines the DRG. For example, hypovolemic shock caused by GI hemorrhage would be coded as DRG 174, GI Hemorrhage with Complication or Comorbidity.

INTRODUCTION

Definition and time focus
Hypovolemic shock is a complex, life-threatening process of microcirculatory dysfunction and altered cellular metabolism resulting from decreased blood volume. Sympathetic stimulation mediates hypovolemic shock's systemic effects, which include constriction of precapillary sphincters and venules. The resulting low capillary pressure promotes an interstitial-to-intravascular fluid shift that temporarily compensates for diminished circulating blood volume and maintains capillary flow. As shock progresses, however, this powerful compensatory mechanism fails. Decompensation results in capillary hypoxemia and acidosis, which promote sphincter relaxation, allowing capillary pressure to rise. Increased capillary permeability permits fluid to leak into the tissues, and the resulting decreased circulating blood volume increases hypoxemia and acidosis, creating a vicious circle that ultimately causes irreparable damage.

On a cellular level, shock disrupts vital processes. Delicate sodium-potassium transport mechanisms are paralyzed, allowing sodium to accumulate inside the cell and produce swelling. Mitochondrial depression impairs energy production; oxygen deprivation causes cells to switch from aerobic to anaerobic metabolism. Anaerobic metabolism, an inefficient energy-generating process, also depletes glucose stores and produces lactic acid, creating metabolic acidosis. As cells die, lysosomal destruction releases proteases, enzymes, and cellular debris. These materials wreak havoc on surrounding cells' integrity and trigger release of vasoactive substances, including myocardial depressant factor, that cause myocardial depression and severe vasodilation, further accelerating the vicious circle. This plan focuses on recognizing the patient in the medical-surgical setting who is at risk for developing hypovolemic shock as well as the critically ill patient with hypovolemic shock.

Etiology and precipitating factors
- Hemorrhage
- Excessive GI fluid losses through emesis and diarrhea
- Severe dehydration
- Excessive diuresis
- Burns
- Trauma
- Diabetes mellitus or diabetes insipidus
- Surgical interventions

FOCUSED ASSESSMENT GUIDELINES

Nursing history (functional health pattern findings)
Health perception–health management pattern
- History of diabetes mellitus, heart failure, pancreatitis, hypertension, hemorrhage (internal or external), or other factors affecting fluid balance
- Recent invasive procedure performed, especially any major surgical procedure, such as open-heart surgery, abdominal resection, or massive trauma repair
- History of recent trauma (particularly to the chest, abdomen, or spinal cord) or burns
Nutritional-metabolic pattern
- Intense thirst
- Inability to verbalize need for fluids
Elimination pattern
- Increased urination or severe diarrhea (early) or oliguria (late)
Activity-exercise pattern
- Weakness and fatigue typical
Cognitive-perceptual pattern
- Reduced alertness or restlessness or anxiety common

Physical findings
Cardiovascular
- Orthostatic hypotension (early)
- Supine hypotension (late)
- Tachycardia
- Arrhythmias
- Decreased or thready peripheral pulses
- Capillary filling time greater than 3 seconds
Neurologic
- Altered level of consciousness, ranging from confusion, irritability, or restlessness (early) to coma (late)

Integumentary
• Altered skin temperature, ranging from coolness (early) to coldness (late)
• Altered skin tone ranging from pallor to mottling to cyanosis

Gastrointestinal
• Pale or cyanotic oral mucous membranes

Renal
• Oliguria or anuria

Diagnostic studies
No laboratory tests are diagnostic for hypovolemic shock. Values will change reflecting end-organ deterioration. Such changes may include:
• complete blood count (CBC) — may vary, depending on shock stage; may be decreased with blood loss; typically, decreased hemoglobin level and increased hematocrit
• blood glucose level — elevated, reflecting stress-induced sympathetic stimulation
• blood urea nitrogen (BUN) and creatinine levels — elevated, reflecting decreased renal perfusion
• serum electrolyte levels — may vary, depending on the underlying problem and shock stage. Commonly, hypernatremia reflects increased renal sodium retention in response to volume losses; hypokalemia reflects urinary potassium losses in exchange for sodium; and hyperkalemia reflects acidosis, decreased glomerular filtration, and cell necrosis

• arterial blood gas (ABG) levels — reveal increased pH level and decreased partial pressure of arterial oxygen ($Paco_2$) in early shock, reflecting respiratory alkalosis caused by hyperventilation that progresses to decreased pH level, increased $Paco_2$, and decreased bicarbonate level in late shock, reflecting respiratory acidosis caused by hypoventilation and metabolic acidosis caused by anaerobic metabolism
• clotting profile — may reveal coagulopathy, shown by decreased platelet level, decreased fibrinogen level, and increased fibrin split products or altered D-dimer results
• serum osmolality — may increase, reflecting fluid loss
• urine osmolality or specific gravity — increase, reflecting volume loss
• 12-lead electrocardiogram (ECG) — may reveal arrhythmias or changes reflecting myocardial ischemia, acute myocardial infarction (AMI), or electrolyte imbalances
• chest X-ray — may reveal pneumothorax or hemothorax

Potential complications
• Acute renal failure
• Adult respiratory distress syndrome (ARDS)
• Disseminated intravascular coagulation (DIC)
• Cardiogenic shock
• Cerebral anoxia
• Multiple organ dysfunction syndrome

CLINICAL SNAPSHOT

HYPOVOLEMIC SHOCK

Major nursing diagnoses and collaborative problems	Key patient outcomes
Risk for fluid volume deficit	Maintain stable vital signs: typically, heart rate, 60 to 100 beats/minute; systolic blood pressure, 90 to 140 mm Hg; and diastolic blood pressure, 50 to 90 mm Hg.
Hypovolemic shock	Have warm dry extremities, indicating sufficient tissue perfusion.
Hypoxemia	Show pulse oximetry and ABG levels within expected limits.
Risk for injury: Complications	Show no signs of end-organ failure.
Risk for ineffective individual coping, ineffective family coping, or both	Use support offered by caregivers.

Cardiovascular disorders

Nursing diagnosis

Risk for fluid volume deficit related to disease processes, surgical interventions, or iatrogenic interventions

Nursing priorities

- Recognize patients at high risk for developing hypovolemia.
- Monitor patient status and prevent progression to shock state.

Patient outcome criteria

Within 48 hours, the patient will:
- show stable vital signs: typically, heart rate, 60 to 100 beats/minute; systolic blood pressure, 90 to 140 mm Hg; and diastolic blood pressure, 50 to 90 mm Hg
- have adequate urine output (greater than 30 ml/hour)
- have strong peripheral pulses
- have normal temperature of skin
- display level of consciousness normal for patient.

Interventions

1. Identify patients at risk for development of hypovolemic shock.

2. If patient is actively bleeding, apply direct continuous pressure and elevate the area, if possible.

3. Assess as accurately as possible the volumes of loss from emesis, diarrhea, drainage tubes, ostomies, fistulas, dressings, and other sources.

4. Assess for changes in:
- pulse quality

- blood pressure
- tachypnea

- urine output

5. Obtain orders for fluid volume replacement, if indicated. Monitor for indications of normalizing volume status, such as normalizing blood pressure, slowing of heart rate to within normal range, and increased urine output.

6. Additional individualized interventions: _____

Rationales

1. Early intervention may prevent progression of hypovolemia to a hypovolemic shock state that may result in end-organ damage. Hemorrhage is the primary reason for development of hypovolemia; excessive GI losses are the second reason.

2. Direct pressure to bleeding sites mechanically controls hemorrhage and aids in clot formation.

3. Measurement of volumes from these sources is commonly inaccurate, leading to inadequate fluid volume replacement therapy.

4. These changes may indicate a potential problem:
- Thin and thready pulse indicates hypovolemia; bounding pulse indicates hypervolemia.
- Orthostatic (postural) changes indicate hypovolemia.
- Increased respiratory rate indicates attempt to increase circulating oxygen.
- A rate of less than 30 ml/hour indicates decreased cardiac output (CO).

5. Early replacement of lost volumes with either crystalloids or colloids may prevent progression of hypovolemia to shock.

6. Rationales: _____

Collaborative problem

Hypovolemic shock related to blood loss, diuresis, dehydration, or third-space fluid shift

Nursing priority

Restore fluid volume.

Patient outcome criteria

Within 48 hours, the patient will:
• show stable vital signs: typically, heart rate, 60 to 100 beats/minute; systolic blood pressure, 90 to 140 mm Hg; and diastolic blood pressure, 50 to 90 mm Hg
• be hemodynamically stable and no longer require hemodynamic monitoring
• show no signs of fluid overload
• have warm, dry extremities indicating sufficient tissue perfusion
• have stable neurologic status—ideally, alert and oriented.

Interventions

1. Observe for signs and symptoms of fluid loss:

• minimal volume loss: slight tachycardia; normal supine blood pressure; positive postural vital signs (systolic blood pressure decrease greater than 10 mm Hg or pulse increase greater than 20 beats/minute); capillary refill time greater than 3 seconds; urine output greater than 30 ml/hour; cool, pale extremities; and anxiety

• moderate volume loss: rapid, thready pulse; supine hypotension; cool truncal skin; urine output 10 to 30 ml/hour; severe thirst; and restlessness, confusion, or irritability

• severe volume loss: marked tachycardia and hypotension; weak or absent peripheral pulses; cold, mottled, or cyanotic skin; urine output less than 10 ml/hour; and unconsciousness.

2. Elevate the patient's legs above heart level, unless there is active bleeding from the head and neck or suspected increased ICP or cardiogenic shock.

3. Obtain initial and serial diagnostic tests, including CBC, blood typing and crossmatching, serum electrolyte levels, ABG levels, urinalysis, 12-lead ECG, and chest X-ray.

4. Insert and maintain the following, as ordered:
• two or more large-bore I.V. lines

• indwelling urinary catheter.

Rationales

1. Signs and symptoms correlate with the approximate percentage of volume loss.
• Powerful compensatory mechanisms produce these signs, which correlate with blood volume loss between 10% and 15%. Medullary vasomotor center stimulation via the baroreceptor reflex causes tachycardia and vasoconstriction. Also, antidiuretic hormone and aldosterone release causes renal retention of sodium and water. All of these mechanisms help to maintain blood volume and normal supine blood pressure. However, postural vital signs are positive because homeostatic mechanisms cannot compensate for the added stress of a position change. Prolonged capillary refill time and slight oliguria reflect decreased circulating volume. Cool, pale skin with normal mental status reflects shunting of blood away from the periphery to preserve function of the brain and heart.
• These signs correlate with a volume loss of approximately 25%. As circulating blood volume drops to this level, compensatory mechanisms are no longer sufficient and decompensation occurs. Oliguria reflects decreased renal perfusion, while mental changes indicate decreased cerebral perfusion.
• These signs reflect a volume loss of at least 40% and severely decreased vital organ perfusion.

2. Elevation promotes venous drainage from the legs and increases circulating blood volume as much as 800 ml. This measure will exacerbate the conditions indicated, however.

3. Serial data provide objective evidence of the disorder's severity and the effectiveness of interventions.

4. These invasive measures will combat shock.
• Large-bore I.V. lines allow rapid infusion of large fluid volumes.
• An indwelling catheter facilitates monitoring of urine output, the most easily assessed indicator of renal perfusion as well as an indicator of CO.

5. Assist with insertion of a central venous pressure (CVP) catheter or pulmonary artery (PA) catheter, if ordered. Monitor CVP or pulmonary artery wedge pressure (PAWP) hourly or according to protocol. Determine the frequency of measurement according to the depth of shock and rapidity of its progression.

5. CVP measurements can be used to guide fluid volume replacement and may be ordered for patients with lesser degrees of shock. For patients with severe shock, a PA catheter is preferred because it allows measurement of PAWP, which reflects left ventricular filling pressures more accurately than CVP does. Frequent measurements help determine the degree of shock and evaluate the effectiveness of interventions.

6. Administer a fluid challenge, if ordered. See *Fluid challenge algorithm,* for details.

6. A fluid challenge involves administration of a fluid bolus over a limited period. It allows assessment of hemodynamic response to rapid volume administration, which helps identify hypovolemic shock.

7. Administer blood products and crystalloid or colloid I.V. solutions, as ordered.

7. Various I.V. solutions may be used; their advantages and drawbacks remain controversial. Blood products should be given to replace direct losses. Colloids—solutions containing protein—help expand intravascular volume through osmosis; however, proteins may leak into the interstitial space, causing such complications as pulmonary edema. Crystalloid solutions—solutions containing salt, sugar, or both—require relatively large volumes because they leave the vascular space quickly. They also move into interstitial and intracellular spaces potentially causing edema as well.

8. Assist with insertion of an arterial line, if ordered. Monitor blood pressure continuously and measure mean arterial pressure (MAP) electronically.

• If an arterial line is not in place, measure cuff blood pressure every 5 to 15 minutes until stable, then every hour. Monitor MAP electronically or calculate it by adding one-third of pulse pressure to diastolic pressure, or by using this formula:

$$\frac{SP + (DP \times 2)}{3}$$

where SP equals systolic pressure and DP equals diastolic pressure.

8. Direct blood pressure measurement is preferred because it provides more accurate data than cuff measurements. MAP reflects the average pressure at which organs are perfused.
• Cuff blood pressure measurements and arithmetic MAP calculation, though less desirable than intra-arterial measurement, provide valuable data. MAP is closer to diastolic blood pressure than to systolic blood pressure because diastole is about twice as long as systole in the cardiac cycle.

• Maintain MAP within the desired range—usually at least 70 mm Hg. Consult with the doctor about the appropriate range for the patient.

• Maintaining MAP within the desired range provides for adequate organ perfusion. In most cases, MAP must be maintained above 70 mm Hg in a previously normotensive patient. A higher MAP is appropriate for the patient with chronic hypertension. An MAP that is too low promotes ischemia; an MAP that is too high contributes to such complications as cerebral and pulmonary edema.

9. During all fluid administration, monitor the trend of hemodynamic measurements and urine output. Observe for signs of fluid overload, such as crackles, neck vein distention, or a third heart sound.

9. Because the shock patient is hemodynamically unstable and has compromised compensatory mechanisms, volume administration may cause rapid progression from fluid depletion to fluid overload. If not detected promptly, fluid overload may cause pulmonary edema, heart failure, or cerebral edema.

10. Additional individualized interventions: _____

10. Rationales: _____

Fluid challenge algorithm

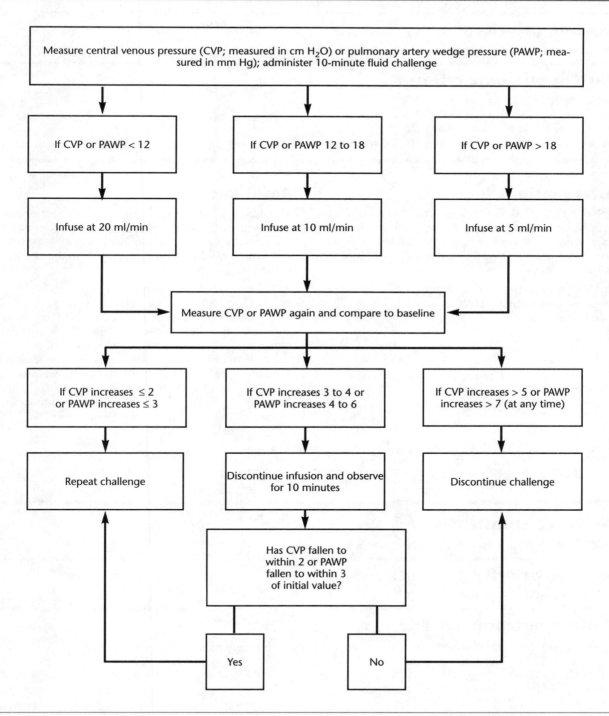

Adapted from M.H. Weil and E.C. Rackow, "A Guide to Volume Repletion," *Emergency Medicine* 16(8):101-10, ©1984 by Cahners Publishing Company. Used with permission.

Cardiovascular disorders

COLLABORATIVE PROBLEM

Hypoxemia related to ventilation-perfusion imbalance and diffusion defect

Nursing priority

Maintain ventilation and oxygenation.

Patient outcome criteria

Within 48 hours, the patient will:
• maintain a patent airway
• have clearing breath sounds bilaterally
• have ABGs within normal limits: pH, 7.35 to 7.45; P_{CO_2}, 35 to 45 mm Hg; HCO_3^-, 23 to 28 mEq/L.

Interventions

1. Provide standard nursing care related to impaired gas exchange: maintain airway patency; monitor respiratory status; suction as necessary; provide supplemental oxygen, as ordered; and assist with intubation and mechanical ventilation, if indicated.

2. Monitor oxygen saturation through continuous pulse oximetry. Monitor ABG levels, as ordered — typically at least every 4 hours.

3. Additional individualized interventions: _____

Rationales

1. Numerous factors may cause ventilation-perfusion imbalance in shock, including atelectasis, microemboli, pulmonary congestion, and impaired capillary perfusion. The general measures listed apply to the care of any critically ill patient.

2. Pulse oximetry determines oxygen saturation rapidly, continuously, and noninvasively. ABG results indicate oxygenation status and degree of acid-base imbalance at the time the sample was drawn. Hyperventilation, a compensatory response to hypoxemia, is common in early hypovolemic shock and can lead to respiratory alkalosis. Combined metabolic acidosis (lactic acid production in anaerobic metabolism from increased capillary perfusion time) and respiratory acidosis (due to hypercarbia) characterize late hypovolemic shock.

3. Rationales: _____

NURSING DIAGNOSIS

Risk for injury: Complications related to ischemia

Nursing priority

Prevent or minimize complications.

Patient outcome criteria

By the time of discharge, the patient will show no signs of end-organ failure of the following systems:
• neurologic
• cardiologic
• mesenteric
• hepatic
• renal
• hematologic.

Interventions

1. Prevent paralytic ileus and stress ulcers. Withhold food and fluids; insert a nasogastric tube connected to suction, as ordered. Administer cimetidine (Tagamet), ranitidine (Zantac), sucralfate (Carafate), or antacids, as ordered. Monitor bowel sounds.

2. Observe for signs and symptoms of ARDS, such as tachypnea, progressive dyspnea, increased inspiratory pressure (if the patient is mechanically ventilated), deteriorating ABG or pulse oximetry values, or lung compliance less than 50 ml/cm H_2O. If you detect these problems, document them and alert the doctor. Implement measures described in the "Adult respiratory distress syndrome" plan, page 240, as appropriate.

3. Observe for signs and symptoms of AMI, such as severe chest pain, shortness of breath, hypotension, diaphoresis, pained facial expression, elevated cardiac isoenzymes, or ECG showing ST-segment displacement, T-wave inversion, or pathologic Q waves. See the "Acute MI: Critical care unit" plan, page 338, for more details.

4. Observe for signs and symptoms of DIC, such as blood oozing from multiple sites, repeated bleeding episodes, oral cyanosis, petechiae, ecchymoses, hematomas, prolonged prothrombin time (PT), prolonged activated partial thromboplastin time, decreased fibrinogen level, decreased platelet count, elevated fibrin split products level or altered D-dimer results. See the "Disseminated intravascular coagulation" plan, page 780, for details.

5. Observe for signs and symptoms of acute renal failure, such as oliguria or anuria, weight gain, neck vein distention, crackles, dependent edema, or elevated BUN and serum creatinine levels. As appropriate, implement measures described in the "Acute renal failure" plan, page 686.

6. Observe for signs and symptoms of liver failure, such as drowsiness, intellectual deterioration, personality changes, septicemia, fever, hyperkinetic circulation, jaundice, hepatomegaly, ascites, easy bruising, increased PT, elevated serum aspartate aminotransferase level, or increased bilirubin level. See the "Liver failure" plan, page 551.

7. Additional individualized interventions: _____

Rationales

1. Paralytic ileus may result from mesenteric ischemia. The resulting gastric distention provokes vomiting, which can lead to chemical pneumonitis if aspiration occurs. Withholding food and fluids reduces stress on the stomach. Nasogastric drainage decompresses the stomach. The medications listed reduce the risk of stress ulcers by decreasing hydrochloric acid secretion or coating the gastric mucosa.

2. Shock ranks as a major potential complication of ARDS because of such factors as decreased perfusion, hypoxemia, increased capillary permeability, and high oxygen levels used in treatment. The plan for ARDS describes this ominous development and related care.

3. Decreased perfusion, catecholamine stimulation, hypoxemia, and increased afterload all may cause AMI. The AMI plan gives details on this complication.

4. Shock is a major risk factor for DIC because of such factors as capillary sludging, acidosis, and sepsis, trauma, or other underlying causes. The "Disseminated intravascular coagulation" plan describes this devastating development in depth.

5. Constriction of renal blood vessels is an early compensatory mechanism in shock. Although this constriction limits glomerular filtration, thus conserving fluid volume, it impairs renal perfusion, which may result in acute renal failure. The "Acute renal failure" plan describes this complication in detail.

6. Although shock may damage hepatic cells, prompt correction of shock may allow these cells to regenerate. Early detection of liver failure may prevent severe damage to this critical organ. The "Liver failure" plan presents the pathophysiology of this disorder and related care.

7. Rationales: _____

Cardiovascular disorders

Nursing diagnosis

Risk for ineffective individual coping, ineffective family coping, or both related to threat to life

Nursing priority

Provide emotional support to the patient and family.

Patient outcome criteria

By the time of discharge, the patient will verbalize increased coping ability, and the family will participate in establishing a family action plan to cope with this crisis.

Interventions

1. Implement measures described in the "Ineffective individual coping" plan, page 67, and the "Ineffective family coping: Compromised" plan, page 63, as appropriate.

2. Additional individualized interventions: _____

Rationales

1. Families (and alert patients) are aware that shock is life-threatening, and they react to the possibility of death in various ways. Measures to help them cope with their realistic fear and other emotional responses are described in these plans.

2. Rationales: _____

Discharge planning

Discharge checklist

Before discharge, the patient shows evidence of:
- ❏ blood pressure within normal limits without I.V. inotrope or vasopressor support
- ❏ pulse and respirations within normal limits
- ❏ ABG levels within expected limits for recovery stage
- ❏ urine output within normal limits
- ❏ no evidence of major complications.

Teaching checklist

Document evidence that the patient and family demonstrate an understanding of:
- ❏ cause and significance of shock
- ❏ expectations for recovery
- ❏ purpose of monitoring devices
- ❏ rationales for therapeutic interventions.

Documentation checklist

Using outcome criteria as a guide, document:
- ❏ clinical status on admission
- ❏ significant changes in status
- ❏ pertinent diagnostic test findings
- ❏ care for invasive monitoring lines
- ❏ fluid administration
- ❏ use of inotropes, vasopressors, or other pharmacologic agents
- ❏ measures to support ventilation and oxygenation
- ❏ emotional support

- ❏ patient and family teaching
- ❏ discharge planning.

Associated plans of care

Adult respiratory distress syndrome
Disseminated intravascular coagulation
Impaired physical mobility
Ineffective family coping
Ineffective individual coping: Compromised
Liver failure
Major burns
Mechanical ventilation
Multiple trauma
Pulmonary embolism

References

Rice, V. "Shock, A Clinical Syndrome: An Update. Part 1. An Overview of Shock," *Critical Care Nurse* 11(4):20-27, April 1991.

Rice, V. "Shock, A Clinical Syndrome: An Update. Part 2. The Stages of Shock," *Critical Care Nurse* 11(5):74-89, May 1991.

Rice, V. "Shock, A Clinical Syndrome: An Update. Part 3. Therapeutic Management," *Critical Care Nurse* 11(6):34-39, June 1991.

Rice, V. "Shock, A Clinical Syndrome: An Update. Part 4. Nursing Care of the Shock Patient," *Critical Care Nurse* 11(7):28-43, July-August 1991.

Thompson, J., et al. *Mosby's Clinical Nursing*, 4th ed. St. Louis: Mosby–Year Book, Inc., 1997.

Weil, M., and Rackow, E. "A Guide to Volume Repletion," *Emergency Medicine* 16(8): 100-5;108-10, April 30, 1984.

Percutaneous transluminal coronary angioplasty

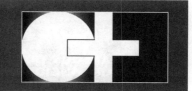

DRG information

DRG 116   Other Permanent Cardiac Pacemaker Implant or Percutaneous Transluminal Coronary Angioplasty with Coronary Artery Stent Implant.
Mean LOS = 5.4 days

DRG 112   Percutaneous Cardiovascular Procedures.
Mean LOS = 4.7 days

The differentiation in the above selections is whether a coronary artery stent is implanted when performing percutaneous transluminal coronary angioplasty (PTCA). It is important to note, however, that if a PTCA is performed during heart catheterization only using intracoronary thrombolytics (such as tissue plasminogen activator or heparin), it is not grouped to DRG 112. DRG 112 is acquired only when a coronary atherectomy or balloon angioplasty is performed. To reiterate, the placement of a coronary artery stent moves the patient to DRG 116.

If the patient fails angioplasty or stent placement and is taken for cardiac surgery, the cardiac surgery performed would then take precedence in DRG selection.

INTRODUCTION

Definition and time focus

PTCA is a therapeutic alternative to coronary artery bypass surgery for patients with coronary artery disease. Over the last 20 years, PTCA has become an effective, widely used treatment for patients with coronary ischemia. In the last decade alone, the number of PTCAs performed has increased more than tenfold. PTCA has several advantages over cardiac surgery: shorter hospital stay, less discomfort for the patient, fewer potential complications, faster convalescence, and lower cost.

The procedure is performed in the cardiac catheterization laboratory and lasts 1 to 4 hours. The cardiac surgical team is on standby in the even of a complication and the need for open-heart surgery. Patients are admitted the evening before or the morning of the procedure and are discharged an average of 28 hours after it.

During PTCA, a cardiologist places an expandable dilatation balloon in the partially obstructed coronary artery and then inflates it to widen the lumen of the vessel. Most PTCAs are performed percutaneously via the femoral artery, which requires insertion of an arterial introducer sheath at the access site in the groin. This approach allows for left-sided heart catheterization, angiography, and angioplasty. A venous sheath is placed only if right-sided heart catheterization is performed. At the end of the procedure, the sheaths are flushed with heparin and capped. The sheaths are then sutured in place. Most patients are admitted to an intensive care unit or telemetry unit after PTCA. Sheaths commonly remain in place several hours or sometimes overnight; they then are removed by a doctor or a specially trained nurse.

This plan focuses on the patient undergoing routine (non–acute myocardial infarction [AMI]) PTCA from the preprocedure stage to discharge.

Etiology and precipitating factors

• Coronary artery disease
• Angina poorly controlled or refractory to conventional medical therapy
• Objective evidence of ischemia
• Good left ventricular function
• Candidate for coronary artery bypass surgery
• Coronary artery lesions amenable to dilatation
  – One or more coronary vessels
  – Proximal lesion
  – Discrete
  – Concentric
  – Noncalcified

Focused assessment guidelines

Because PTCA is performed to relieve angina, findings are the same as in the "Angina pectoris" care plan.

Potential complications

• Rupture of coronary artery
• Major bleeding at access site
• Abrupt closure of the treated vessel
• Myocardial infarction
• Arterial occlusion

PERCUTANEOUS TRANSLUMINAL CORONARY ANGIOPLASTY

Major nursing diagnoses and collaborative problems	Key patient outcomes
Anxiety	Verbalize fears and concerns, if desired, about diagnosis and treatment.
Risk for femoral artery occlusion	Have palpable pedal pulses greater than 2+ on a scale of 0 to 4.
Risk for injury	Display no evidence of excessive bleeding or significant hematoma.
Risk for hypovolemia	Have stable vital signs: heart rate, 60 to 100 beats/minute; systolic blood pressure, 90 to 140 mm Hg; and diastolic blood pressure, 50 to 90 mm Hg.
Pain	Rate pain as less than 3 on a pain rating scale of 0 to 10.
Knowledge deficit (postdischarge care)	Be able to correctly describe site care and what to do for signs and symptoms of complications.

NURSING DIAGNOSIS

Anxiety related to known risks associated with PTCA and to fear of unknown

Nursing priority

Relieve anxiety and foster effective coping.

Patient outcome criteria

Prior to PTCA, the patient will:
• if desired, verbalize fears and concerns related to diagnosis and treatment
• exhibit effective coping behavior, such as asking questions and responding calmly to questions from staff.

Interventions

1. If the patient is admitted to the unit prior to PTCA, assess level of knowledge about the procedure and level of anxiety.

Rationales

1. In some cases, preprocedure teaching will be accomplished on an outpatient basis.

2. Provide preprocedure teaching or reinforce knowledge. Discuss the following with the patient:
• preoperative routine, including nothing by mouth 12 hours prior to procedure, check for allergies, need to empty bladder on call, premedication
• appearance of cardiac catheterization laboratory, such as staff in surgical scrub suits, monitoring equipment and fluorescope
• preparation in catheterization laboratory, including use of cardiac monitor, I.V. lines, site preparation, pretest sedative
• expected sensations with PTCA, especially flushing with dye or chest discomfort with balloon inflation
• description of how to obtain pain medication and how to cope with need to urinate
• intraprocedure and postprocedure monitoring for complications
• explanation of doctor's requests to cough and breathe deeply during procedure
• postprocedure care, including need for bed rest, importance of keeping leg straight, and sheath removal
• where family can wait and how they will be kept informed during procedure.

3. Additional individualized interventions: _____

2. The patient may or may not have detailed teaching before admission. Describing activity and what to expect can lessen fear of the unknown.

3. Rationales: _____

COLLABORATIVE PROBLEM

Risk for femoral artery occlusion related to indwelling sheath

Nursing priority

Promptly detect and report femoral artery occlusion.

Patient outcome criterion

Throughout the post-PTCA period, the patient will have palpable pedal pulses greater than 2+ on a scale of 0 to 4.

Interventions

1. With each assessment of vital signs, check bilateral distal pulses (dorsalis pedis or posterior tibial). Mark pulse locations on feet with a marker for easy identification. Use Doppler ultrasound to verify pulses if they are weak or nonpalpable. If a dorsalis pedis pulse is absent, assess posterior tibial pulses. If pulses are absent or diminished in the catheterized limb, alert the doctor immediately.

Rationales

1. Femoral artery occlusion may occur in the catheterized extremity as a complication of PTCA due to thrombus formation on the catheter or a possible embolism. Presence of normal distal pulses indicates adequate blood flow. Pulses should be equal bilaterally. The dorsalis pedis pulse may be absent bilaterally as a normal variant. Otherwise, a diminished or absent pulse requires prompt medical intervention to restore flow.

Cardiovascular disorders

2. Maintain the heparin infusion, as ordered. To determine dose, use a heparin nomogram dosing chart, such as a heparin dosing flow chart based on weight or activated partial thromboplastin time (APTT) values. Keep APTT values within limits specified by the cardiologist, typically 60 to 90 seconds.

2. A national survey of PTCA care practices (Juran et al., 1996) revealed wide variability in heparin administration post-PTCA. About 41% of the 70 hospitals surveyed maintain a heparin infusion for 12 to 18 hours postprocedure, but 31% don't infuse heparin at all. Using a flowchart helps determine appropriate doses of heparin based on measurement of APTT. Doses are titrated to the specific patient's coagulation status.

3. Discontinue heparin 2 to 4 hours before removal of the sheath, if ordered.

3. Nationally, 54% of hospitals using heparin post-PTCA discontinue it 2 to 4 hours before sheath removal; the remaining 46% discontinue it either before 2 hours or after 4 hours.

4. Additional individualized interventions: _____

4. Rationales: _____

Nursing diagnosis

Risk for injury related to break in skin and presence of foreign body

Nursing priority

Protect the patient from injury.

Patient outcome criterion

Throughout the post-PTCA period, the patient will adhere to activity limitations.

Interventions

1. Maintain complete bed rest, with head of bed flat or elevated up to 30 degrees for prescribed period of time, usually 8 to 24 hours. Consult doctor about acceptability of logrolling to side-lying position.

2. Instruct the patient to report to the nurse bleeding at the site or a warm, wet feeling at the groin site. Also teach the patient to keep the affected leg straight and to avoid straining with turning or bowel movement for 12 to 24 hours.

3. Additional individualized interventions: _____

Rationales

1. The femoral sheath, venous sheath, or both are left in place for several hours after the procedure. Most doctors will allow logrolling, as long as the affected leg is maintained straight and no hip flexion occurs.

2. The patient can serve as a monitor of the integrity of the groin site. If the patient flexes at the groin or strains, the rigid sheath might injure the vessel, triggering bleeding.

3. Rationales: _____

Collaborative problem

Risk for hypovolemia related to bleeding or diuresis

Nursing priorities

• Promptly detect bleeding.
• Restore fluid volume.

Patient outcome criteria

• Immediately following PTCA and thereafter, the patient will have stable vital signs: heart rate, 60 to 100 beats/minute; systolic blood pressure, 90 to 140 mm Hg; and diastolic blood pressure, 50 to 90 mm Hg.
• Within 1 to 2 hours before discharge, the patient will ambulate without assistance, without excessive pain (less than 3 on a 0 to 10 pain rating scale), and with no bleeding.

Interventions

1. Measure pulse and blood pressure four times every 15 minutes, four times every 30 minutes, every hour while the sheath is in place, and then every 4 hours and as necessary. Monitor cardiac rhythm continuously.

2. With each vital sign check, assess access site for bleeding, swelling, or discoloration.

3. If bleeding occurs at the insertion site while the sheath is in place, remove the dressing and evaluate the amount of blood. Apply a sterile dressing over the access site and apply manual pressure above the introducer until bleeding stops. Notify the cardiologist and administer a transfusion, if ordered.

4. Assist with sheath removal according to unit protocol (see *Sheath removal after percutaneous transluminal coronary angioplasty,* page 446).

5. After sheath removal, maintain dressing per unit protocol.

6. Maintain the I.V. line as ordered.

7. Encourage the patient to drink water freely.

8. Monitor urine output.

Rationales

1. The contrast agent used during angiography causes an osmotic diuresis. Frequent vital sign checks allow prompt detection of hypovolemia, which may result from diuresis or from internal bleeding. Continuous cardiac monitoring is necessary to detect arrhythmias, a complication of PTCA.

2. The patient usually receives one or more boluses of heparin or a continuous infusion during the procedure for anticoagulation. Hemorrhage is a constant danger. Swelling and discoloration are indicators of hematoma formation.

3. Removing the dressing allows for adequate observation of the site. Manual pressure stops the bleeding and allows clotting to occur. A transfusion may be needed to replace blood volume.

4. In two-thirds of the hospitals surveyed, a specially trained nurse pulls the sheath; in the remaining hospitals, a doctor performs this action.

5. About two-thirds of all hospitals surveyed apply a pressure dressing after sheath removal. The remainder use a plain dressing, adhesive bandages, or no dressing at all. Sandbags are used by 83% of those surveyed, although they do not decrease bleeding. Sandbags also increase pain.

6. An I.V. line provides emergency access for medication administration, fluid to promote excretion of the contrast medium, and a ready source of additional volume if the patient becomes hypovolemic.

7. Oral intake of water replaces water lost during the osmotic diuresis. Also, the contrast medium is nephrotoxic and may cause renal tubular necrosis and subsequent renal failure.

8. Urine output is an indicator of renal perfusion, and should measure at least 30 ml/hour.

Cardiovascular disorders

Sheath removal after percutaneous transluminal coronary angioplasty

A specially trained nurse or doctor will take the following steps to remove a sheath. In addition to the person removing the sheath, an additional nurse is needed to monitor the patient's tolerance of the procedure.

Before pulling the sheath

• Discontinue the heparin drip, as ordered.

• Nothing by mouth for 1 to 2 hours.

• Explain the procedure to the patient, including the need to avoid holding his breath while intense pressure is exerted on the site after the catheter is removed (to avoid a vasovagal response with bradycardia and hypotension).

• Premedicate the patient as ordered, usually with morphine.

• Evaluate the patient's vital signs, cardiac rhythm, and quality of pedal pulses every 5 minutes during removal.

Pulling the sheath

• Remove dressing.

• Check the groin for ecchymosis and hematoma.

• Instill local anesthetic per protocol.

• Remove sutures, if any.

• Remove the sheath.

After pulling the sheath

• Immediately apply pressure until hemostasis is established (typically 15 to 30 minutes manual pressure, or use a mechanical pressure device such as a C-clamp or other device). Remind the patient to breath freely.

• Assess the patient for chest pain, back pain, and site pain.

• Apply a pressure dressing per unit protocol.

• Remind the patient to keep the leg straight and remain on bed rest another 6 to 8 hours.

• Instruct the patient to call the nurse for any pain or sense of wetness at the groin.

• Document the sheath removal and vital signs, site, and circulatory assessments.

• Maintain complete bed rest for 6 to 8 hours.

• Consult the clinical plan for additional measures for monitoring vital signs and for complications.

---

9. Assess for orthostatic hypotension before allowing the patient out of bed for the first time. Measure blood pressure and pulse while the patient is supine; then have the patient sit up and promptly repeat measurement. Compare values, looking for a systolic blood pressure drop of 10 mm Hg or more or a pulse increase of 20 beats or more per minute. If these symptoms are present, keep patient in bed and increase I.V. fluids as ordered until the supine and sitting blood pressure values are within 10 mm Hg of each other and the pulse rates are within 20 beats of each other.

10. Additional individualized interventions: _____

_____

9. Internal hemorrhage and internal bleeding may also occur, especially retroperitoneal bleeding from perforation of the iliac artery. Orthostatic vital signs can identify a hidden hypovolemia. Although blood pressure and pulse may be normal in the supine position due to compensatory mechanisms for volume loss, the body may be unable to compensate for the additional stress of position change. If blood pressure drops 10 mm Hg or more or pulse increases 20 beats/minute or more, positive orthostatic vital signs are present, indicating an inadequate blood volume.

10. Rationales: _____

_____

NURSING DIAGNOSIS

Pain related to restrictions on mobility and percutaneous puncture at the groin site

Nursing priority

Promptly detect and relieve pain.

Patient outcome criteria

Throughout the post-PTCA period, the patient will:
• experience no chest pain
• rate other pain (such as back pain) as less than 3 on a 0 to 10 pain rating scale.

Interventions

1. On admission to the unit, ask whether the patient has leg or back pain. Also specifically ask about the presence of chest discomfort. Instruct the patient to report any pain or other discomfort to you promptly.

2. If back or leg pain is present, reposition the patient within accepted limits. Use other nonpharmacologic nursing measures, such as back rubs, massage, relaxation, music, or imagery. If necessary, administer pain medication, as ordered.

3. If chest pain is present, assess and treat it according to unit protocol for chest pain. Notify the cardiologist immediately.

4. Additional individualized interventions: _____

Rationales

1. During PTCA, the patient must lie on a hard table for 1 to 4 hours. Following the procedure, bed rest is necessary while the sheaths are in place (a range of 4 to 12 hours) and for an additional 6 to 8 hours after a sheath is removed. As a result, the patient may spend as much as 24 to 36 hours on complete bed rest. The primary discomforts that patients report after PTCA are back and leg pain from the prolonged bed rest and restricted mobility.

2. Recent studies suggest that the head of the bed can safely be elevated up to 60 degrees. A flexible sheath has recently become available, allowing for more liberal positioning. Various nursing measures may help to reduce the patient's perception of pain. Pain medication should successfully control pain that cannot be relieved by other measures.

3. Chest pain may recur as a result of the underlying pathologic condition or from abrupt reocclusion of a coronary artery from vasospasm or thrombus. Angina occurs as a result of decreased coronary blood flow to the myocardium. Prolonged ischemia may result in an AMI.

4. Rationales: _____

Cardiovascular disorders

NURSING DIAGNOSIS

Knowledge deficit (postdischarge care) related to lack of exposure to information

Nursing priority

Teach the patient (and family) about postdischarge care.

Patient outcome criteria

Before discharge the patient will:
• describe site care at home
• describe signs and symptoms of complications and what to do
• verbalize commitment to reduce risk factors.

Interventions

1. Prior to discharge, discuss with the patient and family and evaluate their comprehension of:
• need for follow-up care
• site care and signs and symptoms of infection
• pain management
• signs and symptoms to report to the doctor, such as pain, numbness, tingling, bleeding, difficulty breathing
• discharge medications
• date, time, and place of next appointment
• risk factor modification — including diet, exercise, and smoking cessation.

2. Additional individualized interventions: _____

Rationales

1. The patient and family are more likely to follow through with postprocedure care if they are taught what they need to know and if their understanding of the care is assessed before discharge.

2. Rationales: _____

DISCHARGE PLANNING

Discharge checklist
Before discharge, the patient shows evidence of:
❏ vital signs within normal limits
❏ pain controllable with oral medication
❏ affected leg warm, dry, and of normal color
❏ pulses same as on admission
❏ no signs or symptoms of complications.

Teaching checklist
Document evidence that the patient and family demonstrate an understanding of:
❏ diagnosis
❏ insertion site care
❏ measures for pain control
❏ activity restrictions
❏ symptoms to report to doctor
❏ all discharge medications
❏ activity resumption.

Documentation checklist
Using outcome criteria as a guide, document:
❏ clinical status on admission
❏ significant changes in status
❏ pertinent diagnostic test findings
❏ heparin therapy
❏ adherence to positioning limitations
❏ patient and family teaching
❏ discharge planning.

ASSOCIATED PLANS OF CARE
Acute MI: Critical care unit
Acute MI: Telemetry unit
Angina pectoris
Impaired physical mobility

Ineffective family coping: Compromised
Ineffective individual coping
Knowledge deficit
Pain

REFERENCES

Gregory, S., and Fowler, S. "Removing Femoral Sheaths: A New Nursing Skill," *AJN* Supplement:12-14, May 1996.
Gulanik, M., et al. "Patients' Responses to the Angioplasty Experience: A Qualitative Study," *American Journal of Critical Care* 6(1):25-32, January 1997.
Juran, N., et al. "Survey of Current Practice Patterns for Percutaneous Transluminal Coronary Angioplasty," *American Journal of Critical Care* 5(6):442-48, November 1996.
Mayer, D., and Hendrickx, L. "Comfort and Bleeding After Percutaneous Transluminal Coronary Angioplasty: Comparison of a Flexible Sheath and a Standard Sheath," *American Journal of Critical Care* 6(5):341-47, September 1997.
Seitz, S. "Percutaneous Transluminal Coronary Angioplasty (Non-AMI) Care Trail," Concord, Calif.: Mt. Diablo Medical Center, July 1997.

Permanent pacemaker insertion

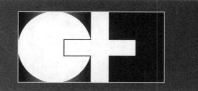

DRG information

DRG 115   Permanent Cardiac Pacemaker Implant with Acute Myocardial Infarction, Heart Failure, or Shock or Automatic Implantable Cardioverter-Defribrillator Lead or Generator Procedure.
Mean LOS = 11.5 days

DRG 116   Other Permanent Cardiac Pacemaker Implant or Percutaneous Transluminal Coronary Angioplasty with Coronary Artery Stent Implant.
Mean LOS = 5.4 days

INTRODUCTION

Definition and time focus

Permanent pacemaker insertion may be required when the patient experiences symptoms of decreased cardiac output (CO) secondary to irreversible or uncontrolled arrhythmias. Irreversible bradycardia results from atrioventricular (AV) heart block (typically, Mobitz Type II second- or third-degree), sinus bradycardia, sinus arrest, or sinoatrial (SA) block. Some tachyarrhythmias unresponsive to other treatments also may benefit from a permanent pacemaker, as may sick sinus (bradycardia-tachycardia) syndrome. This plan focuses on managing the patient who has had a permanent pacemaker inserted transvenously. The lead is inserted through a vein — commonly the cephalic, jugular, or subclavian — and positioned with fluoroscopy in the right atrium or ventricle. Lead attachment to the endocardium is either passive, with fibrosis occurring at the contact point, or active, with the lead screwed into the muscle. A subcutaneous pocket is made in the submammary area, upper chest, or abdominal region, and the pulse generator box is placed in it. The distal end of the lead is connected under the skin to the generator box. The procedure is commonly done under local anesthesia with some additional sedation and pain relief.

Etiology and precipitating factors

• Idiopathic sclerotic degeneration of the SA node
• Coronary artery disease, especially with significant disease or infarction involving the artery to the SA node (right coronary artery in 55% of the population, circumflex in 45%) or the AV node (right coronary artery in 90%, circumflex in 10%)

• Rheumatic heart disease
• Cardiomyopathy
• Congenital heart disease, such as ventricular septal defect or transposition of the great vessels
• Surgical trauma or edema affecting the cardiac conduction system
• Myocarditis
• Hypersensitive carotid sinus syndrome

FOCUSED ASSESSMENT GUIDELINES

Nursing history (functional health pattern findings)

Note: Findings vary, depending on the underlying condition.

Health perception–health management pattern
• Treatment of arrhythmias
• Treatment of angina, atherosclerosis, hypertension, or heart failure
• History of myocardial infarction, congenital heart disease, or cardiac surgery

Nutritional-metabolic pattern
• Swelling of extremities and weight gain

Activity-exercise pattern
• Shortness of breath, fatigue, activity intolerance, and paroxysmal nocturnal dyspnea

Cognitive-perceptual pattern
• Chest pain
• Palpitations
• Syncope, dizziness, and light-headedness (Adams-Stokes disease)

Self-perception–self-concept pattern
• Concern over anticipated changes in body image and functioning
• Concern over follow-up care and restrictions

Physical findings

Physical findings before pacemaker insertion appear below.

Cardiovascular
• Arrhythmias — bradycardia, irregular rhythms, or (uncommonly) tachycardia
• Hypotension
• Venous engorgement or jugular vein distention
• Third or fourth heart sounds
• Decreased peripheral pulses
• Increased capillary refill time

Pulmonary
• Crackles

- Shortness of breath
- Orthopnea

Neurologic
- Dizziness
- Syncope
- Seizures
- Transient ischemic attacks

Integumentary
- Cool, clammy skin
- Edema

Renal
- Weight gain (from fluid retention)

Gastrointestinal
- Liver enlargement
- Positive hepatojugular reflux

Diagnostic studies

- Electrolyte panel — deviations from normal in potassium, magnesium, and calcium may affect cardiac conduction and contractility
- Serum drug levels — may reveal subtherapeutic or toxic medication levels that may affect heart rate and rhythm (medications that may affect heart rate or rhythm include digoxin [Lanoxin], quinidine, procainamide, narcotics, and some psychotropics)
- Blood urea nitrogen and creatinine levels — may reflect low renal perfusion from low CO

- Triiodothyronine and thyroxine levels — may be low, indicating that hypothyroidism may be depressing cardiac impulse formation or conduction
- 12-lead electrocardiogram (ECG) — may reveal electrical activity not obvious in a single-lead rhythm strip and may help identify the arrhythmia
- Holter monitor — may be used to confirm sick sinus syndrome or other transient arrhythmias
- Chest X-ray — may show cardiac enlargement and respiratory status
- Electrophysiology studies — may allow induction and identification of symptom-causing arrhythmias

Potential complications

- Arrhythmias
- Infection
- Thrombosis or embolism
- Tamponade or perforation of myocardium
- Hematoma or hemorrhage
- Lead fracture
- Pneumothorax
- Hiccups (diaphragmatic pacing)
- Tricuspid insufficiency
- Painful subcutaneous pocket or pocket erosion
- Pacemaker syndrome (shortness of breath, dizziness, chest pain resulting from suboptimal pacing mode or inappropriate pacing parameters)

CLINICAL SNAPSHOT

PERMANENT PACEMAKER INSERTION

Major nursing diagnoses and collaborative problems	Key patient outcomes
Risk for arrhythmias	Display ECG evidence of appropriate pacer sensing, firing, and capturing.
Risk for infection	Show no signs of infection.
Bathing, feeding, and toileting self-care deficit	Resume normal self-care activities.
Knowledge deficit (self-care after discharge)	Demonstrate accurate pulse rate measurement.
Risk for body-image disturbance	Ask appropriate questions and show interest in learning about the pacemaker.

COLLABORATIVE PROBLEM

Risk for arrhythmias related to pacemaker malfunction or lead or electrode displacement

Nursing priority

Maintain optimal cardiac rhythm.

Patient outcome criteria

- Immediately after surgery and throughout the hospital stay, the patient will:
  - display a cardiac rate no less than pacemaker setting
  - display ECG evidence of appropriate pacer sensing, firing, and capturing.
- Within 3 days after surgery, the patient will:
  - have decreased or no signs and symptoms of low CO (if present before surgery)
  - visit the pacemaker clinic for a definitive check of pacemaker functioning.

Interventions

1. Initiate constant ECG monitoring until discharged or as ordered. Keep alarms on at all times. Set the low limit at 3 beats/minute less than the pacer setting. Set the high limit 10 beats/minute above the anticipated maximum cardiac rate. Place monitoring electrodes 2" (5 cm) away from the generator box. Change the monitoring electrode sites to obtain another perspective if the pacer appears to be malfunctioning.

2. Document in the plan of care the patient's intrinsic rate and rhythm. Also indicate the pacemaker type and rate (see *Generic pacemaker code*).

Rationales

1. Continuous monitoring facilitates early problem detection. If the pacemaker is functioning properly, the cardiac rate should not go below the pacer setting. The risk of tachyarrhythmias cannot be ignored. Monitoring electrodes placed near the generator box or in lead locations where the ECG amplitude is small may result in failure to record intrinsic beats.

2. This information is necessary for correct ECG interpretation.

Generic pacemaker code

The North American Society of Pacing and Electrophysiology and the British Pacing and Electrophysiology Group have recommended a sequence of five letters to designate pacemaker capabilities. Note that the first three positions are used for antibradyarrhythmia function exclusively.

Chamber paced (Position I)	Chamber sensed (Position II)	Response to sensing (Position III)	Programmability, rate modulation (Position IV)	Antitachyarrhythmia function (Position V)
O = none A = atrium V = ventricle D = dual (A and V)	O = none A = atrium V = ventricle D = dual (A and V)	O = none T = triggered I = inhibited D = dual (T and I)	O = none P = simple programmable M = multiprogrammable C = communicating R = rate modulation	O = none P = pacing (antitachyarrhythmia) S = shock D = dual (P and S)

Adapted from Bernstein, A.D., et al. "The NASPE/BPEG Generic Pacemaker Code for Antibradyarrhythmia and Adaptive Rate Pacing and Antitachyarrhythmia Devices," *PACE* 10:794-99, July-August 1987. Used with permission.

Cardiovascular disorders

3. Record and document rhythm strips every shift and mount them in the patient's chart. Analyze the strips: Appropriately paced beats will show a pacer spike artifact followed by a depolarization wave that differs from the intrinsic waveform. Notify the doctor promptly if problems occur with impulse initiation, conduction, or sensing.
• failure to sense — pacer spikes occur despite the presence of the patient's intrinsic beat

• failure to capture — pacing spikes not followed by cardiac depolarization

• failure to pace — absence of pacing spikes when the intrinsic rate is below the pacer setting.

4. Maintain standby transdermal pacing equipment.

5. Obtain 12-lead simultaneous ECG recordings as ordered.

6. Administer cardiac medications, as ordered, and document their effectiveness and adverse effects.

7. Observe for signs and symptoms of decreased CO. Monitor blood pressure, apical pulse, and respirations.

8. Maintain and document I.V. line patency, as ordered.

9. Maintain the patient on bed rest with turning limitations and with the head of the bed elevated 30 to 45 degrees as ordered.

10. If use of the affected arm is restricted, perform limited passive range-of-motion (ROM) exercises with the arm every hour during the first 24 hours after surgery.

11. Assure chest X-ray is performed as ordered.

12. Additional individualized interventions: _____

3. Systematic documentation provides an objective, organized means of analyzing pacer activity. Waveforms of paced and intrinsic beats differ because of independent conduction paths.

• The sensitivity setting may be such that the pacemaker undersenses and does not consistently detect intrinsic low-amplitude cardiac electrical activity. Failure to sense also may result from fibrosis at the lead tip, lead fracture, or a dislodged lead. Failure to sense may result in inappropriate, unnecessary pacing and may cause R-on-T phenomenon, in which a pacer spike falls on the downslope of the preceding T wave, triggering ventricular tachycardia or ventricular fibrillation.
• Failure to capture results when the voltage of the pacemaker stimulus is insufficient to trigger depolarization. It may result from fibrosis at the lead-myocardial junction, a weak battery, the effect of cardiac drugs, electrolyte imbalance, or a dislodged or malpositioned lead.
• Failure to pace may result from a fractured leadwire, malfunction at the lead-generator connection, power source depletion, or oversensing — the sensing of noncardiac electrical activity, such as muscle activity near the generator box, power lines, other sources of electrical noise, or crosstalk in dual chamber pacemakers.

4. Alternative emergency pacing may be needed.

5. A 12-lead recording shows pacer function and cardiac electrical activity more accurately than a single-lead rhythm strip. Simultaneous tracings help to confirm pacing spikes and intrinsic beats that may vary in amplitude in different leads and therefore may not be obvious in one particular lead.

6. Cardiac medications may be indicated for treatment of underlying cardiac problems, such as coronary artery or valvular disease.

7. Deviation from postoperative baseline vital signs may indicate pacemaker failure or other complications.

8. The I.V. line may be needed to administer emergency medications.

9. With passive lead placement, activity and positioning limitations may be needed temporarily to maintain lead placement until fibrosis develops around the electrode tip and anchors it in place. Limitations may be less restrictive with active lead attachment.

10. Movement restrictions may be ordered to reduce the chance of lead displacement. Passive ROM exercises may prevent frozen shoulder.

11. Chest X-rays may be used to confirm lead placement.

12. Rationales: _____

NURSING DIAGNOSIS

Risk for infection related to surgical disruption of skin barrier

Nursing priorities

• Promote incisional healing by primary intention.
• Prevent or promptly detect infection.

Patient outcome criteria

• Within 1 day after surgery and throughout the hospital stay, the patient will:
  – have a dry and intact incision
  – experience no fever.
• By the time of discharge, the patient will:
  – have a white blood cell (WBC) count within normal limits
  – show no signs of infection.

Rationales

1. Check the primary dressing for drainage. Circle any drainage, and write the date and time when first discovered.

2. Reinforce the primary dressing as needed for 24 hours. Do not change the primary dressing without an order from the doctor.

3. After removal of the primary dressing, check the incision for excessive redness, swelling, warmth, and drainage.

4. Perform wound care, as ordered.

5. Administer antibiotics, as ordered.

6. Monitor body temperature as ordered. Notify the doctor if the patient's oral temperature exceeds 100° F (37.8° C).

7. Monitor the WBC count, as ordered.

8. Culture purulent drainage, if present, as ordered.

9. Additional individualized interventions: _____

Interventions

1. This is an objective method of monitoring for bleeding and incisional drainage.

2. Reinforcement protects the incision and aids hemostasis while providing a protective barrier against microorganisms. Removing the primary dressing increases the risk of accidentally disrupting the incision and causing bleeding.

3. These signs may reflect infection.

4. The pacemaker pocket is the most common entry site for infectious organisms, which can migrate along the pacing wires to the heart. A clean, dry incision promotes healing.

5. Antibiotics may be prescribed prophylactically because pacemaker insertion is an invasive procedure that involves implanting a foreign object into the heart. Also, the disruption of the skin barrier provides a potential portal of entry for infectious organisms into the heart.

6. Commonly, elevated temperature is a systemic response to infection.

7. The WBC count increases in response to infectious organisms.

8. WBCs and cellular debris accumulate locally in response to infectious organisms. Proper treatment requires identifying the causative agent and its medication sensitivity.

9. Rationales: _____

Cardiovascular disorders

Nursing diagnosis

Bathing, feeding, and toileting self-care deficit related to bed rest and activity limitations

Nursing priority

Assist with bathing, feeding, and toileting while bed rest is required.

Patient outcome criteria

- While on bed rest, the patient will:
  - accept self-care assistance
  - observe activity restrictions.
- Within 3 days after surgery, the patient will:
  - resume normal self-care activities
  - perform normal bowel elimination without straining.

Rationales

1. Assist with bathing and oral hygiene daily, as needed.

2. Assist the patient at mealtime. Elevate the head of the bed, as ordered.

3. Assist the patient with a bedpan and urinal, as needed.

4. Administer stool softeners and laxatives judiciously, as ordered, and document their use. Encourage alternatives or supplements to stool softeners and laxatives, such as increased dietary fiber (if possible) and prune juice.

5. If arm use is not restricted, encourage the patient to move the arm and resume self-care.

6. Additional individualized interventions: _____

_____

Interventions

1. Bed rest and arm movement limitations prevent the patient from sitting up and using bathing and oral hygiene supplies.

2. The patient may be unable to reach or manipulate items on the meal tray while on bed rest. Raising the head of the bed facilitates swallowing and minimizes the risk of aspiration.

3. The patient will be unable to use the bathroom.

4. Straining to defecate requires considerable energy and may produce vagal-mediated arrhythmias. Laxative dependence diminishes the urge for normal defecation.

5. The patient may be hesitant to use the arm initially for fear of dislodging the electrode.

6. Rationales: _____

_____

Nursing diagnosis

Knowledge deficit (self-care after discharge) related to unfamiliar therapeutic intervention

Nursing priority

Teach the information and skills necessary for optimal self-care.

Patient outcome criteria

By the time of discharge, the patient will:
- demonstrate accurate pulse rate measurement
- list significant, reportable signs and symptoms
- verbalize activity expectations, limitations, and environmental hazards
- reinforce initial follow-up arrangements or appointments
- state the purpose, dosage, administration schedule, and adverse effects of medications
- verbalize understanding of the need to inform health care providers about the pacemaker.

Rationales

1. Explain potential signs and symptoms of decreased CO that should be reported to the doctor, such as shortness of breath, low or erratic pulse, light-headedness, chest pains, decreased exercise tolerance, prolonged fatigue or weakness, or recurrence of preimplant symptoms.

2. Discuss signs and symptoms of extraneous stimulation that should be reported, such as muscle, arm, or skin twitching near the generator box or prolonged and rapid hiccups.

3. Teach the patient to recognize and report signs and symptoms of pocket infection, such as fever or chills and incisional drainage, redness, swelling, or pain.

4. Teach the patient to check the radial pulse for a full minute at the same time daily after resting for 5 minutes; reinforce guidelines for reporting significant changes, particularly a decrease of 3 to 5 beats/minute below the pacer setting or an erratic, persistent high rate.

5. Emphasize the importance of complying with the follow-up monitoring regimen (by in-person appointments or a telephone monitoring device).

6. Emphasize the need to inform health care providers about the pacemaker. The patient should wear a medical alert bracelet and carry a wallet identification card with pacemaker specifications.

7. Discuss potential environmental hazards, such as power plants, high voltage power lines, radio and television transmitters, and electromagnetic power fields. Potential hazards include antitheft devices, airport security systems, close proximity to the generator of a running car engine, and use of cellular phones close to the pacemaker site. Encourage the patient to discuss limitations and hazards with the doctor.

8. As specified by the doctor, instruct the patient about resuming activity and any limitations on travel, exercise, bathing and showering, tight clothing, and sexual activity.

9. Teach the purpose, dosage, administration schedule, and adverse effects of all medications.

10. Provide written material for all patient-teaching topics.

11. Additional individualized interventions: _____

Interventions

1. These signs and symptoms may indicate pacemaker malfunction.

2. These signs and symptoms may result from electrode or lead malposition and adjacent tissue stimulation.

3. Infection may not be apparent until after discharge.

4. Changes in pacemaker function may be detected by regular assessment.

5. Pacemaker function can be evaluated most accurately by an ECG. Periodic checks using a donut-shaped magnet help determine when a new battery is needed.

6. Certain procedures, such as electrocautery, diathermy, lithotripsy, radiation treatment, transcutaneous epidermal nerve stimulation, and nuclear magnetic resonance imaging, may be contraindicated. A medical alert bracelet and pacemaker specifications will help ensure faster treatment if an emergency occurs.

7. Exposure to electromagnetic power sources has the potential to interfere with some pacemakers depending on the age of the pacemaker, mode of action, and type of lead. Most home electrical appliances, including microwave ovens, are not a problem if in proper working order.

8. Gradual resumption of activities according to patient tolerance generally is encouraged. Activities involving abrupt, forceful arm movement (such as tennis and golf) that may cause lead fracture may be limited for several weeks. Contact sports typically are not allowed. Tight clothing over the incision may impair healing. Activities involving arm pushing create myopotentials that may be interpreted by some pacemakers as intrinsic heartbeats.

9. Knowledge may increase compliance.

10. Written material reinforces and serves as a reference for this detailed information.

11. Rationales: _____

Cardiovascular disorders

NURSING DIAGNOSIS

Risk for body image disturbance related to dependence on pacemaker

Nursing priority

Promote positive incorporation of the pacemaker into the patient's body image.

Patient outcome criteria

By the time of discharge, the patient will:
• participate actively in self-care
• ask appropriate questions and show interest in learning about the pacemaker
• show no evidence of maladaptive coping.

Rationales

1. Assess the patient's adaptation to change, including perceptions and personal meaning of limitations.

2. Encourage the patient to ask questions and verbalize feelings.

3. Encourage the patient to look at the incision and the pacemaker site.

4. Assess for maladaptive coping behaviors, such as manipulating the generator box, verbalizing inability to make lifestyle or health-promoting changes, crying or a flat affect, lack of participation and interest in activities, or anxiety.

5. If indicated, consult the "Grieving" and "Ineffective Individual Coping" plans, pages 44 and 67 respectively.

6. Additional individualized interventions: _____

Interventions

1. The changes caused by pacemaker implantation will vary in significance among patients. Many patients welcome the increased activity tolerance and show signs of improved self-image. For others, however, loss of a body function may trigger the grieving process.

2. Verbalization enables the nurse to listen to, assess, and validate the patient's feelings, thus facilitating adjustment to change.

3. Willingness to view the incision and site may reflect beginning acceptance and adjustment.

4. These behaviors may indicate that the patient is having difficulty adjusting to the physical change and the need for pacemaker dependence.

5. These plans contain generalized interventions related to these problems.

6. Rationales: _____

DISCHARGE PLANNING

Discharge checklist

Before discharge, the patient shows evidence of:
❏ normal body temperature
❏ absence of angina and arrhythmias
❏ ECG within expected parameters, indicating appropriate pacemaker settings, sensing, firing, and capturing
❏ vital signs within acceptable parameters

❏ absence of pulmonary and cardiovascular complications
❏ absence of redness, swelling, and drainage at incision site
❏ WBC count within normal parameters
❏ ability to transfer, ambulate, and perform activities of daily living (ADLs) in the same manner as before hospitalization or better
❏ adequate home support system or referral to home care if indicated by inadequate support system and the patient's inability to perform ADLs.

Teaching checklist

Document evidence that the patient and family demonstrate an understanding of:

❏ symptoms of pacemaker failure or complications
❏ signs and symptoms of infection
❏ type of pacemaker and rate
❏ need for daily pulse rate measurement
❏ how to obtain a wallet pacemaker specification card and medical alert bracelet
❏ need to inform other health care providers about pacemaker
❏ plan for resuming activities
❏ limitations and precautions
❏ all discharge medications' purpose, dosage, administration schedule, and adverse effects requiring medical attention
❏ follow-up monitoring
❏ how to contact the doctor.

Documentation checklist

Using outcome criteria as a guide, document before surgery:

❏ clinical status on admission
❏ 12-lead ECG reading
❏ chest X-ray and results
❏ urinalysis results
❏ blood chemistry studies and complete blood counts
❏ Prothrombin time/international normalized ratio and activated partial thromboplastin time
❏ patient teaching
❏ surgical skin preparation
❏ I.V. line patency and site condition
❏ nothing-by-mouth status

Using outcome criteria as a guide, document after surgery:

❏ clinical status
❏ telemetry findings
❏ 12-lead ECG reading
❏ incision status and care
❏ I.V. line patency and site condition
❏ chest X-ray and results
❏ pacemaker clinic check completed or a clinic appointment
❏ patient and family teaching
❏ discharge planning.

ASSOCIATED PLANS OF CARE

Acute MI: Telemetry unit
Angina pectoris
Geriatric care
Grieving
Heart failure
Ineffective individual coping
Pain

Surgery
Thrombophlebitis

REFERENCES

Bernstein, A.D., et al. "The NASPE/BPEG Generic Pacemaker Code for Antibradyarrhythmia and Adaptive Rate Pacing and Antitachyarrhythmia Devices," *PACE* 10:794-99, July-August 1987.

Hayes, D.L., et al. "Interference with Cardiac Pacemakers By Cellular Telephones." *New England Journal of Medicine*, 336(21):1473-79, May 22, 1997.

Moser, S.A., and Gilbert, C.J. "Nursing Care of Patients Undergoing Interventional Electrophysiology Procedures," in *Interventional Electrophysiology*. Edited by Singer, I. Baltimore: Williams & Wilkins Co., 1997.

Strathmore, N.F. "Interference in Cardiac Pacemakers, " in *Clinical Cardiac Pacing*. Edited by Ellenbogen, K.A., et al. Philadelphia: W.B. Saunders Co., 1995.

Cardiovascular disorders

Septic shock

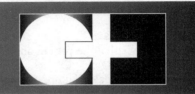

DRG information

DRG 415   Operating Room Procedure for Infectious and Parasitic Diseases.
Mean LOS = 15.8 days
DRG 416   Septicemia; Age 18+.
Mean LOS = 8.8 days
DRG 417   Septicemia; Ages 0 to 17.
Mean LOS = 4.6 days

Additional DRG information: Septic shock is coded as 785.59 in the International Classification of Diseases, from which DRGs are derived. This is a *symptom* code, which cannot be used as a principal diagnosis. Therefore, the cause of the septic shock, the underlying septicemia, the urosepsis (DRGs 320 and 321), the gram-negative pneumonia (DRGs 079 and 080), and so forth would drive the DRG. If sepsis were the principal diagnosis and an operative procedure were performed, this would optimize the DRG of a septic shock patient to DRG 415; in other words, a patient with *Escherichia coli* sepsis and septic shock due to pressure ulcers who has an excisional debridement of these ulcers at bedside once stabilized.

INTRODUCTION

Definition and time focus

Septic shock is one of three forms of distributive shock. It is a complex, life-threatening process of microcirculatory dysfunction and altered cellular metabolism resulting from altered blood flow and capillary permeability at the microcirculatory level. Septic shock usually starts with an infection that progresses to bacteremia (when the infectious agents enter the vascular compartment) and then to sepsis with a systemic response (tachycardia, tachypnea, pyrexia, and leukocytosis). The condition advances to shock when the immune system is overwhelmed and hypotension and altered tissue perfusion are present. Although any type of bacteria (both gram-positive and gram-negative), virus, parasite, or fungus may precipitate the condition, septic shock in adults is typically due to the gram-negative organism.

Much of the shock state is caused by chemical mediators and immunologic responses to the infectious agent. The responses and mediators include significant elevations of white blood cells (WBCs), cytokines, tumor necrosis factor, and interleukins 1 and 6; activation of the complement system with prostaglandins and their metabolites; and other endogenous mediators that exacerbate vasodilation and vascular permeability. As the shock state progresses, the changes in vascular permeability allow the development of edema that may mask hypovolemia. With cytokine release, the patient commonly has a temperature greater than 101° F (38.3° C). Changes in systemic vascular resistance (SVR) and blood pressure may cause flushed skin that can lead to the false assumption that the body is sufficiently perfused, although the cells actually have significant increases in oxygen demand (hypermetabolism). With activation of the complement system, microvascular damage leads to fibrin and platelet clumping in the capillary beds. The development of disseminated intravascular coagulation (DIC) occurs rapidly. Following release of the prostaglandins, blood flow stagnates because of the zones of vasoconstriction and vasodilation, further inhibiting tissue perfusion and allowing for the development of ischemia. With the body under such significant stress, changes in glucose, cortisol, and glucagon occur, resulting in elevated serum glucose levels. The infection overwhelms the body's defenses, and a vicious cycle of destruction occurs as additional systems are activated. This plan focuses on recognizing the patient in the medical-surgical setting who is at risk or develops septic shock as well as the critically ill patient with septic shock.

Etiology and precipitating factors
See *Risk factors for nosocomial infection.*

FOCUSED ASSESSMENT GUIDELINES

Nursing history (functional health pattern findings)
Health perception–health management pattern
• History of heart failure, diabetes mellitus, malnutrition, burns, or other factors affecting fluid balance
• Recent invasive procedure, especially any major surgical procedure, such as abdominal surgery, massive trauma repairs, or placement of invasive hemodynamic monitoring lines or urinary catheters
• Recent history of an infection — bacterial, viral, fungal, or parasitic
• History of recent antibiotic use
Nutritional-metabolic pattern
• History of elevated serum glucose levels unresponsive to treatment
• Altered or decreased intake
• Temperature elevation

Risk factors for nosocomial infection

The table below lists endogenous and exogenous risk factors for nosocomial infection.

Endogenous	Exogenous

• Age greater than 70 years
• Alcoholism
• Cardiopulmonary disease (for example, heart failure or chronic obstructive pulmonary disease)
• Depressed level of consciousness
• Diabetes
• Malnutrition
• Severe underlying disease (for example, acquired immunodeficiency syndrome or cancer)
	• Abdominal or thoracic surgery
	• Conditions favoring aspiration
	  – Endotracheal intubation
	  – Nasogastric intubation
	  – Supine positioning
	• Immobility
	• Prolonged mechanical ventilation
	• Use of antibiotics
	• Use of histamine$_2$ blockers or antacids
	• Use of immunosuppressive drugs (such as steroids)
	• Lapses in aseptic technique
	• Burns
	• Trauma
	• Invasive catheters

Adapted from Tasota, F., et al. "Protecting ICU Patients from Nosocomial Infections: Practical Measures for Favorable Outcomes," *Critical Care Nurse* 18(1):54-65, February 1998.

Cardiovascular disorders

Elimination pattern
• History of recent urinary tract infection
• Diarrhea or alterations in bowel pattern
• Severe abdominal pain
Activity-exercise pattern
• Weakness and fatigue
Cognitive-perceptual pattern
• Restlessness, anxiety, or altered level of consciousness (LOC)

Physical findings
Neurologic
• Altered LOC, ranging from subtle changes (early), restlessness, anxiety, irritability, disorientation, lethargy to coma (late)
• Possible slight decrease in Glasgow Coma Scale score
Cardiovascular
• Hypotension that does not respond to vasopressors
• Tachycardia
• Arrhythmias
• Temperature greater than 101° F (38.3° C)
• Altered hemodynamic parameters (markedly increased cardiac output [CO], decreased ejection fraction, decreased SVR in early stage; decreased CO, ejection fraction, and SVR in late stage)
• Increased capillary refill time (greater than 3 seconds)
• Decreased or thready peripheral pulses

Pulmonary
• Tachypnea (usually greater than 36 breaths/minute)
• Hyperventilation (respiratory alkalosis)
• Altered or decreased oxygen saturation levels
• Dyspnea on exertion
• Increasing presence of crackles
Gastrointestinal
• Abdominal tenderness or pain especially over right upper quadrant
• Pale or cyanotic oral mucous membranes
Hematologic
• Presence of slow bleeding from mucous membranes
• Bleeding from puncture sites, incisions or the GI or genitourinary tract
Renal
• Oliguria to anuria
Integumentary
• Altered skin temperature: warm progressing to cool
• Progression from flushed to mottled to pallor to cyanosis

Diagnostic studies
No laboratory tests are diagnostic for septic shock. Microbiology studies will support the diagnosis.
    Values will change, reflecting end-organ deterioration. Possible changes include:
• complete blood count — may vary, depending on shock stage; significant elevation of WBC count

(>15,000/µl); RBCs may be decreased with blood loss; decreased hemoglobin levels and increased hematocrit
• serum osmolality — may increase, reflecting fluid loss
• urine osmolality or specific gravity — increased, reflecting volume loss
• elevated serum lactate levels — reflect change by cells from aerobic to anaerobic metabolism; the higher the level, the greater the switch
• blood urea nitrogen and creatinine levels — increased, reflecting decreased renal perfusion
• glucose level — increased, reflecting stress-induced sympathetic stimulation
• serum electrolyte levels — may vary, depending on the underlying problem and shock stage. Commonly, hypernatremia reflects increased renal sodium retention in response to volume losses, hypokalemia reflects urinary potassium losses in exchange for sodium, and hyperkalemia reflects acidosis, decreased glomerular filtration, and cell necrosis.
• arterial blood gas (ABG) levels — reveal increased pH level and decreased partial pressure of arterial carbon dioxide ($Paco_2$) in early shock, reflecting respiratory alkalosis caused by hyperventilation and stimulation of the hypothalmic respiratory center by the endotoxin. ABG results progress to decreased pH level, increased $Paco_2$, and decreased bicarbonate level in late shock, reflecting respiratory acidosis caused by hypoventilation and metabolic acidosis caused by anaerobic metabolism.
• clotting profile — may reveal coagulopathy, shown as decreased platelet level, decreased fibrinogen level, increased fibrin split products or altered D-dimer results
• 12-lead electrocardiogram (ECG) — may reveal arrhythmias or changes reflecting myocardial ischemia, acute myocardial infarction (AMI), or electrolyte imbalances

Potential complications
• Acute renal failure
• Adult respiratory distress syndrome (ARDS)
• DIC
• Cardiogenic shock
• Cerebral anoxia
• Pancreatitis
• Hepatic failure
• Multiple organ dysfunction syndrome

CLINICAL SNAPSHOT

SEPTIC SHOCK

Major nursing diagnoses and collaborative problems	Key patient outcomes
Risk for infection	Show no signs of infection, such as elevated temperature.
Risk for hypovolemic shock	Have normal ABG values: pH, 7.35 to 7.45; $Paco_2$, 35 to 45 mm Hg; HCO_3^-, 23 to 28 mEq/L.
Hypoxemia	Maintain normal vital signs: heart rate, 60 to 100 beats/minute; systolic blood pressure, 90 to 140 mm Hg; and diastolic blood pressure, 50 to 90 mm Hg.
Risk for injury: Complications	Display normal organ function of neurologic, cardiovascular, pulmonary, and renal systems, as evidenced by normal LOC, vital signs, capillary refill, ABGs, and urine output.

NURSING DIAGNOSIS

Risk for infection related to increased exposure to pathogens, inadequate defenses, multiple invasive lines, surgical interventions, or multiple other risk factors

Nursing priorities

• Prevent infection when possible.
• Recognize patients at high risk for infection.
• Prevent progression to shock.

Patient outcome criteria

Within 48 to 72 hours of onset of infection, the patient will:
• maintain a temperature normal to him, ideally 98.6° F (37° C) or less
• maintain a LOC normal for him, ideally alert and oriented to person, place, and time
• maintain vital signs within normal limits: typically, heart rate, 60 to 100 beats/minute; systolic blood pressure, 90 to 140 mm Hg; and diastolic blood pressure, 50 to 90 mm Hg
• display a WBC count between 5,000 and 10,000/mm³.

Interventions

1. Be aware of the major sites for infection and constantly protect patients and staff. For example, ensure that invasive devices are removed promptly, following institutional or Centers for Disease Control and Prevention (CDC) guidelines.

2. Be vigilant in applying standard precautions and other infection control measures. Routinely follow principles of medical asepsis, especially hand washing. Teach the patient and family the value of hand washing. Implement strategies to prevent nosocomial pneumonia (such as using sterile technique to suction secretions, providing meticulous mouth care, and elevating the head of the bed for a patient with a nasogastric [NG] tube), nosocomial urinary tract infection (such as using sterile technique to insert a urinary catheter and maintaining a closed drainage system), and I.V. catheter nosocomial infection (such as replacing peripheral catheters and dressings according to institutional or CDC guidelines). Also consult institution policy, the CDC's *Guidelines for Isolation Precautions in Hospitals,* and the latest CDC guidelines for further details.

3. Identify patients at risk for bacteremia, sepsis, or septic shock. Be on the alert for impending infections. Obtain orders to culture suspicious sites, secretions, or drainage. Also consider the need to obtain cultures when the patient has a fever of unknown origin or fails to improve despite antimicrobial therapy.

Rationales

1. In the acute care setting, the three major sites for patient infection are the respiratory system, the urinary tract, and the bloodstream. Pneumonia, urinary tract infections, and septicemia are common diagnoses for infections in these sites. The most important factor related to infections associated with invasive lines is the length of time that catheters are left in place.

2. Because of the high mortality rate for septic shock, prevention remains the most important strategy. Patients may develop infections from exogenous sources (outside the patient) or from endogenous sources (the patient's normal flora). Routine application of infection control measures is critical, because an estimated 33% of nosocomial (hospital-acquired) infections are preventable. People are the major source of nosocomial infection. Pathogens on the hands may survive for several hours, and the spread of most infections can be prevented by simple hand washing. Lapses in sterile technique allow the introduction of organisms into the patient. The CDC's guidelines specify types of precautions appropriate to specific situations.

3. Bacteremia is the asymptomatic presence of bacteria in the bloodstream. Sepsis is present when a systemic inflammatory response occurs, producing systemic signs such as fever. Septic shock is present when a septic patient develops profound hypotension and markedly abnormal tissue perfusion. Early recognition and intervention may prevent infection from progressing to bacteremia, sepsis, or septic shock. Mortality rates from septic shock may be as high as 60% with aggressive early treatment and as high as 90% if early subtle signs are missed.

Cardiovascular disorders

4. Be meticulous in obtaining specimens for culture and sensitivity testing. For example, obtain blood cultures, as ordered, *before* instituting antimicrobial therapy. Ideally, obtain blood cultures from different sites. When obtaining a urine specimen from a patient with a urinary catheter, obtain it from the sampling port. If no sampling port is present, obtain the specimen from the catheter rather than the drainage tubing or bag. Disinfect the catheter, and aspirate the sample with a needle and syringe.

5. Observe for local signs and symptoms of infection, such as erythema, edema, and redness at a particular skin site, or coughing or altered breath sounds. Monitor the patient for classic systemic signs and symptoms, such as fever or an increased WBC count. Consult with the doctor about which level of increased temperature should be treated. Be alert for patients who cannot mount a normal response to infection, such as neutropenic or elderly patients. Monitor these patients for subtle signs of infection, such as confusion, fatigue, or restlessness.

6. Administer antimicrobial drugs empirically, as ordered. When culture and sensitivity reports arrive, make sure the organism is sensitive to the drug in the dose ordered. Consult with the doctor for definitive drug therapy.

7. Monitor closely for expected and adverse effects. Alert the doctor if the drug seems ineffective, as evidenced by continuing or increasing signs of infection, deterioration in vital signs, or other indicators.

8. Additional individualized interventions: _____

4. A contaminated specimen will produce inaccurate results. Treatment may then be inappropriate, and identification and treatment of an appropriate organism will be delayed. Starting antimicrobial therapy before obtaining blood cultures will lessen the number of pathogens in the bloodstream, thus masking infection. Having specimens from different sites increases the doctor's ability to differentiate contaminants from pathogens. Using the urinary sampling port or aspirating from the catheter provides a fresh sample for testing.

5. Elderly patients are at risk because aging impairs numerous defense mechanisms. For example, in the pulmonary system ciliary action decreases, respiratory excursion lessens, and the cough reflex becomes diminished, placing the patient at increased risk for respiratory infections. Protein malnutrition, common in the elderly, depletes energy reserves; it is linked to bacterial movement from the gut, via both bacterial translocation (movement of bacteria through an intact mucosal barrier) and disruption of the intestinal mucosal lining, which allows bacteria to move through the disrupted barrier. Fever, a protective response in a patient with normal immunity, creates a hostile environment for pathogens.

6. Commonly, infection is suspected based on clinical evidence. Before the infecting organism is identified, a broad-spectrum antibiotic usually is used. The choice of drug is based on clinical judgment and experience as well as on the suspected organism and organisms usually found in similar clinical situations in the unit or institution. Common infecting organisms include *Pseudomonas aeruginosa, Staphylococcus aureus, Candida, Enterobacter,* and *Enterococcus.*

When the culture and sensitivity report arrives, check which body area the specimen came from (which will help you distinguish normal flora from pathogens), the colony count (number of organisms), and the identification of a specific pathogen. Then check the drugs to which the organism is sensitive, and double-check the dosage against the dosage the patient is receiving. The doctor may wish to change the empiric medication to one or more specific to the organism.

7. Monitoring drug effects is important not only for the patient but for all patients, because of concern about the emergence of drug-resistant organisms. Drug resistance occurs when a specific pathogen no longer is killed by an antimicrobial to which it used to be effective. Among the greatest concerns are methicillin-resistant *Staphylococcus aureus* and vancomycin-resistant *Enterococcus.* Overuse and misuse of antibiotics allows drug-resistant organisms to emerge.

8. Rationales: _____

COLLABORATIVE PROBLEM

Risk for hypovolemic shock related to inflammatory mediators

Nursing priorities

- Identify the stage of septic shock.
- Intervene to maintain CO.

Patient outcome criteria

Within 48 hours of developing septic shock, the patient will:
- maintain normal vital signs: heart rate, 60 to 100 beats/minute; systolic blood pressure, 90 to 140 mm Hg; diastolic blood pressure, 50 to 90 mm Hg
- display normal hemodynamic values (CO, 4 to 6 L/minute; SVR, 800 to 1,200 dynes/sec/cm^{-5}; and pulmonary artery wedge pressure, 4 to 12 mm Hg)
- produce a normal urine output (60 to 150 ml/hour)
- have warm, dry skin and a capillary refill time of less than 3 seconds, indicating sufficient tissue perfusion
- display a stable neurologic status, ideally alert and oriented.

Interventions

1. Be alert for the signs and symptoms of early stage septic shock: flushed skin, tachycardia, tachypnea, and fever or reduced temperature.

Rationales

1. Septic shock may progress from an early stage to a late stage. Early stage septic shock is characterized by a hyperdynamic cardiovascular function, peripheral vasodilation, systemic edema, and relative hypovolemia. These changes result from excessive vascular mediators released from the cell wall of dying cells. These mediators produce widespread vasodilation, characterized by warm, dry, flushed skin; tachycardia; and good urine output. Hemodynamic values typically reveal decreased SVR, markedly increased CO, hypotension, and widened pulse pressure. The decreased SVR results in decreased resistance to cardiac ejection and shunting of blood to the peripheral tissues, producing the warm, flushed skin. Despite the increased CO, myocardial function decreases, probably due to the release of myocardial depressant factor. Increased vascular permeability results in fluid movement from the vascular system to the interstitium, producing both systemic edema and a relative hypovolemia. Other signs seen during this early stage are tachypnea and a subtly decreased LOC, which appears as confusion, restlessness, or agitation. Fever may be present if the patient has been able to mount an immune response to the organism. If not, hypothermia is present. This can be misleading, because the patient who formerly had a decreased temperature may now have a temperature within the normal range, which represents an increased temperature for him.

Cardiovascular disorders

2. Implement therapy, as ordered, including fluid administration and antimicrobial drugs. See this entry's previous problem, "Risk for infection," for further information on drug administration. Assist the doctor with removal of the infection's source, if possible (for example, drainage of an abcess or wound debridement).

2. Early, aggressive treatment is the key to intervening in septic shock. Because of marked vasodilation and increased vascular permeability, fluid shifts from the vascular system to the periphery, producing a relative hypovolemia. Therefore, treatment of early septic shock includes generous fluid replacement and administration of vasopressors to counteract the decreased SVR, as well as administration of antimicrobials presumed effective against the suspected pathogen. This entry's "Risk for infection" problem details appropriate drug administration in sepsis.

3. Be alert for signs of the late stage of septic shock: severe hypotension, cold mottled extremities, poor peripheral pulses, markedly decreased LOC, systemic and pulmonary edema, and oliguria or anuria. Monitor hemodynamic values for decreased CO and further decreased SVR. As ordered, implement standard hypovolemic shock measures, as detailed in the "Hypovolemic shock" plan, page 432.

3. The late stage of septic shock is decompensation. Hypodynamic cardiac function produces decreased CO, responsible for such signs as severe hypotension and oliguria or anuria. Treatment of this stage is similar to that of hypovolemic shock, with increased emphasis on monitoring the patient for signs of fluid overload and cautious titration of vasopressors to maximize CO. The "Hypovolemic shock" plan details further management of this stage.

4. Additional individualized interventions: _____

4. Rationales: _____

COLLABORATIVE PROBLEM

Hypoxemia related to ventilation-perfusion imbalance and diffusion defects

Nursing priority

Maintain ventilation and oxygenation.

Patient outcome criteria

- Within 48 hours, the patient will:
  - show ABG levels within expected limits
  - have clearing breath sounds bilaterally
  - show no or limited signs of ARDS progression.
- By discharge, the patient will:
  - maintain a patent airway
  - be free from mechanical ventilation support
  - have normal ABG results and pulmonary function values
  - have stabilized oxygen consumption values.

Interventions

1. Provide standard nursing care related to impaired gas exchange. Maintain airway patency and monitor respiratory status. Suction as necessary. Provide supplemental oxygen, as ordered, and assist with intubation and mechanical ventilation if indicated.

Rationales

1. Numerous factors may cause ventilation-perfusion imbalance in shock, including atelectasis, microemboli, pulmonary congestion, and impaired capillary perfusion. The general measures listed apply to the care of any critically ill patient.

2. Monitor oxygen saturation through continuous pulse oximetry. Monitor ABG levels, as ordered, typically at least every 4 to 12 hours.

2. Pulse oximetry determines oxygen saturation rapidly, continuously, and noninvasively. ABG results indicate oxygenation status and degree of acid-base imbalance. Hyperventilation, a compensatory response to hypoxemia, is common in early septic shock and can lead to respiratory alkalosis. Late septic shock is characterized by combined metabolic acidosis from decreased capillary perfusion (lactic acid production and anaerobic metabolism) and respiratory acidosis (due to hypercarbia).

3. Observe for signs and symptoms of ARDS, such as tachypnea, progressive dyspnea, increasing inspiratory pressure, lung compliance less than 50 ml/cm H_2O (if mechanically ventilated), deteriorating ABG or pulse oximetry values, or hypoxemia. If you detect these problems, document them and alert the doctor. Implement measures described in the "Adult respiratory distress syndrome" plan, page 240, as appropriate.

3. Septic shock ranks as a major risk factor for ARDS due to such factors as decreased perfusion, hypoxemia, increased capillary permeability, and high oxygen levels used in treatment. The plan for ARDS describes this ominous complication and related care.

4. Assist with insertion of pulmonary artery catheter, if ordered. Monitor hemodynamic parameters as well as oxygen delivery and oxygen consumption (VO_2).

4. With the progression of septic shock there are changes in the hemodynamic parameters as well as in cellular VO_2 and oxygen delivery. The tissues have increased demand, yet altered cellular metabolism prevents the cells from extracting sufficient oxygen to meet metabolic needs; therefore, mixed venous saturation is greater than 80% (normal is 60% to 80%).

5. Additional individualized interventions: _____

5. Rationales: _____

NURSING DIAGNOSIS

Risk for injury: complications related to ischemia or bleeding

Nursing priority

Prevent or minimize complications.

Patient outcome criteria

By the time of discharge, the patient will:
• be alert and oriented to person, place, and time, moving all extremities spontaneously
• maintain normal vital signs: heart rate, 60 to100 beats/minute; systolic blood pressure, 90 to140 mm Hg; diastolic blood pressure, 50 to 90 mm Hg; and normal perfusion (evidenced by capillary refill less than 3 seconds)
• have normal ABG values: pH, 7.35 to 7.45; $Paco_2$, 35 to 45 mm Hg; HCO_3^-, 23 to 28 mEq/L
• have a urine output of 60 to 150 ml/hour.

Interventions

1. Prevent paralytic ileus and stress ulcers. Withhold food and fluids; insert an NG tube connected to suction, as ordered. Administer cimetidine (Tagamet), ranitidine (Zantac), sucralfate (Carafate), or antacids, as ordered. Monitor bowel sounds.

Rationales

1. Paralytic ileus may result from mesenteric ischemia. The resulting gastric distention provokes vomiting, which can lead to chemical pneumonitis if aspiration occurs. Withholding food and fluids reduces stress on the stomach. NG drainage decompresses the stomach. The medications listed reduce the risk of stress ulcers by decreasing hydrochloric acid secretion or coating the gastric mucosa.

2. Administer antibiotics by mouth or NG tube if indicated. Attempt enteral feedings if the patient is able to tolerate food and there is adequate bowel motility. If not, use parenteral feedings to provide nutrients. (See the "Nutritional deficit" plan, page 80.)

2. This antibiotic regimen may prevent translocation of GI bacteria from the lumen of the gut into the vascular compartment, thereby limiting an additional source of infection. Food in a mobile gut is thought to prevent translocation of bacteria. If the patient is unable to tolerate enteral feedings, use parenteral feedings to support hypermetabolic tissue demands. The "Nutritional deficit" plan provides detailed information on this problem.

3. Observe for signs and symptoms of AMI, such as severe chest pain, shortness of breath, hypotension, diaphoresis, pained facial expression, elevated cardiac isoenzymes, or ECG showing ST-segment displacement, T-wave inversion, or pathologic Q waves. See the "Acute MI: Critical care unit" plan, page 338.

3. Decreased perfusion of the heart, catecholamine stimulation, hypoxemia, and increased afterload all may cause AMI. Decreased perfusion of the pancreas may release myocardial depressant factor, which also may cause AMI. The AMI plan gives details on this complication.

4. Observe for signs and symptoms of DIC, such as blood oozing from multiple sites, repeated bleeding episodes, oral cyanosis, petechiae, ecchymoses, hematomas, prolonged prothrombin time (PT), prolonged partial thromboplastin time, decreased fibrinogen level, decreased platelet count, or elevated fibrin split products level. Refer to the "Disseminated intravascular coagulation" plan, page 780 for further information.

4. Shock is a major risk factor for DIC because of such factors as capillary sludging, acidosis, sepsis, trauma, or other underlying causes. The "Disseminated intravascular coagulation" plan describes this devastating development in depth.

5. Observe for signs and symptoms of acute renal failure, such as oliguria or anuria, weight gain, neck vein distention, crackles, dependent edema, or elevated BUN and serum creatinine levels. As appropriate, implement measures described in the "Acute renal failure" plan, page 686.

5. Renal blood vessel constriction is an early compensatory mechanism in shock. Although this constriction limits glomerular filtration, thus conserving fluid volume, it impairs renal perfusion, which may result in acute renal failure. The "Acute renal failure" plan describes this complication in detail.

6. Observe for signs and symptoms of liver failure, such as drowsiness, intellectual deterioration, personality changes, septicemia, fever, hyperkinetic circulation, elevated serum ammonium levels, jaundice, hepatomegaly, ascites, easy bruising, increased PT, elevated serum aspartate aminotransferase level, or increased bilirubin level. See the "Liver failure" plan, page 551.

6. Although shock may damage hepatic cells, prompt correction of shock may allow these cells to regenerate. Early detection of liver failure may prevent severe damage to this critical organ. The "Liver failure" plan presents the pathophysiology of this disorder and related care.

7. Additional individualized interventions: _____

7. Rationales: _____

NURSING DIAGNOSIS

Risk for ineffective individual coping, ineffective family coping, or both, related to threat to life

Nursing priority

Provide emotional support to the patient and family.

Patient outcome criterion

By the time of discharge, the patient will meet outcome criteria identified in the "Ineffective individual coping" plan.

Interventions

1. Implement measures described in "Ineffective individual coping," page 67, and "Ineffective family coping: Compromised," page 63, as appropriate.

2. Additional individualized interventions: _____

Rationales

1. Families (and alert patients) are aware that shock is life-threatening, and they react to the possibility of death in various ways. These plans describe measures to help them cope with their realistic fear and other emotional responses.

2. Rationales: _____

DISCHARGE PLANNING

Discharge checklist
Before discharge, the patient shows evidence of:
❐ blood pressure within normal limits without I.V. inotrope or vasopressor support
❐ pulse and respirations within normal limits
❐ ABG levels within expected limits for recovery stage
❐ urine output within normal limits
❐ freedom from infection
❐ freedom from major complications.

Teaching checklist
Document evidence that the patient and family demonstrate an understanding of:
❐ cause and significance of shock
❐ expectations for recovery
❐ purpose of monitoring devices
❐ rationales for therapeutic interventions.

Documentation checklist
Using outcome criteria as a guide, document:
❐ clinical status on admission
❐ significant changes in status
❐ pertinent diagnostic test findings
❐ care for invasive monitoring lines
❐ fluid administration
❐ use of inotropes, vasopressors, or other pharmacologic agents
❐ measures to support ventilation and oxygenation
❐ emotional support
❐ patient and family teaching
❐ discharge planning.

ASSOCIATED PLANS OF CARE

Acute MI: Critical care unit
Acute renal failure
Adult respiratory distress syndrome
Cardiogenic shock
Disseminated intravascular coagulation
GI hemorrhage
Hypovolemic shock
Impaired physical mobility
Ineffective family coping: Compromised
Ineffective individual coping
Liver failure
Major burns
Mechanical ventilation
Multiple trauma
Pulmonary embolism

REFERENCES

Crowley, S.R. "The Pathogenesis of Septic Shock," *Heart & Lung* 25(2):124-36; March-April 1996.

DeGroot-Kosolcharoen, J. "Solving the Infection Puzzle with Culture and Sensitivity Testing," *Nursing96* 26(9):33-38, September 1996.

Hoppe, B. "Control of Infections Caused by Drug-Resistant Organisms in Critical Care," *American Journal of Critical Care* 6(2):141-44, March 1997.

Tasota, F, et al. "Protecting ICU Patients from Nosocomial Infections: Practical Measures for Favorable Outcomes." *Critical Care Nurse* 18(1):54-65, February 1998.

Thompson, J., et al. *Mosby's Clinical Nursing,* 4th ed. St. Louis: Mosby—Year Book, Inc., 1997.

Wardle, E. "Prevention and Treatment of Septic Shock, SIDS, ARDS, and Multi-Organ End Failure, Part I," *Care of the Critically Ill* 12(5):177-80, 1996.

Wardle, E. "Experimental and Futuristic Approaches to Treatment of Septic Shock, Part 2," *Care of the Critically Ill* 25(2):124-36, 1996.

Wiessner, W.H., et al. "Treatment of Sepsis and Septic Shock: A Review," *Heart & Lung* 24(5):380-93, September-October 1995.

Cardiovascular disorders

Thrombophlebitis

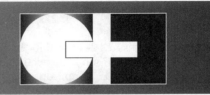

DRG information
DRG 128   Deep Vein Thrombophlebitis.
           Mean LOS = 6.7 days
DRG 130   Peripheral Vascular Disorders with Compli-
           cation or Comorbidity (CC).
           Mean LOS = 6.7 days
DRG 131   Peripheral Vascular Disorders without CC.
           Mean LOS = 5.2 days

INTRODUCTION

Definition and time focus
Thrombophlebitis is the severe, acute inflammation of small- and medium-sized veins associated with secondary thrombus formation. It can occur in superficial or deep veins. The most common site of superficial thrombophlebitis is the saphenous vein; the most common sites of deep vein thrombosis are the iliofemoral vein, popliteal veins, and small calf veins. This plan focuses on the patient admitted for diagnosis and management of acute lower-extremity thrombophlebitis.

Etiology and precipitating factors
• Venous stasis from prolonged bed rest, sitting, or standing; varicose veins; low cardiac output; obesity; or limb paralysis
• Hypercoagulability from dehydration or oral contraceptive use
• Vessel wall trauma from venipunctures, leg injury, venous disease, infection, or chemical irritants, such as I.V. antibiotics or potassium chloride
• Vascular narrowing or degeneration from hypertension, hypercholesterolemia, diabetes, kidney disease, cerebrovascular accident, or smoking

FOCUSED ASSESSMENT GUIDELINES

Nursing history (functional health pattern findings)
Health perception–health management pattern
• Acute onset of local pain (relieved by elevation of extremity), tenderness, edema, erythema, warmth, induration, or febrile reaction
• Known risk factors for thrombophlebitis, such as prolonged bed rest
• History of recent vessel cannulation or vessel trauma

Activity-exercise pattern
• Sedentary lifestyle or occupation that requires standing for long periods
• Recent prolonged bed rest or immobility
Role-relationship pattern
• Family history of cardiac risk factors

Physical findings
Cardiovascular
• Local edema
• Engorged vessel
• Positive Homans' sign
Integumentary
• Local erythema
• Warmth
• Local induration
• Ulceration

Diagnostic studies
• Complete blood count — white blood cell count may reflect inflammatory response and systemic infection
• Activated partial thromboplastin time (APTT) and prothrombin time/international normalized ratio (PT/INR) — may be prolonged, indicating clotting defects or hypercoagulability
• Cholesterol levels — may be elevated, suggesting increased risk for atherosclerosis
• Triglyceride levels — may be elevated, indicating increased risk of atherosclerosis
• Serum glucose levels — may be elevated, reflecting stress response or diabetes
• Doppler ultrasound blood flow detector test — determines venous return, may identify thrombolic occlusion
• Plethysmography — may show segmental occlusion
• Venography — may indicate loss of significant venous return
• [125]I fibrinogen leg scanning — may reflect vascular insufficiency

Potential complications
• Venous ulcer
• Pulmonary embolus
• Phlegmasia cerulea dolens (sudden, marked leg swelling and cyanosis related to iliofemoral venous thrombosis)

CLINICAL SNAPSHOT

THROMBOPHLEBITIS

Major nursing diagnoses and collaborative problems	Key patient outcomes
Acute venous insufficiency	Show improved color and temperature of affected area.
Pain	Rate pain as less than 3 on a 0 to 10 pain rating scale.
Risk for thromboembolism	Show no signs of pulmonary embolism.
Knowledge deficit (postdischarge care)	Be able to correctly describe details of anticoagulant administration, if prescribed, and how to minimize bleeding risk.

COLLABORATIVE PROBLEM

Acute venous insufficiency related to obstruction and stasis

Nursing priority

Promote venous blood flow.

Patient outcome criteria

Within 3 days of admission, the patient will:
• show normal color (for example, pink and warm for a white patient) and temperature of affected area
• have decreased measurement of calf
• show no evidence of bleeding
• rate pain as less than 3 on a 0 to 10 pain rating scale.

Interventions

1. Assess calves and thighs daily for signs and symptoms of thrombophlebitis. Early signs include swelling, erythema, edema, tenderness, venous patterning, or engorgement along the vein. Later signs include pain, cording (vein has a cordlike feeling), and a positive Homans' sign (not always present). Avoid deep palpation. If swelling is suspected or present, measure and record calf circumference, placing a reference mark on the leg. Repeat the measurement daily, comparing the latest measurement with previous values.

2. Notify the doctor immediately if new signs and symptoms develop or existing ones worsen, such as onset of new pain of increased swelling.

Rationales

1. Early signs and symptoms result from vessel wall inflammation; later ones, from thrombus formation. Homans' sign (pain in the calf on dorsiflexion of the foot), commonly believed to indicate deep vein thrombosis, is an unreliable indicator. Absent in many cases of deep vein thrombosis, Homans' sign can be produced in any painful calf condition. Deep palpation may dislodge a clot. Leg circumference monitoring provides an objective method to evaluate swelling; using a reference mark ensures consistency.

2. New or worsening signs of thrombophlebitis require prompt medical attention. Superficial thrombophlebitis, although not dangerous, is painful. Untreated deep vein thrombophlebitis can be life-threatening if the thrombus moves to the lungs.

Cardiovascular disorders

3. Implement activity restrictions:
• Maintain complete bed rest, usually for 3 to 7 days.
• Elevate the extremity at least 30 degrees continuously, unless contraindicated.
• Avoid using the knee gatch, pillows under the knees, and, when the patient is allowed out of bed, leg crossing and prolonged sitting.

4. Encourage the patient to perform gentle foot and leg exercises every hour. Consult the doctor about appropriate exercises, which may include isometric exercises (quadriceps setting or plantar flexion against a footboard) or isotonic exercises (active or passive foot and leg flexion and extension and ankle rotation).

5. Increase fluid intake to eight 8-oz glasses (2,000 ml) a day, unless contraindicated.

6. Consult the doctor about using antiembolism stockings or an intermittent pneumatic compression device.

7. Teach the patient stress-control measures, as needed, such as progressive relaxation techniques, breathing exercises, and visualization. Encourage smoking cessation and refer the patient to appropriate resources for help.

8. Administer medications, as ordered: anti-inflammatory agents, such as ibuprofen (Advil) and indomethacin (Indocin), and anticoagulants, such as heparin, warfarin sodium (Coumadin), or aspirin.

9. Monitor clotting studies, as ordered: APTT if the patient is receiving heparin, PT/INR if the patient is receiving warfarin sodium. Report values outside the desired range to the doctor before the next scheduled anticoagulant dose.

10. Observe for signs of bleeding, such as oozing at intravenous or intramuscular injection sites, epistaxis, bleeding gums, ecchymoses, hematuria, or melena.

11. Increase the patient's activity level, as ordered.

12. Observe for signs of chronic venous insufficiency: dependent ankle edema, induration, shiny skin, varicosities, and stasis ulcers. Consult the doctor if these signs are present.

3. Bed rest and elevation improve venous flow by using gravity to reduce the pressure gradient between the extremity and the heart. Also, bed rest reduces oxygen requirements, limits the risk of thrombus dislodgement, and promotes fibrinolytic breakdown and clot absorption. The remaining measures avoid increased popliteal pressure, which compresses veins and impedes venous return.

4. The pumping effect of muscle action promotes venous return. Gentle exercise minimizes further thrombus formation, but overly vigorous exercise may dislodge clots. Isometric exercises, generally recommended after surgery, increase venous flow but also may increase blood pressure. Because this effect may be detrimental, particularly to the patient with cardiovascular disease, some doctors prefer isotonic exercises, which cause a more desirable cardiovascular response.

5. Increased fluid intake increases vascular volume and reduces viscosity, thus improving blood flow.

6. Superficial veins may be dilated and tortuous, particularly in the older patient. Antiembolism stockings or intermittent pneumatic compression devices may support venous return by compressing superficial veins and redirecting blood flow to deeper veins.

7. Stress-related catecholamine release and smoking induce vasoconstriction.

8. Anti-inflammatory agents are the primary treatment for superficial thrombophlebitis. Anticoagulants may be used if a superficial thrombus extends or threatens the deep venous system in the groin. Anticoagulants are the mainstay of treatment for deep venous thrombophlebitis. Heparin interferes with platelet aggregation, conversion of prothrombin to thrombin, and conversion of fibrinogen to fibrin, thereby minimizing further clot formation. Warfarin sodium interferes with the vitamin K activity necessary for clotting. Aspirin interferes with platelet aggregation.

9. Dosages are adjusted to maintain PT/INR and APTT within a therapeutic range. The typical ranges desired are 2 to 2 times control values.

10. Excessive anticoagulant dosages increase the risk of bleeding.

11. Muscle movement compresses vessels, improving venous return.

12. Repeated episodes of deep vein thrombosis can cause chronic venous insufficiency from venous valvular destruction.

13. Additional individualized interventions: _____ | **13.** Rationales: _____

Nursing diagnosis

Pain related to vessel obstruction, inflammation, and edema

Nursing priority

Relieve pain.

Patient outcome criterion

Within 1 hour of reporting pain, the patient will rate pain level as less than 3 on a 0 to 10 pain rating scale.

Interventions

1. See the "Pain" plan, page 88.

2. Implement measures to promote venous flow (such as bed rest and leg elevation), as described in the previous problem.

3. Handle the affected extremity gently. Use a bed cradle.

4. Apply warm, moist heat to the affected area, as ordered.

5. Administer analgesics, as ordered, observing for therapeutic and adverse effects. Question the use of indomethacin or aspirin if the patient is receiving an anticoagulant.

6. Administer anti-inflammatory agents, as ordered.

7. Additional individualized interventions: _____

Rationales

1. The "Pain" plan contains multiple interventions for pain relief.

2. Eliminating the pain's cause is the most effective relief measure.

3. The thrombophlebitic extremity is extremely sensitive; even slight pressure or movement may be painful. A bed cradle keeps the weight of linens off the extremity.

4. Heat is soothing and causes vasodilation, improving blood flow.

5. The appropriate type and amount of analgesic depends on the degree of pain and the use of anticoagulants. Indomethacin and aspirin, which may be used to control pain, increase anticoagulant activity and may be inappropriate for the patient taking heparin or warfarin.

6. Reducing inflammation and edema reduces stimulation of nerve fibers and thus reduces pain.

7. Rationales: _____

Collaborative problem

Risk for thromboembolism related to dislodged thrombus

Nursing priority

Prevent or promptly detect thromboembolism.

Patient outcome criteria

Within 24 hours of thrombophlebitis onset, the patient will show no signs of pulmonary embolism, as evidenced by absence of tachypnea, cyanosis, dyspnea or chest pain.

Cardiovascular disorders

Interventions

1. Monitor for signs and symptoms of either a massive pulmonary embolism (profound shock, cyanosis, diaphoresis, and a sense of impending doom) or a lesser pulmonary embolism (tachypnea, dyspnea, pleuritic chest pain [sharp, stabbing pain that worsens on inspiration or coughing], and restlessness).

2. Alert the doctor promptly if any signs or symptoms of pulmonary embolism appear. If signs of massive pulmonary embolism occur, place the patient in the high Fowler position, administer oxygen at 6 L/minute by nasal prongs, monitor vital signs, and summon immediate medical assistance. Refer to the "Pulmonary embolism" plan, page 308.

3. During acute thrombophlebitis, maintain bed rest as ordered. Request an order for graduated compression stockings or an intermittent pneumatic compression device for patients at risk for thrombophlebitis.

4. Caution the patient against rubbing the painful area.

5. Help the patient avoid Valsalva's maneuver. Teach the patient to exhale during defecation, and provide fluid, high-fiber foods, prune juice, or other measures to promote passage of soft stool.

6. Observe for persistent or recurrent thrombophlebitis. If present, consult with the doctor about further treatment.

7. Additional individualized interventions: _____

Rationales

1. Pulmonary embolism is the most common pulmonary complication in hospitalized patients. Deep venous thrombosis is the primary risk factor for embolus development.

2. Pulmonary emboli can cause local areas of pulmonary dysfunction and increase the risk of massive embolism. Massive pulmonary embolism, in which 50% or more of the pulmonary vascular bed is occluded, is a medical emergency. Treatment may include full cardiopulmonary support, surgical intervention, I.V. streptokinase (Kabikinase), and heparin. The "Pulmonary embolism" plan contains further details on this disorder.

3. Bed rest decreases the likelihood that muscle contractions will dislodge a clot, while compression improves venous flow.

4. Rubbing may cause the clot to break free and embolize.

5. A sudden increase in intrathoracic pressure, such as that produced by Valsalva's maneuver, may dislodge the clot.

6. Persistent or recurrent thrombophlebitis increases the risk of pulmonary embolism. Treatment may include prolonged anticoagulant therapy or insertion of an inferior vena caval umbrella to trap clots.

7. Rationales: _____

NURSING DIAGNOSIS

Knowledge deficit (postdischarge care) related to unfamiliar therapeutic regimen

Nursing priority

Educate the patient and family about continuing therapy and preventing recurrence.

Patient outcome criteria

By the time of discharge, the patient will:
• be able to list personal risk factors
• be able to list the signs and symptoms of thrombophlebitis
• be able to identify five ways to improve venous flow
• be able to correctly describe the details of anticoagulant administration, if prescribed, and how to minimize bleeding risk
• verbalize the importance of regular medical follow-up
• verbalize intent to obtain a medical alert bracelet or necklace.

Interventions

1. Teach the patient and family about factors that may increase the risk of recurrence. Discuss measures that may reduce or eliminate risk factors, including weight control through diet and exercise, smoking cessation, drug therapy for hypertension, and careful diabetes control.

2. Teach the patient ways to improve venous flow: exercising feet and legs hourly while awake; increasing fluid intake to at least eight 8-oz glasses (2,000 ml) a day (unless contraindicated); elevating extremity when sitting or lying down; participating in prescribed activity program; avoiding girdles, garters, knee-high stockings, and other constricting clothing; using antiembolism stockings; avoiding leg crossing; and avoiding oral contraceptives.

3. Teach the patient and family to observe for signs and symptoms of recurrence.

4. Teach the patient how to care for extremities: maintaining clean, dry skin; carefully monitoring any skin lesions; and protecting skin from injury.

5. Teach the patient and family about oral anticoagulant therapy, if prescribed. Also teach ways to minimize the risk of bleeding, such as using an electric shaver and avoiding aspirin. (See the "Cerebrovascular accident" plan, page 127, for further details.)

6. Emphasize the importance of following the doctor's recommendations for regular medical follow-up, including laboratory test monitoring. Also stress the value of wearing a medical alert bracelet or necklace, and tell the patient how to obtain one.

7. Additional individualized interventions: _____

Rationales

1. Thrombophlebitis commonly recurs, particularly if risk factors are not eliminated. Teaching measures to eliminate or reduce risk factors may avert further problems.

2. These methods prevent the classic causes of thrombophlebitis: venous stasis, vessel trauma, and hypercoagulability.

3. Early detection promotes early treatment.

4. Impaired circulation in the extremities predisposes the patient to stasis ulcers.

5. A patient with uncomplicated deep venous thrombophlebitis usually takes warfarin for 4 to 6 weeks after discharge. Complications may warrant lifelong anticoagulant therapy. The "Cerebrovascular accident" plan contains further details related to anticoagulant therapy.

6. Thrombophlebitis may recur or develop into chronic venous insufficiency. Conscientious medical follow-up provides the greatest protection against future life-threatening episodes or chronicity. Monitoring laboratory parameters, such as PT/INR for the patient taking warfarin, helps the doctor maintain therapeutic dosage. A medical alert bracelet or necklace increases the likelihood of appropriate treatment should the patient be unable to communicate in a medical emergency.

7. Rationales: _____

DISCHARGE PLANNING

Discharge checklist
Before discharge, the patient shows evidence of:
❏ absence of heat, pain, swelling, or inflammation at affected site
❏ APTT or PT/INR within acceptable parameters
❏ absence of pulmonary or cardiovascular complications
❏ absence of fever
❏ vital signs within normal parameters
❏ absence of bowel or bladder dysfunction
❏ heparin therapy discontinued for 24 hours
❏ anticoagulation controlled with oral medication
❏ presence of bilateral pedal pulses
❏ absence of pain and pallor in the affected lower extremity
❏ ability to perform activities of daily living (ADLs), transfers, and ambulation same as before hospitalization
❏ adequate home support system, or referral to home care or a nursing home if indicated by lack of home support system or inability to perform ADLs, transfers, and ambulation.

Cardiovascular disorders

Teaching checklist

Document evidence that the patient and family demonstrate an understanding of:

❏ signs and symptoms of recurring thrombophlebitis
❏ continued use of antiembolism stockings
❏ all discharge medications' purpose, dosage, administration schedule, all food and drug interactions and adverse effects requiring medical attention (usual discharge medications include oral anticoagulants and anti-inflammatory medications)
❏ allowable activity level
❏ importance of wearing medical alert identification if the patient remains on anticoagulant therapy
❏ need to modify risk factors
❏ procedure for obtaining follow-up laboratory tests such as PT
❏ date, time, and location of follow-up appointment
❏ reportable signs and symptoms (such as those of pulmonary embolism) and how to contact the doctor.

Documentation checklist

Using outcome criteria as a guide, document:

❏ clinical status on admission
❏ significant changes in status
❏ pertinent laboratory data and diagnostic test findings
❏ pain-relief measures
❏ effect of position changes and extremity elevation
❏ application and effect of warm, moist compresses
❏ anticoagulant administration
❏ any change in clotting studies
❏ any bleeding tendencies
❏ administration of other pharmacologic agents, such as an anti-inflammatory, antibiotic, or fibrinolytic medication (such as streptokinase or urokinase)
❏ level of activity and the patient's response to progressive ambulation
❏ patient and family teaching
❏ discharge planning.

ASSOCIATED PLANS OF CARE

Cerebrovascular accident
Ineffective individual coping
Knowledge deficit
Pain
Pulmonary embolism
Surgery

REFERENCES

Black, J.M., and Matassarin-Jacobs, E. *Medical-Surgical Nursing: Clinical Management for Continuity of Care,* 5th ed. Philadelphia: W.B. Saunders Co., 1997.

Bright, L.D. "Clinical Snapshot: DVT," *AJN* 95(6):48-49, June 1995.

Chernecky, C.C., and Berger, B.J. *Laboratory Tests and Diagnostic Procedures*. 2nd ed. Philadelphia: W.B. Saunders Co., 1997.

Launius, B.K., et al. "Understanding and Preventing Deep Vein Thrombosis and Pulmonary Embolism," *AACN Clinical Issues* 9(1):91-99, February 1998.

Schlant, R., et al., eds. *The Heart*, 9th ed. New York: McGraw-Hill Book Co., 1997.

Part 7

Gastrointestinal disorders

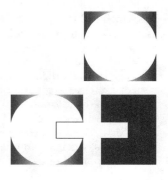

Anorexia nervosa and bulimia nervosa

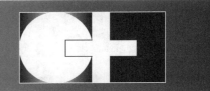

DRG information

Anorexia nervosa:

DRG 428   Disorders of Personality and Impulse Control.

         Mean LOS = 8.4 days

Bulimia nervosa:

DRG 432   Other Diagnoses of Mental Disorders.

         Mean LOS = 6.5 days

INTRODUCTION

Definition and time focus

Anorexia nervosa and bulimia nervosa are complex psychiatric disorders characterized by abnormal eating patterns and eating-related behaviors. The defining criterion for anorexia nervosa are the refusal to maintain body weight at the expected normal minimal range for age and height, accompanied by the fear of becoming fat, body image problems, amenorrhea, and denial of the dangers of low body weight. Two categories of anorexia nervosa exist, the binge-eating–purging type and the restrictive type without binge-eating–purging behaviors. Bulimia nervosa is defined as recurrent episodes of binge eating and recurrent inappropriate actions to control weight gain. Bulimia nervosa can be categorized as the purging type with self-induced vomiting and abuse of laxatives, or the nonpurging type with the use of excessive fasting or exercise (American Psychiatric Association, 1994). Because many patients move between the diagnostic categories over time, a patient may not fit neatly into either category. The following information is based on current definitions and understanding of the disorders.

Anorexia nervosa involves dramatic weight loss unrelated to organic causes: intentional starvation, ritualistic or compulsive eating behaviors, and bizarre delusional disturbances in body image are part of the typical picture. Although the patient is obsessed by thoughts of food, the need for control overrides the desire to eat. Limiting food intake provides a sense of control. Bulimia nervosa is characterized by binge-purge cycles in which the patient consumes large quantities of high-calorie food, then uses laxatives or purgatives, fasts or exercises excessively, or induces vomiting to rid the body of the calories consumed. The binges usually occur at least twice weekly, during periods of stress. Anorexia nervosa involves weight loss of dangerous proportions, whereas bulimia nervosa may be characterized by normal or even above-normal weight with frequent, sometimes abrupt fluctuations. Usually, the bulimic patient displays more insight into the abnormal character of threatening behaviors and hides them from family and friends. The anorexic patient is less able to recognize potentially harmful eating behaviors because of a severely altered body image. In either disorder, life-threatening physical complications related to the physiologic effects of malnutrition may occur.

Anorexia nervosa has been reported to have the highest death rate of any psychiatric disorder. Up to 25% of bulimics also suffer from clinical depression; a similar number attempt suicide. Many patients with eating disorders also have substance abuse problems and characteristics typical of personality disorders. Treatment recommendations also vary widely. Some clinicians advocate rigorous behavior-modification techniques; others use in-depth psychotherapy, psychoanalysis, family therapy, or a combination of approaches. Because the etiology and perpetuating factors for eating disorders vary among individuals, multiple treatment approaches are needed. When the patient with an eating disorder is admitted to an inpatient medical-surgical unit, the immediate focus is likely to be controlled nutritional replenishment, prevention of complications, restoration of physiologic equilibrium, and initiation or continuation of appropriate psychiatric treatment.

This plan focuses on the anorexic or bulimic patient admitted for diagnosis and management of severely disruptive and potentially dangerous eating patterns.

Etiology and precipitating factors

No clear-cut or consistent factors have been identified as causing these disorders. Instead, a combination of complex psychodynamic, familial, and societal factors appears to be involved.

Psychodynamic

• Developmental deficits related to issues of loss, separation, sexuality, autonomy, and power

• Sense of powerlessness or lack of control

Familial

• With anorexia nervosa, perfectionistic or overprotective families, pattern of avoiding family conflicts, lack of conflict-resolution skills

• With bulimia nervosa, perfectionistic or overprotective families, families lacking clear interpersonal boundaries or roles

Societal

• Emphasis on being thin and exercising as a basis for peer acceptance

• Thinness as societal image of female beauty

–seen in all economic, cultural, and religious groups
–less common among blacks and southern Europeans
–predominantly affects adolescent girls and young women

Focused assessment guidelines

Nursing history (functional health pattern findings)

Health perception–health management pattern

Anorexia nervosa

• Onset that may have followed a successful diet taken to extremes (a typical finding in adolescent girls)
• Pleading, punitive measures, or arguments by others to eat, with no effect on eating patterns
• Frequent pressure to seek treatment

Bulimia nervosa

• Onset that may have followed actual or impending separation from home (a typical finding in young adult women ages 18 to 25)
• Quick weight-loss attempt that may have escalated to a compulsive need to binge, followed by vomiting
• Undiagnosed anorexic episode in adolescence
• History of drug or alcohol abuse

Nutritional-metabolic pattern

Anorexia nervosa

• Absence of hunger likely
• Restriction of food intake for various reasons, such as GI discomfort, food allergies, or dislike of certain foods
• Encouragement of others (such as brothers or sisters) to eat
• Mealtime rituals, with an excessive amount of time spent over each meal
• Expressed interest in recipes and cooking
• Consumption of low-calorie, low-fat, low-carbohydrate, and "diet" foods
• Hiding or hoarding of food

Bulimia nervosa

• Difficulty breathing after bingeing
• Planning of, or preoccupation with, bingeing and purging
• Secretive binge eating but may binge with others (a group binge)
• History of hiatal hernia
• Esophageal or GI discomfort
• Consumption of high-carbohydrate foods during a binge but eating balanced meals or "diet" food at regular meals

Elimination pattern

Anorexia nervosa

• Chronic constipation
• Self-induced or spontaneous vomiting

Bulimia nervosa

• Constipation or diarrhea
• Constipation if laxative abuse is discontinued

• Permanent loss of bowel reactivity once laxatives are discontinued (rare)
• Vomiting, most commonly self-induced and not usually accompanied by nausea
• Spontaneous regurgitation

Activity-exercise pattern

Anorexia nervosa

• High energy level
• Exercising done secretly after meals
• History of rigidly scheduled and compulsive exercise
• Emotional distress when exercise is not possible or is interrupted
• Extremely structured and active lifestyle

Bulimia nervosa

• All of the above, plus may report lethargy after bingeing

Sleep-rest pattern

• Sleep disturbances
• Dreams about food or eating
• Nocturnal binges after delaying food intake during the day

Cognitive-perceptual pattern

Anorexia nervosa

• Dichotomous thinking—that is, an all-or-nothing attitude toward many issues and "good-bad" perception of staff members
• Preoccupation with food, weight, and diets
• Denial of feelings of hunger, along with any other needs
• Denial of seriousness of weight loss, weight loss itself, and body-image distortion
• Blurred vision
• Difficulty concentrating
• Auditory disturbances
• Dizziness or headaches

Bulimia nervosa

• Dichotomous thinking
• Preoccupation with food, weight, or diets
• Acknowledgment of need for treatment and report distress over bingeing; less commonly, reports distress about purging behavior

Self-perception–self-concept pattern

• Guilt over worrying others or being a burden because of disorder
• Body-image distortion: for example, may report "feeling fat" despite being at normal or below-normal weight
• Feelings of inadequacy, hopelessness, rejection, and self-loathing

Role-relationship pattern

Anorexia nervosa

• Compliance, introversion, shyness; may avoid socializing with peers
• Reputation as being "a good child" who had no problems before the onset of the eating disorder

Bulimia nervosa
- Same as above; also possible temper outbursts followed by guilt

Sexuality-reproductive pattern

Anorexia nervosa
- Sexual inactivity
- Denial of masturbation
- Feelings of shame, guilt, or disgust regarding sexuality or sexual functioning
- Denial of sexual desires
- Amenorrhea
- History of sexual abuse by others

Bulimia nervosa
- Same as above, or reports episodes of sexual promiscuity that are impulsive or compulsive in nature

Coping–stress tolerance pattern

Anorexia nervosa
- Perfectionistic, obsessive, and compulsive personality
- Feeling of well-being from control of body size through food restriction and exercise
- Attempted manipulation of staff in an effort to gain control

Bulimia nervosa
- Same as above, or exhibition of a pattern of losing control through impulsive behaviors, then regaining control through purging, vigorous exercise, or (less commonly) self-mutilation

Value-belief pattern

Anorexia nervosa
- Belief that to negate needs and desires is "good" and that to "give in" to needs and desires is "bad"
- Thinness equated with happiness

Bulimia nervosa
- Same as above
- Anorexic inclination, shameful over loss of control
- Distress over symptoms and behaviors, more commonly than anorexic patients

Physical findings

General appearance

Anorexia nervosa
- 20% to 25% below normal weight for height and frame (common)
- Absence of secondary sexual characteristics

Bulimia nervosa
- Low-normal to high-normal weight range (common)
- Obesity (less common)

Cardiovascular

Anorexia nervosa
- Hypotension
- Bradycardia
- Hypothermia
- Dehydration
- Edema, possibly generalized

Bulimia nervosa
- Arrhythmias
- Finger clubbing
- Dehydration
- Rebound water retention (on cessation of purging)

Gastrointestinal

Anorexia nervosa
- Abdominal distention
- Constipation or diarrhea

Bulimia nervosa
- Vomiting
- Erosion of dental enamel
- Irritation of esophagus or chronic hoarseness
- Reddened throat
- Swollen salivary glands, especially parotids
- Steatorrhea
- Constipation or diarrhea

Neurologic

Anorexia nervosa
- Hyperactivity
- Poor motor control
- Paresthesia
- Hypersensitivity to noise and light

Bulimia nervosa
- Seizures
- Weakness and lethargy

Integumentary

Anorexia nervosa
- Pallor
- Hair loss
- Growth of lanugo
- Poor skin turgor

Bulimia nervosa
- Dry skin and hair
- Pale color

Musculoskeletal

Anorexia nervosa
- Emaciated appearance
- Loss of muscle mass, muscle weakness

Bulimia nervosa
- Tetany (rare)

Genitourinary

Anorexia nervosa
- Chronic or persistent vaginal and urinary tract infection

Diagnostic studies

Initial laboratory data may reflect no abnormalities or may reflect signs of malnutrition or starvation.
- Complete blood count (CBC) with differential — may indicate anemias or leukopenia, blood dyscrasias associated with malnutrition, or leukopenia
- Urinalysis and culture and sensitivity testing — may indicate renal dysfunction, dehydration, or infection related to malnourished state

• Chemistry panel—may indicate electrolyte imbalances, such as hypokalemia, hypocalcemia, hypernatremia, hypoglycemia, or hypercholesterolemia
• Growth hormone level—may be high
• Luteinizing hormone level—may be low because of decreased body fat
• Follicle-stimulating hormone level—may be low
• Thyroid function (triiodothyronine [T_3], thyroxine, renal uptake, and plasma T_3 levels)—may be underactive
• Fasting plasma cortisol levels—may be high
• Testosterone levels (in males)—may be low
• Dexamethasone suppression test (if indicated)—may show nonsuppression of adrenal response
• Chest X-ray—may indicate pulmonary edema or heart failure
• Electrocardiography—may indicate arrhythmias

Potential complications
• Cardiac arrest (from hypokalemia)
• Arrhythmias
• Starvation
• Amenorrhea or irregular menses (exact cause unknown)
• Dental caries or erosion (from vomiting)
• Peripheral myopathy and cardiomyopathy (with ipecac syrup use)
• Bone decalcification
• Gastric dilation and perforation (from refeeding)
• Heart failure
• Blood disorders (from malnutrition)
• Osteoporosis (from hypocalcemia)
• Insulin-dependent (type 1) diabetes (relationship to eating disorders is not clearly understood)
• Liver damage
• Renal damage

CLINICAL SNAPSHOT

ANOREXIA NERVOSA AND BULIMIA NERVOSA

Major nursing diagnoses and collaborative problems	Key patient outcomes
Nutritional deficit	Ingest food according to plan.
Powerlessness	Identify one personal non-food-related goal.
Self-esteem disturbance	Identify three positive characteristics of self.

Gastrointestinal disorders

NURSING DIAGNOSIS
Nutritional deficit related to inadequate food intake or purging behavior

Nursing priority
Establish and monitor safe and controlled refeeding.

Patient outcome criteria
Throughout the hospital stay, the patient will:
• verbalize an understanding of the diet plan and feeding alternatives
• ingest food according to plan
• show improving vital signs as refeeding progresses
• show no evidence of arrhythmias.

Interventions

1. On admission, perform a baseline nutritional assessment, noting weight in relation to height, body protein stores, skin and hair condition, and fluid and electrolyte status. See the "Nutritional deficit" and "Total parenteral nutrition" plans, pages 80 and 527, respectively, for further details.

2. With the doctor and dietitian, plan the type, amount, and route of refeeding based on the patient's nutritional needs and ability to comply with the refeeding plan. Discuss the plan in advance with the patient and consider using a written contract. Include a clear explanation of the alternatives (tube feeding or total parenteral nutrition) if the patient does not comply with the plan for oral food intake. If a nasogastric (NG) tube is used, remove it after each feeding.

3. Provide emotional support while closely monitoring intake and output of food and fluids. Avoid authoritative attitudes. Convey an attitude of warm yet firm support and consistent expectations.

4. Set and maintain specific limits regarding the amount of time allowed for meals or tube feedings, the amount of intake, and the privileges linked to compliance. Ensure that the patient and all personnel working with or around the patient are aware of these limits.

5. Provide one-to-one supervision during and for 1 to 2 hours after meals if the patient has a history of purging.

6. Weigh the patient before breakfast and after voiding, ensuring that the patient is wearing only a hospital gown. Reward meeting weight goals by increasing privileges. Weight gain increases the patient's anxiety. Increasing privileges reinforces healthy behavior.

7. Monitor vital signs at least every 8 hours.

8. Observe for signs and symptoms of hypokalemia and hypovolemia: weakness, irregular pulse, paresthesia, and hypotension. Maintain a normal fluid and electrolyte balance, including administering I.V. electrolyte replacements, as ordered by the doctor. See Appendix C, Fluid and Electrolyte Imbalances, for details.

9. When the patient refuses to eat, avoid excessive attentiveness while carrying out alternative feeding measures.

Rationales

1. Baseline assessment of nutritional status is essential to developing a refeeding plan. The "Nutritional deficit" and "Total parenteral nutrition" plans contain detailed information on nutritional assessment.

2. Refeeding must be carefully controlled in order to avoid too-rapid weight gain with subsequent psychological and physiologic trauma. Resistance to eating may be so strong that tube feeding or total parenteral nutrition (TPN) must be instituted. A written contract and clear understanding of the alternatives to oral intake provide choices and may minimize manipulative behavior. If the patient does not eat, an NG tube may be inserted for feeding of a previously specified amount of liquid nutrients. This method is controversial. If it is used, a matter-of-fact, nonpunitive attitude is essential to minimize feelings of powerlessness. The patient may try to siphon food out of the stomach if the tube is left in place.

3. Feelings of powerlessness increase as refeeding begins. A careful tally of intake and output is essential in assessing the feeding plan's adequacy. Consistency reduces manipulative behavior.

4. Limit-setting conveys caring and clear expectations, minimizing manipulative behavior. If all personnel (including housekeepers and laboratory technicians) are not made aware of the limits, the patient may be able to circumvent the diet plan.

5. The patient may refuse to eat, hide or hoard food, or purge in an attempt to control weight gain. Being with the patient during times of stress is a way to provide emotional support.

6. Weight gain provides an objective measurement of nutritional status improvement. Weighing at the same time daily ensures consistency. The patient may try to hide objects in street clothes to simulate weight gain.

7. Hypotension and bradycardia can result from malnourishment and dehydration. Vital signs should improve as refeeding is instituted.

8. Hypokalemia-induced arrhythmias may be fatal, and severe hypovolemia can provoke cardiovascular collapse. Specific signs, symptoms, and interventions associated with hypokalemia and hypovolemia are contained in the Fluid and Electrolyte Imbalances appendix.

9. Providing extra attention, even if negative, when the patient refuses food may be perceived as an indirect reward for such behavior, contributing to the self-destructive cycle.

10. Ensure that the patient is referred for psychiatric care from an eating disorders specialist.

11. Additional individualized interventions: _____
_____

10. Treating the nutritional deficit and other life-threatening manifestations is essential, but ongoing psychiatric therapy is also necessary for definitive treatment of these complex disorders.

11. Rationales: _____
_____

NURSING DIAGNOSIS

Powerlessness related to inability to identify and meet emotional, physical, sexual, and social needs and to familial and societal expectation to focus on others' needs

Nursing priorities

• Help the patient identify emotional, physical, sexual, and social needs.
• Explore ways to meet these needs.

Patient outcome criteria

• Within 1 week of admission, the patient will identify one personal, non-food-related goal.
• Several weeks to months after discharge, the patient will:
  – establish a regular pattern of socializing and sharing with others without undue anxiety
  – engage spontaneously in self-nurturing behaviors without trying to sabotage any progress made
  – respond to familial and societal expectations in ways that do not negate personal goals
  – participate in creative activity.
Because of their long-term nature, the last four criteria will not be met during one hospital stay. They are included here so that the nurse is aware of them and can recognize and reward steps toward meeting them.

Interventions

1. Be aware that the issue of control permeates all aspects of the patient's personal life.

2. Encourage the patient to participate in unit activities that foster socialization and mutual sharing.

3. Encourage self-nurturing behaviors while discouraging self-destructive behaviors. Observe for signs of depression, anxiety, or suicide potential, such as withdrawal, lack of eye contact, agitation, frequent references to death or self-destructive activities, or sudden improvement in a previously depressed patient. Ask if the patient has a plan for suicide.

Rationales

1. Fear of losing control may relate to anxiety over many issues. Controlling food intake may be the only way the patient knows how to control the self or others.

2. The patient with an eating disorder tends to be isolated because of feelings of shame or a fear of "not measuring up" to others. If these feelings are explored in a group setting as they occur, the patient will receive and learn to seek feedback from others. This learning process increases the patient's sense of power and control.

3. Once needs are identified and attempts are made to meet them, the patient may try to sabotage any progress. The patient with an eating disorder believes that personal needs are "bad" and that wanting needs to be fulfilled is also "bad." The patient may be so uncomfortable with these needs that suicide seems an acceptable option. Sudden improvement of mood in a previously depressed patient may indicate the patient has decided to commit suicide. Most patients are honest about their plans for self-harm.

Gastrointestinal disorders

4. Give the patient positive reinforcement for expressing and meeting personal needs in spite of fears of losing control.
• Encourage expression of anger, and help the patient learn assertive conflict-resolution skills, especially in family interactions.
• Help the patient identify non-food-related goals.
• Provide opportunities for creative expression.

5. Additional individualized interventions: _____
_____

4. Once needs can be identified and met without a loss of control, the patient will be able to achieve a sense of satisfaction from self-nurturing behaviors.
• The family may need guidance to react supportively to expressions of anger instead of withdrawing affection.
• Identifying goals promotes a sense of self-control.
• Creative expression may facilitate recognition of previously "unacceptable" feelings.

5. Rationales: _____
_____

NURSING DIAGNOSIS

Self-esteem disturbance related to perfectionism, sense of inadequacy, or dysfunctional family dynamics

Nursing priority

Promote a healthy self-image.

Patient outcome criteria

Within 1 week of admission, the patient will:
• identify three positive characteristics of self
• participate in unit activities
• communicate feelings spontaneously.

Interventions

1. Provide a positive role model for the patient by displaying a consistent, caring, truthful attitude and realistic self-acceptance.

2. Relate to the patient as a person with positive characteristics and interests apart from eating behaviors and food.

3. Promote activities that have a high probability of success, beginning with simple tasks and gradually increasing the amount of effort required. Making the bed, cleaning the room, and helping another patient with room-cleaning are examples of related tasks that require increasing effort. Praise and recognize successes.

4. Refer the patient to an occupational or physical therapist as appropriate. Consult with other therapists to ensure consistency in the treatment plan.

5. If family dysfunction is identified, encourage family members to consider family therapy.

6. Observe the patient's interactions with others, and provide support and positive reinforcement when the patient is able to identify emotions and express them clearly, particularly "negative" feelings such as anger. Encourage assertiveness.

Rationales

1. If the family unit is dysfunctional, the patient may have had limited opportunity for role or behavior testing. A "safe" setting such as the hospital may encourage healthful identification and experimentation.

2. Emphasizing other personal aspects helps the patient to base self-esteem on factors other than physical characteristics.

3. Success, even in simple activities, provides a sense of satisfaction and helps decrease depression and feelings of inadequacy. Helping others involves increased effort and promotes realistic self-appraisal as the patient receives positive feedback from others.

4. Diversionary activity decreases boredom and improves the patient's general feeling of well-being. Adjunctive therapies may also provide opportunities for goal achievement.

5. The patient's behavior usually reflects the family's underlying psychopathology.

6. The patient with an eating disorder may be using eating behaviors as a means of self-assertion, even though this is self-destructive. Learning that it is acceptable to express feelings directly and forcefully may decrease attachment to eating behaviors as a coping device and promote a more positive self-image.

7. Encourage the patient to explore family and societal beliefs and attitudes about food, eating, and body image.

8. Additional individualized interventions: _____
_____

7. The family and society can teach unrealistic and perfectionistic attitudes. The patient needs support to question such attitudes.

8. Rationales: _____
_____

DISCHARGE PLANNING

Discharge checklist
Before discharge, the patient shows evidence of:
- ❏ stable vital signs
- ❏ stabilizing weight
- ❏ electrolytes and CBC within normal parameters
- ❏ I.V. lines or TPN, if used, discontinued for at least 48 hours
- ❏ adequate oral intake
- ❏ ability to comply with refeeding regimen
- ❏ absence of cardiovascular or pulmonary complications
- ❏ motivation to continue psychiatric treatment on an outpatient basis
- ❏ referral for ongoing psychiatric follow-up.

Teaching checklist
Document evidence that the patient and family demonstrate an understanding of:
- ❏ physical status at time of discharge
- ❏ warning signs of hypokalemia, dehydration, or any other physical complications of fasting, bingeing, or purging
- ❏ all discharge medications' purpose, dosage, administration schedule, and adverse effects requiring medical attention
- ❏ diet plan
- ❏ community support resources
- ❏ helpful attitudes and behaviors family members can exhibit toward the patient
- ❏ attitudes and behaviors to avoid
- ❏ awareness that treatment for an eating disorder is long-term and involves the family as well as the patient
- ❏ date, time, and location of follow-up appointments
- ❏ emergency telephone numbers to use when the patient or family is in crisis.

Documentation checklist
Using outcome criteria as a guide, document:
- ❏ clinical status on admission and discharge
- ❏ significant changes in clinical status
- ❏ completion of all diagnostic studies and laboratory tests indicated by clinical status on admission, with repeat testing of all abnormal findings
- ❏ eating pattern before and at discharge
- ❏ exercise pattern

- ❏ daily weights
- ❏ any occurrence of vomiting, prohibited exercise, or unprescribed use of laxatives or diuretics
- ❏ daily mental status checks, including assessment for depression, suicide potential, and body-image distortion
- ❏ sleep patterns
- ❏ complete intake and output records, especially use of I.V., total parenteral nutrition, or tube feeding
- ❏ patient and family teaching, including medication teaching
- ❏ discharge planning.

ASSOCIATED PLANS OF CARE
Chronic renal failure
Heart failure
Ineffective family coping: Compromised
Ineffective individual coping
Nutritional deficit
Total parenteral nutrition

REFERENCES
Ammerman, S.D., et al. "Unique Considerations for Treating Eating Disorders in Adolescents and Preventive Intervention," *Topics in Clinical Nutrition* 12(1):79-85, December 1996.
Burgess, A.W. *Psychiatric Nursing, Promoting Mental Health*. Stamford, Conn.: Appleton & Lange, 1997.
Diagnostic and Statistical Manual of Mental Disorders, 4th ed. Washington D.C.: American Psychiatric Association, 1994.
Haber, J., et al. *Comprehensive Psychiatric Nursing*, 5th ed. St. Louis: Mosby–Year Book, Inc., 1997.
Lego, S., ed. *Psychiatric Nursing : A Comprehensive Reference*, 2nd ed. Philadelphia: Lippincott-Raven Pubs., 1996.

Gastrointestinal disorders

Colostomy

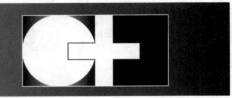

DRG information

DRG 146   Rectal Resection with Complication or Comorbidity (CC).
Mean LOS = 11.2 days

DRG 147   Rectal Resection without CC.
Mean LOS = 7.3 days

DRG 148   Major Small and Large Bowel Procedure
with CC.
Mean LOS = 13.5 days

DRG 149   Major Small and Large Bowel Procedure
without CC.
Mean LOS = 7.7 days

INTRODUCTION

Definition and time focus

A colostomy is a surgically created opening (stoma) between the abdominal wall and the colon that permits fecal diversion. A colostomy may be created because of
trauma, inflammation, or obstruction of the distal bowel or when the distal bowel is resected, as in procto-
colectomy (excision of colon and rectum) or ab-
dominoperineal resection (APR; removal of rectum).

The stoma's location in the GI tract determines stool
consistency and frequency and affects selection of a
management approach. With a descending or sigmoid
colostomy, output is soft to solid, frequency is similar to
preoperative patterns, and output may be regulated by
irrigation. With a transverse colostomy, output is
mushy, occurs after meals and unpredictably, and cannot be regulated by irrigation.

Colostomies may be designated according to location, construction, or duration.

Location
Although a colostomy may be constructed anywhere in
the large bowel, the two most common locations are the
transverse colon and the descending colon.

Construction
Common surgical construction methods include:
• end colostomy (bowel is divided; proximal bowel is
brought out as a stoma and distal bowel is either removed—as in APR of the distal colon and rectum—or
"oversewn" and left in place—as in Hartmann's procedure)
• double-barreled colostomy (bowel is divided and both
ends are brought out as stomas; the proximal stoma
drains stool and the distal stoma drains only mucus)
• loop colostomy (entire loop of bowel is brought out
through the abdominal wall and stabilized over a rod,

bridge, or catheter until granulation to the abdominal
wall occurs; the bowel's anterior wall is opened to provide fecal diversion; the posterior bowel wall remains
intact).

Duration
A colostomy is classified as permanent (no potential for
reversal) if the rectum and anus are removed or as temporary (potential for reversal) if the rectum and anus remain.

This plan focuses on preoperative assessment of
teaching needs and on the postoperative phase, the "active teaching" phase, between initial recovery or stabilization and discharge.

Etiology and precipitating factors
• Disease conditions requiring removal of the distal
bowel (for example, colorectal cancer or pelvic malig-
nancies)
• Infectious or inflammatory conditions of the distal
bowel requiring fecal diversion (for example, diverticulitis or Crohn's disease)
• Trauma to the distal bowel requiring fecal diversion
(as in a gunshot or stab wound)
• Extensive surgery of the distal bowel requiring protective fecal diversion (for example, low anterior colon resection)
• Obstruction of the distal bowel (as in obstructing tumor)

FOCUSED ASSESSMENT GUIDELINES

Nursing history (functional health pattern findings)
Because a colostomy may be performed for widely varied conditions, no typical presenting picture exists;
therefore, the nursing history and physical findings sections are omitted in this plan. The following are guidelines for preoperative assessment.

Health perception–health management pattern
• Determine the diagnosis or reason for colostomy. Determine the planned procedure, prognosis, and the patient's potential for independence as a basis for discharge planning and teaching.
• Explore the patient's perceptions concerning colostomy and its impact on health status and lifestyle. (Note:
Previous contact with a person with an ostomy will affect the patient's expectations and adaptation.)

• Identify any allergies, particularly to topical agents such as tape; the patient with such allergies may react to colostomy products.

Nutritional-metabolic pattern

• Assess diet and fluid intake when planning patient teaching. Assess the home diet for adequate fiber and fluid intake and for consumption of gas-producing foods.

• Assess nutritional status (skin turgor, mucous membranes, hair condition, height and weight, and recent weight loss). Be alert to signs of nutritional deficiency that may predispose the patient to postoperative complications, such as wound infection or delayed healing.

Elimination pattern

• Determine usual bowel patterns. Assess the preoperative frequency and character of bowel movements as a basis for colostomy management and patient teaching (particularly important in selecting a management approach for a descending or sigmoid colostomy).

Activity-exercise pattern

• Assess independence and any limitations in activities of daily living (ADLs). The amount of independence is significant in planning for colostomy management and patient-family teaching. The patient's manual dexterity and coordination are particularly significant in selecting appropriate equipment, such as a pouch system or clip.

Cognitive-perceptual pattern

• When planning teaching, assess the patient's understanding of the diagnosis, prognosis, surgical procedure, and management of colostomy.

• Assess for any sensory deficits, such as in visual and auditory acuity, when planning self-care instruction; most patients requiring colostomy are over age 60, so sensory loss is common.

Self-perception–self-concept pattern

• Self-concept and self-esteem correlate with adaptation potential; be alert to consistent self-derogatory statements or inappropriate affect, which may indicate low self-esteem.

• Emotional response is variable. It is common for a patient to have negative feelings regarding colostomy.

• Openness in expressing feelings is affected by the patient's personality and the nurse's communication skills.

Role-relationship pattern

• Assess areas of concern about roles and relationships. Patients commonly express concern about a colostomy's effect on relationships, with major concern relating to spouse or partner reaction.

• Young and middle-aged adults commonly express concern about their ability to resume preoperative roles and responsibilities.

• Older adults commonly express concern about their ability to maintain independence and to manage the cost of ostomy supplies.

• Assess family dynamics, particularly dependence-independence issues. Older patients may desire their spouse's or a family member's involvement in care, while younger adults may value independence and privacy.

Sexuality-reproductive pattern

• Assess the patient's and partner's openness with each other and in discussing sexuality, preoperative sexual patterns, and other major concerns.

• A common concern is how the colostomy affects intimate relationships — that is, sexual attractiveness and function.

Coping–stress tolerance pattern

• The patient's and family's responses to colostomy are highly variable and reflect coping patterns.

• Assess the patient's feelings about support groups, to determine the appropriateness of referral to the United Ostomy Association.

Value-belief pattern

• Response to colostomy is affected by cultural beliefs and familial response to illness, surgery, and elimination.

Diagnostic studies

Studies vary according to the patient's condition and the underlying disorder; they may include:

• complete blood count — may reveal low hemoglobin level or hematocrit that indicate continuing or unreplaced blood loss; may also reveal elevated white blood cell count indicating infection, usually intra-abdominal

• electrolyte panel — detects or rules out electrolyte abnormalities that affect fluid balance (for example, hyponatremia or hypernatremia) and GI tract function (for example, hypokalemia or hyperkalemia)

• chemistry panel — detects electrolyte imbalances and nutritional deficits that affect wound healing (for example, hypoproteinemia) and monitors liver and kidney function, which may be affected by underlying disease, such as metastatic disease, or by treatment, such as antibiotic therapy

• serum drug levels — peak and trough levels may detect toxic or subtherapeutic levels of prescribed antibiotics or other drugs

• carcinoembryonic antigen (CEA) levels — may be done before and after surgery for comparison; if elevated before surgery, effective surgical resection should result in decreased CEA level

• flat plate or upright abdominal X-ray — may be done before surgery to rule out colon perforation (in a trauma patient) or colon obstruction (in a patient with suspected malignancy); done after surgery as needed to differentiate postoperative ileus (visualized as air-filled loops of bowel) from mechanical obstruction (visualized as air-fluid levels and dilated proximal bowel)

• transrectal ultrasound — may be done before surgery to determine lymph node involvement, tumor depth, and adherence to adjacent structures

• computed tomography scan of abdomen — may be used before or after surgery to rule out intra-abdominal abscess or to detect metastatic lesions

Gastrointestinal disorders

• stool guaiac (Hemoccult) test — preliminary study to rule out GI bleeding; positive study requires further workup to rule out malignancy, hemorrhoidal bleeding, inflammatory bowel disease, or upper tract bleeding; negative study inconclusive because of high incidence of false-negative results

• barium enema with air and contrast — rules out diverticular disease and detects filling defects that indicate colon lesions (such as polyps and tumors)
• sigmoidoscopy or colonoscopy — rules out colon lesions and allows removal of polyps or biopsy of suspicious lesions

---

CLINICAL SNAPSHOT

COLOSTOMY

Major nursing diagnoses and collaborative problems	Key patient outcomes
Risk for stomal necrosis	Display a pink and viable stoma.
Risk for stomal retraction	Display a stoma granulated to the abdominal wall.
Risk for impaired skin integrity: Peristomal breakdown	Display peristomal skin free from breakdown.
Knowledge deficit (care of descending or sigmoid colostomy)	Select a preferred bowel management approach.
Risk for body-image disturbance	Discuss feeling about stoma.
Risk for sexual dysfunction	Describe any alteration in sexual function (if applicable).

COLLABORATIVE PROBLEM

Risk for stomal necrosis related to the surgical procedure, bowel wall edema, or traction on the mesentery

Nursing priorities
• Optimize blood flow to the bowel wall.
• Prevent complications related to circulatory impairment.

Patient outcome criterion
Within the first 4 days after surgery, the patient will display a pink and viable stoma.

Interventions

1. Assess and document stoma color every 8 hours during the first 4 days after surgery (or until the stoma remains pink for 3 days).

2. If the stoma is ischemic or necrotic, check the viability of the proximal bowel by inserting a test tube into the stoma and using a flashlight to assess the mucosa for ischemia. Document your findings.

3. Document and notify the doctor promptly if necrosis extends to the end of the test tube (see above).

Rationales

1. Healthy bowel tissue is pink; a dusky blue color indicates ischemia; a brown or black color indicates necrosis. Ischemia may or may not progress to necrosis.

2. A distal stoma is most likely to necrose because it is farthest from the mesenteric blood supply. Stomal necrosis does not necessarily represent a surgical emergency (the stoma may be allowed to "slough" as long as the proximal bowel is viable).

3. Necrosis extending to the fascia represents a surgical emergency because of the threat of perforation and peritonitis.

4. Implement measures to prevent or minimize abdominal distention:
• Examine the abdomen for distention every 8 hours during the first 4 days after surgery.
• If distention is present, monitor its degree by measuring abdominal girth at the umbilicus.
• If distention is present, notify the doctor and request an order to insert a nasogastric (NG) tube.
• If an NG tube is present, irrigate as needed to maintain patency.

5. Additional individualized interventions: _____

_____

4. Severe abdominal distention may cause mesenteric stretching, which places blood vessels under tension; this stress may decrease blood flow to the distal bowel and stoma. Using the umbilicus as the reference point for measuring abdominal girth promotes consistency and accuracy of measurements.

5. Rationales: _____

_____

COLLABORATIVE PROBLEM

Risk for stomal retraction related to mucocutaneous separation

Nursing priorities
• Optimize wound healing and granulation of the stoma to the abdominal wall.
• Prevent stomal retraction.

Patient outcome criteria

By the time of discharge, the patient will:
• display a stoma granulated to the abdominal wall
• exhibit a healed mucocutaneous suture line
• show no stomal retraction.

Interventions

1. Assess and document the integrity of the mucocutaneous suture line at each pouch change.

2. Initiate and document nutritional support measures for the patient at risk for nutritional deficiency, based on the recommendations of a nutritional resource nurse or dietitian.

3. Request vitamin A supplements for the patient receiving steroids.

4. For the patient with a loop colostomy stabilized by a rod or bridge, expect that the loop support will not be removed until the stoma granulates to the abdominal wall.

5. If mucocutaneous separation occurs, alter the pouch system to prevent fecal contamination of exposed subcutaneous tissue. Fill the separated area with absorptive powder or granules; cover with tape strips, then pectin-based paste. Apply a pouch sized to fit closely around the stoma.

6. Additional individualized interventions: _____

_____

Rationales

1. Breakdown of the stoma or skin suture line is a major contributing factor to stomal retraction.

2. Nutritional deficiency causes negative nitrogen balance. Because wound repair depends on adequate protein stores, the suture line may break down.

3. Vitamin A partially compensates for corticosteroids' negative effects on wound healing; by supporting macrophage activity and wound repair, vitamin A helps prevent suture line breakdown.

4. Loop support removal before abdominal wall attachment may cause stomal retraction.

5. An optimal environment for healing includes protection from secondary infection, absorption of exudate, and maintenance of a clean, moist surface. The absorptive agent and tape strips prevent fecal contamination and absorb exudate. Using paste and a pouch sized for the stoma provides a secure seal.

6. Rationales: _____

_____

Gastrointestinal disorders

NURSING DIAGNOSIS

Risk for impaired skin integrity: Peristomal breakdown related to fecal contamination of skin

Nursing priorities
• Maintain an intact pouch seal.
• Prevent peristomal skin breakdown.

Patient outcome criteria
• Throughout the postoperative phase, the patient will display peristomal skin free from breakdown.
• By the time of discharge, the patient will have had an intact pouch for 2 days.

Interventions

1. Have an enterostomal therapy nurse mark the optimal stoma site before surgery, if possible.

2. Assess the patient's abdominal contours and select a pouch system that matches those contours: for example, try an all-flexible system for a stoma in a crease or fold.

3. Use the following principles in preparing and applying the pouch:
• Use a drainable pouch.

• Remove peristomal hair with safety razor and shaving cream. Rinse and dry skin.
• Use a skin sealant (such as Skin Prep) under the tape.

• Use a pouch with a barrier ring sized to fit closely around the stoma; apply a thin layer of barrier paste (such as Stomahesive) around the stoma to fill in gaps and prevent leakage.
• If an adhesive-only pouch is used, size it to clear the stoma by ⅛″ (3 mm); use a pouch with a barrier ring and paste.

4. Change the pouch routinely every 5 to 7 days and as needed if leakage or complaints of peristomal burning or itching occur.

5. Inspect the skin at each pouch change, and treat any denudation by dusting the area with absorptive powder (such as Stomahesive). Seal the area by blotting it with water or sealant (such as Skin Prep).

6. Additional individualized interventions: _____

Rationales

1. For best results, the stoma should be located in an area free from creases or folds, within the patient's view, and within the rectus muscle. Site selection is best done before surgery, when the patient can be evaluated lying down, sitting, and standing.

2. Accurately matching the pouch system to abdominal contours optimizes the pouch-to-skin seal and minimizes leakage.

3. Good technique provides maximum security and skin protection.
• A drainable pouch can be emptied as needed without being removed.
• Hair removal prevents folliculitis.

• The copolymer film prevents epidermal stripping with pouch removal.
• This procedure prevents fecal material from contacting skin and causing breakdown.

• Inflexible pouch edges placed too close to the stoma can damage it during peristalsis. Exposed skin must be protected.

4. Routine changes before leaks can occur protect skin and provide the patient with a sense of control. Burning or itching may indicate fecal contamination of skin.

5. Powder provides an absorptive protective layer over the area of breakdown; sealing provides a surface for pouch adherence.

6. Rationales: _____

NURSING DIAGNOSIS

Knowledge deficit (care of descending or sigmoid colostomy) related to unfamiliarity with altered bowel

Nursing priority

Help the patient select options most appropriate for personal physical status and lifestyle.

Patient outcome criterion

By 2 days before discharge, the patient will describe options considered and select a preferred approach.

Interventions

1. Assess the patient's candidacy for bowel function regulation by irrigation. Consider the following factors:
• Is the colostomy permanent?

• Do stomal complications, such as hernia or prolapse, exist?

• Is the patient mentally and physically able to learn and perform the procedure?
• What were the preoperative bowel patterns?

• Is the patient to receive radiation?

• Does the patient have adequate home facilities?

2. If the patient meets feasibility criteria, discuss management options:
• wearing a pouch continuously, emptying as needed, and changing every 5 to 7 days
• daily or every-other-day irrigations to stimulate bowel movements, wearing a security pouch between irrigations.

3. Help the patient explore the options based on personal priorities, such as tolerance of the pouch versus the time required for regular irrigations.

4. Establish a teaching plan based on the patient's decision. Base teaching strategies on the patient's learning style and sensory strengths; for example, if a patient with diminished visual acuity learns best by doing, self-care instruction should involve much practice (with a magnifying mirror) but minimal reading.

5. Additional individualized interventions: _____

Rationales

1. Irrigation is usually contraindicated if:

• the colostomy is temporary (because of the time factor and potential for bowel dependence)
• the patient has a peristomal hernia (potential for perforation) or prolapse (potential for worsening of prolapse)
• the patient has coordination problems or learning difficulties
• the patient has a preoperative history of diarrhea (less likely to achieve control than the patient with a preoperative history of regular stools or constipation)
• the patient is to receive radiation therapy (because diarrhea is a usual adverse effect)
• the patient has no running water or indoor plumbing in the home.

2. Colostomy irrigations are not necessary because peristalsis and bowel movements continue; however, regular irrigations induce evacuation and promote colonic "dependence" on their stimulating effects, providing increased control over bowel function. Thus, regulation by irrigation is a management option.

3. Exploring the pros and cons of various options and discussing the patient's concerns and priorities facilitates decision making and increases the patient's sense of self-control.

4. The patient must be able to perform colostomy care before discharge.

5. Rationales: _____

NURSING DIAGNOSIS

Risk for body-image disturbance related to loss of control over fecal elimination

Nursing priorities

• Prevent or minimize alteration in body image.
• Enhance the patient's sense of control over bowel functions.

Patient outcome criteria

- By 2 days before discharge, the patient will:
  - observe and perform stoma care
  - discuss feelings about the stoma.
- By the time of discharge, the patient will:
  - describe the colostomy as manageable
  - describe plans for resuming preoperative lifestyle.

Interventions

1. Teach the patient measures for odor control, such as performing regular pouch care; using an odor-proof pouch; using pouch deodorant, if desired; using a room deodorant when the pouch is emptied; altering diet to reduce fecal odor, if desired; and using over-the-counter internal deodorants, if desired, such as bismuth subgallate.

2. Teach the patient measures to reduce and control flatus, such as identifying gas-forming foods; understanding the "lag time" between ingestion and flatulence; muffling sounds of flatus; and using pouch filters that deodorize flatus.

3. Teach the patient how to conceal the pouch under clothing; wearing a knit or stretchy layer next to the skin holds the pouch close to the body and helps conceal large or bulky stomas.

4. Discuss the normal emotional response to colostomy with the patient and family. Allow the patient and family to explore their feelings about the colostomy. Assess the patient's usual coping strategies. Present helpful coping strategies, such as discussing feelings and seeking information.

5. Offer information on the United Ostomy Association; arrange for an ostomy visitor if the patient wishes.

6. Discuss colostomy management during occupational, social, and sexual activity. Help the patient to role-play difficult situations, such as telling someone about the stoma.

7. Additional individualized interventions: _____

_____

Rationales

1. Odor control is a major concern of most patients; instruction in odor-control methods increases feelings of control and confidence and reduces feelings of embarrassment and shame. Onions, garlic, beans, and cabbage generally increase odor; orange juice, buttermilk, and yogurt may decrease odor. Bismuth reduces flatus and odor and thickens stool; it is contraindicated in the patient with renal failure or on anticoagulant therapy.

2. Inability to control flatus may lead to social embarrassment and self-deprecation. The patient can time the intake of any gas-forming foods so that flatulence occurs during "safe" periods. Filters keep the pouch flat by allowing flatus to escape and prevent odor by first deodorizing flatus.

3. The ability to dress normally and look the same as before surgery diminishes alterations in body image and enhances self-concept.

4. Discussing the normal emotional response and accepting negative feelings gives the patient and family permission to explore their feelings. Accepting feelings enhances self-concept and promotes adaptation. Discussing various coping strategies may provide the patient with new or more effective ways to handle emotions.

5. Contact with others who have ostomies reduces isolation and increases perception of the colostomy as manageable, thus enhancing the patient's sense of control.

6. Preparing for such activities increases coping skills and the likelihood that the patient will manage them successfully. Role playing helps the patient prepare for difficult situations, which increases the sense of control and enhances self-concept.

7. Rationales: _____

_____

NURSING DIAGNOSIS

Risk for sexual dysfunction related to change in body image or damage to autonomic nerves (applies to the patient with rectal resection, particularly wide resection for cancer treatment)

Nursing priorities
• Facilitate the resumption and maintenance of intimate relationships.
• Minimize alteration in sexual function.

Patient outcome criteria
By the time of discharge, the patient will:
• share feelings about stoma with spouse or partner
• describe any alteration in sexual function (if applicable)
• describe measures for pouch management during sexual activity (if applicable).

Interventions

1. Discuss with the patient (and spouse or partner, if possible) the importance of openness and honesty as well as the fact that both must adapt to the ostomy.

2. Teach the patient measures for securing and concealing the pouch during sexual activity, such as using a small pouch or wearing a pouch cover, a "tube top" or cummerbund around the midriff, or crotchless panties.

3. For a female with a wide rectal resection, discuss the possible need for artificial lubrication.

4. For a male with a wide rectal resection, explain potential interference with erection and ejaculation; explain that no loss of sensation or orgasmic potential will occur; explore alternatives to intercourse as indicated; explain the availability of penile injections, urethral inserts, penile prostheses, and vacuum devices to restore erectile function. Reinforce the importance of intimacy, whether or not it involves intercourse.

5. Additional individualized interventions: _____

Rationales

1. Both the patient and spouse (or partner) may have concerns and negative feelings that can affect their sexual relationship. Openness in discussing feelings may help resolve these.

2. The stoma and pouch affect overall body image and feelings of sexual attractiveness. Securing and concealing the pouch help prevent leakage and allow the patient to focus on sexuality and sharing rather than on the pouch and stoma.

3. Wide rectal resection may damage parasympathetic nerves thought to mediate vaginal lubrication.

4. Wide rectal resection may damage parasympathetic nerves controlling erection and sympathetic nerves controlling ejaculation. Sensation and orgasm, mediated by the pudendal nerve, remain intact. Intimacy—emotional closeness—is a human need separate from the desire for sexual expression. It can be met in ways other than sexual behavior, such as sharing feelings and affectionate touching. A number of medical and surgical interventions are now available that restore erectile function.

5. Rationales: _____

DISCHARGE PLANNING

Discharge checklist
Before discharge, the patient shows evidence of:
❏ absence of fever
❏ stable vital signs
❏ absence of pulmonary or cardiovascular complications
❏ healing wound with no signs of redness, swelling, or drainage
❏ ability to change and empty pouch using proper technique
❏ ability to tolerate diet
❏ absence of skin problems around stoma
❏ absence of bladder dysfunction
❏ absence of abdominal distention
❏ restored bowel function
❏ ability to perform ADLs and ambulate same as before surgery
❏ ability to control pain with oral medications
❏ adequate home support system or referral to home care if indicated by inadequate home support system or inability to manage colostomy care at home.

Teaching checklist
Document evidence that the patient and family demonstrate an understanding of:
❏ reason for colostomy
❏ colostomy's impact on bowel function

Gastrointestinal disorders

❏ normal stoma characteristics and function
❏ pouch-emptying procedure
❏ pouch-changing procedure
❏ peristomal skin care
❏ colostomy irrigation procedure (if applicable)
❏ management of mucous fistula stoma (if applicable)
❏ flatus and odor control
❏ management of diarrhea and constipation
❏ normal adaptation process and feelings after colostomy
❏ community resources available for support
❏ recommendations affecting resumption of preoperative lifestyle
❏ potential alteration in sexual function (if applicable)
❏ sources of colostomy supplies and reimbursement procedures for them
❏ signs and symptoms to report to the doctor
❏ need for follow-up appointment with the doctor (and enterostomal therapy nurse, if available)
❏ how to contact the doctor.

Documentation checklist
Using outcome criteria as a guide, document:
❏ clinical status on admission
❏ significant changes in clinical status
❏ GI tract function (bowel sounds, NG tube output, and colostomy output)
❏ stoma color and status of mucocutaneous suture line
❏ oral intake and tolerance
❏ episodes of abdominal distention, nausea, and vomiting
❏ incision status (any signs of infection)
❏ stoma location and abdominal contours
❏ management plan, including pouch system selected (and decision about irrigation for the patient with a descending or sigmoid colostomy)
❏ peristomal skin status
❏ emotional response to colostomy and discussion of coping strategies
❏ patient and family teaching
❏ discharge planning.

Associated plans of care
Grieving
Ineffective family coping: Compromised
Ineffective individual coping
Knowledge deficit
Pain
Surgery

References
Arnell, T., and Stamos, M. "Alternatives in Therapy for Low Rectal Cancer," *Journal of Wound, Ostomy, Continence Nursing* 23(3):150-55, May 1996.

Golis, A. "Sexual Issues for the Person with an Ostomy," *Journal of Wound Ostomy, Continence Nursing* 23(1):33-37, January 1996.

Hampton, B., and Bryant, R., eds. *Ostomies and Continent Diversions: Nursing Management*. St. Louis: Mosby–Year Book, Inc., 1992.

O'Keefe, M., and Hunt, D. "Assessment and Treatment of Impotence," *Medical Clinics of North America* 79(2):415-30, March 1995.

Pieper, B., and Mikols, C. "Predischarge and Postdischarge Concerns of Persons with an Ostomy," *Journal of Wound, Ostomy, Continence Nursing* 23(2):105-09, March 1996.

Duodenal ulcer

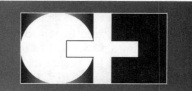

DRG information

DRG 174   GI Hemorrhage with Complication or Comorbidity (CC).
Mean LOS = 5.6 days
Principal diagnoses include:
• acute or chronic duodenal ulcer with
hemorrhage
• acute or chronic duodenal ulcer with or
without obstruction.

DRG 175   GI Hemorrhage without CC.
Mean LOS = 3.5 days

INTRODUCTION

Definition and time focus

Duodenal ulcer results from an inflammatory and ulcerative process that affects the first portion of the duodenum within 1⅛″ (3 cm) of the gastroduodenal junction. This plan focuses on the duodenal ulcer patient admitted with signs and symptoms that have not been controlled through outpatient management. Long-term maintenance medication therapy is generally recommended instead of surgical treatment; therefore, the plan focuses on medical treatment.

Etiology and precipitating factors

Gastric acid secretion is necessary for duodenal ulcers to develop. Pathophysiologic abnormalities that influence gastric acid secretion are:
• increased parietal cell and chief cell mass (related to gastrinomal gastrin-secreting tumor or familial or genetic factors)
• increased basal secretory or postprandial secretory drive (related to gastrinoma or antral G cell hyperfunction)
• rapid gastric emptying (related to familial or genetic factors)
• *Helicobacter pylori* infection (present in 90% of all duodenal peptic ulcers and 70% of all gastric ulcers)
• impaired mucosal defense (related to ingestion of aspirin, corticosteroids, or phenylbutazone and to other factors, such as stress or infectious agents).

FOCUSED ASSESSMENT GUIDELINES

Nursing history (functional health pattern findings)

Health perception–health management pattern
• Steady, gnawing, burning, aching, or hungerlike discomfort high in the right epigastrium; pain occurs 2 to 4 hours after meals, usually does not radiate, and is relieved by food or antacids
• Increased risk if male, ages 40 to 60, with type O blood, a cigarette smoker, or with chronic emotional stress
• Ingestion of certain drugs that contribute to duodenal ulceration, such as aspirin-containing compounds, corticosteroids, phenylbutazone, or indomethacin (Indocin)
• Family history of ulcers

Nutritional-metabolic pattern
• History of excessive alcohol consumption
• Nausea (vomiting not common)
• Appetite usually good

Elimination pattern
• Feeling of fullness, gaseous indigestion, or constipation

Activity-exercise pattern
• Fatigue
• Exacerbation of pain following unusual physical exertion
• Orthostatic hypotension if actively bleeding

Sleep-rest pattern
• Sleep disturbances from pain, commonly occurring between 12 and 3 a.m.

Coping–stress tolerance pattern
• Stressful life events—such as occupational, educational, or financial problems or family illness—preceding development or exacerbation of signs and symptoms
• Denial of signs and symptoms during pain-free periods (symptoms commonly disappear for weeks or months and then recur)

Physical findings

Gastrointestinal
• Localized tenderness in epigastrium over ulcer site

Diagnostic studies
• Routine laboratory studies—add little to the workup
• More sophisticated GI studies, such as serum pepsinogen I or fasting gastrin levels—may be ordered

based on the suspected cause of the duodenal ulcer; a high serum pepsinogen I level and a high fasting gastrin level provide evidence for gastrinoma or antral G cell hyperfunction
• Endoscopy — reveals the ulcer's location and allows for biopsy and cytology
• Abdominal films — reveals free air due to perforation
• Screening test for *H. pylori* — likely to be positive
• Single - or double-contrast radiography — may be ordered along with endoscopy to locate ulcer

• Hemoglobin level and hematocrit if bleeding is occurring

Potential complications
• Duodenal obstruction
 – Gastric atony
 – Mechanical obstruction
• Perforation

CLINICAL SNAPSHOT

DUODENAL ULCER

Major nursing diagnoses and collaborative problems	Key patient outcomes
Risk for GI hemorrhage	Show stable vital signs: typically, heart rate, 60 to 100 beats/minute; systolic blood pressure, 90 to 140 mm Hg; and diastolic blood pressure, 50 to 90 mm Hg.
Pain	Rate pain as less than 3 on a pain rating scale of 0 to 10.

COLLABORATIVE PROBLEM
Risk for GI hemorrhage related to extension of duodenal ulcer into the submucosal layer of the intestinal lining

Nursing priority
Observe for, prevent, or promptly treat hemorrhage.

Patient outcome criteria
Within 24 hours of admission, the patient will:
• show evidence that any bleeding has ceased, such as normal nasogastric (NG) drainage and normal guaiac testing
• show stable vital signs: typically, heart rate, 60 to 100 beats/minute; systolic blood pressure, 90 to 140 mm Hg; and diastolic blood pressure, 50 to 90 mm Hg.

Interventions
1. Observe for and report signs of GI hemorrhage. Describe any hematemesis, melena, or other signs of intestinal bleeding, including amount, consistency, and color. Test all stools and vomitus with a guaiac reagent strip (Hemoccult). See the "Gastrointestinal hemorrhage" plan on page 505.

2. Institute NG intubation, if ordered. Keep the tube patent by instilling 30 ml of saline solution every 2 to 4 hours, then removing the same amount by mechanical suction.

Rationales
1. Hematemesis of frank red blood indicates active bleeding, while coffee-ground vomitus indicates old bleeding. Guaiac testing unmasks occult bleeding. The "Gastrointestinal hemorrhage" care plan covers this disorder in detail.

2. NG intubation reveals the presence or absence of blood in the stomach, helps assess the rate of bleeding, and provides a route for saline lavage. If the tube is not patent, the patient may vomit stomach contents.

3. Institute continuous saline lavage, if ordered. Instill aliquots of room-temperature fluid (500 to 1,000 ml); then remove the same amount by gentle suction and gravity drainage.

4. If the patient is bleeding actively, check vital signs hourly (more frequently if unstable). Alert the doctor immediately to any deterioration, as indicated by decreasing alertness, dropping systolic blood pressure, tachycardia, narrowing pulse pressure, or restlessness or agitation, or decreasing hemoglobin level.

5. Treat hypovolemia, if present. Keep the patient warm, administer I.V. fluids and blood transfusions, as ordered, and provide oxygen at 2 to 6 L/minute via nasal cannula.

6. Prepare the patient for surgery, if indicated.

7. Maintain the patient on bed rest after the bleeding episode. Begin the prescribed medication regimen, as ordered.

8. Additional individualized interventions: _____

3. Continuous lavage indicates the rapidity of bleeding and cleans the stomach should endoscopy be necessary. Iced saline may impair coagulation. Experimental evidence suggests that room-temperature water lavage may be as effective as iced saline lavage.

4. Loss of blood volume leads rapidly to hypovolemic shock. Untreated, shock may progress to irreversible tissue ischemia; death follows quickly. Early detection of active bleeding and aggressive fluid replacement are essential to prevent shock.

5. Restoring intravascular volume and supplementing oxygen transport reduce the effects of blood loss on tissues until bleeding can be controlled.

6. Surgery may be indicated if bleeding continues longer than 48 hours, recurs, or is associated with perforation or obstruction. The preferred surgery is parietal cell vagotomy.

7. Rest aids hemostasis and decreases GI tract activity. A medication regimen (as in the following nursing diagnosis) is the usual therapy before surgery is considered.

8. Rationales: _____

Nursing diagnosis

Pain related to increased hydrochloric acid secretion or increased spasm, intragastric pressure, and motility of upper GI tract

Nursing priorities
• Promote stomach and intestinal healing.
• Teach about risk factors and measures to prevent recurrence.

Patient outcome criteria
Within 2 days of admission, the patient will:
• rate pain as less than 3 on a 0 to 10 pain rating scale
• identify dietary intolerances
• observe dietary recommendations in menu selection
• identify personal stressors, on request
• demonstrate interest in stress-reduction measures
• list signs and symptoms of ulcer recurrence and bleeding
• state understanding of prescribed medications.

Gastrointestinal disorders

Interventions

1. Administer ulcer-healing medications and document their use, as ordered. Medications may include one or a combination of the following:
• histamine (H_2)-receptor antagonists (cimetidine [Tagamet], ranitidine [Zantac], famotidine [Pepcid], and nizatidine [Axid]), usually given with meals and at bedtime
• antacids, given after meals and at bedtime unless otherwise ordered
• anticholinergics
• sucralfate (Carafate)
• anti-infectives.

2. Provide bed rest and a quiet environment, minimizing visitors and telephone calls.

3. Teach and reinforce the role of diet in ulcer healing. Help the patient identify specific foods that may increase discomfort.

4. Encourage adequate caloric intake from the basic food groups at regular intervals. Encourage frequent small meals.

5. Teach and reinforce required lifestyle changes to reduce physical and emotional stress. Help the patient identify specific personal stressors and recognize the relationship between increased stress and ulcer pain. As appropriate, present information on relaxation techniques, exercise, priority setting, time management and personal organization, building and nurturing relationships, the importance of "play" time, and assertiveness techniques.

6. Encourage the patient who smokes to quit.

7. Teach the patient signs and symptoms indicating ulcer recurrence and bleeding, including pain, hematemesis, dark or tarry stools, pallor, increasing weakness, dizziness, or faintness.

8. Additional individualized interventions: _____

Rationales

1. Increased hydrochloric acid secretion results in edema and inflammation of gastric mucosa. H_2-receptor antagonists inhibit gastrin release, antacids buffer hydrochloric acid, anticholinergics decrease hydrochloric acid secretion, and sucralfate binds to proteins at the base of the ulcer to form a protective barrier against acid and pepsin. An effective treatment for *H. pylori* in duodenal peptic ulcer disease is a 14-day regimen of bismuth subsalicylate, metronidazole tetracycline hydrochloride, and omeprazole. It is important for the patient to complete the entire therapy to eradicate the *H. pylori* infection. Eradication of *H. pylori* normally results in healing of a duodenal peptic ulcer and resolution of gastritis.

2. Ulcer symptoms are usually reduced by rest and a quiet environment.

3. Dietary restrictions other than avoidance of excessive alcohol and caffeine are not currently recommended. Promotion of specific diets is highly controversial; none has been scientifically proven to promote healing. Identifying personal food intolerances aids diet planning.

4. Food itself acts as an antacid, neutralizing stomach acid 30 to 60 minutes after ingestion.

5. Stressful life situations, such as occupational, financial, or family problems, are reported more commonly in patients with duodenal ulcers that require longer than 6 weeks to heal. Identifying cause-and-effect relationships helps the patient make necessary lifestyle changes.

6. Research indicates that patients who smoke have impaired ulcer healing and a higher mortality rate when compared to nonsmokers.

7. Early identification of ulcer recurrence and bleeding may permit intervention before bleeding becomes severe.

8. Rationales: _____

DISCHARGE PLANNING

Discharge checklist
Before discharge, the patient shows evidence of:
❏ stable vital signs
❏ absence of signs and symptoms of GI hemorrhage
❏ hemoglobin level within expected parameters
❏ absence of pain
❏ ability to tolerate nutritional intake as ordered
❏ ability to verbalize diet and medication instructions
❏ ability to perform activities of daily living and ambulate as before hospitalization
❏ adequate home support system or referral to home care if indicated by inadequate home support system or inability to perform self-care.

Teaching checklist
Document evidence that the patient and family demonstrate an understanding of:
❏ nature and implications of disease
❏ pain-relief measures
❏ all discharge medications' purpose, dosage, administration schedule, and adverse effects requiring medical attention (usual discharge medications include antacids or H_2-receptor antagonists, or both)
❏ recommended dietary modifications
❏ need for smoking-cessation program (if applicable)
❏ stress reduction measures
❏ signs and symptoms of ulcer recurrence and GI bleeding
❏ date, time, and location of follow-up appointment
❏ how to contact the doctor.

Documentation checklist
Using outcome criteria as a guide, document:
❏ clinical status on admission
❏ significant changes in status
❏ pain-relief measures
❏ nutritional intake and intolerances
❏ pertinent diagnostic test findings
❏ medication administration
❏ patient and family teaching
❏ discharge planning.

ASSOCIATED PLANS OF CARE

Esophagitis and gastroenteritis
Gastrointestinal hemorrhage
Ineffective individual coping
Knowledge deficit
Pain

REFERENCES

al-Assi, M.T., et al. "Ulcer Site and Complications: Relation to Helicobacter pylori Infection and Nonsteroidal Anti-inflammatory Drug Use," Endoscopy, 28(2):229-33, February 1996.

Guthann, S.P., et al. "Individual Nonsteroidal Anti-inflammatory Drugs and Other Risk Factors for Upper Gastrointestinal Bleeding and Perforation," Epidemiology 8(1):18-24, January 1997.
Heslin, J. "Peptic Ulcer Disease: Making a Case Against the Prime Suspect," Nursing97 27(1):34-39, January 1997.
Jaspersen, D., et al. "Helicobacter pylori Eradication Reduces the Rate of Rebleeding in Ulcer Hemorrhage," Gastrointestinal Endoscopy 41(1):5-7, January 1995.
Jutabha, R., and Jensen, D.M. "Management of Upper Gastrointestinal Bleeding in the Patient with Chronic Liver Disease," Medical Clinics of North America 80(5):1035-68, September 1996.
Roth, S.H. "Nonsteroidal Anti-inflammatory Drug Gastropathy. A New Understanding," Archives of Internal Medicine 156(15):1623-28, August 1996.
Wilcox, C.M., et al. "A Prospective Characterization of Upper Gastrointestinal Hemorrhage Presenting with Hematochezia," American Journal of Gastroenterology 92(2):2331-35, February 1997.

Gastrointestinal disorders

Esophagitis and gastroenteritis

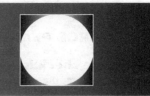

DRG information

DRG 182   Esophagitis, Gastroenteritis, and Miscellaneous Digestive Disorders; Age 17+ with Complication or Comorbidity (CC).
Mean LOS = 5.0 days

DRG 183   Esophagitis, Gastroenteritis, and Miscellaneous Digestive Disorders; Ages 0 to 17 without CC.
Mean LOS = 3.4 days

DRG 184   Esophagitis, Gastroenteritis, and Miscellaneous Digestive Disorders; Ages 0 to 17.
Mean LOS = 2.8 days

INTRODUCTION

Definition and time focus

Esophagitis and gastroenteritis are nonspecific inflammatory conditions of the mucosa of the esophagus and the stomach and small bowel, respectively. Esophagitis is usually related to inadequate cardiac sphincter tone, resulting in gastric reflux and subsequent irritation. Gastroenteritis is most commonly caused by bacteria or viruses that produce severe vomiting, diarrhea, and abdominal cramping. Both conditions may cause temporary discomfort (which can be treated on an outpatient basis) or serious, even life-threatening, illness if the patient is elderly, debilitated, or otherwise at increased risk. This plan focuses on the patient admitted for diagnosis and treatment of acute esophagitis or gastroenteritis.

Etiology and precipitating factors

• Infectious agents — fungal (candidiasis), viral (herpes simplex), and bacterial (staphylococcus, *Helicobacter pylori*)
• Drugs and chemical agents — gastric acid reflux; bile reflux; ingestion of caustic substances (such as lye); medications such as aspirin, steroids, indomethacin (Indocin), or antibiotics
• Dietary factors — excessive ingestion of alcohol, spicy foods, mint, coffee, or caffeine-containing products; cigarette smoking; ingestion of very hot or cold substances
• Physical or trauma factors — hiatal hernia; obesity; nasogastric intubation; radiation therapy; severe physical stress from surgery, sepsis, burns, accidents, or heavy weight-lifting; excessive emotional stress

FOCUSED ASSESSMENT GUIDELINES

Nursing history (functional health pattern findings)

Health perception–health management pattern
• Various nonspecific symptoms; may be acute (as from infection or ingestion of a caustic substance) or gradual (reflux esophagitis)
• Delay in seeking medical attention because of vagueness of symptoms (reflux esophagitis)
• Tendency to self-medicate with multiple over-the-counter remedies for GI upset
• Radiation therapy for scleroderma or other disease that makes esophageal or gastric mucosa more susceptible to infection and inflammation
• Treatment of sepsis, trauma, burns, immunologic disorder, endocrine disorder, liver disease, pancreatitis, or pulmonary disease

Nutritional-metabolic pattern
• With esophagitis, may report heartburn, dysphagia, or odynophagia (pain on swallowing); with gastroenteritis, typically complains of epigastric or abdominal discomfort, nausea, vomiting, diarrhea, or fever
• Hematemesis and food regurgitation
• Eructation and epigastric fullness after meals
• Anorexia or weight loss
• Swollen and inflamed mouth
• History of excessive alcohol consumption, aspirin ingestion, cigarette smoking, or ingestion of caustic substance
• Habitually eating excessive amounts of spicy foods, consuming very hot or cold substances, and eating late at night

Elimination pattern
• Cramping, abdominal distention, diarrhea, increased flatus, or melena

Activity-exercise pattern
• Sudden or chronic fatigue

Sleep-rest pattern
• Restlessness
• Awakening at night because of pain or with regurgitated food on pillow

Cognitive-perceptual pattern
• Pain of varying intensity, depending on cause of problem (for example, acute gastritis may cause epigastric discomfort and abdominal cramping, and caustic chemical ingestion may cause immediate localized pain and odynophagia)
• Morning hoarseness (laryngitis)

• Salty salivary secretions (water brash)
• Altered taste (from damage of salivary glands) if symptoms result from ingestion of caustic substance
Coping–stress tolerance pattern
• High levels of stress at work or home

Physical findings
Gastrointestinal
Esophagitis
• Hematemesis
• Eructation
• Dysphagia
Gastroenteritis
• Vomiting
• Diarrhea
• Eructation
• Hyperactive bowel sounds
• Flatulence
• Hematemesis
• Melena
Cardiovascular
(if hypovolemia present)
• Hypotension
• Tachycardia
Neurologic
(if hypovolemia present)
• Dizziness
• Restlessness
• Irritability
Integumentary
(if hypovolemia present)
• Pallor
• Cool, clammy skin
• Poor skin turgor
Musculoskeletal
(when in pain)
• Tense posture
• Facial grimacing

Diagnostic studies
For esophagitis and gastroenteritis:
• complete blood count (CBC) — may show decreased hemoglobin level or hematocrit, possibly indicating GI blood loss; elevated white blood cell count may indicate infection or inflammation
• serum electrolyte levels — may be studied to detect signs of fluid imbalance from blood loss, vomiting, or diarrhea (hypokalemia common with significant vomiting or diarrhea)
• serum amylase and lipase levels — elevations indicate pancreatitis as cause of symptoms
• cultures — may be taken to identify specific causative organism (especially for immunocompromised patients)
For esophagitis:
• barium swallow — detects inflammation, ulceration, esophageal strictures, and gastric reflux

• esophagoscopy — allows direct visualization of the esophagus to detect inflammation, ulceration, strictures, and hiatal hernia; biopsy of mucosa or brushing for cytology may be used for tissue diagnosis
• esophageal manometry — may reveal decreased esophageal sphincter pressure, as seen with gastro-esophageal reflux; may detect peristaltic abnormalities responsible for infections or inflammatory changes in the esophagus
• acid perfusion test (Bernstein test) — if the patient has pain or burning during perfusion of acid (via a tube) into esophagus, may indicate esophagitis
• pH reflux test — a pH less than 4 may indicate gastroesophageal reflux (normal esophageal pH is greater than 5)
For gastroenteritis:
• esophagogastroduodenoscopy — allows direct visualization of esophagus, stomach, and duodenum; biopsy of mucosa or brushing for cytology may be performed for tissue diagnosis; *Campylobacter*-like organism test (CLOtest) may be performed to detect the urease enzyme of *H. pylori*
• upper GI series — radiographically visualizes lining of esophagus, stomach, and duodenum; may detect inflammation, ulcerations, or strictures
• guaiac test — occult blood in stool may indicate blood loss

Potential complications
Esophagitis
• Ulcerative esophagitis
• Esophageal bleeding
• Hemorrhage
• Esophageal stricture
• Aspiration pneumonia
• Barrett's epithelium — columnar (gastric) epithelium in the esophagus resulting from chronic gastroesophageal reflux; places the patient at great risk for adenocarcinoma of the esophagus
• Esophageal carcinoma
• Inflammatory polyps of the vocal cords
• Lung abscess
Gastroenteritis
• Hemorrhage
• Ulceration — gastric or duodenal
• Gastric outlet obstruction
• Perforation of the GI lumen

Gastrointestinal disorders

ESOPHAGITIS AND GASTROENTERITIS

Major nursing diagnoses	Key patient outcomes
Risk for fluid volume deficit	Show stable vital signs: typically, heart rate, 60 to 100 beats/minute; systolic blood pressure, 90 to 140 mm Hg; and diastolic blood pressure, 50 to 90 mm Hg.
Pain	Rate pain as less than 3 on a 0 to 10 pain rating scale.
Nutritional deficit	Discuss nutritional needs with the dietitian.

NURSING DIAGNOSIS

Risk for fluid volume deficit related to vomiting, diarrhea, or GI hemorrhage

Nursing priority

Reestablish and maintain fluid and electrolyte balance.

Patient outcome criteria

Within 2 hours of admission, the patient will:
• show stable vital signs: typically, heart rate, 60 to 100 beats/minute; systolic blood pressure, 90 to 140 mm Hg; and diastolic blood pressure, 50 to 90 mm Hg
• experience no vomiting
• maintain adequate urine output (greater than 60 ml/hour).

Interventions

1. Monitor and record the patient's vital signs every 15 minutes if bleeding or every 4 hours if stable. Unless the patient is syncopal, frankly hypotensive, or severely tachycardic when supine, assess for orthostatic blood pressure and pulse rate changes every 8 hours: Take the patient's blood pressure and pulse while supine; then have the patient sit up and measure blood pressure and pulse rate again. Document your findings.

2. Withhold oral foods and fluids until vomiting has subsided. Begin I.V. fluids, as ordered. Monitor CBC and serum electrolyte levels, as ordered, and report abnormalities. See Appendix C, Fluid and Electrolyte Imbalances.

Rationales

1. Tachycardia and hypotension may indicate hypovolemia or shock. Orthostatic changes (a blood pressure decrease of 10 mm Hg or more or a pulse rate increase of 20 beats/minute or more) may indicate hypovolemia.

2. Allowing the patient to eat and drink may cause more vomiting and lead to metabolic alkalosis, hypokalemia, or hyponatremia. The Fluid and Electrolyte Imbalances appendix provides details related to specific abnormalities.

3. Administer antiemetics, antidiarrheals, and anticholinergics, as ordered.

3. Antiemetics, such as prochlorperazine (Compazine), promethazine (Phenergan), and chlorpromazine (Thorazine), prevent activation of the vomiting center in the brain stem. Adverse reactions include sedation, blurred vision, and restlessness.

Antidiarrheals, such as diphenoxylate with atropine (Lomotil), loperamide (Imodium), and kaolin and pectin (Kaopectate), may be used to decrease fluid loss from diarrhea. Diphenoxylate with atropine and loperamide are synthetic opium alkaloids that decrease intestinal motility, thereby decreasing diarrhea. They are contraindicated in patients with obstruction or diarrhea caused by infectious agents. Because kaolin and pectin act by adsorbing liquids, bacteria, toxins, nutrients, and drugs, loss of essential nutrients may occur with prolonged use.

Anticholinergics, such as dicyclomine hydrochloride (Bentyl) and propantheline bromide (Pro-Banthine), decrease gastric acid secretion and GI tone and motility and effectively control nausea and vomiting in acute gastritis. Adverse reactions include urine retention, dryness of mucous membranes (including dry mouth), dizziness, flushing, and headache.

4. Monitor and record the effectiveness of medications.

4. Lack of effectiveness may indicate the need to reevaluate the pharmacologic regimen.

5. Assess the patient's skin for signs of dehydration — poor skin turgor, dry skin and mucous membranes, and pallor. Also assess for thirst, especially in the elderly or debilitated patient.

5. Poor skin turgor, dry skin and mucous membranes, and increased thirst may indicate hypovolemia resulting from decreased extracellular fluid volume.

6. Monitor and record intake and output each shift. Include all vomitus, diarrhea, tube drainage, and blood loss in output, and all blood products and I.V. fluids in input. Record hourly urine outputs in the unstable patient. Record daily weights. Test all GI output with guaiac reagent strips (Hemoccult).

6. Accurate monitoring of intake and output alerts caregivers to imbalances that may cause hypovolemic shock. Oliguria (less than 30 ml of urine per hour) indicates decreased glomerular filtration rate; this may result from decreased blood flow, as in hypovolemia. Weight loss may reflect fluid loss. Checking GI output for occult blood may provide early detection of bleeding.

7. Assess and record the patient's level of consciousness (LOC), muscle strength, and coordination at least every 8 hours. Report changes promptly.

7. Confusion, dizziness, or stupor may indicate hypovolemia and electrolyte imbalance. A decreased LOC reflects cerebral hypoxemia caused by decreased circulating blood volume. Vomiting and diarrhea can cause electrolyte loss. Sodium loss may cause confusion and delirium; potassium loss may cause muscle weakness.

8. If the patient develops a GI hemorrhage, consult the "Gastrointestinal hemorrhage" plan, page 505.

8. The "Gastrointestinal hemorrhage" plan contains detailed information on this complication.

9. Additional individualized interventions: _____

9. Rationales: _____

NURSING DIAGNOSIS

Pain related to inflammation of the esophagus, stomach, and duodenum

Gastrointestinal disorders

Nursing priority

Relieve pain.

Patient outcome criteria

Within 2 hours of admission, the patient will:
• rate pain as less than 3 on a 0 to 10 pain rating scale
• rest comfortably
• show stable vital signs: typically, heart rate, 60 to 100 beats/minute; systolic blood pressure, 90 to 140 mm Hg; and diastolic blood pressure, 50 to 90 mm Hg.

Interventions

1. See the "Pain" plan, page 88.

2. Assess and document the pain's characteristics: onset, location, duration, and severity; radiation to back, neck, or shoulder; relationship to activity or position changes; relationship to eating patterns and bowel movements; and relationship to ingestion of spicy foods, coffee, alcohol, hot or cold liquids, or certain medications. Notify the doctor of any findings. Assess and document pain-relief measures.

3. Administer antacids (typically hourly and 1 hour after meals), histamine (H_2)-receptor antagonists (1 hour before meals and at least 30 minutes before sucralfate administration), sucralfate (Carafate), antibiotics, and antifungal medication, as ordered. In cases of severe pain, analgesics, such as viscous lidocaine or other topical agents, may be used. More potent analgesics may also be required.

4. Monitor and record the effectiveness of medications.

5. Assist and instruct the patient to rest, physically and emotionally. Help the patient identify personal stressors and ways to minimize their effects. Limit the number of visitors. Coordinate patient care to minimize interruptions. Keep room lights low. Teach stress-relieving techniques, such as deep-breathing and relaxation exercises.

Rationales

1. Pain associated with esophagitis and gastroenteritis may be subtle, as in abdominal cramping or heartburn, or may be more acute, such as sharp substernal pain similar to angina. The "Pain" plan provides general interventions for pain. This plan contains additional information related to esophagitis and gastroenteritis.

2. Accurate assessment is important in determining the pain's cause and formulating a medical diagnosis. Substernal burning pain (heartburn) and odynophagia are commonly associated with esophagitis. Epigastric pain while eating and abdominal cramping and tenderness are associated with acute gastritis.

3. Antacids are effective for about 30 minutes in the fasting stomach and should be given hourly for optimum neutralization of gastric acid. In case of severe pain, antacids may be given every 30 to 60 minutes. Antacids are most effective if given 1 hour after meals to neutralize increased gastric acid secretion stimulated by food ingestion.

H_2-receptor antagonists decrease gastric acid secretions and lower gastric pH by blocking H_2. They are poorly absorbed if given with meals, antacids, or sucralfate.

Sucralfate provides a protective coating for the gastric lining and is not absorbed. It may be ordered crushed and mixed with water to form a slush that coats the esophagus.

Antibiotics should be given after meals. Combination therapy (two different antibiotics and bismuth salt) is given to treat *H. pylori* infection.

4. Lack of effectiveness may indicate improper administration, inadequate dosage, the need to change medications, or new or complicating factors.

5. Stress stimulates the vagus nerve, which increases gastric mucosal blood flow, gastric acid secretion, and gastric motility. These factors may increase pain and inhibit healing.

6. Instruct the patient and family about pain-prevention measures. If pain causes the patient to awake at night or if the pain is worse on awakening, instruct the patient to sleep with the head of the bed elevated and to avoid eating for 3 hours before bedtime. Advise the patient to avoid bending, lifting heavy objects, and wearing constrictive clothing. Administer stool softeners, if prescribed, to avoid straining during bowel movements. Assess the patient's diet and habits to identify known causes of pain, such as spicy foods, alcohol, caffeinated products, aspirin, and smoking.

7. Additional individualized interventions: _____
_____

6. Eating stimulates gastric acid secretion. The patient with esophagitis should avoid eating for 3 hours before bedtime and elevate the head of the bed to prevent gastric reflux during sleep. Bending, lifting, wearing constrictive clothing, and straining decrease esophageal pressure and increase intra-abdominal pressure. Spicy foods, alcohol, caffeinated products, and aspirin irritate the gastric lining, increasing discomfort, and should be avoided. Cigarette smoking stimulates increased gastric secretion, which may contribute to further inflammation.

7. Rationales: _____
_____

NURSING DIAGNOSIS

Nutritional deficit related to nausea and vomiting, dysphagia, and mouth soreness

Nursing priority

Reestablish nutritional balance.

Patient outcome criteria

• Within 2 hours of admission, the patient will verbalize relief of nausea and vomiting.
• Within 24 hours of admission, the patient will discuss nutritional needs with the dietitian.

Interventions

1. Assess the patient's ability to retain oral food and fluids, noting any nausea, vomiting, or regurgitation; dysphagia for solids, liquids, or both; and complaints of mouth pain or soreness. Record all observations.

2. Monitor intake and output. Withhold oral foods and fluids until vomiting subsides. If total parenteral nutrition (TPN) is ordered, infuse the solution at the prescribed rate. (See the "Total parenteral nutrition" plan, page 527.) Administer oral nutritional and vitamin supplements as ordered. Record daily weights and calorie counts.

3. Explain the dilatation procedure, if ordered, for dysphagia, and assist when needed.

Rationales

1. Careful assessment of symptoms aids differential diagnosis. Mouth pain or soreness may indicate fungal infection or occur after ingestion of a caustic substance. Dysphagia may result from stricture formation from reflux esophagitis or ingestion of a caustic substance.

2. Food and fluids may cause further vomiting, increasing the risk of such complications as Mallory-Weiss tears (tearing of the esophageal mucosa, usually after forceful or prolonged vomiting). TPN may be necessary if oral intake is contraindicated for an extended period. The TPN plan contains details about this therapy. Nutritional supplements are indicated for the patient with esophageal strictures who is unable to swallow solid foods or for the patient who is unable to maintain metabolic balance because of anorexia, nausea, or mouth soreness.

3. Esophageal strictures, a common cause of dysphagia in esophagitis, can result from ingestion of a caustic substance, gastric reflux, or chronic infection (such as candidiasis). Carefully explaining the dilatation procedure helps alleviate the patient's anxiety. (Because dilatation procedures vary widely, consult institution protocol for details.)

Gastrointestinal disorders

4. Assist the dietitian in teaching the patient how to plan a well-balanced, nutritious diet. Teach the patient with esophageal strictures who cannot eat solids to puree foods and drink nutritional supplements. Instruct the patient with acute gastritis to eat frequent small meals instead of three large meals a day. Tell the patient to restrict or avoid spicy foods, alcohol, and caffeinated products, if necessary. Record all patient teaching.

5. Additional individualized interventions: _____

4. Dietary instruction aims to establish a balanced diet and ultimately return the patient's weight to normal. Thorough teaching may prevent subsequent problems and complications. Careful documentation of teaching provides a record for other caregivers so that reinforcement and review may be provided, as appropriate.

5. Rationales: _____

DISCHARGE PLANNING
Discharge checklist
Before discharge, the patient shows evidence of:
❏ stable vital signs
❏ absence of pulmonary or cardiovascular complications
❏ hemoglobin levels and hematocrit within expected parameters
❏ ability to tolerate adequate nutritional intake
❏ adequate hydration
❏ absence of pain
❏ urine output and bowel function same as before onset of acute illness
❏ stabilizing weight
❏ ability to follow prescribed diet
❏ ability to ambulate and perform activities of daily living same as before hospitalization.

Teaching checklist
Document evidence that the patient and family demonstrate an understanding of:
❏ disease and its implications
❏ all discharge medications' purpose, administration schedule, dosage, and adverse effects requiring medical attention (usual discharge medications include antacids, H_2-antagonists, anticholinergics, antibiotics, or antifungal medications)
❏ recommended dietary modifications or TPN administration, if patient is being discharged on TPN.
❏ recommended lifestyle modifications, including smoking cessation and stress reduction
❏ importance of medical follow-up, which may include weekly visits for dilatation
❏ how to contact the doctor
❏ signs and symptoms of complications
❏ available community resources such as Alcoholics Anonymous, as indicated.

Documentation checklist
Using outcome criteria as a guide, document:
❏ clinical status on admission
❏ significant changes in status
❏ description of pain
❏ pain-relief measures and effectiveness
❏ episodes of nausea and vomiting
❏ description of vomitus
❏ description of stools
❏ bleeding episodes
❏ fluid intake and output
❏ stress-relief measures
❏ pertinent laboratory and diagnostic test findings
❏ nutritional status
❏ patient and family teaching
❏ discharge planning.

ASSOCIATED PLANS OF CARE
Gastrointestinal hemorrhage
Ineffective individual coping
Knowledge deficit
Pain
Total parenteral nutrition

REFERENCES
Black, J. M., and Matassarin-Jacobs, E. *Medical-Surgical Nursing: Clinical Management for Continuity of Care,* 5th ed. Philadelphia: W.B. Saunders Co., 1997.
Thompson, J., et al. *Mosby's Clinical Nursing,* 4th ed.. St. Louis: Mosby–Year Book, Inc., 1997.

Gastrointestinal hemorrhage

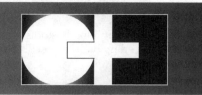

DRG information
DRG 174   Gastrointestinal Hemorrhage with Complication or Comorbidity (CC).
Mean LOS = 5.6 days
Principal diagnoses include:
• GI hemorrhage — site or etiology unspecified
• hemorrhage of anus or rectum
• acute ulcer (gastric, peptic, duodenal, je-
junal, or a combination of sites) with hemorrhage
• esophageal varices with hemorrhage.
DRG 175   Gastrointestinal Hemorrhage without CC.
Mean LOS = 3.5 days
Principal diagnoses include selected principal diagnoses listed under DRG 174. The
distinction is that patients grouped under
DRG 175 have no CC.

INTRODUCTION

Definition and time focus
In the acute care setting, severe GI bleeding is most
commonly associated with upper GI pathology; although bleeding can occur anywhere in the GI tract,
lower GI bleeding is usually less severe. Bleeding may
result from an underlying condition, such as ulcers, invasive tumors, or esophageal varices. (Gastritis and gastric ulcers are estimated to account for up to 80% of all
GI bleeding episodes.) Bleeding may also develop as an
untoward effect of therapeutically administered medications, such as anti-inflammatory drugs or anticoagulants. Trauma, burns, sepsis, and other conditions may
cause stress ulcers, which usually manifest as sudden,
severe, and painless bleeding. Regardless of the cause,
acute GI bleeding may be life-threatening without
prompt diagnosis and treatment. Delay in diagnosis is
associated with a higher mortality rate and increased
complications. This plan focuses on the patient experiencing an acute episode of upper GI bleeding.

Etiology and precipitating factors
• Gastric irritation or altered gastric pH, as with medication use (for example, salicylates, steroids, or other
anti-inflammatory drugs), alcohol or caffeine abuse,
toxic or allergic reactions, ingestion of corrosive substances, peptic or gastric ulcer, gastritis, and stress reactions

• Altered gastric function or circulation, as with tumors,
portal hypertension or esophageal varices, or
Mallory-Weiss laceration of gastric mucosa
• Altered blood coagulation, as with anticoagulant use,
blood dyscrasias, cancer, shock, sepsis, uremia, and disseminated intravascular coagulation (DIC)

FOCUSED ASSESSMENT GUIDELINES

Nursing history (functional health pattern findings)
Health perception–health management pattern
• History of gastric ulcer or gastritis
• History of heavy alcohol intake or cigarette smoking
(associated with gastritis and esophageal varices)
• History of long-term steroid, salicylate, or other
anti-inflammatory therapy
Nutritional-metabolic pattern
• Nausea
• Fullness in the abdomen
• Thirst
• Heartburn
Elimination pattern
• Dark or tarry stools
• History of coffee-ground vomitus
Activity-exercise pattern
• Weakness and easy fatigability
Cognitive-perceptual pattern
• With bleeding related to ulcer disease: gnawing,
aching, or burning abdominal pain, which may be re-
lieved by eating
• With bleeding related to stress ulcer: no pain
Coping–stress tolerance pattern
• Extreme fear in reaction to sight of own blood

Physical findings
General appearance
• Frightened or anxious facial expression
Cardiovascular
• Tachycardia
• Orthostatic hypotension
• Weak, thready peripheral pulse
Gastrointestinal
• Melena
• Hematemesis (associated with upper GI bleeding)
• Coffee-ground vomitus (indicates slower upper GI
bleeding)

• Hematochezia (bright, bloody stools — usually indicates lower GI bleeding but may occur with rapid upper GI hemorrhage)

Pulmonary
• Hyperventilation

Neurologic
• Restlessness
• Decreased alertness (with shock)

Integumentary
• Pallor
• Diaphoresis

Diagnostic studies

• Blood urea nitrogen (BUN) levels — elevated because of digestion of blood proteins in the GI tract and accumulated blood breakdown by-products
• Complete blood count (CBC) — obtained for baseline; may reflect minimal abnormalities for up to 36 hours if bleeding is slow. Eventually, reduced hemoglobin level, hematocrit, and red blood cell (RBC) count reflect overall blood loss; reticulocyte count may be elevated in response to bleeding
• Blood typing and crossmatching — obtained in anticipation of blood replacement; in acute bleeding, type-specific, noncrossmatched blood may be administered as an emergency measure
• Prothrombin time/international normalized ratio, activated partial thromboplastin time — obtained for baseline and for evaluation of altered coagulation status as cause of bleeding. Further clotting studies may also be obtained if coagulation defects are suspected

• Gastric aspiration — provides information regarding amount and time of bleeding; results are used to guide further intervention. For example, a small aspiration of material resembling coffee grounds may indicate "old" bleeding that only warrants close observation of the patient; aspiration of fresh bright red blood is evidence of active hemorrhage and demands prompt intervention
• Endoscopic examination, including flexible fiber-optic endoscopy — provides visualization of bleeding site and associated pathology; may permit tissue biopsy or direct coagulation of bleeding sites via endoscope
• Abdominal angiography — allows visualization of abdominal vasculature; used to locate bleeding sites and may be used for localized treatment by infusion of vasopressin (Pitressin) or injection of clot formation material (embolization)
• Computed tomography scan — may be used to detect tumors or polyps
• Barium studies — may be used to identify gastric erosions or tumors as bleeding source if angiography is not available; used as a last resort in patients with active bleeding because barium obscures the field for subsequent endoscopic or angiographic assessment

Potential complications
• Shock
• Renal failure
• DIC
• Hepatic encephalopathy
• Myocardial ischemia or myocardial infarction (MI)

CLINICAL SNAPSHOT

GASTROINTESTINAL HEMORRHAGE

Major nursing diagnoses and collaborative problems	Key patient outcomes
Risk for hypovolemic shock	Show stable vital signs: typically, heart rate, 60 to 100 beats/minute; systolic blood pressure, 90 to 140 mm Hg; and diastolic blood pressure, 50 to 90 mm Hg.
Risk for injury: Complications	Remain alert and oriented.
Fear	Verbalize feelings related to the condition, if desired.
Knowledge deficit (potential recurrent bleeding)	Describe signs and symptoms of possible recurrent bleeding.

COLLABORATIVE PROBLEM

Risk for hypovolemic shock related to blood loss

Nursing priorities

- Assess amount of blood loss.
- Restore blood and fluid volume.
- Help identify the source or cause and provide treatment.

Patient outcome criteria

Within 24 hours of detection of bleeding, the patient will:
- show stable vital signs: typically, heart rate, 60 to 100 beats/minute; systolic blood pressure, 90 to 140 mm Hg; and diastolic blood pressure, 50 to 90 mm Hg
- show no orthostatic changes in vital signs
- have urine output of at least 60 ml/hour
- show no signs of frank bleeding
- have warm, dry skin
- exhibit gastric pH greater than 4.

Interventions

1. See the "Hypovolemic shock" plan, page 432.

2. Assess the amount of blood loss using the following procedures:
- Maintain accurate intake and output records, including precise measurement of all vomitus and stools. Unless output is visibly bloody, guaiac-test it.

- Evaluate vital signs every 4 hours, or more frequently if indicated; include evaluation of orthostatic changes unless the patient is syncopal, frankly hypotensive, or severely tachycardic when supine. Note and report promptly to the doctor a systolic blood pressure decrease of more than 10 mm Hg or a pulse increase of more than 20 beats/minute.

- If the patient is in a critical care unit, evaluate hemodynamic pressures and electrocardiography (ECG) findings according to Appendix A, Monitoring Standards, or unit protocol.

Rationales

1. The "Hypovolemic shock" plan provides detailed interventions for assessment and treatment of the patient in actual or impending shock.

2. Prevention of shock depends on accurate status assessment.
- Direct measurement of bloody output is essential to guide replacement therapy. Guaiac testing provides objective assessment for the presence of occult blood. Careful monitoring of urine output is vital because a drop in hourly urine output (less than 60 ml/hour) may signal the development of shock.
- Compensatory neurovascular mechanisms may be able to maintain normal supine blood pressure when blood loss is less than 500 ml. Moving from a supine to a sitting position adds an orthostatic stress that may unmask hidden hypotension. A pulse increase of 20 to 30 beats/minute with no change in blood pressure correlates with a blood loss of 500 ml, while a pulse increase of more than 30 beats/minute and systolic blood pressure drop of more than 10 mm Hg may indicate a blood loss of 1,000 ml or more. Although many critically ill patients are too unstable to tolerate orthostatic assessment, it may provide useful data in the stable patient. However, when clear evidence of hypotension already exists, the test may accelerate shock progression.
- These parameters provide additional data useful in judging the degree of shock present.

• Obtain appropriate laboratory studies, as ordered, including CBC, BUN, and creatinine for baseline and ongoing monitoring.

• Hemoglobin level and hematocrit reflect blood volume status but may show no changes initially. BUN and creatinine levels are of greater diagnostic value. An elevated BUN level in the presence of normal creatinine level indicates a likely blood loss of more than 1,000 ml.

• Assess the patient frequently for clinical signs of hypovolemia. Note constellations of signs and symptoms, such as those of mild shock (for example, anxiety, perspiration, or weakness); moderate shock (for example, hyperactive bowel sounds, tachycardia, or thirst); or severe shock (for example, pallor, cool and clammy skin, decreased level of consciousness (LOC), decreased urine output, and thready pulse).

• Clinical parameters help define stages of blood loss. Signs and symptoms of mild shock (less than 500 ml blood loss) are nonspecific. Signs of moderate shock (500 to 1,000 ml blood loss) reflect progressive activation of sympathetic nervous system compensatory mechanisms and other homeostatic mechanisms. Signs of severe shock (more than 1,000 ml blood loss) reflect ischemia of core organ systems.

• Insert and maintain a gastric tube, as ordered, and check drainage for blood.

• Gastric intubation permits removal and accurate measurement of accumulated blood from the stomach. It is also therapeutic because blood in the stomach may stimulate vomiting and excess gastric acid secretion, both of which may cause or accelerate bleeding. Finally, blood that passes into the intestines is broken down into ammonia, which may have toxic metabolic effects.

3. Replace blood loss, as ordered, by:

3. Replacement therapy is essential to prevent hypovolemia and hypoxemia related to reduced hemoglobin level.

• establishing and maintaining I.V. access with one or two large-bore cannulas

• A large-bore cannula is necessary for rapid infusion of blood and fluids.

• rapidly administering I.V. crystalloid solution (such as lactated Ringer's solution)

• Crystalloid solutions effectively expand plasma volume. Rapid administration averts cardiovascular collapse.

• administering and monitoring the response to transfusion of packed RBCs, fresh frozen plasma, or other blood components as well as volume expanders, such as plasma protein fraction (Plasmanate) or albumin.

• Restoration of circulating volume and replacement of blood components are essential to minimize cell death from hypoxemia. If heart failure is present, packed cells may be administered with minimal additional fluid to avert fluid overload. The hematocrit should increase with each unit of packed cells administered. Persistent bleeding is present if hematocrit does not improve. For other patients, volume expanders may be indicated. Albumin, for example, provides an osmotically induced fluid expansion equal to five times its volume. Blood that has been stored for a period of time may be deficient in some clotting factors, so the administration of fresh frozen plasma or other components may be needed.

• Prepare the patient for emergency surgery if blood pressure does not increase in response to 1 L of fluid given over 10 minutes or if hemoglobin level and hematocrit fail to increase in response to blood product administration.

• Emergency surgery is indicated to identify and correct the cause of massive bleeding.

4. Initiate measures to stop bleeding, as ordered, such as:

4. As many as 90% of upper GI hemorrhages cease spontaneously, but severe bleeding constitutes a medical or surgical emergency, and prompt corrective treatment is warranted.

• maintaining activity restrictions, which usually include strict bed rest

• Activity may increase intra-abdominal pressure and accelerate bleeding.

• performing gastric lavage, usually with room temperature or iced normal saline solution, with or without addition of norepinephrine (Levophed) to the solution. If norepinephrine is used, the usual dilution is 2 ampules to 1,000 ml normal saline solution in a continuous irrigation.

• administering vasopressin I.V., unless the patient has a history of coronary artery disease or other vascular problems. The dose range is 0.02 to 0.06 mcg/minute I.V. or through an arterial catheter placed near the bleeding site. Monitor the ECG during administration.

• preparing the patient with uncontrollably bleeding esophageal varices, if a poor surgical risk, for injection sclerotherapy; after injection, observe for rebleeding, chest pain, fever, and other complications

• preparing the patient for laser therapy, if ordered

• assisting with insertion, monitoring, and maintaining the placement of a Sengstaken-Blakemore tube or other compression tubes. Elevate the head of the bed. Suction the oropharynx, nasopharynx, and upper esophagus frequently. Irrigate the tube at least every 2 hours. Maintain proper balloon pressures. Maintain proper positioning by verifying balloon placement by X-ray, as ordered, and maintaining traction on the balloon. Cut and remove the tube immediately if airway compromise occurs.

• as an alternative to sclerotherapy, administering somatostatin in a 250-mg bolus followed by an I.V. infusion of 250 mg/hour or octreotide 50 mcg I.V. bolus followed by an I.V. infusion of 25 to 50 mcg/hour over 1 to 5 days.

• Gastric lavage removes accumulated blood and clots and clears the stomach for endoscopic examination. Iced lavage, which was traditionally ordered based on the theory that gastric cooling decreased blood flow, has become controversial as a therapeutic measure. Some studies have demonstrated prolonged clotting times in response to iced irrigation. Norepinephrine may be added for its local vasoconstrictive effects, although its value has not been proven. Systemic effects are minimized when norepinephrine is administered in this way because the drug is metabolized in the liver immediately after gastric absorption.

• Vasopressin causes vasoconstriction and contraction of smooth muscle in the GI tract. It also increases reabsorption of water in the renal tubules. However, its use may cause myocardial ischemia, MI, or hypertension, particularly in a patient with cardiovascular disease.

• Injection sclerotherapy is a definitive treatment involving injection of a coagulating substance into a bleeding vessel. This produces intense inflammation and scarring, and stops bleeding in approximately 80% of cases. Hemorrhage may recur, requiring multiple treatments. Chest pain and fever (typically appearing within 6 hours and lasting 3 days) result from the inflammatory process.

• Laser coagulation therapy may be used when endoscopy indicates active bleeding, fresh clots, or a duodenal ulcer or gastric erosion with a visible vessel.

• Compression balloon tubes, such as the Sengstaken-Blakemore tube, may be used to control hemorrhage temporarily in patients with esophageal varices. However, the high rebleeding rate, significant discomfort, and risk of aspiration limit the tubes' usefulness. The balloon applies direct pressure against bleeding vessels, while the gastric tube permits continued decompression and aspiration. Elevating the head of the bed helps prevent esophageal reflux and associated irritation. When the tube is in place, the patient is unable to swallow salivary secretions. Also, nasal secretions may be increased because of local irritation from the tube. Irrigation ensures patency of the tube and prevents gastric distention.

Excessive pressure may result in perforation, inflammation, or ulceration of the esophagus or gastric mucosal lining, while insufficient pressure may render the tube ineffective or contribute to its displacement.

X-ray verification and maintenance of traction help ensure correct positioning. If the tube becomes displaced, it may obstruct the airway. Cutting the tube deflates the gastric and esophageal balloons and permits immediate removal.

• Somatostatin and octreotide are as effective as vasopressin with fewer systemic complications. Patients with known ischemic heart disease, peripheral vascular disease or cardiac arrhythmias will benefit from somatostatin or octreotide.

Gastrointestinal disorders

• administering vitamin K₁ (phytonadione, AquaME-PHYTON) intramuscularly, as ordered

• preparing the patient for surgery if medical treatment is unsuccessful (bleeding requires more than 2 units of blood per hour to maintain blood pressure, requires more than 6 to 8 units of blood within 24 hours, exceeds more than 2,500 ml in the first 24 hours, or recurs during therapy).

5. Administer medications to control gastric acidity, typically histamine (H_2)-blockers such as cimetidine (Tagamet) or ranitidine (Zantac) I.V. during acute bleeding episodes. Monitor gastric aspirate pH and adjust dosage, as ordered, to maintain a pH greater than 4.0. Observe for drug interactions, especially if the patient is also receiving theophylline (Slo-Phyllin), procainamide (Pronestyl), or warfarin (Coumadin). Observe for signs of toxicity if cimetidine and lidocaine (Xylocaine) are administered concurrently.

6. Prepare the patient and family for and assist with diagnostic procedures, as ordered, such as endoscopic examination, angiography, or other studies.

7. Additional individualized interventions: _____

• The patient receiving I.V. feedings or multiple antibiotics for a prolonged period may develop vitamin K deficiency because this catalyst for clotting factor production is either obtained through a normal diet or synthesized by intestinal bacteria. Replacement therapy may be necessary to restore normal clotting status.
• If bleeding does not stop, surgery is indicated to identify and correct the problem.

5. Gastric hyperacidity, indicated by a low pH, is a primary contributor to ulcer development and the need for dosage increases. H_2 blockers inhibit the action of histamine, raising gastric pH. Cimetidine and ranitidine reduce theophylline clearance, increasing the risk of theophylline toxicity; impair metabolism of procainamide, possibly producing toxicity; and impair metabolism of warfarin, increasing the risk of bleeding. Cimetidine reduces liver clearance of lidocaine.

6. Identification of the site and cause of the bleeding is essential because delay in diagnosis is associated with a higher mortality rate.

7. Rationales: _____

NURSING DIAGNOSIS

Risk for injury: Complications related to undetected bleeding, inadequate organ perfusion, accumulation of toxins, electrolyte imbalance, release of procoagulants, or ulcer perforation

Nursing priority

Prevent or promptly detect and treat complications.

Patient outcome criteria

Throughout the hospital stay, the patient will:
• exhibit decreasing BUN and normal creatinine values
• display electrolyte levels within normal limits
• maintain urine output greater than 60 ml/hour
• remain alert and oriented.

Interventions

1. Continue to perform guaiac tests on all gastric contents and stools at least daily, even after the patient's condition has stabilized.

2. Immediately report and thoroughly investigate any complaint of chest pain, particularly in a patient with preexisting cardiac disease.

Rationales

1. As much as 200 ml of blood may be lost daily without detectable clinical signs. Early detection allows prompt treatment.

2. Blood loss reduces the level of circulating hemoglobin, thus compromising normal delivery of oxygen to tissues. If coronary circulation is already impaired, this reduction may cause ischemic changes or MI.

3. Monitor renal and hepatic function, including hourly urine output, LOC every 2 hours, daily BUN and creatinine levels, and daily weight. Note daily serum electrolyte values, including serum calcium, particularly if the patient has received multiple blood transfusions.

4. Observe for bleeding from other sites, such as epistaxis or petechiae. See the "Disseminated intravascular coagulation" plan, page 780.

5. Immediately report any complaint of sudden, severe abdominal pain or rigidity, and prepare the patient for surgery if these occur.

6. Additional individualized interventions: _____

3. Hemorrhage and the resulting hypovolemia may cause renal and hepatic hypoperfusion, eventually leading to kidney or liver failure. Liver dysfunction, commonly associated with esophageal varices, contributes to elevated blood ammonia levels and can result in hepatic encephalopathy. Hypocalcemia is a common adverse effect of multiple transfusions because calcium binds with the preservative in stored blood.

4. Bleeding from other sites may signal the development of DIC, a grave complication of hemorrhage. The plan for this disorder contains detailed interventions.

5. These signs and symptoms may indicate gastric perforation, which causes peritonitis, sepsis, and shock unless promptly treated. Immediate surgical intervention is warranted to remove gastric contents from the peritoneal cavity.

6. Rationales: _____

Nursing diagnosis

Fear related to sight of blood and distressing physical symptoms

Nursing priority

Reduce the patient's fear.

Patient outcome criterion

After initial stabilization, the patient will verbalize feelings related to the condition, if desired.

Interventions

1. Provide care promptly, explaining all interventions to the patient in simple terms. Avoid expressing dismay or revulsion at the sight of bleeding; assume a calm, confident, matter-of-fact manner. Acknowledge the patient's fear by saying, for example, "I know it must be pretty scary to see all this blood, but we treat this condition often. We will be replacing your blood by giving you transfusions and extra fluids."

2. Encourage verbalization of feelings by using active listening skills. See the "Ineffective individual coping" plan, page 67.

3. Accept expressions of anxiety related to the possibility of death. See the "Dying" plan, page 20.

4. Additional individualized interventions: _____

Rationales

1. The sight of blood is normally extremely threatening to the patient, who justifiably may fear bleeding to death. Anxiety may interfere with the patient's ability to comprehend, but simple explanations about what is happening may reassure the patient that needed care is being given. Recognizing the normalcy of the patient's fear reduces the patient's sense of isolation. Patients typically are quite concerned about bloody excreta and losing bowel control. Calm acceptance may minimize shame related to these losses of bodily control.

2. Verbalizing feelings helps the patient identify specific fears and begin to mobilize coping strategies. The "Ineffective individual coping" plan details interventions that may be helpful in promoting coping behaviors.

3. Issues of death are always of acute importance for the patient with a critical condition. The "Dying" plan contains specific interventions useful in caring for patients and families confronting issues of mortality.

4. Rationales: _____

Gastrointestinal disorders

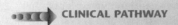

Managing GI hemorrhage

Patient problem	Day 1
Tests and procedures Risk of increased instability of condition related to delay in tests or procedures	• Goal: Tolerates tests and procedures; endoscopy/colonoscopy completed – Type and screen – PT/PTT – CBC – Hct q 6 hr – Renal profile – Upper endoscopy – Colonoscopy – Patient preparation as ordered
Medications and treatments Risk of recurrence of GI bleeding related to irritation or ulceration of site	• Goal: Exhibits appropriate therapeutic response to drugs; no adverse reactions – I.V. H_2 blockers – Transfuse per doctor's orders – I.V. fluids
GI problem Risk for altered bowel function	• Goal: Stable GI function; no active bleeding; NG tube patent – NG tube – Document color, amount, character of aspirate, vomitus, stool – Collect specimens as ordered
Nutrition Risk for altered nutrition: Less than body requirements	• Goal: Stable digestive processes; no vomiting, diarrhea – NPO
Activity Risk for activity intolerance related to weakness	• Goal: Compliant with activity restriction – Bed rest
Cardiovascular Risk for fluid volume deficit related to GI blood loss	• Goal: Stable CV function; adequate fluid balance, stable LOC, skin warm and dry, urine output > 60ml/hr, normal vital signs (SBP > 90, HR 60 to 100) – Vital signs q 4 hr – I&O q shift – Indwelling urinary catheter
Psychosocial and spiritual needs Risk for ineffective coping related to illness or bleeding	• Goal: Effective coping patterns; patient and family verbalize thoughts and feelings about illness and demonstrate compliance with care – Allow patient and family to verbalize thoughts and feelings about illness – Assess response to care and treatment
Patient teaching Knowledge deficit related to illness, procedures, or preventive measures	• Goal: Patient and family participate in identification of learning needs and verbalize understanding of procedure, prep, and post-procedure care • Assess knowledge deficit and begin teaching as indicated: – procedures – treatments – medications
Discharge planning	• Goal: Discharge planning needs identified and addressed – Discharge planning assessment – Consult case manager to evaluate discharge needs

Day 2	Day 3	Day 4

• Goal: Tests normal; Hct stable, no hematemesis, melena, or rectal bleeding
  – Hct q 8 hr
	• Goal: Tests normal: Hct normal or baseline x 48 hr; no hematemesis, melena, or rectal bleeding
	  – Hct q a.m.
		• Goal: Tests normal

• Goal: Exhibits appropriate therapeutic response to drugs; no adverse reactions
  – I.V. H_2 blockers
  – I.V. fluids
	• Goal: Exhibits appropriate therapeutic response to drugs; no adverse reactions
	  – Change to P.O. meds
	  – Discontinue I.V. fluids
	  – Change I.V. to S.L.
		• Goal: Exhibits appropriate therapeutic response to drugs; no adverse reactions
		  – Discontinue saline lock

• Goal: Stable GI function; no active bleeding
  – Discontinue NG tube
  – Collect specimens as ordered
	• Goal: Stable GI function; normal bowel pattern	• Goal: Stable GI function; normal bowel pattern; benign abdomen

• Goal: Stable digestive processes; tolerates P.O. intake; no vomiting, diarrhea
  – Clear liquids, advance as tolerated
	• Goal: Stable digestive processes: P.O. intake ⩾50% of meals; no nausea, vomiting, diarrhea
	  – Advance diet as tolerated
		• Goal: Stable digestive processes; tolerates 100% of meals; nutritional intake meets body requirements
		  – Diet as tolerated

• Goal: Tolerates activity progression
  – Chair t.i.d.
	• Goal: Tolerates activity progression
	  – Up in room
		• Goal: Patient and family or significant other able to manage care
		  – Up ad lib

• Goal: Stable CV function: adequate fluid balance, stable LOC, skin warm and dry, urine output > 60 ml/hr, normal vital signs (SBP > 90, HR 60 to 100)
  – Vital signs q 8 hr
  – I&O q shift
  – Discontinue indwelling urinary catheter
	• Goal: Stable CV function: adequate fluid balance, stable LOC, skin warm and dry, urine output > 60 ml/hr, normal vital signs (SBP > 90, HR 60 to 100)
	  – Vital signs q 8 hr
	  – I&O q shift
		• Goal: Stable CV function; adequate fluid balance, stable LOC, skin warm and dry, urine output > 60 ml/hr, vital signs normal (SBP > 90, HR 60 to 100)
		  – Vital signs q 8 hr
		  – I&O q shift

• Goal: Effective coping patterns: patient and family verbalize thoughts and feelings about illness and demonstrate compliance with care
  – Allow patient and family to verbalize thoughts and feelings about illness
  – Assess their response to care and treatment
	• Goal: Effective coping patterns: patient and family verbalize thoughts and feelings about illness and demonstrate compliance with care
	  – Allow patient and family to verbalize thoughts and feelings about illness
	  – Assess their response to care and treatment
		• Goal: Effective coping patterns; patient and family verbalize thoughts and feelings about illness and demonstrate compliance with care
		  – Allow patient and family to verbalize thoughts and feelings about illness
		  – Assess response to care and treatment

• Goal: Identified learning needs met; patient and family verbalize understanding of progression of care
• Continue teaching:
  – diet
  – medications
  – activity
  – assessment and preventive measures
	• Goal: Identified learning needs met; patient and family verbalize understanding of progression of care
	  – Continue/reinforce teaching
		• Goal: Identified learning needs met; patient and family verbalize understanding of:
		• _____
		• _____
		• _____
		• _____

• Goal: Discharge planning needs identified and addressed; discharge planning assessment completed	• Goal: Discharge planning completed, needs identified, arrangements completed	• Goal: Discharge planning completed, needs identified, arrangements completed

Gastrointestinal disorders

NURSING DIAGNOSIS

Knowledge deficit (potential recurrent bleeding) related to unfamiliarity with disorder

Nursing priority

Teach assessment techniques and preventive measures.

Patient outcome criteria

Before discharge, the patient will (as condition allows):
• list any precipitating or contributing factors identified
• describe signs and symptoms of possible recurrence of bleeding
• verbalize understanding of any dietary recommendations.

Interventions

1. See the "Knowledge deficit" plan, page 72.

2. Defer detailed teaching until the patient is alert and physiologically stable. Then, as indicated by condition, discuss with the patient:
• precipitating or contributing factors of bleeding episode (for example, alcohol consumption or medication use)
• signs and symptoms indicating possible recurrence (for example, melena, coffee-ground vomitus, weakness, or dizziness)
• other causes of dark stools (for example, intake of iron, beets, berries, or greens)
• dietary recommendations, as ordered (for example, avoidance of caffeine).

3. Additional individualized interventions: _____
_____

Rationales

1. The "Knowledge deficit" plan contains detailed interventions related to patient and family teaching.

2. The patient's condition may limit teaching, but abbreviated teaching may lay the groundwork for more detailed education before discharge.
• Awareness of contributing factors over which the patient has control may decrease the likelihood of a recurrence.
• Early medical attention if bleeding recurs may avert the need for a prolonged hospital stay.

• Knowing other causes may avert undue alarm.

• Careful dietary management may be the primary preventive therapy for some conditions.

3. Rationales: _____
_____

DISCHARGE PLANNING

Discharge checklist

Before discharge, the patient shows evidence of:
❏ stable vital signs within normal limits
❏ urine output of at least 60 ml/hour
❏ normal or decreasing BUN values
❏ normal serum electrolytes
❏ normal skin perfusion
❏ gastric pH of 4.0 or greater
❏ normal guaiac test of stools or vomitus
❏ stable LOC for more than 12 hours
❏ balanced fluid intake and output.

Teaching checklist

Document evidence that the patient and family demonstrate an understanding of:
❏ cause and site of bleeding
❏ precipitating or contributing factors
❏ signs and symptoms indicating possible recurrence of bleeding
❏ dietary recommendations, if any.

Documentation checklist

Using outcome criteria as a guide, document:
❏ clinical status on admission
❏ significant changes in status
❏ pertinent diagnostic test findings
❏ bleeding episodes
❏ fluid and blood replacement measures
❏ fluid intake and output
❏ emotional response
❏ pharmacologic interventions
❏ procedures to stop bleeding
❏ patient and family teaching
❏ discharge planning.

ASSOCIATED PLANS OF CARE

Acute renal failure
Disseminated intravascular coagulation
Dying
Hypovolemic shock
Impaired physical mobility
Ineffective individual coping
Knowledge deficit
Liver failure
Nutritional deficit
Pancreatitis

REFERENCES

Besson, I., et al. "Sclerotherapy With or Without Octreotide for Acute Variceal Bleeding," *New England Journal of Medicine* 333(9):555-60, February 1995.

Gostout, C.J. "Evaluation and Management of Esophogeal Variceal Bleeding," *Clinical Update* 4(1):1-4, July 1996 (supplement of American Society for Gastrointestinal Endoscopy) .

Gastrointestinal disorders

Inflammatory bowel disease

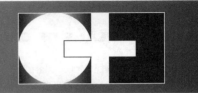

DRG information
DRG 179 Inflammatory Bowel Disease.
Mean LOS = 7.2 days
Principal diagnoses include:
- proctocolitis
- regional enteritis.

DRG 182 Esophagitis, Gastroenteritis, and Miscellaneous Digestive Disorders; Age 17+ with Complications or Comorbidity (CC).
Mean LOS = 5.0 days
Principal diagnoses include:
- diverticulitis
- infectious diarrhea.

DRG 183 Esophagitis, Gastroenteritis, and Miscellaneous Digestive Disorders; Age 17+ without CC.
Mean LOS = 3.4 days

DRG 184 Esophagitis, Gastroenteritis, and Miscellaneous Digestive Disorders; Ages 0 to 17.
Mean LOS = 2.8 days

INTRODUCTION

Definition and time focus
Inflammatory bowel disease (IBD) is a broad diagnostic category that includes ulcerative colitis, Crohn's disease (regional enteritis), appendicitis, diverticulitis, infectious diarrhea, functional bowel disorders, and humorally mediated diarrheal syndromes. Hospitalized IBD patients may be acutely ill and may demonstrate similar management problems. This plan focuses on the problems associated with acute exacerbations of ulcerative colitis and regional enteritis.

Ulcerative colitis and regional enteritis involve local defects characterized by excavation of the bowel surface from sloughing of necrotic inflammatory tissue. The ulcerations in regional enteritis are transmural, involving all layers of the bowel; those of ulcerative colitis begin in the crypts of Lieberkühn and usually involve the mucosa and submucosa. The lesions in ulcerative colitis are usually confined to the descending large bowel and sigmoid colon and are continuous in nature; the defects in regional enteritis occur predominantly in, but are not confined to, the terminal ileum and tend to alternate with areas of normal bowel surface.

Etiology and precipitating factors
- Exact cause unknown—infectious agents, genetic or familial tendencies, immunologic mechanisms, and stress-related psychological factors may be involved
- Stressful event, possibly preceding an acute attack by 4 to 6 months
- Bacterial infection, possibly occurring several weeks before an acute attack
- Age—attacks are more severe, with a higher mortality rate, after age 40 in regional enteritis and after age 60 with ulcerative colitis

FOCUSED ASSESSMENT GUIDELINES

Nursing history (functional health pattern findings)
Health perception–health management pattern
- Gradual or acute onset of abdominal cramping, anorexia, and weight loss related to fear of intake of food and fluids that increase cramping; low-grade fever (may be high-grade if perforation present); change in bowel habits with increasing frequency of stools (in ulcerative colitis, stools may exceed 15 per day, be accompanied by urgency and tenesmus [the frequent, painful, unproductive urge to defecate], and contain blood, mucus, or pus)
- History of acute exacerbations
- Drug regimen that includes corticosteroids or immunosuppressants
- Family history of disorder
- White, typically, but an unexplained increase in regional enteritis among blacks has been observed
- Growth retardation (seen in childhood onset of IBD)

Nutritional-metabolic pattern
- Anorexia with weight loss
- Signs and symptoms of chronic malnutrition
- Intake of fatty foods or other dietary indiscretions; if disease is chronic, may report being on a low-residue, low-fiber, bland diet

Elimination pattern
- Increasing frequency of bowel movements (may have been gradual or acute in onset)
- Abdominal pain and possible audible bowel sounds (borborygmi) before onset of discomfort
- Bright red rectal bleeding with fecal incontinence, particularly with ulcerative colitis
- Visible peristaltic waves over the abdomen

Activity-exercise pattern
- Malaise and fatigue

- Muscle weakness
Sleep-rest pattern
- Sleep disturbance related to abdominal discomfort and nocturnal defecation
Self-perception–self-concept pattern
- Low self-esteem, compensated for by ambitious, hard-driving lifestyle
Role-relationship pattern
- Use of dependent behavior to cope with feelings of anger, hostility, and anxiety
- may report family history of similar GI problems
Sexuality-reproductive pattern
- Altered ability to cope with human relationships (with chronic disease)
- Delayed development of secondary sex characteristics and sexual function if IBD begins before puberty
- Decreased fertility
Coping–stress tolerance pattern
- Feelings of hopelessness and despair
- Use of somatization (recurrent, multiple physical complaints with no organic cause), expressions of helplessness, crying, excessive demands on staff time, and excessive praise as mechanisms for individual coping

Physical findings
Cardiovascular
- Hypotension
- Tachycardia
- Arrhythmias
Renal
- Decreased output
- Fecal material in urine (if bladder fistula present)
Gastrointestinal
- Diarrhea
- Weight loss
- Hyperactive or hypoactive bowel sounds
- Abdominal tenderness and mass
- Abdominal distention and rigidity
- Rectal bleeding
- Liver tenderness
Neurologic
- Restlessness
- Irritability
- Blurred vision (uncommon)
- Iritis (uncommon)
- Conjunctivitis (uncommon)
- Uveitis (uncommon)
Integumentary
- Poor skin turgor
- Pallor
- Pustules (uncommon)
- Erythematous lesions (uncommon)
- Pyoderma gangrenosum (uncommon skin infection)
- Icterus (if hepatitis present)

- Draining fistulas (particularly around umbilicus or surgical scars)
- Ecchymoses
Musculoskeletal
- Muscle weakness
- Joint pain and tenderness
- Ankylosing spondylitis (uncommon)

Diagnostic studies
- Complete blood count — may reveal moderate elevation in white blood cell (WBC) count, unless perforation is present (which causes a major elevation above normal); hemoglobin level and hematocrit are decreased with chronic blood loss; if blood loss is sudden and dramatic, hemoglobin level and hematocrit may not immediately reflect the change in blood volume; the red blood cell (RBC) count may reflect megaloblastic anemia if the part of the ileum responsible for vitamin B absorption is affected
- Electrolyte profile — sodium, potassium, and chloride may be deficient with persistent or acute loss of fluids from the GI tract with inadequate replacement
- Total protein levels — decreased because a significant amount of protein is lost in inflammatory exudate in the bowel and through bleeding of damaged tissues, which can deplete albumin and other plasma proteins
- Blood urea nitrogen (BUN) level — decreased because significant nutritional deficits cause the catabolism of body proteins; reflected in negative nitrogen balance
- Bleeding and clotting time — prolonged because vitamin K synthesis decreases as bowel surfaces are destroyed; liver involvement may disturb clotting factor synthesis, altering clotting mechanisms
- Stool studies — culture and sensitivity testing and examination for ova and parasites and fecal leukocyte count are usually ordered to rule out an infectious origin for the symptoms; a guaiac test is usually abnormal for occult blood; fat may also be found in stools (steatorrhea) if destruction of bowel surfaces impairs bile reabsorption
- Liver function tests — hepatitis is a complication of IBD; consequently, elevated bilirubin and liver enzyme levels may be observed
- Alkaline phosphatase levels — increased if arthritic skeletal involvement or hepatitis is present
- Urine studies — culture and sensitivity testing may be ordered if a fistula to the bladder is suspected; opportunistic infections may also occur in the genitourinary tract from overall immunosuppression
- Tuberculin skin test — tuberculosis of the cecum may mimic symptoms of IBD
- Antibody titers — anticolon antibodies are demonstrated commonly in patients with ulcerative colitis but not usually observed in other IBD patients

Gastrointestinal disorders

• Carcinoembryonic antigen — may be ordered for patients with ulcerative colitis because they tend to develop colon cancer after 10 years with the disorder
• Barium enema — in ulcerative colitis, demonstrates the characteristic obliteration of haustral folds, blurring of bowel margins, and narrowing and stenosis of the large bowel; in regional enteritis, changes usually found in the small bowel but may occur in the large bowel, so distinguishing between the two disorders on the basis of a barium enema is difficult; procedure may be omitted if abscess or fistula is suspected because the bowel preparation for the procedure, and the procedure itself, may aggravate the condition
• Carotene and Schilling tests — reflect the intestine's absorptive capacity; estimate degree of damaged bowel surface in regional enteritis
• Proctoscopy or colonoscopy — demonstrates hyperemic, edematous, friable bowel mucosa; if lesion is beyond the ileocecal valve, narrowing and stenosis of the valve may be evident
• Rectal biopsy — inflammation and abscesses of the crypts are evident in ulcerative colitis; biopsy usually does not contribute to regional enteritis diagnosis
• Computed tomography scan — reveals abdominal masses that could be fistulas or abscesses

• Upper GI series — lesions in regional enteritis can occur at any point along the GI tract and tend to alternate with segments of normal tissue; upper GI series reveals the extent of involvement and indicates segments where scarring and stenosis may obstruct intestinal flow
• Skeletal X-rays — used to demonstrate the presence and extent of arthritic changes and ankylosing spondylitis, which can occur with IBD

Potential complications
• Malnutrition
• Bowel obstruction
• Arrhythmias
• Peritonitis
• Hepatitis
• Sepsis
• Toxic megacolon
• Malabsorption syndrome
• Gangrenous skin lesions
• Ankylosing spondylitis
• Exudative retinopathy
• Kidney stones
• Pericarditis
• Carcinoma of the colon

CLINICAL SNAPSHOT

INFLAMMATORY BOWEL DISEASE

Major nursing diagnoses and collaborative problems	Key patient outcomes
Risk for cardiac arrhythmias	Show stable vital signs: typically, heart rate, 60 to 100 beats/minute; systolic blood pressure, 90 to 140 mm Hg; and diastolic blood pressure, 50 to 90 mm Hg.
Risk for fluid volume deficit	Maintain urine output within normal limits.
Nutritional deficit	Tolerate diet without undue distress.
Risk for infection	Show no signs of infection.
Pain	Rate pain as less than 3 on a 0 to 10 pain rating scale.
Sleep pattern disturbance	Experience adequate rest and sleep.
Impaired perianal skin integrity	Show no evidence of skin breakdown.
Social isolation	Decrease use of ineffective coping behaviors.
Risk for altered sexuality patterns	Identify techniques for minimizing physical demands of sexual activity.

COLLABORATIVE PROBLEM

Risk for cardiac arrhythmias related to electrolyte depletion

Nursing priority

Maintain electrolyte levels within normal limits.

Patient outcome criteria

• Within 24 hours of admission, the patient will show vital signs within normal limits: typically, heart rate, 60 to 100 beats/minute; systolic blood pressure, 90 to 140 mm Hg; and diastolic blood pressure, 50 to 90 mm Hg.
• Within 3 days of admission, the patient will:
  – have serum electrolyte levels within normal limits
  – display normal cardiac rate and rhythm.

Interventions

1. Monitor and record fluid losses. Evaluate serum electrolyte levels daily, as ordered. Monitor apical and radial pulses, changes in tendon reflexes, and muscle strength every 4 hours or more frequently, depending on the severity of the patient's condition.

2. Administer and document electrolyte replacement therapy.

3. Notify the doctor immediately of any evidence of arrhythmias (for example, pulse irregularity, syncopal episodes, or altered level of consciousness [LOC]). See Appendix C, Fluid and Electrolyte Imbalances.

4. Additional individualized interventions: _____

Rationales

1. Diarrhea and internal fluid sequestration can cause significant electrolyte loss. Frequent observations for signs of alterations in the cellular membrane potential are necessary. Reminders to the doctor to order electrolyte determinations may also be necessary.

2. Normal saline or lactated Ringer's solution and potassium supplements usually are ordered during the acute stage, when oral replacement may be contraindicated.

3. Cardiac arrest can occur without warning in severe hypokalemia or hyperkalemia. The Fluid and Electrolyte Imbalances appendix provides details on specific imbalances.

4. Rationales: _____

NURSING DIAGNOSIS

Risk for fluid volume deficit related to decreased fluid intake, increased fluid loss through diarrhea or internal sequestration of fluid, or hemorrhage

Nursing priority

Maintain fluid balance or replace fluid loss to improve cellular perfusion.

Patient outcome criteria

• Within 24 hours of admission, the patient will:
  – show stable vital signs: typically, heart rate, 60 to 100 beats/minute; systolic blood pressure, 90 to 140 mm Hg; and diastolic blood pressure, 50 to 90 mm Hg
  – maintain urine output of at least 30 ml/hour
  – show good skin turgor.
• Within 3 days of admission, the patient will maintain urine output within normal limits.

Gastrointestinal disorders

Interventions

1. Measure and document hourly urine output with specific gravity determinations for the acutely ill patient. Report a urine output of less than 30 ml/hour. Weigh the patient daily.

2. Maintain accurate records of the type and amount of fluid lost.

3. Monitor and record skin color, turgor, and temperature; LOC; body temperature; and vital signs every 1 to 4 hours, depending on the severity of the patient's condition. Note trends.

4. Auscultate and palpate the abdomen, and observe for increasing pain. Document evidence of distention and changes in bowel sounds.

5. Administer and document fluid replacement, as ordered.

6. Additional individualized interventions: _____

Rationales

1. Urine output and specific gravity determinations provide an immediate, objective indication of the need for volume replacement. Weight loss may indicate loss of fluid volume.

2. The type and amount of fluid lost will guide replacement therapy.

3. A persistent or dramatic change in the parameters listed indicates either sequestration of fluid or blood volume loss. Hypovolemia is indicated by hypotension, tachycardia, and signs of decreased peripheral perfusion.

4. Sudden, acute distention, increased pain, and loss of or diminished bowel sounds can be early indications of serious bowel injury. Increased bowel activity may also indicate early obstruction or increasing tissue damage and inflammation.

5. The preferred route for fluid replacement is by mouth. However, the IBD patient may be too ill or oral replacement may increase distressing symptoms. I.V. fluids usually include volume expanders such as normal saline solution. Whole blood or packed RBCs may also be ordered if hypotension is related to blood loss.

6. Rationales: _____

NURSING DIAGNOSIS

Nutritional deficit related to decreased nutrient intake, increased nutrient loss, and possible decreased bowel absorption

Nursing priorities
• Maintain or increase body weight.
• Improve general nutritional status.

Patient outcome criteria
• Within 2 days of admission, the patient will comply with the agreed-upon treatment plan.
• By the time of discharge, the patient will:
  – gain mutually agreed-upon weight
  – perform activities of daily living (ADLs)
  – tolerate diet without undue distress.

Interventions

1. Estimate and document the extent of the nutritional deficit based on body weight; character, color, and texture of hair and skin; the presence or absence of corneal plaques, cracked and bleeding gums and mucous membranes, muscle wasting and weakness, and anemia; changes in visual acuity; and decreased BUN level.

Rationales

1. Rapidly reproducing cells, such as those of the hair, skin, mucous membranes, and retinas, tend to be the first to demonstrate the changes characteristic of nutritional deficit. Later manifestations of a severe deficit include muscle wasting, weakness, decreased BUN level, and anemia.

2. Collaborate with the patient, family, and other health team members to set goals and plan for normal nutritional maintenance.

2. The IBD patient tends to ignore dietary recommendations and may eat irritating foods. The IBD patient also learns to associate food and fluid intake with unpleasant sensations and may voluntarily decrease intake to avoid distressing symptoms. The patient must have the support of both family and caregivers for the dietary plan to succeed.

3. Administer medications, as ordered, to control peristalsis before meals.

3. The presence of food in the gut stimulates peristalsis and causes increased discomfort and diarrhea. Diphenoxylate hydrochloride with atropine sulfate (Lomotil) or camphorated opium tincture (paregoric) are commonly used to control peristalsis.

4. Serve small, frequent meals rather than three large meals a day. Assess patient response.

4. Small, frequent meals tend to be better tolerated and cause fewer distressing symptoms.

5. Administer I.V. nutritional supplements, such as fat emulsions (Intralipid) and vitamins, or total parenteral nutrition, as ordered. See the "Total parenteral nutrition" plan, page 527, for further details.

5. I.V. nutritional supplements or total parenteral nutrition may be indicated for the IBD patient who cannot take anything by mouth, to rest the gut and promote healing, and for the patient too malnourished to tolerate surgery. Vitamin B_{12} is useful in reversing anemia associated with decreased blood cell formation and for treating immunosuppression associated with chronic inflammation. The "Total parenteral nutrition" plan contains details about this therapy.

6. Additional individualized interventions: _____

6. Rationales: _____

Nursing diagnosis

Risk for infection related to bowel perforation, immunosuppression, and general debilitation

Nursing priority

Prevent opportunistic infections.

Patient outcome criteria

By the time of discharge, the patient will:
• have a normal body temperature
• show no signs of infection.

Interventions

1. Monitor and record vital signs, body temperature, bowel sounds, breath sounds, urine character and odor, and the presence or absence of abdominal distention, joint pain, hepatic tenderness, icterus, increasing malaise, and exudative skin or eye lesions.

2. Administer antibiotics, as ordered.

3. Obtain specimens for culture and sensitivity testing, as ordered, before beginning antibiotic therapy.

Rationales

1. The patient with IBD is susceptible to many opportunistic infections. Close observation is necessary because such infections may not produce the usual dramatic rise in body temperature and WBC count as a result of medication-related immunosuppression and the condition's chronicity.

2. Typically, broad-spectrum antibiotics such as sulfasalazine (Azulfidine) are ordered as a prophylactic measure.

3. Culture and sensitivity testing tend to be inaccurate when performed after initiation of antibiotic therapy.

Gastrointestinal disorders

4. Practice careful aseptic technique for all nursing procedures.

5. Question orders for extensive bowel preparation for the patient with abdominal tenderness or masses, decreased or absent bowel sounds, or abdominal distention or rigidity.

6. Additional individualized interventions: _____

_____

4. The IBD patient tends to be immunosuppressed, as noted previously.

5. Enemas and purgatives are irritants that can cause or exacerbate detrimental changes in the patient with acute abdominal pathology.

6. Rationales: _____

_____

NURSING DIAGNOSIS

Pain related to abdominal and possible skeletal pathology

Nursing priority

Prevent or control pain.

Patient outcome criteria

Within 3 days of admission, the patient will verbalize pain relief.
By the time of discharge, the patient will:
• verbalize rationale for pain-control measures
• use nonpharmacologic pain-control methods, as appropriate
• rate pain as less than 3 on a 0 to 10 pain rating scale.

Interventions

1. Assess and document complaints of pain, using a 0 to 10 pain rating scale. Be especially alert for sudden and severe abdominal pain, guarding, rigidity, or distention, and for vomiting, and report their occurrence to the doctor immediately.

2. Administer appropriate analgesic medication, as ordered. Teach the patient about nonpharmacologic pain control measures. See the "Pain" plan, page 88.

3. Administer anti-inflammatory medications, as ordered, and document their therapeutic and adverse effects.

4. Additional individualized interventions: _____

_____

Rationales

1. Changes in the character and severity of abdominal pain may indicate a life-threatening condition, such as perforation of the GI tract.

2. Narcotic analgesics are administered judiciously in IBD because they tend to mask potentially life-threatening conditions. Medications that inhibit GI motility and abdominal cramping, such as diphenoxylate hydrochloride with atropine sulfate or camphorated opium tincture, may be ordered. Skeletal discomfort related to arthritis is best handled with gentle exercise, warm soaks, and frequent repositioning because many of the oral anti-inflammatory medications used to control skeletal pain are GI irritants. The "Pain" plan contains general interventions for pain control.

3. Control of IBD reduces distressing and painful symptoms. Common medications used to suppress inflammation include hydrocortisone sodium succinate (Solu-Cortef), methylprednisolone sodium succinate (Solu-Medrol), and dexamethasone (Decadron).

4. Rationales: _____

_____

NURSING DIAGNOSIS

Sleep pattern disturbance related to uncomfortable sensations, possible anxiety related to hospitalization, nocturnal defecation, or change in usual sleep environment

Nursing priority

Promote adequate rest and sleep.

Patient outcome criteria

• Within 2 days of admission, the patient will verbalize feelings of being rested.
• Throughout the hospital stay, the patient will experience adequate rest and sleep.

Interventions

1. Ask the patient to describe the usual sleep environment; when possible, modify the patient's surroundings to match that environment.

2. Avoid performing prolonged or painful procedures within the hour before bedtime.

3. Group all nursing procedures that must be done while the patient sleeps.

4. Encourage the patient to express fears. Offer reassurance as appropriate.

5. Allow the patient to follow rituals that promote sleep at home.

6. Reposition the patient for comfort, and offer soothing back rubs.

7. Provide a bedside commode for night use. Administer antidiarrheal medication at bedtime.

8. Additional individualized interventions: _____

Rationales

1. An unfamiliar environment may inhibit sleep.

2. Autonomic nervous system stimulation, with increased catecholamine secretion, may interfere with sleep.

3. The sleep cycle is 90 to 120 minutes long. Grouping nursing procedures allows the patient to complete sleep cycles.

4. Some patients may equate sleep with death. They may need to be reassured that the staff will be available to meet their needs.

5. At home, most individuals follow sleep rituals such as reading that help them fall asleep.

6. If the patient is on bed rest, immobility can increase discomfort.

7. These measures help minimize sleep disturbance related to nocturnal defecation.

8. Rationales: _____

NURSING DIAGNOSIS

Impaired perianal skin integrity related to frequent stools and altered nutritional status

Nursing priority

Prevent skin breakdown.

Patient outcome criterion

By the time of discharge, the patient will show no evidence of skin breakdown.

Gastrointestinal disorders

Interventions

1. Provide and document perianal care after each bowel movement.

2. Institute and document a skin care routine, based on the patient's general condition, to be performed every 2 to 4 hours.

3. Promote and document food and fluid intake, paying special attention to protein consumption.

4. Additional individualized interventions: _____

Rationales

1. The acid secretions and digestive enzymes from diarrhea quickly excoriate the perianal area. A protective ointment, such as lanolin and petroleum jelly (A&D), is commonly used because the skin is vulnerable to breakdown.

2. Anticipating and preventing skin breakdown on other body surfaces is important because tissue damage heals slowly, if at all, in the critically ill IBD patient.

3. Adequate intake of nutrients (especially protein) and fluids is necessary for tissue repair.

4. Rationales: _____

Nursing diagnosis

Social isolation related to dependent behavior

Nursing priorities

• Decrease use of dependent behavior.
• Facilitate direct expression of feelings.

Patient outcome criteria

By the time of discharge, the patient will:
• decrease use of ineffective coping behaviors
• express anger, hostility, and anxiety appropriately.

Interventions

1. Identify dependent behavior for patient, self, staff, and family.

2. Collaborate with staff and family to set limits on unacceptable behavior. Ensure that all staff members agree to maintain the limits and to share concerns with each other.

3. Avoid bargaining about or justifying limits. Enforce them without apology.

4. Discuss the patient's feelings concerning limits. Encourage expression of feelings of anxiety, hostility, and anger.

5. Investigate somatic complaints immediately and matter-of-factly.

Rationales

1. Dependent behavior may be manifested by crying, expressions of hopelessness, endless requests for staff attention, or excessive praise of staff. Although such behavior represents an attempt to control and manage underlying feelings of anger, hostility, and anxiety, it commonly provokes social isolation, reinforcing negative feelings.

2. Limit setting and consistent enforcement allow the patient to know exactly what is expected and interrupts the cycle of dependency and isolation. The dependent patient may attempt to turn staff members against each other through manipulative behavior.

3. Engaging in dialogue concerning limits creates doubt about their enforcement.

4. The patient may have difficulty identifying feelings. A nonjudgmental atmosphere provides a way to recognize and discuss uncomfortable emotions.

5. Somatization is an attention-getting behavior used by people with inadequate coping skills. The seriousness of the illness warrants investigation of complaints; avoid prolonged discussions of physical complaints, however, and focus instead on the patient's feelings.

6. If behavioral problems persist, consult a psychiatric clinical nurse specialist or other mental health professional.

7. Additional individualized interventions: _____

6. A mental health professional can offer expertise for dealing with manipulative behavior and the staff's negative response to such behavior.

7. Rationales: _____

NURSING DIAGNOSIS

Risk for altered sexuality patterns related to diminished physical energy and persistence of uncomfortable physical symptoms

Nursing priority

Encourage the discussion and expression of sexual desires.

Patient outcome criteria

By the time of discharge, the patient will:
• discuss sexual feelings openly with partner, if desired
• identify techniques for minimizing physical demands of sexual activity.

Interventions

1. Initiate discussion about values, beliefs, and feelings concerning sexuality. Assess for sexual dysfunction. Include the patient's spouse or partner in discussions, if possible.

2. Allow the patient to discuss feelings, values, and beliefs concerning sexuality in a nonjudgmental atmosphere. It is important to be aware of personal feelings about sexuality. If you are too uncomfortable to counsel the patient and spouse or partner effectively, make an appropriate referral.

3. To the extent possible, allow the patient and spouse or partner uninterrupted private time together.

4. Construct a teaching plan for sexual expression. Address energy-conserving positions for intercourse, timing activity to coincide with peak energy levels, alternatives to intercourse, specific patient concerns, and potential interactions between contraceptives and medications used to treat IBD.

Rationales

1. Discussions concerning sexuality are difficult for many patients to initiate, although the topic may be of considerable importance. The nurse must anticipate that altered sexual function is common in patients who have chronic or debilitating illnesses and who have diminished energy and persistent, uncomfortable physical sensations. The IBD patient may also be facing surgery for fecal diversion; thus, body-image changes and altered sexual function should be anticipated. The patient may or may not communicate openly with the spouse or partner. Both may welcome frank discussions of sexual matters.

2. The nurse's values and beliefs concerning sexual behavior may interfere with the ability to provide professional care. If this occurs, referral to another professional may provide acceptance and counsel to benefit the patient and partner.

3. Sexuality can be expressed in many forms besides sexual intercourse, such as cuddling and fondling. The IBD patient may be hospitalized for prolonged periods and needs privacy to express intimate feelings.

4. The sexual intercourse guidelines for cardiac patients can be modified to meet the needs of the patient with chronic IBD who has diminished physical energy and uncomfortable physical sensations. Patient teaching should also cover the potential interactions between various types of contraceptives and the medications used to treat chronic IBD to prevent unexpected contraceptive failure.

Gastrointestinal disorders

5. Additional individualized interventions: _____

5. Rationales: _____

DISCHARGE PLANNING

Discharge checklist
Before discharge, the patient shows evidence of:
- ❑ absence of fever
- ❑ absence of signs and symptoms of infection
- ❑ stable vital signs
- ❑ ability to tolerate oral nutritional intake
- ❑ I.V. lines discontinued for at least 24 hours before discharge
- ❑ stabilized weight
- ❑ ability to control pain using oral medications
- ❑ ability to perform perianal care
- ❑ controlled bowel movements
- ❑ absence of skin breakdown
- ❑ electrolyte levels within acceptable parameters
- ❑ ability to ambulate and perform ADLs
- ❑ adequate home support system, or referral to home care if indicated by inability to perform ADLs and perianal care independently, by inadequacy of the home support system, or by the need to reinforce teaching.

Teaching checklist
Document evidence that the patient and family demonstrate an understanding of:
- ❑ extent of disease
- ❑ all discharge medications' purpose, dosage, administration schedule, and adverse effects requiring medical attention (usual discharge medications include steroids and immunosuppressants)
- ❑ recommended dietary modifications (usual diet is low-fiber, low-residue, and bland)
- ❑ community support groups and resources, including an ostomy club, when appropriate
- ❑ resumption of normal role activity
- ❑ signs and symptoms indicating exacerbation of illness
- ❑ date, time, and location of follow-up appointments
- ❑ how to contact the doctor.

Documentation checklist
Using outcome criteria as a guide, document:
- ❑ clinical status on admission
- ❑ significant changes in status
- ❑ pertinent laboratory and diagnostic findings
- ❑ pain-relief measures
- ❑ I.V. line patency
- ❑ fluid intake
- ❑ acute abdominal pain episodes
- ❑ use of emergency protocols

- ❑ nutritional intake
- ❑ other therapies
- ❑ patient and family teaching
- ❑ discharge planning.

ASSOCIATED PLANS OF CARE
Colostomy
Grieving
Ineffective individual coping
Pain
Total parenteral nutrition

REFERENCES
Corbett, J. *Laboratory Tests and Diagnostic Tests with Nursing Diagnoses.* Stamford, Conn.: Appleton & Lange, 1997.
Guyton, A., and Hall, J. *Textbook of Medical Physiology,* 9th ed. Philadelphia: W.B. Saunders Co., 1996.
Luckman, J., and Sorenson, K. *Medical Surgical Nursing.* Philadelphia: W.B. Saunders Co., 1996.
Noble, J., ed. *Textbook of Primary Care Medicine,* 2nd ed. St. Louis: Mosby Year–Book, Inc., 1996.
Spencer, R., et al. *Clinical Pharmacology and Nursing Management.* Philadelphia: Lippincott-Raven Pubs., 1996.

Total parenteral nutrition

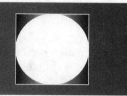

DRG information

DRG 296   Nutritional and Miscellaneous Metabolic Disorders; Age 17+ with Complication or Comorbidity (CC).
Mean LOS = 6.1 days

DRG 297   Nutritional and Miscellaneous Metabolic Disorders; Age 17+ without CC.
Mean LOS = 4.1 days

DRG 298   Nutritional and Miscellaneous Metabolic Disorders; Ages 0 to 17.
Mean LOS = 3.2 days
Principal diagnoses include:
- anorexia
- dehydration
- malnutrition.

Additional DRG information: Total parenteral nutrition (TPN) is used to treat numerous disorders. The diagnosis necessitating its use determines the DRG assigned. Examples of diagnoses and DRGs that may require TPN are listed above. Several others associated with cancer could also require TPN but were omitted here for brevity.

INTRODUCTION

Definition and time focus

TPN is the delivery of nutrients through a venous infusion of glucose, amino acids, fats, vitamins, and trace elements in sufficient quantities to promote growth, weight gain, anabolism, and wound healing. The patient requiring TPN typically exhibits one of four problems:

- cannot eat — the patient may have an obstruction or ileus at any point along the GI tract or may be at risk for aspiration if fed orally
- will not eat — the geriatric, cancer, or anorexic patient may be unwilling to ingest food
- should not eat — the patient may have a disease or condition aggravated by oral intake, such as intestinal fistula, severe pancreatitis, small-bowel obstruction, or inflammatory bowel disease
- cannot eat enough — the patient has such a severe disease or degree of injury that sufficient nutrients cannot be provided enterally. Examples are short-bowel syndrome, multiple trauma, and major burns.

  TPN is indicated when:
- the patient has a nonfunctioning GI tract
- the patient is in a stressed state or preexisting state of malnutrition that precludes waiting until the GI tract is available

- the patient has an irreversible condition that will preclude using the GI tract in the foreseeable future.

  Safe delivery of TPN depends on four basic principles of care:
- aseptic technique in catheter placement
- aseptic technique in catheter care
- proper preparation and delivery of the TPN solution
- careful patient monitoring.

  This plan focuses on the patient who requires TPN to maintain nutritional status during the hospital stay.

FOCUSED ASSESSMENT GUIDELINES

Nursing history (functional health pattern findings)

Health perception–health management pattern
- Chronic illness or have an acute condition that increases nutritional needs

Activity-exercise pattern
- Decreased energy level
- Generalized weakness or weak extremities related to muscle wasting

Nutritional-metabolic pattern
- Nausea, vomiting, diarrhea, or constipation
- Lack of appetite
- Recent weight loss
- Lack of interest in food
- Improperly fitting dentures
- Chronically thirsty
- Change in the taste of food

Physical findings

Clinical signs of malnutrition are rarely observed and may not be recognized as clinically significant.

Musculoskeletal
- Generalized muscle wasting and weakness (muscle mass and major organs are spared unless the patient has moderate to severe malnutrition)
- Edematous extremities

Integumentary
- Skin — subcutaneous fat loss, scaly dermatitis (primarily on legs and feet), pellagrous dermatitis, seborrheic dermatitis of face, nasolabial seborrhea (greasy and scaly skin of the nasolabial folds of the nose, from riboflavin deficiency), thinning of the innermost layer of the epidermis (possibly from vitamin A deficiency), dilated veins, petechiae, purpura, poor skin turgor, dry mucous membranes

• Hair—increased pluckability, lack of luster, alopecia, sparsity, decreased pigmentation
• Nails—brittle, lined, increased rigidity, thin, flattened or spoon-shaped

Eye
• Xerosis (dryness) of conjunctivae
• Keratomalacia (a condition linked to vitamin A deficiency that causes softening of the cornea; early signs include xerotic spots on conjunctivae and xerotic, insensitive, and hazy cornea)
• Corneal vascularization
• Blepharitis (scaly inflammation of eyelid edges)
• Bitot's spots (gray, triangular conjunctival spots, linked to vitamin A deficiency)
• "Spectacle eye" (inflammation of the periorbital skin associated with a vitamin B [biotin] deficiency)

Neurologic
• Lethargy
• Hyporeflexia
• Decreased proprioception
• Disorientation
• Confabulation
• Paresthesia
• Weakness of legs
• Irritability
• Seizures
• Flaccid paralysis
• Confusion

Gastrointestinal
• Tongue—baldness, glossitis, edema
• Lips—cheilosis, angular stomatitis

Glandular
• Parotid enlargement
• Thyroid enlargement

Diagnostic studies
See *Major elements monitored in TPN.*

Potential complications
• Sepsis
• Mechanical injury from catheter
  – Pneumothorax, hemothorax
  – Arterial puncture
  – Air emboli
  – Catheter emboli
  – Catheter and venous thrombosis
• Metabolic disorders
  – Hypoglycemia
  – Fluid and electrolyte abnormalities
  – Hyperglycemia
  – Essential fatty acid deficiency

CLINICAL SNAPSHOT

TOTAL PARENTERAL NUTRITION

Major nursing diagnoses and collaborative problems	Key patient outcomes
Risk for injury	Show no signs of catheter-related injury.
Nutritional deficit	Exhibit increased weight, muscle strength, and energy level.
Risk for fluid volume excess or deficit	Manifest no signs or symptoms of fluid imbalance.
Knowledge deficit (TPN care)	List signs and symptoms of potential TPN complications.
Risk for infection	Show no signs or symptoms of infection.

NURSING DIAGNOSIS

Risk for injury related to complications of TPN catheter insertion, displacement, use, or removal

Nursing priority

Prevent or promptly treat complications that may result from TPN catheter.

Patient outcome criteria

While the central venous catheter (CVC) is in place, the patient will:
• exhibit unrestricted, pain-free inhalation and exhalation
• exhibit symmetrical chest movement
• exhibit normal respirations
• present a normal chest X-ray
• have a patent catheter
• show no fluid infiltration
• show no evidence of catheter emboli.

Interventions

1. Observe for signs and symptoms of respiratory distress and shock during insertion of the CVC, including tachypnea, tachycardia, dropping systolic blood pressure, dyspnea, use of accessory muscles for respiration, and decreased or absent breath sounds on side of insertion.

2. Maintain the patient in Trendelenburg's position during CVC insertion.

3. After CVC insertion, assess for bilateral breath sounds in all lung fields and ensure that a chest X-ray is obtained. Monitor the patient's respiratory status and breath sounds at least every 8 hours thereafter.

Rationales

1. After using a local anesthetic, the doctor inserts the catheter into the subclavian or internal jugular vein and positions the tip in the superior vena cava. He then sutures the catheter in place and applies an occlusive dressing. The lungs or an artery may be punctured during subclavian venous cannulation. The artery may bleed to the point of compressing the trachea, causing life-threatening respiratory distress. A puncture of the lung creates a pneumothorax, causing respiratory compromise from entry of air into the pleural space and collapse of all or part of the lung on the venipuncture side.

2. Trendelenburg's position increases venous pressure in the upper half of the body. This prevents air influx into the venous system through the insertion needle or I.V. catheters when their lumens are open to air.

3. Bilateral breath sounds and symmetrical pain-free chest movement indicate fully inflated lungs. Chest X-ray confirms placement of the catheter tip in the superior vena cava and rules out hemothorax, chylothorax (from puncture of a lymph vessel), and pneumothorax.

Major elements monitored in TPN

Glucose — serum levels may be elevated above 200 mg/dl when total parenteral nutrition (TPN) infusion is begun, decreasing to 150 to 200 mg/dl after 24 to 48 hours as body adjusts to increased glucose load. (Serum glucose levels greater than 200 mg/dl indicate glucose intolerance or hyperglycemia. Levels less than 60 mg/dl indicate hypoglycemia, the more dangerous of the two states; without glucose, the brain cannot function and death is imminent if hypoglycemia continues.)

Electrolytes — sodium, potassium, and chloride levels obtained for baseline and as guide for replacement therapy. (Fluid and electrolyte management is the most important aspect of TPN because the patient requiring nutritional repletion typically has fluid and electrolyte abnormalities. Electrolytes are provided as needed to replace loss from fistulas, nasogastric [NG] drainage, diarrhea, or excessive output or — in an appropriate ratio — to promote lean muscle mass, nutritional repletion, and positive nitrogen balance.)

Magnesium — low serum levels may occur in intestinal malabsorption syndrome, bowel resection, intestinal fistula, or in patients with extended NG suction. (Magnesium requirements increase with nutritional repletion related to new tissue synthesis: 0.35 to 0.45 mEq/kg/day is sufficient to prevent magnesium depletion in patients receiving TPN. Magnesium levels need to be monitored at least every week and twice a week for patients in renal failure. The normal range of magnesium is 1.4 to 2.2 mEq/L.)

Phosphorus — low serum levels occur in patients receiving TPN because of increased use of phosphorus for glucose metabolism. (For each kilocalorie of TPN administered, 2 mEq/dl of phosphorus is required. Serum levels should be measured weekly. Serum phosphorus levels below 1 mg/dl will produce clinical signs and symptoms of hypophosphatemia. The normal range is 2.5 to 4.5 mg/dl.)

4. Do not begin administering the TPN solution until the position of the catheter tip is confirmed by chest X-ray.

5. Use locking (luer-lock) connections, or tape the connections securely.

6. Before opening the I.V. system to the air, instruct the patient to perform Valsalva's maneuver (hold the breath and bear down), or clamp the catheter. If the patient is unable to perform Valsalva's maneuver, change the tubing only during exhalation.

7. Observe for signs and symptoms of air emboli, such as extreme anxiousness, sharp chest pain, cyanosis, or churning precordial murmur. If air emboli are suspected, position the patient in Trendelenburg's position on the left side, administer oxygen, and notify the doctor immediately.

8. During dressing changes, observe for a suture at the insertion site of a temporary CVC, a suture at the exit site of a permanent CVC, or increased external catheter length.

9. Observe for inability to withdraw blood; complaints of chest pain or burning; leaking fluid; and swelling around the insertion site, shoulder, clavicle, and upper extremity.

10. Observe for visible collateral circulation on the chest wall.

11. When the catheter is being removed, be sure that:

• the patient is supine

• the patient performs Valsalva's maneuver before the catheter is removed

• a completely sealed airtight dressing is applied over the insertion site after the CVC is removed.

12. When the catheter is removed, measure its length and observe for jagged edges.

13. Additional individualized interventions: _____

---

4. The hyperosmolar TPN solution irritates veins smaller than the superior vena cava. Thrombophlebitis can result if the TPN solution is infused into the jugular, subclavian, or innominate vein.

5. Secure connections are essential to prevent accidental tubing disconnection. Accidental disconnection may cause bleeding, loss of catheter patency from clot formation, air emboli, hub contamination, and sepsis.

6. Valsalva's maneuver increases intrathoracic pressure, forcing blood through the area of least resistance (in this case, the catheter) and preventing inflow of air. Air will enter the catheter only as the patient inhales. (Negative intrathoracic pressure allows the lungs to fill with air. If the I.V. catheter is open to the air during inhalation, air can be pulled into the bloodstream as well.)

7. Small amounts of air may produce no symptoms. Large amounts, however, may cause an air lock in the heart, in which case no blood can pass through the heart. The patient may die from cardiac arrest related to blocked blood flow and resultant ischemia.

Trendelenburg's and the left lateral recumbent positions allow air to collect at the apex of the right ventricle. Small amounts of air may pass into the pulmonary circulation and be reabsorbed. Large amounts of air in the heart may need to be aspirated through a catheter passed into the right atrium.

8. A suture at the insertion or exit site stabilizes the catheter. Increased external catheter length indicates movement and possible catheter displacement.

9. These signs and symptoms may indicate catheter displacement and vein thrombosis.

10. Development of collateral circulation on the chest wall is a sign of vein thrombosis.

11. Conscientious attention to the details of catheter removal is important for several reasons:
• The supine position allows a clear view while removing stitches and the catheter and applying a sealed dressing.
• Air can be sucked in through the CVC sinus tract if the catheter is pulled out during inhalation, causing air emboli.
• The CVC sinus tract allows air to enter the venous system with each inhalation if an airtight dressing is not applied.

12. To ensure that the entire catheter was removed, the catheter should be measured and inspected for breaks.

13. Rationales: _____

NURSING DIAGNOSIS

Nutritional deficit related to inability to ingest nutrients orally or digest them satisfactorily, or to increased metabolic need

Nursing priority

Provide for adequate nutritional intake.

Patient outcome criteria

- Within 24 hours of starting TPN and throughout TPN therapy, the patient will:
  - maintain normal urine glucose level
  - maintain serum glucose level of 100 to 200 mg/dl
  - show no signs or symptoms of hypoglycemia, hyperglycemia, hyperosmolar hyperglycemic nonketotic syndrome (HHNS), electrolyte imbalance, or vitamin or trace metal deficiencies.
- Within 7 days of starting TPN, the patient will:
  - exhibit weight gain of less than ½ lb (0.2 kg)/day
  - exhibit increased muscle strength
  - exhibit increased energy level
  - verbalize increased sense of well-being.

Interventions

1. Administer the appropriate TPN solution via peripheral or central venous route, including tunneled catheters and peripherally inserted central catheter.

2. Infuse TPN solution at a constant rate with an infusion pump.

- Check the volume of solution, flow rate, and patient tolerance every half hour.

- Do not interrupt the flow of TPN solution.

Rationales

1. TPN solution composition is based on the individual patient's calculated needs. Usual nutrient requirements for critically ill patients include calories, 1,500 to 2,000 kcal/day; protein, 1.2 to 1.5 g/kg/day; fat, 30% of nonprotein calories; trace elements; and vitamins. Peripheral parenteral nutrition contains a lesser concentration of the same ingredients found in central formula TPN. Solutions containing higher concentrations of dextrose (greater than 10%) must be delivered via a central vein because chemical phlebitis may result if a peripheral vein is used.

2. The infusion pump regulates the flow rate with greater accuracy than a standard I.V. set, decreasing the likelihood of accidentally infusing a bag of TPN solution too quickly.
- This prevents a hyperglycemic, hyperosmolar load. (The hyperosmolar state results in osmotic diuresis that can lead to dehydration, lethargy, and coma.)
- Turning TPN on and off at intervals creates fluctuations in the serum glucose level. The pancreas responds to high or low serum glucose by altering the secretion of glucagon and insulin. This system keeps the serum glucose level within the normal range; if changes in flow rate are made too quickly, the body cannot adjust and signs and symptoms of hypoglycemia or hyperglycemia may occur.

Gastrointestinal disorders

• Do not attempt to "catch up" if the TPN infusion is behind schedule or "slow down" if it is ahead of schedule. Set the I.V. infusion to the ordered rate.

• If TPN on gravity drip has fallen behind the ordered drip rate, there will be less glucose circulating in the blood and less insulin secreted to handle the glucose (insulin decreases serum glucose levels by transporting glucose into the cells to be converted to glycogen for storage). A rapid infusion of TPN solution results in a rapid rise in serum glucose to above normal levels without a corresponding increase in insulin production. (The body takes 30 to 60 minutes to sense the high serum glucose level and respond by increasing insulin production.)

The physiologic effect of high serum glucose levels is dehydration. Water is drained out of the interstitial spaces into the vascular system in an attempt to equalize serum and interstitial glucose levels. This results in dehydrated interstitial spaces, causing excessive thirst and hunger. The kidneys sense the increased vascular volume and excrete the excess fluid and glucose. Dehydration, if not treated, will lead to lethargy, confusion, and coma.

• When discontinuing central formula TPN, lower the rate to 50 ml/hour for 3 to 4 hours.

• Slowing the TPN rate to 50 ml/hour for 3 to 4 hours allows the body to sense the lower serum glucose level and adjust to it. The pancreas responds by decreasing insulin production. These mechanisms prevent development of hypoglycemia, which can occur if TPN is discontinued too rapidly.

3. Ensure that the TPN infusion does not stop suddenly, or take appropriate corrective action:

3. If the TPN infusion stops suddenly, another source of glucose must be supplied to prevent hypoglycemia. The high levels of insulin in the bloodstream will deplete the serum glucose level to less than 60 mg/dl within an hour.

• For a clotted catheter, hang dextrose 10% in water at another I.V. site to infuse at the ordered TPN rate.

• Brain cells cannot function without glucose as an energy source. Another source of I.V. glucose prevents a rapid drop in the serum glucose level.

• During cardiopulmonary arrest, stop the TPN infusion and provide one or more boluses of dextrose 50% in water, as ordered.

• This precaution prevents accidentally giving a bolus of TPN solution during an emergency. One or more boluses of dextrose prevents hypoglycemia and allows more control. In an emergency situation, a rapidly decreasing serum glucose level may otherwise go unnoticed.

4. Monitor fingerstick glucose levels and laboratory serum glucose levels every 6 hours, as ordered. Maintain serum glucose level at 100 to 200 mg/dl.

4. Monitoring serum glucose levels evaluates the patient's tolerance of the glucose load being infused. Levels greater than 200 mg/dl may indicate that the body is not using glucose, and additional insulin may be necessary to increase conversion of glucose to glycogen. Levels greater than 200 mg/dl also may indicate new stressors: Medications, surgery, and sepsis all can cause hyperglycemia. To handle the stress, the body increases the amount of glucose available for energy. Blood glucose checks may be less frequent if hyperglycemia does not exist.

5. Observe for signs and symptoms of the following problems:
• hypoglycemia—weakness; agitation; tremors; cold, clammy skin; serum glucose level less than 60 mg/dl

• hyperglycemia—thirst, acetone breath, diuresis, dehydration; serum glucose level above 200 mg/dl

• protein overload—elevated blood urea nitrogen and creatinine levels
• hyperosmolar overload—thirst, headache, lethargy, seizures, and urine positive for glucose and negative for acetone

• electrolyte imbalances (see Appendix C, Fluid and Electrolyte Imbalances)—hypocalcemia (numbness and tingling), hypokalemia (muscle weakness, cramps, paresthesia, lethargy, confusion, ileus, and arrhythmias), hypomagnesemia (confusion, positive Chvostek's sign, and tetany), hyponatremia (lethargy and confusion), and hypophosphatemia (weakness, signs of encephalopathy, and poor resistance to infection). Monitor serum electrolyte levels as ordered, typically daily until stable and then 2 to 3 times a week. Obtain 24-hour urine for urine urea nitrogen once a week for nutritional assessment.

• vitamin and trace mineral deficiencies (see *Signs and symptoms of vitamin and trace mineral deficiencies,* page 534).

6. Infuse I.V. fat emulsion as ordered through one of two infusion methods:

5. The complex nature of TPN therapy places the patient at risk for numerous complications:
• The brain cannot survive without glucose. Death may occur within an hour if glucose levels are not restored to normal.
• Monitoring for signs and symptoms of hyperglycemia promotes early identification of glucose intolerance and its cause. This may be related to a new stress such as sepsis. Unchecked, hyperglycemia leads to osmolar diuresis, causing dehydration, thirst, confusion, lethargy, seizures, and coma.
• Protein overload can cause osmotic diuresis.

• HHNS may occur if the TPN solution is infused over too short a time. A serum osmolar level above 300 mOsm/kg water pulls fluid into the vascular bed to dilute the osmolar load. The excess vascular fluid results in osmotic diuresis. Also, HHNS may occur with simultaneous infusion of TPN solution and tube feeding. To prevent this problem, decrease the TPN rate as the tube feeding rate is increased.
• The Fluid and Electrolyte Imbalances appendix contains general information on these disorders; this section covers information specific to TPN. Fluid and electrolyte status requires careful monitoring for several reasons:
– Increased glucose metabolism and protein synthesis tend to deplete potassium and phosphate; if they are not replaced appropriately with TPN, a deficit may result.
– The primary diagnosis may alter fluid and electrolyte balance. Fluid and electrolyte losses from fistulas, diarrhea, or nasogastric tubes can cause electrolyte and acid-base abnormalities.
– To promote lean body mass repletion and positive nitrogen balance, electrolytes have to be supplied in a specific ratio: phosphorus 0.8 g, sodium 3.9 mg, potassium 3 mEq, chloride 2.5 mEq, and calcium 1.2 mEq for every gram of nitrogen infused.
• Vitamins and trace minerals are necessary for vital processes. Vitamins may function as hormones and as catalysts in enzyme systems. Minerals serve as coenzyme activators and as major factors in the regulation of acid-base and fluid and electrolyte balance.
    Deficiencies of vitamins and minerals result from inadequate intake, inability to digest and absorb, poor utilization of nutrients, excess losses, and increased requirements related to medication or severity of illness.

6. Fat emulsions are used as an adjunct to TPN therapy to prevent essential fatty acid deficiency. Fats also can be used as a source of calories if calories from TPN alone are not sufficient. For example, if hyperglycemia is a consistent problem and insulin cannot control the serum glucose level, the glucose infusion is decreased and the lost calories are supplied as fat.

Gastrointestinal disorders

• through a Y-connector added between the TPN catheter and the I.V. tubing

• as a 3-in-1 solution or total nutrient admixture.

• The Y-connector allows fats to infuse with minimal mixing with the TPN solution, preventing breakdown of the fat emulsion and decreasing the risk of fat emboli. Fats appear to float on top of the TPN solution when administered through a Y-connector.

• The pharmacy can mix carbohydrates, protein, and fat in one bag to hang over a 24-hour period. This method saves nursing time because there is no Y-connector to add and pharmacy time because only one bag must be mixed and dispensed. These solutions are also cost-effective because they use less I.V. tubing and fewer I.V. catheters. They also have the potential for decreased contamination because the catheter requires less manipulation. Most important, the patient is spared the pain of venipuncture for a fat emulsion I.V.

7. If 3-in-1 solution is used, ensure that it is mixed in a ratio of calcium, less than or equal to 15 mEq/L; phosphorus, less than or equal to 30 mEq/L; and magnesium, less than or equal to 10 mEq/L.

7. The milky color of 3-in-1 solutions obscures particulate matter. The ratio listed prevents precipitate formation.

8. Check that the infusion pump delivers the correct volume of 3-in-1 solution. Adjust the infusion rate as needed to ensure delivery of the desired volume.

8. When fats are added to a TPN solution, the solution's increased viscosity may alter infusion pump delivery.

Signs and symptoms of vitamin and trace mineral deficiencies

Vitamin deficiencies are avoided by adding 1 unit of a multivitamin preparation to the TPN solution every day. Trace mineral deficiencies will usually not develop until 2 to 4 weeks after oral intake has stopped.

Water-soluble vitamins	Fat-soluble vitamins	Trace mineral deficiencies
vitamin B complex blepharitis, periorbital fissures, cheilosis, glossitis, weakness, paresthesia of legs, dermatoses	**vitamin A** night blindness, Bitot's spots	**chromium** glucose intolerance, mental confusion
vitamin C (ascorbic acid) bleeding gums, joint and muscle aching	**vitamin D** bone tenderness	**copper** depigmentation of skin and hair within 2 to 4 weeks, kinky hair
	vitamin E myopathy, creatinuria	**iodine** enlarged thyroid, impaired memory, hoarseness, hearing loss
	vitamin K prolonged blood clotting	**manganese** transient dermatitis
		molybdenum night blindness, irritability
		selenium muscle pain and tenderness
		zinc hypogeusia (abnormally diminished sense of taste); moist, excoriated rash in paranasal, anal, and groin areas

9. Observe for fat separation in the 3-in-1 solution as indicated by a yellow ring around the edges of the solution. Stop the infusion if this occurs, and replace the solution bag with a fresh one.

9. The 3-in-1 solution can separate if it is not mixed properly or if it hangs for more than 24 hours. Separation may cause fat emboli.

10. Culture the 3-in-1 solution if the patient develops sepsis.

10. If it becomes contaminated, the 3-in-1 solution is more likely to support microbial growth than a TPN solution without fat.

11. If a separate fat infusion is used, administer it slowly over the first 15 to 20 minutes (1 ml/minute for a 10% fat infusion or 0.5 ml/minute for a 20% fat infusion). Observe for dyspnea, pain at the I.V. site, or chest or back pain. If any of these signs or symptoms occur, stop the infusion and notify the doctor. Otherwise, increase the rate as ordered.

11. Allergic reactions to the fat emulsion may be local or systemic. Slow administration allows time to observe for an allergic reaction before a dangerous amount of antigen is administered. Signs and symptoms listed indicate possible allergic reactions.

12. If the fat emulsion is to be infused separately, infuse it over 4 hours (for a 10% fat emulsion) or 8 hours (for a 20% fat emulsion). Do not allow fat emulsions to hang more than 12 hours unless mixed in a 3-in-1 solution.

12. The patient with renal failure or heart failure may not tolerate an additional 500 ml of fluid 2 to 3 times per week. The slower infusion rate allows the body to assimilate the emulsion and prevents hyperlipidemia.

13. Do not use I.V. filters with separate fat emulsion infusions. When infusing fats on a long-term basis (longer than 3 months), ensure that thiosalicylate-free tubing is used.

13. The fat emulsion particle size exceeds the filter pore size, so the solution will not infuse through the filter. Fats leach thiosalicylate from ordinary tubing; it can accumulate in the body, with unknown effects.

14. Encourage walking or mild exercise to promote nitrogen retention and nutrient use.

14. Exercise improves use of nutrients and promotes lean muscle mass development rather than the storage of fatty acids. Exercise also prevents muscle wasting, which occurs with inactivity.

15. Weigh the patient daily, at the same time, with the same amount of clothing, and using the same scale.

15. Weighing is necessary to determine if nutritional goals are being met. Weight is also used to assess the patient's fluid status. Weight gain of more than ½ lb (0.2 kg) a day may indicate fluid retention.

16. When oral intake resumes, initiate a daily calorie count and measure fat intake. Observe for nausea, vomiting, or diarrhea.

16. Daily monitoring of fat intake and calories provides guidelines for therapy. If used for essential fatty acid deficiency only, I.V. fat emulsions can be discontinued when the patient is taking 10 g of fat per day orally. When the patient can consume 1,000 calories/day or half of the estimated caloric intake without nausea, vomiting, or diarrhea, TPN can be discontinued.

17. Observe for changes in muscle strength, wound healing, and energy level.

17. Increased strength, energy level, sense of well-being, and tissue granulation indicate that TPN is meeting the body's nutritional needs.

18. Additional individualized interventions: _____

18. Rationales: _____

NURSING DIAGNOSIS

Risk for fluid volume excess or deficit related to fluid retention, altered oral intake, or osmotic diuresis

Gastrointestinal disorders

Nursing priority

Maintain optimal fluid balance.

Patient outcome criteria

Throughout TPN therapy, the patient will:
• maintain fluid intake that approximately equals output
• exhibit no signs or symptoms of fluid imbalance
• maintain urine output greater than 200 ml/8 hours
• exhibit weight gain less than ½ lb (0.2 kg)/day.

Interventions

1. See Appendix C, Fluid and Electrolyte Imbalances.

2. Observe for edema, increased pulse rate, and increased blood pressure. If any of these signs are present, consult with the doctor about decreasing overall fluid administration.

3. Observe for thirst, dry mucous membranes, dry skin, decreased urine output, and increased urine specific gravity.

4. Assess breath sounds each shift.

5. Record fluid intake and output each shift. Maintain approximate balance.

6. Weigh the patient daily. For every liter lost or gained, weight should change approximately 2 lb (1 kg). Generally, maintain weight gain at less than ½ lb/day.

7. Additional individualized interventions: _____

Rationales

1. The Fluid and Electrolyte Imbalances appendix contains further details related to fluid and electrolyte disorders.

2. Edema, increased pulse rate, and increased blood pressure may be signs of excess fluid volume. This may result from the body's inability to tolerate the increased cardiac and renal workload imposed by TPN or from the underlying disease itself (for example, heart failure or renal failure). Edema in the malnourished patient is also commonly related to protein depletion, in which circulating serum protein levels are lower than protein levels in the interstitial spaces. This inequality causes fluids to shift into the interstitial spaces to equalize protein-to-fluid ratios.

3. These may be signs and symptoms of fluid deficit or dehydration.

4. Crackles or gurgles may indicate fluid overload.

5. An intake consistently lower than output indicates a fluid deficit and the need for additional fluid to prevent dehydration and renal failure. An intake higher than output may reflect fluid overload and result in pulmonary complications.

6. Daily weight is another way to determine whether the patient is being given too much or too little fluid. Weight gain over ½ lb/day is too rapid and reflects fluid retention.

7. Rationales: _____

NURSING DIAGNOSIS

Knowledge deficit (TPN care) related to lack of experience with TPN

Nursing priority

Teach the patient and family about TPN.

Patient outcome criteria

Within 48 hours of starting TPN, the patient or family will:
• describe TPN on request
• discuss medical reasons for TPN
• discuss the role of the nutrition support service staff
• use appropriate problem-solving skills for hypothetical problems with TPN
• list signs and symptoms of complications and what to do about them.

Interventions

1. Briefly explain the purpose and method of TPN therapy.

• Explain that in TPN calories and nutrients infuse directly into the bloodstream until the patient can resume oral intake.
• Define the roles of the dietitian, nurse, pharmacist, doctor, and other health care team members in TPN.
• Explain that the TPN solution contains carbohydrate, protein, fat, vitamins, and electrolytes and will provide all the calories and protein the patient needs.
• Describe the route and equipment used, the length of time TPN may be infused, and the patient's responsibilities.
• Provide the patient and family with written material on TPN therapy.

2. If the patient is to receive TPN at home, take the following steps:

• Collaborate with the nutrition support service to determine appropriate teaching strategies.

• Teach the signs, symptoms, and necessary actions for managing complications, such as infection, abnormal serum glucose levels, air emboli, clotted catheter, and displaced catheter. Ask the patient to report any signs or symptoms to the nutrition support team.
• Review the information, and answer questions. Ask the patient "what if" questions.

• Provide written instructions on home TPN protocols.

3. See the "Knowledge deficit" plan, page 72, for further details.

4. Additional individualized interventions: _____

Rationales

1. A general understanding of TPN provides a framework within which to understand the specific details of therapy.
• This defines TPN in terms the patient can understand.

• Describing the roles of the health care team members ensures patient awareness of resources.
• Describing the TPN solution may reassure the patient and family.

• A thorough understanding of TPN administration, clear expectations, and acceptance of responsibility for self-monitoring promote optimum therapeutic benefit.
• Written material reinforces the nurse's explanation.

2. TPN is a complex therapy requiring substantial expertise on the patient's part for successful home management.
• The nutrition support service can provide expert advice on adapting teaching to the home setting. The patient receiving TPN at home will need to be followed by the service (or by a home care agency specializing in TPN management).
• Knowledge of how to detect and manage complications may increase the patient's confidence about managing this therapy at home. Prompt reporting facilitates timely intervention.

• Reviewing, clarifying, and using practical "what if" examples promote understanding and boost problem-solving skills.
• Written information reinforces teaching and provides a permanent reference.

3. The "Knowledge deficit" plan contains interventions related to patient teaching.

4. Rationales: _____

Gastrointestinal disorders

NURSING DIAGNOSIS

Risk for infection related to invasive CVC, leukopenia, or damp dressing

Nursing priority

Prevent or detect and promptly treat infection.

Patient outcome criteria

Throughout TPN therapy, the patient will:
• be afebrile
• present urine negative for glucose
• show no infection or inflammation at the catheter site
• maintain serum glucose level between 100 and 200 g/dl.

Interventions

1. Follow hospital protocol for dressing changes. Use sterile technique and standard precautions. Apply a clear, completely sealed dressing.

2. Inspect the dressing every 8 hours, and change it any time it is unsealed or damp.

3. Observe the insertion site every 8 hours for signs and symptoms of infection. Report any redness, swelling, pain, or purulent drainage.

4. Follow hospital protocol for tubing changes and antibacterial preparation at all connections before changing I.V. tubing.

5. Use filter appropriate for type of solution.

6. Infuse only TPN solution through the TPN catheter. Do not use the TPN line for injecting medications or drawing blood samples.

7. Use only solutions prepared in the pharmacy under a laminar flow hood. Do not make any additions on the unit. If additions are necessary, request that they be made in the pharmacy under a laminar flow hood.

8. Return cloudy or precipitated solution to the pharmacy.

9. Allow each bag or bottle to hang no more than 24 hours.

Rationales

1. Good technique decreases the risk of infection. Dressing change frequency ranges from every day to once a week.

2. Moisture and exposure to air encourage microbial growth at the insertion site. Colonization may lead to sepsis.

3. These signs and symptoms may indicate infection of the insertion site.

4. Using proper technique when changing and disconnecting tubing decreases the risk of TPN line contamination. Tubing changes usually are performed every 24 hours.

5. The reason for use of in-line filters centers on removal of microprecipitates rather than microorganisms. Using a 0.22 micron filter for dextrose–amino acid solution with lipids piggybacked below the filter will effectively retain bacteria, fungi, and particulate matter. The total nutrient admixture or 3:1 solution requires the use of a 1.2 micron filter.

6. Using the TPN catheter for other solutions provides another possible source of contamination and increases the risk of sepsis.

7. Preparing the solution in a sterile area decreases the risk of contamination. The laminar flow hood minimizes contamination from airborne microorganisms.

8. Cloudy solution indicates possible bacterial contamination. Precipitate may occlude the catheter or cause thrombus formation.

9. Infusing solutions over longer periods allows for rapid multiplication of any microorganisms inadvertently introduced during mixing of the TPN solution.

10. Monitor for signs and symptoms of infection:
• increased pulse and respiratory rates
• temperature above 101° F (38.3° C)
• white blood cell (WBC) count over 10,000/μl
• serum glucose level over 200 mg/dl
• glycosuria
• chills, diaphoresis, or lethargy.

11. Notify doctor if signs and symptoms of infection are present.

12. Additional individualized interventions: _____
_____

10. A change in vital signs or WBC count, hyperglycemia, glycosuria, chills, or diaphoresis may indicate developing infection.

11. Prompt notification allows the doctor to identify source of infection and order appropriate therapy. Infection may require removal of venous catheter and culture of the tip and any other potential source of infection.

12. Rationales: _____
_____

DISCHARGE PLANNING

Discharge checklist
Before discharge, the patient shows evidence of:
❏ absence of fever
❏ stabilizing weight
❏ absence of pulmonary or cardiovascular complications
❏ electrolytes within acceptable parameters
❏ WBC counts within normal parameters
❏ absence of redness, swelling, pain, and drainage at catheter site
❏ absence of nausea and vomiting
❏ ability to perform activities of daily living (ADLs), transfer, and ambulate same as before hospitalization
❏ adequate home support system, or referral to home care or a nursing home if indicated by an inadequate home support system or the patient's inability to perform ADLs, transfers, and ambulation
❏ a plan for follow-up by nutrition support service or home care agency specializing in TPN for the patient receiving TPN at home.

Teaching checklist
If the patient is to receive TPN at home, document evidence that the patient and family demonstrate an understanding of:
❏ preventing complications
❏ actions to take if complications do occur
❏ where and how to obtain supplies
❏ catheter site care
❏ procedure for TPN administration
❏ community resources
❏ date, time, and location of follow-up appointments
❏ how to contact the doctor.

Documentation checklist
Using outcome criteria as a guide, document:
❏ nutritional status on admission
❏ any significant changes in status
❏ CVC insertion — difficulties or complications; length of catheter; position and any change in position; signs and symptoms of infection, thrombosis, emboli, or other postinsertion complication
❏ dressing and tubing changes
❏ TPN solution and fat emulsion — for each bag or bottle, record date, time, name of nurse hanging solution; all ingredients; rate of infusion
❏ patient and family teaching
❏ discharge planning.

ASSOCIATED PLANS OF CARE
Knowledge deficit
Nutritional deficit

REFERENCES
Anderson, C. "Metabolic Complications of Total Parenteral Nutrition: Effects of a Nutrition Support Service," *Journal of Parenteral and Enteral Nutrition* 20(3):206-10, May-June 1996.

Centers for Disease Control and Prevention. "Intravascular Device-Related Infections Prevention; Guideline Availability," *Federal Register*, 60:49978-50006, September 27, 1995.

Crow, S. "Prevention of Intravascular Infections Way and Means," *Journal of Intravenous Nursing* 19(4):175-81, July 1996.

Dudek, S. *Nutrition Handbook for Nursing Practice*, 3rd ed. Philadelphia: Lippincott-Raven Pubs., 1997.

Klein, S. "Nutrition Support in Clinical Practice: Review of Published Data and Recommendations for Future Research Directions," *Journal of Parenteral and Enteral Nutrition* 21(3):133-47, May-June 1997.

Krzyuda, E.A." Administering TPN Safely," *Nursing96* 26(9):661, September 1996.

Rombeau, J., and Caldwell, M. "Enteral and Tube Feeding," in *Clinical Nutrition: Enteral and Tube Feeding*, 3rd ed. Edited by Rombeau, J. Philadelphia: W.B. Saunders Co., 1997.

Gastrointestinal disorders

Terry, J. *Intravenous Therapy: Clinical Principles and Practice.* Philadelphia: W.B. Saunders Co., 1995.

Torosian, M. *Nutrition for the Hospitalized Patient.* New York: Marcel Dekker, Inc., 1995.

Viall, C. "Taking the Mystery out of TPN," *Nursing95* 25(5):56-59, May 1995.

Weinstein, S. *Plumer's Principles and Practice of Intravenous Therapy,* 6th ed. Philadelphia: Lippincott-Raven Pubs., 1997.

Wilson, J. "Nutritional Assessment and its Application," *Journal of Intravenous Nursing* 19(6):307-14, November 1996.

Part 8

Hepatobiliary and pancreatic disorders

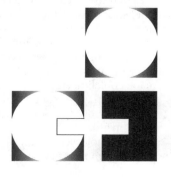

Cholecystectomy

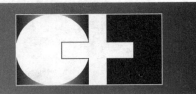

DRG information

DRG 195   Cholecystectomy with Common Bile Duct Exploration with Complication or Comorbidity (CC).
Mean LOS = 10.5 days

DRG 196   Cholecystectomy with Common Bile Duct Exploration without CC.
Mean LOS = 6.7 days

DRG 197   Cholecystectomy Except by Laparoscope without Common Bile Duct Exploration with CC.
Mean LOS = 9.2 days

DRG 198   Cholecystectomy Except by Laparoscope without Common Bile Duct Exploration without CC.
Mean LOS = 4.9 days

DRG 493   Laparoscopic Cholecystectomy without Common Bile Duct Exploration with CC.
Mean LOS = 5.9 days

DRG 494   Laparoscopic Cholecystectomy without Common Bile Duct Exploration without CC.
Mean LOS = 2.4

Other than the usual CCs that differentiate many DRGs, the two main factors in the differentiation of cholecystectomy patients' DRGs are the use of laparoscopic procedures and common bile duct exploration (CBE). Acalculus cholecystitis discovered at the time of cholecystectomy carries a high mortality rate and greatly increases the LOS. There is no DRG for laparoscopic cholecystectomy with common bile duct exploration. Failed laparoscopic cholecystectomies (due to such conditions as adhesions) revert then to open cholecystectomies and the DRGs that include them.

INTRODUCTION

Definition and time focus

Cholecystitis (inflammation of the gallbladder) is an extremely common disorder usually associated with cholelithiasis (gallstone formation). Cholelithiasis may be symptomatic or asymptomatic. Cholecystitis may be acute or chronic. Some patients who have asymptomatic cholelithiasis or short, infrequent periods of biliary colic may be treated with oral bile salts. Prophylactic cholecystectomy for asymptomatic persons is not recommended.

Acute cholecystitis may be associated with transient gallstone impaction at the gallbladder–cystic duct junc-

tion, infections such as cytomegalovirus, ischemic changes after critical illness or major surgery, or rapid weight loss. Most gallstones are composed predominantly of cholesterol or calcium bilirubinate. Cholecystectomy is the treatment of choice for symptomatic cholecystitis.

Laparoscopic cholecystectomy is now more commonly performed than the traditional, or open, cholecystectomy. Although the only absolute contraindication to laparoscopic cholecystectomy is third trimester normal pregnancy, relative contraindications include bleeding or coagulopathy, abscess or fistula formation, peritonitis, multiple abdominal surgeries or gallbladder malignancy. Approximately 5% of laparoscopic cholecystectomies convert to open cholecystectomy due to technical problems or excessive bleeding encountered during surgery. Laparoscopic cholecystectomy may be performed in an outpatient surgery setting or as a short-stay procedure.

For laparoscopic cholecystectomy, several small incisions are made. Carbon dioxide is instilled through the umbilical incision to inflate the abdomen; then the laparoscope is inserted. Instruments, such as the cautery, laser, and operative instruments, are inserted through other small skin incisions in the upper right abdomen. After the procedure is completed, adhesive bandages are placed over the small incisions; sutures are usually unnecessary. The traditional, or open, cholecystectomy generally requires a 5″ to 8″ (13 to 20 cm) incision that is sutured after the procedure. Biliary drains are more commonly used in postoperative care of the open cholecystectomy patient. Bile leaks are a more common complication after laparoscopic cholecystectomy.

This plan focuses on preoperative and postoperative care for the patient with acute cholecystitis who requires traditional, or open, cholecystectomy.

Etiology and precipitating factors
Cholecystitis
• Critically ill patients may develop acalculus (no gallstones) cholecystitis related to localized ischemic reactions.
• HIV-positive patients may develop either calculus or acalculus cholecystitis. Gallbladder infections resistant to antibiotic therapy may develop.
• Patients with sickle cell disease may develop cholecystitis related to hemolysis of the sickled cells.
• Ninety percent of all cases of cholecystitis are related to impaction of gallstones in the cystic duct causing inflammation and obstruction. Gangrene may develop or

perforation may occur. Repeated episodes of biliary colic may result in chronic cholecystitis and the development of a scarred, nonfunctional gallbladder.

Cholelithiasis
• Diabetes (also contributes to higher complication and comorbidity rates postoperatively)
• Obesity
• Significant weight loss or extensive fasting
• Oral contraceptive use
• For women, more than one child

FOCUSED ASSESSMENT GUIDELINES

Nursing history (functional health pattern findings)

Health perception–health management pattern
• Pain, initially situated in midepigastrium, that becomes pronounced in the right upper quadrant (RUQ); pain is initially mild but persistent and intensifies as inflammation spreads; pain may be referred to the right scapula or right shoulder and is exacerbated by movement, coughing, and deep breathing
• History of diabetes, extensive bowel resections, or hemolytic anemia
• Increased risk if over age 50
• Ethnic background: Native American, Jewish, Asian, Italian

Nutritional-metabolic pattern
• Ingestion of heavy or fatty meal
• Intolerance of heavy meals or fatty foods
• Indigestion leading to anorexia
• Nausea, possibly with vomiting
• Recent weight loss

Elimination pattern
• Flatulence
• Change in color of urine or stool (indicates obstructed bile flow)
• Pruritus

Activity-exercise pattern
• Sedentary lifestyle; increases risk for gallstones and therefore cholecystitis

Sleep-rest pattern
• Pain that disturbs sleep

Physical findings

General
• Elevated temperature
• Obesity

Eyes
• Icteric sclera

Mouth
• Jaundiced mucous membranes

Cardiovascular
• Tachycardia
• Hypertension

Pulmonary
• Short and shallow respirations

Abdomen
• Pain in RUQ, referred to right scapula and intensified by deep breathing or percussion above right costal margin
• Localized rebound tenderness in RUQ
• Distention
• Light-colored stools
• Murphy's sign (tenderness in subcostal area with deep aspiration)

Urinary
• Dark, frothy urine

Integumentary
• Jaundice, especially on inner aspects of forearms
• Bruising

Diagnostic studies
• White blood cell count — typically 10,000 to 15,000/µl, although it may not be elevated
• Serum bilirubin level (direct and indirect) — may be elevated when gallstones obstruct the bile duct
• Prothrombin time/international normalized ratio (PT/INR) — may be prolonged because bile is necessary for vitamin K absorption (prothrombin synthesis depends on vitamin K)
• Alkaline phosphatase level — may be elevated because normal excretion through the biliary system may be impeded
• Oral cholecystogram — may not visualize gallbladder because of biliary duct obstruction or inability of the gallbladder to concentrate the dye; repetition may be ordered to rule out inadequate preparation
• Cholangiogram — may show gallstones or strictures in biliary tree
• Ultrasonography — may show gallstones, gallbladder wall thickness

Potential complications
• Perforation of the gallbladder
• Hemorrhage
• Empyema of the gallbladder
• Subphrenic or hepatic abscess
• Fistulas
• Pancreatitis
• Cholangitis
• Pneumonia
• Cancer of the gallbladder

Hepatobiliary and pancreatic disorders

CHOLECYSTECTOMY

Major nursing diagnoses and collaborative problems	Key patient outcomes
Risk for peritonitis	Show stable vital signs: heart rate, 60 to 100 beats/minute; systolic blood pressure, 90 to 140 mm Hg; diastolic blood pressure, 50 to 90 mm Hg.
Risk for hemorrhage	Show no evidence of bleeding.
Pain	Have no abdominal pain or distention, nausea, vomiting, or anorexia.
Risk for postoperative infection	Show no signs of infection.
Risk for postoperative ineffective breathing pattern	Display nonlabored, deep respirations.
Risk for nutritional deficit	Have a sufficient caloric intake by mouth.
Risk for altered oral mucous membrane	Have an intact, moist mucous membrane.

COLLABORATIVE PROBLEM

Risk for peritonitis related to possible preoperative perforation of the gallbladder

Nursing priorities

• Detect perforation.
• Minimize possible complications.

Patient outcome criteria

Within 24 hours of admission, the patient will:
• display stable vital signs: typically, heart rate, 60 to 100 beats/minute; systolic blood pressure, 90 to 140 mm Hg; and diastolic blood pressure, 50 to 90 mm Hg
• verbalize reduction of pain
• show lessening of abnormal abdominal signs.

Interventions

1. Monitor vital signs every 2 hours for 12 hours, then every 4 hours if stable. Document and report abnormalities, especially fever, tachycardia, or dropping blood pressure.

2. Assess the abdomen during vital sign checks, particularly noting bowel sounds, distention, firmness, and presence or absence of a mass in the RUQ. Document and report any changes.

3. During vital sign checks, note the location and character of pain. Document and report any changes.

Rationales

1. Early detection of changes in vital signs will alert caregivers to possible perforation and the need for emergency surgery. Temperature changes indicate further inflammation or a response to antibiotics.

2. Muscle rigidity and a palpable mass in the RUQ suggest peritonitis. In peritonitis, an initial period of hypermotility is followed by hypoactive or absent bowel sounds.

3. RUQ pain that becomes generalized may indicate perforation.

4. Maintain antibiotic therapy as ordered.

4. Antibiotics excreted through the biliary tree are given to prevent or treat infection and to decrease the risk of perforation from a friable or necrotic gallbladder wall.

5. Additional individualized interventions: _____

5. Rationales: _____

COLLABORATIVE PROBLEM

Risk for hemorrhage related to decreased vitamin K absorption and decreased prothrombin synthesis

Nursing priorities

• Prevent hemorrhage.
• Detect clotting abnormalities so that they can be corrected before surgery.

Patient outcome criteria

Within 48 hours of admission, the patient will:
• have PT/INR level approaching normal
• show no evidence of bleeding.

Interventions

1. Monitor PT/INR, as ordered. Alert the doctor to an abnormally prolonged PT/INR.

2. Administer vitamin K as ordered.

3. Observe for bleeding from the gums, nose, or injection sites and for blood in the urine or stool. Document and report bleeding.

4. Give injections using small-gauge needles. If an increased bleeding tendency is noted, limit the number of injections or venipunctures as much as possible, and apply direct pressure for at least 5 minutes after such procedures.

5. Apply gentle pressure to injection sites instead of massaging them.

6. Additional individualized interventions: _____

Rationales

1. Prothrombin is manufactured in the liver and depends on vitamin K for synthesis. Bile is necessary for vitamin K absorption; thus, PT may be prolonged and INR level may be elevated if an obstruction interferes with bile excretion.

2. Administration of vitamin K will correct any deficiency and promote prothrombin synthesis.

3. Observing for bleeding aids in detecting coagulation problems.

4. Small-gauge needles reduce the risk of bleeding at injection sites. Minimizing the number of punctures reduces the risk of significant blood loss. Direct pressure controls bleeding and allows clot formation.

5. Gentle pressure reduces the trauma at injection sites and controls bleeding.

6. Rationales: _____

NURSING DIAGNOSIS

Pain related to gallbladder inflammation

Nursing priority

Relieve RUQ pain.

Hepatobiliary and pancreatic disorders

Patient outcome criteria

Within 1 hour of admission, and then continuously, the patient will:
• verbalize pain relief
• with pain medications, rate pain as less than 3 on a 0 to 10 pain rating scale.

Interventions

1. See the "Pain" plan, page 88.

2. Maintain nothing by mouth (NPO) status.

3. Administer medications, as ordered, and document their effectiveness. Meperidine (Demerol) is the analgesic of choice; papaverine hydrochloride (Pavabid) may be used.

4. Additional individualized interventions: _____

Rationales

1. Generalized interventions regarding pain management are included in the "Pain" plan.

2. NPO status decreases stimulation of the gallbladder.

3. Specific medications are most appropriate for pain from cholecystitis. Meperidine is less likely than morphine to cause spasm of the sphincter of Oddi. Papaverine hydrochloride exerts a nonspecific spasmolytic effect on smooth muscle.

4. Rationales: _____

COLLABORATIVE PROBLEM

Risk for postoperative infection related to obstruction or dislodgment of external biliary drainage tube

Nursing priorities

• Prevent or promptly detect complications.
• Maintain patency of the drainage system.

Patient outcome criteria

Throughout the period of external biliary drainage, the patient will:
• be afebrile
• show no signs of infection or peritonitis
• show no signs of tube obstruction
• show no signs of tube dislodgment.

Interventions

1. Monitor vital signs every 4 hours. Document and report abnormalities.

2. Assess the abdomen every shift, noting any abdominal pain or rigidity. Document and report any changes.

3. Assess for signs of infection at the T-tube insertion site. Document and report any redness, swelling, warmth, or purulent drainage. Teach the patient and family to recognize and report signs of infection.

4. Assess for signs of T-tube obstruction. Document and report pain in the RUQ, biliary drainage around the T-tube, nausea and vomiting, clay-colored stools, jaundice, or dark yellow urine.

Rationales

1. Elevated temperature may indicate infection (either wound infection or biliary peritonitis).

2. Generalized abdominal pain and rigidity, combined with an elevated temperature, may indicate biliary peritonitis.

3. Early detection of infection facilitates prompt treatment.

4. These signs indicate the backup of bile into the common bile duct and liver.

5. Assess for signs of tube dislodgment: decreased drainage or a change in tube position.

6. Using sterile technique, connect the T-tube to a closed gravity drainage system, and attach sufficient tubing so it does not kink or pull as the patient moves.

7. Monitor the amount and character of any drainage. Measure and record the drainage every 4 hours for 12 hours, then once per shift and as needed.

8. Monitor and record the patient's stool color.

9. Place the patient in low Fowler's position upon return from surgery.

10. If the patient will be discharged with a T-tube in place, teach the patient and family how to care for the drainage system, including the expected amount of drainage, frequency of bag emptying and dressing changes, techniques for site care and dressing changes, and signs to report to the doctor (excessive drainage, leakage, and signs of obstruction).

11. Additional individualized interventions: _____

5. Prompt detection and treatment of tube dislodgment reduces the risk of complications (such as peritonitis) from bile leakage.

6. After choledochostomy, a T-tube is inserted into the hepatic duct and the common bile duct to allow biliary drainage and maintain patency until edema subsides. A closed biliary drainage system ensures sterility. Providing enough tubing reduces the risk of obstructing or dislodging the T-tube.

7. Initially, all bile output (500 to 1,000 ml/day) may flow through the T-tube. Within 7 to 10 days, however, most of the bile should flow into the duodenum. Monitoring the amount of drainage permits early detection of an obstructed or dislodged tube.

8. Stools will be light-colored initially, when most of the bile is flowing out through the T-tube. Stools should gradually become normal in color as bile passes into the duodenum. Persistence of light-colored stools for more than 7 days may indicate tube obstruction.

9. Low Fowler's position facilitates T-tube drainage.

10. To successfully manage the T-tube at home, the patient and family need to know about routine care as well as what to do about potential complications.

11. Rationales: _____

NURSING DIAGNOSIS

Risk for postoperative ineffective breathing pattern related to high abdominal incision and pain

Nursing priorities
• Maintain optimal air exchange.
• Prevent atelectasis.

Patient outcome criteria
Throughout the postoperative period, the patient will:
• maintain a respiratory rate of 12 to 24 breaths/minute
• display nonlabored, deep respirations
• have clear breath sounds in all lobes.

Interventions

1. Monitor respiratory rate and character every 4 hours. Note the depth of respirations. Document and report abnormalities. If indicated, obtain oxygen saturation (SaO_2) and report SaO_2 less than 95%.

Rationales

1. After cholecystectomy, the patient may breathe shallowly to avoid pain associated with deep breathing. SaO_2 less than 95% may indicate the need for supplemental oxygen and more aggressive spirometry.

2. Auscultate for breath sounds once per shift. Document and report changes.

3. Instruct and coach the patient in diaphragmatic breathing.

4. Assist the patient to use the incentive spirometer — 10 breaths/hour during the day and every 2 hours at night.

5. Turn the patient every 2 hours.

6. Assess pain and administer pain medication, as needed, before breathing exercises and ambulation.

7. Assist the patient to splint the incision with a pillow or bath blanket while coughing.

8. Encourage the patient to increase ambulation progressively.

9. Additional individualized interventions: _____

2. Breath sounds may be diminished at the bases, especially on the right side.

3. Diaphragmatic breathing increases lung expansion by allowing the diaphragm to descend fully.

4. Using the incentive spirometer promotes sustained maximal inspiration, which fully inflates alveoli.

5. Position changes promote ventilation of all lung lobes and drainage of secretions.

6. The pain-free patient is better able to take deep breaths, and therefore is more likely to cooperate with prescribed pulmonary hygiene measures and activity level.

7. Splinting relieves stress and pulling on the incision.

8. Ambulation promotes adequate ventilation by increasing the depth of respirations.

9. Rationales: _____

Nursing diagnosis

Risk for nutritional deficit related to preoperative nausea and vomiting, postoperative NPO status, nasogastric suction, altered lipid metabolism, and increased nutritional needs during healing

Nursing priorities

• Maintain optimal nutritional status.
• Teach the patient and family about postoperative dietary recommendations.

Patient outcome criteria

• Throughout the hospital stay, the patient will have normal fluid and electrolyte status.
• By the time of discharge, the patient will:
  – list three general dietary considerations
  – identify specific foods that may need to be restricted.

Interventions

1. Maintain I.V. fluid replacement, as ordered. (See Appendix C, Fluid and Electrolyte Imbalances.)

2. Once peristalsis returns, remove the NG tube and encourage a progressive dietary intake, as ordered.

3. Clamp the T-tube during meals, as ordered.

Rationales

1. During the immediate postoperative period, the patient will receive nothing by mouth until peristalsis returns. The patient may also have a nasogastric (NG) tube in place to reduce distention and minimize the pancreatic stimulation normally triggered by gastric juices. Gastric suction and NPO status increase the risk of fluid and electrolyte disorders.

2. Patients usually are able to take clear liquids 24 to 48 hours after surgery and gradually increase to a full diet, with fat restrictions as ordered.

3. Clamping the T-tube during meals may aid fat absorption by allowing additional bile to flow into the duodenum.

4. Teach the patient and family about a fat-restricted diet, as ordered. Involve a dietitian in meal planning and home care teaching.

4. After cholecystectomy, the liver must store and release all bile for lipid digestion; thus, fat absorption may be altered, especially if postoperative edema limits hepatic bile excretion. Fat intake is usually limited for $1\frac{1}{2}$ to 6 months, depending on the doctor's preference and the patient's response to gradual increases in fat intake. A dietitian can help ensure that the patient's diet compensates for the calories normally provided by fats.

5. Suggest small, frequent meals.

5. Large meals may contribute to distention and increase discomfort.

6. Instruct the patient to minimize alcohol intake during recovery.

6. Pancreatitis is a common complication after cholecystectomy. Alcohol intake commonly triggers acute pancreatic inflammation.

7. Prepare the patient for the possibility of persistent flatulence.

7. Flatulence is common after surgery. Typically, these patients have other gastrointestinal disorders (such as hiatal hernia or ulcer) that may cause persistent symptoms, such as bloating and nausea. Dietary modifications and treatment of the underlying disorder may reduce symptoms.

8. Additional individualized interventions: _____

8. Rationales: _____

NURSING DIAGNOSIS

Risk for altered oral mucous membrane related to NPO status and possible NG suction

Nursing priority

Maintain integrity of the oral mucous membrane.

Patient outcome criteria

Throughout the period of NPO status, the patient will:
• have an intact, moist oral mucous membrane
• display no evidence of an inflamed oral mucosa.

Interventions

1. Assess the oral mucous membrane once per shift for dryness, cracks, coating, or lesions.

2. Assist the patient with gentle mouth care at least twice daily or as needed. Make sure that water and oral hygiene materials are within the patient's reach.

3. Apply lubricant to the lips every 2 hours while the patient is awake or more frequently as needed.

4. Additional individualized interventions: _____

Rationales

1. Early identification of potential problems facilitates prompt treatment.

2. NPO status and NG suction (as well as any previously existing nutritional deficits) may contribute to fragility of the oral mucosa and increase the risk of infection or injury. Frequent mouth care reduces accumulation of bacteria and decreases discomfort associated with NPO status.

3. Lubricant keeps lips smooth and moist.

4. Rationales: _____

Discharge planning

Discharge checklist

Before discharge, the patient shows evidence of:
❏ absence of wound infection
❏ absence of fever
❏ stable vital signs
❏ absence of pulmonary and cardiovascular complications
❏ ability to tolerate diet as ordered
❏ same ability to ambulate as before surgery
❏ ability to perform activities of daily living (ADLs) independently
❏ adequate support system after discharge, or referral to home care if indicated by inadequate home support system or inability to perform ADLs.

Teaching checklist

Document evidence that the patient and family demonstrate an understanding of:
❏ signs and symptoms of wound infection
❏ dietary modifications (patient may be on a low-fat diet for up to 6 months; a normal diet is resumed as soon as tolerated)
❏ resumption of normal activities (lifting restricted to less than 10 lb for 3 to 4 weeks)
❏ resumption of sexual activity (when cleared by doctor, usually after 2 weeks or when pain-free)
❏ all discharge medications' purpose, dosage, administration schedule, and adverse effects (postoperative patients may be discharged with oral analgesics)
❏ if discharged with a T-tube, routine care and signs to report to the doctor
❏ date, time, and location of follow-up appointment
❏ how to contact the doctor.

Documentation checklist

Using outcome criteria as a guide, document:
❏ clinical status on admission
❏ significant changes in status
❏ pertinent laboratory and diagnostic test findings
❏ wound assessment
❏ amount and character of T-tube drainage
❏ pain-relief measures
❏ pulmonary hygiene measures
❏ observations of oral mucous membrane
❏ nutritional intake
❏ gastrointestinal assessment
❏ patient and family teaching
❏ discharge planning.

Associated plans of care

Knowledge deficit
Pain
Pancreatitis
Surgery

References

Black, J.M., and Matassarin-Jacobs, E. *Medical-Surgical Nursing: Clinical Management for Continuity of Care*, 5th ed. Philadelphia: W.B. Saunders, Co., 1997.

Kelley, W.N., ed. *Textbook of Internal Medicine*, 3rd ed. Philadelphia: Lippincott-Raven, Pubs., 1997.

Rakel, R.E., ed. *Conn's Current Therapy, 1997*. Philadelphia: W.B. Saunders Co., 1997.

Tierney, L.M., et al., eds. *Current Medical Diagnosis and Treatment*. Stamford, Conn.: Appleton & Lange, 1996.

Liver failure

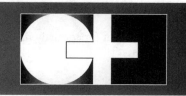

DRG information
DRG 205   Disorders of Liver Except Malignancy, Cirrhosis, or Alcoholic Hepatitis with Complications or Comorbidity (CC).
Mean LOS = 7.3 days
Principal diagnoses include:
- acute or chronic liver failure
- various types of hepatitis
- hepatomegaly
- jaundice, unspecified etiology
- hepatic infarction
- liver abscess.

DRG 206   Disorders of Liver Except Malignancy, Cirrhosis, or Alcoholic Hepatitis without CC.
Mean LOS = 4.7 days
Principal diagnoses include selected principal diagnoses listed under DRG 205. The distinction is that a case assigned DRG 206 has no CC.

INTRODUCTION

Definition and time focus
The liver is an organ essential for life, with metabolic, secretory, excretory, and vascular functions. Metabolic functions include glycogen formation, storage, and breakdown; glucose formation; fat storage, breakdown, and synthesis; amino acid deamination; ammonia conversion; and synthesis of plasma proteins, including clotting factors. Secretory functions include bile production and bilirubin conjugation. Excretory functions include detoxification of hormones and drugs. Vascular functions include blood storage and filtration.

In liver failure, which can result from almost all forms of liver disease, parenchymal cells are progressively destroyed and replaced with fibrotic tissue. Once chronically damaged, the liver will never regain normal structure. However, because liver cells retain an enormous regenerative capacity, functional compensation may be attained if precipitating factors are eliminated. This plan focuses on the critically ill patient presenting with acute symptoms of liver failure. These symptoms include hepatic encephalopathy, fluid and electrolyte imbalance from ascites, and related complications of liver failure.

Etiology and precipitating factors
- Laënnec's (alcoholic) cirrhosis with an acute episode of alcohol ingestion, hypovolemia from rapid diuresis or shock, gastrointestinal bleeding, or infection
- Acute hepatic failure caused by fulminant hepatitis, hepatotoxic chemicals, or biliary obstruction
- Primary biliary cirrhosis

FOCUSED ASSESSMENT GUIDELINES

Nursing history (functional health pattern findings)
Health perception–health management pattern
- Commonly complains about weakness and fatigue
- Treatment for chronic alcoholism, hepatitis, or biliary obstructive disease

Nutritional-metabolic pattern
- Diet history that includes excessive alcohol consumption and fat intolerance
- Anorexia and resulting weight loss
- Ingestion of certain drugs, such as large doses of acetaminophen (Tylenol), tetracycline (Tetracyn), or antituberculosis drugs such as isoniazid (Laniazid)

Elimination pattern
- Clay-colored stools or dark urine resulting from jaundice

Activity-exercise pattern
- Psychomotor defects

Sleep-rest pattern
- Increased drowsiness

Cognitive-perceptual pattern
- Intellectual deterioration and slurred speech in beginning stages of hepatic encephalopathy commonly reported by patient's family
- Personality changes or altered moods reported by patient's family

Sexuality-reproductive pattern
- Impotence in male patients because of endocrine changes
- Erratic menstruation among female patients

Role-relationship pattern
- Job involving hepatotoxic chemicals such as vinyl chloride

Physical findings
General appearance
- Fever unaffected by antibiotics; reason for fever is unknown

Cardiovascular
- Hyperkinetic circulation: flushed extremities, bounding pulse, and capillary pulsations that result primarily from liver cell failure but also may occur with the open-

ing of many normal but functionally inactive arteriovenous anastomoses

Pulmonary
- Cyanosis

Neurologic
- Hyperactive reflexes, positive Babinski's reflex
- Various stages of encephalopathy with resultant altered level of consciousness (LOC)

Gastrointestinal
- Fetor hepaticus: sweetish, slightly fecal breath smell, presumably intestinal in origin
- Hepatomegaly, splenomegaly
- Ascites
- Distant bowel sounds and muffled percussion notes

Endocrine
- Male: hypogonadism, gynecomastia
- Female: gonadal atrophy

Integumentary
- Jaundiced skin, sclera, and mucous membranes from failure to metabolize bilirubin
- Vascular spiders: consist of central arteriole with radiating small vessels; usually in vascular territory of superior vena cava (above nipple line)
- Palmar erythema: hands warm, palms bright red from estrogen excess
- Easy bruising from inadequate clotting factors
- "Paper money skin": numerous small blood vessels that resemble silk threads in a dollar bill

Diagnostic studies
- Complete blood count—may reveal decreased hematocrit and hemoglobin values, which reflect the liver's inability to store hematopoietic factors (such as iron, folic acid, and vitamin B_{12}); decreased white blood cell (WBC) and thrombocyte levels, which appear with splenomegaly; and elevated WBC count, which may indicate infection
- Prolonged prothrombin time/international normalized ratio (PT/INR)—reflects decreased synthesis of prothrombin, impaired vitamin K absorption, or both
- Enzyme tests—may show elevated serum aspartate aminotransferase, serum alanine aminotransferase, alkaline phosphatase, and lactate dehydrogenase values, which reflect hepatocellular or biliary tissue dysfunction and necrosis
- Protein metabolite tests (serum albumin and total protein levels)—may reflect impaired protein synthesis
- Lipid and carbohydrate tests—may reveal decreased serum cholesterol levels, reflecting impaired hepatic synthesis, or increased levels, reflecting obstructive pathology; elevated serum ammonia values, reflecting impaired hepatic synthesis of urea; and decreased serum glucose levels, which accompany malnutrition
- Bilirubin levels—increased in liver disease
- Urine and stool tests—may reveal increased urine urobilinogen and reduced fecal urobilinogen values, which accompany jaundice
- Testosterone level — reduced
- Abdominal ultrasound—may be performed if biliary obstruction is suspected
- Abdominal X-rays—may reveal liver enlargement
- Angiography or superior mesenteric arteriography—important for evaluation of portal hypertension
- Liver scan—reveals abnormalities in hepatic structure
- Liver biopsy—indicates extent of hepatic tissue changes
- Electroencephalography (EEG)—may show generalized slowing of frequency, which substantiates encephalopathy
- Endoscopy—helps locate gastrointestinal bleeding site

Potential complications
- Hepatorenal failure
- Disseminated intravascular coagulation
- Bleeding esophageal varices

CLINICAL SNAPSHOT

LIVER FAILURE

Major nursing diagnoses and collaborative problems	Key patient outcomes
Deteriorating neurologic status	Display improved neurologic status.
Risk for fever	Have a temperature of 97.5° to 99.5° F (36.4° to 37.5° C).
Fluid and electrolyte imbalance	Show lessened ascites and edema.
Risk for gastrointestinal hemorrhage	Show stable vital signs: typically, heart rate, 60 to 100 beats/minute; systolic blood pressure, 90 to 140 mm Hg; and diastolic blood pressure, 50 to 90 mm Hg.
Nutritional deficit	Tolerate protein intake without encephalopathy recurring.
Risk for impaired skin integrity	Have no apparent skin breakdown.

COLLABORATIVE PROBLEM

Deteriorating neurologic status related to hepatic encephalopathy syndrome

Nursing priorities

- Monitor changes in psychomotor skills, mental status, and speech.
- Eliminate factors that decrease hepatocellular function.

Patient outcome criteria

Within 24 to 48 hours of admission, the patient will:
- display improved neurologic status
- display a decreased need for respiratory support.

Interventions

1. Assess neurologic status hourly. Assess and implement safety measures.
Describe the changes observed, typically:
- Stage 1: confusion, altered mood or behavior, psychomotor deficits
- Stage 2: drowsiness, inappropriate behavior
- Stage 3: stupor, marked confusion, and inarticulate speech (although the patient may speak or obey simple commands)
- Stage 4: coma, but response to painful stimuli still present
- Stage 5: deep coma; no response to painful stimuli.

2. Assess for asterixis (flapping tremor of the wrist).

3. Auscultate the chest and assess respiratory rate hourly. Administer oxygen therapy using nasal prongs, as ordered. Monitor pulse oximetry continuously. Anticipate more aggressive measures, such as intubation, if the encephalopathy progresses to coma.

4. Stop intake of dietary protein. Also stop administration of all drugs containing nitrogen, such as ammonium chloride, urea (Ureaphil), and methionine, as ordered.

5. Administer neomycin (Mycifradin) by nasogastric (NG) tube, if ordered. The usual dose is 1 g.

6. Administer lactulose (Cephulac) by NG tube, if ordered. The usual dose is 10 to 30 ml. Expect frequent bowel movements due to lactulose. Keep patient clean and comfortable. Monitor closely for skin breakdown due to excessive bowel movements. Monitor for diarrhea; if it occurs, consult with the doctor about reducing the dose.

Rationales

1. Symptoms vary; therefore, close monitoring and implementation of appropriate safety measures is important. The encephalopathy syndrome results from impaired nitrogen metabolism, passage of toxic substances of intestinal origin (ammonia, active amines, and short-chain fatty acids) to the brain, and numerous other metabolic abnormalities occurring in hepatocellular failure. The toxic substances are thought to interfere with glucose metabolism and cerebral blood flow. Chronic exposure of brain cells to these substances through repeated bouts of encephalopathy results in irreversible damage.

2. This sign, caused by impaired flow of proprioceptive information to the brain stem reticular formation, indicates that the patient is in the early stages of encephalopathy.

3. The patient with long-standing liver disease will have developed decreased oxygen saturation and decreased diffusing capacity before the onset of encephalopathy. Therefore, respiratory support measures are commonly required.

4. Intake of dietary protein and drugs containing nitrogen increase the accumulation of nitrogenous substances that the liver can't break down.

5. Neomycin decreases the intestinal bacteria that produce ammonia.

6. Although lactulose's exact mechanism of action is unclear, it may be instrumental in chelating ammonia (NH_3), acting as an osmotic agent for inducing diarrhea, changing gut pH resulting in excretion of ammonium (NH_4^+), or changing gut flora to decrease the growth of NH_3-forming bacteria. Diarrhea is a sign of excessive dosage.

Hepatobiliary and pancreatic disorders

7. Stop any diuretic therapy, as ordered.

7. If the patient has hepatic cirrhosis, the most common cause of hepatic encephalopathy is excessive diuresis from diuretic therapy. The resulting hypovolemia further reduces hepatic perfusion, causing the encephalopathy.

8. Administer neutral, acid-free enema solutions, as ordered.

8. Purging the intestines reduces NH_4^+ absorption and may result in improvement of clinical symptoms and EEG readings.

9. Avoid all sedatives metabolized primarily by the liver. If the patient is uncontrollable, administer half the usual dose of barbiturate, as ordered. Morphine and paraldehyde (Paral) are contraindicated.

9. The patient in impending coma is extremely sensitive to sedatives. Drugs metabolized primarily by the liver are particularly dangerous because toxic accumulations can occur rapidly from impaired hepatic perfusion. Some sedation may be necessary, however, if the patient becomes agitated as hepatic failure worsens and toxic metabolic substances accumulate. Long-acting, short-chain barbiturates that are excreted largely by the kidney are preferred. Morphine and paraldehyde may cause coma.

10. Teach the patient and family about necessary interventions, as appropriate. Emphasize causes of changes in neurologic status and rationales for methods to reduce encephalopathy.

10. Although patient teaching may be of limited success because of altered LOC, brief and repeated explanations may help the patient feel more secure psychologically. Teaching family members may help them understand mood swings and behavior changes.

11. Additional individualized interventions: _____

11. Rationales: _____

COLLABORATIVE PROBLEM

Risk for fever related to liver disease or infection

Nursing priority

Assist in determining the cause of the fever.

Patient outcome criterion

Within 24 to 48 hours of admission, the patient will have a temperature less than 100.4° F (38° C).

Interventions

1. Assess temperature every 4 hours. If elevated, assess more frequently. Consult with the doctor about abnormal readings.

Rationales

1. Continuous, low-grade fever rarely exceeding 100.4° F (38° C) is seen in about one-third of patients with liver disease. This fever is unaffected by antibiotics and attributable to liver disease alone, although the reason for it is unknown. However, the patient may have fever from infection. The liver normally is bacteriologically sterile and filters bacteria from the bloodstream. Cirrhosis allows bacteria to pass into the circulation. Differentiation of possible causes of fever is necessary for effective treatment.

2. Observe for cloudy, concentrated urine and pain upon urination, if a catheter is not in place. Avoid catheterization, if possible.

2. These signs indicate urinary tract infection. Avoiding catheterization reduces the risk of infection. However, accurate measurement of input and output is crucial for the critically ill patient with liver disease. An indwelling urinary catheter may be necessary to monitor accurate hourly urine output. Remember, urine may be dark amber because of jaundice.

3. Auscultate lung fields at least every 2 hours. Also assess respiratory rate, skin color, and level of cyanosis.

3. Respiratory difficulties may indicate aspiration pneumonia. Pulmonary arteriovenous shunting from liver disease and the resultant decreased oxygen saturation place the patient at increased risk for pneumonia.

4. Auscultate bowel sounds at least every 4 hours. Observe for abdominal rigidity, increased abdominal girth, or vomiting.

4. Spontaneous peritonitis is known to occur in patients with liver disease.

5. If infection is diagnosed, assist with treatment, as ordered; for example, administer antibiotics. If the fever stems solely from liver disease, provide symptomatic care such as frequent linen changes.

5. Infection requires prompt, aggressive treatment because it promotes protein accumulation from tissue catabolism. Low-grade fever may remain if fever results solely from liver disease. Frequent linen changes reduce discomfort from diaphoresis.

6. Additional individualized interventions: _____

6. Rationales: _____

COLLABORATIVE PROBLEM

Fluid and electrolyte imbalance related to ascites

Nursing priority

Restore a normal fluid balance (as described in outcome criteria).

Patient outcome criteria

Within 4 days of admission, the patient will:
• manifest urine output of at least 60 ml/hour
• display urinary sodium excretion greater than 10 mEq/day
• show lessened ascites and edema, as evidenced by decreased weight and improved respiratory status.

Interventions

1. Closely monitor fluid and electrolyte status, including strict intake and output measurements, hourly determination of urine specific gravity, daily weights, and assessment of lung fields at least every 2 hours for crackles or gurgles.

Rationales

1. Close monitoring of fluid status is necessary to judge the degree of cardiovascular and pulmonary compromise imposed by ascites. In liver failure, ascites develops from lowered plasma oncotic pressure, portal venous hypertension, and sodium and water retention. The lowered plasma oncotic pressure results from the liver's failure to synthesize albumin. This lowered oncotic pressure, combined with increased hydrostatic pressure from portal hypertension, causes fluid to shift into interstitial spaces (third spacing) in the peritoneal cavity. The resulting depletion of effective intravascular volume causes the renal tubules to retain sodium and water through the aldosterone effect.

Hepatobiliary and pancreatic disorders

2. Percuss and palpate the abdomen every 4 hours. Don't rely solely on abdominal girth measurements.

2. Percussion and palpation allow evaluation of changes in fluid shifting. Dullness on percussion in the flanks is the earliest sign of ascites and indicates approximately 2 L of fluid. The liver and spleen may be palpated if only moderate amounts of fluid are present; with tense ascites, it is difficult to palpate abdominal viscera. A fluid thrill indicates a large amount of free fluid. It is a very late sign of fluid under tension. Abdominal girth measurements are unreliable as gaseous distention is common.

3. Maintain strict bed rest.

3. Bed rest increases renal perfusion and the kidneys' ability to excrete excess fluid. Placing the patient with ascites in the semi-Fowler's or Fowler's position may impair ventilation due to excessive pressure on the diaphragm.

4. Implement therapy, as ordered:
• dietary restrictions, typically sodium intake of 0.5 g/day and fluid intake of 1 L/day
• diuretic administration, typically furosemide (Lasix) or spironolactone (Aldactone)
• postoperative care after peritoneovenous (LeVeen) shunt insertion.

4. The rate of ascitic fluid reabsorption is limited to 700 to 900 ml/day. Limiting sodium and water intake reduces ascitic fluid production, while diuretic administration increases fluid excretion. Shunt insertion controls ascites in less than 5% of patients with liver failure.

5. Teach the patient and family about necessary interventions, as appropriate.

5. Understanding the effects of ascites and treatment methods improves the patient and family's cooperation with the treatment plan, increasing the likelihood of its effectiveness.

6. Additional individualized interventions: _____

6. Rationales: _____

COLLABORATIVE PROBLEM

Risk for gastrointestinal hemorrhage related to esophageal varices

Nursing priority

Monitor for, prevent, or promptly treat hemorrhage.

Patient outcome criteria

Within 24 hours of detection of bleeding, the patient will:
• exhibit stable vital signs: typically, heart rate, 60 to 100 beats/minute; systolic blood pressure, 90 to 140 mm Hg; and diastolic blood pressure, 50 to 90 mm Hg
• have warm, dry skin.

Interventions

1. Observe for and report signs of esophageal bleeding such as hematemesis. Anticipate drug treatment with vasopressin (Pitressin), propranolol (Inderal), or octreotide (Sandostatin), or insertion of a gastric compression tube. See the "Gastrointestinal hemorrhage" plan, page 505, for specific nursing interventions.

2. Additional individualized interventions: _____

Rationales

1. The mechanism of esophageal varices formation is unclear; they are thought to be caused by excessive portal venous backflow into the esophageal vasculature. Hematemesis of frank red blood indicates active bleeding. Vasopressin constricts blood vessels and smooth muscle in the GI tract. Octreotide suppresses secretion of serotonin and gastroenteropancreatic peptides, while propranolol lowers blood pressure. A compression tube may control bleeding varices temporarily. The "Gastrointestinal hemorrhage" plan contains detailed information on detecting and treating bleeding varices.

2. Rationales: _____

NURSING DIAGNOSIS

Nutritional deficit related to catabolism from liver disease

Nursing priority

Restore metabolism to an anabolic state.

Patient outcome criterion

Within 96 hours of admission, the patient will tolerate protein intake without recurrence of encephalopathy.

Interventions

1. Implement dietary restrictions, as ordered. Maintain high caloric intake, usually 1,600 calories/day, by administering high carbohydrate I.V. infusions, as ordered. If jaundice is present, do not administer oral fat or fat infusions.

2. If encephalopathy is present, stop protein intake, as ordered. Once encephalopathy has subsided, start protein intake at 20-g/day increments. Monitor closely for recurrence of encephalopathy.

3. Emphasize to the patient and family the importance of dietary restrictions.

4. Additional individualized interventions: _____

Rationales

1. Dietary control of precursors to toxic metabolites plays an important role in the control of symptoms. High-caloric intake is necessary to meet energy needs. Jaundice indicates decreased bile salt levels, which impair fat absorption.

2. Inability to metabolize protein causes the blood ammonia level to rise, producing encephalopathy. Restricting protein intake helps eliminate symptoms. Gradual reintroduction of protein helps determine the amount the patient can metabolize safely. Recurrence of symptoms indicates the need for permanent protein restriction.

3. The necessary restrictions may make the diet unpalatable and difficult to accept. Understanding the rationale increases the patient's motivation to follow recommendations and the likelihood of family support.

4. Rationales: _____

NURSING DIAGNOSIS

Risk for impaired skin integrity related to jaundice, increased bleeding tendencies, malnutrition, and ascites

Hepatobiliary and pancreatic disorders

Nursing priority
Maintain or restore skin integrity.

Patient outcome criterion
Within 48 hours of admission, and then continuously, the patient will have no apparent skin breakdown.

Interventions

1. Monitor skin condition. Particularly note the presence of vascular spiders.

2. Monitor PT/INR as ordered.

3. Turn the patient and rub bony prominences every 2 hours. Implement additional measures found in the "Impaired physical mobility" plan, page 50, as appropriate.

4. Provide symptomatic treatment of pruritus, as necessary; for example, bathe the skin with cool water.

5. Additional individualized interventions: _____

Rationales

1. Careful monitoring of skin status, commonly overlooked, allows early detection of skin problems that liver failure patients are particularly susceptible to. Vascular spiders can bleed profusely.

2. Liver failure impairs the synthesis of clotting factors. A prolonged PT increases the risk of skin bruising and breakdown.

3. Malnutrition and ascites predispose the patient to pressure ulcer formation. The "Impaired physical mobility" plan itemizes detailed information on potential skin problems.

4. Pruritus, which results from jaundice, can cause extreme discomfort. Treatment may be limited because phenothiazides and antihistamines are contraindicated if the patient has encephalopathy.

5. Rationales: _____

Discharge planning

Discharge checklist
Before discharge, the patient shows evidence of:
❏ improved neurologic status
❏ absence of respiratory complications
❏ adequate urine output
❏ reduction of ascites and weight
❏ normal temperature or stable low-grade fever
❏ resumption of I.V. or oral protein and fat intake.

Teaching checklist
Document evidence that the patient and family demonstrate an understanding of:
❏ relationship between alcohol consumption and exacerbation of liver disease
❏ causes of changes in neurologic status and relationship to liver disease
❏ effects of ascites and methods of treatment
❏ importance of diet in liver disease.

Documentation checklist
Using outcome criteria as a guide, document:
❏ clinical status on admission

❏ significant changes in status
❏ pertinent laboratory and diagnostic test findings
❏ weight
❏ fluid intake and output measurements
❏ fluctuations in fever and associated symptoms
❏ skin integrity
❏ any signs of GI bleeding
❏ patient and family teaching
❏ discharge planning.

Associated plans of care
GI hemorrhage
Impaired physical mobility
Nutritional deficit
Sensory-perceptual alteration

References
Brown, R.S., Jr., and Lake, J.R. "Transjugular Intrahepatic Portosystemic Shunt as a Form of Treatment of Portal Hypertension: Indications and Contraindications," *Advances in Internal Medicine* 42(P):485-504, 1997.

Lee, W.M. "Management of Acute Liver Failure," *Seminars in Liver Disease* 16(4):369-378, November 1996.

Pancreatitis

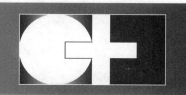

DRG information

DRG 204   Disorder of Pancreas Except Malignancy.
Mean LOS = 6.8 days
Principal diagnoses include:
- pancreatitis
- benign neoplasm of pancreas, except islets of Langerhans
- injury to any portion of the pancreas.

INTRODUCTION

Definition and time focus

Pancreatitis (inflammation of the pancreas) is an autodigestive disorder in which premature activation of pancreatic proteolytic enzymes damages the organ itself. The exact physiologic mechanism is unknown but, theoretically, duodenal reflux or spasm, or blockage of pancreatic ducts by gallstones or edema, may result in the backup of pancreatic secretions. Pancreatitis may be a complication of surgery for other biliary tract or GI disease; numerous other causative factors have also been implicated.

Depending on the nature and severity of the disorder, significant edema, tissue necrosis, and life-threatening hemorrhage may result. Pancreatitis may be either acute or chronic. Chronic pancreatitis causes progressive loss of pancreatic function and may be associated with repeated bouts of acute pancreatitis. This plan focuses on the care of the patient who is admitted for diagnosis and management of an episode of acute pancreatitis.

Etiology and precipitating factors

- Alcohol abuse
- Cholecystitis or cholelithiasis
- Abdominal surgery
- Trauma
- Peptic or duodenal ulcer
- Hyperparathyroidism
- Viral hepatitis
- Mumps
- Hyperlipidemia
- Anorexia nervosa
- Ischemia related to shock
- Metabolic disorders
- Use of certain medications: thiazide diuretics, steroids, sulfonamides, oral contraceptives, tetracycline, acetaminophen (in excessive doses)

FOCUSED ASSESSMENT GUIDELINES

Nursing history (functional health pattern findings)

Health perception–health management pattern
- Severe abdominal pain in epigastric or umbilical region that radiates into back or flank
- Pain that increases when supine or when food is taken and after administration of certain narcotics
- History of gallbladder disease or alcoholism with recent dietary indiscretion or drinking binge

Nutritional-metabolic pattern
- Nausea or vomiting
- Anorexia
- Recent weight loss

Elimination pattern
- Increased flatus
- Steatorrhea (associated with chronic disease)

Activity-exercise pattern
- Preference for a hunched sitting position because of pain
- Dizziness or faintness when standing

Cognitive-perceptual pattern
- Shoulder pain or frequent hiccups (if diaphragmatic irritation is present)
- Pleuritic-like pain that increases with deep inspiration

Coping–stress tolerance pattern
- Habitual use of unhealthy coping mechanisms (such as alcoholism)

Physical findings

General appearance
- Hunched posture
- Restlessness

Cardiovascular
- Fever
- Tachycardia
- Hypotension

Pulmonary
If pleural effusion is present:
- reduced chest excursion
- crackles
- tachypnea

Gastrointestinal
- Abdominal distention
- Guarding
- Reduced or absent bowel sounds
- Ascites

Neurologic
- Seizures
- Stupor
- Neuromuscular irritability

Integumentary
- Jaundice
- Pallor
- Diaphoresis
- Cullen's sign (ecchymosis around umbilicus)
- Turner's sign (ecchymosis in flank, retroperitoneal, and groin area)
- Cool extremities
- Cyanosis (if advanced shock)

Musculoskeletal
If hypocalcemia is present:
- tetany
- positive Chvostek's sign
- positive Trousseau's sign

Renal
- Oliguria (if acute tubular necrosis is present)

Diagnostic studies
- Serum amylase level—elevated in acute pancreatitis; although not specific for pancreatitis, increased enzyme levels occur during pancreatic inflammation
- amylase-creatinine-clearance ratio—indicates acute pancreatitis if greater than 5%
- Urine amylase level—elevated for the first 3 to 5 days of illness; it reflects pancreatic secretion better than serum value; in acute pancreatitis, renal clearance of amylase is markedly increased
- Serum calcium level—decreased, usually less than 8 mg/dl (unless hyperparathyroidism is present, in which instance value may be normal)
- Complete blood count (CBC)—likely to reveal leukocytosis; hemoglobin and hematocrit values vary depending on fluid status, hemorrhage, or degree of compensation
- Serum and urine glucose levels—may be elevated because of altered insulin production

- Serum lipase level—elevated
- Serum and urine bilirubin levels—elevated
- Serum albumin value—usually less than 3.2 g/dl
- Serum triglyceride levels—may be elevated
- Serum electrolyte levels—may reveal hypokalemia or hyponatremia
- Computed tomography (CT) scan—visualizes tumors, dilated pancreatic ducts, calcification, or pseudocyst
- Abdominal ultrasound—may provide evidence of inflammation, edema, gallstones, calcified pancreatic ducts, abscess, organ enlargement, hematoma, or pseudocyst (cavities of exudate, blood, and pancreatic products that may expand and compress other organs)
- Abdominal X-rays—may reveal areas of calcification or adhesion, or identify indicators of reduced bowel motility
- Upper GI X-rays—may show enlarged pancreas or may reveal stomach displacement from pseudocyst formation
- Chest X-ray—may reveal diaphragmatic elevation if abscess formation or peritonitis is present; may identify areas of atelectasis or effusion
- I.V. cholangiography—used to rule out acute cholecystitis as cause of symptoms
- Paracentesis—may reveal elevated amylase levels or blood, both associated with acute pancreatitis

Potential complications
- Hypovolemic shock
- Hemorrhage
- Adult respiratory distress syndrome
- Renal failure
- Pulmonary edema
- Myocardial infarction
- Peritonitis or sepsis
- Pleural effusion
- Abscess formation
- Hyperglycemia or diabetes mellitus
- Paralytic ileus
- Pseudocyst formation

CLINICAL SNAPSHOT

PANCREATITIS

Major nursing diagnoses and collaborative problems	Key patient outcomes
Risk for hypovolemic shock	Show stable vital signs: typically, heart rate, 60 to 100 beats/minute; systolic blood pressure, 90 to 140 mm Hg; and diastolic blood pressure, 50 to 90 mm Hg.
Pain	Rate pain as less than 3 on a 0 to 10 pain rating scale.
Risk for injury: Complications	Display no evidence of complications.
Nutritional deficit	Maintain prescribed nutritional intake.

COLLABORATIVE PROBLEM

Risk for hypovolemic shock related to hemorrhage, fluid shifts, hyperglycemia, or vomiting

Nursing priority

Maintain fluid volume.

Patient outcome criteria

Within 24 hours of admission and then continuously, the patient will:
- have stable vital signs: typically, heart rate, 60 to 100 beats/minute; systolic blood pressure, 90 to 140 mm Hg, and diastolic blood pressure, 50 to 90 mm Hg
- display serum glucose, urine glucose, and ketone levels returning to normal
- have serum electrolyte levels returning to normal.

Interventions

1. Monitor vital signs, fluid intake and output, hemodynamic pressures, and electrocardiography findings according to Appendix A, Monitoring Standards, or unit protocol. Immediately report any findings indicating hypovolemia.

2. Maintain I.V. access through peripheral or central lines. Monitor I.V. fluid replacement, usually with lactated Ringer's solution, dextran, or albumin. If hemorrhage is suspected, anticipate and monitor transfusion, as ordered.

3. Assess serum glucose or fingerstick glucose and urine ketone levels every 4 to 6 hours or more frequently if severe hyperglycemia is present. Administer regular insulin, as ordered, and monitor and document effects.

4. Monitor serum electrolytes daily, as ordered, including serum calcium. (See Appendix C, Fluid and Electrolyte Imbalances.) Stay alert for characteristic signs of severe hypocalcemia: neuromuscular irritability and tetany.

Rationales

1. The damaged pancreas releases several substances that have systemic vasoactive effects. Kinins increase vascular permeability and cause vasodilation, increasing the likelihood of shock. Elastase and chymotrypsin cause necrosis and damage blood vessels, which may cause hemorrhage. In addition, pancreatic fluid and blood entering the peritoneum may cause chemical irritation of the bowel and bowel atony, resulting in fluid shift into interstitial spaces (third spacing) as fluid leaks out of the damaged intestine. Reduced renal blood flow may lead to acute tubular necrosis.

2. Rapid I.V. infusion of large volumes of fluid or blood is the primary immediate treatment indicated for hypovolemia. Untreated, hypovolemia quickly results in circulatory collapse and tissue death.

3. Injury to the insulin-producing islet cells of the pancreas commonly decreases insulin production and causes at least transient hyperglycemia. If damage is severe, particularly if chronic pancreatitis is also present, overt diabetes mellitus may develop. Hyperglycemia may contribute further to functional hypovolemia as the body responds to the hyperosmolar state with further fluid shifts.

4. Fluid shifts associated with acute pancreatitis may result in various electrolyte imbalances, including hypokalemia and hyponatremia. Hypocalcemia is a common finding, possibly caused by the bonding of calcium with fatty substances. Clinically significant hypocalcemia is associated with a poor prognosis.

Hepatobiliary and pancreatic disorders

5. Maintain continuous gastric drainage with low suction, as ordered, preferably with a double-lumen tube. Administer anticholinergic medications, if ordered. Test gastric drainage for blood at least every 8 hours. Withhold food and fluids.

5. Draining gastric secretions removes a stimulus for pancreatic secretions, thus reducing the release of vasoactive substances and allowing the damaged pancreas to rest. A double-lumen tube is preferable for continuous suction because the air vent minimizes the risk of damage to the gastric mucosa. Anticholinergic use is controversial because such medication may contribute to ileus; some practitioners believe anticholinergics effectively reduce pancreatic secretions, but this is unproven. Withholding food and fluids prevents stimulation of gastric secretions.

6. Administer I.V. dopamine (Intropin) or other vasopressor, as ordered, if hypotension persists.

6. In acute pancreatitis, the release of myocardial depressant factor from the pancreas is thought to reduce cardiac output. Dopamine increases blood pressure and cardiac output by increasing heart rate and peripheral vasoconstriction. Low-dose dopamine (2 to 5 mcg/kg/minute) causes increased blood flow to renal arteries, thus increasing urinary output. The patient must be well hydrated prior to administration of any vasoactive agent.

7. Prepare the patient for surgery if hemodynamic parameters don't stabilize in response to therapeutic interventions.

7. Persistent shock indicates the need for surgical intervention to stop bleeding, relieve duct obstruction, drain an abscess or pseudocyst, or evaluate other possible intra-abdominal pathology

8. Additional individualized interventions: _____

8. Rationales: _____

Nursing diagnosis

Pain related to edema, necrosis, autodigestive processes, abdominal distention, abscess formation, ileus, or peritonitis

Nursing priorities

Monitor, evaluate, and relieve pain and treat underlying cause.

Patient outcome criteria

• Within 1 hour of the onset of pain, and then continuously, the patient will rate pain as less than 3 on a 0 to 10 pain rating scale.
• Within 2 days, the patient will, upon request, state two recommended dietary or lifestyle changes.

Interventions

1. Assess pain, noting location, character, severity, radiation, frequency, and any accompanying symptoms. Immediately report changes in pain quality or location, particularly if abdominal rigidity, reduced or absent bowel sounds, palpable abdominal mass, or other indications of generalized peritonitis or abscess occur. See the "Pain" plan, page 88.

Rationales

1. Evaluating the nature of the patient's pain is essential for early detection of complications. Typically, the pain accompanying acute pancreatitis is severe, steady, and felt across the entire abdomen, and it commonly radiates to the back or flank. Tenderness on deep palpation may occur; however, the abdomen usually remains soft. Abdominal rigidity and reduced bowel sounds may indicate peritonitis; a mass may indicate abscess or pseudocyst. Prompt surgical intervention is warranted if these occur. The "Pain" plan contains general interventions for any patient in pain.

2. Ensure that blood samples for serum amylase and lipase levels are obtained before administering analgesics.

3. Medicate, as ordered, with narcotic analgesics, usually meperidine. Observe for increased pain after narcotic administration and collaborate with the doctor to adjust pain control regimen, as indicated.

4. Administer antacids, as ordered, clamping the gastric tube for 30 minutes after administration. When oral intake is resumed, avoid simultaneous administration of antacids with oral cimetidine (Tagamet).

5. If the patient's condition permits, begin teaching dietary and lifestyle measures that reduce discomfort and help avert recurrence of acute attacks. Include family members in all teaching. Address the following considerations:
• need for lifelong avoidance of alcohol
• low-fat diet, depending on presence of gallbladder disease
• avoidance of caffeine or other substances linked to increased gastric secretions.

6. Additional individualized interventions: _____

2. Many analgesics, including meperidine (Demerol) and morphine, may elevate serum amylase and lipase levels, limiting the usefulness of these findings in diagnosis.

3. The severity of pain associated with acute pancreatitis generally warrants narcotic analgesia. Morphine is thought to increase spasm of Oddi's sphincter and, thus, is usually avoided for these patients. However, other analgesics, including meperidine, may also have such effects to some degree.

4. Antacids reduce gastric acidity and associated discomfort; some products may also act to relieve flatulence and distention. Antacids may impair cimetidine absorption if given at the same time.

5. The patient's condition may limit teaching, but introductory material can lay the groundwork for more thorough discussion after the patient has stabilized. Alcohol is a common factor in the recurrence of acute pancreatitis, although the exact physiologic mechanism is not known. Gallbladder disease may indicate the need for a low-fat diet to avoid exacerbating symptoms. Caffeine causes increased gastric acid secretion, thus increasing pancreatic activity.

6. Rationales: _____

NURSING DIAGNOSIS

Risk for injury: Complications related to pulmonary insults, hypovolemia, alcoholism, or other factors

Nursing priority

Prevent or detect and promptly treat complications.

Patient outcome criteria

Throughout the hospital stay, the patient will:
• perform pulmonary hygiene measures as instructed
• show no evidence of complications.

Interventions

1. Assess lung sounds, sputum production, skin color, and respiratory rate and effort frequently, at least every 2 hours. Report decreased breath sounds, crackles, productive cough, increased respiratory rate or effort or other signs of respiratory complications immediately. Monitor arterial blood gas levels daily or as ordered and report abnormal results.

Rationales

1. The patient with acute pancreatitis is at increased risk for pulmonary complications from edema, fluid shifts, diaphragmatic irritation, and possible decreased myocardial contractility. Adult respiratory distress syndrome, pulmonary edema, pleural effusion, or pneumonia may occur. Endotracheal intubation and mechanical ventilation may be required for adequate oxygenation if respiratory impairment is a factor. Early intervention reduces the risk of significant hypoxic damage.

2. Encourage deep breathing, coughing, incentive spirometer use, and position changes at least every 2 hours.

3. Assess for indicators of paralytic ileus, perforated viscus, or peritonitis, such as reduced or absent bowel sounds, vomiting, increased abdominal distention, rigid or boardlike abdomen, and tympany.

4. Monitor for signs and symptoms of pseudocyst development, such as increasing tenderness, palpable mass, upper abdominal pain, diarrhea, and worsening of general condition despite interventions.

5. After surgical intervention, assess for and report indications of colonic, enteric, or pancreatic fistula. Observe for signs of a fistula opening to the skin: pinpoint openings at wound edges or within the wound, green or yellow wound drainage, and excoriated wound edges. If the fistula opens to the skin, collect drainage; provide frequent, meticulous skin care; measure drainage pH; and replace fluids and electrolytes as ordered. Also observe for signs of an internal fistula: electrolyte imbalance, hypovolemia, fever, and peritonitis. If the fistula is internal, anticipate surgery.

6. Assess for and report indications of disseminated intravascular coagulation (DIC), such as bleeding or oozing from wounds, drains, or puncture sites; purpura of the chest or abdomen; petechiae; hematuria; melena; or epistaxis. Guaiac test all drainage. See the "Disseminated intravascular coagulation" plan, page 780, for details.

7. Assess for early indications of renal impairment, such as oliguria or anuria, increased urine osmolality, and elevated blood urea nitrogen level.

8. Be alert for indications of alcohol withdrawal syndrome, such as agitation, tremors, insomnia, hypertension, and anxiety. If alcoholism is a likely contributing factor to the patient's condition, consult with the doctor regarding measures to prevent or minimize alcohol withdrawal syndrome.

9. Additional individualized interventions: _____

2. Abdominal distention, pain, and the use of narcotic medications may contribute to reduced chest expansion, predisposing the patient to pulmonary abnormalities. These measures help reexpand atelectatic areas and improve clearance of pulmonary secretions.

3. These conditions may arise as a result of chemical irritation of the bowel, necrosis, and abscess formation associated with acute pancreatitis. Without immediate surgical intervention, sepsis may develop.

4. Pseudocysts are pockets left in the pancreas after tissue necrosis, in which blood, tissue debris, and pancreatic secretions accumulate. They may resolve spontaneously, rupture and cause chemical peritonitis, or grow so large that they compress other organs. Intervention may include drainage with percutaneous aspiration guided by CT scan, or surgical resection.

5. Fistulas (abnormal openings from body cavities or hollow organs to other cavities or the skin surface) can result from impaired wound healing around surgical anastomosis sites or an anastamotic leak. Pancreatic fistulas are more common when necrosis of the head or midportion of the pancreas leaves a viable, pancreatic-juice-secreting tail behind. Because pancreatic secretions have a high enzyme content, drainage collection minimizes skin excoriation; it also helps predict fluid replacement needs. The pancreas produces bicarbonate, so an alkaline pH confirms pancreatic fistula drainage. Fluid and electrolyte loss from fistula drainage can cause dehydration, hypokalemia, and hyponatremia.

6. DIC is a major potential complication associated with acute pancreatitis, possibly from release of tissue fragments, toxins associated with shock, or other physiologic mechanisms. Early detection allows prompt treatment. The "Disseminated intravascular coagulation" plan contains interventions for this disorder.

7. Hypovolemia may decrease renal perfusion and lead to acute renal failure. Renal impairment may also occur in acute pancreatitis when volume status is normal; the mechanism involved is unclear, but may involve DIC.

8. Because excessive alcohol intake is a common factor in acute pancreatitis, always consider the possibility of overt or hidden alcoholism. Untreated, the withdrawal syndrome may progress rapidly to seizures, hallucinations, hyperthermia, other severe complications, or death.

9. Rationales: _____

NURSING DIAGNOSIS

Nutritional deficit related to vomiting, pain, gastric suction, nothing by mouth (NPO) status, and impaired digestion

Nursing priority

Maintain or restore adequate nutritional intake.

Patient outcome criterion

Throughout the hospital stay, the patient will maintain prescribed nutritional intake (see the "Nutritional deficit" plan, page 80, for specific criteria).

Interventions

1. Assess nutritional status. See the "Nutritional deficit" plan, for details.

2. Administer total parenteral nutrition (TPN), as ordered, and monitor patient response, including careful monitoring of glucose levels. Consult the "Total parenteral nutrition" plan, page 527, for details.

3. As the patient's condition permits, institute dietary teaching, as indicated, including:
• diabetic diet
• use of pancreatic enzymes, if recommended
• avoidance of alcohol and caffeine.

4. Additional individualized interventions: _____

Rationales

1. Baseline assessment of nutritional status is essential for planning appropriate maintenance or replacement therapy. The "Nutritional deficit" plan provides details on evaluating nutritional status.

2. Oral nutrient intake during an acute pancreatitis episode tends to exacerbate pain and increase pancreatic activity. In the patient requiring prolonged NPO status, TPN may be indicated to avert malnutrition. Increased protein and calories are necessary for healing and for maintenance of the body's immunologic defenses. In pancreatitis, glucose levels may be elevated because of damage to the insulin-producing islet cells in the pancreas; if hyperglycemia has been present, the additional glucose in the TPN solution makes insulin dosage adjustment necessary. Enteral products may be contraindicated during the initial phases of pancreatitis.

3. Careful dietary teaching may help the patient avoid recurrences. A diabetic diet may be necessary because of reduced insulin production. Oral intake of pancreatic enzymes helps correct deficiencies. Alcohol and caffeine avoidance eliminates common triggers of acute pancreatitis.

4. Rationales: _____

DISCHARGE PLANNING

Discharge checklist

Before discharge, the patient shows evidence of:
❏ stable vital signs
❏ normal electrolyte values
❏ serum glucose controlled by medication, as needed
❏ pain controlled by medication
❏ absence of pulmonary or cardiovascular complications
❏ normal bowel sounds and elimination
❏ normal urine output
❏ adequate nutritional intake.

Teaching checklist

Document evidence that the patient and family demonstrate an understanding of:
❏ disease, precipitating factors, and prognosis
❏ dietary considerations
❏ diabetic teaching, as required
❏ signs and symptoms indicating recurrence or complications
❏ pain-relief measures.

Hepatobiliary and pancreatic disorders

Documentation checklist

Using outcome criteria as a guide, document:
- ❐ clinical status on admission
- ❐ significant changes in status
- ❐ pertinent laboratory and diagnostic test findings
- ❐ fluid intake and output
- ❐ bowel function
- ❐ patient and family teaching
- ❐ discharge planning.

ASSOCIATED PLANS OF CARE

Adult respiratory distress syndrome
Diabetic ketoacidosis
Disseminated intravascular coagulation
Ineffective individual coping
Knowledge deficit
Nutritional deficit
Pain
Pulmonary embolism
Total parenteral nutrition

REFERENCES

Banks, P.A., "Acute Pancreatitis: Medical and Surgical Management," *American Journal of Gastroenterology* 89(9):S78-85, August 1994.

Bartholomew, M., and Barkin, J. "Early Antibiotic Treatment in Acute Necrotizing Pancreatitis," *Gastrointestinal Endoscopy* 44(6):763-64, December 1996.

Di Francesco, V., et al. "Effect of Octreotide on Sphincter of Oddi Motility in Patients with Acute Recurrent Pancreatitis: A Manometric Study," *Digest of Disease Sciences* 41(12)2392-96, December 1996.

Skaife, P. and Kingsnorth, A.N. "Acute Pancreatitis: Assessment and Management," *Journal of Postgraduate Medicine* 72(847):277-83, May 1996.

Tsiotos, G.G., et al. "Intraabdominal Hemorrhage Complicating Surgical Management of Necrotizing Pancreatitis," *Pancreas* 12(2):26-30, March 1996.

Part 9

Musculoskeletal and integumentary disorders

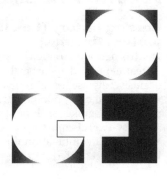

Amputation

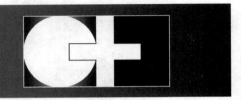

DRG information

DRG 213   Amputation for Musculoskeletal System
            and Connective Tissue Disorders.
            Mean LOS = 9.7 days
Additional DRG information: DRG 213 is only provided
as a rough guideline. Determining the correct DRG for
amputations depends on the underlying disease or type
of trauma, and the site and level of amputation.

INTRODUCTION

Definition and time focus
Amputation is the surgical removal of an irreparably
damaged or diseased limb. An amputation may be immediate because of the nature of an injury (such as
from a motor vehicle accident or burn), or offered together with a prosthesis to improve function. The
stump is closed with sutures or staples unless massive
infection was present before surgery, in which case a
guillotine-like surgery is performed and the wound is
left unsutured. Traction may be applied to prevent skin
retraction and to allow healing.
    This plan focuses on providing care after amputation
of an upper or lower extremity.

Etiology and precipitating factors
• Advanced peripheral vascular disease (especially
when associated with diabetes mellitus, infection, or
smoking)
• Trauma (such as that from crushing injuries, motor
vehicle accidents, or industrial accidents)
• Thermal injury (such as that from frostbite, chemical
exposure, or burns)
• Tumor
• Congenital anomaly

FOCUSED ASSESSMENT GUIDELINES

Nursing history (functional health pattern findings)
Health perception–health management pattern
• Treatment for diabetes mellitus, atherosclerotic arterial
occlusive disease, or osteomyelitis
• Likelihood of amputation is significantly increased if
patient is a smoker with peripheral vascular disease
Activity-exercise pattern
• Difficulty in ambulation if lower limb is involved,
leading to an altered exercise pattern

• Severe pain associated with exercise in lower limbs if
peripheral vascular disease is present
Sleep-rest pattern
• Interrupted sleep pattern associated with discomfort
Cognitive-perceptual pattern
• Tingling or burning sensation or paresthesia
Self-perception–self-concept pattern
• Difficulty accepting body-image change
• Verbalized concern about returning to work
Role-relationship pattern
• Concern about relationships and rejection by others
• Verbalized fear of role change
Coping–stress tolerance pattern
• Failure to seek or follow medical treatment for prob-
lem, necessitating amputation
• Denial to deal with current experience

Physical findings
Integumentary
(in affected extremity)
• Shiny skin
• Skin atrophy
• Skin cool to touch
• Cyanosis or redness of extremities when in dependent
position
• Thickened nails
• Stasis ulcer
• Edema
• Nonhealing wound
• Palpable mass
Cardiovascular
• Capillary refill time greater than 3 seconds
• Severe, cramping pain with exercise, usually relieved
by rest
• Decreased pulse amplitude
• Diminished or absent peripheral pulses
Musculoskeletal
• Limited limb movement
• Limited ambulation
• Pain
• Contractures
• Protective holding of affected extremity

Diagnostic studies
• Wound culture and sensitivity — if infection is present, may identify causative microorganism and identify
appropriate antibiotics
• Complete blood count — elevated white blood cell
count indicates infection

• Erythrocyte sedimentation rate — elevation indicates an inflammatory response
• X-rays — may reveal skeletal trauma, anomalies, or a mass
• Computed tomography scan — may reveal primary and metastatic tumors, infection, or trauma
• Arteriography and Doppler flow studies — may confirm circulatory inadequacy in major arteries or veins
• Biopsy — confirms presence of a malignant or benign mass

• Physical and occupational therapy evaluation — extent of gross and fine motor function determines ability to use assistive devices (such as prosthesis, crutches, and walker)

Potential complications
• Hemorrhage
• Infection
• Flexion contracture
• Psychopathologic adaptation to limb loss

CLINICAL SNAPSHOT

AMPUTATION

Major nursing diagnoses and collaborative problems	Key patient outcomes
Risk for hemorrhage	Have stable vital signs: typically, heart rate, 60 to 100 beats/minute; systolic blood pressure, 90 to 140 mm Hg; and diastolic blood pressure, 50 to 90 mm Hg.
Pain	Rate pain as less than 3 on a 0 to 10 pain rating scale.
Risk for infection	Show no signs or symptoms of infection.
Risk for disuse syndrome (loss of joint function)	Demonstrate independent use of transfer techniques.
Body-image disturbance	Verbalize feelings and concerns regarding amputation.

COLLABORATIVE PROBLEM

Risk for hemorrhage related to amputation

Nursing priority

Maintain circulatory volume.

Patient outcome criteria

• Within 1 day after surgery and then continuously, the patient will have normal vital signs: typically, heart rate, 60 to 100 beats/minute; systolic blood pressure, 90 to 140 mm Hg; and diastolic blood pressure, 50 to 90 mm Hg.
• Within 3 days after surgery, the patient will have decreased drainage.

Interventions

1. Assess the surgical site immediately upon the patient's arrival on the unit after surgery. Document your findings, including the type of dressing and a description of any drainage and drainage devices such as a Hemovac.

Rationales

1. Baseline assessment permits comparison of data, which assists in the ongoing status evaluation. A drain or portable wound suction device may be in place to remove fluid or blood that might interfere with granulation. Observed drainage will be minimal and serosanguineous. Increased amounts of bright red drainage may indicate hemorrhage.

2. Observe and document signs of oozing on the dressing. Reinforce the dressing as required. Don't remove the dressing until ordered. Document the amount of supplies used and the frequency of reinforcement.

3. Maintain an I.V. line. Document its site, appearance, and patency.

4. Keep a tourniquet at the bedside. Apply it to the limb or apply direct pressure to the artery if significant bleeding occurs. Notify the doctor immediately, remain with the patient until the doctor arrives, and document the events.

5. Additional individualized interventions: _____

2. A small amount of oozing from the incision is normal. Documenting the supplies used and drainage characteristics helps other caregivers assess status changes. Initially, most postamputation dressings are pressure or pressure-cast dressings; premature removal may result in undesirable edema and bleeding.

3. Loss of circulating blood volume results in vessel constriction, increasing the difficulty of venipuncture. An established line provides a route for rapid fluid replacement if necessary.

4. If hemorrhage occurs, immediate tourniquet application prevents significant blood loss and shock. If bleeding is severe, direct arterial pressure may be necessary. The patient may be frightened by the amount of blood lost; the nurse's presence can be reassuring.

5. Rationales: _____

NURSING DIAGNOSIS

Pain related to postoperative tissue, nerve, and bone trauma

Nursing priorities

Relieve pain, provide reassurance, and teach about phantom limb phenomena.

Patient outcome criteria

• Within 4 hours after surgery, the patient will:
 – show no associated pain behaviors
 – rate pain (with pain medication) as less than 3 on a 0 to 10 pain rating scale.
• Within 1 day after surgery, the patient will verbalize understanding of phantom limb pain and sensation.
• Within 3 days after surgery, the patient will decrease requests for pain medication.

Interventions

1. See the "Pain" plan, page 88.

2. Monitor for pain continually. Listen to complaints of discomfort and observe for tense posture, tightening fists, diaphoresis, and increased pulse rate. Have patient rate pain level using a 0 to 10 pain rating scale.

3. Document pain episodes, noting location, characteristics, radiation, frequency, severity, and associated findings.

4. When pain occurs, administer medication promptly, as ordered. Evaluate and document the patient's response. Taper the frequency of intramuscular medication administration after the third or fourth postoperative day, as ordered; substitute oral medication, as ordered and as needed.

Rationales

1. The "Pain" plan provides general guidelines and interventions for pain.

2. Pain is what the patient states it is; early detection and intervention promote patient comfort. Pain stimulates the sympathetic nervous system, resulting in physical symptoms.

3. Documentation provides a baseline to help others interpret pain-related behaviors.

4. Early administration of pain medication is more effective in controlling pain than waiting until the pain becomes severe. Pain normally begins to diminish in intensity 3 or 4 days after surgery.

5. Evaluate the dressing or cast for tightness each time the patient complains of pain and every 3 to 4 hours. Document the findings. If circulation, sensation, or movement is impaired, notify the doctor and reapply the dressing more loosely.

6. Reposition the patient or the affected limb every 2 to 3 hours. Document repositionings.

7. Gently massage the stump every 4 hours after the surgeon removes the dressing. Avoid using emollients. Evaluate and document the patient's response.

8. Explain the cause of phantom limb sensation and pain. Inform the patient that this may last as long as 6 months (rarely longer), although phantom limb pain may arise again even years later.

9. Use nonpharmacologic pain relief measures between doses of pain medication and when the patient does not experience pain relief. Consider diversion, activity, backrub, relaxation techniques, imagery, or cutaneous stimulation (such as counterirritation with oil of wintergreen). Consider consulting the doctor about a transcutaneous electrical nerve stimulation device.

10. Additional individualized interventions: _____
_____

5. Decreased circulation causes tissue hypoxia and increases the pain response.

6. Pain increases with external pressure or fatigue. Changing position relieves pressure and the risk of complications from immobility.

7. Massage increases circulation to the traumatized area. Emollients can cause skin maceration.

8. Phantom limb sensation is the feeling or perception of the amputated limb's presence. Phantom limb pain, a separate phenomenon, is the awareness of pain in the amputated body part. Unfortunately, treatment methods for persistent phantom limb pain are of limited value. The cause of these relatively uncommon phenomena is unknown. Knowing that phantom limb sensation and pain are normal responses to amputation may reassure the patient.

9. These methods decrease awareness of painful stimuli.

10. Rationales: _____
_____

NURSING DIAGNOSIS

Risk for infection related to interrupted skin integrity

Nursing priority

Promote wound healing.

Patient outcome criteria

By the time of discharge, the patient will:
• show no signs or symptoms of infection
• list signs of stump breakdown
• demonstrate stump-toughening exercises.

Interventions

1. Observe the incision line for redness, edema, or exudate during each dressing change. Document all findings. If a plaster cast is in place, check for signs of tissue necrosis: "hot" spots, drainage on the cast, unrelieved pain, or foul odor.

Rationales

1. Assessment of the incision line during the first dressing change provides baseline data for future comparison. Histamine release causes the classic signs of inflammation. Diminished tissue perfusion, resulting from decreased circulation secondary to external pressure, causes cell death. Tissue necrosis results in pain, a sensation of local heat, drainage, and odor.

2. Protect the stump from contamination and trauma. If the patient is incontinent, protect the limb with a plastic covering. Always use sterile technique during dressing changes.

3. Always rewrap dressings securely but not tightly. Do not apply tape to skin.

4. Encourage the patient to follow the prescribed diet. Document the patient's likes and dislikes, and assist with menu selection. Promote intake of foods high in protein, vitamins, calories, and minerals.

5. After a dressing is no longer necessary, bathe the stump daily with mild soap and water. Dry it thoroughly and leave it exposed to air twice daily for at least 20 minutes.

6. Teach the signs and symptoms of stump breakdown. Examine the stump daily for edema, redness, and skin breaks. Teach the patient to examine the stump regularly after discharge, such as during exercise or bathing.

7. Teach stump-toughening exercises. Have the patient push the stump against a soft pillow four to six times daily. Increase resistance gradually. Document progress.

8. Additional individualized interventions: _____
_____

2. Exposing the stump to microorganisms increases the risk of infection. Trauma causes tissue death and slows healing.

3. Tight dressings may inhibit blood flow to the healing wound, reducing the availability of oxygen and essential nutrients. Tape can cause tissue trauma during removal.

4. Preexisting diseases, such as diabetes, may require that the patient follow a specific diet. Additional amounts of protein, calories, vitamins, and minerals are needed for wound healing.

5. Hygiene is essential to maintaining healthy skin that can tolerate a prosthesis. Moist skin allows maceration to occur.

6. Early detection of stump breakdown allows prompt treatment. Undetected complications jeopardize the patient's rehabilitation program and may make further amputation necessary.

7. Fragile, delicate skin will not withstand the pressure a prosthesis will apply. Toughening the skin prepares the patient to wear a prosthesis and reduces the chance of infection related to skin breakdown.

8. Rationales: _____
_____

NURSING DIAGNOSIS

Risk for disuse syndrome (loss of joint function) related to impaired physical mobility

Nursing priority

Maintain range of motion (ROM) in affected joint.

Patient outcome criteria

By the time of discharge, the patient will:
- display no signs of joint contracture
- demonstrate independent use of transfer techniques
- use assistive devices independently
- demonstrate muscle-strengthening exercises
- initiate discussion of follow-up plans.

Interventions

1. Promote joint extension. Don't use pillows under a lower-extremity stump; raise the foot of the bed instead. Use slings and pillows under an upper-extremity stump.

2. Place the patient in the prone position for 30 minutes four times daily and for sleep (for lower-limb amputation), if not contraindicated.

Rationales

1. Proper positioning promotes venous return and decreases edema without causing flexion contracture.

2. The prone position facilitates normal joint alignment in extension.

3. Don't allow the knee to bend over the edge of the chair or bed if the patient had a below-the-knee amputation.

4. Institute ROM exercises for the affected limb two to three times daily, beginning on the first day after surgery. Gradually increase the frequency on subsequent days. Evaluate and document the patient's response.

5. Provide a trapeze bar over the patient's bed.

6. Plan activities around the time of pain medication administration. Be alert for medication effects that can decrease alertness or increase the patient's potential for injury.

7. Position personal belongings, water, the telephone, and the call light within the patient's reach at all times, particularly if an arm was amputated.

8. Instruct a patient with a lower-extremity amputation to call for assistance when getting out of bed. Keep the bed in the low position at all times.

9. Teach transfer techniques appropriate to the patient's amputation (for example, repositioning in bed, or bed-to-chair or bed-to-wheelchair transfer). Document the teaching and the patient's use of the techniques.

10. Teach muscle-strengthening exercises specific to the limb amputated. Gluteal-setting exercises for above-the-knee amputation, hamstring-setting exercises for below-the-knee amputation, and straightening the flexed proximal joint against resistance are examples of valuable exercises. Include exercises for increasing triceps strength, such as pushing against the bed with the fists and raising the buttocks off the bed. Tell the patient to exercise twice daily, gradually increasing frequency as muscle strength increases.

11. Explain that stance will be altered. Teach abdominal and gluteal muscle-tightening exercises to perform while standing. Have the patient practice balancing on the toes. Teach him to bend the knee and hop while holding onto a chair. Remain with the patient during these exercises.

12. Consult with the doctor concerning physical therapy or occupational therapy referrals.

13. After a lower-extremity amputation, reinforce skills of ambulation, crutch walking, or use of assistive devices learned during physical therapy. Encourage the patient to use these techniques whenever ambulating.

3. Allowing the stump to hang in a dependent position decreases venous return and increases edema. Flexion contracture may occur if the stump remains bent.

4. ROM exercises are directed toward maintaining normal joint mobility. Disuse can cause permanent shortening of the muscles, resulting in contractures.

5. A trapeze increases mobility in bed, allows the patient to be more independent, and prevents exclusive use of the heel or elbow for pushing when the patient moves (which may contribute to skin breakdown).

6. Pain prevents full participation in activities. Narcotics may cause orthostatic hypotension and fainting from vascular dilation.

7. Being able to reach needed items promotes independence and increases self-confidence in a patient with an altered self-concept.

8. Muscle weakness and impaired balance after a lower-limb amputation may result in an injury.

9. Learning transfer techniques reestablishes the patient's independence and promotes a feeling of security when moving in and out of bed.

10. Optimal muscle strength is required to maintain balance while using assistive devices, such as crutches, a walker, and a prosthesis.

11. An altered center of gravity requires increased muscle strength, balance, and coordination to compensate for the amputated extremity. Remaining with the patient during practice provides reassurance and helps prevent injury related to loss of balance.

12. Early intervention by physical and occupational therapy specialists increases the patient's rehabilitation potential.

13. Consistent use of learned methods increases the patient's skill, self-confidence, and awareness of their importance.

14. Ensure appropriate referral for home care if self-care ability or motivation is a problem. Emphasize the importance of ongoing rehabilitative follow-up.

15. Additional individualized interventions: _____

14. Inadequate follow-up may lead to functional limitations or further limb compromise. Ongoing follow-up allows early detection of problems.

15. Rationales: _____

NURSING DIAGNOSIS

Body-image disturbance related to loss of a body part

Nursing priority

Promote acceptance of the loss of a body part.

Patient outcome criteria

By the time of discharge, the patient will:
• verbalize feelings and concerns regarding amputation
• participate in stump care
• express knowledge about the availability of a prosthesis (if appropriate).

Interventions

1. Show an accepting attitude toward the patient. Anticipate a period of mourning for the lost limb. See the "Grieving" plan, page 44.

2. Spend time with the patient each shift. Encourage verbalization of feelings about the amputation. Clarify areas of misunderstanding and reassure the patient that feelings are normal.

3. Encourage family and friends to interact with the patient. Explain the patient's response, if necessary. Refer family members to a counselor, as needed.

4. Encourage the patient to look at the stump and to help in its care during the early postoperative period. Do not force this, however, if the patient is hesitant.

5. Introduce the patient to others with similar amputations who have adapted successfully.

Rationales

1. Acceptance helps the patient feel valued as an individual. The patient may experience various manifestations of the grieving process, such as directing anger and frustration toward staff and family members. The "Grieving" plan contains detailed information on assisting with the grieving process.

2. Clarifying knowledge and encouraging expression of feelings helps the patient pass through the stages of grief.

3. The demonstration of acceptance and love by family and friends is essential to completing the grieving process.

4. Acknowledging the stump helps the patient recognize reality and promotes acceptance of an altered body image. Acceptance is a highly individualized process; forcing the patient to look at the stump may provoke undue distress.

5. Seeing someone who has adapted successfully demonstrates that the amputation doesn't have to interfere with a normal lifestyle. Peers may provide realistic encouragement and practical help in adapting to the change.

6. Provide information about an appropriate prosthesis and its use, reinforcing the teaching of the prosthetist or physical therapist.

7. Consult a member of the clergy, psychiatric clinician, or social worker if the patient is unable to progress through the grieving process. See the "Ineffective individual coping" plan, page 67.

8. Additional individualized interventions: _____

6. Replacement of the amputated body part with a prosthesis gives the body a more normal appearance and increases the patient's participation in daily activities. Knowing that a prosthesis is available provides the patient with a goal to work toward.

A prosthesis may be applied immediately after surgery. This reduces residual limb edema, loss of muscle strength, and complications of immobility and also promotes healing through increased tissue perfusion at the operative site as a result of early ambulation. More importantly, immediate application of a prosthesis improves the patient's psychological outlook.

A prosthesis may also be applied 1 to 6 months after surgery. This occurs when wound healing is delayed because of infection, peripheral vascular disease, or the patient's debilitated status.

7. Special assistance may be necessary to help the patient accept the amputation. Maladaptation to amputation may result in severe depression or suicidal behavior.

8. Rationales: _____

DISCHARGE PLANNING

Discharge checklist
Before discharge, the patient shows evidence of:
- ❑ stable vital signs
- ❑ absence of pulmonary or cardiovascular complications
- ❑ a healing incision with no signs of swelling, redness, inflammation, or drainage
- ❑ absence of fever
- ❑ absence of contractures
- ❑ pain controlled by oral medication
- ❑ ability to tolerate diet
- ❑ ability to perform stump care independently or with minimal assistance
- ❑ ability to perform activities of daily living (ADLs) independently or with minimal assistance
- ❑ completion of initial physical therapy program with appropriate assistive devices
- ❑ ability to transfer and ambulate independently or with minimal assistance (with a lower-extremity amputation)
- ❑ adequate home support or referral for home care or to a rehabilitation setting if indicated by lack of home support system; inability to perform ADLs, stump care, and safe transfers; or continued need for physical therapy.

Teaching checklist
Document evidence that the patient and family demonstrate an understanding of:
- ❑ underlying disease and implications
- ❑ all discharge medications' purpose, dosage, administration schedule, and adverse effects requiring medical attention (discharge medications are prescribed only if the patient has an infection or a preexisting condition such as diabetes mellitus; patient may be prescribed pain medication to be taken as needed)
- ❑ prescribed diet
- ❑ necessary equipment and supplies
- ❑ care of stump and prosthesis
- ❑ phantom limb sensation and pain
- ❑ signs of wound inflammation and infection that require medical attention
- ❑ prescribed exercises for the residual limb
- ❑ need for smoking cessation program (if appropriate)
- ❑ name and telephone number of contact person for additional information or answers to questions
- ❑ date, time, and location of follow-up appointments
- ❑ how to contact the doctor
- ❑ available community resources.

Documentation checklist
Using outcome criteria as a guide, document:
- ❑ clinical status on return from surgery
- ❑ significant changes in status
- ❑ pertinent laboratory and diagnostic test findings
- ❑ pain at surgical site
- ❑ phantom limb pain

❏ phantom limb sensation
❏ pain-relief measures
❏ mobility and positioning
❏ dressing changes
❏ appearance of wound
❏ drainage devices
❏ I.V. line patency
❏ oxygen therapy
❏ nutritional intake
❏ psychological status
❏ physical therapy, occupational therapy, or both
❏ assistive devices, such as a walker, crutches, and prosthesis
❏ patient and family teaching
❏ discharge planning.

ASSOCIATED PLANS OF CARE

Diabetes mellitus
Grieving
Ineffective individual coping
Knowledge deficit
Pain
Surgery

REFERENCES

Guyton, A.C. *Textbook of Medical Physiology*, 9th ed. Philadelphia: W.B. Saunders Co., 1994.
Lewis, S.M., and Collier, I.C. *Medical-Surgical Nursing: Assessment and Management of Clinical Problems,* 4th ed. New York: Mc-Graw-Hill Book Co., 1996.
Phipps, W.J., et al. *Medical-Surgical Nursing: Concepts and Clinical Practice,* 5th ed. St. Louis: Mosby–Year Book, Inc., 1995.

Fractured femur

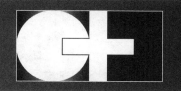

DRG information
DRG 210   Hip and Femur Procedures, Except Major
          Joint; Age 17+ with Complication or Co-
          morbidity (CC).
          Mean LOS = 8.6 days
DRG 211   Hip and Femur Procedures, Except Major
          Joint; Age 17+ without CC.
          Mean LOS = 6.3 days
DRG 212   Hip and Femur Procedures, Except Major
          Joint; Ages 0 to 17.
          Mean LOS = 11.1 days
Principal procedures for DRGs 210, 211, and 212 in-
clude:

> • fixation of bone without fracture reduc-
> tion
> • closed and open reduction with internal
> fixation
> • open reduction without internal fixation.

PRO alert: DRG 210 is a frequently occurring DRG.
Professional review organizations (PROs) are scrutiniz-
ing discharge planning criteria for this category because
patients assigned this DRG commonly complain of premature discharge. Therefore, daily nursing documentation must describe the patient's progress with activities
of daily living (ADLs), transfers, and ambulation. Upon
discharge, the patient's ability to perform ADLs and
transfers must be documented carefully.

INTRODUCTION

Definition and time focus
The femur, which connects the hip joint and the knee
joint, is the longest and strongest bone in the body. Because of its strength, most fractures of the femur are the
result of traumatic accidents involving considerable
force.
    The two primary classifications of femur fractures are:
• proximal end fractures, involving the portion of the
femur that engages with the acetabulum (These fractures may be further classified into two subtypes: intra-
capsular, involving the head and neck of the femur
within the hip joint, and extracapsular, involving the
area from the femoral neck distally to about 2″ [5 cm]
below the lesser trochanter.)
• femoral shaft fractures, involving the distal portion of
the femur.
    This plan focuses on preoperative and postoperative
care of the patient admitted to the hospital for treat

ment of a femur fracture. See the "Total joint replacement in a lower extremity" plan, page 643, for more information on fractures involving the hip joint.

Etiology and precipitating factors
• Proximal end fractures — fall injuries most common,
with osteoporosis a significant contributing factor in
older patients
• Femoral shaft fractures — high-impact traumatic accidents, most often in younger patients
• Related fractures of sacrum or lumbar spine.

FOCUSED ASSESSMENT GUIDELINES

Nursing history (functional health pattern findings)
Health perception–health management pattern
• If older, history of coexisting medical conditions
(such as heart disease, diabetes, and hypertension) that
caused or contributed to the fall
• If younger, may be the first contact with an inpatient
setting
Activity-exercise pattern
• Ability to walk (in proximal end fractures) but more
typically, can't bear weight
• Inability to bear weight (in femoral shaft fractures)
Cognitive-perceptual pattern
• Severe, localized pain in the affected limb
• Numbness or tingling in the affected limb
Value-belief pattern
• Disbelief that injury is severe (in proximal end frac-
tures); an older patient may insist that only pain relief is
necessary; may deny need for surgical intervention

Physical findings
Cardiovascular
• Edema at injury site or distally
• Tachycardia
• Hypotension
• If severe vascular involvement: absent pulse, reduced
pulse rate, or reduced or absent pulse amplitude in the
affected limb
Pulmonary
• Hyperventilation, tachypnea
Musculoskeletal
• Deformity at injury site (for example, external rotation
or shortening)
• Severe pain with movement of affected limb
• Ecchymosis

- Crepitus

Integumentary
- Diaphoresis
- Pallor (if significant blood is lost)

Diagnostic studies

Diagnostic studies may reveal no significant abnormalities initially, unless related to a coexisting condition.
- Complete blood count — performed before surgery to establish baseline; may reveal extent of blood loss associated with the injury (loss of up to 1.5 L may occur); decreased hemoglobin and hematocrit values result from dilution by crystalloid fluid replacement during resuscitation; white blood cell count may be elevated in response to injury
- Blood typing and cross-matching — performed in preparation for blood replacement if significant blood loss is present or incurred during surgery
- Chemistry panel — obtained before surgery to establish baseline and assess for underlying imbalances that may have contributed to the injury or that may affect intraoperative care (for example, potassium imbalances, which can cause increased cardiac irritability during anesthesia); blood urea nitrogen and creatinine levels evaluate renal function
- Prothrombin time, international normalized ratio (PT/INR), and activated partial thromboplastin time (APTT) — performed before surgery to establish baseline; usually are normal unless an underlying bleeding disorder is present; older patients may be started on anticoagulant therapy after surgery to minimize the risk of thromboembolism

- Urinalysis — performed for baseline evaluation of renal function
- Serum drug levels — performed if medication overdose or noncompliance is suspected as contributing factor to injury
- Femur X-ray — identifies location and type of fracture
- Chest X-ray — routinely obtained before surgery to rule out associated injuries or preexisting conditions affecting surgical care (such as cardiomegaly and heart failure)
- 12-lead electrocardiography (ECG) — obtained before surgery to establish baseline and to identify preexisting cardiac abnormalities, if any; may be especially significant in older patients or in those with blunt trauma to the chest (possible cardiac contusion) in addition to the leg injury

Potential complications
- Shock
- Hemorrhage
- Pulmonary embolism
- Fat embolism
- Thrombophlebitis
- Aseptic necrosis of the femoral head
- Nonunion of the affected portions
- Osteomyelitis
- Pneumonia
- Arthritic deformities
- Hemoglobin depletion related to iron depletion or deprivation

---

CLINICAL SNAPSHOT

FRACTURED FEMUR

Major nursing diagnoses and collaborative problems	Key patient outcomes
Risk for preoperative complications	Show stable vital signs: typically, heart rate, 60 to 100 beats/minute; systolic blood pressure, 90 to 140 mm Hg; and diastolic blood pressure, 50 to 90 mm Hg.
Risk for postoperative complications	Have no signs of excessive bleeding, neurovascular impairment, or infection.
Knowledge deficit (home care)	Identify signs and symptoms of complications.

COLLABORATIVE PROBLEM

Risk for preoperative complications related to nature of traumatic injury

Nursing priorities

• Prepare the patient to undergo surgery in optimal physical condition.
• Prevent or identify and promptly treat preoperative complications.

Patient outcome criteria

Before surgery, the patient will:
• have normal respirations or, if abnormal, receive treatment for respiratory problems
• show stable vital signs: typically, heart rate, 60 to 100 beats/minute; systolic blood pressure, 90 to 140 mm Hg; and diastolic blood pressure, 50 to 90 mm Hg
• have no uncontrolled bleeding
• have neurovascular findings within expected limits
• rate pain (with pain medications) as less than 3 on a 0 to 10 pain rating scale
• have received initial tetanus and infection prophylaxis, if indicated.

Interventions

1. Ensure adequacy of respirations. Auscultate the lungs and note any evidence of unequal chest excursion, unequal or diminished breath sounds, pain on respiration, cyanosis, restlessness, or dyspnea. Report any respiratory difficulty to the doctor immediately, and prepare to support ventilation or assist with insertion of chest tubes, if indicated.

2. Assess for signs of bleeding, and maintain circulatory volume. Report increasing pulse rate, decreasing blood pressure, pallor, diaphoresis, or decreasing alertness. Establish and maintain an I.V. line as ordered, usually with lactated Ringer's solution initially. If an open fracture is bleeding, apply direct, continuous pressure to the area and notify the doctor.

3. Assess the limb's neurovascular status. Note weakened or absent pulses, mottling, cyanosis, paresthesia, or loss of sensation. Compare pulse rates bilaterally. Avoid moving the limb unnecessarily. Report deficits to the doctor immediately.

4. Control pain. Assess level of pain using a 0 to 10 pain rating scale. Administer analgesics as ordered during the preoperative period, making sure all medications are noted on the surgical checklist. Apply cold packs to the fracture area. Maintain traction or splinting as ordered.

Rationales

1. High-impact accidents, such as those which cause femoral fractures, have a high incidence of multisystem injuries, including chest trauma. Pulmonary or chest abnormalities may indicate tracheal injury, pneumothorax, rib fractures, or other complications. In older patients, pre-existing medical conditions may involve cardiac or central nervous system functions, affecting respiratory capability and adequacy.

2. Femoral fractures are associated with significant blood loss because of the vascularity of long bones and the proximity of large vessels. The parameters noted are signs of shock and require immediate intervention. Intravenous infusions help replace fluids lost from bleeding; Ringer's lactate expands blood volume and replaces electrolyte losses. Direct pressure controls active bleeding until it can be stopped surgically.

3. Blood vessels and nerves in the fracture area may be displaced or severed by bone fragments or by edema and deformity. Movement may cause further injury. Inadequate perfusion of the limb may result in permanent functional impairment or loss of the affected portion.

4. Pain contributes to increasing anxiety, stresses the cardiovascular system, and may contribute to increased muscle tension and associated displacement at the injury site. Noting medications on the checklist ensures that their effects are considered in the administration of anesthetics. Cold packs help minimize edema by causing local vasoconstriction. Traction and splints may help reduce muscle spasms and pain.

5. If an open fracture is present, make sure tetanus and infection prophylaxis is considered before surgery. Cover the wound with a sterile dressing.

5. Tetanus immunization, if not current, should be updated because open wounds associated with trauma are considered tetanus-prone. Any break in skin integrity predisposes the patient to infection. Covering the wound minimizes further contamination from airborne bacteria.

6. Prepare the patient for surgery, if indicated. See the "Surgery" plan, page 103, for details.

6. Depending on the location and type of fracture, a femoral fracture may be treated with traction or a cast; however, surgery is usually the treatment of choice. Various surgical procedures are used to repair these fractures, including placement of a prosthesis, pins, intramedullary rods, or nails and bone grafts. Proper preoperative preparation helps minimize postoperative problems. General interventions for the surgical patient are included in the "Surgery" plan.

7. Additional individualized interventions: _____

7. Rationales: _____

COLLABORATIVE PROBLEM

Risk for postoperative complications related to the initial trauma injury, surgical intervention, or immobility

Nursing priorities

Prevent, or identify and promptly treat, postoperative complications and promote healing.

Patient outcome criteria

Within 2 hours of arrival on the unit after surgery, the patient will:
• maintain vital signs within normal limits: typically, heart rate, 60 to 100 beats/minute; systolic blood pressure, 90 to 140 mm Hg; and diastolic blood pressure, 50 to 90 mm Hg
• have no signs of excessive bleeding, neurovascular impairment, or infection
• rate pain (with pain medication) as less than 3 on a 0 to 10 pain rating scale
• manage coughing and deep breathing well
• maintain proper positioning.
Within 24 hours after surgery, the patient will:
• perform exercises as permitted
• show no signs of skin breakdown
• show no signs of embolism
• verbalize awareness of positioning restrictions
• take adequate food and fluids by mouth, if permitted.

Interventions

1. See the "Pain" plan, page 88, and the "Surgery" plan, page 103.

2. Assess vital signs according to postoperative protocol or more often if unstable. Check dressings and drains for bleeding. Report abnormalities in vital signs; excessive bleeding from the wound, surgical sites, drains, or graft sites; increasing edema; or ecchymosis. Assess for associated injuries if a high-impact trauma was involved.

Rationales

1. General guidelines for care of the surgical patient and for pain management are included in these plans.

2. As noted previously, femoral fractures may cause massive bleeding. Tachycardia and hypotension may indicate inadequate fluid replacement, excessive blood loss related to injury and repair, or other undetected injuries.

3. Assess neurovascular status at least once every hour and more often if compromised. Note weakened or absent pulses, mottling, cyanosis, paresthesia, loss of sensation, or a significant increase in edema after surgery. Be especially alert for signs and symptoms of compartment syndrome: increasing pain exacerbated by stretching, sensory deficits, paralysis, tense or hard swelling, or decreasing distal pulses. Notify the doctor immediately if neurovascular status becomes impaired.

4. Maintain a patent I.V. line and administer fluids as ordered, usually for at least 24 hours after surgery.

5. Administer antibiotics, if ordered. Observe the wound carefully and report increases in erythema or swelling, fever, purulent drainage, and other signs and symptoms of infection. Assess pH, transferrin, and free iron levels.

6. Prevent complications associated with immobility.

• Encourage the patient to perform gentle range-of-motion exercises for unaffected extremities; encourage alternate flexion and extension or quadriceps-setting exercises for the affected limb, as permitted. Increase activity level as permitted and as tolerated.
• Apply antiembolism stockings or sequential compression pants, as prescribed.

• Provide a trapeze to assist movement.

• Encourage coughing and deep breathing hourly while the patient is awake.

• Urge adequate fluid intake, when allowed, forcing fluids unless contraindicated. Document intake and output.

• Provide clean, dry bedding and a special bed or mattress as needed; reposition the patient at least every 2 hours, and provide frequent skin care, with special attention to bony prominences.
• Encourage verbalization of feelings. Provide diversionary activities.

• Consult the "Impaired physical mobility" plan on page 50.

3. Careful assessment ensures prompt intervention should the limb's neurovascular status be compromised after surgery. Increasing edema may put pressure on surrounding vascular structures, impairing oxygenation of tissue. Immediate intervention is needed to restore circulation. Compartment syndrome is a complication caused by muscle swelling in which increased tissue pressure causes circulatory impairment and ischemia. This condition may occur immediately after injury or may develop over several days. Immediate treatment (fasciotomy) may prevent permanent damage.

4. I.V. infusions replace fluid losses related to bleeding, restricted oral intake, preexisting dehydration, or tissue loss during surgery. Also, maintaining venous access allows administration of I.V. medication.

5. I.V. antibiotics are usually ordered during the initial postoperative period, particularly for the patient with an open fracture or increased susceptibility to infection. Infected bone wounds can be particularly serious; untreated, they may lead to osteomyelitis and bone disintegration. If the patient is already on antibiotic therapy when the infection develops, a different antibiotic may be indicated because the causative organism may be resistant to current therapy. An effort may be made to decrease free iron availability.

6. Immobility predisposes the patient to serious complications.
• Exercise, as allowed, decreases venous stasis and helps maintain muscle tone.

• Antiembolism stockings or sequential compression pants increase venous return and may help prevent thrombus formation.
• A trapeze allows the patient to assist with repositioning.
• Pulmonary hygiene measures help prevent postoperative lung infections related to immobility, anesthesia, decreased respiratory effort, and accumulation of secretions.
• Forcing fluids helps maintain hydration, liquefy secretions, maintain renal function, and minimize risk of urinary infection from stasis. Documenting intake and output identifies fluid imbalances.
• The immobilized patient is at increased risk for skin breakdown from constant pressure. A warm, moist environment encourages bacterial growth. Special beds and careful skin care prevent pressure ulcers.
• Prolonged immobilization contributes to depression, anxiety, and frustration. Verbalizing feelings to an accepting caregiver may help decrease stress. Diversionary activities decrease boredom and give the patient some sense of self-control.
• This plan provides further information about this condition.

7. Observe for signs and symptoms of embolism, as follows:

• fat embolism—tachycardia, dyspnea, pleuritic pain, pallor and cyanosis, petechiae, crackles, wheezing, nausea, syncope, weakness, altered mentation, ECG changes, or fever; in the affected limb, pallor, numbness, and coldness to touch
• pulmonary embolism—sudden chest pain, dyspnea, tachycardia, cough, hemoptysis, anxiety, syncope, ECG changes, hypotension, and fever

• thrombophlebitis—positive Homans' sign, pain in calf, swelling, and local redness in the limb. Report any signs to the doctor immediately, and initiate treatment, as ordered.

8. Maintain proper immobilization of the affected limb, depending on the fracture site and the type of repair. Usually, adduction, external rotation, and acute hip flexion should be avoided in a patient with a proximal end fracture; lateral pressure or overpulling with traction must be avoided in a patient with a femoral shaft fracture. Verify specific positioning orders with the doctor.

9. Observe for and immediately report any sudden, sharp pain, shortening or rotation of the affected limb, or persistent muscle spasm.

10. Encourage adequate nutritional intake, especially of protein-rich foods and foods high in vitamins and minerals.

11. Additional individualized interventions: _____

7. The nature of the injury and the period of postoperative immobility predispose the patient to this complication.
• Fat embolism occurs most often with long-bone fractures, usually within the first 3 days after injury. The exact physiologic mechanism is unknown. Fat emboli may lodge in the lungs, heart, brain, or extremities, and associated lipase release may cause tissue irritation.
• Pulmonary embolism is usually a later complication, occurring 10 to 24 days after injury. Signs may be related to obstruction from a blood clot that travels to the lungs and from reflex vasoconstriction.
• Thrombophlebitis usually occurs in the lower extremities as the result of clot formation and obstruction of superficial veins, although thrombi can occlude major vessels as well. Immediate intervention is required because these complications may be life-threatening. Treatment may include ventilatory support, corticosteroids, anticoagulants, or thrombolytic agents.

8. Movement of the fracture site may displace bone fragments and interfere with healing. Positioning of the affected limb depends on the fracture location and the surgical approach; common rules don't hold true for all patients. Verifying positioning recommendations and careful positioning prevent dislocation during turning.

9. These signs and symptoms may indicate dislocation of the joint or necrosis of the femoral head in a patient with a proximal end fracture. Immediate intervention is needed to prevent permanent damage.

10. Healing requires additional calories and protein. Deficits in vitamins and minerals (particularly vitamins B and C and calcium) retard healing and can contribute to long-term bone disorders such as osteomalacia. Careful dietary assessment and monitoring may be required for the patient with impaired renal, hepatic, or pulmonary function.

11. Rationales: _____

Nursing diagnosis

Knowledge deficit (home care) related to lack of exposure to information and ongoing care of injury after discharge

Nursing priorities

Reinforce the doctor's recommendations for home care, and identify potential problems related to home care and intervene as appropriate.

Patient outcome criteria

By the time of discharge, the patient and family will:
• verbalize and demonstrate understanding of positioning, activity restrictions, and care of the injury
• verbalize understanding of the recommended diet and medication regimen
• identify signs and symptoms of complications.

Interventions

1. See the "Knowledge deficit" plan, page 72.

2. Provide patient and family teaching related to positioning, activity restrictions, cast care, crutch walking, use of a cane or walker, diet, complications, and medications. Verify recommendations with the doctor, and incorporate teaching throughout the hospital stay.

3. Assess available resources for home care and make appropriate referrals.

4. Additional individualized interventions: _____
_____

Rationales

1. General interventions for patient and family teaching are included in this plan.

2. Home care recommendations vary widely depending on the nature of the fracture and repair, the patient's age and condition, and any associated or preexisting conditions. The patient may be more responsive to continuous, repetitive instruction during inpatient care routines than to a large amount of information just before discharge.

3. Depending on the factors mentioned above and on the family support structure, the patient may require home medical or nursing assistance or other follow-up care to ensure an uncomplicated recovery.

4. Rationales: _____
_____

DISCHARGE PLANNING

Discharge checklist

Before discharge, the patient shows evidence of:
❑ stable vital signs
❑ absence of pulmonary or cardiovascular complications
❑ healing incision with no signs of swelling, redness, inflammation, or drainage
❑ ability to control pain using oral medication
❑ absence of fever
❑ hemoglobin levels within expected parameters
❑ ability to perform activities of daily living (ADLs) independently or with minimal assistance
❑ ability to transfer independently or with minimal assistance
❑ ability to demonstrate weight-bearing restrictions when transferring
❑ ability to verbalize activity restrictions
❑ completion of initial ambulation training with the appropriate assistive device
❑ ability to tolerate diet
❑ normal voiding and bowel movements
❑ referral to home care if indicated by inability to perform ADLs or safe transfer technique or by continued need for physical therapy

❑ adequate home support or, if home support isn't adequate, ability to verbalize agreement with temporary placement in a nursing home to convalesce and continue physical therapy.

Teaching checklist

Document evidence that the patient and family demonstrate an understanding of:
❑ site and nature of injury and repair
❑ implications of injury
❑ all discharge medications' purpose, dosage, administration schedule, and adverse effects requiring medical attention (discharge medications may include antibiotics, analgesics, anticoagulants, and antispasmodics)
❑ signs and symptoms of complications
❑ activity and positioning recommendations
❑ care of cast, if present
❑ dietary recommendations
❑ when and how to access the emergency medical system
❑ home care and follow-up referrals
❑ date, time, and location of follow-up appointments, and availability of transportation, if indicated
❑ how to contact the doctor.

Documentation checklist

Using outcome criteria as a guide, document:
❏ clinical status on admission
❏ preoperative assessment and treatment
❏ postoperative assessment and treatment
❏ significant changes in status
❏ pertinent laboratory and diagnostic findings
❏ pain-relief measures
❏ recommendations for and tolerance of activity and positioning
❏ nutritional intake
❏ fluid intake and output
❏ bowel status
❏ patient and family teaching
❏ discharge planning.

ASSOCIATED PLANS OF CARE

Geriatric care
Impaired physical mobility
Knowledge deficit
Pain
Pulmonary embolism
Surgery
Thrombophlebitis
Total joint replacement in a lower extremity

REFERENCES

Black, J.M., and Matassarin-Jacobs, E. *Medical-Surgical Nursing: Clinical Management for Continuity of Care*, 5th ed. Philadelphia: W.B. Saunders, Co. 1997.
Butcher, J. "Long-Term Outcomes after Lower Extremity Trauma," *Journal of Trauma* 41(1):4-9, 1996.
Clochesy, J. *Critical Care Nursing*, 2nd ed. Philadelphia: W.B. Saunders Co., 1996.
Duis, H., "The Fat Embolism Syndrome," *Injury: International Journal of the Care of the Injured* 28(2):77-83, 1997.
Kiely, N. "Sexual Dysfunction in Women Following Pelvic Fractures with Sacro-Iliac Disruption," *Injury: International Journal of the Care of the Injured* 27(1):45-46, January 1997.
Lewis, S. *Medical Surgical Nursing*, 4th ed. St Louis: Mosby–Year Book, Inc., 1996.
Litwack, K. *Post Anesthesia Care Nursing*, 2nd ed. St. Louis: Mosby–Year Book, Inc., 1995.
Mattox, K. *Complications of Trauma*. New York: Churchill Livingstone, Inc., 1994.
Rokkanen, P. "Absorbable Devices in the Fixation of Fractures," *Journal of Trauma* 40(3):S123-25, 1996.
Ruppert, S., et al. *Dolan's Critical Care Nursing: Clinical Management Through the Nursing Process,* 2nd ed. Philadelphia: F.A. Davis, Co., 1997.
Shoemaker, W. *Textbook of Critical Care*, 3rd ed. Philadelphia: W.B. Saunders Co., 1995.
Starr, A. "Treatment of Femur Fracture with Associated Vascular Injury," *Journal of Trauma* 40(1):17-21, 1996.
Thompson, J. *Mosby's Clinical Nursing*, 4th ed. St. Louis: Mosby–Year Book, Inc., 1997.
Ward, C. "Iron and Infection: New Developments and Their Implications," *Journal of Trauma* 41(2):356-64, 1996.
Wilson, R. *Management of Trauma: Pitfalls and Practice*, 2nd ed. Baltimore: Williams & Wilkins, 1996.

Major burns

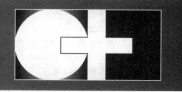

DRG information

DRGs involving burns may be assigned based on specific sites, percent of body surface burned, percent of third-degree burns, and surgical procedures. The following are examples of some DRG classifications for burns.

DRG 458 Nonextensive Burns With Skin Grafts.
Mean LOS = 16.9 days
Principal diagnoses include first-, second-, or third-degree burns of face, scalp, head, or neck (with or without loss of body part). Usually includes burns involving 10% to 49% of body surface, with 10% to 19% third-degree burns.

This diagnosis must be accompanied by one or more of the following principal procedures:
• graft (free skin, full-thickness, or split-thickness) to breast, hand, or other site
• heterograft or homograft to skin.

DRG 459 Nonextensive Burns With Wound Debridement and Other Operating Room Procedures.
Mean LOS = 10.3 days
Principal diagnoses include selected principal diagnoses listed under DRG 458.

This diagnosis must be accompanied by one or more of the following selected principal procedures:
• debridement of infection or burn
• amputation of penis or upper or lower limb
• revision of amputation stump
• closure of oral, bronchial, tracheal, thoracic, or gastric fistula
• reconstruction, repair, or plastic operations and reattachments of body parts or organs.

INTRODUCTION

Definition and time focus

A burn is a traumatic skin injury caused by exposure to heat, chemicals, or electricity. A burn's severity depends on its depth and the body surface area affected. Partial-thickness burns can be superficial (first-degree), involving only the epidermis, or deep (second-degree), involving the epidermal and dermal layers of the skin. Because some epithelial tissue, such as the hair follicles, is uninjured, the skin can regenerate. Full-thickness burns (third and fourth-degree) involve the epidermis, dermis, subcutaneous tissues and, sometimes, underly-

ing muscle, tendon, and bone. Full-thickness burns require skin grafting to heal.

The total body surface area (TBSA) burned is estimated using the Rule of Nines or the Lund-Browder classification system. Both the burn's depth and area are used to determine the initial treatment and if admission to a burn unit is necessary. Treatment in a burn unit is indicated for patients with a partial thickness burn involving more than 25% of TBSA; a full-thickness burn involving more than 10% of TBSA; burns complicated by trauma, chronic illness, or inhalation or electrical injuries; or burns affecting such special areas as the face, eyes, ears, hands, feet, or perineum. Treatment in a burn unit is also indicated for children under age 2 and adults over age 60.

Minor burns can be treated in the emergency department or in the doctor's office. Patients with moderate burns without complications can be treated in a general critical care setting. This plan focuses on the patient admitted for treatment of superficial and deep partial-thickness burns involving more than 25% of TBSA.

Etiology and precipitating factors
• Occupational exposure to causes of burns, such as fuels, chemicals, electricity, or hot substances
• Home exposure to causes of burns, such as stoves, hot water, electricity, heaters, chemicals, matches, or cigarettes
• Outdoor exposure to causes of burns, such as ultraviolet light, lightning, barbecues, or flammable liquids
• High-risk populations, such as young children, older adults, drug or alcohol abusers, chronically ill or debilitated patients, or those working in high-risk jobs

FOCUSED ASSESSMENT GUIDELINES

Nursing history (functional health pattern findings)
Health perception–health management pattern
• High occupational risk for burns
• High-risk activity that caused the burn
• Chronic illness or debilitation
Nutritional-metabolic pattern
• Thirst
• Nausea, vomiting, and loss of appetite
• Feelings of abdominal fullness
Elimination pattern
• Decreased or absent urination

Activity-exercise pattern
• Pain and stiffness when moving involved area
• Difficulty breathing at rest and during movement

Cognitive-perceptual pattern
• Pain
• Repeated discussion of the circumstances of the burn, or confusion and loss of memory about burn incident

Self-perception–self-concept pattern
• Fear of disfigurement or loss of body part
• Fear of dying

Role-relationship pattern
• Concern about whereabouts and condition of others involved in the burn incident
• Fear about maintaining role in family and in relationships
• Concern over effects of injury on family
• Fear about not being able to work again

Sexuality-reproductive pattern
• Fear about future sexual performance
• Fear about lack of sexual attractiveness because of injury

Coping–stress tolerance pattern
• Initial lack of concern about burn
• Fear and anxiety
• Expressed feelings of being overwhelmed by burn

Value-belief pattern
• Expressed need to see member of clergy

Physical findings

Physical findings may vary depending on the burn's type, depth, surface area, and location.

Pulmonary
• Tachypnea, dyspnea, shortness of breath on exertion
• Soot in nostrils or sputum, with an inhalation injury
• Stridor
• Wheezing
• Hoarse voice
• Diminished breath sounds
• Mucosal edema, vesicles, redness

Cardiovascular
• Tachycardia
• Hypotension
• Arrhythmias
• Pale, clammy, diaphoretic, or cool skin
• Cardiac arrest (from an electrical injury) with ventricular fibrillation, chest pain, or cardiac irritability

Neurologic
• Agitation
• Memory loss
• Confusion
• Headache
• Mentation changes

Gastrointestinal
• Decreased or absent bowel sounds
• Distention
• Vomiting

• Dry mouth and mucous membranes

Genitourinary
• Oliguria or anuria
• Cloudy or tea-colored urine

Musculoskeletal
• Pain and stiffness on movement of affected areas
• Tetany (from an electrical injury) and bone fractures caused by tetany or fall

Integumentary
• Bright red to pink color, glistening blisters, blanching on pressure, and pain (with a superficial partial-thickness burn)
• Pink to white color, blanching, pain, sensitivity to pressure, and blisters (with a deep partial-thickness burn)
• White, gray, brown, or black skin color (with a full-thickness burn); eschar (coagulated and necrotic tissue) formation; no pain or pressure sensations; no blanching; dry, easily pulled out hair
• Massive edema
• Hypothermia
• Shivering

Diagnostic studies

• Complete blood count—determines red blood cell count, hemoglobin level, and hematocrit, reflecting any blood loss or destruction and indicating the blood's oxygen-carrying ability; the white blood cell (WBC) count reflects the ability of the WBCs to respond to the inflammatory process; baseline data and serial evaluations may reflect the seriousness of the fluid shifts and cell destruction accompanying major burns
• Serum electrolyte level—monitors fluid, electrolyte, and acid-base status; hyperkalemia initially occurs because of the release of potassium into the serum during cell destruction and the hemoconcentration caused by fluid shifts into the interstitium; hypokalemia may occur during the second day after injury as electrolytes are excreted into the urine; other electrolytes may be low during the initial period after injury because of the massive shifts of fluid and electrolytes into the interstitium
• Blood glucose level—monitors the effect of the catabolic burn state on sugar metabolism and insulin production
• Blood urea nitrogen and creatinine levels—monitor the adequacy of kidney function; acute tubular necrosis is a common complication after major tissue destruction
• Clotting time (prothrombin time/international normalized ratio and activated partial thromboplastin time)—prolonged clotting time may reflect coagulation problems associated with major tissue destruction
• Serum proteins (albumin and globulin) and serum osmolality—may reflect movement of intravascular colloids in and out of the interstitium.
• Arterial blood gas (ABG) values—monitor oxygena-

tion, ventilation, and acid-base status, especially with a suspected inhalation injury; initially, ABG values may reveal respiratory alkalosis, reflecting hyperventilation; later, metabolic acidosis, reflecting hypoxemia and shock
• Carboxyhemoglobin level — may be elevated, confirming carbon monoxide poisoning and smoke inhalation
• Urinalysis, specific gravity, urine electrolytes, and urine myoglobin levels — monitor kidney status; total urine output monitors hydration status
• Blood and tissue cultures — provide baseline data and monitor infections
• Chest X-ray — usually normal at first; in 1 to 2 days, may reveal atelectasis or pulmonary edema
• Electrocardiogram — may reveal arrhythmias
• Ventilation-perfusion pulmonary scan — may reveal areas of nonventilation and nonperfusion
• Bronchoscopy — may reveal abnormalities of the bronchial tree such as redness, blistering, edema, or soot

• Tissue biopsies and repeat cultures — may reveal excessive wound contamination

Potential complications
• Hypovolemic shock
• Cardiac arrhythmias
• Cardiac arrest
• Respiratory arrest
• Atelectasis, pneumonia
• Pulmonary edema
• Infection, sepsis, septic shock
• Acute tubular necrosis
• Acute renal failure
• Conversion of partial-thickness burns to full-thickness burns
• Contractures
• Loss of mobility and function
• Scarring
• Social and emotional isolation
• Hematologic disorders

CLINICAL SNAPSHOT

Major burns

Major nursing diagnoses and collaborative problems	Key patient outcomes
Risk for further injury	Display minimal or no continuing tissue damage.
Risk for hypoxemia	Maintain a patent airway and show no signs of respiratory distress.
Hypovolemia	Have stable vital signs: typically, heart rate, 60 to 100 beats/minute; systolic blood pressure, 90 to 140 mm Hg; and diastolic blood pressure, 50 to 90 mm Hg.
Risk for peripheral ischemia	State that pain relief is adequate.
Risk for burn infection	Display signs of adequate tissue perfusion such as warm, dry skin.
Pain	Rate pain as less than 3 on a 0 to 10 pain rating scale.
Risk for impaired skin integrity	Display an intact and healing graft.
Nutritional deficit	Manifest minimal or no signs of nutritional deficit.
Impaired physical mobility	Display active range-of-motion of affected extremity.
Body-image disturbance	Express fears and concerns openly.

NURSING DIAGNOSIS

Risk for further injury related to continued exposure to heat or chemicals

Nursing priority

Stop the burn from expanding.

Patient outcome criteria

Within the 1st hour after admission, the patient will:
• display minimal or no continuing tissue damage, such as additional areas of redness, blistering, or sensation loss
• manifest no signs of chemical residue on skin.

Interventions

1. Remove any jewelry, belts, coins, or other metal objects from the patient and then immediately flush the burn with cool water for 10 to 15 minutes. Document your actions.

2. For a chemical burn, quickly remove the patient's clothes, brush off dry chemicals, and flush the burns with large amounts of water. Observe the site for chemical residues. After flushing, use a neutralizer, if appropriate, on any remaining chemicals; consult a burn center or poison control center for the appropriate agent. Assess the site hourly and as needed for continuing damage, such as spreading redness, blistering, or loss of sensation. Document your findings.

3. Temporarily cover the flushed burn with a clean or sterile dressing or sheet while other interventions continue.

4. Additional individualized interventions: _____

Rationales

1. Metal items retain heat and permit continued thermal burning. Immediate flushing with cool water will cool the tissue and may limit the damage. Prolonged flushing or using ice water may cause such complications as arrhythmias, hypothermia, or shock.

2. Clothes may contain chemical residues and should be removed to prevent further injury. Thorough flushing with water will remove most chemicals. Neutralization may be helpful, but flushing is a higher initial priority than finding an appropriate neutralizer. Some chemicals, such as alkalies, may continue to cause damage even when neutralized, making ongoing assessments necessary.

3. Covering the burn may limit contamination and decrease pain from air exposure. Further burn care, such as debridement and application of topical antibiotics, has a low priority compared with stabilization of airway, breathing, and circulation.

4. Rationales: _____

COLLABORATIVE PROBLEM

Risk for hypoxemia related to airway burns and carbon monoxide inhalation

Nursing priority

Promote ventilation and gas exchange.

Patient outcome criteria

Within 24 hours of admission, the patient will:
• maintain a patent airway
• display no signs of respiratory distress
• display improving breath sounds
• remain alert and oriented.

Interventions

1. Maintain a patent airway. Anticipate the possible need for endotracheal intubation and mechanical ventilation.

2. Assess the patient's respiratory status on admission, then every 15 minutes until stable, then every 1 to 2 hours. Monitor respiratory rate; chest movements; use of accessory muscles; signs of anxiety or restlessness; color; breath sounds; adventitious sounds, such as crackles, gurgles, or wheezes; hoarseness when speaking; and soot around the nostrils. Notify the doctor and document findings. Be prepared to assist with chest wall escharotomy, if necessary.

3. Monitor ABG values initially and then every shift and as needed for changes in respiratory status. Monitor initial and serial carboxyhemoglobin levels. Monitor pulse oximetry oxygen saturation levels continuously for 24 hours and then every 2 hours or as needed. Document and notify doctor of abnormalities.

4. Provide 100% humidified oxygen therapy, as needed and ordered, especially for smoke inhalation or respiratory distress. Document oxygen administration.

5. Obtain initial and serial chest X-rays, as ordered.

6. Encourage deep-breathing and coughing exercises every hour and as needed. Assist with incentive spirometer use. Document pulmonary hygiene measures.

7. Administer bronchodilators every 4 to 8 hours, if ordered. Document their use.

8. Assess the amount, color, and consistency of sputum, including the presence of soot, every shift. Notify the doctor and document your findings.

9. Assist with bronchoscopy.

10. After stabilization, assist with intermittent positive pressure breathing (IPPB) therapy every 4 hours, if ordered. Document all treatments.

11. Additional individualized interventions: _____

Rationales

1. Airway burns or inhalation of hot air can cause laryngospasm, progressive edema, and rapid airway occlusion up to 8 hours after the burn. Intubation is usually performed before progressive edema occludes the airway.

2. Abnormal findings, including hoarseness, crackles, wheezes, gurgles, signs of hypoxemia, restlessness, and soot around the nostrils, may indicate an inhalation injury and impending respiratory failure. Circumferential chest burns can restrict chest wall expansion and require escharotomy to allow ventilation.

3. ABG values reflect general oxygenation and acid-base levels. Low oxygen and high carbon dioxide levels may indicate a need for oxygen therapy or mechanical ventilation. Carbon monoxide interferes with oxygen transport because of its strong affinity for hemoglobin. Carboxyhemoglobin levels reflect the amount of abnormal hemoglobin present. Pulse oximetry measures provide noninvasive monitoring of oxygenation.

4. Oxygen therapy may be required during the initial postinjury period to maintain desirable ABG levels, help eliminate carbon monoxide, and assist burn healing.

5. Pulmonary involvement may not appear on X-ray for up to 24 hours.

6. Regular deep-breathing and coughing exercises promote lung expansion, mobilize secretions, and prevent atelectasis. Incentive spirometry encourages deep inspiratory efforts that expand the alveoli more effectively than forceful expiratory efforts.

7. Bronchodilators may interrupt bronchospasms and counteract the narrowing effect of airway edema.

8. Soot in the sputum may confirm an inhalation injury. Excessive sputum may indicate an infection.

9. Bronchoscopy is used diagnostically to locate soot in smaller airways, airway burns, and pulmonary inflammation. It is also used therapeutically to remove soot and secretions, minimizing the risk of later infection and atelectasis.

10. IPPB therapy promotes lung expansion by the deep delivery of bronchodilators and positive pressure breaths.

11. Rationales: _____

COLLABORATIVE PROBLEM

Hypovolemia related to movement of vascular fluids to the interstitium and water evaporation from burns

Nursing priority

Maintain vascular fluid volume.

Patient outcome criteria

Within 24 hours of admission, the patient will:
• maintain normal vital signs: typically, heart rate, 60 to 100 beats/minute; systolic blood pressure, 90 to 140 mm Hg; and diastolic blood pressure, 50 to 90 mm Hg
• have a urine output of 50 to 100 ml/hour
• stay within normal ranges for urine specific gravity, serum electrolytes, serum osmolality, and hematocrit
• have no observable changes in mentation.
Within 48 to 72 hours of admission, the patient will manifest a weight loss of no more than 2% per day.

Interventions

1. On admission, place one or two large-bore I.V. lines in large veins in the arms, as ordered, using sterile technique. Document your actions.

2. Collaborate with the doctor on fluid replacement therapy. Administer fluids, as ordered, and document their use.
• On admission, assess the patient's fluid needs. Use the Rule of Nines or the Lund-Browder classification system to determine the TBSA burned; use a fluid replacement formula, preferably the Parkland formula (4 ml lactated Ringer's solution × kg body weight × % TBSA), to determine the volume of fluid needed in the first 24 hours after injury.
• Give crystalloid fluid replacements during the first 24 hours after injury. According to the Parkland formula, administer half the volume in the first 8 hours, a quarter in the next 8 hours, and a quarter in the last 8 hours.
• After 24 to 48 hours, administer colloids and dextrose in water solutions.

3. Assess adequacy of fluid replacement every 1 to 2 hours and as needed, including vital signs, urine output, urine specific gravity, mentation, weight, serum electrolytes and osmolality, and hematocrit. Document your findings.

Rationales

1. Large I.V. access lines are needed to give the large amount of fluids required during the fluid resuscitation period.

2. Appropriate fluid therapy is critical to the patient's survival.

• Fluid replacement formulas, in conjunction with the TBSA burned, estimate the fluid replacement needed every 24 hours. Numerous fluid replacement formulas are available. The American College of Surgeons and the American Burn Association recommend the Parkland formula.

• Large amounts of crystalloid fluids are needed to replace the massive amounts of vascular fluids that leak into the interstitium during the first 24 hours, a result of inflammation and increased capillary permeability.

• After the capillary membranes stabilize, colloids such as plasma can be administered to replace colloid losses. Dextrose in water solutions are also given to replace evaporative fluid loss and as a maintenance solution.

3. Normal vital signs, urine output (50 to 100 ml/hour), specific gravity and osmolality, mental status, serum electrolyte levels, and hematocrit all reflect adequate fluid replacement. Diuresis commonly begins on the third day after injury. A weight loss of less than 2% a day during this time reflects adequate fluid replacement.

4. Assess serum electrolyte levels and administer replacements, as ordered. Document your actions. See Appendix C, Fluid and Electrolyte Imbalances, for general assessments and interventions.

5. After fluid resuscitation is complete and the patient's GI function returns, begin enteral feedings and remove the I.V. lines, as ordered. Document your actions.

6. Additional individualized interventions: _____

4. During the first 24 to 48 hours, electrolytes follow the fluid shifts into the interstitium, reducing the amounts available in the intravascular areas. Electrolyte replacement may be necessary except for potassium, whose serum levels increase because of cell destruction during the immediate postburn period. Careful monitoring guides electrolyte replacement. Appendix C, Fluid and Electrolyte Imbalances, includes general assessments and interventions for electrolyte imbalances.

5. Enteral feedings should begin as soon as possible to decrease the risk of infection at the I.V. insertion sites.

6. Rationales: _____

COLLABORATIVE PROBLEM

Risk for peripheral ischemia related to circumferential eschar formation on arms and legs, compartment syndrome, or vascular disruption

Nursing priority

Maintain adequate tissue perfusion.

Patient outcome criteria

Within 1 to 2 days of admission, the patient will:
• display signs of adequate tissue perfusion distal to the burned area, such as pink color, capillary refill less than 3 seconds, normal sensation, adequate function, minimal pain, and warm, dry skin
• display minimal bleeding or other complications at eschar site.

Interventions

1. When possible, elevate burned areas, but not above the level of the heart.

2. Assess tissue perfusion distal to the burn site every 1 to 2 hours, noting color, temperature, capillary refill, pulses, sensation, function, and pain. Notify the doctor of and document any abnormalities.

3. Assist the doctor in performing an escharotomy, if necessary. Assess the escharotomy site for bleeding and circulation return. Apply dressings to the site. Document your actions.

4. If ordered, apply proteolytic enzymes to eschar. Assess and document their effect.

5. Additional individualized interventions: _____

Rationales

1. Elevation may decrease edema by using gravity to optimize venous return.

2. As eschar hardens, it may constrict circulation, particularly if it is circumferential. The patient with arm or leg burns is also at great risk for compartment syndrome, in which edema increases pressure in a fascial compartment and compresses nerves, blood vessels, and muscle. Early recognition of impaired circulation allows early intervention and minimizes the risk of permanent damage.

3. Incisions across areas of eschar formation release tissue tension and allow circulation to return to constricted areas. Assessment provides for early identification and correction of complications.

4. Proteolytic enzymes selectively digest necrotic tissue. By softening the eschar, they decrease its constricting effects.

5. Rationales: _____

Nursing diagnosis

Risk for burn infection related to loss of protective integument, exposure to contamination, decreased perfusion, and impaired immunologic response

Nursing priorities
- Protect the burn.
- Prevent or minimize infection.

Patient outcome criteria

Within 1 week of admission, the patient will:
- display clean and healing superficial burns, including scab formation
- display development of red granulation tissue over deeper partial-thickness wounds that are also free from odor, purulent drainage, and elevations or depressions
- display no complications of topical antibiotic use, such as pain, leukopenia, tissue damage, electrolyte or fluid loss, and secondary infections
- display intact wound covers
- manifest vital signs, WBC count, urine output, and mentation within normal ranges.

Interventions

1. Explain the purpose and methods of burn care to the patient and family.

2. Use strict sterile technique, including cap, mask, gown, and sterile gloves, during all burn care. Wash the burn once or twice daily with a mild soap or normal saline solution. A hydrotherapy tub, shower stretcher, or basins at the bedside may be used. Use a gentle circular scrubbing motion. Debride with scissors if necessary. Shave hair over involved areas, except for the eyebrows. Rinse with water. Document your actions.

3. During washing and debridement, assess the burn for color, drainage, size, odor, elevations or depressions, and pain. Document your findings.

4. Apply topical antibiotics, if ordered, after washing and debridement, typically silver nitrate, mafenide acetate (Sulfamylon), silver sulfadiazine (Silvadene), or povidone-iodine (Betadine). Use sterile technique including mask, cap, gown, and sterile gloves. Cover the burn with gauze or stretch bandages after applying antibiotics. Monitor for medication-related complications, such as pain, leukopenia, tissue damage, or electrolyte depletion. If signs of medication-related complications occur, notify the doctor and document your findings.

5. Leave partial-thickness burns exposed to air, if ordered. Document scab formation and condition of the burn.

Rationales

1. Understanding the purpose of wound care may help the patient cope with the inevitable pain such care causes, while understanding the general methods may decrease fear of the unknown. Involving family members in teaching and care, when appropriate, acknowledges their learning needs and the importance of their emotional support to the patient.

2. To reduce the risk of infection, strict sterile technique must be used when the burn is uncovered. Regular washing and debridement removes dead tissue and stimulates the development of granulation tissue, which serves as the base for skin grafts. Shaving excess hair removes a medium for bacterial growth. Eyebrows are not shaved because they may not grow back, leaving the patient with an odd facial appearance.

3. Regular assessment may identify early signs of infection and allow timely treatment.

4. Topical antibiotics are commonly used to prevent massive bacterial colonization of burns from the patient's skin flora or contaminants. Strict sterile technique reduces the risk of infection. Monitoring for adverse effects or complications of antibiotic therapy helps avoid further compromise of the patient's status.

5. Partial-thickness burns may heal in a week without complications when left exposed to air.

6. Monitor temporary wound covers, such as biologic, biosynthetic, or synthetic dressings, if used. Change as needed, observing for infection and excessive exudate. Remove excess liquid, as necessary. Document your actions.

7. Maintain patient warmth during washing, debridement, and dressing changes. Limit procedures to 30 minutes or less. Document the procedure and the patient's tolerance.

8. Assist in obtaining needle biopsy cultures from burns, as ordered. Document the procedure.

9. Assess for signs of sepsis, including increased pulse rate, respiratory rate and temperature, decreased blood pressure, decreased urine output, and mentation changes, every 2 to 4 hours and as needed. Document and notify the doctor of abnormal findings.

10. Administer tetanus toxoid on admission, as ordered. Administer tetanus immunoglobulin in another site, if tetanus toxoid has not been given during the preceding 10 years. Document their administration.

11. Give I.V. antibiotics, as ordered, if major wound sepsis occurs. Observe for secondary infections of the mouth, GI tract, and the genitalia. Monitor for resistance to topical and systemic antibiotics. Document your findings.

12. Additional individualized interventions: _____

_____

6. Temporary wound covers used early in treatment prevent infection and evaporative losses and promote granulation tissue development. The dressings are left in place for varying amounts of time. Usually, excessive exudate should be removed to enhance the dressing's adherence.

7. Evaporative water loss during procedures may increase the risks of volume deficit, electrolyte loss, and shock.

8. Needle biopsy cultures are more accurate monitors of wound infection than surface cultures. Early detection of wound infection allows timely treatment and may prevent sepsis.

9. Loss of the skin barrier, frequent manipulation of burn wounds, and the general catabolic state place the patient at high risk for sepsis. Early recognition and treatment may prevent irreversible sepsis and septic shock, a major cause of death in burn patients.

10. Burns are at high risk for anaerobic infections, including tetanus. Tetanus toxoid stimulates antibody production. Tetanus immunoglobulin provides protection until tetanus antibodies develop. Using different sites prevents inactivation of the immunoglobulin.

11. I.V. antibiotics usually are given only for major wound sepsis because areas of eschar have poor circulation and are better treated with topical antibiotics. Secondary infections may result from overgrowth of normally suppressed pathogens. Development of resistant strains of microorganisms is a common result of long-term topical antibiotic use.

12. Rationales: _____

_____

NURSING DIAGNOSIS

Pain related to tissue destruction and exposure of nerves in partially destroyed tissue

Nursing priority

Relieve pain.

Patient outcome criteria

Within 1 to 2 days of admission, the patient will:
• rate pain (with pain medications) as less than 3 on a 0 to 10 pain rating scale
• verbalize pain relief from pain medication.

Interventions

1. See the "Pain" plan, page 88.

Rationales

1. The "Pain" plan includes general assessments and interventions for a patient with pain. This plan contains additional information specific to the burn patient.

2. Administer I.V. analgesics 10 to 20 minutes before burn cleaning, debridement, and dressing changes. Medicate frequently and liberally within the ordered parameters. Document administration and degree of pain relief achieved.

2. Burn care is excruciatingly painful and may need to be repeated several times daily. Anticipation increases the patient's perceived pain. Frequent and liberal analgesic administration may prevent the pain from reaching intolerable levels. Addiction to pain medication is rare in burn patients. The I.V. route is preferred because massive edema and inflammation reduce medication absorption through the subcutaneous and intramuscular routes.

3. Decrease anxiety and fear by explaining procedures and treatments thoroughly. Document teaching. See the "Knowledge deficit" plan, page 72, and the "Ineffective individual coping" plan, page 67.

3. Fear of the unknown, helplessness, and powerlessness may increase pain. Burn care is complex and long term. Thorough teaching and emotional support may allay fear of the unknown and provide the patient some sense of control over treatment, which may lessen the pain experience. The "Knowledge deficit" and "Ineffective individual coping" plans contain general assessments and interventions applicable to any patient.

4. Additional individualized interventions: _____

4. Rationales: _____

Nursing diagnosis

Risk for impaired skin integrity related to nonadherence of graft and impaired donor site healing

Nursing priority

Optimize burn healing.

Patient outcome criteria

Within 2 to 5 days after grafting, the patient will:
• display an intact and healing graft without redness, swelling, exudate formation, bleeding, or foul odor
• display a dry and healed donor site
• maintain normal vital signs: typically, heart rate, 60 to 100 beats/minute; systolic blood pressure, 90 to 140 mm Hg; and diastolic blood pressure, 50 to 90 mm Hg
• display no signs of wound sepsis
• maintain activity limitations.

Interventions

1. Apply homografts or heterografts in single sheets to freshly cleaned burns, as ordered, using sterile technique. Trim to prevent overlapping. Smooth the graft, removing wrinkles and air. Apply thin gauze (with or without antibiotic ointment) over the graft, as ordered. Apply a dressing over the gauze. Protect the site from movement or trauma. Document your actions.

Rationales

1. Homografts and heterografts are temporary biological dressings that protect burns and stimulate formation of granulation tissue until autografts can be applied. Removing wrinkles and air pockets promotes adherence. Gauze and dressings protect the graft. Freshly grafted sites must be protected from accidental dislodgment until circulation has been established with underlying tissue.

2. After surgery for autografting, immobilize the graft and protect it from injury for at least 48 hours. Keep the large, bulky dressings in place. Use a bed cradle. Prevent prolonged pressure over the graft. Elevate the graft site to the highest position possible. Use splints and elastic bandages over graft sites, particularly when the patient walks. Discontinue activities, such as hydrotherapy or active physical therapy, for several days after grafting. Document your actions.

3. Protect the donor site from infection or trauma. If outer dressings are used, keep them in place by using splints and limiting exercise for several days. Leave the inner gauze dressing in place until it falls off, usually in 2 to 3 weeks. Use a heat lamp or hair dryer to dry the site for 15 to 20 minutes four times daily or as ordered. Leave the site exposed to air, as ordered. Document treatments and the condition of the site every shift.

4. Observe the homograft, heterograft, or autograft for signs of adherence; monitor all grafts and donor sites for signs of infection. Report immediately any redness, exudate, blood under the graft, swelling, separation, drainage, foul odor, or increased temperature, pulse rate, or respirations. Document your findings.

5. Apply moist, warm compresses to the donor site, if ordered, for 20 to 30 minutes four times a day. Document your actions.

6. Apply topical antibiotics to the burn and donor site and administer systemic antibiotics I.V., if ordered. Document your actions.

7. Additional individualized interventions: _____

2. The graft must be immobilized and protected from trauma and movement for several days to prevent dislodgment and promote circulation until it adheres. Large dressings provide protective padding. A bed cradle prevents pressure from bed linens. Elevation limits edema. Splints and elastic bandages provide support, maintain dressing placement, prevent excessive movement of the graft site, and allow some activity. Excessive moisture or exercise may dislodge the graft in the first days after grafting.

3. The donor site must be protected to prevent its conversion from a partial-thickness wound to a deeper-thickness wound. Using dressings and splints and limiting exercise may protect the site and promote tissue regeneration. The inner gauze is left in place to stabilize and cover the site during tissue regeneration; early removal could traumatize the new tissue. Heat increases circulation and promotes healing. Air exposure promotes drying and scab formation.

4. Regular assessment may permit early detection of graft rejection or wound sepsis.

5. Warmth and moisture may increase circulation and promote epithelization.

6. As previously described, topical antibiotics are commonly used to prevent wound sepsis from the patient's skin flora. Systemic antibiotics are used when major wound sepsis occurs.

7. Rationales: _____

NURSING DIAGNOSIS

Nutritional deficit related to increased metabolic needs of burn healing

Nursing priority

Provide adequate nutrition to promote burn healing.

Patient outcome criteria

Within 1 week of admission, the patient will:
• display minimal or no signs of nutritional deficit
• manifest expected wound healing
• display no more than a 10% weight loss.

Interventions

1. See the "Nutritional deficit" plan, page 80.

2. Upon the patient's admission, insert a nasogastric tube and withhold food and fluids until bowel sounds return. Provide I.V. fluids and total parenteral nutrition continuously, as ordered. Assess patient tolerance, including weights, intake and output, edema, and blood glucose, electrolyte, and protein levels. Document your findings.

3. After bowel function returns, collaborate with the dietitian or nutritional support nurse to provide a high-calorie, high-protein diet with vitamin supplements, as ordered. Provide high-calorie liquids, such as milk shakes or prepared liquid diet supplements, instead of water. Take the patient's food preferences into consideration whenever possible. Document daily intake.

4. Additional individualized interventions: _____

Rationales

1. The "Nutritional deficit" plan contains general assessments and interventions for a patient with a nutritional deficit. This section provides additional information pertinent to the burn patient.

2. A burn commonly causes paralytic ileus, which prevents oral intake for 2 to 4 days. Nutritional requirements are met through I.V. administration during this time. Regular assessments monitor the adequacy of fluid and nutrient intake.

3. A high-calorie, high-protein diet (between 5,000 and 6,000 calories daily) may be required to meet the increased metabolic needs for tissue healing. All intake must help meet these increased needs, so milk shakes are preferable to water. Because the burn patient commonly experiences loss of appetite, offering favorite foods may improve intake. Extra vitamins are needed to meet tissue-healing needs.

4. Rationales: _____

NURSING DIAGNOSIS

Impaired physical mobility related to prescribed position and movement limitations

Nursing priority

Maintain mobility within the range of limitations.

Patient outcome criteria

Within 2 weeks of admission, the patient will:
• have no contractures
• maintain proper anatomic and functional positions of arms and legs
• perform range-of-motion (ROM) and other exercises
• experience minimal pain during activities.

Interventions

1. Implement measures in the "Impaired physical mobility" plan, page 50, as appropriate.

2. Provide active and passive ROM exercises to arms and legs with a healing graft every 2 hours and as needed, as ordered. Document patient tolerance.

3. Promote self-care within the patient's limitations.

Rationales

1. The "Impaired physical mobility" plan covers general information about this problem. This section provides additional information pertinent to burn patients.

2. ROM exercises prevent contractures and promote circulation, healing, and a sense of well-being.

3. Self-care increases the patient's activity level and promotes a sense of well-being and control over the environment.

4. Provide protective devices, such as splints and dressings, during exercise, as ordered. Document their use.

5. Position body parts in anatomic and functional alignment. Document your actions.

6. Provide pain medication, as needed and ordered. Document its administration.

7. Additional individualized interventions: _____

_____

4. Protective devices allow mobility while maintaining the integrity of the graft site.

5. Anatomic and functional alignment prevents contracture formation and promotes eventual return to normal activities.

6. Pain relief encourages movement and activity.

7. Rationales: _____

_____

NURSING DIAGNOSIS

Body-image disturbance related to extensive burns and potential scarring

Nursing priority

Promote adjustment to body changes.

Patient outcome criteria

Throughout the recovery period, the patient will:
• express fears and concerns openly
• set small, realistic goals for recovery
• participate in recovery.

Interventions

1. See the "Ineffective individual coping" plan, page 67, and the "Grieving" plan, page 44.

2. Encourage verbalization of feelings about the burn, potential scarring, and loss of function. Document concerns.

3. Provide information about procedures and expected results. Document teaching and the patient's response.

4. Encourage realistic goals.

5. Additional individualized interventions: _____

_____

Rationales

1. The extensive emotional adjustments necessary to recover from the burn may severely tax the patient's and family's coping abilities. Grieving for lost appearance or the function of body parts is a necessary first step in emotional recovery. The plans listed provide multiple interventions helpful to recovery.

2. Verbalization of concerns decreases anxiety and fear and encourages self-appraisal to determine realistic goals.

3. Knowledge of procedures and expected results decreases fear of the unknown and encourages patient participation and cooperation during recovery.

4. Focusing on realistic goals, such as small, obtainable daily goals, may prevent disappointment and despair during recovery

5. Rationales: _____

_____

DISCHARGE PLANNING

Discharge checklist
Before discharge, the patient shows evidence of:
- ❐ stable vital signs and monitoring parameters
- ❐ healing graft and donor sites
- ❐ absence of wound or systemic sepsis
- ❐ stable fluid and electrolyte status
- ❐ renal status within normal limits
- ❐ adequate nutrition and fluid intake
- ❐ ability to perform ROM and other exercises
- ❐ ability to maintain proper anatomic and functional positions of arms and legs
- ❐ absence of such complications as shock, cardiac arrhythmias, renal failure, contractures, or bleeding
- ❐ minimal edema.

Teaching checklist
Document evidence that the patient and family demonstrate an understanding of:
- ❐ grafting and wound care procedures, including expected course of healing
- ❐ signs and symptoms of such complications as shock, bleeding, infection, and graft rejection
- ❐ importance of ROM exercises and proper anatomic and functional positioning of affected arms and legs
- ❐ nutritional needs
- ❐ comfort measures for pain
- ❐ protective measures, such as splints and dressings, for wounds
- ❐ long-term recovery goals.

Documentation checklist
Using outcome criteria as a guide, document:
- ❐ clinical status on admission
- ❐ significant changes in status
- ❐ pertinent diagnostic test findings
- ❐ status of graft and donor sites
- ❐ complications, such as shock, arrhythmias, sepsis, renal failure, or contractures
- ❐ oxygen therapy
- ❐ ROM and other exercises
- ❐ tolerance of tubbing, debridement, and wound care
- ❐ pain and effect of medication
- ❐ mental and emotional status
- ❐ patient and family teaching
- ❐ discharge planning.

ASSOCIATED PLANS OF CARE
Impaired physical mobility
Ineffective individual coping
Knowledge deficit
Nutritional deficit
Pain

REFERENCES
Greenfield, E., and Jordan, B. "Advances in Burn Wound Care," *Critical Care Nursing Clinics of North America* 8(2):203-15, June 1996.

Greenhalgh, D.G. "The Healing of Burn Wounds," *Dermatology Nursing* 8(1):13-25, February, 1996.

LeMone, S.M., et al. *Medical-Surgical Nursing: Assessment and Management of Clinical Problems.* St. Louis: Mosby–Year Book, Inc., 1996.

Roberts, S.L. *Critical Care Nursing: Assessment & Intervention.* Stamford, Conn.: Appleton & Lange, 1996.

Ruppert, S.D., et al. *Dolan's Critical Care Nursing: Clinical Management through the Nursing Process.* 2nd ed. Philadelphia: F.A. Davis Co., 1996.

Multiple trauma

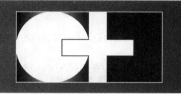

DRG information

DRG 484   Craniotomy for Multiple Significant Trauma.
Mean LOS = 15.9

DRG 485   Limb Reattachment, Hip and Femur Procedures for Multiple Significant Trauma.
Mean LOS = 11.7

DRG 486   Other OR Procedures for Multiple Significant Trauma.
Mean LOS = 9.1

DRG 487   Other Multiple Significant Trauma.
Mean LOS = 9.1

To attain the correct DRG for a Multiple Trauma patient, the injuries must include significant trauma to different significant trauma body site categories as outlined by DRG guidelines. It is important to document all injuries sustained and procedures (surgical and nonsurgical) performed because, for example, a bedside excisional debridement could enhance the DRG; similarly, an injury to a separate body site that seems minor might be the injury that prompts the multiple injury DRGs.

INTRODUCTION

Definition and time focus

Multiple trauma results from accidental or intentional injury to more than one body part, organ, or system. Trauma usually can be described as either blunt or penetrating, depending on whether the skin is broken.

This plan focuses on the first few days after trauma — the critical care phase. It assumes that the patient has been moved from the field to the emergency department for stabilization, to surgery where essential repairs have been accomplished, and then to the unit. If the patient is not already stable, plan and implement appropriate cardiopulmonary support and cervical spine protection, and provide preoperative care based on institution policies. Although every possible complication can't be included, this plan reviews major complications in detail and refers to other plans where appropriate. Long-term rehabilitation is not covered here, but prevention of long-term disability — the focus of nursing care — is discussed. The plan refers to special equipment used to care for the trauma patient, but no endorsement of a specific product or manufacturer is implied.

Etiology and precipitating factors

- Chemical impairment of mentation and judgment, such as by alcohol, narcotics, cocaine, or other street drugs
- Suicide attempts
- Assaults
- Falls
- Industrial accidents
- Motor vehicle accidents
- Pedestrian-vehicle collisions
- Sports injuries
- Underlying physical problems, such as acute myocardial infarction (MI) and cerebrovascular accident
- Major psychiatric disorders
- Recent personal stress

FOCUSED ASSESSMENT GUIDELINES

Nursing history (functional health pattern findings)

Health perception–health management pattern
- Male (likely) ages 15 to 35; about 75% of trauma patients are male

Nutritional-metabolic pattern
- Well-nourished

Activity-exercise pattern
- History of athletic competition

Cognitive-perceptual pattern
- Complaints of pain, if conscious
- Reported or displayed confusion, anxiety, or amnesia, if conscious

Coping–stress tolerance pattern
- Situational or maturational life crisis
- History of psychiatric problems

Physical findings

Alcohol, drugs, anxiety, restlessness, decreased level of consciousness (LOC), or altered sensory function commonly interfere with accurate assessment. Serial observations and analysis of trends in findings are critical. Physical findings vary with the particular trauma present.

Cardiovascular
- Hypotension and tachycardia (if shock is present)
- Hypertension and tachycardia (if shock is absent)
- Diminished or absent pulse (if trauma is to an extremity)
- Arrhythmias
- Jugular vein distention (if cardiac tamponade is present)

• Muffled heart sounds (if cardiac tamponade is present)
• Capillary refill time greater than 3 seconds (if shock or vascular disruption is present)

Pulmonary
• Tachypnea
• Shallow respirations
• Paradoxical chest movement (if flail chest is present)
• Crepitus and ecchymoses (if chest trauma is present)

Gastrointestinal
• Cullen's sign (ecchymoses around umbilicus) and Turner's sign (ecchymoses in flanks) if intra-abdominal or retroperitoneal bleeding present (a late sign)

Neurologic
• Decreased LOC
• Rhinorrhea or otorrhea (if cerebrospinal fluid [CSF] leak is present)
• Pupillary changes
• Sensory or motor impairment (if trauma is to the head, the spinal cord, or an extremity)

Integumentary
• Abrasions
• Lacerations
• Ecchymoses
• Road burns
• Battle's sign (ecchymoses over mastoid area) and raccoon eyes (periorbital ecchymoses) if basilar skull fracture or facial fracture is present
• Pallor, mottling, or cyanosis
• Cool, cold, or clammy skin

Musculoskeletal
• Fractures
• Amputations

Diagnostic studies

• Complete blood count — commonly reveals decreased hemoglobin level and hematocrit secondary to hemorrhage; white blood cell count may be elevated
• Serum electrolytes — monitors fluid and electrolyte status
• Blood urea nitrogen and serum creatinine levels — may be elevated secondary to decreased renal perfusion in shock
• Lactate levels — may be elevated, reflecting anaerobic metabolism in shock; high initial levels are associated with low probability of survival
• Serum bilirubin — assesses hepatic damage
• Cardiac isoenzymes — determine acute MI, a common cause of trauma, or cardiac injury
• Arterial blood gas (ABG) levels — vary, depending on cardiopulmonary status; generally, respiratory alkalosis occurs if tachypnea is present; respiratory acidosis occurs if respiratory depression is present; metabolic acidosis occurs if shock is present
• Coagulation pane — monitors for disseminated intravascular coagulation (DIC)

• Serum aspartate aminotransferase, alanine aminotransferase, and lactic dehydrogenase levels — monitor for liver damage
• Anteroposterior, odontoid, and lateral cervical spine radiography — an essential procedure to visualize cervical vertebrae C1 to C7; can detect spinal injury or "clear" the cervical spine of fractures
• 12-lead electrocardiography (ECG) — can help evaluate MI or contusion, arrhythmias, electrolyte imbalance, or antiarrhythmic agent effects
• Chest X–ray — can detect fractured ribs, widened mediastinum, pneumothorax, hemothorax, or other life-threatening chest injuries; a chest X–ray can also confirm placement of an endotracheal tube and central lines and monitor for adult respiratory distress syndrome (ARDS), pneumonia, and other complications
• Anteroposterior pelvic X–ray, including both hips — can detect pelvic ring disruption or hip dislocation
• Diagnostic peritoneal lavage — may reveal blood, feces, bile, or amylase, indicating abdominal injury
• Excretory urogram, cystogram, or ureterogram — used to identify the size, location, and filling of the renal pelvis, ureters, and urethra
• Computed tomography (CT) scan — can visualize injuries to the head, neck, spine, abdomen, and kidneys
• Arteriography — determines vessel integrity
• Radionuclide scanning and sonography — assists in the identification of organ structure and function; especially useful in suspected chest, abdominal, or pelvic injuries

Potential complications

• Infection or sepsis
• Pulmonary embolism
• Atelectasis or pneumonia
• ARDS
• DIC
• Renal failure
• Cardiac failure
• Liver failure
• Increased intracranial pressure (ICP)
• Paralysis
• Fat embolism
• Compartmental syndrome
• Malnutrition
• Multisystem organ failure
• Posttraumatic stress disorder

CLINICAL SNAPSHOT

MULTIPLE TRAUMA

Major nursing diagnoses and collaborative problems	Key patient outcomes
Risk for hypoxemia	Display ABGs within normal limits (pH, 7.35 to 7.45; P_{CO_2}, 35 to 45 mm Hg; HCO_3^-, 23 to 28 mEq/L) and pulse oximetry levels 90% or higher.
Risk for shock	Show stable vital signs: typically, heart rate, 60 to 100 beats/minute; systolic blood pressure, 90 to 140 mm Hg; and diastolic blood pressure, 50 to 90 mm Hg.
Risk for undetected injury	Have no signs or symptoms of previously unapparent injury.
Impaired physical mobility	Have no new evidence of skin breakdown or other hazards of immobility.
Risk for posttrauma response	Discuss feelings about the traumatic incident.
Risk for injury: complications	Show no signs or symptoms of complications.

COLLABORATIVE PROBLEM

Risk for hypoxemia related to pulmonary injury, head injury, shock, or other factors

Nursing priority

Maintain optimal airway, ventilation, and oxygenation.

Patient outcome criteria

According to individual readiness, the patient will:
• display ABGs within normal limits (pH, 7.35 to 7.45; P_{CO_2}, 35 to 45 mm Hg; HCO_3^-, 23 to 28 mEq/L) and pulse oximetry levels 90% or higher
• have clear breath sounds bilaterally
• have clear lung fields on chest X-ray.

Interventions

1. Maintain a patent airway. Maintain cervical spine precautions until radiologic or tomographic findings have ruled out ligamentous injury or fracture.

Rationales

1. Although airway patency will have been evaluated before unit admission, trauma to the head, face, neck, or torso can compromise a previously patent airway at any time. Although cervical spine clearance is usually done before unit admission, general precautions may still be required while awaiting the official radiologic reading. The C6 and C7 vertebrae may be difficult to clear in a patient with large shoulders, and CT scan may be required.

2. Monitor ventilatory status. Observe respiratory rate, rhythm, effort of breathing, and tidal volume. Monitor trends in pulse oximetry and ABG values. Consult doctor about acceptable limits. Prepare for intubation and mechanical ventilation, as ordered, particularly if the patient has flail chest, pulmonary contusion, or shock. See the "Mechanical ventilation" plan, page 283.

2. If the patient's condition deteriorates, ventilatory status may change abruptly. Deterioration also may be insidious (for example, if the patient tires), so close monitoring is essential. The "Mechanical ventilation" plan presents comprehensive information on indications for mechanical ventilation, types of ventilators, and associated nursing care.

3. Provide supplemental oxygen as ordered.

3. All multiple-trauma patients need supplemental oxygenation. Hypoxemia involves many factors and may result from pulmonary injury, depressed LOC, decreased cardiac output (CO), ischemia, acidosis, and other factors. Supplemental oxygen elevates arterial oxygen tension, ensuring that the blood reaching the tissues provides the maximum amount of oxygen possible.

4. Obtain serial chest X-rays at least daily, as ordered.

4. Serial chest X-rays can detect complications in time for corrective action.

5. Additional individualized interventions: _____

5. Rationales: _____

COLLABORATIVE PROBLEM

Risk for shock related to hypovolemia, cardiac injury, spinal cord injury, or sepsis

Nursing priorities

Monitor for shock, and restore circulating blood volume and tissue perfusion if shock occurs.

Patient outcome criteria

Within 24 hours of the onset of therapy, the patient will:
• display stable vital signs: typically, heart rate, 60 to 100 beats/minute; systolic blood pressure, 90 to 140 mm Hg; and diastolic blood pressure, 50 to 90 mm Hg
• have an adequate circulating volume, as manifested by warm, dry skin; urine output within normal limits; and strong, bilaterally equal peripheral pulses
• have a core temperature within normal limits.

Interventions

1. Implement measures in the "Hypovolemic shock" plan, page 432, as appropriate, such as monitoring LOC, vital signs, urine output, ECG pattern, hemodynamic measurements, and laboratory values; maintaining patency of two large-bore I.V. lines; and administering fluids and positive inotropic agents, as ordered.

Rationales

1. The "Hypovolemic shock" plan covers assessment and interventions for this potential problem in detail. This plan provides additional information specific to the trauma patient.

2. Implement autotransfusion, when possible. Follow the manufacturer's directions for acid-citrate-dextrose (ACD) anticoagulant, if used, and reinfusion.

2. The patient's blood, when captured in drainage, is an ideal source of blood replacement because it decreases the possibility of transfusion reactions and infection. ACD may be used to prevent the retrieved blood from coagulating in the autotransfusor.

3. Monitor continually for new or ongoing bleeding.

3. Commonly, restoration of adequate blood pressure reverses peripheral vasoconstriction and dislodges fragile clots, so additional bleeding becomes apparent.

4. Collaborate with the doctor to adjust blood replacement needs according to the sites of suspected or obvious bleeding and estimated amount lost.

5. Warm I.V. fluids before administration.

6. Additional individualized interventions: _____

4. Rough guidelines exist for the amount of blood loss to expect with particular injuries, such as for the following closed orthopedic injuries: humerus, 1 to 2 units; ulna-radius, ½ to 1 unit; pelvis, 2 to 12 units; tibia-fibula, ½ to 4 units; and ankle, ½ to 2 units. With open injuries, an estimated 1 to 3 additional units may be lost per site. Such guidelines, when used with clinical findings, help determine appropriate blood replacement.

5. The volume of fluid required in a major trauma resuscitation is so massive that infusing room temperature solutions and cold blood products may cause hypothermia and shivering. Shivering requires an extraordinary energy expenditure the patient can ill afford.

6. Rationales: _____

COLLABORATIVE PROBLEM

Risk for undetected injury related to mechanism of injury

Nursing priorities

• Correlate the mechanism of injury with the patient's clinical presentation.
• Remain alert for new signs of injury.

Patient outcome criterion

Throughout the unit stay, the patient will have no signs or symptoms of previously unapparent injury.

Interventions

Blunt head trauma
1. Implement measures in the "Increased intracranial pressure" plan, page 169, as appropriate.

2. Monitor LOC, pupillary reactions, motor function, and sensory function. Alert the doctor immediately to any signs of neurologic deterioration.

Rationales

1. Brain damage may not reflect velocity and duration of the injuring force because a contrecoup injury (which is opposite the site of injury) may be worse than the coup injury (the injury at point of contact) to the head. Preadmission health status, the specific injury, and immediate detection and treatment of increased ICP are critical to survival. The "Increased intracranial pressure" plan discusses these problems in detail.

2. Brain damage may not be apparent until days or weeks after injury. An epidural hematoma, usually from arterial bleeding secondary to blows to the temple that tear the middle meningeal artery, is life-threatening and requires immediate surgical evacuation. Signs of acute subdural hematoma usually appear within 24 hours of injury. Signs of concussion usually reverse within 24 hours, while those from contusion may persist for several days. Failure to recover within the expected time may indicate ongoing pathology or previously undetected injury and requires medical evaluation.

Blunt chest trauma

1. Notify the doctor promptly of the onset of subcutaneous emphysema in the chest or neck, gastric contents in tracheal secretions, severe chest pain, deteriorating ABG values, or dyspnea.

2. Monitor for indicators of cardiac tamponade, such as rising central venous pressure, falling blood pressure, neck vein distention, or muffled heart sounds. Notify the doctor immediately and prepare for pericardiocentesis.

3. Monitor for signs and symptoms of cardiac contusion, including tachycardia, chest pain, arrhythmias, elevated pulmonary artery wedge pressure, and indicators of heart failure. Obtain serial ECGs, cardiac enzymes, and a Doppler echocardiogram during the diagnostic phase, as ordered. Provide care, as ordered, depending on the contusion's effect on the patient.

4. Monitor for signs of pulmonary contusion, such as dyspnea, increasing pulmonary secretions (usually bloody), increasing inspiratory pressure while on a volume ventilator, and hypoxemia. Follow serial ABG measurements and chest X-ray results.

5. Additional individualized interventions: _____

_____

Blunt abdominal trauma

1. Lap belt restraints may produce intraperitoneal, retroperitoneal, or pelvic disruption, resulting in life-threatening hemorrhage. These acceleration-deceleration injuries may not appear immediately after injury but hours or even days later.

2. Maintain placement and patency of gastric and urinary catheters, as ordered. Avoid nasogastric (NG) tube placement if facial fractures or cribriform plate injury is suspected. Avoid urinary catheter insertion if blood is present at the urinary meatus; notify the doctor.

3. Additional individualized interventions: _____

_____

1. These signs and symptoms may indicate tracheal disruption or esophageal or bronchial tears. The trachea, esophagus, and bronchi are attached to other body structures by "stalks" that are prone to tearing from direct impact, deceleration, and shearing or rotary forces associated with blunt trauma.

2. When the chest strikes the steering wheel in a motor vehicle accident, for example, the heart is compressed between the sternum and vertebrae. The abrupt increase in intracardiac pressure may cause cardiac rupture. Damage may also occur to great vessels, especially to the venae cavae and pulmonary veins, which are thought to have different deceleration rates than the atria. Cardiac damage may occur even without thoracic injury, if a lap belt compresses the abdomen and the knees strike the dashboard. Abdominal and leg compression creates a "hydraulic ram" effect, displacing abdominal viscera and blood upward, increasing intracardiac pressure and causing cardiac damage.

3. Cardiac contusion may result from horizontal or vertical deceleration, compression, or shock wave damage in a gunshot wound to the chest or abdomen. Some controversy exists over management of cardiac contusion. Recent studies show little risk for most patients. If an ECG and Doppler echocardiogram don't reveal electrical or mechanical dysfunction, this disorder may not be critical. If function is impaired or arrhythmias threaten CO, however, treatment should be similar to that for acute MI.

4. Pulmonary insufficiency from contusions increases within the first several hours after injury. Contusion creates swelling, a natural inflammatory process, and a capillary leak, which is worsened by the aggressive fluid resuscitation necessary for the multiple-trauma patient.

5. Rationales: _____

_____

1. Report changes in abdominal pain, tenderness, rebound tenderness, absent bowel sounds, and increased abdominal distention.

2. A gastric catheter decompresses the stomach and helps detect gastric bleeding; a urinary catheter does the same for the bladder. Attempts to insert an NG tube when facial fractures or cribriform plate injury is present may result in catheter placement into the brain. Bleeding at the urinary meatus may indicate urethral transection and requires medical evaluation.

3. Rationales: _____

_____

Blunt spinal cord injury

1. Mechanisms of spinal cord injury include horizontal loading, vertical loading, and acceleration or deceleration. Horizontal loading is lateral cord motion, such as when the patient hits the ground after being ejected from an automobile. Vertical loading results in cord compression, such as with a vertical fall or diving injury. Acceleration or deceleration injuries are common in falls.

2. Additional individualized interventions: _____

1. Perform and document a motor and sensory examination every shift.

2. Rationales: _____

Penetrating wounds

1. Bullet wounds usually are explored surgically because of the erratic path the bullet may take as it moves through tissue and because the bullet's kinetic energy (which depends on its mass and velocity) creates a much larger internal wound than the surface may indicate.

2. With stab wounds, observe distal vascular supply and tissue integrity, and assess signs of underlying organ function. Assume underlying vessel, tissue, and organ damage until proven otherwise.

3. Additional individualized interventions: _____

1. With bullet wounds, observe the wound edge for necrosis and distal tissue for perfusion. Also inspect carefully for other wounds.

2. Depending on the length of the weapon and the direction of penetration, body areas other than that of the surface wound may be injured. For example, an abdominal stab wound may penetrate the diaphragm and involve the chest cavity, or a buttock stab wound may enter the abdomen. Maintain suspicion regarding the extent of the wound.

3. Rationales: _____

All injuries

1. Assess and report to the doctor if the apparent mechanism of injury and observed injuries don't match.

2. Additional individualized interventions: _____

1. Inconsistencies between the apparent mechanism of injury and pattern of observed injuries may indicate previously undetected mechanisms of injury or abuse.

2. Rationales: _____

NURSING DIAGNOSIS

Impaired physical mobility related to orthopedic injury

Nursing priorities

- Restore maximum mobility.
- Strengthen muscle groups involved in weight bearing and range of motion (ROM).
- Prevent orthopedic complications.

Patient outcome criterion

By the third day after traumatic injury, the patient will have no new evidence of skin breakdown or other hazards of immobility.

Interventions

1. Implement measures in the "Impaired physical mobility" plan, page 50, as appropriate.

2. Elevate casted extremities. Check neurovascular function every 1 to 2 hours. Report to the doctor altered sensation, increased pain, decreased ability to move fingers or toes, and capillary refill time greater than 3 seconds.

3. Observe uncasted extremities for crepitus, deformity, swelling, discoloration, pain, paralysis, pulse loss, and muscle spasms. If present, splint the extremity and notify the doctor.

4. If reimplantation is planned for a severed body part, maintain the part in a sealed plastic bag on ice; don't soak, wrap, or pack in ice. Prepare the patient for reimplantation surgery.

5. Maintain traction and immobilization of all cervical spine injuries and all other unstable spinal fractures. Besides halo traction, methods include using Gardner-Wells or Crutchfield tongs.

6. Prevent skin breakdown and other hazards of immobility by obtaining turning orders and restrictions, as appropriate, instituting a program of diligent side-to-side turning, at least every 2 hours as ordered, or using trauma beds. Trauma beds include:
• Roto Rest bed

• air bag beds (avoid these for the patient in spinal traction)

• Stryker Frame and CircOlectric beds.

7. Apply, monitor, and maintain continuous passive ROM or sequential compression devices, if ordered.

8. Additional individualized interventions: _____
_____

Rationales

1. The "Impaired physical mobility" plan presents comprehensive information on the hazards of immobility and their prevention. This plan provides additional information pertinent to the trauma patient.

2. Extremities in casts commonly swell from tissue edema; elevation decreases the amount of swelling. Altered sensation, increased pain, limited movement, and prolonged capillary refill time indicate that the swelling is causing neurovascular compromise. Unrecognized damage can threaten limb survival or function.

3. Occasionally, injuries may be missed during resuscitation, especially if other life-threatening injuries require immediate surgery.

4. Several hours may elapse before reimplantation. Maintaining the body part as described preserves viability.

5. Maintaining traction prevents further injury to the spinal cord. Although cervical spine injuries require immediate treatment along with other life-threatening injuries, treatment of thoracolumbar injuries can be deferred until the patient is stable.

6. Skin breakdown, thromboembolism, and other complications of immobility may threaten life or markedly prolong recovery. Preventive methods depend on the injury and degree of activity allowed.

• A Roto Rest bed cycles automatically and continuously to 90-degree positions and has been used with various injuries, including cervical spine fractures. A patient on a ventilator can be cared for easily on this bed.
• Various air bag beds are available. Benefits include side-to-side turning, bacterial filtration, and prevention of skin breakdown. Because of the potential for deflation with air bag beds, they are contraindicated for the patient with an unstable spine. A Roto Rest bed is better suited for the patient in spinal traction.
• Although these beds facilitate turning, they don't automatically change the patient's position and thus require more nursing supervision. They're no longer recommended.

7. These devices are designed to maintain leg ROM and prevent deep vein stasis and thromboembolism.

8. Rationales: _____
_____

NURSING DIAGNOSIS

Risk for posttrauma response related to overwhelming psychological assault from sudden, unexpected injury

Nursing priority

Facilitate effective coping.

Patient outcome criteria

According to individual readiness, the patient will:
• discuss feelings about the traumatic incident
• learn to cope with flashbacks and other signs of the posttraumatic response.

Interventions

1. Refer to the "Ineffective individual coping" plan, page 67, the "Grieving" plan, page 44, and the "Dying" plan, page 20.

2. Observe for indications that the patient is reexperiencing the traumatic incident, such as flashbacks, intrusive thoughts, nightmares, guilt over survival, and excessive talking about the event. Also observe for indications of psychic numbing, such as confusion, amnesia, limited affect, misinterpretation of reality, and poor impulse control.

3. Encourage the patient to discuss feelings and reach out to others for help in coping with them. Explicitly acknowledge the intense feelings involved and the difficulty in coping with them.

4. Reassure the patient about being safe now. Praise behaviors contributing to survival, if appropriate.

5. Support the family and help them understand the patient's response.

6. With the patient's and family's consent, call in counseling professionals, such as a spiritual advisor, social worker, or trauma stress specialist. Refer the patient and family to a trauma support group, if available.

7. Additional individualized interventions: _____
_____

Rationales

1. These plans contain helpful interventions for any trauma patient and the family. This section provides additional specific information.

2. These signs and symptoms characterize the posttraumatic response that may follow a sudden event over which the victim felt powerless, such as a motor vehicle accident, natural disaster, or act of violence.

3. Retelling the incident and verbalizing feelings are important steps toward psychic integration of the experience. Reaching out to others provides comfort and reestablishes psychological security. By recognizing the powerful feelings involved and acknowledging the patient's difficulty in coping with the experience, the nurse conveys respect and establishes rapport and trust.

4. The posttraumatic syndrome can be so intense that the patient becomes absorbed in reexperiencing the terrifying incident. Reassurance helps reorient the patient to reality and brings closure to the terrifying incident. Praise for survival behaviors helps restore a sense of control.

5. Distress at seeing the patient upset may cause the family to shut off verbalizations, crying, and other expressions of emotion. Although well intentioned, such blocking may ultimately interfere with the patient's ability to integrate the experience.

6. Counseling professionals offer special skills that may facilitate coping. Calling them in without consent, however, may reinforce the powerless feeling the patient experienced during the traumatic incident.

7. Rationales: _____
_____

NURSING DIAGNOSIS

Risk for injury: Complications related to impaired immunologic defenses, hypermetabolic state, stress, and other factors

Nursing priority

Prevent or minimize complications.

Patient outcome criterion

Throughout the hospital stay, the patient will show no signs or symptoms of complications.

Interventions

1. Identify and minimize potential sources of infection. For example, use strict sterile technique when opening invasive lines; provide care at the insertion site of skeletal pins, wires, and tongs, as ordered; and administer antibiotics, as ordered. If a CSF leak is present, avoid suctioning and packing the nose or ears, and tell the patient to avoid nose blowing. Ideally, remove and replace I.V. lines and urinary catheters within 24 hours of insertion in the field or emergency department.

2. Verify that tetanus prophylaxis was administered, if needed.

3. Provide adequate nutrition within 24 hours of admission as ordered. See the "Nutritional deficit" plan, page 80, for details.

4. Prevent stress ulcers by administering antacids, titrated to gastric pH, and histamine antagonists or anticholinergic agents, as ordered. Monitor gastric drainage for occult blood.

5. Monitor for signs and symptoms of compartmental syndrome, such as unrelievable pain, muscle tension, and neurovascular compromise. If any of these signs and symptoms are present, alert the doctor and assist with measurement of compartmental pressure or transfer to surgery for fasciotomy.

Rationales

1. Breach of the skin barrier, ischemia and necrotic tissue, inadequate inflammatory response, chronic disease, many invasive procedures, malnutrition, and pharmacologic agents contribute to the high risk of infection for the trauma patient. The measures listed prevent or treat infection. Lines and catheters placed hurriedly tend to become contaminated and serve as a wick for infection. Early replacement minimizes the infection risk.

2. Although tetanus prophylaxis usually is accomplished in the emergency department, it may have been overlooked if life-threatening injuries required immediate surgery.

3. Adequate nutrition is critically important to recovery because trauma induces a hypermetabolic response. Commonly, paralytic ileus or facial, airway, esophageal, chest, or abdominal injuries preclude oral nutrition. If these injuries are substantial, a jejunostomy tube is placed during the initial chest or abdominal surgery. If the enteral route is unavailable, parenteral nutrition should be started. Nutritional goals include achieving positive nitrogen balance and preventing complications from inadequate nutrition, such as sepsis, delayed wound healing, and multiple organ failure. The "Nutritional deficit" plan discusses this potential complication in detail.

4. The trauma patient is at increased risk for stress ulcers. Prevention is the best therapy. The medications indicated reduce the secretion and acidity of gastric fluids, and gastric drainage monitoring can detect incipient stress ulcers.

5. Compartmental syndrome, also called low-velocity crush syndrome, results from excessive pressure within a fascial compartment caused by swollen tissue or blood confined within the compartment. Soft-tissue injury, burns, pneumatic antishock garment use, and tight casts or dressings increase the risk of compartmental syndrome. Neurovascular compromise results and, if the pressure is not relieved by fasciotomy, the end result may be nerve damage or paralysis.

6. Monitor for signs and symptoms of myoglobinuric renal failure, such as decreased urine output and elevated specific gravity. Notify the doctor and obtain plasma creatine kinase (CK) and urine myoglobin levels, as ordered. If myoglobinuria is present, administer fluids and mannitol, as ordered.

6. Myoglobinuria reflects myoglobin release from muscle damage associated with crush injury or compartmental syndrome. When circulation is restored to the damaged tissue, a flood of myoglobin enters the central circulation. Myoglobinuria peaks about 3 hours after circulation is restored and may persist for as long as 12 hours after the ischemic event. If myoglobin precipitates in the renal tubules, it may cause acute renal failure. Elevated plasma CK and urine myoglobin levels confirm the diagnosis. Fluid administration and osmotic diuresis maintain renal tubular flow and lessen the risk of myoglobin clogging the renal tubules.

7. If musculoskeletal, soft tissue, burn, arterial, or multisystem trauma is present, observe for signs of fat embolism, such as sudden onset of respiratory distress, tachypnea, tachycardia, decreased LOC, and personality changes. If any of these signs or symptoms are present, alert the doctor.

7. Fat embolism results from mobilization of fat globules (for example, fat escaping from a fractured bone) or altered fat metabolism. The signs and symptoms from fat globules lodging in the lungs, brain, and kidneys usually occur 24 to 48 hours after injury. The early signs listed may be followed by petechiae (which appear 2 to 4 days after injury), retinal changes, and hematuria. Untreated, fat embolism may result in ARDS. Treatment is controversial but usually includes mechanical ventilation with positive end-expiratory pressure and possibly corticosteroids.

8. If death is imminent, consult with the doctor, family, and organ transplant team about possible organ donation.

8. Because trauma commonly involves young, previously healthy people, the trauma patient may be a suitable organ donor. Although contemplating the end of a loved one's life is naturally distressing, donating the patient's organs may bring meaning and comfort to the family.

9. Additional individualized interventions: _____

9. Rationales: _____

DISCHARGE PLANNING

Discharge checklist
Upon the patient's discharge, documentation shows evidence of:
❏ stable vital signs
❏ stable laboratory values
❏ absence of major complications, such as sepsis, renal failure, and increased ICP.

Teaching checklist
Document evidence that the patient and family demonstrate an understanding of:
❏ extent of injuries
❏ prognosis
❏ treatments
❏ pain management
❏ posttrauma response
❏ coping resources
❏ organ donation process, if appropriate.

Documentation checklist
Using outcome criteria as a guide, document:
❏ clinical status on admission
❏ significant changes in status
❏ pertinent laboratory and diagnostic test findings
❏ airway and ventilation support
❏ fluid administration
❏ medication administration
❏ nutritional support
❏ emotional support
❏ measures to prevent or treat complications
❏ patient and family teaching
❏ discharge planning.

ASSOCIATED PLANS OF CARE

Acute renal failure
Adult respiratory distress syndrome
Disseminated intravascular coagulation
Dying
Grieving

Hypovolemic shock
Impaired physical mobility
Increased intracranial pressure
Ineffective individual coping
Knowledge deficit
Mechanical ventilation
Nutritional deficit
Pain
Sensory-perceptual alteration
Septic shock

REFERENCES

Black, J.M., and Matassarin-Jacobs, E. *Medical-Surgical Nursing: Clinical Management for Continuity of Care*, 5th ed. Philadelphia: W.B. Saunders Co., 1997.

Burch, J. "New Concepts in Trauma," *American Journal of Surgery* 173(1):44-48, January 1997.

Clochesy, J. *Critical Care Nursing,* 2nd ed. Philadelphia: W.B. Saunders Co., 1996.

Litwack, K. *Post Anesthesia Care Nursing*, 2nd ed. St. Louis: Mosby–Year Book, Inc., 1995.

Lowdermilk, D. *Maternity & Women's Health Care*, 6th ed. St. Louis: Mosby–Year Book, Inc., 1995.

Mattox, K. *Complications of Trauma*. New York: Churchill Livingstone, Inc. 1994.

Mattox, K. "Red River Anthology," *Journal of Trauma* 42(1):353-68, March 1997.

Reeder, S. *Maternity Nursing: Family, Newborn, and Women's Health Care*, 18th ed. Philadelphia: Lippincott-Raven Pubs., 1997.

Shoemaker, W. *Textbook of Critical Care,* 3rd ed. Philadelphia: W.B. Saunders Co., 1995.

Thompson, J. *Mosby's Clinical Nursing,* 4th ed. St. Louis: Mosby–Year Book, Inc., 1997.

Victarino, G. "Jehovah's Witnesses: Unique Problems in a Unique Trauma Population," *Journal of the American College of Surgeons* 184(5): 458-67, May 1997.

Ward, C. "Iron and Infection: New Developments and Their Implications," *Journal of Trauma* 41(2):356-64, August 1996.

Wijngaarden, M. "Blunt Cardiac Injury: A 10-Year Institutional Review," *Injury: International Journal of the Care of the Injured* 28(1):51-55, 57-61, January 1997.

Wilson, R. *Management of Trauma Pitfalls and Practice,* 2nd ed. Baltimore: Williams & Wilkins Co., 1996.

Woods, S. *Cardiac Nursing,* 3rd ed. Philadelphia: Lippincott-Raven Pubs., 1995.

Osteomyelitis

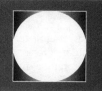

DRG information
DRG 238   Osteomyelitis.
          Mean LOS = 10.1 days
Principal diagnoses include:
- acute osteomyelitis
- chronic osteomyelitis
- unspecified osteomyelitis.

INTRODUCTION

Definition and time focus
Osteomyelitis is a bone infection that may be classified as primary, secondary, or chronic. *Primary osteomyelitis* occurs from compound fractures, penetrating wounds, or surgery. *Secondary osteomyelitis* may be hematogenous (bloodborne) or may represent extension of nearby infections (especially pressure ulcers). *Chronic osteomyelitis,* a persistent bone infection manifested by draining sinus tracts, is rare.

    This section focuses on the patient receiving nonsurgical treatment of osteomyelitis for which postdischarge antibiotic therapy is anticipated.

Etiology and precipitating factors
- Bone infection (either bloodborne or from an open wound) with sufficient numbers of pathogenic bacteria, most commonly *Staphylococcus aureus*
- Sufficient bone and soft-tissue trauma and hematoma to provide growth media for the infecting agent
- Implantation of foreign material (joint replacements or metallic internal fixation devices) that may impair the body's ability to control bacterial growth
- Infection near bone or joints
- I.V. drug abuse

FOCUSED ASSESSMENT GUIDELINES

Nursing history (functional health pattern findings)
Health perception–health management pattern
- Lack of knowledge about basic health care practices, especially hand washing and signs and symptoms of infection
- History of unreported local infection
- Unreported systemic indicators of infection, such as fever, malaise, weakness, irritability, anorexia, and generalized sepsis (rare)
- Recent upper respiratory tract infection, urinary tract infection, otitis media, impetigo, tonsillitis, or dental procedure
- History of disinterest in learning about care of an immobilization device or devices (for example, cast, splint, external fixator, or brace) needed previously

Activity-exercise pattern
- Weakness and fatigue

Cognitive-perceptual pattern
- Pain in affected limb, increasing with movement

Sleep-rest pattern
- Night sweats
- Pain affecting sleep

Physical findings
General
- Emotional irritability

Cardiovascular
- Tachycardia

Integumentary
- Localized edema and erythema in infection area
- Localized tenderness in infection area
- Draining wound, with either serous or gross purulent drainage (may not be present in all patients)
- Diaphoresis and flushing with fever
- Chronically draining sinus tracts (rare)

Musculoskeletal
- Pseudoparalysis (inability to move joints adjacent to area of osteomyelitis because of anticipated pain)
- Muscle spasm in infected extremity

Diagnostic studies
- Wound aspirate or bone biopsy of sequestrum (involved bone) — demonstrates the infecting organism
- Complete blood count — reveals leukocytosis and, after prolonged infection, anemia related to associated decrease in erythropoietin production and reduced red blood cell life span
- Erythrocyte sedimentation rate — elevated; degree of elevation relates to extent of infection
- Blood cultures — may reveal infecting organism when shaking chills and temperature spikes are associated with osteomyelitis
- X-rays of involved bones — may eventually show evidence of osteonecrosis and new bone formation
- Radioisotope scanning — may reveal areas of increased vascularity, indicating infection
- Sinograms of draining sinus tract — may outline involved areas of chronic osteomyelitis

• Computed tomography scan — may reveal changes indicating osteonecrosis
• Magnetic resonance imaging — may reveal soft-tissue inflammation
• Myelogram — may be required for vertebral infections

Potential complications
• Chronic osteomyelitis
• Sepsis
• Dysfunctional limb
• Refractory, life-threatening infection requiring amputation
• Pathologic fractures
• Nonunion of existing fractures

CLINICAL SNAPSHOT

OSTEOMYELITIS

Major nursing diagnoses	Key patient outcomes
Pain	Rate pain severity as less than 3 on a 0 to 10 pain rating scale.
Risk for recurrent or spreading infection	List, on request, local and systemic signs and symptoms of infection.
Risk for injury	Monitor responses as needed for specific antibiotics.
Risk for disuse syndrome	Independently perform prescribed exercises. Show no signs or symptoms of complications.

NURSING DIAGNOSIS

Pain related to inflammation

Nursing priority

Relieve pain.

Patient outcome criteria

• Within 1 day of admission, the patient will:
 – show no indications of uncontrolled pain, such as facial grimacing, tachycardia, increased blood pressure, or groaning
 – verbalize pain control
 – rate pain severity as less than 3 on a 0 to 10 pain rating scale while using pain medications.
• Within 2 days of admission, the patient will:
 – verbalize or demonstrate an understanding of at least two personally effective nonpharmacologic methods of pain control
 – verbalize an understanding of the need to report increasing or uncontrolled pain.

Interventions

1. See the "Pain" plan, page 88.

2. Clearly identify and document the source and degree of pain. Aid the patient in rating pain, using a scale of 0 to 10 (0 = no pain, 10 = severe pain).

Rationales

1. General interventions for pain are detailed in this plan.

2. Continuing or increasing severe pain may indicate increasing inflammation.

3. Medicate the patient with narcotics and nonsteroidal anti-inflammatory drugs (NSAIDs), as ordered, and carefully document their effectiveness. Monitor for adverse reactions.

4. Instruct the patient in nonpharmacologic pain control methods, including relaxation, enhanced relaxation, guided imagery, distraction (verbal, auditory, visual, or tactile), rhythmic breathing, cutaneous stimulation (such as with oil of wintergreen), massage, transcutaneous electrical nerve stimulation, use of heat and cold, and biofeedback. Document methods that the patient finds helpful.

5. Elevate and support the affected extremity.

6. Schedule necessary activity of the involved extremity to coincide with the peak effectiveness of analgesics or NSAIDs.

7. Instruct the patient to report increasing or uncontrolled pain.

8. Use adjunctive devices (such as a bed cradle, antirotation boots, or a mechanical bed) to aid in pain control.

9. Maintain traction and support devices (such as a cast, a splint, or internal fixators), as ordered.

10. Additional individualized interventions: _____

3. Bone pain is usually severe.

4. Nonpharmacologic pain control allows self-control of pain without possible adverse drug reactions to medications. Ice, for example, acts as a tactile distraction, stimulates large-diameter cutaneous sensory neurons, which decreases deeper pain sensation (the gate control theory), and causes vasoconstriction, which reduces edema that contributes to pain.

5. Elevation enhances venous return to reduce inflammatory edema; supportive positioning protects against muscle strain and spasm.

6. Scheduling activity to coincide with the peak of medication action decreases discomfort while allowing necessary mobility.

7. Increasing or uncontrolled pain may indicate worsening osteomyelitis, ineffective therapy, or both.

8. Reducing direct pressure, rotational force, and discomfort from turning may help control pain in some circumstances.

9. Immobilization and external support devices aid fracture healing, protect the infected bone from excessive stress, and decrease pain.

10. Rationales: _____

NURSING DIAGNOSIS

Risk for recurrent or spreading infection related to lack of knowledge of infection control

Nursing priority

Teach the patient to recognize local and systemic indicators of infection.

Patient outcome criteria

Within 2 days of admission, the patient will:
• list, on request, local and systemic signs and symptoms of infection
• verbalize an understanding of the need to alert health care providers promptly if infection occurs.

Interventions

1. Instruct about signs and symptoms of local infection (erythema, edema, localized tenderness, serous or purulent discharge, and local warmth) and systemic infection (fever, chills, malaise, weakness, and irritability). Teach the need to report limited range of motion (ROM) as a possible indication of spreading infection. Stress the need to report these findings promptly; provide a phone number for postdischarge contact.

Rationales

1. Prompt reporting of these signs and symptoms ensures early identification and treatment of infection.

2. Evaluate learning by having the patient list the signs and symptoms of infection, preferably in writing. Document learning. See the "Knowledge deficit" plan, page 72.

3. Provide the patient with a written list of local and systemic signs and symptoms of infection for periodic review. Document the material provided.

4. When necessary, establish continuity for continued education or evaluation of learning through community health nurse referrals.

5. Additional individualized interventions: _____

2. Having the patient list signs and symptoms provides feedback about learning and an opportunity to identify omissions and correct misconceptions. The "Knowledge deficit" plan contains further details related to patient teaching.

3. Readily accessible review materials help the patient retain new knowledge.

4. Some patients will not benefit from the patient education provided and will require continued instruction or appropriate follow-up care.

5. Rationales: _____

NURSING DIAGNOSIS

Risk for injury related to use of antibiotics with high potential for toxic effects

Nursing priority

Prevent or minimize toxic effects of antibiotic therapy.

Patient outcome criteria

- Within 2 days after initiation of therapy, the patient will:
  - (with aminoglycoside therapy) list signs and symptoms of ototoxicity, nephrotoxicity, and superimposed infections
  - (with penicillin therapy) list signs and symptoms of anemia, hypersensitivity reaction, and opportunistic infections
  - (with cephalosporin therapy) list signs and symptoms of photosensitivity, hepatotoxicity, nephrotoxicity, and opportunistic infections
  - (with sulfonamide therapy) list signs and symptoms of nephrotoxicity, agranulocytosis, crystalluria, and hemorrhagic tendencies
  - (with fluoroquinolone therapy) list the signs and symptoms of nephrotoxicity and potential drug interactions
  - (with vancomycin therapy) list the signs and symptoms of ototoxicity, nephrotoxicity, hypersensitivity reactions and "red neck" syndrome.
  - verbalize the importance of rapidly reporting signs and symptoms of untoward effects.
- By the time of discharge, the patient will:
  - monitor responses as needed for specific antibiotics.

Interventions

1. Teach the patient about antibiotic administration, especially monitoring for significant antibiotic adverse effects. See *Minimizing adverse effects of antibiotic therapy.*

2. Instruct the patient to report any adverse effects promptly.

3. Additional individualized interventions: _____

Rationales

1. A patient's knowledgeable participation in self-care while in the hospital improves the quality of care, allows for rapid identification of complications, and prepares the patient for self-care after discharge.

2. Prompt identification and notification reduce the potential for long-term complications.

3. Rationales: _____

Minimizing adverse effects of antibiotic therapy

The following chart lists common antibiotics and appropriate interventions.

Drugs	Nursing considerations
aminoglycosides (gentamicin, neomycin, streptomycin, and tobramycin)	• Teach the potential for ototoxicity (as shown by high-frequency hearing loss [for example, decreased ability to hear a ticking wristwatch], tinnitus, vertigo, and dizziness); superimposed infections (especially fungal infections of mucous membranes or at the site of indwelling vascular access catheters); and nephrotoxicity (as shown by oliguria, polyuria, abnormal specific gravity, and rapid weight gain). • Explain the rationale for baseline and weekly audiograms and serum creatinine and blood urea nitrogen (BUN) studies. • Explain the need for laboratory assessment of serum peak and trough levels (respectively the highest and lowest drug levels). These specimens are collected to ensure the lowest effective dose to maintain bactericidal levels while reducing the potential for adverse effects. • Monitor and document fluid intake and output and urine specific gravity while the patient is hospitalized. Report oliguria, polyuria, and specific gravity extremes (less than 1.010 and greater than 1.030). When appropriate, instruct the patient about continuing this monitoring after discharge. • Weigh the patient twice weekly and document. Teach him about twice weekly weight measurement after discharge. Report weight gain exceeding 3 lb (1.4 kg). • Teach the patient to closely monitor mucous membranes for indications of fungal infection (redness, tenderness, cheesy white discharge, black or furry tongue, fever, nausea, and diarrhea) and the need to report any that occur.
penicillins (ampicillin, carbenicillin, dicloxacillin, methicillin, nafcillin, and oxacillin)	• Teach the potential for anemia (as shown by weakness, paleness, and malaise), hypersensitivity reactions (as shown by asthmatic reactions, erythematous-maculopapular rash, urticaria, and anaphylaxis), and overgrowth of nonsusceptible organisms leading to opportunistic infection (as shown by fever, chills, and continuing or increasing indications of infection or inflammation).
cephalosporins (cefamandole, cefazolin, cefepime, cefoxitin, cephalothin, cephapirin, and cephradine)	• Teach the potential for opportunistic infections (as shown by fever, chills, and continuing or increasing indications of infection or inflammation), photosensitivity (unusual skin sensitivity to sunlight) and, in the patient with suspected renal or hepatic disease, nephrotoxicity (as shown by oliguria, polyuria, abnormal specific gravity, and rapid weight gain) and hepatotoxicity (as shown by jaundice, icteric sclera, dark brown urine, and pale, pasty stools). • Explain the rationale for baseline and weekly measurement of serum creatinine, BUN, lactic dehydrogenase, serum aspartate aminotransferase, and serum alanine aminotransferase levels. • Monitor and instruct the patient about nephrotoxicity and weight gain, as discussed under "aminoglycosides" above. • When oral medications are used, teach the patient to avoid concurrent intake of iron products or dairy foods because they decrease cephalosporin absorption. • Instruct the patient to avoid direct sunlight and to use sun-blocking agents when sun exposure is unavoidable.
sulfonamides (sulfadiazine, sulfamethoxazole, and sulfisoxazole)	• Teach the potential for nephrotoxicity (as shown by polyuria, oliguria, abnormal specific gravity, and rapid weight gain), agranulocytosis (as shown by fever and lesions of the mucous membranes, GI tract, and skin), crystalluria (as shown by evidence of renal calculi—hematuria, pyuria, frequency, urgency,

(continued)

Minimizing adverse effects of antibiotic therapy *(continued)*

Drugs	Nursing considerations
sulfonamides *(continued)*	retention, and pain in the flank, lower back, perineum, thighs, groin, labia, or scrotum), and hemorrhagic tendencies (as shown by epistaxis, bleeding gums, prolonged bleeding from wounds, ecchymoses, melena, hematuria, hemoptysis, and hematemesis from disruption of intestinal flora and synthesis of vitamin K). • Explain the rationale for baseline and weekly measurement of serum creatinine, BUN, and granulocyte levels. • Monitor and instruct the patient about nephrotoxicity and weight gain, as discussed under "aminoglycosides" above. • Instruct the patient taking oral sulfonamides to drink 8 oz (237 ml) of fluid with each dose. Encourage total fluid intake of at least 8 8-oz glasses daily.
fluoroquinolones *(ciprofloxacin and enoxacin)*	• Teach the potential for adverse reactions (such as nausea, vomiting, diarrhea, abdominal discomfort, dizziness, headaches, insomnia, slit lamp eye changes, and skin disorders). Nausea associated with enoxacin may be decreased by taking the medication within 1 hour of a meal. • Teach the potential for drug interactions, especially when taking theophylline, because these agents slow the clearance of theophylline and increase its potential for toxicity. Under the doctor's supervision, the theophylline dosage may need to be decreased. Similarly, concurrent use of antacids may decrease absorption of fluoroquinolones. • Explain the need to take ciprofloxacin 2 hours after meals and to drink plenty of fluids while taking this agent. • Monitor for and instruct the patient about nephrotoxicity and weight gain, as discussed under "aminoglycosides" above.
vancomycin *(Vancocin, Vancoled)*	• Teach the potential for ototoxicity (high frequency hearing loss [for example decreased ability to hear a ticking wristwatch], tinnitus, vertigo, or dizziness), nephrotoxicity (as shown by oliguria, polyuria, abnormal specific gravity, and rapid weight gain), hypersensitivity reactions (urticaria, chills, fever, skin rash, and anaphylactoid reaction with accompanying vascular collapse) and, following too-rapid I.V. infusion, "red neck" syndrome (flushing and erythematous rash on the upper thorax and face accompanied by hypotension.) • Explain the need for laboratory assessment of serum peak and trough levels (respectively the highest and lowest drug levels). These specimens are collected to ensure the lowest effective dose to maintain bactericidal levels while reducing the potential for adverse effects. • Monitor for nephrotoxicity and weight gain, as discussed under "aminoglycosides" above.
I.V. antibiotics	• When indwelling vascular access catheters are used for antibiotic administration, closely monitor the insertion sites for inflammation or irritation that doesn't respond to treatment with topical antibiotics. Teach the patient to monitor for this complication and promptly report it to the health care provider. • Teach close monitoring of wounds for indications of unresolving or increasing inflammation or infection (which are evidence of opportunistic infection).
Any oral antibiotic	• Instruct the patient about the need to take medication as ordered. Although some antibiotic therapy (such as with fluoroquinolones) may be administered orally, this doesn't decrease the need to ensure that medications are administered on schedule to provide adequate serum drug levels.

NURSING DIAGNOSIS

Risk for disuse syndrome with risk factors of prolonged infection, pain, and immobilization

Nursing priority

Help the patient regain or exceed usual activity level.

Patient outcome criteria

- Within 2 days of admission, the patient will:
  - verbalize an understanding of the need for exercise when mobility is restricted
  - list exercise goals
  - demonstrate the exercise regimen.
- By the time of discharge, the patient will:
  - independently perform prescribed exercises
  - show no signs or symptoms of complications.

Interventions

1. Assess and document the patient's baseline activity level, including muscle strength and ability to perform activities of daily living (ADLs).

2. Document activity goals set in collaboration with the patient.

3. Teach the patient about the need to maintain muscle strength and endurance while immobilized. Provide instruction in isotonic and isometric exercises that can be accomplished within the patient's activity limitations.

4. Have the patient demonstrate the exercises, and evaluate and document the patient's learning. Establish and monitor an exercise regimen throughout the hospital stay. Help the patient establish a home exercise program as well, and ensure community health care follow-up after discharge, when needed.

5. Provide abundant positive reinforcement. Develop goals of increasing strength (increasing increments of resistance or weight) and endurance (increasing numbers or repetitions or longer exercise periods), when feasible.

6. Provide written materials on exercises for review as needed. Document the materials provided.

7. Additional individualized interventions: _____

Rationales

1. Adequate baseline information allows determination of individualized goals.

2. Involving the patient in planning increases the potential for success. Goals provide focus.

3. Maintenance exercise programs decrease loss of muscle strength and endurance during immobilization by maintaining adequate blood flow to muscle and by stressing bone to ensure continued balance in bone remodeling.

4. Return demonstration of exercises allows effective evaluation of patient learning. Monitoring the exercise regimen ensures that the patient will maintain strength and endurance.

5. Positive reinforcement helps establish health-promoting behaviors. Isometric and isotonic exercises performed within activity restrictions may increase strength and endurance in unaffected body areas.

6. Written materials increase understanding of exercises and the potential for doing exercises as required.

7. Rationales: _____

DISCHARGE PLANNING

Discharge checklist
Before discharge, the patient shows evidence of:
- ❏ wound drainage within expected parameters, with little or no purulent or bloody drainage
- ❏ stable vital signs
- ❏ absence of fever
- ❏ absence of pulmonary or cardiovascular complications
- ❏ no erythema, edema, or tenderness at wound site
- ❏ no loss of ROM in joints adjacent to the infection
- ❏ ability to control pain using oral medications
- ❏ stabilizing weight and adequate nutritional intake
- ❏ ability to perform ADLs at usual level
- ❏ ability to transfer, ambulate, and perform prescribed exercise regimen at usual level or with minimal assistance
- ❏ ability to perform wound care and dressing changes as prescribed, with minimal assistance
- ❏ hemoglobin level and blood cultures within normal parameters
- ❏ white blood cell count within expected parameters
- ❏ normal bowel and bladder function
- ❏ adequate home support system, or referral to home care if indicated by inadequate home support system or inability to perform self-care.

If the patient is discharged with an indwelling vascular access catheter, documentation also shows:
- ❏ evidence of automatic referral to home care or arrangements for short-term stay in a nursing home (depending on the patient's home support system and ability to care for catheter and administer medications independently)
- ❏ knowledge of where to obtain additional supplies
- ❏ knowledge of signs and symptoms indicating catheter dysfunction or infection
- ❏ ability to follow prescribed medication regimen and I.V. administration technique
- ❏ ability to monitor weight and follow instructions for oral intake, as directed
- ❏ knowledge of signs and symptoms indicating fungal or other systemic infection.

Teaching checklist
Document evidence that the patient and family demonstrate an understanding of:
- ❏ disease and implications
- ❏ hand-washing techniques
- ❏ dressing changes, pin site care, cast care, or care of braces or splints, as appropriate
- ❏ nonpharmacologic pain-control interventions
- ❏ use of elevation and supportive positioning
- ❏ ROM exercise of the affected extremity, as appropriate
- ❏ dietary requirements
- ❏ all discharge medications' purpose, dosage, administration schedule, precautions, and adverse effects re-

quiring medical attention (usual discharge medications include antibiotics, analgesics, and NSAIDs)
- ❏ need to report increasing or uncontrolled pain
- ❏ care of indwelling vascular access catheters
- ❏ self-administration of I.V. antibiotics
- ❏ vascular access complications
- ❏ patient exercise regimen
- ❏ how to obtain clarification of instructions or further information
- ❏ date, time, and place of follow-up appointments
- ❏ referral agencies and medical supply resources
- ❏ how to contact the doctor.

Documentation checklist
Using outcome criteria as a guide, document:
- ❏ clinical status on admission
- ❏ significant changes in status
- ❏ pertinent laboratory and diagnostic test findings
- ❏ baseline information on muscle strength, ADLs performed, endurance, and collaborative goals established with the patient
- ❏ source and degree of pain, especially if persistent or increasing
- ❏ effective pain-relief measures
- ❏ daily or biweekly measurement of weight, intake, output, and urine specific gravity, when appropriate
- ❏ appearance of indwelling vascular access catheter site, and catheter care
- ❏ patient and family teaching
- ❏ discharge planning.

ASSOCIATED PLANS OF CARE

Chronic renal failure
Ineffective individual coping
Knowledge deficit
Pain
Surgery
Urolithiasis

REFERENCES
Chambers, H.F. "Infections Diseases: Bacterial and Chlamydial," in *Current Medical Diagnosis and Treatment,* 36th ed. Edited by Tierney, L.M., et al. Stamford, Conn.: Appleton & Lange, 1997.

Gray, M.A. "Local Application of Antibiotics in Orthopaedic Infections," *Orthopaedic Nursing* 14(5):69-79, September 1995.

Hellmann, D.B. "Arthritis and Musculoskeletal Disorders," in *Current Medical Diagnosis and Treatment,* 36th ed. Edited by Tierney, L.M., et al. Stamford, Conn.: Appleton & Lange, 1997.

Karch, A.M. *1997 Lippincott's Nursing Drug Guide.* Philadelphia: Lippincott-Raven Pubs., 1997.

Laughlin, R.T., et al. "Osteomyelitis," *Current Opinion in Rheumatology* 7(4):315-21, July 1995.

Shannon, M.T., et al. *Drugs and Nursing Implications,* 8th ed. Norwalk, Conn.: Appleton & Lange, 1995.

Yandrich, T.J. "Preventing Infection in Total Joint Replacement Surgery," *Orthopaedic Nursing* 14(2):15-19, March-April 1995.

Radical neck dissection

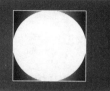

DRG information

DRG 076   Other Respiratory System Operating Room (OR) Procedures with Complication or Co-morbidity (CC).
Mean LOS = 12.5 days

DRG 077   Other Respiratory System OR Procedures without CC.
Mean LOS = 5.5 days

Principal diagnoses include:
- • excision of regional lymph nodes
- • excision or repair of larynx
- • tracheostomy.

DRG 400   Lymphoma or Leukemia with Major OR Procedure.
Mean LOS = 10.4 days

Principal diagnoses include:
- • malignant neoplasm of lymph nodes
- • lymphosarcoma.

Additional DRG information: Radical neck dissection has a number of alternative DRGs. The DRG assigned depends on the cause of the surgery (where the cancer is located), not on its extent (tracheostomy or laryngectomy) or how radical a dissection is performed.

INTRODUCTION

Definition and time focus

Radical neck dissection (RND) is a surgical procedure performed for cancers of the head and neck. Normally, RND involves the surgical removal of:
- • lymph nodes in the neck
- • lymphatic vessels
- • the sternocleidomastoid muscle
- • the internal jugular vein
- • the spinal accessory nerve (innervates the trapezius muscle)
- • the submandibular salivary gland
- • the tail of the parotid gland.

When RND is combined with removal of a tumor located in the mouth, pharynx, or larynx (a common occurrence), a tracheostomy is usually created. If a total laryngectomy is performed, the tracheostomy will be permanent, and the opening between the trachea and the pharynx will be surgically closed. A patient who doesn't require total laryngectomy may have a temporary tracheostomy until surgical or radiation-related edema subsides. After surgery, the patient is commonly admitted to the intensive care unit initially. This clinical plan focuses on preoperative and postoperative care for the patient undergoing RND.

Etiology and precipitating factors

RND is performed to remove:
- • primary malignant tumors of the mouth, pharynx, or larynx
- • skin lesions (melanomas).
    Risk factors associated with these cancers include:
- • heavy use of alcohol and cigarettes (oral and laryngeal cancer)
- • pipe or cigar smoking (oral cancer)
- • tobacco chewing (oral cancer)
- • exposure to nickel or wood dust or woodworking chemicals (nasopharyngeal cancer)
- • fair complexion and long-term or frequent sun exposure (melanoma).

FOCUSED ASSESSMENT GUIDELINES

Nursing history (functional health pattern findings)

Health perception–health management pattern
- • History of heavy cigarette smoking, alcohol abuse, or both
- • Past radiation or chemotherapy (for head and neck cancer)
- • History of previous head or neck cancer

Nutritional-metabolic pattern
- • Weight loss
- • Dysphagia, sore throat, or difficulty chewing
- • Lack of appetite
- • History of skin lesions (basal cell)

Sleep-rest pattern
- • Fatigue

Cognitive-perceptual pattern
- • Change in taste sensation
- • Neck pain (rare)

Self-perception–self-concept pattern
- • Strong, active, and easy going, or possibly passive
- • Voice change

Role-relationship pattern
- • may describe self as independent of others
- • may be head of household
- • may have a history of sporadic employment related to alcoholism

Coping–stress tolerance pattern
- • may have delayed seeking treatment (denial)

• may tend to avoid issues requiring a decision
• may have only spouse or friend as major support system

Value-belief pattern
• Disease viewed as life-threatening
• Desire to have surgery in order to return to usual activities
• Difficulty accepting seriousness of disease (with melanoma) and need for radical surgery

Physical findings
Pulmonary
• Productive cough or wheezing
• Hoarseness
• Difficulty breathing
Gastrointestinal
• Nonhealing ulcer in oral cavity
• Toothless or poor oral hygiene
Neurologic
• Otalgia (ear pain)
Integumentary
• Melanoma
Musculoskeletal
• Lump on neck

Diagnostic studies
• Blood studies, including complete blood count and electrolyte determinations — establishes preoperative baseline; findings usually within normal limits; decreased albumin levels indicate altered nutrition; elevated or depressed white blood cell (WBC) count may indicate immune system's response to the disease or stage of recovery from radiation therapy or chemotherapy
• Liver function test — rules out liver disease before surgery
• Chest X-ray — may show metastasis or pulmonary disease
• Head and neck X-rays or computed tomography (CT) scan — identify location and extent of tumor and metastasis to sinuses, neck, or brain
• Panendoscopy and biopsy — define tumor type and extension of tumor
• Barium swallow — if dysphagia is present, defines involvement of pharynx, epiglottis, or esophagus
• Lymphoscintigraphy (for melanoma) — identifies involved lymph nodes and drainage pathways
• Laryngogram — if hoarseness is present, defines area of involvement in larynx and extent of airway obstruction
• Abdominal CT scan — may demonstrate metastasis to abdominal organs
• Upper or lower GI series — may demonstrate metastasis to esophagus or digestive system

Potential complications
• Airway obstruction
• Carotid artery rupture
• Cutaneous or tracheoesophageal fistula formation

CLINICAL SNAPSHOT

RADICAL NECK DISSECTION

Major nursing diagnoses	Key patient outcomes
Knowledge deficit (preoperative)	State on request the reason for the surgery and expected outcomes.
Risk for ineffective denial	State on request one action to decrease the risk of recurrence of head and neck cancer.
Altered role performance	Return to functional role within family or society.
Risk for ineffective airway clearance	Maintain a patent airway.
Impaired swallowing	Use a modified eating technique effectively.
Risk for injury	Protect the wound site effectively during activities of daily living.
Pain	Rate pain (with pain medication) as less than 3 on a 0 to 10 pain rating scale.
Nutritional deficit	Have nutritional intake meeting calculated calorie and protein requirements.
Altered oral mucous membrane	Exhibit no signs or symptoms of oral infection.
Impaired verbal communication	Maintain communication with others.
Bathing-hygiene or dressing-grooming self-care deficit	Be able to bathe and dress with minimal help.
Body-image disturbance	Show beginning acceptance of body changes and limitations.
Family coping: Potential for growth	(The family will) demonstrate skills needed for home care.

NURSING DIAGNOSIS

Knowledge deficit (preoperative) related to unfamiliar diagnosis and surgical procedure

Nursing priority

Supplement the patient's and family's knowledge of impending surgery.

Patient outcome criteria

- Before surgery, the patient will:
  - state on request the reason for surgery and expected outcomes
  - exhibit a decreased anxiety level.
- Before surgery, family members will describe their greatest concern and at least one way they will deal with it.

Interventions

1. See the "Knowledge deficit" plan, page 72, and the "Surgery" plan, page 103.

Rationales

1. These plans contain general interventions for the surgical patient who has a nursing diagnosis of knowledge deficit.

2. On admission, assess the patient's knowledge base. Encourage questions. Help the patient and family to identify concerns and methods to cope with them. As appropriate, explain and illustrate the signs and symptoms of head and neck cancer, the planned treatment, and the expected postoperative outcomes. After surgery, the patient can expect a bulky neck dressing, intensive care unit care until stable, a nasogastric tube, intubation or tracheostomy, skin catheters, and skin graft and donor sites. Document the patient's and family's level of understanding and their response.

3. Additional individualized interventions: _____

_____

2. Knowledge of expected events may decrease anxiety and give a sense of control. Providing information helps the patient and family focus questions on topics they don't understand. Individuals differ in the amount of detail desired: Some may want only minimal descriptions while others may request to see pictures or equipment. Airway management after surgery varies, but most patients have a temporary tracheostomy until edema subsides. The temporary tracheostomy is usually closed within 2 weeks after surgery, depending on the patient's status. If the patient will be undergoing radiation therapy, the tracheostomy may be maintained longer. The patient undergoing total laryngectomy will have a permanent tracheostomy.

3. Rationales: _____

_____

NURSING DIAGNOSIS

Risk for ineffective denial related to inaccurate perception of health status

Nursing priority

Promote accurate perception of health status and available resources for health promotion.

Patient outcome criterion

By the time of discharge, the patient will state on request one action to decrease the risk of recurrence of head and neck cancer.

Interventions

1. On admission, determine the time between initial symptoms and when treatment was sought. Explain the common signs and symptoms. Allow expression of guilt, resentment, and regret if treatment was delayed because of denial or avoidance. Emphasize that treatment is occurring now.

2. Evaluate for alcohol dependence. As part of the admission interview, question the patient specifically, directly, and in a matter-of-fact manner about alcohol consumption patterns, noting the time of the last drink. Observe for periorbital edema and ecchymoses or abrasions in various stages of healing. Be alert to any excessive use of such toiletries as mouthwash.

Rationales

1. If the time between when symptoms appeared and the patient sought help is lengthy, denial may be the patient's primary coping method. Initial symptoms are commonly mild and may be easily overlooked. Verbalization decreases unnecessary guilt if treatment was delayed.

2. Alcohol dependence is a typical finding in this patient group and must be identified for early assessment and treatment of withdrawal symptoms. Specific questions may unmask hidden alcoholism; although these patients tend to underestimate their consumption, they usually can and will accurately identify the time of their last drink. Periorbital edema suggests fluid retention, possibly related to excessive alcohol consumption. Lesions in various stages may be a sign of frequent falls because of intoxication. The patient may attempt to fend off withdrawal symptoms by using alcohol-laden toiletries while in the hospital.

3. Assess for signs and symptoms of alcohol withdrawal delirium as follows:
• mild (4 to 16 hours after the last drink) — tremors, agitation, tachycardia, vomiting, hypertension, diarrhea
• moderate (1 to 3 days later) — profuse diaphoresis, seizures, hallucinations, incontinence
• severe (variable onset, usually about 72 hours after the last drink) — delirium tremens, hyperthermia, violent behavior, extreme blood pressure changes, disorientation.
Notify the doctor if withdrawal is suspected, and institute sedative therapy, as ordered, along with any other medical measures.

4. After surgery, teach risk factors for head and neck cancer, and document the patient's level of understanding.

5. Before discharge, offer resources available for smoking cessation and alcohol rehabilitation, if appropriate, and document the plan for follow-up.

6. Additional individualized interventions: _____

3. Severe alcohol withdrawal delirium is a potentially life-threatening occurrence that may be prevented with early intervention. Sedation (usually with benzodiazepines) may prevent the syndrome's progression. Untreated, severe alcohol withdrawal delirium may result in myocardial infarction, cerebrovascular accident, or other serious complications.

4. A review of risk factors provides a baseline for discussion and planning to eliminate known risks.

5. Major lifestyle changes require support and follow-up. Smoking and alcohol intake are major risk factors for the recurrence of head and neck cancer.

6. Rationales: _____

NURSING DIAGNOSIS

Altered role performance related to muscle weakness and job disruption

Nursing priority

Advise the patient of available resources for job adjustment.

Patient outcome criteria

• Before surgery, the patient will express minimal anxiety about work and finances.
• By the time of discharge, the patient will state a plan for vocational rehabilitation.

Rationales

1. Before surgery, assess the physical requirements of the patient's job, especially noting any heavy lifting or use of shoulder muscles. Have the patient and family discuss work options with the patient's employer. Involve a social worker or vocational rehabilitation specialist.

2. Before discharge, document a referral to Social Services for a plan for alternative employment or disability follow-up.

3. Additional individualized interventions: _____

Interventions

1. The patient may be unaware of surgery's effect on job performance. Planning minimizes postoperative distress about changed abilities or activity restrictions. A social worker or vocational rehabilitation specialist may offer new options.

2. Financial concerns and the need for job security may be major obstacles to compliance with the total treatment plan if not addressed.

3. Rationales: _____

NURSING DIAGNOSIS

Risk for ineffective airway clearance related to edema and excessively thick secretions

Nursing priorities

- Prevent airway obstruction.
- Facilitate secretion removal.

Patient outcome criteria

- Throughout the postoperative period, the patient will maintain patent airway.
- Within 48 hours after surgery, the patient will effectively clear the airway with minimal assistance.
- By the time of discharge, the patient and family will:
  - demonstrate the correct technique for suctioning and cleaning the tracheostomy tube
  - verbalize a plan for emergency airway maintenance.
- By the time of discharge, the patient will:
  - identify ways to avoid aspiration
  - verbalize the intent to obtain medical alert identification.

Interventions

1. In the immediate postoperative period, assess and document upper airway patency, the presence and consistency of secretions, and the patient's ability to clear the airway.

2. If a tracheostomy is present, provide humidification and oxygen, as ordered. Suction the patient according to amount and consistency of secretions, possibly as often as every hour in the first 24 hours after surgery.

3. Assess the wound site for increasing edema, reevaluating upper airway patency and documenting changes at least hourly for the first 24 hours after surgery. Note and report any choking sensation, sense of apprehension, change in respiratory rate or depth, and increased upper airway sounds or tracheal shift.

4. If the patient has a permanent tracheostomy, teach the patient and at least one family member the skills necessary for home care. Include the following points:
- need for adequate humidification
- suctioning
- tube cleaning
- emergency reinsertion of the tube if it dislodges
- stoma covering
- need to cover the stoma when showering
- need to carry medical alert identification.

5. Additional individualized interventions: _____

Rationales

1. The effects of surgery and intubation alter airway patency and secretion consistency. Patients vary in their ability to expectorate secretions.

2. A tracheostomy bypasses the normal humidification function of the nose, so the patient requires supplemental humidity to liquefy secretions. The need for suctioning varies, depending on the duration of intubation, preoperative lung status, and the patient's response to the tracheostomy.

3. Early signs of upper airway obstruction are subtle and progressive and may be related to pressure on the trachea from increasing edema at the wound site. If edema compromises the airway, immediate medical intervention is required.

4. Skill at tracheostomy care reduces the patient's and family's anxiety and increases their confidence in coping with the lifestyle changes the surgery creates. Suctioning and cleaning are necessary to maintain airway patency. An emergency plan for tube dislodgment may help avert panic if this complication occurs. A stoma covering prevents aspiration of dust or insects, and covering the stoma during showers and avoiding water sports prevents aspiration of water. Medical alert identification will help emergency medical personnel quickly establish an appropriate airway if the patient suffers cardiac arrest or airway compromise.

5. Rationales: _____

Nursing diagnosis

Impaired swallowing related to decreased strength of muscles involved in mastication or to edema, tracheostomy tube, or esophageal sutures (applies to the patient who has had combined surgery, including RND)

Nursing priorities
- Prevent aspiration.
- Promote adequate food intake.

Patient outcome criteria

Throughout the postoperative period, the patient will:
- exhibit no aspiration
- use suction equipment effectively.

By the time of discharge, the patient will:
- control oral secretions without using suction
- use a modified eating technique effectively.

Interventions

1. Teach the patient to use oral suction equipment, and keep it at the bedside continuously.

2. Be present during meals, and teach the patient to use the "supraglottic swallow" (if the patient has a tracheostomy); eat soft foods in frequent, small feedings (if the patient underwent total laryngectomy); and place food in the area of the mouth unaffected by surgery. Encourage persistence in swallowing, and document progress. Obtain a speech therapy consult to assist in evaluating swallowing ability.

3. Additional individualized interventions: _____

Rationales

1. An increase in the amount of secretions is common after RND and difficult to handle if swallowing is impaired. Saliva flows continually; the ability to suction secretions decreases the patient's anxiety and minimizes the risk of choking.

2. The "supraglottic swallow" protects the airway and decreases the potential for aspiration. The sequence is usually cough, take a breath, take food, swallow, cough, swallow, and breathe. Soft foods and frequent feedings gradually stretch the esophageal incision site and encourage muscle relaxation. Swallowing success is increased when the patient can control food in the mouth; inspecting the mouth after swallowing indicates areas of weakness and helps determine the optimal site for food placement. Initial attempts may be unsuccessful and discouraging unless support is given. New techniques require practice to be effective.

3. Rationales: _____

Nursing diagnosis

Risk for injury related to impaired tissue integrity and sensory alterations (decreased sense of temperature, touch, and hearing on side of surgery)

Nursing priorities
- Prevent injury.
- Maintain sensory function.

Patient outcome criteria

- Within 5 days after surgery, the patient will:
  - exhibit less than 20 ml of drainage every 8 hours
  - exhibit decreased redness, no pallor, no increased edema, and minimal areas of crusting at the wound site.
- Throughout the postoperative period, the patient will support the shoulder and arm effectively.
- By the time of discharge, the patient will:
  - protect the wound site effectively during activities of daily living (ADLs)
  - identify areas of numbness and state protective measures for each area.

Interventions

1. See the "Skin grafts" plan, page 634.

2. Maintain continuous suction on drainage catheters: the recommended level is 100 to 120 mm Hg. When the patient ambulates, use a portable drainage collector. Interrupt suction, using standard precautions, to assess the system's patency every 1 to 2 hours for the first 48 hours, then every 4 hours until drains are removed.

3. Observe and document wound drainage every 8 hours. Report abnormalities, especially any sudden increase in the amount of drainage. Instruct the patient and family on the importance of careful observation.

4. If infection or a fistula occurs, determine the need for instituting carotid artery rupture precautions. These vary between facilities but always include avoidance of coughing, sudden head movements, and Valsalva's maneuver.

Make sure supplies are placed at the bedside as follows:
- towels, packing, and dressings
- hemostats and clamps
- gowns and gloves
- suture materials
- a light source
- a laryngoscope, cuffed endotracheal and tracheostomy tubes, and a 10 ml syringe
- suction equipment.

5. If carotid rupture occurs, stay with the patient, call for help, apply direct pressure if the hemorrhage site is visible, and maintain airway patency by orotracheal suctioning if hemoptysis is present.

6. Inspect and document changes at the wound site, especially noting redness, pallor, and increasing edema. Report abnormalities.

Rationales

1. This plan contains interventions for skin graft care.

2. Negative pressure is required to remove clots and fluid from the surgical wound. Inadequate suction may cause drain blockage and result in excessive edema, airway obstruction, or both.

3. A dramatic increase in bloody drainage may indicate impending carotid artery rupture. This is most likely in the immediate postoperative period, or later if infection or fistula formation occurs near the carotid artery. An increase in clear fluid or a change to milky drainage may indicate infection or fistula formation. Typically, drainage is less than 100 ml every 8 hours for the first 2 days, then less than 20 ml every 8 hours on successive days.

4. The carotid artery may be exposed if surrounding tissues are damaged by infection or if fistula formation delays healing. Artery rupture is a life-threatening complication requiring immediate medical intervention. Keeping needed supplies at the bedside facilitates prompt intervention if rupture occurs.

5. Most patients remain awake during carotid artery rupture. External pressure on a visible site controls the hemorrhage temporarily until help arrives. The trachea is a common pathway for internal hemorrhage.

6. Redness or pallor may indicate tension on the area, requiring arm, shoulder, or neck repositioning or adjustment of tracheostomy ties or the oxygen collar. Increasing edema may indicate inadequate or blocked drainage tubes.

7. Clean the suture line, as ordered, and document changes. Usual care involves removing crust with hydrogen peroxide and sterile swabs three or four times daily, followed by a thin application of bactericidal ointment to the suture line.

8. Assess for and document any hearing loss on the side of surgery. If hearing loss is evident, speak to the patient on the unaffected side. Don't shout. Use active listening skills at the bedside.

9. Support the patient's shoulder and arm at all times. Begin range-of-motion exercises, as ordered.

10. Teach the patient to protect the surgical site when performing ADLs. Also teach the male patient to look at the neck when shaving rather than depending on touch. Emphasize the importance of testing food temperatures before eating. Discourage the use of heat for relief of shoulder pain.

11. Additional individualized interventions: _____

7. Cleaning facilitates healing and decreases the potential for infection. Controversy continues, however, regarding the relative effectiveness of available bactericidal preparations.

8. Edema may temporarily block the ear canal. Shouting may intimidate or annoy the patient. Standing near the patient when speaking or listening facilitates communication.

9. Proper body alignment promotes healing and decreases tension on the surgical site. Innervation to the muscle is lost, but muscle mass remains and requires exercise to prevent atrophy.

10. Numbness increases the risk of accidental injury while shaving and eating. Heat should not be used to treat shoulder pain because temperature awareness in that area is impaired after surgery.

11. Rationales: _____

NURSING DIAGNOSIS

Pain related to edema, intubation, and the surgical wound

Nursing priority

Relieve postoperative pain.

Patient outcome criteria

Throughout the postoperative period, the patient will:
• rate pain (with pain medications) as less than 3 on a 0 to 10 pain rating scale
• exhibit relaxed posture and facial expression.

Interventions

1. See the "Pain" plan, page 88.

2. For headache, administer medication as ordered and document promptly. Keep the head of the bed elevated at all times.

3. For a sore throat, administer mouth care before meals, and offer fluids every 1 to 2 hours.

Rationales

1. This plan contains general interventions for pain management.

2. Edema related to loss of lymphatics and the jugular vein can cause postoperative headache. The semi-upright position facilitates fluid drainage and decreases pressure.

3. Fluids bathe the oral mucosa and stimulate salivary flow.

4. For shoulder pain, support the arm and shoulder at all times; teach the patient support methods; and administer medication promptly, as ordered, at the onset of pain and before ambulation or ADLs. Document all measures taken.

5. Additional individualized interventions: _____

4. Adequate support decreases tension on the wound site and maintains body alignment. Analgesics decrease pain, facilitating resumption of therapeutic activity.

5. Rationales: _____

NURSING DIAGNOSIS

Nutritional deficit related to anorexia and impaired swallowing

Nursing priority

Optimize nutritional intake.

Patient outcome criteria

Throughout the postoperative period, the patient will:
• experience no further weight loss
• have nutritional intake meeting calculated calorie and protein requirements.

Interventions

1. On admission, document the patient's height, weight, weight loss, intake pattern, and food consistency tolerances. See the "Nutritional deficit" plan, page 80.

2. Consult a dietitian for a thorough nutritional assessment to calculate calorie and protein requirements.

3. Monitor and document intake at each meal. Assess and document changes in chewing and swallowing ability. Supplement the diet as needed. Administer enteral feedings, as ordered, and document the patient's response.

4. Weigh the patient twice weekly and document.

5. Administer mouth care or an analgesic, as ordered, before meals.

6. Additional individualized interventions: _____

Rationales

1. Weight and weight loss help establish the patient's current nutritional status. Intake patterns and food consistency tolerances provide a focus for dietary planning. The "Nutritional deficit" plan provides further details.

2. Nutritional requirements are increased in disease and during treatment. The dietitian's expertise helps meet individual patient needs.

3. To achieve the required calorie and protein intake, additional feedings are commonly necessary. Changes in chewing and swallowing ability require dietary modifications. Individual patients respond differently to enteral feedings, and frequent adjustment is required.

4. Weight changes indicate progress or the need for adjustment to meet body requirements.

5. Good oral hygiene enhances food appeal when appetite is poor. Analgesics may be indicated if pain keeps the patient from eating.

6. Rationales: _____

NURSING DIAGNOSIS

Altered oral mucous membrane related to intake restrictions and nasogastric tube

Nursing priorities

• Minimize mucous membrane damage.
• Promote healing.

Patient outcome criteria

Throughout the postoperative period, the patient will:
• exhibit pink and moist mucous membranes
• exhibit no signs or symptoms of oral infection.

Interventions

1. While the patient is restricted from taking food or fluids, provide mouth care every 2 hours, as ordered.

2. After oral intake is resumed, provide mouth care after meals and at bedtime.

3. If oral suture lines are present, perform mouth care using a power spray, according to protocol and as ordered. Document the appearance of the oral cavity, and note changes.

4. Additional individualized interventions: _____

Rationales

1. Mouth care stimulates saliva flow and removes pooled secretions, which foster bacterial growth. Usually, care involves half-strength hydrogen peroxide and normal saline solution.

2. Food trapped in the altered oral cavity serves as a medium for bacterial growth and must be removed to prevent infection.

3. Crusting requires the pressure of a power spray for adequate removal.

4. Rationales: _____

NURSING DIAGNOSIS

Impaired verbal communication related to oral surgery and tracheostomy (applies to the patient who has had combined surgery, including RND)

Nursing priorities

• Maximize communication.
• Minimize patient frustration.

Patient outcome criteria

Throughout the hospital stay, the patient will:
• maintain communication with others
• experience minimal frustration with communication.

Interventions

1. Before surgery, help the patient select postoperative methods of communication. Document the methods chosen; options include:
• pencil and paper on a clipboard
• a "magic slate"
• a communication board or set of cards with pictures of commonly needed items
• an electrolarynx device (for later postoperative stages).

2. After surgery, tag the call system "patient cannot talk." Explain to the patient and family that the patient can still use the call system.

Rationales

1. Using alternative communication methods of the patient's choosing decreases anxiety and facilitates communication. The patient may prefer pencil and paper because the "magic slate" may be associated with child-like feelings of helplessness. The patient can help prepare a communication board or picture cards before surgery, increasing self-control. An electrolaryngeal device for the patient undergoing laryngectomy usually isn't used until 5 to 7 days after surgery, so another method will be needed initially.

2. This alerts the secretary or nurse that the patient's call must be attended to quickly. The patient is assured that personal needs will be met.

3. Address the patient in a normal conversational tone.

4. Allow the patient using a communication device to finish writing before replying.

5. Obtain a speech therapy consultation, as ordered.

6. Teach the patient with a tracheostomy to cover the opening when speaking, according to protocol or as ordered.

7. Additional individualized interventions: _____

3. Inability to speak doesn't necessarily indicate deafness.

4. Waiting prevents incorrect second-guessing and allows the patient to express feelings adequately.

5. Speech therapy exercises improve speech clarity.

6. Covering the tracheostomy prevents air leakage around the trachea, improving speech clarity and volume.

7. Rationales: _____

NURSING DIAGNOSIS

Bathing-hygiene or dressing-grooming self-care deficit related to muscle weakness, pain, and uncompensated neuromuscular impairment

Nursing priorities
• Maximize the patient's self-care ability.
• Encourage the use of affected muscles.

Patient outcome criterion
Within 5 days after surgery, the patient will be able to bathe and dress with minimal help.

Interventions

1. After surgery, demonstrate methods to compensate for loss of function, such as using the unaffected arm and shoulder to bathe, comb hair, and dress by putting clothing on the affected side first.

2. Administer an analgesic, as ordered, before activities.

3. Teach strengthening exercises, as ordered, and document progress. Refer the patient to a physical therapist for an ongoing activity plan.

4. Additional individualized interventions: _____

Rationales

1. Initial weakness may discourage the patient from using the unaffected arm and shoulder to the fullest advantage.

2. Relieving pain encourages arm use.

3. The muscle can be trained to tense, offsetting some of the shoulder drop that occurs with lost innervation. The physical therapist's expertise helps in planning rehabilitation.

4. Rationales: _____

NURSING DIAGNOSIS

Body-image disturbance related to change in physical appearance and to functional limitations

Nursing priority
Encourage acceptance of change and limitations.

Patient outcome criteria

• Within 2 days after surgery, family members will show beginning acceptance of the patient's appearance and give positive support.
• By the time of discharge, the patient will:
– show beginning acceptance of body changes and limitations
– verbalize a method for dealing with rejection.

Interventions

1. See the "Grieving" plan, page 44, and the "Ineffective individual coping" plan, page 67.

2. After surgery, demonstrate acceptance by looking directly at the patient when speaking and giving care.

3. Discuss and document family reactions to appearance changes and the level of acceptance the patient needs.

4. By the second postoperative day, help the patient to ambulate outside the room.

5. Prepare the patient for the wound's appearance, and discuss the healing process.

6. Prepare the patient for possible social rejection after discharge. Discuss and document feelings and responses.

7. Encourage prescribed exercises to strengthen the shoulder muscle.

8. Additional individualized interventions: _____

_____

Rationales

1. These plans contain interventions that are helpful in coping with potential body-image disturbance.

2. The patient can sense nonverbal communication. An initial positive response to the patient's changed appearance strengthens self-esteem.

3. Awareness of patient needs helps the family give adequate support.

4. Early ambulation outside the room encourages adjustment to changes.

5. Initial appearance is distorted until healing is complete. Preparing the patient in advance minimizes distress over the wound's appearance.

6. Acquaintances may have limited experience with facial surgery, and the patient should be prepared for their responses. Discussion of possible reactions may help minimize the painfulness of such encounters.

7. The muscle can be strengthened to offset shoulder drop.

8. Rationales: _____

_____

NURSING DIAGNOSIS

Family coping: Potential for growth related to successful management of situational crisis (prolonged treatment for head and neck cancer)

Nursing priority

Support the family.

Patient outcome criteria

By the time of discharge, family members will:
• state the plan for support after discharge
• demonstrate skills needed for home care—dietary management, wound care, and mouth care
• verbalize plans for required lifestyle modifications related to current or future treatments
• identify the most common complication and state the plan of action should this complication occur.

Interventions

1. Assess and document the family's reactions to and feelings about the patient's illness, care, and future needs. Allow the family time and space away from the patient to verbalize their feelings and concerns.

2. Discuss with the patient and family the dietary, activity, and lifestyle modifications needed as a result of surgery or any future treatment, such as radiation therapy or chemotherapy. Document the course of action the patient and family choose.

3. After surgery, encourage the patient and family to look at the graft site, if appropriate. Teach the patient and family skills needed after discharge, such as preparing a high-calorie, high-protein diet; enteral feeding; changing dressings (if a fistula develops); performing special mouth care, as ordered; and providing tracheostomy care and suctioning. Discuss signs and symptoms of possible complications and a plan of action should complications occur. If a tracheostomy is present, provide referral for home care follow-up.

4. Arrange for a person who has undergone similar surgery to visit, if the patient desires. Document the patient's and family's response to the visit.

5. Initiate and document referral to appropriate community resource groups, such as home health care, a cancer support group, a smoking-cessation group, or an alcoholism support group.

6. Additional individualized interventions: _____

Rationales

1. Verbalization facilitates the family's ability to identify strengths and plan for the patient's postoperative care.

2. Planning decreases anxiety surrounding discharge. Typically, the initial symptoms of head and neck cancer require changes in diet. Family members may have already made these changes and identified others; in this case, the family may simply need reassurance that plans are appropriate.

3. Instruction, demonstration, and practice of home care skills enable the patient and family to effectively meet needs after discharge. Familiarity with procedures increases self-care abilities and the confidence of both the patient and family. Explanation of potential problems and possible solutions relieves anxiety and encourages early assessment and prompt treatment of complications.

4. A peer can identify common problems and helpful solutions, and act as a positive role model, benefiting both the patient and family.

5. Support groups strengthen and expand the patient's and family's coping resources.

6. Rationales: _____

DISCHARGE PLANNING

Discharge checklist
Before discharge, the patient shows evidence of:
- ❏ stable vital signs
- ❏ absence of fever
- ❏ absence of life-threatening dysphagia
- ❏ absence of pulmonary and cardiovascular complications
- ❏ hemoglobin level and WBC count within normal parameters
- ❏ a healing wound with drainage amount within expected parameters and no evidence of bloody or purulent drainage
- ❏ completion of a diagnostic workup for evidence of cancer
- ❏ ability to tolerate adequate oral nutrition
- ❏ ability to perform wound care, dressing changes, and exercise program independently or with minimal assistance
- ❏ ability to perform ADLs and ambulate at usual level
- ❏ ability to control pain using oral medications
- ❏ adequate home support system or referral to home care if indicated by patient's inability to perform ADLs, ambulate, and care for wound as directed.

The following additional information should be documented if the patient has undergone a laryngectomy or a tracheotomy:
- ❏ ability to communicate adequately
- ❏ ability to perform tracheostomy care independently or with minimal assistance
- ❏ ability to perform emergency tracheostomy care if the entire tracheostomy apparatus dislodges
- ❏ automatic referral to home care or nursing home care if indicated by inadequate home support system and patient's inability to perform tracheostomy care.

Teaching checklist
Document evidence that the patient and family demonstrate an understanding of:
- [ ] extent of disease and surgery, and implications
- [ ] caloric requirements and dietary modifications
- [ ] wound care
- [ ] mouth care
- [ ] schedule for resuming activities and returning to work
- [ ] common changes in feelings after RND
- [ ] signs and symptoms of disease recurrence
- [ ] all discharge medications' purpose, dose, administration schedule, and adverse effects requiring medical attention (usual discharge medications include an analgesic and an antibiotic)
- [ ] date, time, and location of follow-up appointments
- [ ] how to contact the doctor
- [ ] need for smoking-cessation program or alcoholism rehabilitation, as needed
- [ ] community resources for speech rehabilitation, physical therapy, and support
- [ ] when and how to seek emergency medical care.

Documentation checklist
Using outcome criteria as a guide, document:
- [ ] clinical status on admission
- [ ] significant changes in status
- [ ] pertinent laboratory and diagnostic test findings
- [ ] pain-relief measures
- [ ] wound appearance and drainage
- [ ] mouth care and wound care
- [ ] nutritional intake
- [ ] patient and family teaching
- [ ] discharge planning.

ASSOCIATED PLANS OF CARE

Dying
Grieving
Ineffective family coping: Compromised
Ineffective individual coping
Knowledge deficit
Nutritional deficit
Pain
Skin grafts
Surgery

REFERENCES
Groenwald, S.L. *Cancer Nursing Principles and Practice,* 4th ed. Boston: Jones & Bartlett Pubs., Inc., 1997.
McCorkle, R., et al., eds. *Cancer Nursing: A Comprehensive Textbook,* 2nd ed. Philadelphia: W.B. Saunders Co., 1996.
Murphy, G.P., et al. *American Cancer Society Textbook of Clinical Oncology.* Atlanta: American Cancer Society, 1995.

Skin grafts

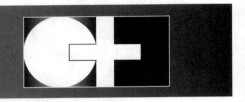

DRG information
DRG 263   Skin Grafts or Debridement for Skin Ulcer
           or Cellulitis with Complication or Comor-
           bidity (CC).
           Mean LOS = 13.9 days
DRG 264   Skin Grafts or Debridement for Skin Ulcer
           or Cellulitis without CC.
           Mean LOS = 8.3 days
DRG 439   Skin Grafts for Injuries.
           Mean LOS = 8.9 days

INTRODUCTION

Definition and time focus
Skin grafting is the process of covering damaged tissue,
such as burns or pressure ulcers, with healthy skin
transplants. The skin transplants may be autografts
from the patient's body, allografts or homografts from
another person, or heterografts from a different species
(such as porcine grafts). Grafts vary in thickness, depending on the extent of the wound, the availability of
donor sites, the mobility and vascularity of the area to
be covered, and the desired cosmetic results. The usual
types are:
• split-thickness grafts — epidermis and part of the dermis, varying from thin to thick, meshed or nonmeshed;
thinner grafts are used for large, hidden areas; thicker
grafts, large, visible areas
• full-thickness grafts — epidermis and dermis, used
for visible, mobile areas, such as the eyelids and hands
• flap grafts — autografts of skin and subcutaneous tissue where part of the flap is left attached to the donor
site; used for large areas with a poor blood supply
• allogenic or autologous cultured epithelial sheets —
healthy skin cell biopsies minced and cultured into thin
sheets over 3 to 4 weeks; sheets can cover large body
surface areas.
    This plan focuses on the patient with any large, open
skin wound who is admitted for preoperative wound
preparation and skin grafting with a split-thickness autograft.

Etiology and precipitating factors
• Burns of sufficient extent or depth to require grafting
for protection and healing
• Large pressure ulcers, particularly over bony, avascular areas, that can't heal effectively through normal ep-
ithelialization and granulation from the wound edges
inward

• Major trauma, such as avulsion of an extremity, that
may require grafting for protection and to preserve
function

FOCUSED ASSESSMENT GUIDELINES

Nursing history (functional health pattern findings)
Because skin grafts are performed for different reasons,
such as burns, pressure ulcers, and trauma, a typical
presenting picture doesn't exist. However, the nurse
must assess all patients undergoing skin grafting for
preoperative preparedness to ensure optimal outcomes;
therefore, this section presents preoperative assessment
guidelines instead.

Health perception–health management pattern
• Determine the purpose for grafting, including the
cause and extent of the injury; the grafting procedure;
expectations for successful graft adherence; and the potential for return of function as the basis for care, patient teaching, and discharge planning.
• Determine the patient's perceptions regarding potential disfigurement and its impact on health status and
lifestyle.

Nutritional-metabolic pattern
• Assess typical nutritional intake for adequate fluids,
calories, proteins, and vitamins.
• Assess nutritional status for signs of nutritional deficiency, such as weight loss and poor skin and hair condition, that may increase the risk of graft loss and infection.
• Assess for general conditions that may contribute to
poor healing, such as general debilitation, immobility,
age, prolonged bed rest, skin and circulatory problems,
and inability to perform activities of daily living (ADLs).
• Assess the graft site for the presence of healthy granulation tissue and the absence of necrotic areas, drainage,
and odor. Grafts will adhere only to healthy granulated
tissue.

Elimination pattern
• Assess for elimination problems, such as frequent
bowel and bladder incontinence, that may contribute to
skin breakdown and poor healing.

Activity-exercise pattern
• Assess normal activity and exercise habits to determine the patient's potential for adjusting to position and
activity limitations.
• Establish a baseline assessment of present musculoskeletal and neurologic functions for comparison to

potential postoperative changes in function and sensation.

Sleep-rest pattern
• Assess normal sleep patterns to guide postoperative management of pain and rest.

Cognitive-perceptual pattern
• Determine the patient's readiness for treatment by assessing understanding of the injury's extent, the prognosis for return of function, the surgical procedure, and rehabilitation phases during the hospital stay and home care.

Self-perception–self-concept pattern
• Assess the patient's usual self-perception–self-concept pattern to determine ability to adapt positively during the hospital stay and recovery at home.
• Assess the impact of body changes on the patient's feelings of self-worth.

Role-relationship pattern
• Assess the patient's concerns regarding the impact of current or potential disfigurement on relationships with family and others.
• Assess family members' and friends' ability to support the patient.

Sexuality-reproductive pattern
• Assess the patient's concerns regarding alterations in physical attractiveness, ability to feel sensations, and ability to perform sexually. (Note: Grafted tissue may have a decreased touch sensation.)

Coping–stress tolerance pattern
• Assess for anxiety, anger, and depression related to changes in body image and potentially permanent disfigurement. (Note: Regression is a common coping pattern for the patient with large wounds needing grafting.)

Value-belief pattern
• Assess the effect of cultural and value-belief systems on the patient's response to illness.

Physical findings
Cardiovascular
• Poor capillary refill

Neurologic
• Diminished sensation, including pain response, over wound
• Increased pain response around wound edges

Integumentary
• Fragile skin
• Poor skin turgor
• Ulcerated area (damage may extend to subcutaneous tissue, underlying fat, and muscle; tissue may be reddened, draining, and necrotic)
• Bleeding and clot formation from early excision of eschar and necrotic tissue

Musculoskeletal
• Limited mobility
• Limited range of motion (ROM)

Diagnostic studies
• Culture and sensitivity testing of wound drainage — may indicate infecting organism and help determine the most desirable antibiotic treatment
• White blood cell (WBC) count — may be elevated in presence of inflammation and infection
• Complete blood count — may show a low hematocrit, which may affect tissue healing
• Clotting time — may be prolonged, affecting tissue healing
• Serum protein (albumin and globulin) and fat (cholesterol and triglyceride) levels — may be depressed in poor nutritional status
• Postoperative tissue biopsy — may show infection or indicate degree of graft success
• Ultrasound — may determine size of wound, particularly if deep

Potential complications
• Nonadherence of graft
• Infection
• Contractures
• Hypertrophic scar formation at donor or recipient site

SKIN GRAFTS

Major nursing diagnoses and collaborative problems	Key patient outcomes
Risk for nonadherence of graft	Have a healing graft free from infection, swelling, and accumulation of blood or exudate.
Risk for infection of donor site	Exhibit a dry, infection-free donor site.
Impaired physical mobility	Perform activities of daily living, position changes, range-of-motion exercises, and other activities as allowed.
Body-image disturbance	Verbalize feelings about the wound and healing on request.
Nutritional deficit	Exhibit no signs or symptoms of inadequate nutritional intake.
Knowledge deficit (home care of donor and graft sites)	Describe appropriate graft and donor site appearance and care.

COLLABORATIVE PROBLEM

Risk for nonadherence of graft related to inadequate wound preparation

Nursing priority

Prepare the wound properly for grafting.

Patient outcome criteria

Within 2 days of admission, the patient will:
• exhibit signs of wound healing
• exhibit no redness over pressure points.

Interventions

1. Assess and document wound condition on admission and at least every shift. Indicate the wound's size, color, and depth and the presence or absence of odor, drainage, necrotic tissue, and swelling.

2. Change dressings every shift, as ordered, using good hand-washing and sterile technique. Use wet-to-dry dressings.

3. Clean the wound and surrounding skin with soap and water, as ordered, every shift. Apply topical agents such as povidone-iodine (Betadine), as ordered, according to recommended guidelines.

4. Irrigate the wound with sterile water every shift, as ordered.

5. Apply hydrophilic agents such as dextranomer (Debrisan) every shift, as ordered.

Rationales

1. Initial documentation provides baseline data concerning wound condition. Regular assessment and documentation provide data on the pattern of healing.

2. Conscientious attention to technique helps prevent infection. Wet-to-dry dressings aid healing by debriding the wound, keeping the tissue moist, and applying antiseptics.

3. Cleaning the skin prevents bacterial colonization and spread. Topical microbicidal agents such as povidone-iodine may help prevent infections.

4. Wound irrigation with large amounts of sterile water removes drainage, debriding agents, and contaminants.

5. Hydrophilic agents absorb drainage and aid in wound debridement.

6. Apply enzymes such as fibrinolysin and desoxyribonuclease (Elase) to the wound every shift, as ordered. Apply only to the wound, protecting healthy tissue with an ointment such as zinc oxide.

7. Assist the doctor, as needed, with surgical debridement of necrotic tissue.

8. Apply barrier dressings, if ordered, every 3 to 4 days or as needed for leakage.

9. Change the patient's position every 2 hours, protecting the affected area from pressure by using rubber rings, extra padding, or special positioning.

10. Additional individualized interventions: _____

_____

6. Enzymes soften necrotic tissue by fibrinolytic action, breaking up clots and exudates. Although enzymes act primarily on necrotic tissue, healthy tissue may be irritated unless protected.

7. Removal of necrotic tissue speeds healing and granulation tissue development.

8. Barrier dressings maintain a moist environment, which promotes granulation tissue formation.

9. Position changes promote circulation and prevent tissue damage from prolonged pressure.

10. Rationales: _____

_____

COLLABORATIVE PROBLEM

Risk for nonadherence of graft related to postoperative exudate or blood accumulation, movement, or infection

Nursing priorities

Maintain graft integrity and promote graft healing.

Patient outcome criteria

• Within 2 days after surgery, the patient will:
  – exhibit an intact graft
  – exhibit a graft free from injury
  – keep the dressing intact.
• Within 2 weeks after surgery, the patient will:
  – exhibit a graft free from infection, swelling, and exudate or blood accumulation
  – exhibit graft adherence and blood supply formation.

Interventions

1. Maintain movement restrictions for 3 days or as ordered. Use splints, restraints, pillows, or other devices to maintain the desired position. Teach patient about position and activity limitations.

2. Elevate the grafted area, if possible, for 1 week after surgery.

3. Continuously protect the graft from injury, using splints or bed cradles.

4. Assist the doctor during initial removal of inner dressings and graft inspection, usually 1 to 2 days after surgery. Document findings. Thereafter, carefully assess the graft every 8 hours and document its appearance. Report immediately any swelling, redness, and exudate or blood under the graft.

Rationales

1. Movement of the tissue under the graft may dislodge it. Adherence will be evident several days after surgery, although 2 to 3 weeks are needed for vascularization.

2. Elevation prevents swelling, which could cause graft separation.

3. Jarring or pressure may dislodge the graft.

4. Initial dressing removal must be done with utmost care to prevent separating the graft from the underlying tissue. Regular inspections allow prompt treatment of complications. Any substance, such as exudate or blood, coming between the graft and underlying tissue may cause separation. Swelling or redness may indicate infection, which can dislodge the graft. The doctor must carefully remove any drainage by aspiration or by rolling an applicator toward a nicked area.

5. Maintain dressings continuously, as ordered. Report unusual drainage or dislodged dressings.

5. Various dressings — including petroleum gauze, nonadhesive gauze, coarse mesh gauze, and moist saline-soaked gauze — are used to maintain gentle pressure on the graft. Drainage or dislodged dressings may prevent adherence.

6. Apply moist, warm compresses for 20 to 30 minutes four times daily, as ordered.

6. Warmth and moisture increase circulation and enhance epithelial tissue formation and blood supply to the graft.

7. Administer topical or systemic antibiotics, or both, as ordered.

7. Antibiotics may be used to prevent or treat graft infection.

8. Additional individualized interventions: _____

8. Rationales: _____

NURSING DIAGNOSIS

Risk for infection of donor site related to surgical excision of half of the skin layer

Nursing priority

Promote healing of the donor site.

Patient outcome criteria

- Within 2 days after surgery, the patient will exhibit a dry, infection-free donor site.
- Within 2 weeks after surgery, the patient will:
  – exhibit a reepithelialized donor site
  – exhibit soft and unscarred skin.

Interventions

1. Maintain dressings over the donor site for 1 to 2 days. Document your actions. Then replace the outer layers or remove them and leave the inner layer exposed, as ordered. Leave the inner dressing in place until it falls off spontaneously.

2. Promote drying by leaving the donor site exposed to air or by cautiously applying heat from a heat lamp or hair dryer for 15 to 30 minutes four times daily or as ordered.

3. Promote air circulation to the donor site by using a cradle to keep bedding and clothing away from the site.

4. If infection occurs, apply wet antiseptic dressings such as acetic acid four times daily, as ordered.

5. After healing (usually in 2 to 3 weeks), apply lotion to the site four times daily or as ordered.

6. Additional individualized interventions: _____

Rationales

1. Dressings are left over the site until serum dries. The inner dressing is either a nonadherent dressing or fine mesh gauze; it is left in place until it falls off (usually 2 to 3 weeks).

2. Drying, such as from evaporation or heat, enhances serum formation and helps prevent infection. (Note: Skin at the donor site is sensitive to excess heat.)

3. Air circulation aids drying and healing.

4. Antiseptic dressings decrease microorganism growth and aid healing.

5. Lotions keep the skin soft and help prevent scarring.

6. Rationales: _____

NURSING DIAGNOSIS

Impaired physical mobility related to position and movement limitations

Nursing priority

Promote maintenance of muscle tone and skin integrity.

Patient outcome criteria

Within 8 hours after surgery, the patient will:
- have no uncontrolled pain or discomfort
- exhibit an intact graft
- perform ADLs, position changes, ROM exercises, and other activities as allowed.

Interventions

1. Provide active and passive ROM exercises to unaffected areas every 2 hours, as ordered.

2. Promote self-care according to the patient's tolerance and the doctor's orders.

3. Apply splints and other devices, as ordered, either continuously or as needed during activities or ambulation.

4. Provide relief as needed for discomfort or pain. See the "Pain" plan, page 88.

5. Additional individualized interventions: _____

Rationales

1. ROM exercises promote muscle tone, circulation, and a feeling of well-being; they also help prevent contractures.

2. Self-care enhances feelings of independence and control over the course of recovery.

3. Protective devices allow some mobility while protecting the graft site.

4. The patient will experience pain from the graft and donor sites and discomfort from immobility. Relief from pain or discomfort encourages movement, as allowed, and aids healing by promoting a sense of well-being. The "Pain" plan contains general interventions for pain management.

5. Rationales: _____

NURSING DIAGNOSIS

Nutritional deficit related to increased metabolic needs secondary to tissue healing

Nursing priority

Provide adequate calories and protein to promote tissue healing.

Patient outcome criteria

Within 1 week after surgery, the patient will:
- exhibit no signs or symptoms of inadequate nutritional intake
- exhibit a healing wound.

Interventions

1. Assess and document nutritional status daily, including weight, wound healing, and condition of skin, hair, and mucous membranes. Note baseline serum total protein findings.

Rationales

1. Baseline and ongoing assessment data help guide dietary intake.

2. Provide a high-calorie, high-protein diet along with vitamin supplements. Document calorie intake and fluid intake and output daily.

3. Additional individualized interventions: _____

2. A diet high in calories, protein, and vitamins aids tissue healing. Maintaining fluid balance is necessary for supple skin.

3. Rationales: _____

NURSING DIAGNOSIS

Body-image disturbance related to wound and potential scarring

Nursing priority

Optimize adjustment to body changes.

Patient outcome criteria

Within 8 hours after surgery, the patient will:
• verbalize feelings about the wound and healing, on request
• express appropriate expectations regarding healing.

Interventions

1. Allow expression of fears and concerns related to wounds and scarring. Document patient concerns. Encourage continuity of discussion by all health team members on all shifts by documenting the patient's current psychological status on the plan of care.

2. Provide information about the expected stages of graft healing during nursing care and as needed.

3. Additional individualized interventions: _____

Rationales

1. Sharing concerns releases tension and opens discussion, which may lead to more realistic self-appraisal of body changes.

2. Knowing what to expect decreases fear of the unknown and allows the patient to participate in assessment of healing. Initially, the area will be reddened, swollen, and different in appearance from surrounding tissue. After 6 months, the area will be more normal in appearance as swelling decreases and color matches other tissue.

3. Rationales: _____

NURSING DIAGNOSIS

Knowledge deficit (home care of donor and graft sites) related to lack of exposure to information

Nursing priority

Provide information to optimize long-term healing of donor and graft sites.

Patient outcome criteria

By the time of discharge, the patient will:
• demonstrate ointment and dressing application
• describe specific activity and position limitations
• explain skin protection methods
• identify diet requirements
• describe appropriate graft and donor site appearance and care
• list two risk factors for poor healing
• list four signs of complications and what to do about them.

Interventions

1. See the "Knowledge deficit" plan, page 72.

2. Teach the patient and family the following care measures:
• Apply topical ointments, such as corticosteroids (as ordered) and skin softeners (lanolin and mineral oil), to the donor and graft sites.
• Maintain pressure and protective dressings as ordered.

• Avoid sun exposure by wearing protective clothing and using sunscreen lotions until the graft heals completely (usually in 6 to 12 months).
• Maintain activity and position limitations as ordered.
• Perform ROM exercises and maintain a positioning program, as ordered, until the tissue heals and matures in 6 to 12 months.
• Maintain a diet high in calories, protein, and vitamins.

• Avoid smoking. Attend a smoking-cessation program, if needed.
• Assess the donor and graft sites daily for healing progress and absence of such complications as redness or other discolorations, swelling, drainage, bad odor, pain, and excessive warmth. Promptly report signs of complications to the doctor.

3. Additional individualized interventions: _____
_____

Rationales

1. The "Knowledge deficit" plan contains general interventions related to patient teaching.

2. These measures provide the following benefits:

• Corticosteroids prevent inflammation, which can compromise circulation and healing. Grafted tissue may lack lubricating glands and may dry more readily.
• Pressure dressings inhibit excessive scar formation. Protective dressings may be necessary because new tissue is very sensitive and easily injured.
• New tissue lacks melanin-producing cells and is more susceptible to sunburn. Melanin-producing cells may regenerate in 6 to 12 months.
• Premature or excessive activity may dislodge the graft.
• ROM exercises and positioning extend the affected area and prevent contractures.

• Additional calories, protein, and vitamins are necessary for tissue healing because the stresses of an open wound, surgery, and hospitalization create a catabolic state.
• Smoking decreases blood flow and oxygen supply to peripheral tissues, thus inhibiting healing.
• Healing tissue should be warm, flat, only slightly more reddened than the surrounding tissue, and flexible, and it should have a capillary refill time of less than 3 seconds. Such signs and symptoms as redness, swelling, and pain may indicate an infection, which could prevent permanent graft adherence. Prompt reporting of complications allows early intervention and preservation of the graft.

3. Rationales: _____
_____

DISCHARGE PLANNING

Discharge checklist
Before discharge, the patient shows evidence of:
❏ healing and intact donor and graft sites with no evidence of abnormal drainage or swelling
❏ ability to control pain using oral medications
❏ stable vital signs
❏ absence of fever
❏ absence of pulmonary or cardiovascular complications
❏ hemoglobin level and WBC count within normal parameters
❏ ability to perform proper graft and donor-site care independently or with minimal assistance
❏ ability to tolerate adequate nutritional intake
❏ absence of hospital-acquired contractures
❏ ability to verbalize and demonstrate activity and position limitations

❏ absence of bowel and bladder dysfunction
❏ ability to perform ADLs, transfers, and ambulation at usual level with minimal assistance
❏ an adequate home support system or referral to home care or a nursing home if indicated by an inadequate home support system, inability to perform ADLs, or inability to care for graft and donor sites independently.

Additional information: The patient undergoing skin grafts for pressure ulcers is commonly disabled, not independently mobile, and dependent on others for care. Because of this, the patient is considered a "vulnerable adult." Any patient with pressure ulcers should automatically be referred to the social services department so that the ulcers' cause can be investigated. Most states have an automatic reporting mechanism for vulnerable adults, and nurses should be aware of this.

The patient with this diagnosis commonly lives in a nursing home, in which case the nursing home staff should be contacted to ascertain their ability to care for the patient during convalescence. Important questions to consider include: Does the nursing home have adequate staff to care for the patient? Does the nursing home have access to a special mattress or bed that promotes healing? What is the charge for such equipment? Where can the patient be discharged if the nursing home can't provide adequate care or supply needed equipment?

Under Medicare, the cost of special equipment — such as a Clinitron bed — is covered in an acute care setting but is not covered in a nursing home at the per diem rate. This creates a problem if the patient is discharged to a nursing home that can't supply the necessary equipment. Another issue to consider is whether the patient meets Medicare's criteria for extended care benefits. Many patients who undergo skin grafting are eligible for care in extended care facilities upon discharge. If the patient lives at home with a capable, willing caregiver, obtaining and paying for equipment and supplies must be addressed. All of these issues must be considered early in the hospital stay to prevent a delay in discharge. Although these are all nursing considerations, the social services department will probably address them, which is why a social services referral should be automatic.

Teaching checklist
Document evidence that the patient and family demonstrate an understanding of:
❏ care of the graft and donor sites
❏ signs and symptoms of complications
❏ activity and position limitations
❏ all discharge medications' purpose, dosage, administration schedule, and adverse effects requiring medical attention (usual discharge medications include topical ointments, such as corticosteroids and skin softeners (such as lanolin or mineral oil)
❏ recommended dietary modifications
❏ date, time, and location of follow-up appointments
❏ how to contact the doctor.

Documentation checklist
Using outcome criteria as a guide, document:
❏ clinical status on admission
❏ significant changes in status
❏ pertinent laboratory and diagnostic test findings
❏ wound condition (donor and graft sites)
❏ pain episodes
❏ pain-relief measures
❏ activity and position limitations
❏ resumption of ADLs
❏ nutritional intake

❏ psychological adjustment
❏ patient and family teaching
❏ discharge planning.

ASSOCIATED PLANS OF CARE
Grieving
Ineffective family coping: Compromised
Ineffective individual coping
Knowledge deficit
Pain
Surgery

REFERENCES
Hansbrough, W., et al. "Management of Skin-Grafted Burn Wounds with Xeroform and Layers of Dry Coarse Mesh Gauze Dressing Results in Excellent Graft Take and Minimal Nursing Time," *Journal of Burn Care & Rehabilitation* 16(5):531-34, September-October, 1995.

Hastings, B., et al. "Wound Coverage: Is There a Difference?" *Journal of Burn Care & Rehabilitation* 17(5):4116-20, September-October, 1996.

LeMone, P., and Burke, K.M. *Medical-Surgical Nursing: Critical Thinking in Client Care.* Menlo Park, Calif.: Addison-Wesley-Longman Publishing Co., 1996.

Lewis, S.M., et al. *Medical-Surgical Nursing: Assessment and Management of Clinical Problems.* St. Louis: Mosby–Year Book, Inc., 1996.

Rennekampff, H.O., et al. "Growth Peptide Release from Biologic Dressings: A Comparison," *Journal of Burn Care & Rehabilitation* 17(6, part 1):522-27, November-December 1996.

Roberts, S.L. *Critical Care Nursing: Assessment & Intervention.* Stamford, Conn.: Appleton & Lange, 1996.

Ruppert, S.D., et al. *Dolan's Critical Care Nursing: Clinical Management through the Nursing Process,* 2nd ed. Philadelphia: F.A. Davis Co., 1996.

Total joint replacement in a lower extremity

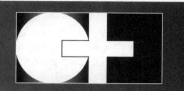

DRG information

DRG 209   Major Joint and Limb Reattachment Procedure.
          Mean LOS = 10.6 days
DRG 471   Bilateral or Multiple Major Joint Procedures of the Lower Extremity.
          Mean LOS = 14.2 days

Additional DRG information: These DRGs have been significant money losers because of the cost of surgical components and the rehabilitation time. Although the surgeon may inform the patient before surgery about transfer to a nursing home or extended care facility (ECF), most patients want to stay in the hospital until they feel ready to go home. Nurses can help prepare the patient for an early discharge and transfer.

INTRODUCTION

Definition and time focus

Total joint replacement involves the surgical implantation of a prosthesis, which replaces the damaged articulating surfaces of the joint. Joint damage may result from debilitating arthritis or from traumatic degenerative bone disease. In the lower extremity, total joint replacement entails removing the damaged tissues, including bone, synovium, and cartilage. An acrylic cement may be used to attach a metallic prosthesis, which replaces the femoral head or the femoral condyle, or a polyethylene prosthesis, which replaces the acetabulum or tibial plateau. Porous, coated metal implants have been developed that allow bone to grow into the joint area; this method may be used instead of the acrylic cement.

This plan focuses on preoperative and postoperative care of the patient admitted for total hip or knee replacement.

Etiology and precipitating factors

• Factors contributing to joint debilitation, including arthritis, infection, trauma, and obesity
• Causes of degenerative joint incongruity, including hormonal imbalance, instability related to dysplasia, calcium deficiency from menopause, and physiologic changes from aging
• Femoral head irregularities from Legg-Calvé-Perthes disease or avascular necrosis

FOCUSED ASSESSMENT GUIDELINES

Nursing history (functional health pattern findings)

Health perception–health management pattern
• Decreased motivation to carry out a previously prescribed rehabilitation program for an injured or painful joint
• History of misconceptions about care of injured or painful joint — for example, may report exercise during acute pain episodes or inappropriate use of mobility aids
• Accompanying problems, such as obesity, excessive involvement in sports, neurologic deficits, arthritis, or evidence of osteoporosis
• History of problems with or surgical procedures involving this or other joints
• Need for specific aids (such as a knee immobilizer) to prevent falls or further damage
• Short- or long-term use of prescribed corticosteroids

Nutritional-metabolic pattern
• Inadequate nutrient intake before admission, indicating poor tissue state for wound healing

Elimination pattern
• Constipation (related to decreased mobility)

Activity-exercise pattern
• Inability to ambulate, sit up, change position, move extremities, or get in and out of bed
• Inability to tolerate an exercise program because of unusual fatigue and weakness before or after exercise
• Some soreness over bony prominences
• History of unusual swelling around affected joint
• Decreased ability to perform activities of daily living (ADLs)
• Decreased leisure activity related to joint problems

Sleep-rest pattern
• Ineffective rest and sleep patterns, with frequent waking because of pain or stiffness
• Stiffness after sleep or periods of rest

Cognitive-perceptual pattern
• Pain, stiffness, or both, usually chronic and associated with movement or weight bearing
• Lack of knowledge about the specific joint condition, causes of the condition, aggravating factors, ways this procedure will change the condition, stages of recovery and rehabilitation, and personal responsibility during recovery and rehabilitation

• Displayed inability to recognize needs related to healing of affected joint, especially concerning nutrition needed for healing and limitations on ADLs and planned exercise

Role-relationship pattern
• Inadequate support system during planned rehabilitation program

Coping–stress tolerance pattern
• Concern about recovery of full function in affected joint

Physical findings
Physical findings vary, depending on the joint involved and the nature and extent of the injury or disease.

Cardiovascular
• Normal peripheral pulses in affected extremity

Neurologic
• Decreased bilateral patellar and Achilles reflexes

Musculoskeletal
• Pain on active or passive range-of-motion (ROM) exercise of affected joint
• Limited ROM or contracture of affected joint
• Varus, valgus, or flexion deformity of knees
• Decreased leg strength
• Shortening of affected limb
• Impaired gait
• Joint enlargement, inflammation, or tenderness
• Distorted posture from pain or effort to maintain balance
• Crepitation on movement

Integumentary
• Ischemic blanching or redness over bony prominences

Diagnostic studies
• Serum electrolytes — may show hypokalemia from corticosteroid use
• Fasting blood glucose — may show hyperglycemia from corticosteroid use
• Bilateral X-ray of hip or knee joints — demonstrates extent of degenerative changes
• Chest X-ray — may demonstrate presence of lung disease, indicating that the patient is a poor surgical risk during anesthesia and the first 3 to 5 postoperative days

Potential complications
• Hemorrhage
• Thrombophlebitis
• Infection (systemic, wound, or joint)
• Disarticulation of prosthesis
• Pulmonary embolus
• Atelectasis
• Pneumonia
• Neurovascular damage in the extremity
• Fat embolism
• Osteomyelitis

CLINICAL SNAPSHOT

TOTAL JOINT REPLACEMENT IN A LOWER EXTREMITY

Major nursing diagnoses and collaborative problems	Key patient outcomes
Risk for postoperative complications (hypovolemic shock, neurovascular damage, or thromboembolic phenomena)	Exhibit stable vital signs: typically, heart rate, 60 to 100 beats/minute; systolic blood pressure, 90 to 140 mm Hg; and diastolic blood pressure, 50 to 90 mm Hg.
Impaired physical mobility	Perform self-care activities independently and ambulate 50 feet with a walker and prescribed amount of weight bearing.
Impaired skin integrity	Exhibit clean wound healing with well-approximated edges.

COLLABORATIVE PROBLEM
Risk for postoperative complications (hypovolemic shock, neurovascular damage, or thromboembolic phenomena) related to surgical trauma, bleeding, edema, improper positioning, or immobility

Nursing priority
Prevent or promptly detect complications.

Patient outcome criteria

Within 2 hours after surgery and then continuously, the patient will exhibit stable vital signs: typically, heart rate, 60 to 100 beats/minute; systolic blood pressure, 90 to 140 mm Hg; and diastolic blood pressure, 50 to 90 mm Hg.

For hypovolemic shock
- Within 2 hours after surgery, the patient will:
  - exhibit drainage changing from frank bleeding to serosanguineous drainage.
- Within 1 day after surgery, the patient will:
  - exhibit drainage less than 300 ml/day
  - exhibit serosanguineous drainage.
- Within 2 days after surgery, the patient will exhibit drainage less than 100 ml/day.

For neurovascular damage
Throughout the hospital stay, the patient will:
- exhibit bilaterally equal pedal pulses and toe temperature
- exhibit capillary refill time less than 3 seconds
- have no foot numbness or tingling
- be able to move the toes spontaneously and dorsiflex the ankle.

For thromboembolic phenomena
- Within 3 days after surgery, the patient will exhibit no signs or symptoms of fat embolism:
  - be alert and oriented
  - experience no respiratory distress
  - exhibit no petechiae
  - have a partial pressure of arterial oxygen level of 80 to 100 mm Hg.
- Throughout the hospital stay, the patient will exhibit no signs or symptoms of thromboembolism. The patient will:
  - present bilaterally clear breath sounds
  - exhibit vital signs within normal limits
  - experience no calf pain on foot dorsiflexion (negative Homans' sign).

Interventions

1. For hypovolemic shock, implement these measures:
- See the "Surgery" plan, page 103, and the "Hypovolemic shock" plan, page 432.
- Maintain patency of the wound drainage device (such as a Hemovac). Assess, measure, and record the amount of drainage every 8 hours or as needed to maintain continuous suction. Monitor the amount of bleeding, and report unusual increases. Monitor results of hematocrit studies.

Rationales

1. Usual postoperative factors and the unique nature of joint replacement place the patient at risk for hypovolemic shock.
- The "Surgery" and "Hypovolemic shock" plans contain general interventions related to postoperative shock. This plan presents information pertinent to the patient undergoing hip or knee replacement.
- The hip area is highly vascular. Also, the patient may be taking an anticoagulant to prevent thromboembolism. Initial drainage may be frankly bloody but should become serosanguineous within a few hours. A typical amount is 200 to 300 ml in the first 24 hours after surgery, decreasing to less than 100 ml within 48 hours. The drainage device usually is removed by the second postoperative day.

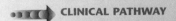

Managing joint replacement (elective)

DRG: 209
Estimated LOS: 4 days

Plan	Before surgery	Day 1	Day 2
Laboratory studies	• Complete blood count (CBC) • Labwork, chest X-ray, ECG as indicated per anesthesia protocol requirements		• PT/INR, if on warfarin • Chem 7 profile • CBC
Tests		• Vital signs, neurologic and circulatory checks per policy • Pain scale q 2 h while awake	• Vital signs q shift, if stable • Check pain scale q 2 h while awake
Consults	• Medical co-management, if ordered	• Physical therapy • Occupational therapy • Respiratory care • Pharmacist consult for warfarin teaching • Case management social work • Medical co-management, if ordered	• Diet consult if < 80% ideal body weight or >120% ideal body weight (Use HAMWI formula: 106 lb for 5 ft plus 6 lb for q in;100 lb for 5 ft plus 5 lb for q in) • ET nurse regarding skin care
Medication/ I.V.	• Bring all medications to hospital	• PCA • Epidural • Pain controlled (< 4 on pain scale) • Enoxaparin • Warfarin • Home medications • Nausea controlled with antiemetics	• Maintenance I.V. – PCA/Epidural • Pain controlled (< 4 on pain scale) • Enoxaparin • Warfarin
Treatments	• SCDs	• Drain • THR: abductor pillow • Granulex/ET mix • Spenco boots	• Drain • Nurse to check heels, sacrum, and elbows every shift
Nutrition	• Nothing by mouth after midnight	• Tolerating diet without N/V	• Diet consistent with diagnosis and condition
Elimination		• Indwelling urinary catheter • u.l. >60 ml/2°×16 hr • Voiding without difficulty	• D/C indwelling urinary catheter in a.m. or when D/C epidural and patient is out of bed
Activity		• Hips: reposition q 2 h to unoperative side with abductor pillow between legs • Knee: immobilizer if ordered • Knee: CPM if ordered	• Exercise program per rehabilitation • Activity wall chart posted • Dangle • THR: transfer to chair, if tolerated • TKR: transfer to chair, if tolerated

Patient teaching	• Pain management
	• 0-10 pain scale
	• Cough and deep breathe
	• Incentive spirometry
		• Pre-admission: video, class, tour
		• Exercise sheets
		• Hip or knee folder during class
		• Pain management (0-10 pain scale)
		• PCA, if receiving PCA
		• Incentive spirometry
			• Joint precautions
			• Demonstrate adaptive equipment Review:
			  – Incentive spirometry
			  – Pain management
			  – PCA review if indicated

Discharge planning	• High risk cases referred to case management via doctor's office	• Interdisciplinary consultation with case management if high risk case	• Interdisciplinary consultation with case management if high risk case

Day 3	Day 4	Outcome goals met
• PT/INR, if on warfarin	• PT/INR, if on warfarin • CBC • If discharged on warfarin, F/U PT/INR planned	• Lab results normal • PT/INR therapeutic, if on warfarin
• Check pain scale q 2 h while awake • Rehab performs functional independence measure (FIM) scores		• Temp <101° F (38.3° C)
• D/C PCA/epidural • Pain controlled (<4 on pain scale) by P.O. analgesics • D/C I.V. • Saline well • Warfarin • Enoxaparin	• Warfarin dose before discharge • Enoxaparin, continue for __ days	• Adequate pain control and anticoagulation
• Drain D/C • Nurse to check heels, sacrum, and elbows q shift • No skin breakdown	• D/C SCDs when fully ambulatory • 1st dsg change per doctor within 72h • Independent with wound care • Nurse to check heels, sacrum, and elbows q shift	• Wounds without infection • No skin breakdown
• Diet consistent with diagnosis and condition	• Diet consistent with Dx and condition	• Tolerating food
• If no bowel movement, give laxative	• Last BM date:	• Normal elimination
• Initiate gait training • Progressive exercise • Occupational therapy instruction on use of adaptive equipment and home recommendations • Up in chair for meals/t.i.d.: breakfast, lunch, dinner, other	• Transfers to commode, bed, chair with standby assist • Ind. with exercise program • Bathing, dressing, tub w/SBA • Transfer with assistive device • Functional gait • Ind. with usage/knowledge of adaptive equipment	• >70° flexion (knee) • Independent ADLs, transfer, functional gait with equipment • Independent with home exercises • Demonstrates safety precautions

• Pharmacist to teach about: warfarin
• Nursing to instruct on:
  – S.C. injection of enoxaparin, if ordered
  – Rehabilitation to dispense hip/knee booklet
	• Drug/nutrient interaction sheet (if applicable)
	• Incision care
	• Anticoagulant therapy
	• Medications
	• Patient/family provide wound care with supervision
	• Home care precautions with pain medications
	• Car transfers
		• Patient and family verbalize:
		  – signs and symptoms of complications
		  – name, dose, adverse effects, purpose, schedule, food/drug interactions of medications
		  – wound care

• Case management assessment and planning for discharge needs	• Appropriate follow-up scheduled • Durable medical equipment needs met • Interventions on home health, outpatient therapy, rehabilitation unit or ECF	• Discharge disposition/plan is appropriate and meets patient's needs • Discharge information completed: discharge date, length of stay

2. For neurovascular damage, implement these measures:

• Perform neurovascular checks every hour for the first 4 hours after the patient's return from surgery, then every 2 hours for 12 hours, and then every 4 hours until ambulatory. Assess pedal pulses, capillary refill time, toe temperature, skin color, foot sensation, and ability to move the toes and dorsiflex the ankle. Compare findings to the other extremity as well as to earlier findings. Once the patient is ambulatory, reassess at least daily.
• Notify the doctor immediately if pedal pulses are absent or unequal bilaterally; if capillary refill time is greater than 3 seconds; if the patient has cold toes, pale skin, foot numbness, tingling, or pain; or if the patient cannot move the toes.
• Maintain positioning as recommended. See the "Impaired physical mobility" nursing diagnosis in this plan for further details.
• Apply ice packs to the affected joint for 24 to 48 hours after surgery, if ordered.
• Maintain patency of the drainage device as previously described.

3. For thromboembolic phenomena, implement these measures:

• Instruct and coach preoperative exercises for calves, quadriceps, gluteals, and ankles. After surgery, supervise performance of exercises 5 to 10 times hourly while the patient is awake.
• Monitor for signs of thromboembolism, assessing daily for calf pain, a positive Homans' sign, redness, and swelling. See the "Surgery" plan, page 103, and the "Thrombophlebitis" plan, page 468, for details.

• Apply elastic stockings to both legs (to the affected extremity only after the dressing is removed). Remove daily for 1 hour every 8 hours. Check the skin for signs of pressure. Use pneumatic compression devices as ordered.
• Monitor for signs of fat embolism daily. Immediately report sudden onset of dyspnea, tachycardia, pallor or cyanosis, or pleuritic pain. See the "Surgery" plan for details.
• Administer prophylactic anticoagulants (aspirin, heparin, or warfarin [Coumadin]), as ordered. Monitor clotting studies and report findings outside the recommended therapeutic range. Observe for (and advise the patient and family to report) melena, petechiae, epistaxis, hematuria, ecchymoses, or other unusual bleeding.

4. Additional individualized interventions: _____

_____

2. Altered neurovascular status may be associated with trauma to the nerves or blood vessels as a result of surgery, joint dislocation, edema, improper positioning, or excessive tightness of abduction pillow straps.
• Early detection of neurovascular damage facilitates prompt intervention to correct the underlying cause and minimize the chance of permanent damage.

• Early medical intervention can prevent permanent damage in the affected extremity.

• Proper positioning is critical to prevent prosthesis dislocation, which can trap and irreparably damage nerves or blood vessels.
• Ice packs promote vasoconstriction, thereby decreasing inflammation, edema, and bleeding.
• Drainage must be maintained because fluid accumulation could exert pressure on nearby nerves and vessels.

3. The patient undergoing total joint replacement is at particular risk for thrombophlebitis, embolism, and fat embolism because of immobility-induced venous stasis and possible surgical trauma to veins.
• Practice before surgery enhances the patient's ability to perform exercises later. These exercises are designed to promote venous return, minimizing the risk of thromboembolic phenomena.
• Calf pain, redness, or swelling may indicate thrombus formation. The "Surgery" plan contains general interventions related to various thrombotic and embolic phenomena. The "Thrombophlebitis" plan provides additional details on assessing for this complication.
• Elastic support stockings and pneumatic compression devices may promote venous return by redirecting flow from superficial veins to deeper veins.

• The patient undergoing total joint replacement is at particular risk for fat embolism because of bone marrow release from surgical disruption of flat (pelvic) or long bones.
• Prophylactic anticoagulants may reduce the risk of thrombophlebitis or thromboembolism. However, the patient must be monitored carefully because anticoagulant use may cause uncontrolled bleeding.

4. Rationales: _____

_____

NURSING DIAGNOSIS

Impaired physical mobility related to hip or knee surgery

Nursing priorities

- Maintain proper alignment of the affected extremity to prevent dislocation of the prosthesis.
- Increase mobility in the extremity through implementation of the rehabilitation plan.
- Educate the patient concerning rehabilitation needs.

Patient outcome criteria

- By the time of discharge, the patient will:
  – maintain mobility of unaffected joints equal to or greater than preoperative level
  – perform self-care activities independently
  – verbalize an understanding of the rehabilitation plan.
- By the time of discharge, the patient with a hip replacement will:
  – ambulate 50 feet with a walker and partial weight bearing on the affected side, as tolerated
  – observe ROM restrictions — flexion of the affected joint limited to 90 degrees during the rehabilitation phase.
- By the time of discharge, the patient with a knee replacement will:
  – ambulate with an assistive device and light weight bearing, as tolerated
  – flex the knee up to 90 degrees of flexion
  – not extend the knee (0-degree extension).

Interventions

1. Before surgery, instruct the patient about the correct postoperative positioning of the affected extremity:
• hip — maintain flexion of the hip joint at a 45-degree angle or less. Don't rotate the hip joint externally. Don't adduct the hip joint (don't cross the legs).
• knee — do not flex or hyperextend the leg. Maintain the leg slightly elevated from the hip, using a pillow or continuous passive motion machine as ordered, typically for 48 to 72 hours.

2. Before surgery, teach the patient how to use the appropriate walking device (walker or crutches). Provide practice with the device, if possible.

3. After surgery, maintain the patient on bed rest as ordered, usually for 12 to 24 hours. Place the affected joint in the prescribed position (usually in the neutral position), using rolls, splints, pillows, or abduction pillows, as ordered and appropriate. Observe position and activity precautions, as noted above.

4. At least every 8 hours, observe for shortening of the extremity, a sudden increase in pain, a bulge over the femoral head on the affected side (in hip replacement), and decreased neurovascular status of the affected extremity. Report any such findings to the doctor immediately.

5. Supervise position changes at least every 2 hours. Have the patient use a trapeze and either shift weight in bed or turn to the unaffected side. Assist only as necessary.

Rationales

1. Preoperative teaching provides information that helps the patient maintain proper positioning of the joint after surgery. The positions described help prevent prosthesis dislocation.

2. Preoperative instruction and practice, if possible, allow the patient to feel more secure when using the device.

3. The affected joint must be stabilized to prevent dislocation. Excessive flexion, internal rotation, or adduction will cause postoperative hip dislocation. Knee elevation helps reduce swelling and pain.

4. These signs indicate prosthesis dislocation, a common occurrence in hip replacement that requires immediate attention.

5. Self-propelled movement helps the patient maintain muscle tone and reduces the risk of skin breakdown.

6. Implement a planned and progressive daily ambulation schedule, as ordered, 1 to 3 days after surgery. Use either crutches or a walker to allow weight bearing as recommended. Coordinate this activity with the physical therapy program.

7. Ensure that unaffected joints are put through at least ten repetitions of full ROM exercises, three to four times daily.

8. Help the patient maintain preferred rest and sleep routines. Use back rubs, other skin care measures, positioning, and ordered medications, as necessary.

9. Collaborate with the health care team to design an appropriate rehabilitation plan that includes:
• muscle-strengthening activities until maximum potential strength is reached
• increasing ROM of the affected joint until full ROM is attained
• return to occupational and leisure activities.

10. Identify, with the patient, the specific methods that will be used to implement the plan.

11. Additional individualized interventions: _____

6. Progressive daily ambulation promotes the patient's return to increased physical activity and self-care.

7. ROM exercises of unaffected joints must be maintained during periods of decreased activity. Arthritic joints lose function more rapidly when activity is restricted.

8. Uninterrupted periods of full relaxation and deep sleep help maintain the energy needed for remobilization of the affected joint.

9. An effective rehabilitation plan requires input from the doctor, physical therapist, occupational therapist, and professionals from other appropriate disciplines to maximize the patient's rehabilitation potential.

10. For a rehabilitation program to be successful, the patient must agree to the plan and be able to describe its implementation.

11. Rationales: _____

Nursing diagnosis

Impaired skin integrity related to surgery

Nursing priorities
• Promote wound healing.
• Prevent infection.

Patient outcome criteria

By the time of discharge, the patient will:
• exhibit clean wound healing with well-approximated edges
• be afebrile
• exhibit warm and dry skin
• exhibit no bleeding
• exhibit no signs or symptoms of infection
• list signs and symptoms to report.

Interventions

1. Maintain the patency of the drainage device, as previously described. Avoid contaminating the drainage port when emptying the device.

2. Don't administer injections in the affected extremity. Teach the patient to take precautions to minimize the risk of injury.

Rationales

1. Adequate suction with a self-controlled vacuum must be maintained to prevent blood collection in the joint — an excellent medium for bacterial growth. Contamination of the device may lead to wound infection.

2. Any break in the skin may predispose the patient to infection.

3. Assess daily for signs and symptoms of infection: fever, chills, purulent drainage, incisional swelling, redness, and increasing tenderness. Teach the patient which signs and symptoms to report.

4. Additional individualized interventions: _____
_____

3. Infection is devastating to a patient with total joint replacement because the joint cannot be saved once infection and prosthetic loss occur.

4. Rationales: _____
_____

DISCHARGE PLANNING

Discharge checklist
Before discharge, the patient shows evidence of:
❏ absence of fever
❏ vital signs within acceptable limits
❏ absence of signs and symptoms of infection at the incision
❏ absence of contractures or skin breakdown
❏ administration of oral anticoagulant medication for at least the previous 48 to 72 hours and activated partial thromboplastin time within acceptable parameters
❏ ability to control pain using oral medications
❏ absence of bowel or bladder dysfunction
❏ absence of pulmonary or cardiovascular complications
❏ ability to perform ADLs independently or with minimal assistance
❏ adherence to hip flexion and adduction restrictions when transferring and ambulating
❏ adherence to weight-bearing restrictions when transferring or ambulating
❏ ability to transfer and ambulate independently or with minimal assistance, using appropriate assistive devices
❏ ability to tolerate adequate nutritional intake
❏ absence of signs and symptoms of prosthesis dislocation
❏ adequate home support system or referral to home care or nursing home if indicated by an inadequate home support system; inability to perform ADLs, transfers, and ambulation independently; or inability to adhere to flexion or weight-bearing restrictions
❏ demonstration of maximum hospital rehabilitation benefit.

One of the peer review organization criteria used when reviewing total joint replacement is whether the patient received maximum hospital benefit. The major criteria are whether the patient had a physical therapy evaluation and whether discharge planning was appropriate. The discharge would be deemed premature if a rehabilitation program had not been designed and if the patient showed evidence of medical instability.

Discharge planning for a patient who undergoes total hip or knee replacement should include automatic referral to the social services department. Most patients cannot function at their usual level after this procedure, especially if it's bilateral. Documentation should indicate plans for long-term rehabilitation. The nurse isn't necessarily responsible for this documentation; the physical therapist, occupational therapist, or discharge planner–social worker may provide it.

After discharge, many patients are eligible for care in a nursing home or ECF until they can ambulate 50′ to 80′ (15 to 24 m) independently or with minimal assistance. Because the discharge plan commonly includes early discharge with transfer to an ECF, timely referral to the social services department is essential to allow adequate time to find an opening at an appropriate facility.

Teaching checklist
Document evidence that the patient and family demonstrate an understanding of:
❏ implications of joint replacement
❏ rationale for continued use of antiembolism stockings
❏ all discharge medications' purpose, dosage, administration schedule, and adverse effects requiring medical attention (discharge medications typically include analgesics, antibiotics, anti-inflammatories, and anticoagulants)
❏ need for laboratory and medical follow-up if discharged on warfarin
❏ schedule for progressive ambulation and weight bearing
❏ additional activity restrictions
❏ signs and symptoms of infection, bleeding, and dislocation
❏ use of self-help devices, such as a raised toilet seat
❏ appropriate resources for posthospitalization care
❏ diet to promote healing
❏ wound care
❏ date, time, and location of follow-up appointments
❏ how to contact the doctor
❏ need for antibiotic prophylaxis prior to dental and GI or genitourinary procedures

Documentation checklist

Using outcome criteria as a guide, document:
- [ ] clinical status on admission
- [ ] significant changes in status
- [ ] preoperative and postoperative teaching
- [ ] position of affected extremity
- [ ] exercises and ROM achieved
- [ ] neurovascular checks
- [ ] calf pain
- [ ] wound drainage
- [ ] progressive ambulation
- [ ] pain-relief measures
- [ ] presence or absence of disabling fatigue
- [ ] nutritional intake
- [ ] patient and family teaching
- [ ] discharge planning and referrals.

ASSOCIATED PLANS OF CARE

Ineffective individual coping
Knowledge deficit
Pain
Surgery

REFERENCES

Black, J.M., and Matassarin-Jacobs, E. *Medical-Surgical Nursing: Clinical Management for Continuity of Care*, 5th ed. Philadelphia: W.B. Saunders Co., 1997.

Callaghan, J.J. "Total Hip Arthroplasty: Clinical Perspectives," *Clinical Orthopedics and Related Research* 276:33-40, March 1992.

Crutchfield, J., et al. "Preoperative Pain in Total Knee Replacement Patients," *Orthopaedic Nurse* 19 (supplement):6-8, August 1996.

Lewis, S.M., and Collier, I.C. *Medical-Surgical Nursing: Assessment and Management of Clinical Problems*, 4th ed. New York: McGraw-Hill Book Co., 1996.

Maher, A.B., et al. *Orthopedic Nursing.* Philadelphia: W.B. Saunders Co., 1998.

Monahan, F., and Neighbors, M. *Medical-Surgical Nursing: Foundations for Clinical Practice.* Philadelphia: W.B. Saunders Co., 1998.

Moskowitz, R.W., et al. *Osteoarthritis: Diagnosis and Medical-Surgical Management,* 2nd ed. Philadelphia: W.B. Saunders Co., 1992.

Quinat, R.J., and Winters, E.G. "Total Joint Replacement of the Hip and Knee," *Medical Clinics of North America* 76:1235, September 1992.

Ranawat C.S., et al. "Long-term Results of the Total Knee Arthroplasty: A 15-Year Survivorship Study," *Clinical Orthopedics and Related Research,* January 1993.

Part 10

Endocrine disorders

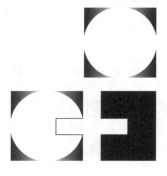

Diabetes mellitus

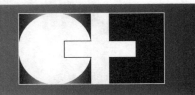

DRG information

DRG 294   Diabetes; Age 35+.
               Mean LOS = 5.7 days
DRG 295   Diabetes; Ages 0 to 35.
               Mean LOS = 4.3 days
               Principal diagnoses for DRGs 294 and 295
               include:

- diabetes mellitus (DM) without complication
- DM with coma
- DM with ketoacidosis
- DM with other manifestations
- DM with unspecified complications
- glycosuria.

INTRODUCTION

Definition and time focus

DM is a chronic metabolic disorder in which an absolute or relative lack of endogenous insulin causes abnormal metabolism of carbohydrates, proteins, and fats. The clinical hallmark of diabetes is hyperglycemia. Altered glucose metabolism provokes a pattern of associated acute and chronic complications. This plan focuses on the two most common types of diabetes, type 1 (insulin-dependent DM) and type 2 (non-insulin-dependent DM), their diagnosis, and initiation of a treatment and management regimen.

Note: Although type 2 is commonly called non-insulin-dependent DM, these patients may require insulin as part of their management plan, either initially or later in the course of the disease.

Etiology and precipitating factors

Type 1 (10% of cases): primary defect is inadequate or absent insulin production secondary to autoimmune destruction of beta (insulin-producing) cells in the pancreas by islet-cell antibodies and insulin antibodies
- genetic predisposition, probably related to genes of human leukocyte antigen affecting immune system
- viral infections

    Type 2 (approximately 90% of cases): primary defect is insulin resistance by skeletal muscle, fat, and liver receptors for insulin; hyperglycemia leads to increased insulin production and eventual beta cell secretory exhaustion
- strong genetic predisposition, not yet as clearly defined as in type 1
- obesity (in 80% to 90% of patients at diagnosis)
- sedentary lifestyle

- possibly other environmental factors
- higher incidence in Native Americans and blacks than in whites

FOCUSED ASSESSMENT GUIDELINES

Nursing history (functional health pattern findings)

Type 1 DM is commonly diagnosed when the patient presents in diabetic ketoacidosis (DKA); type 2 is commonly diagnosed on routine examination or when the patient seeks treatment for one of the many associated symptoms. Many medications may be associated with impaired glucose tolerance, including steroids, some diuretics, oral contraceptives, anticonvulsants, and psychoactive medications. The doctor who suspects diabetes should ensure that medication-related factors are identified and ruled out before making the diagnosis.

Health perception–health management pattern
Type 1
- Family history of diabetes
- Patient usually under age 30
- Acute onset of symptoms (flulike syndrome)

Type 2
- Family history of diabetes
- Patient usually over age 40
- Gradual onset of symptoms
- Patient may report multiple minor symptoms

Nutritional-metabolic pattern
Type 1
- Increased thirst (polydipsia)
- Increased appetite (polyphagia)
- Weight loss
- Ketosis
- Nausea (occasionally)

Type 2
- Polydipsia and polyphagia
- History of diet high in refined carbohydrates and calories
- Usually overweight (possibly recent weight gain)

Elimination pattern
Type 1
- Polyuria
- Constipation or diarrhea

Type 2
- Nocturia
- Polyuria
- Constipation or diarrhea
- Diuretics taken for another condition

Activity-exercise pattern
Type 1
• Sudden weakness
• Increased fatigue or sleepiness
Type 2
• Gradually increasing weakness and fatigability
• History of lack of regular exercise

Sleep-rest pattern
Type 1
• Sleep disturbance related to nocturia
Type 2
• Nocturia
• Drowsiness after meals

Cognitive-perceptual pattern
Type 1
• Dizziness or orthostatic hypotension
• Abdominal pain
Type 2
• Pruritus, acute or recurrent urinary tract infections (UTIs), recurrent vaginitis, or vaginal infection
• Poorly healing skin infections
• Myopia or blurred vision
• Muscle cramping
• Abdominal pain
• Numbness, pain, or tingling in extremities
• Irritability

Physical findings
Cardiovascular
• Tachycardia
• Postural hypotension
• Cool extremities and decreased pulses

Pulmonary
• Deep, rapid (Kussmaul's), respirations; fruity breath odor (in DKA)

Gastrointestinal
• Abdominal distention
• Decreased bowel sounds
• Abdominal tenderness

Integumentary
• Poorly healing skin wounds, especially on feet
• Skin infections
• Warm, flushed, dry skin (in DKA)

Neurologic
• Drowsiness
• Confusion
• Coma (in DKA)
• Altered reflexes

Genitourinary
• Vaginal discharge
• Perineal irritation
• Impotence or decreased libido

Diagnostic studies
• Random serum glucose test — a level greater than or equal to 200 mg/dl plus classic signs and symptoms confirms DM
• Fasting serum glucose test — elevation greater than or equal to 126 mg/dl
• Urinalysis — reveals glycosuria and (in type 1) ketonuria
• Glucose tolerance test — confirms DM if levels are greater than or equal to 200 mg/dl in the 2-hour sample. This test should be performed after a glucose load dose of 75 g anhydrous glucose.
• Blood insulin level — type 1, absent or minimal; type 2, low, normal, or high
• Glycosylated hemoglobin — evaluates overall glucose control over previous 120 days (life of red blood cell) by detecting elevations or wide fluctuations in blood glucose over time; 2% or more above normal laboratory values indicates poor glucose control in either type 1 or type 2
• Arterial blood gas levels — may reveal metabolic acidosis, particularly common in type 1, with compensatory respiratory alkalosis
• Electrolyte panel — may be normal or may reveal hyponatremia or hyperkalemia associated with dehydration or DKA (type 1); needed to establish baseline
• Blood urea nitrogen (BUN) and creatinine levels — BUN may be normal or elevated in DKA or hyperosmolar hyperglycemic nonketotic syndrome (HHNS); both may be normal or elevated in presence of renal involvement; needed to establish baseline
• Thyroid function studies — may be ordered to rule out coexisting thyroid dysfunction, which could increase need for insulin and contribute to hyperglycemia (thyroid disorders more common in type 1)
• Electrocardiography — commonly ordered to establish baseline and to rule out underlying cardiac disorders
• Lipid profile — needed to establish baseline

Potential complications
• Coma related to DKA, hypoglycemia, or HHNS
• Renal failure (nephropathy)
• Conditions related to degenerative vascular disease: accelerated atherosclerosis, cerebrovascular accident, myocardial infarction, thrombophlebitis, peripheral vascular disease
• Retinopathy, blindness, or cataracts
• Neuropathies, autonomic and especially peripheral
• Microangiopathies

DIABETES MELLITUS

Major nursing diagnoses and collaborative problems	Key patient outcomes
Hyperglycemia	Maintain blood glucose levels between 70 and 110 mg/dl.
Knowledge deficit (self-care)	Discuss disease management in relation to medication, diet, exercise, and stress.
Risk for altered health maintenance	Have resource deficits resolved or appropriate referrals completed.

COLLABORATIVE PROBLEM

Hyperglycemia related to inadequate endogenous insulin (type 1 DM) or inadequate endogenous insulin and insulin resistance (type 2 DM)

Nursing priority

Prevent or minimize complications when establishing treatment regimen to control altered glucose metabolism.

Patient outcome criteria

- Within 2 hours of admission, the patient will:
  – have an improved blood glucose level
  – be awake and alert
  – maintain vital signs within normal limits: typically, heart rate, 60 to 100 beats/minute; systolic blood pressure, 90 to 140 mm Hg; and diastolic blood pressure, 50 to 90 mm Hg.
- Within 24 to 48 hours of admission, the patient will:
  – show no signs of dehydration
  – maintain blood glucose levels between 70 and 110 mg/dl
  – have no hypoglycemia, or have promptly treated hypoglycemic episodes with no associated complications.

Interventions

1. Administer insulin (I.V., I.M., or subcutaneously [S.C.]) or oral hypoglycemics.

• Monitor fingerstick blood glucose levels according to unit protocol, typically every 6 hours or before meals and at bedtime. Always check the blood glucose level before giving hypoglycemic medications. Follow established protocol for withholding the dose based on normal values.

• Be aware of differences in peak action and duration of action for various hypoglycemic medications:

– Rapid-acting insulins (Regular, Semilente) peak between 2 and 4 hours; intermediate-acting insulins (NPH, Lente) peak between 6 and 12 hours; and long-acting insulins (Ultralente, PZI) peak between 10 and 30 hours.

– Oral hypoglycemics peak on the average between 3 and 4 hours.

2. Establish and maintain an I.V. fluid infusion (usually normal saline solution), as ordered. Monitor for dry mucous membranes, poor skin turgor, cracked lips, abdominal pain, elevated urine specific gravity, elevated hematocrit, and other signs or symptoms of dehydration. Keep an accurate intake and output record. Document daily weight.

Rationales

1. Insulin increases cellular glucose uptake and decreases gluconeogenesis. Exogenous insulin is essential for controlling type 1 DM and may also be used in type 2 DM. In initial treatment of type 1 or 2, especially if DKA is present, I.V. infusion of regular insulin may be ordered concurrently with aggressive fluid replacement. The I.V. route is preferred because it offers the fastest absorption rate, but too-rapid lowering of blood glucose without adequate fluid replacement may cause vascular collapse or cerebral edema. Alternatively, the slower-acting I.M. route may be used. Circulatory insufficiency can make insulin uptake from S.C. sites unpredictable; however, it is the route of choice for ongoing therapy. Oral hypoglycemics are indicated only in type 2 DM because their effectiveness depends on endogenous insulin. Two types of oral hypoglycemics exist: Sulfonylureas (such as glipizide [Glucotrol] and glyburide [Micronase]) stimulate beta cells to secrete insulin; the newer biguanide drug metformin increases glucose use in peripheral tissue and can be used alone or in conjunction with other oral agents or insulin.

• In the initial diagnosis and treatment of DM, frequent assessment of glucose levels is essential for monitoring the patient's response. Checking the glucose level and withholding the dose if the level is acceptable prevents medication-induced hypoglycemia. Protocols for withholding doses vary depending on the hypoglycemic ordered and patient status.

• Awareness of these characteristics helps the nurse correlate onset and duration of signs and symptoms with peaks and troughs in serum drug levels.

– Insulins differ according to onset, peak, and duration of action. The type of insulin, timing of injections, and individual response influence when a reaction is most likely to occur. With insulins given in the morning, a reaction from a short-acting insulin is most likely between breakfast and lunch; an intermediate-acting insulin, between midafternoon and dinner; and a long-acting insulin, between 2 a.m. and 7 a.m.

– Because duration of action is more prolonged with oral agents, a single daily or divided dose is usually sufficient for control. Reactions are most likely to coincide with peak action.

2. Hyperglycemia causes dehydration through hyperosmolality. Water is drawn from the cells into the vascular system and then into the urine in an attempt to maintain homeostasis. Normal saline is the preferred solution to prevent further elevation of blood glucose (and to replace sodium in DKA). Accurate intake and output documentation and daily weights are essential for assessing fluid status and for early detection of inadequate renal function. Daily weight is a gross indicator of general fluid and nutritional status.

3. Observe for signs or symptoms of medication-induced hypoglycemia: pallor, confusion, diaphoresis, headache, weakness, shallow respirations, irritability, and restlessness or stupor. Reactions are most likely to coincide with peak insulin effect or late or missed meals, depending on the type of insulin and the patient's response. If a reaction occurs, notify the doctor, measure blood glucose level, and treat immediately with I.V. glucose, glucagon, or oral glucose, depending upon protocol and the patient's responsiveness. Once the patient is stable, use the episode as an example for teaching.

4. Make sure the patient is served the prescribed therapeutic diet at consistent times.

5. Observe for signs of DKA (in type 1 DM only):
• early — nausea; fatigue; polyuria; dry, flushed skin; dry mucous membranes; thirst; and tachycardia
• late — vomiting, poor skin turgor, lethargy, Kussmaul's respirations, acetone breath, hypotension, and abdominal pain.

If the patient's condition suggests DKA, notify the doctor immediately. Obtain a blood glucose level (usually 300 to 800 mg/dl), and check urine ketones (typically positive). Treat according to protocol (usually rapid hypotonic or isotonic I.V. fluid replacement, I.V. insulin, and — as hyperglycemia and dehydration resolve — potassium replacement; ensure that the patient has had some urine output before adding potassium to I.V. fluids). Once the patient is stable, use the episode as an example for teaching. See the "Diabetic ketoacidosis" plan, page 664, for details.

3. Insulin reactions can occur with relative suddenness. If the newly diagnosed diabetic patient is unaware of the symptoms' significance and does not seek treatment, a hypoglycemic reaction may be life-threatening.

4. The patient with DM — especially type 1 DM — needs diet guidelines tailored to meet his specific needs. Generally, concentrated sweets and alcohol are avoided for patients with either type of DM.
• The patient with type 1 DM adjusts insulin to dietary intake and exercise and distributes carbohydrate consumption equally throughout the day. If necessary, the patient's diet may include bedtime snacks, depending on insulin use. (If the patient needs intensive therapy, frequent blood glucose monitoring and multiple daily injections of insulin or an insulin pump allow adjustment of insulin to compensate for the patient's diet.)
• The patient with type 2 DM restricts calories to achieve moderate weight loss (usually necessary), lowers fat intake, spaces meals, and avoids snacks.
• Insulin and oral hypoglycemics are prescribed to fit the normal diet schedule; a missed or delayed meal can lead to hypoglycemia.

5. Inadequate pharmacologic control, increased dietary intake, infection, stress, or the interaction of other factors may cause DKA in type 1 DM. Hyperglycemia causes osmotic diuresis, which provokes compensatory mechanisms to maintain blood volume and pressure. In DKA, incomplete breakdown of fatty acids leads to accumulation of ketones in the bloodstream in addition to high (unusable) glucose levels. This leads to a state of metabolic acidosis, usually with a compensatory respiratory alkalosis. I.V. fluids correct dehydration and insulin facilitates glucose metabolism. As hyperglycemia and dehydration resolve, potassium shifting from the plasma back into the cells may unmask hypokalemia related to urinary potassium loss. The "Diabetic ketoacidosis" plan contains comprehensive information on managing this complication.

6. Observe for signs of HHNS (in type 2 DM): lethargy or stupor, fatigue, drowsiness, confusion, coma, seizures, intense thirst, and very dry mucous membranes. If the patient's condition suggests HHNS, notify the doctor immediately. Obtain a blood glucose level (typically over 800 mg/dl), check urine ketones (usually negative), and obtain a serum osmolality level, as ordered (characteristically over 350 mOsm/kg). Treat according to protocol, typically vigorous hypotonic fluid replacement, low-dose insulin, and potassium repletion. Once the patient is stable, use the episode as an example for teaching. Refer to the "Hyperosmolar hyperglycemic nonketotic syndrome" plan, page 673, for further details.

6. HHNS, a complication that occurs over days to weeks, develops most commonly in the older and infirm type 2 diabetic patient who does not recognize (or does not react to) fluid loss. It usually is caused by infection or massive fluid loss. The pathophysiology includes severe hyperglycemia and profound dehydration in the absence of ketosis. Perhaps because of pancreatic exhaustion, not enough insulin is produced to metabolize glucose, so glucose accumulates. However, enough insulin is produced to prevent adipose tissue breakdown, so ketosis does not occur. Blood glucose and osmolality levels are much more elevated in HHNS than in DKA.

Hypotonic fluids help reverse high serum osmolality; vigorous replacement is necessary because of the extent of dehydration. The patient with HHNS may be more sensitive to insulin than the patient with DKA. Urinary potassium loss may require earlier replacement in HHNS than in DKA. The "Hyperosmolar hyperglycemic nonketotic syndrome" plan contains detailed guidance on managing this complication.

7. Additional individualized interventions: _____

7. Rationales: _____

NURSING DIAGNOSIS

Knowledge deficit (self-care) related to newly diagnosed complex chronic disease

Nursing priority

Coordinate self-care teaching with establishment of a diabetes control regimen.

Patient outcome criteria

• Within 48 hours of diagnosis, the patient will:
 – initiate diet planning with dietitian
 – observe and practice injection technique (if insulin is ordered)
 – practice blood glucose and urine ketone testing (type 1 DM only).
• By the time of discharge, the patient will:
 – demonstrate proficiency in injection technique
 – produce evidence of site rotation documentation
 – discuss disease management in relation to medication, diet, exercise, and stress
 – demonstrate proper foot care
 – discuss hypoglycemia and appropriate treatment
 – discuss hyperglycemia and appropriate treatment
 – plan adequate diet for 3-day period
 – perform and interpret blood glucose and urine ketone tests accurately.

Interventions

1. See the "Knowledge deficit" plan, page 72.

Rationales

1. The "Knowledge deficit" plan provides general guidelines for patient teaching. This plan provides additional information pertinent to diabetes.

Endocrine disorders

2. Emphasize that DM control involves coordinating many aspects of daily living with prescribed interventions. Teach the significance of insulin or oral hypoglycemics for disease control. Demonstrate injection techniques, and observe patient performance. Rotate sites for S.C. injections every 7 to 10 days (abdominal sites are preferred over arms or legs). Document site rotation. Link medication needs to other factors, such as diet and exercise. Ensure that the patient and family are aware of signs and treatment of hypoglycemia as well as the protocol for managing persistent hyperglycemia, DKA (for type 1 DM), and HHNS (for type 2 DM). Involve family members in all teaching. Use the patient's symptomatic episodes as teaching tools. Where possible, link changes in habits to the prevention of complications.

2. Patient understanding is essential for home management of DM. A patient may mistakenly believe that attention to a single factor (for example, medication) will control the disorder. Compliance may increase if the patient links control with personal preventive efforts. Observing the patient's injection technique and providing opportunities for supervised practice help ensure accuracy. Rotating injection sites (after using same site for 7 to 10 days) minimizes lipodystrophy and helps prevent scar tissue formation; documentation serves as a reminder. Insulin absorption is fastest from abdominal sites (followed by arm sites, then leg sites) and abdominal sites are minimally affected by exercise. The need for medication increases with stress, infection, and higher caloric intake but may decrease with excessive activity, decreased caloric intake, or vomiting. Awareness of hyperglycemia and hypoglycemia (signs and symptoms, possible causes, treatment, and prevention) decreases patient anxiety and increases self-control; using the patient's personal experiences as teaching tools helps the patient identify and recognize personal responses to the disease.

3. Involve the patient, family, and dietitian in planning a therapeutic diet. Reinforce nutritional guidelines. Encourage supervised weight loss if the patient is overweight. Ensure the patient has written diet guidelines before discharge. Provide referral for further questions and special situations (such as "sick day" management, pregnancy, dining out, exercise, use of alcohol, or complications).

3. Involving the patient and family with dietary planning helps ensure compliance at home. Diet is specific for each patient. For the patient with type 2 DM, diet alone or diet with weight loss may be sufficient to control hyperglycemia. Written materials help minimize misunderstanding. Referral ensures an ongoing source of dietary information. The registered dietitian is an important member of the health care team and the best professional to provide nutrition counseling. The nurse's role typically is to provide reinforcement and support.

4. For type 1 or certain cases of type 2 DM, teach blood glucose and urine ketone testing methods for home use. Observe patient demonstrations for accuracy of testing, interpretation of results, and documentation. Provide target glucose ranges. Be aware that the patient may think "the lower the better" regarding blood glucose; ensure that the patient understands the body's need for glucose in regulated amounts. Encourage the patient to keep a daily record of glucose monitoring. At least annually, evaluate the patient's technique and provide revised target glucose ranges, if necessary.

4. Successful home management of DM requires that the patient perform self-monitoring to ensure that the prescribed regimen of medication, diet, and exercise remains appropriate to needs. Stressors (or disease progression) may change body requirements; blood and urine testing alerts the patient to such changes and helps avert complications. Misconceptions about the disease may have disastrous consequences. Keeping a record of glucose levels helps identify trends. Periodic evaluation helps detect errors in the testing methods and ensures that target glucose ranges reflect the patient's current needs.

5. Emphasize the importance of regular activity and exercise and of maintaining the same level of activity from day to day.

5. Regular, consistent exercise is an essential part of DM management. Exercise stimulates carbohydrate metabolism, lowers blood pressure, aids in weight control, and may help avert or minimize circulatory complications by increasing levels of high-density lipoproteins. Increases or decreases in activity may require dietary or medication changes.

6. Teach or review "sick day" management techniques: testing blood glucose and urine ketones more often, increasing fluids, continuing to take diabetes medication, contacting the doctor early in illness, and postponing exercise. Explain the importance of contacting the doctor if fever, nausea, or vomiting lasts for more than 24 hours or if blood glucose levels rise above 250 mg/dl.

7. Tell the patient to be aware of increased susceptibility to infections; discuss ways to avoid exposure. Review signs of infection: redness, swelling, exudate, and fever. Emphasize the importance of prompt, appropriate treatment of even minor injuries to avoid serious complications.

8. Discuss ways to prevent the vascular complications of DM:

• Discuss leg and foot care. Teach the patient how to perform foot care, skin care, leg exercises, and to assess circulatory status; observe return demonstration of all techniques. If the patient smokes, emphasize the importance of quitting and provide a referral to a smoking cessation program. Ensure that the patient and family receive a written plan of foot care.
• Discuss potential eye complications of DM. Help the patient understand the significance of careful disease control (especially glucose and blood pressure) in preventing or slowing diabetic retinopathy. Emphasize the importance of early reporting of vision changes and annual ophthalmologic evaluation.

• Teach the symptoms of UTI and renal impairment — flank pain, fever, dysuria, pyuria, frequency, urgency, and oliguria — and emphasize the importance of prompt treatment. Emphasize the importance of an annual kidney function evaluation (24-hour urine collection for protein and creatinine). Help the patient understand the importance of glucose and blood pressure control in preventing nephropathy.

9. Discuss the implications of diabetic neuropathy (autonomic and peripheral). Explain peripheral symptoms, such as paresthesia, pain, and sensory loss. Emphasize the importance of foot care. Instruct the patient and family to report urine retention or incontinence, orthostatic hypotension, decreased perspiration, diarrhea, or impotence.

10. Additional individualized interventions: _____

6. Unless managed carefully, even minor illnesses can quickly lead to such diabetic emergencies as hyperglycemia, hypoglycemia, DKA, or HHNS.

7. A compromised state of health may make the diabetic patient more susceptible to some infections; also, healing may be impaired or prolonged because of associated vascular insufficiency. Awareness of signs of infection may help ensure prompt treatment. Because of impaired healing from DM, even minor cuts or scratches may develop into gangrenous lesions. Infection also affects medication and dietary needs.

8. DM is characterized by degenerative vascular changes that predispose the patient to infections, ulcerations, and gangrene, particularly of the legs and feet.
• Careful skin care may help avert serious problems. Leg exercises may help develop collateral circulation and promote venous return. Nicotine causes vasoconstriction and contributes to circulatory impairment; additionally, smoking greatly increases the risk of significant heart disease. Written instructions help ensure full compliance.
• The retina consumes oxygen at a higher rate than other body tissues; thus, it is sensitive to the effects of vascular degeneration (microangiopathy) associated with DM. These effects may eventually lead to retinopathy, retinal detachment, and blindness. Although some treatment is available, the most effective deterrent to blindness is careful disease control. Early reporting of vision changes may permit palliative treatment.
• Glycosuria predisposes the patient to UTIs; recurrent severe UTIs or pyelonephritis may increase the likelihood of renal failure. Nephropathy is a long-term complication related to vascular changes in the small vessels of the glomerulus. Proteinuria is the hallmark of changes in renal function.

9. Gradual degeneration of peripheral nerves may cause paresthesia and pain, followed by loss of sensation, particularly in the legs and feet; the patient may thus be unaware of injuries. The signs listed may indicate autonomic nerve dysfunction; if so, the patient may not exhibit the usual signs of hypoglycemia.

10. Rationales: _____

NURSING DIAGNOSIS

Risk for altered health maintenance related to lack of material resources, lack of support, or ineffective coping

Nursing priority

Optimize health maintenance.

Patient outcome criteria

By the time of discharge, the patient will:
• verbalize understanding of need for lifestyle changes
• ask appropriate questions
• verbalize feelings about diagnosis
• participate actively in disease control planning
• have resource deficits resolved or appropriate referrals completed
• have a home visit or outpatient follow-up appointments scheduled.

Interventions

1. Assess the patient's resources, including financial management capabilities and family support system.

2. Involve the family in all teaching and planning.

3. Arrange appropriate follow-up home health visits before the patient's discharge.

4. Link the patient and family with community resources and mutual support groups.

5. Encourage verbalization of feelings, and support healthy coping behaviors. See the "Ineffective individual coping" plan, page 67.

6. Additional individualized interventions: _____
_____

Rationales

1. Independent home management of DM requires the ability to organize activities in a relatively stable setting. Patients are commonly admitted to the hospital "out of control" because of poor financial management and lack of a support system.

2. Family members may help reinforce teaching and encourage compliance.

3. Transferring new knowledge and skills for disease management from the hospital to the home may be difficult. Home visits allow assessment of environmental factors that may contribute to noncompliance.

4. Diagnosis of DM commonly involves major patient reeducation and lifestyle changes. Community or mutual support groups can offer ongoing education and support. Because hospitalization for DM is less frequent than in the past, or of short duration, outpatient diabetes education programs are essential.

5. As with the diagnosis of any serious chronic disease, the patient with DM may experience denial, anger, grief, and other emotions as part of a normal response. Expression of feelings is a necessary prelude to acceptance of the disease and active, responsible management. Supporting healthy coping behaviors helps maintain the patient's independence and sense of self-control — both essential for compliance. The "Ineffective individual coping" plan contains detailed interventions related to this problem.

6. Rationales: _____
_____

DISCHARGE PLANNING

Discharge checklist

Before discharge, the patient shows evidence of:
❏ blood glucose level less than 200 mg/dl
❏ ability to manage medication administration
❏ ability to understand and follow dietary guidelines
❏ ability to follow and perform exercise regimen
❏ ability to perform foot and skin care
❏ ability to perform and interpret results of blood glucose and urine ketone testing (type 1 DM only)
❏ adequate home support system
❏ referral to home care or outpatient services for reinforcement of teaching or if home support is unavailable (because patients with DM are rarely admitted to the hospital unless the disease is out of control or is causing complications, always consider a referral to home care or an outpatient or community diabetes program to reinforce hospital teaching and to allow further observation)
❏ no signs of infection
❏ stable vital signs
❏ ability to describe emergency measures for managing hyperglycemia and hypoglycemia.

Teaching checklist

Document evidence that the patient and family demonstrate an understanding of:
❏ disease and implications
❏ for all medications: purpose, dosage, administration schedule, and adverse effects requiring medical attention (usual discharge medications include insulin or oral hypoglycemics)
❏ blood glucose and urine ketone testing (type 1 DM only)
❏ interrelationship of diet, exercise, and other factors in disease management
❏ hypoglycemia (signs and symptoms, possible causes, treatment, and prevention)
❏ hyperglycemia (signs and symptoms, possible causes, treatment, and prevention)
❏ diet management
❏ exercise regimen
❏ foot care
❏ signs of infection and appropriate treatment
❏ signs and implications of neuropathy
❏ symptoms of retinopathy and need to report them
❏ signs and symptoms of urinary and renal complications and need to report them
❏ community resources
❏ when and how to access emergency medical treatment
❏ date, time, and location of follow-up appointments
❏ how to contact the doctor
❏ written materials, insulin, and syringes, as provided.

Documentation checklist

Using outcome criteria as a guide, document:
❏ clinical status on admission
❏ significant changes in status
❏ pertinent laboratory and diagnostic test findings
❏ episodes of hyperglycemia and hypoglycemia
❏ dietary intake and planning
❏ activity and exercise regimen
❏ medication therapy
❏ I.V. line patency
❏ patient and family teaching
❏ discharge planning and availability of community resources.

ASSOCIATED PLANS OF CARE

Chronic renal failure
Diabetic ketoacidosis
Grieving
Hyperosmolar hyperglycemic nonketotic syndrome
Hypoglycemia
Ineffective individual coping
Knowledge deficit
Retinal detachment
Thrombophlebitis

REFERENCES

Capriotti, T. "Nursing Pharmacology: Beyond Sulfonylureas: New Oral Medications in the Treatment of NIDDM (type II DM)," *Medical-Surgical Nursing* 6(3):166-69, June 1997.

Drass, J., and Peterson, A. "Type II Diabetes: Exploring Treatment Options," *AJN* 96(11):45-50, November 1996.

Dunning, T. *Care of People with Diabetes: A Manual of Nursing Practice.* Cambridge, Mass.: Blackwell Scientific Pubns., 1994.

Guthrie, D., and Guthrie, R. *Nursing Management of Diabetes Mellitus,* 4th ed. New York: Springer Publishing Co., 1997.

Lewis, S., et al. *Medical-Surgical Nursing: Assessment and Management of Clinical Problems,* 4th ed. St. Louis: Mosby–Year Book, Inc., 1996.

Maffeo, R. "Back to Basics: Helping Families Cope with Type I Diabetes," *AJN* 97(6):36-39, June 1997.

McConnell, E. "Clinical Do's and Don'ts. Monitoring Blood Glucose Levels at the Bedside," *Nursing* 27(4):28, April 1997.

Savinetti, R., and Bolmer, L. "Understanding Continuous Subcutaneous Insulin Infusion Therapy," *AJN* 97(3):42-49, March 1997.

Endocrine disorders

Diabetic ketoacidosis

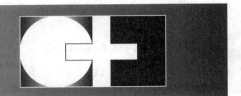

DRG information
DRG 294   Diabetes; Age 35+.
             Mean LOS = 5.7 days
DRG 295   Diabetes; Ages 0 to 35.
             Mean LOS = 4.3 days

INTRODUCTION

Definition and time focus
Diabetic ketoacidosis (DKA) is a life-threatening endocrine emergency in which an acute or absolute insulin deficiency produces metabolic acidosis. Clinical
hallmarks include hyperglycemia, dehydration, ketosis,
and electrolyte imbalance. DKA is most commonly seen
in type 1 (insulin-dependent) diabetes and may be present at the time of diagnosis.

Diabetes mellitus (DM), the disease of insulin deficiency, alters the metabolism of carbohydrates, fats, and
proteins, resulting in various physiologic derangements
that may become life-threatening. Insulin, an anabolic
hormone secreted by pancreatic islet cells, facilitates
glucose transport across cell membranes. It thus promotes glucose uptake, metabolism, and storage (as
glycogen). Insulin also promotes fatty acid synthesis
and amino acid transport while inhibiting excessive
breakdown of fats and proteins. In type 1 DM, the basic
defect is thought to be inadequate or absent insulin secretion, whereas in type 2 (non-insulin-dependent)
DM, inadequate insulin secretion or insulin resistance
or both are thought to be responsible.

This plan focuses on the critically ill diabetic patient
admitted with ketoacidosis.

Etiology and precipitating factors
• Most commonly occurs in type 1 DM
• Mortality rate reported at 4%
• Most common causes include newly diagnosed type 1
DM; incorrect exogenous insulin dosage (omitted or de-
creased); and stressful states (such as acute illness, in-
fection, myocardial infarction, or trauma), which stimu-
late the release of counterregulatory hormones, such as
epinephrine, cortisol, and glucagon
• Occasionally, cause isn't identified

FOCUSED ASSESSMENT GUIDELINES

Nursing history (functional health pattern findings)
Health perception–health management pattern
• New diagnosis or known history of type 1 DM
• Insulin, diet, and exercise to control blood glucose
level in patient with known type 1 DM
• Insulin secretion level cannot prevent ketosis in pa-
tient with known type 2 DM and severe illness or stress
• Recent onset of infection
• Onset of symptoms usually occurring over hours to
days

Nutritional-metabolic pattern
• Anorexia, nausea, abdominal pain, and vomiting
• Increased thirst (polydipsia) reported or displayed
• Increased hunger (polyphagia) reported or displayed
• Weight loss

Elimination pattern
• Excessive urination (polyuria) and nighttime urina-
tion (nocturia) common
• Diarrhea or constipation

Activity-exercise pattern
• Weakness, fatigue, or lethargy

Sleep-rest pattern
• Disturbed sleep (from nocturia)

Cognitive-perceptual pattern
• Dizziness or confusion
• Blurred vision

Physical findings
Cardiovascular
• Postural (orthostatic) hypotension
• Weak, rapid pulse
• Low to normal blood pressure
• Hyperthermia
• Capillary refill time greater than 3 seconds

Pulmonary
• Deep, rapid (Kussmaul's) respirations
• Ketotic, acetone breath odor
• Dyspnea, tachypnea

Gastrointestinal
• Abdominal distention
• Decreased bowel sounds
• Abdominal tenderness or pain
• Dry mucous membranes

Integumentary
• Dry skin and mucous membranes
• Warm, flushed skin, especially on face
• Poor or decreased skin turgor
• Sunken eyes
• Skin infections or poorly healing skin wounds

Neurologic
• Lethargy, stupor, or coma
• Fatigue, drowsiness, disorientation, or confusion
• Normal, decreased, or absent reflexes

Genitourinary
• Polyuria initially; oliguria and anuria may follow
• Underlying renal involvement

Musculoskeletal
• Weakness

Diagnostic studies

• Serum glucose level — elevated (300 to 800 mg/dl or higher)
• Arterial blood gas (ABG) levels — may reveal mild to severe metabolic acidosis with respiratory compensation (pH less than 7.35 and bicarbonate less than 10 mEq/L)
• Electrolyte panel — levels may be low, normal, or elevated depending on severity of dehydration and DKA; sodium and potassium imbalances common; acidosis causes potassium shifts in and out of cells, but a total body potassium deficit exists no matter what current serum level is
• Blood urea nitrogen and creatinine levels — may be normal or elevated depending on severity of dehydration and DKA and presence of underlying renal disease
• Osmolality — usually less than 350 mOsm/kg
• Complete blood count and white blood cell count — may be elevated in presence of infection; hemoglobin levels and hematocrit may be elevated secondary to dehydration
• Ketones — positive in urine and serum
• Electrocardiography — used to rule out myocardial infarction and evaluate potassium abnormalities
• Chest X-ray — rules out infection
• Cardiac enzymes — rule out myocardial infarction
• Blood, urine, sputum cultures — detect infection's source

Potential complications

• Long-term complications of DM (retinopathy, neuropathy, nephropathy, cardiovascular disease, and peripheral vascular disease) that will influence nursing interventions and treatment strategies
• Coma and death if DKA untreated
• Fluid overload
• Hypoglycemia if DKA overtreated
• Hypovolemic shock

Endocrine disorders

CLINICAL SNAPSHOT

Diabetic ketoacidosis

Major nursing diagnoses and collaborative problems	Key patient outcomes
Hypovolemia	Maintain vital signs within normal limits: typically, pulse rate, 60 to 100 beats/minute; systolic blood pressure, 90 to 140 mm Hg; and diastolic blood pressure, 50 to 90 mm Hg.
Hyperglycemia	Display a blood glucose level of less than 250 mg/dl or within therapeutic limits as specified by the doctor.
Sensory-perceptual alteration	Return to baseline level of consciousness (LOC).
Acidosis	Maintain ABG levels within normal limits: pH, 7.35 to 7.45; partial pressure of carbon dioxide, 35 to 45 mm Hg; and bicarbonate, 23 to 28 mEq/L.
Knowledge deficit (self-care)	On request, state plan of care for "sick day" management.

COLLABORATIVE PROBLEM

Hypovolemia related to osmotic diuresis or vomiting, or both

Nursing priority

Restore fluid volume rapidly.

Patient outcome criteria

- Within 12 hours after the onset of therapy, the patient will:
  - maintain vital signs within normal limits: typically, heart rate, 60 to 100 beats/minute; systolic blood pressure, 90 to 140 mm Hg; and diastolic blood pressure, 50 to 90 mm Hg
  - display adequate peripheral perfusion, as manifested by strong peripheral pulses and capillary refill time less than 3 seconds.
- Within 24 hours after the onset of therapy, the patient will:
  - have urine output of 60 to 100 ml/hour
  - have a balanced input and output (I&O)
  - have normal skin turgor, mucous membrane moisture, and other clinical signs of adequate hydration
  - show no signs or symptoms of electrolyte imbalances.

Interventions

1. Monitor for signs and symptoms of dehydration and shock, such as tachycardia; hypotension; weak peripheral pulses; capillary refill time greater than 3 seconds; warm, dry, flushed skin; poor skin turgor; and polyuria or oliguria. Continuously monitor blood pressure and cardiac rate and rhythm.

2. Observe for signs and symptoms of electrolyte imbalances (see Appendix C, Fluid and Electrolyte Imbalances, for details):
- hyperkalemia in the first 1 to 4 hours of treatment

- hypokalemia after 1 to 4 hours of treatment

- hyponatremia early in treatment

- hypernatremia later in treatment

Rationales

1. In DKA, the blood glucose level is elevated because of decreased cellular uptake and use of glucose. The resulting hyperglycemia increases serum osmolality and triggers a fluid shift from the intracellular to the extracellular space, producing intracellular dehydration. Compensatory renal glucose spillage, a powerful control mechanism to prevent excessive hyperglycemia, produces intense, obligatory osmotic diuresis resulting in extracellular dehydration. Eventually, severe dehydration decreases glomerular filtration. The resulting oliguria aggravates hyperglycemia and hyperosmolality. Signs and symptoms indicate the severity of the deficit and the adequacy of fluid replacement. As volume is restored, signs and symptoms should gradually resolve; failure to do so indicates inadequate fluid replacement or continuing fluid losses.

2. Electrolyte status may change rapidly, so monitor closely to identify any imbalances.

- Buffering of excess hydrogen ions released in acidosis displaces intracellular potassium into the serum.
- Renal excretion of potassium accelerates because of hyperkalemia, and the high serum level masks the resulting total body potassium deficit. As therapy reduces acidosis, potassium ions move into the cells from the serum, unmasking the underlying deficit.
- Diuresis and ketone excretion cause hyponatremia from urinary sodium losses.
- As metabolic control is restored, the kidneys begin to conserve sodium. This sodium retention, added to sodium administration in I.V. fluids, may produce hypernatremia.

3. Monitor serum osmolality and electrolyte values, as ordered. Report abnormal values to the doctor.

4. On admission, establish and maintain one or more I.V. lines in large peripheral veins, as ordered.

5. Monitor I&O and urine specific gravity meticulously. Weigh the patient daily, and document findings. Insert an indwelling urinary catheter, as ordered.

6. Administer I.V. solutions, as ordered. Replacement may include 4 to 9 L in the first 24 hours, typically:

• normal saline solution, 1 to 2 L in the first 2 hours

• half normal saline, after the first few hours, or half normal saline with 5% dextrose in water when blood glucose level reaches 250 mg/dl

• plasma volume expanders such as albumin if dehydration is severe (administer only after normal saline solution administration is underway).

7. Administer therapy for electrolyte imbalances, as ordered.

8. For at least 24 hours after rapid fluid repletion, observe for signs and symptoms of pulmonary edema, such as crackles, dyspnea, cough, or frothy sputum. If any are present, alert the doctor immediately.

9. Additional individualized interventions: _____

3. Laboratory values provide objective data on the type and degree of physiologic derangements present. In addition, serum osmolality values guide fluid replacement, while electrolyte values guide electrolyte repletion.

4. Dehydration is the most immediately life-threatening aspect of DKA. In addition, the body must be adequately hydrated for insulin to be effective. Large veins permit rapid administration of the large amounts of fluid necessary to reverse severe dehydration.

5. I&O, specific gravity, and weight records reflect the degree of fluid imbalance and effectiveness of therapy. Initially, output greatly exceeds intake, unless severe dehydration and oliguria are present. As the patient is rehydrated, fluid losses continue for the first several hours until glycosuria and osmotic diuresis are controlled. An indwelling catheter facilitates accurate measurement of urinary fluid loss. An indwelling catheter is rarely used in a conscious patient.

6. The selection of I.V. fluid depends on the patient's blood glucose and electrolyte levels, whereas the amount depends on the existing fluid deficit and ongoing fluid losses. The average fluid deficit on admission ranges from 4 to 9 L. Volume repletion is essential in reversing hypovolemia and allowing continued renal glucose excretion, an important compensatory mechanism in restoring glucose levels to normal.
• Normal saline solution replaces lost volume and sodium without increasing the blood glucose level.
• As the serum sodium level returns to normal, the saline concentration of I.V. solutions is reduced to prevent sodium overload. As the blood glucose level returns to normal, a solution containing glucose may be used to prevent hypoglycemia.
• Usually, normal saline administration is sufficient to reverse volume depletion. Although rarely used, plasma volume expanders may be necessary in severe dehydration. If they are administered before normal saline solution, however, their hypertonicity increases cellular dehydration.

7. Hyperkalemia, hyponatremia, and hypernatremia usually resolve with appropriate fluid administration and control of hyperglycemia. Hypokalemia usually requires I.V. administration of supplemental potassium. Do not add potassium until urine output is established. Potassium replacement usually includes potassium chloride alternated with potassium phosphate.

8. Rapid fluid repletion causes hemodilution. Lowered plasma oncotic pressure may allow fluid to leak into the pulmonary interstitial space, producing pulmonary edema. Pulmonary edema requires prompt aggressive medical intervention.

9. Rationales: _____

Endocrine disorders

COLLABORATIVE PROBLEM

Hyperglycemia related to decreased cellular glucose uptake and use

Nursing priority

Restore glucose control gradually.

Patient outcome criteria

• Within 2 hours of the onset of therapy, the patient's blood glucose level will be decreasing toward normal at a rate of approximately 100 mg/dl/hour.
• Within 24 to 48 hours of the onset of therapy, the patient will:
  – display a blood glucose level between 70 and 110 mg/dl
  – have a small or negative urine ketone level.

Interventions

1. Assess blood glucose levels on admission and as ordered. Perform bedside fingerstick monitoring of blood glucose every hour until normal, then every 6 hours; then before meals and at bedtime; or as ordered.

2. Assess blood ketone level on admission and as ordered. Perform bedside urine monitoring every void until ketone level is low, then every 6 hours or before meals and at bedtime.

3. Administer insulin, as ordered, typically a continuous I.V. infusion of regular insulin; before starting the infusion, flush the I.V. line with 100 ml of the insulin solution. Occasionally, boluses of regular insulin may be given by I.V., I.M., or subcutaneous (S.C.) injection in conjunction with the I.V. infusion.

Rationales

1. Blood glucose levels are the most direct indicators of deranged glucose metabolism and are used to determine therapy. As glomerular filtration of glucose exceeds the transport maximum, glucose spills into the urine. Because blood glucose levels are much more accurate than urine glucose levels, bedside fingersticks are the favored monitoring method. The goal is to reduce the glucose level approximately 100 mg/dl an hour.

2. When carbohydrate metabolism is impaired, the body uses fat as a fuel source. Lipolysis produces free fatty acids, which when oxidized produce ketone bodies. Blood ketone levels directly reflect the degree of ketogenesis. The body initially compensates by buffering ketoacids with bicarbonate. When ketoacid production exceeds buffering, ketoacids accumulate in the blood, producing acidosis. Some of the excess ketoacids are excreted in the urine (largely as sodium salts). Urine ketone levels measure ketone excretion. Urine ketones may be positive for 24 to 48 hours after DKA resolves.

3. Exogenous insulin controls gluconeogenesis and ketogenesis and increases cellular glucose uptake. In profound dehydration, medication absorption may be erratic, so the I.V. route is most reliable. A small amount of insulin may bind to I.V. tubing and bottles; flushing the line first limits the amount of insulin absorbed by the tubing during administration. The optimal dose and type of I.V. administration are controversial. High-dose insulin therapy, although effective, increases the risks of hypoglycemia and cerebral edema by lowering the blood glucose level too rapidly. Low-dose therapy, although equally effective in many cases, carries the risk of undertreatment. Periodic boluses may allow swings in blood glucose level; the goal is to lower the glucose level 75 to 100 mg/dl/hour. Continuous infusion allows delivery of low dosage. Remember, I.V. insulin absorption is greater than I.M. absorption, which in turn is greater than S.C. absorption.

4. Alert the doctor when the blood glucose level reaches 250 mg/dl and again when it reaches 150 mg/dl.

5. Observe for signs and symptoms of medication-induced hypoglycemia, such as headache, confusion, irritability, restlessness, trembling, pallor, diaphoresis, and stupor. If these signs and symptoms are present, notify the doctor, obtain a bedside fingerstick blood glucose level without delay, and treat immediately with food, oral glucose gel, or I.V. glucose or glucagon, depending upon unit protocol and the patient's LOC.

6. Additional individualized interventions: _____

4. As metabolic control is reestablished, the blood glucose level may drop precipitously from the combined effects of therapy and continuing glycosuria. At 250 mg/dl, the I.V. infusion should be changed from normal saline solution to one containing glucose, or the insulin dose should be decreased to avoid hypoglycemia. At 150 mg/dl, administration should be switched from the I.V. to the S.C. route.

5. The brain depends on glucose almost exclusively for energy. Hypoglycemia produces dramatic cerebral dysfunction and a profound stress response. The longer hypoglycemia persists, the greater the chance of transient or permanent neurologic damage. Hypoglycemic reactions may be fatal if left untreated. Mild reactions should be treated with protein and carbohydrates (such as milk and crackers). Simple sugars should be reserved for severe reactions.

6. Rationales: _____

NURSING DIAGNOSIS

Sensory-perceptual alteration related to cerebral dehydration, decreased perfusion, hypoxemia, or acidosis

Nursing priorities

• Ensure patient safety.
• Monitor return to the patient's usual LOC.

Patient outcome criterion

Within 24 hours of the onset of therapy, the patient will return to baseline LOC.

Interventions

1. Implement standard safety precautions such as keeping side rails up for the critically ill patient.

2. Monitor LOC constantly. Alert the doctor if LOC does not return to normal within 2 hours of the onset of therapy.

3. Additional individualized interventions: _____

Rationales

1. A decreased LOC makes the patient unable to guard against accidental injury.

2. Decreased LOC in early DKA may result from hyperosmolality, marked cellular dehydration from osmotic diuresis, altered cellular function from anaerobic metabolism, or acidotic cerebrospinal fluid. Persistently decreased or worsening LOC may result from cerebral edema caused by a precipitous lowering of the blood glucose level. A substantial difference between blood glucose concentration and the concentration of glucose metabolites in the brain creates an osmotic gradient, drawing water into the brain and producing cerebral edema. LOC should return to normal with therapy; failure to do so suggests another disorder and requires further medical evaluation.

3. Rationales: _____

COLLABORATIVE PROBLEM

Acidosis related to altered LOC, ketosis, and decreased tissue perfusion

Nursing priorities

- Maintain optimal ventilation and oxygenation.
- Restore normal acid-base balance.

Patient outcome criteria

- Within 24 hours of the onset of therapy, the patient will:
  – breathe at a rate of 12 to 24 respirations/minute
  – display eupnea.
- Within 36 hours of the onset of therapy, the patient will:
  – have ABG levels within normal limits: pH, 7.35 to 7.45; $Paco_2$, 35 to 45 mm Hg; and HCO_3^-, 23 to 28 mEq/L
  – have normal bowel sounds
  – be able to take oral food and fluids safely.

Interventions

1. Maintain a patent airway.

2. Monitor respiratory status every hour, including:

- respiratory rate and depth

- breath odor

- breath sounds.

3. Anticipate intubation and mechanical ventilation if increasing respiratory distress is present.

4. Administer oxygen, as ordered.

5. Monitor ABG levels, as ordered.

6. Administer I.V. sodium bicarbonate, as ordered, if pH is less than 7.1 or bicarbonate is less than 10 mEq/L.

Rationales

1. Decreased LOC increases risk of aspiration.

2. Serial assessments allow timely detection of respiratory abnormalities.
- The body responds to ketoacidosis, a form of metabolic acidosis, by increasing the rate and depth of ventilation to blow off carbon dioxide and induce a compensatory respiratory alkalosis. The presence of Kussmaul's respirations indicates severe acidosis.
- Acetone breath indicates respiratory excretion of ketones.
- Breath sounds indicate the adequacy of ventilation. Abnormal sounds may suggest pneumonia (an infection that can cause DKA) or fluid overload.

3. Although rarely needed, these measures may be necessary to maintain airway patency and ventilatory adequacy.

4. Acidosis impairs oxygen delivery to tissues. Hypoxia provokes anaerobic metabolism, which produces lactic acid and further worsens the metabolic acidosis. Supplemental oxygen elevates arterial oxygen tension, reducing the need for anaerobic metabolism.

5. ABG levels document the type and degree of acid-base imbalances present and the effectiveness of therapy for DKA. Abnormalities normally resolve with fluid and electrolyte replacement and insulin therapy.

6. These parameters indicate severe acidosis. Bicarbonate administration replenishes bicarbonate ions, which buffer excess hydrogen ions, thus returning pH to normal. Use of I.V. sodium bicarbonate is uncommon.

7. While the patient is acutely ill, withhold food and fluids, even if the patient is extremely thirsty. Auscultate bowel sounds every 8 hours. Insert a gastric tube, as ordered, and connect to suction. Remove the gastric tube and allow oral intake of food and fluids only after LOC and bowel sounds return to normal.

7. Intense thirst is a compensatory mechanism for dehydration, but oral fluid intake can be dangerous. Because hyperglycemia decreases bowel motility, abdominal pain, nausea, and vomiting are common. Vomiting increases the risk of aspiration. Bowel sounds reflect GI motility. Allowing oral intake only after bowel sounds and LOC are normal reduces the risk of aspiration. Use of gastric tubes is rare, unless the patient is unconscious.

8. Additional individualized interventions: _____
_____

8. Rationales: _____
_____

Nursing diagnosis

Knowledge deficit (self-care) related to lack of exposure to complex disease and therapy

Nursing priority

Identify and meet immediate learning needs.

Patient outcome criteria

By the time of discharge, the patient and family will:
• identify learning needs
• show beginning involvement in learning, if appropriate
• on request, state plan of care for "sick day" management.

Interventions

1. Refer to the "Knowledge deficit" plan, page 72.

2. When the patient's condition allows, determine learning needs. Ascertain whether DM is a new or previously identified diagnosis. If the patient is a known diabetic, assess for possible causes of DKA, for example, a missed insulin dose or undetected infection.

3. When the patient's condition allows, begin a teaching program that reviews principles of "sick day" management, including:
• continuing to take insulin or oral hypoglycemic agents
• changing diet to frequent small meals of soft or liquid foods
• contacting the doctor early in the illness
• checking blood glucose level every 1 to 4 hours
• checking urine ketones every void
• increasing sugar-free fluids to more than 4 oz (120 ml) per hour
• postponing exercise.

4. Use the patient's symptomatic episode as a teaching tool. Involve the family members in all teaching sessions.

Rationales

1. The "Knowledge deficit" plan provides general guidelines for patient teaching.

2. Learning needs vary depending on whether the patient is a new or known diabetic. If the patient is newly diagnosed, extensive teaching is necessary. With a known diabetic, DKA episodes are usually preventable, and instruction may focus on unmet learning needs or areas needing reinforcement.

3. Although teaching is crucial to successful management of DM, physiologic needs take precedence in the critically ill patient. Extensive teaching may need to be deferred until after the patient's condition stabilizes. Understanding principles of "sick day" management may avert future crises.

4. The immediacy of the DKA episode makes it a powerful teaching tool for actively involving the patient and family.

Endocrine disorders

5. As appropriate, initiate teaching about the cause of diabetes, signs and symptoms, significance of insulin, injection techniques, factors affecting medication needs (such as food intake and exercise), therapeutic diet, blood and urine testing, importance of consistent level of daily exercise, increased susceptibility to infections, recognition and management of hyperglycemic and hypoglycemic episodes, and long-range complications, such as neuropathy and retinopathy. Refer to the "Diabetes mellitus" plan, page 654.

6. Document learning needs and teaching. When the patient is discharged, communicate learning needs and arrange for teaching to continue on an outpatient basis.

7. Additional individualized interventions: _____
_____

5. Although the patient's and family's knowledge of all these topics is essential for ongoing home management of DM, only initial teaching is feasible for the critically ill patient. The "Diabetes mellitus" plan contains detailed information on these topics.

6. The patient's condition, extensiveness of learning needs, and the hectic unit atmosphere may mean that the patient is likely to be discharged before learning is complete. Documentation and communication enhance continuity of care.

7. Rationales: _____
_____

DISCHARGE PLANNING

Discharge checklist
Before discharge, the patient shows evidence of:
❑ stable vital signs within normal limits
❑ blood glucose level within normal limits without I.V. insulin
❑ return to premorbid LOC — ideally, alert and oriented
❑ ABG levels within normal limits
❑ patient's active participation in self-care.

Teaching checklist
Document evidence that the patient and family demonstrate an understanding of initial teaching related to:
❑ "sick day" management
❑ cause and implications of DM
❑ causes of DKA, including signs and symptoms and appropriate responses
❑ significance of insulin
❑ signs, symptoms, and interventions for hyperglycemia and hypoglycemia
❑ dietary management
❑ exercise plan
❑ blood glucose and urine ketone testing
❑ plan for completing unmet learning needs, including use of community and outpatient resources.

Documentation checklist
Using outcome criteria as a guide, document:
❑ clinical status on admission
❑ significant changes in status
❑ pertinent diagnostic test findings
❑ I.V. fluid therapy
❑ pharmacologic intervention

❑ oxygen administration
❑ patient and family teaching
❑ discharge planning.

ASSOCIATED PLANS OF CARE
Acute renal failure
Diabetes mellitus
Hyperosmolar hyperglycemic nonketotic syndrome
Hypoglycemia
Hypovolemic shock
Knowledge deficit
Sensory-perceptual alteration

REFERENCES
Bowers, R., and Smitter, R. "Diabetic Ketoacidosis," *Emergency* 28(9):42-47, September 1996.
Butkiewicz, F., et al. "Insulin Therapy for Diabetic Ketoacidosis: Bolus Insulin Injection Versus Continuous Insulin Infusion," *Diabetes Care* 18(8):1187-90, August 1995.
Dunning, T. *Care of People with Diabetes: A Manual of Nursing Practice.* Cambridge, Mass.: Blackwell Scientific Pubns., 1994.
Guthrie, D. "Patients with Disorders of Glucose Metabolism," in *Critical Care Nursing*, 2nd ed. Edited by Clochesy, J.M., et al. Philadelphia: W.B. Saunders Co., 1996.
Guthrie, D., and Guthrie, R. *Nursing Management of Diabetes Mellitus*, 4th ed. New York: Springer Publishing Co., 1997.
Jones, T. "From Diabetic Ketoacidosis to Hyperglycemic Hyperosmolar Nonketotic Syndrome: The Spectrum of Uncontrolled Hyperglycemia in Diabetes Mellitus," *Critical Care Nursing Clinics of North America* 6(4):703-21, December 1994.
LeMone, P. "Differentiating and Treating Altered Glycemic Responses," *Medical-Surgical Nursing* 5(4):257-61, 268, August 1996.
Lewis, S., et al. *Medical-Surgical Nursing: Assessment and Management of Clinical Problems*, 4th ed. St. Louis: Mosby–Year Book, Inc., 1996.
Peraglallo-Dittko, V. "Diabetes 2000: Acute Complications," *RN* 58(8):36-42, August 1995.

Hyperosmolar hyperglycemic nonketotic syndrome

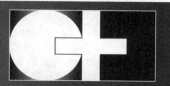

DRG information
DRG 294   Diabetes; Age 35+.
          Mean LOS = 5.7 days
DRG 295   Diabetes; Ages 0 to 35.
          Mean LOS = 4.3 days

INTRODUCTION

Definition and time focus
Hyperosmolar hyperglycemic nonketotic syndrome (HHNS) is an endocrine emergency with a mortality rate as high as 70%, if left untreated. Like diabetic ketoacidosis (DKA), it produces profound hyperglycemia and dehydration, but unlike DKA, ketosis and acidosis are absent. It presents a diagnostic puzzle because its clinical picture is similar to both DKA and cerebrovascular accident (CVA). It may occur in type 1 (insulin-dependent) or type 2 (non-insulin-dependent) diabetes mellitus (DM) but is more common in type 2 and may be present at the time of diagnosis.

The basic defect in HHNS is a relative insulin deficiency in which enough insulin is secreted to prevent ketoacidosis but not enough to prevent hyperglycemia. Failure to recognize or respond to the thirst mechanism, which signals developing dehydration, exacerbates the problem. A precipitating factor (such as infection, new diagnosis of DM, CVA, or myocardial infarction) also is common. Clinical hallmarks include hyperglycemia, dehydration, hyperosmolality, and electrolyte imbalance without ketosis. This plan focuses on the critically ill patient admitted with HHNS.

Etiology and precipitating factors
• Usually only occurs in type 2 DM, but up to 50% of episodes occur in persons with no previous history of DM
• Acute illness (such as myocardial infarction or CVA)
• Treatments (such as dialysis or total parenteral nutrition)
• Infection (such as pneumonia or urinary tract infection)
• Surgery
• Newly diagnosed DM
• Drugs (such as steroids, thiazides, or beta blockers)
• Loss of thirst mechanism
• Pancreatitis

FOCUSED ASSESSMENT GUIDELINES

Nursing history (functional health pattern findings)
Health perception–health management pattern
History typically is obtained from a family member or friend because the patient's level of consciousness is decreased.
• Patient newly diagnosed or has known history of type 2 DM
• Family history of DM common
• More common in older patients (over age 50)
• Slow onset of symptoms, typically over days to weeks
Nutritional-metabolic pattern
• Increased thirst (polydipsia) or loss of thirst mechanism
• Anorexia
• Weight loss
Elimination pattern
• Possible polyuria, nocturia, and incontinence
• Possible diarrhea or constipation
Activity-exercise pattern
• Possible weakness, fatigue, or lethargy
Sleep-rest pattern
• Sleep disturbance related to nocturia
Cognitive-perceptual pattern
• Possible dizziness or orthostatic hypotension
• Confusion
• Possible blurred vision
• Decreased or altered sensorium

Physical findings
Neurologic
• Lethargy or stupor
• Fatigue, drowsiness, disorientation, or confusion
• Seizures
• Normal, decreased, or absent reflexes
Pulmonary
• Tachypnea or dyspnea
• Absence of Kussmaul's respirations (differential finding from DKA)
• Absence of acetone breath (differential finding from DKA)
Cardiovascular
• Tachycardia
• Postural hypotension
• Other cardiovascular disease (such as hypertension or heart failure)
• Hyperthermia

• Capillary refill time greater than 3 seconds
Renal
• Polyuria (early stage)
• Oliguria (late stage)
• Nocturia
• Incontinence
Integumentary
• Dry skin and mucous membranes
• Poor skin turgor
• Warm, flushed skin
• Sunken or soft eyes
• Skin infections or poorly healing wounds
Gastrointestinal
• Abdominal distention
• Decreased bowel sounds

Diagnostic studies
• Serum glucose levels — usually greater than 800 mg/dl, may be as high as 3,000 mg/dl
• Arterial blood gas levels — usually normal
• Electrolyte panel — levels may be low, normal, or elevated depending on severity of dehydration and HHNS
• Blood urea nitrogen (BUN) and creatinine levels — BUN levels may be normal to elevated depending on severity of dehydration and HHNS; both may be normal to elevated in presence of underlying renal disease

• Urine ketones — usually negative
• Serum osmolality — usually greater than 350 mOsm/kg
• Complete blood count and white blood cell count — may be elevated in presence of infection
• Hemoglobin levels and hematocrit — may be elevated secondary to dehydration
• Electrocardiography — may reveal underlying cardiac disorder or arrhythmias
• Chest X-ray — needed to establish baseline and rule out infection
• Blood, urine, and sputum cultures — used to detect infection's source
• Serum amylase — rules out pancreatitis

Potential complications
• Diabetes-related complications (retinopathy, neuropathy, nephropathy, cardiovascular disease, and peripheral vascular disease) that will influence nursing interventions and treatment strategies
• Fluid overload, heart failure, or pulmonary edema
• Disseminated intravascular coagulation
• Hypoglycemia (if HHNS overtreated)
• Hypovolemic shock
• Cerebral edema
• Coma and death if untreated

CLINICAL SNAPSHOT

HYPEROSMOLAR HYPERGLYCEMIC NONKETOTIC SYNDROME

Major nursing diagnoses and collaborative problems	Key patient outcomes
Hypovolemia	Maintain stable vital signs: typically, heart rate, 60 to 100 beats/minute; systolic blood pressure, 90 to 140 mm Hg; and diastolic blood pressure, 50 to 90 mm Hg.
Hyperglycemia	Display a blood glucose level of 70 to 110 mg/dl or within therapeutic limits as specified by the doctor.
Sensory-perceptual alteration	Return to baseline level of consciousness (LOC).
Knowledge deficit (self-care)	On request, state plan of care for "sick day" management.

COLLABORATIVE PROBLEM
Hypovolemia related to osmotic diuresis

Nursing priority
Restore fluid volume.

Patient outcome criteria

Within 24 hours of the onset of therapy, the patient will:
• maintain vital signs within normal limits, typically with heart rate of 60 to 100 beats/minute, systolic blood pressure 90 to 140 mm Hg, and diastolic blood pressure 50 to 90 mm Hg
• peripheral perfusion within normal limits, as evidenced by warm, dry skin and bilaterally equal pedal pulses
• maintain a urine output of 60 to 100 ml/hour
• manifest serum osmolality levels within normal limits
• manifest serum electrolyte levels within normal limits.

Interventions

1. Monitor for signs and symptoms of dehydration and shock, such as tachycardia; hypotension; weak peripheral pulses; capillary refill time greater than 3 seconds; warm, dry, flushed skin; poor skin turgor; polyuria or oliguria; increased hematocrit; increased urine specific gravity; and increased serum osmolality. Monitor blood pressure and cardiac rate and rhythm continuously.

2. Observe for signs and symptoms of electrolyte imbalances, particularly hypernatremia and hypokalemia (see Appendix C, Fluid and Electrolyte Imbalances, for details). Monitor serum electrolyte levels, as ordered, and report abnormal values to the doctor. Administer electrolyte replacements, as ordered.

3. Monitor serum osmolality, as ordered. Report levels greater than 295 mOsm/kg.

4. Implement standard measures for hypovolemia, as ordered. Maintain patency of one or more I.V. lines, insert an indwelling urinary catheter, and monitor intake and output and daily weights. Refer to the "Diabetic ketoacidosis" plan, page 664, for details.

Rationales

1. Impaired insulin release or peripheral insulin resistance causes hyperglycemia, which in turn causes hyperosmolality. To compensate for the hyperosmolality, fluid shifts from the intracellular to the extracellular space, dehydrating cells. Renal glucose spillage, an important compensatory mechanism for hyperglycemia, triggers an intense osmotic diuresis. This diuresis causes obligatory fluid and electrolyte losses, reflected in an elevated hematocrit and increased serum osmolality. Severe hypovolemia decreases glomerular filtration, aggravating the hyperglycemia and hyperosmolality and eventually producing oliguria and increased specific gravity. Fluid loss is usually greater in HHNS than in DKA, so signs of dehydration may be severe. As volume is restored, signs and symptoms should resolve gradually; failure to do so indicates inadequate fluid replacement or continuing losses.

2. Electrolyte status may change rapidly in response to fluid shifts, so close observation for signs and symptoms of imbalances is essential. Hypernatremia results from the large water deficit. In contrast to DKA, where acidosis causes hyperkalemia that commonly masks a low total body potassium, urinary losses in HHNS result in hypokalemia. Hypernatremia usually resolves with fluid administration, while hypokalemia usually requires earlier potassium replacement than with DKA. Potassium doses depend on serum potassium levels.

3. Laboratory values document the extent of hyperosmolality, which usually is more marked than in DKA because of the failure of the thirst mechanism and the intense osmotic diuresis. Values greater than 320 mOsm/kg indicate severe hyperosmolality.

4. These measures are the same as with DKA. The "Diabetic ketoacidosis" plan describes these interventions and associated rationales in detail. Because HHNS is seen more commonly in older patients, an indwelling urinary catheter is useful; it is necessary in the unconscious patient.

Endocrine disorders

5. Administer I.V. solutions, as ordered, typically 6 to 8 L in the first 12 hours:
• normal saline solution if serum sodium level is less than 130 mEq/L

• half-normal saline solution if serum sodium level is greater than 145 mEq/L

• dextrose in water when blood glucose levels reach 250 mg/dl or serum osmolality reaches 300 mOsm/kg.

6. During fluid replacement, monitor closely for signs and symptoms of fluid overload, including crackles, S_3 heart sound, neck-vein distention, dyspnea, or persistently depressed LOC. If any indicators are present, notify the doctor.

7. Additional individualized interventions: _____

5. Aggressive fluid repletion is necessary because of the severity of dehydration in HHNS.
• A very low serum sodium level reflects large urinary sodium losses. Isotonic saline solution replaces sodium and replenishes volume.
• An elevated serum sodium level reflects decreased glomerular filtration and sodium retention in severe hypovolemia. Hypotonic fluid provides free water to reverse hyperosmolality.
• As blood glucose or serum osmolality approaches normal, changing to a glucose-containing solution prevents hypoglycemia.

6. Because the patient with HHNS usually is older and has significant preexisting disease, the risk for heart failure, pulmonary edema, or cerebral edema is higher than in DKA. These signs and symptoms require prompt nursing intervention and medical evaluation.

7. Rationales: _____

COLLABORATIVE PROBLEM

Hyperglycemia related to inadequate insulin secretion or peripheral insulin resistance, or both

Nursing priority

Lower blood glucose level.

Patient outcome criterion

Within 24 to 48 hours of the onset of therapy, the patient will display a blood glucose level between 70 and 110 mg/dl.

Interventions

1. Implement measures for this problem contained in the "Diabetic ketoacidosis" plan, page 664, but with the following modifications:
• Judiciously administer low-dose insulin I.V., as ordered. Discontinue the infusion if the blood glucose level drops more than 100 mg/dl in 1 hour and alert the doctor.
• Monitor closely for medication-induced hypoglycemia.

2. If the patient developed HHNS while on high-carbohydrate enteral nutrition or hyperosmolar dialysis, consult with the doctor about revising orders for these therapies.

3. Additional individualized interventions: _____

Rationales

1. Care for hyperglycemia is similar in both HHNS and DKA, but with different emphasis on two points.

• Because some endogenous insulin is produced, the patient with HHNS is more sensitive to exogenous insulin than a patient with DKA, and lower insulin doses are usually needed.
• Because the patient with HHNS retains some control of glucose metabolism, the risk for developing hypoglycemia in response to measures that lower blood glucose is high.

2. Modifying or discontinuing these causes of HHNS removes an unnecessary glucose load for the patient.

3. Rationales: _____

NURSING DIAGNOSIS

Sensory-perceptual alteration related to cerebral dehydration, decreased perfusion, hypoxemia, glucose deprivation, or cerebral edema during rapid rehydration

Nursing priorities
• Restore the patient's baseline LOC.
• Protect the patient from injury.

Patient outcome criterion

Within 24 hours, the patient will display baseline LOC; ideally, alert, oriented, and able to move all extremities.

Interventions

1. Evaluate neurologic status every 1 to 4 hours, as indicated by the rapidity of other changes in the patient's condition. Alert the doctor to deepening coma or other indications of deteriorating neurologic functioning.

2. Institute seizure precautions. Promptly report any seizures to the doctor.

3. Additional individualized interventions: _____

Rationales

1. Neurologic changes, which are characteristic of this disorder, correlate closely with the degree of hyperosmolality. Deteriorating neurologic function may indicate serious pathophysiologic derangements, other previously undetected disorders, or inadequate therapy, and it requires medical evaluation.

2. Seizures occur commonly with HHNS, as a result of cerebral dehydration, cerebral edema (during rehydration), or glucose deprivation (if hypoglycemia occurs).

3. Rationales: _____

NURSING DIAGNOSIS

Knowledge deficit (self-care) related to lack of exposure to complex disease and management

Nursing priority

Teach the patient and family to avoid recurrence of HHNS, if appropriate.

Patient outcome criteria

By the time of discharge, the patient and family will:
• identify learning needs, if appropriate, as manifested by curiosity, asking questions, and attentiveness to teaching
• show beginning involvement in learning, if appropriate
• state plan of care for "sick day" management on request.

Interventions

1. Identify cause of HHNS. If it is DM, implement measures contained in the "Diabetic ketoacidosis" plan (with the exception of ketone testing), page 664, as appropriate.

2. Additional individualized interventions: _____

Rationales

1. The "Diabetic ketoacidosis" plan details measures that also apply to teaching some HHNS patients. It is pertinent to patients with uncontrolled DM in whom HHNS may recur. It is inappropriate when HHNS results from high-carbohydrate nutrition or hyperosmolar dialysis; in those instances, HHNS should not recur once the cause has been removed.

2. Rationales: _____

DISCHARGE PLANNING

Discharge checklist

Before discharge, the patient shows evidence of:
❏ stable vital signs within normal limits
❏ blood glucose level within normal limits without I.V. insulin
❏ return to baseline LOC
❏ arterial blood gas levels within normal limits
❏ electrolyte levels within normal limits.

Teaching checklist

Document evidence that the patient and family demonstrate an understanding of:
❏ cause and significance of HHNS
❏ methods to decrease risk, if appropriate.
If the patient has DM, also document understanding of the following items:
❏ oral hypoglycemic agents and insulin, if appropriate
❏ hyperglycemia and hypoglycemia (signs and symptoms, possible causes, treatment, and prevention)
❏ "sick day" management plan
❏ dietary plan
❏ exercise and activity plan
❏ blood glucose testing
❏ learning needs at time of discharge
❏ community resources.

Documentation checklist

Using outcome criteria as a guide, document:
❏ clinical status on admission
❏ significant changes in status
❏ pertinent laboratory and diagnostic test findings
❏ I.V. fluid therapy
❏ pharmacologic intervention
❏ patient and family teaching
❏ discharge planning.

ASSOCIATED PLANS OF CARE

Acute renal failure
Diabetic ketoacidosis
Disseminated intravascular coagulation
Hypovolemic shock
Knowledge deficit

REFERENCES

Dunning, T. *Care of People with Diabetes: A Manual of Nursing Practice.* Cambridge, Mass.: Blackwell Scientific Pubns., 1994.
Guthrie, D. "Patients with Disorders of Glucose Metabolism," in *Critical Care Nursing,* 2nd ed. Edited by Clochesy, J.M., et al. Philadelphia: W.B. Saunders Co., 1996.
Guthrie, D., and Guthrie, R. *Nursing Management of Diabetes Mellitus,* 4th ed. New York: Springer Publishing Co., 1997.
Jones, T. "From Diabetic Ketoacidosis to Hyperglycemic Hyperosmolar Nonketotic Syndrome: The Spectrum of Uncontrolled Hyperglycemia in Diabetes Mellitus," *Critical Care Nursing Clinics of North America* 6(4):703-21, December 1994.
Lemone, P. "Differentiating and Treating Altered Glycemic Responses," *Medical-Surgical Nursing* 5(4):257-61, 268, August 1996.
Lewis, S., et al. *Medical-Surgical Nursing: Assessment and Management of Clinical Problems,* 4th ed. St. Louis: Mosby–Year Book, Inc., 1996.
O'Hanlon-Nichols, T. "Hyperglycemic Hyperosmolar Nonketotic Syndrome," *AJN* 96(3):38-39, March 1996.
Peraglallo-Dittko, V. "Diabetes 2000: Acute Complications," *RN* 58(8):36-42, August 1995.

Hypoglycemia

DRG information
DRG 296   Nutritional and Miscellaneous Metabolic Disorders with Complication or Comorbidity (CC); Age 17+.
Mean LOS = 4.7 days
DRG 297   Nutritional and Miscellaneous Metabolic Disorders without CC; Ages 0 to 17.
Mean LOS = 4.3 days
DRG 298   Nutritional and Miscellaneous Metabolic Disorders; Ages 0 to 17.
Mean LOS = 3.4 days

INTRODUCTION

Definition and time focus
Diabetes mellitus (DM) is a chronic metabolic condition involving an absolute (as in type 1 DM) or relative (as in type 2 DM) lack of endogenous insulin. A delicate balance of diet, medicine (insulin or oral hypoglycemics), and exercise is needed to achieve glucose homeostasis. Alterations in glucose metabolism can provoke acute complications. This plan focuses on one of the most common acute complications of DM: hypoglycemia. Also called low blood sugar, insulin reaction, and insulin shock, it occurs when the serum glucose level falls below 50 mg/dl (normal is 70 to 110 mg/dl). Symptoms can also occur when a high blood glucose level is lowered rapidly to 180 mg/dl.

Hypoglycemia can be life-threatening if left untreated. Usually, it is an acute complication of type 1 (insulin-dependent) DM, with a prevalence ranging from 4% to 26%, and is seen more commonly with attempts to establish normoglycemia to diminish chronic complications of DM. It also can occur in type 2 (non-insulin-dependent) DM, especially with use of the oral agent chlorpropamide (Diabinese), but is less common.

Etiology and precipitating factors
• Excessive or unplanned exercise
• Delayed or missed meal
• Tight serum glucose control
• Inappropriate insulin regimen
• Too much insulin or oral hypoglycemic medicine
• Renal failure
• Alcohol use
• Underlying renal disease (nephropathy)
• Pancreatic tumor (rare)

FOCUSED ASSESSMENT GUIDELINES

Nursing history (functional health pattern findings)
Health perception–health management pattern
• History of diabetes
• Use of oral hypoglycemics or insulin
Nutritional-metabolic pattern
• Feeling of hunger
• Nausea
Elimination pattern
• Increased perspiration
Activity-exercise pattern
• Weakness, lethargy
• Feeling of faintness
Sleep-rest pattern
• Bizarre dreams or nightmares
• Restless sleep
• Difficulty waking in the morning
Cognitive-perceptual pattern
• Headache or lack of concentration
• Blurred vision

Physical findings
Cardiovascular
• Tachycardia
• Palpitations
• Syncope
Integumentary
• Pallor
• Flushing
• Sweating (diaphoresis)
Neurologic
• Irritability and mood swings
• Confusion or uncontrollable behavior
• Seizures
• Glazed stare
Musculoskeletal
• Weakness

Diagnostic studies
• Random serum glucose level — less than 50 mg/dl

Potential complications
• Chronic complications of DM (retinopathy, neuropathy, nephropathy, cardiovascular disease, or peripheral vascular disease)
• Rebound hyperglycemia (if hypoglycemia overtreated)
• Coma, brain damage, or death, if untreated

Endocrine disorders

HYPOGLYCEMIA

Major nursing diagnoses	Key patient outcomes
Risk for injury	Have a serum blood glucose level above 70 mg/dl.
Knowledge deficit (self-care)	On request, state the signs and symptoms, possible causes, treatment, and preventive strategies related to hypoglycemia.

NURSING DIAGNOSIS

Risk for injury related to inappropriate exogenous insulin use, lack of food, or excessive exercise

Nursing priority

Restore serum glucose level to normal.

Patient outcome criteria

Within 15 minutes of the onset of treatment, the patient will:
• have a serum glucose level above 70 mg/dl
• be alert, oriented, and able to communicate.

Interventions

1. Observe for signs and symptoms of hypoglycemia constantly:
• adrenergic signs and symptoms (anxiety, tremor, nervousness, flushing, numbness, weakness, hunger, nausea, pallor, irritability, sweating, palpitations)
• neuroglycopenic signs and symptoms (moderate: headache, mental dullness, confusion, fatigue; or severe: glazed stare, bizarre dreams, difficulty waking, nightmares, coma, seizures).
Document findings.

2. Document suspected hypoglycemia with bedside glucose fingerstick or serum glucose, following hospital protocol.

Rationales

1. With hypoglycemia, adrenergic signs and symptoms occur first because low blood glucose stimulates the sympathetic nervous system to release catecholamines. In mild hypoglycemia, these may be the only signs and symptoms that occur. If hypoglycemia remains untreated, neuroglycopenic symptoms emerge because of starvation of cerebral neurons, which are only able to use glucose for energy. Symptoms may be moderate or severe. In long-standing type 1 DM, many patients have "hypoglycemia unawareness," where they experience none of the usual symptoms of hypoglycemia until they suddenly lose consciousness. This is a dangerous and life-threatening situation.

2. Most institutions request a serum glucose level if the fingerstick glucose is less than 50 mg/dl and before treatment. A patient may complain of symptoms of hypoglycemia when the glucose level is normal or elevated. Symptoms may occur with a normal glucose level if the glucose level is quickly lowered or if the patient has had a high glucose level recently brought under control.

3. Treat hypoglycemia promptly:
• If the patient is alert and the glucose level is less than 60 mg/dl (or below normal level specified by your institution), give a simple carbohydrate such as glucose gel by mouth. For mild symptoms, give 10 to 20 g; for moderate symptoms, 20 to 30 g. Follow with a complex carbohydrate and protein snack, such as one-half glass of milk with two graham crackers or four soda crackers (unless a meal will be eaten within an hour).

• If the patient is alert and the glucose level is greater than 80 mg/dl, do not treat. Check on and reassure the patient frequently.

• If the patient is unconscious with a glucose level less than 60 mg/dl, ensure airway patency, check pulse rate, and administer 50% dextrose (25 g by I.V. push) or glucagon (1 mg I.M. or subcutaneously), according to protocol.

3. Prompt treatment reduces the risk of injury.
• Glucose gel or liquids containing simple sugars provide a measured amount of simple, rapidly acting glucose. Using fruit juice is no longer recommended because it provides a variable amount of fructose, a concentrated form of glucose that is absorbed very rapidly and may cause rebound hyperglycemia. However, 4 to 6 oz of orange juice can be used if glucose gel is not available. Other concentrated forms of glucose such as sugared soda or candy also cause an unreliable rise in blood glucose and may cause rebound hyperglycemia. Carbohydrates and protein cause a gradual rise in the glucose level to prevent recurrence of hypoglycemia.
• This is a normal glucose level. The goal of diabetes management is to keep the glucose level as near to normal as possible to prevent, reverse, or delay DM-related complications.
• The patient with DM may also have cardiac disease, so it is important to recognize that unconsciousness may not be related to hypoglycemia. The patient's airway and pulse should be assessed immediately to detect emergency cardiac conditions. The unconscious hypoglycemic patient usually suffers from severe hypoglycemia. Because of the effect of glucose deprivation on cerebral neurons, immediate measures must be taken to reverse the hypoglycemic state. I.V. dextrose supplies glucose most rapidly. Glucagon administration stimulates glycogenolysis, the release of glucose from liver glycogen stores. Never give an unconscious patient liquids by mouth because of the risk of aspiration.

4. Recheck the glucose level 15 minutes after treatment. Repeat treatment if glucose level remains low. If the patient was unconscious, give a protein and carbohydrate snack when fully awake.

4. Blood glucose may drop again rapidly. Rechecking may indicate the need for further treatment. Carbohydrates and protein will cause a sustained rise in blood glucose.

5. If hypoglycemia occurs frequently, consult the doctor.

5. The patient's medication, diet, and activity regimens may need adjustment.

6. Additional individualized interventions: _____

6. Rationales: _____

NURSING DIAGNOSIS

Knowledge deficit (self-care) related to complexity of disease and therapeutic regimen

Nursing priority

Teach the patient and family how to avoid and appropriately manage hypoglycemia.

Patient outcome criteria

By the time of discharge, the patient and family will be able to:
• recognize the risk of hypoglycemia
• state signs and symptoms, possible causes, treatment, and preventive strategies related to hypoglycemia.

Endocrine disorders

Interventions

1. Once the hypoglycemic episode is over, use it as a learning experience. Involve family members in all teaching sessions. Help them to identify the causes of hypoglycemia, if possible.

2. Review the signs and symptoms of hypoglycemia with the patient and family. If possible, have the patient identify personal signs and symptoms. Stress the importance of early recognition and treatment.

3. Discuss appropriate treatment strategies for hypoglycemia with the patient and family:
• If symptoms are mild and the blood glucose level is less than 60 mg/dl, eat a carbohydrate and protein snack.
• If symptoms are severe, eat a simple sugar.
• If the patient is unconscious, a family member should administer glucagon and call for emergency medical assistance.

4. Review strategies to prevent hypoglycemia with the patient and family. Encourage the patient to:
• wear a medical identification bracelet and carry a medical identification card
• have a source of food available at all times at home, in the car, at work, and any other place the patient frequents
• monitor glucose level regularly and record results
• work closely with the doctor and health care team if a pattern of hypoglycemia develops.

5. Additional individualized interventions: _____
_____

Rationales

1. The patient needs to realize that occasional episodes of hypoglycemia can and will happen. By being prepared, the patient and family will be able to alleviate symptoms quickly. Common causes of hypoglycemia usually involve too much insulin or oral hypoglycemic, missed or delayed meals and snacks, or excessive exercise. In the hospital, the patient who can take nothing by mouth because of tests, procedures, surgery, or nausea and vomiting is also at risk for hypoglycemia. Identifying causes may help the patient avoid future episodes.

2. Each patient responds individually to hypoglycemia. Symptoms may be mild to severe. Some patients have no symptoms. Early identification of symptoms promotes prompt treatment and possibly a less severe hypoglycemic episode. Repeated severe episodes can lead to memory loss and learning impairment.

3. A protein and carbohydrate snack causes a gradual rise in the glucose level. Because the goal of management is a normal glucose level, rebound hyperglycemia can occur if the patient eats too much food or uses simple sugars. If the episode occurs close to a meal, the patient may elect to eat a little earlier as treatment. Family members may need one-on-one teaching before administering glucagon.

4. Carrying and wearing medical identification will alert others to the potential for hypoglycemia if the patient is unable to speak. Having food available at all times ensures quick treatment of hypoglycemia. Regularly monitoring glucose level and recording the results helps identify patterns of hypoglycemia. These records should be reviewed at each outpatient visit. Correct insulin administration is essential for optimal effectiveness.

5. Rationales: _____
_____

DISCHARGE PLANNING

Discharge checklist
Before discharge, the patient shows evidence of:
❏ stable vital signs within normal limits
❏ blood glucose level within normal limits without I.V. glucose
❏ return to usual level of consciousness.

Teaching checklist
Document evidence that the patient and family demonstrate an understanding of:
❏ cause and significance of hypoglycemia
❏ signs and symptoms
❏ preventive measures
❏ treatment strategies
❏ proper use of insulin or oral agents
❏ dietary management
❏ exercise and activity plan

- ❏ blood glucose monitoring
- ❏ urine ketone testing (for type 1 DM only)
- ❏ chronic complications related to DM
- ❏ learning needs at time of discharge
- ❏ community resources.

Documentation checklist
Using outcome criteria as a guide, document:
- ❏ clinical status on admission
- ❏ significant changes in status
- ❏ pertinent laboratory and diagnostic test findings
- ❏ I.V. fluid therapy
- ❏ pharmacologic intervention
- ❏ patient and family teaching
- ❏ discharge planning.

ASSOCIATED PLANS OF CARE
Diabetic ketoacidosis
Hyperosmolar hyperglycemic nonketotic syndrome
Hypovolemic shock
Knowledge deficit

REFERENCES
Dunning, T. *Care of People with Diabetes: A Manual of Nursing Practice.* Cambridge, Mass.: Blackwell Scientific Pubns., 1994.

Guthrie, D. "Patients with Disorders of Glucose Metabolism," in *Critical Care Nursing,* 2nd ed. Edited by Clochesy, J.M., et al. Philadelphia: W.B. Saunders Co., 1996.

Guthrie, D., and Guthrie, R. *Nursing Management of Diabetes Mellitus,* 4th ed. New York: Springer Publishing Co., 1997.

Lewis, S., et al. *Medical-Surgical Nursing: Assessment and Management of Clinical Problems,* 4th ed. St. Louis: Mosby–Year Book, Inc., 1996.

Peraglallo-Dittko, V. "Diabetes 2000: Acute Complications," *RN* 58(8):36-42, August 1995.

Endocrine disorders

Part 11

Renal disorders

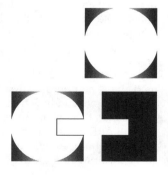

Acute renal failure

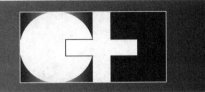

DRG information
DRG 316   Renal Failure.
Mean LOS = 7.6 days
Principal diagnoses include:
- chronic or unspecified renal failure
- acute renal failure (unspecified, with renal cortical necrosis, renal medullary necrosis, or tubular necrosis, or with other specified pathologic lesion in kidney)
- oliguria or anuria.

Renal failure accompanied by any operative procedure will not be classified under DRG 316.
DRG 317   Admit for Renal Dialysis.
Mean LOS = 2.9 days
Principal diagnoses include aftercare involving intermittent dialysis.

Renal failure without intermittent dialysis is coded differently from renal failure with intermittent dialysis. For the latter, the principal diagnosis is actually admission for dialysis; renal failure becomes a secondary diagnosis.

INTRODUCTION

Definition and time focus
Acute renal failure (ARF) is a sudden cessation or decrease in renal function. In ARF, the kidneys cannot maintain fluid and electrolyte balance or filter metabolic waste products. ARF disrupts all body systems and may cause problems in cardiac, respiratory, GI, neurologic, musculoskeletal, integumentary, genitourinary, and endocrine-metabolic functions. The mortality rate can be high depending on the cause, the patient's age, and related physical problems.

Most ARF patients who recover progress through three stages: oliguria, diuresis, and recovery. The oliguric stage lasts about 2 weeks (a shorter period represents a better prognosis). The diuretic stage may last several weeks. The recovery stage may last up to a year, with initial rapid improvement and a continuing slow return to near-normal function. In some cases, patients have nonoliguric ARF with increasing azotemia and urine volumes for 12 days and a return to normal in another 12 days. If the patient does not recover, long-term hemodialysis, peritoneal dialysis, continuous renal replacement therapy, or kidney transplantation is necessary.

This plan focuses on the patient admitted for treatment of ARF, including identification of its cause and support of body systems until the kidneys begin to recover, or evaluation for dialysis or transplantation.

Etiology and precipitating factors
- Prerenal problems leading to decreased renal perfusion, such as hemorrhage, all forms of shock, excessive vomiting or diarrhea, heart failure or other causes of decreased cardiac output, burns, excessive diuresis, third-spacing of fluids, hypotension, vasodilation, or obstruction of the aorta or renal arteries
- Renal (parenchymal) problems leading to destruction of kidney tissue, such as acute tubular necrosis from ischemia or nephrotoxins, glomerulonephritis, emboli, allergic inflammation, or infections
- Postrenal problems leading to obstruction of urine flow, such as calculi, prostate enlargement, tumors, or retroperitoneal fibrosis
- Preexisting multisystem problems increase risk of ARF, especially in an older patient

FOCUSED ASSESSMENT GUIDELINES

Nursing history (functional health pattern findings)
Health perception–health management pattern
- Decreased amount and frequency of urination
- Headaches, swelling of feet and ankles, and palpitations
- Recent high-risk episode such as infection; cardiac, aortic, or biliary surgery; trauma; ingestion of aspirin, antibiotics, or other drugs; exposure to toxins; or an allergic response to food, drugs, or blood transfusions
- History of urinary tract infections, diabetes mellitus, hypertension, kidney disease, or cardiac or liver problems
- Pain around the flank or costal margin areas

Nutritional-metabolic pattern
- Loss of appetite, nausea
- Weight gain or loss
- Odd taste in mouth
- Increased saliva or a dry mouth

Elimination pattern
- Decreased or absent urination
- Change in urine color and smell
- Abdominal cramps, a feeling of fullness, diarrhea, or constipation
- Pruritus

Activity-exercise pattern
- Difficulty in breathing at rest and during exercise
- Weakness and fatigue
- Muscle cramps

Sleep-rest pattern
• Longer sleep periods than usual

Cognitive-perceptual pattern
• Periods of dizziness
• Memory loss and inability to concentrate

Role-relationship pattern
• Job-related exposure to nephrotoxic chemicals, such as carbon tetrachloride, dyes, fungicides, pesticides, or heavy metals

Sexuality-reproductive pattern
• Loss of sexual drive, impotence, or loss of menstruation

Coping–stress tolerance pattern
• Increased irritability and decreased ability to handle stress

Physical findings

Physical findings may vary, depending on the cause, type, and stage of ARF.

Genitourinary
• Oliguria (less than 400 ml/day)
• Less commonly, anuria (less than 50 ml/day) or high urine output (1 to 2 L/day in nonoliguric ARF)
• Abnormal urine color, clarity, or smell (such as red or brown color, cloudiness, or foul smell)

Neurologic
• Lethargy, apathy
• Tremors, seizures
• Memory loss, confusion
• Coma

Cardiovascular
• Arrhythmias
• Bounding, rapid pulse; normal or high blood pressure; and distended neck veins (with hypervolemia)
• Tachycardia, low blood pressure, or orthostatic hypotension (with hypovolemia)
• Pericardial-type chest pain (mild to severe pain that may increase with movement or decrease with leaning forward)
• Anemia

Pulmonary
• Rapid respirations, dyspnea, or crackles (with hypervolemia)
• Tachypnea (with hypovolemia)
• Kussmaul's respirations (with acidosis)

Gastrointestinal
• Moist tongue and increased saliva (with hypervolemia)
• Dry tongue and mucous membranes (with hypovolemia)
• Vomiting
• Diarrhea
• Stomatitis

Musculoskeletal
• Muscle spasms (tetany)
• Weakness
• Asterixis

Integumentary
• Moist, warm skin and pitting edema over bony areas (with hypervolemia)
• Decreased skin turgor and dry skin (with hypovolemia)
• Bruises
• Thin, brittle hair and nails
• Pallor

Diagnostic studies

• 24-hour urine output and serum creatinine and blood urea nitrogen (BUN) levels — monitor the kidneys' ability to excrete fluid and waste products. Oliguric ARF is characterized by oliguria and rising BUN and creatinine levels. Patients with nonoliguric ARF exhibit a urine output of 1 to 2 L/day and rising BUN and creatinine levels. The diuretic stage is characterized by increasing urine output (2 to 3 L/day), indicating returning glomerular filtration. BUN and creatinine levels remain high during this stage because the kidneys cannot concentrate the urine effectively. As the kidneys regain concentrating ability during the recovery stage, the BUN and creatinine levels begin to fall and stabilize at normal or near normal levels depending upon the residual damage to the kidneys.
• Serum electrolyte panel — monitors fluid, electrolyte, and acid-base status. Elevated potassium, sodium, and phosphate levels; decreased calcium level; and a decreased pH level indicate poor renal function.
• Urinalysis — monitors renal excretion and concentration abilities. Sodium and potassium concentrations may vary, depending on the cause and type of ARF. Casts, crystals, hematuria, and proteinuria may be present. White blood cells (WBCs) may indicate infection. With prerenal conditions, specific gravity and osmolality may be high; with renal conditions, they may be constant at 1.010 and approximately 300 mOsm/kg respectively.
• Creatinine clearance — reflects glomerular filtration rate (GFR) and is an accurate indication of renal function. A decrease indicates a poor GFR. A value of 50 to 84 ml/minute indicates mild failure; 10 to 49 ml/minute, moderate failure; and less than 10 ml/minute, severe failure.
• Fractional sodium excretion or renal failure index — compares the clearance of sodium to the clearance of creatinine; indexes greater than 1 may indicate non-functioning tubules.
• Urine-plasma creatinine concentration ratios and urine-plasma urea concentration ratios — reflect the kidneys' ability to save water and excrete wastes. Values vary depending upon the cause and type of ARF. In prerenal failure, ratios are high, reflecting kidney conservation of sodium and water; in acute tubular insufficiency, the kidneys' inability to perform these functions results in low urine-plasma ratios.

Renal disorders

• BUN-creatinine ratio — reflects GFR and tubular function. In prerenal failure, the ratio is high (usually greater than 20:1), reflecting increased tubular reabsorption of urea. In acute tubular insufficiency, the ratio remains approximately 10:1, reflecting increased reabsorption of both urea and creatinine by the damaged tubules.
• Complete blood count (CBC) — may reveal low red blood cell (RBC) count, hemoglobin, and hematocrit, reflecting anemia. An elevated WBC count may reflect infection.
• Coagulation studies — may be abnormal if disseminated intravascular coagulation causes ARF
• Renal concentration tests — may show the kidneys' inability to concentrate solutes in urine
• Electrocardiography (ECG) — may show arrhythmias or high peaked T waves, flattened P waves, and widened QRS complexes associated with high potassium levels
• Kidney-ureter-bladder X-rays — show size, structure, and position of kidneys, ureters, and bladder. The kidneys may be normal or enlarged in ARF. Changes in bladder or ureters suggest postrenal ARF.
• Computed tomography scan — shows cross-sectional views of renal structures
• Magnetic resonance imaging — differentiates normal from abnormal cells
• Ultrasound scan — may show internal and external abnormalities in kidney size and shape
• I.V. or retrograde pyelogram — may show obstruction, constriction, or masses

• Renal biopsy — may help differentiate among parenchymal kidney diseases
• renal angiography — may show renal artery abnormalities, cysts, or tumors
• Radionuclide tests (renal scan and renogram) — may show abnormal distributions of radioactive compounds, indicating structural abnormalities or impaired perfusion or uptake
• Cystoscopy — may show urethra and bladder abnormalities

Potential complications
Most complications result from the uremic syndrome — the accumulation of waste products in the blood. Some complications result from the kidneys' inability to maintain the normal hormonal functions of stimulating RBC production, regulating calcium absorption, and controlling the renin-angiotensin-aldosterone system.
• Infection (sepsis is the most dangerous complication of ARF)
• Stress ulcer
• Heart failure
• Pericarditis
• Pneumonitis
• Encephalopathy
• Peripheral neuropathy
• Coagulation defects
• Pathologic fractures from bone demineralization
• GI bleeding

CLINICAL SNAPSHOT

ACUTE RENAL FAILURE

Major nursing diagnoses and collaborative problems	Key patient outcomes
Electrolyte imbalance	Maintain serum electrolyte levels within acceptable limits for the patient.
Fluid volume excess	Maintain vital signs and hemodynamic readings within acceptable limits for the patient.
Risk for injury	Display no signs or symptoms of uremia such as mentation changes.
Risk for infection	Have clean, dry access sites for lines and catheters.
Nutritional deficit	Have only limited weight loss, muscle wasting, or edema.
Knowledge deficit (ARF and dialysis)	Express commitment to comply with treatments, including dialysis, dietary modifications, and activity restrictions.

COLLABORATIVE PROBLEM

Electrolyte imbalance related to decreased electrolyte excretion, excessive electrolyte intake, or metabolic acidosis

Nursing priority

Prevent complications of electrolyte imbalance.

Patient outcome criteria

- Within 8 hours after treatment for hyperkalemia, the patient will:
  - have a serum potassium level within normal limits (3.5 to 5.5 mEq/L)
  - show no tented T waves or other signs of hyperkalemia on ECG
  - display arterial blood gas (ABG) levels within normal limits: pH, 7.35 to 7.45; $Paco_2$, 35 to 45 mm Hg; HCO_3^-, 23 to 28 mEq/L.
- Within 24 hours of admission and then continuously, the patient will:
  - maintain serum electrolyte levels within acceptable limits
  - have normal sinus rhythm.

Interventions

1. Monitor and document electrolyte levels every 8 to 12 hours, as ordered, particularly potassium, phosphate, calcium, and magnesium. See Appendix C, Fluid and Electrolyte Imbalances, for general assessment parameters and interventions for abnormal electrolyte levels. Consult the nephrologist about acceptable electrolyte levels for the patient.

2. Continuously monitor the ECG and document your findings. See Appendix A, Monitoring Standards. Note and promptly report peaked, high ("tented") T waves; prolonged PR interval; or a widened QRS complex.

3. If hyperkalemia is present, administer and document the following, as ordered:

- I.V. glucose (50%) and insulin solution

- I.V. calcium chloride or calcium gluconate

- cation-exchange resins such as sodium polystyrene sulfonate (Kayexalate) with sorbitol, orally or rectally (do not give oral doses with fruit juices)

- I.V. sodium bicarbonate solution.

Rationales

1. The kidneys' inability to regulate electrolyte excretion and reabsorption may result in high potassium and phosphate levels, a low calcium level, and a high or low magnesium level. These levels can change quickly and result in such complications as cardiac arrhythmias, muscle response changes, mentation changes, skin irritation, and even death. General assessment parameters and interventions are included in the Fluid and Electrolyte Imbalances appendix. The nephrologist can help determine appropriate electrolyte levels for each patient.

2. Electrolyte abnormalities can trigger arrhythmias and cardiac arrest. The Monitoring Standards appendix contains general assessments for arrhythmias. The signs listed indicate hyperkalemia severe enough to cause a cardiac emergency.

3. The kidneys' inability to excrete the potassium released into the serum by normal cellular metabolism results in dangerously high potassium levels.
- Glucose and insulin may transport potassium into cells temporarily, thus lowering serum potassium in an emergency.
- Calcium competes with potassium for entry into heart cells, thus decreasing the dangerous effect of hyperkalemia on cardiac rhythm.
- Sodium polystyrene sulfonate removes potassium at the rate of 1 mEq/g of drug by exchanging it for sodium in the bowel. Sorbitol helps remove the exchanged and bound potassium from the bowel by acting as an osmotic diarrheic. Fruit juices may bind with sodium polystyrene sulfonate and decrease its effectiveness.
- ARF causes metabolic acidosis, which may increase the release of potassium from cells in exchange for hydrogen ions. Sodium bicarbonate corrects acidosis by combining with hydrogen ions, allowing potassium to move back into the cells.

4. Limit dietary and drug intake of potassium; for example, avoid juices high in potassium and drugs such as potassium penicillin (Penicillin VK) or potassium-containing antacids.

5. Give aluminum hydroxide antacid (Amphojel) with meals and every 4 hours, as ordered. Document administration.

6. Give calcium and vitamin supplements as needed and ordered. Document their administration.

7. Limit intake of magnesium, as from magnesium-containing antacids.

8. Give sodium chloride I.V., as needed and ordered. Document its administration.

9. Additional individualized interventions: _____
_____

4. When the kidneys cannot excrete potassium, excess intake can push serum potassium to dangerously high levels.

5. The kidneys cannot excrete the phosphates released from normal cellular metabolism or from dietary phosphate intake. Aluminum hydroxide binds with phosphate in the bowels and prevents absorption into the bloodstream, thus decreasing hyperphosphatemia.

6. The kidneys' inability to stimulate the absorption of calcium in the bowel results in hypocalcemia and bone demineralization. High phosphate levels also cause hypocalcemia. Calcium and vitamin D supplements increase the serum calcium levels, helping to prevent bone demineralization and other adverse effects of hypocalcemia.

7. The kidneys cannot excrete magnesium.

8. Usually, sodium intake is restricted to prevent fluid overload. However, major losses through vomiting, diarrhea, and wound drainage may create a need for sodium replacement.

9. Rationales: _____
_____

NURSING DIAGNOSIS

Fluid volume excess related to sodium and water retention

Nursing priorities

• Maintain adequate hydration.
• Prevent fluid overload.

Patient outcome criteria

By the time of discharge, the patient will:
• maintain vital signs and hemodynamic readings within acceptable parameters
• have clear lungs
• display minimal or absent peripheral edema
• manifest normal skin turgor
• have moist and clean mucous membranes
• experience weight loss of no more than 1 lb (0.5 kg) per day.

Interventions

1. See Appendix C, Fluid and Electrolyte Imbalances.

Rationales

1. Appendix C contains general information on fluid and electrolyte imbalances. This plan presents additional information specific to ARF.

2. Assess for signs of fluid overload and document findings.

• Assess vital signs, breath sounds, and peripheral edema every 4 hours, or more frequently if appropriate. Assess weight and CBC, especially hematocrit, daily. If the patient has an invasive hemodynamic monitoring line, measure right atrial pressure, pulmonary artery pressures, pulmonary artery wedge pressure, mean arterial pressure, and cardiac output according to hospital protocol.
• Report the following promptly: high blood pressure, rapid pulse, rapid respirations, high hemodynamic parameters, crackles or gurgles, peripheral edema, increasing daily weight, or low hematocrit.
• Also report the following promptly: low hemodynamic monitoring parameters, rapid pulse, low blood pressure, dry skin and mucous membranes, poor skin turgor, decreased weight, or high hematocrit.

3. Measure and document intake and output (I&O) every 8 hours.

4. Restrict fluid intake to measured losses plus 400 ml/day, unless fluid or weight losses are excessive. Correlate the I&O record with daily weights. Consult the doctor about increasing fluid replacement if excessive fluid losses are present or if weight loss exceeds 1 lb (0.5 kg) per day. Document fluid administration.

5. Give I.V. infusions continuously through an infusion pump, as ordered.

6. Provide hard candies, ice chips, and mouth care every 2 hours as needed and ordered. Document your actions.

7. Give diuretics, such as mannitol, furosemide (Lasix), or ethacrynic acid (Edecrin), as needed and ordered. Document administration and results. Administer vasodilators, as ordered, such as low-dose dopamine (Intropin).

8. Additional individualized interventions: _____
_____

2. Inability to maintain normal fluid homeostasis results in fluid overload during the oliguric stage and potential dehydration during the diuretic stage.
• Regular assessment of indicated parameters provides for early detection of imbalances.

• Prompt medical intervention is necessary to resolve imbalances. These signs indicate fluid overload. A low hematocrit may reflect hemodilution from overhydration.
• These signs reflect a low circulating fluid volume. High hematocrit may reflect hemoconcentration.

3. A careful comparison of I&O is necessary to prevent fluid overload or dehydration.

4. Because the kidneys cannot eliminate excess fluids, intake must be restricted to replacement of lost fluids. The additional 400 ml represents insensible fluid losses (through lungs, skin, and stool). Although such losses are estimated at 400 ml/day, excess losses from high temperatures, wound drainage, diarrhea, or vomiting may require increasing this amount. Daily weight may help guide fluid replacement because the ARF patient usually loses ¾ lb (0.3 kg) to 1 lb/day from catabolism. A loss of more than 1 lb/day may indicate a need for additional fluids.

5. The patient with ARF is susceptible to fluid overload. An infusion pump prevents accidental administration of fluid boluses.

6. Fluid restrictions cause dry mouth and thirst. These measures aid mouth comfort by stimulating salivation and removing debris during fluid restriction.

7. Diuretics may be given initially in prerenal conditions to increase fluid volume through the kidneys in an attempt to prevent ARF. However, diuretics may cause ARF in marginally functioning kidneys and are not effective in nonfunctioning kidneys. Vasodilators expand the vascular bed, lessening vascular congestion and the risk of pulmonary edema. Low-dose dopamine causes dopaminergic stimulation of renal blood vessels, thus increasing renal perfusion.

8. Rationales: _____
_____

Renal disorders

NURSING DIAGNOSIS

Risk for injury related to uremic syndrome

Nursing priorities

• Assess for signs and symptoms of uremia.
• Monitor for complications.
• Prevent injuries.

Patient outcome criteria

• Immediately at the start of dialysis, the patient will:
  – have a patent dialysis shunt or catheter
  – display no signs of infection
  – manifest no signs of hemorrhage.
• Within 3 days of admission, the patient will:
  – have an acceptable blood pressure
  – display strong, regular peripheral pulses
  – show a level of consciousness within normal limits
  – manifest a normal temperature.
• Within 7 days of admission, the patient will:
  – have BUN, creatinine, uric acid, and pH values within expected limits
  – display ABG levels within normal limits
  – manifest no signs or symptoms of uremia
  – maintain therapeutic drug levels
  – have a hemoglobin level and hematocrit within expected limits
  – display no signs of pericarditis, such as pericardial friction rub and chest pain.

Interventions

1. See Appendix B, Acid-Base Imbalances.

2. Monitor BUN, creatinine, uric acid, and pH levels once daily or as needed and ordered. Monitor ABG levels once daily or as needed and ordered. Document your findings.

3. Assess for and document signs and symptoms of uremia every 2 to 4 hours and as needed. Note headache, mentation changes, fatigue, confusion, lethargy, pruritus, uremic frost, stomatitis, nausea and vomiting, ammonia breath odor, weight loss, muscle wasting, Kussmaul's respirations, seizures, or coma. Report significant findings to the doctor.

4. Give sodium bicarbonate I.V. as needed and ordered, typically if the plasma bicarbonate level is 10 to 15 mEq/L or less. Document administration.

Rationales

1. Appendix B contains general information on acid-base imbalances. This plan presents additional information specific to ARF.

2. Accumulation of the metabolic waste products in the blood and increasing acidosis reflect worsening failure and may indicate the need for dialysis.

3. Uremia affects every system and may cause subtle changes as the condition worsens. Careful assessments are valuable in determining the need for dialysis and gauging its frequency.

4. Acidosis is commonly treated by dialysis, but severe cases may be treated with sodium bicarbonate.

5. Assess the hemodialysis access site, if present, every 2 hours for patency, warmth, color, thrill, and bruit. Check circulation above and below the access site. Do not use the access site for I.V. infusions or to draw blood. Do not take blood pressures on an arm or leg with an access site. Inject heparinized normal saline solution into the catheter every 12 hours to maintain patency, as ordered. Document access site status and report abnormalities promptly to the doctor.

5. The access site must remain patent because of the limited number of large vessels available for dialysis. Early discovery of a clotted catheter may allow clot removal and salvaging of the site. Using the site for purposes other than dialysis increases the risk of infection and loss of the site. Regular heparinization prevents clotting.

6. Assess the peritoneal dialysis access catheter site, if present, every 24 hours and as needed for signs and symptoms of infection, including redness, swelling, excess warmth, and drainage. Also assess for general signs and symptoms of infection, including fever, malaise, abdominal pain, and cloudy drainage. Maintain surgical aseptic technique when manipulating the site, changing dressings, or adding medication to the dialysate.

6. The patient undergoing peritoneal dialysis is at high risk for peritonitis, a life-threatening complication. Early detection of infection permits aggressive intervention and increases the likelihood of its success.

7. Prepare the patient for dialysis, as needed and ordered, when potassium, BUN, and creatinine levels, and other parameters indicate worsening uremia, usually every 1 to 3 days.

7. Both hemodialysis and peritoneal dialysis remove serum waste products and excess fluids and electrolytes, allowing a more homeostatic metabolic state.

8. Monitor drug administration and blood levels, as ordered. Assess potential nephrotoxicity, electrolyte content, dosage, and timing with dialysis.

8. Renal dysfunction may decrease drug excretion, resulting in excessive blood levels and varying durations of drug effects. Certain drugs, including antibiotics, may be nephrotoxic and may worsen kidney damage. Drugs containing electrolytes should be limited to prevent undesirable effects. Dialysis may remove some drugs from the blood, so drug administration should be timed with dialysis treatments. Monitoring blood levels provides accurate guidelines for drug therapy.

9. Monitor hematocrit and hemoglobin level daily for signs of anemia. Give packed RBCs, folic acid, and iron supplements as needed and ordered. Document your findings and actions.

9. Erythropoietin, a hormone manufactured by the kidneys, normally stimulates RBC production. Diminished erythropoietin production in ARF results in anemia. Folic acid and iron supplements stimulate RBC production and may correct the anemia. Administering packed cells instead of whole blood provides oxygen-carrying RBCs without exacerbating fluid overload.

10. Assess continually for signs and symptoms of hemorrhage, including changes in vital signs, CBC, and coagulation panel. If present, alert the doctor immediately. Give vitamin K, packed RBCs, and other blood components as needed and ordered, and document their use. See the "Gastrointestinal hemorrhage" plan, page 505.

10. Uremic syndrome places the patient at high risk for stress ulcers and coagulation problems. General interventions for the patient with GI bleeding are included in the "Gastrointestinal hemorrhage" plan.

11. Assess daily for signs and symptoms of pericarditis, including tachycardia, fever, friction rub, and pleuritic pain that is relieved by sitting forward. If these indicators are present:
• Notify the doctor. Administer steroids or nonsteroidal anti-inflammatory agents, as ordered. Document their use.

11. About 20% of patients with ARF develop pericarditis (inflammation of the pericardial sac).

• Untreated, pericarditis can lead to pericardial effusion and cardiac tamponade. The medications listed relieve inflammation.

Renal disorders

• Monitor every 4 hours for indicators of pericardial effusion and a small cardiac tamponade: weak peripheral pulses, paradoxical pulse greater than 10 mm Hg, or a decreased level of consciousness. If present, alert the doctor immediately.
• Monitor continually for indicators of a large cardiac tamponade: distended neck veins, profound hypotension, and rapid loss of consciousness. Summon immediate medical assistance and prepare for emergency pericardial aspiration.
12. Additional individualized interventions: _____

• Pericardial effusion can range from mild to major. Mild effusion produces a small cardiac tamponade and mildly decreased cardiac output. Increased dialysis may be used to remove the uremic toxins causing mild effusion.
• A large cardiac tamponade — a medical emergency — compromises cardiac output severely. Immediate removal of pericardial fluid is necessary to allow ventricular filling and prevent cardiac arrest.
12. Rationales: _____

Nursing diagnosis

Risk for infection related to decreased immune response and skin changes secondary to uremia

Nursing priority

Assess for and prevent infection.

Patient outcome criteria

Within 72 hours of admission and then continuously, the patient will:
• have a normal temperature
• have clean, dry access sites for lines and catheters
• have negative cultures
• if taking antibiotics, have a therapeutic blood level.

Interventions

1. Assess continually for signs of infection, such as increased temperature, redness, swelling, warmth, and drainage. Document findings and report them to the doctor.

2. Continually protect the patient from cross-contamination by practicing medical and surgical asepsis.

3. Give antibiotics every 4 to 12 hours, as ordered, and document their use. Follow the guidelines for drug administration in the "Risk for injury" nursing diagnosis above.

4. Provide site care and dressing changes for central and peripheral I.V. lines, catheters, and dialysis access every 12 to 48 hours, according to policy. Assess and document condition of skin and puncture sites; document date and care given.

Rationales

1. Uremic syndrome suppresses normal cell metabolism and immune response, resulting in an increased risk for infection, a major cause of death for ARF patients. Continuous assessment is necessary to identify infection and to begin early treatment, reducing the risk of life-threatening sepsis and septicemia.

2. Carefully washing hands and using aseptic technique during procedures and when handling equipment may prevent infection.

3. Antibiotics are a potent weapon against infection; however, many are nephrotoxic. Because the kidneys may be unable to excrete antibiotics normally, lower-than-normal doses may be needed. Coordination with dialysis is important to minimize drug removal and maintain therapeutic blood levels.

4. Site care may prevent the accumulation of secretions that could serve as growth media for infective organisms, while regular assessment may allow the early identification of infection. Careful documentation of site care promotes continuity of care.

5. Provide skin care at frequent intervals. Use preventive measures such as position changes, range-of-motion exercises, massage, wrinkle-free linens, and protective pads and mattresses. Document skin condition and nursing care given. See the "Impaired physical mobility" plan, page 50.

6. Avoid continuous invasive procedures such as indwelling urinary catheterization. Catheterize intermittently, as needed and as ordered.

7. Collect urine, blood, and secretion specimens for culture and sensitivity laboratory tests, as needed and ordered. Document your actions.

8. Additional individualized interventions: _____

5. Skin integrity is compromised in the patient with ARF and uremia because of altered metabolism and the accumulation of fluid and waste products in the tissues. Frequent skin care may counteract the increased risk of skin breakdown and infection. The "Impaired physical mobility" plan provides further detail on preventing skin breakdown.

6. Continuous invasive procedures provide reservoirs for infective organisms in a patient already at high risk for infection.

7. Careful monitoring of body secretions for infection may allow timely and appropriate treatment if needed.

8. Rationales: _____

Nursing diagnosis

Nutritional deficit related to anorexia, nausea and vomiting, and restricted dietary intake

Nursing priorities
• Maintain nutritional status.
• Minimize protein catabolism.

Patient outcome criteria

Upon discharge, the patient will:
• be free from nausea and vomiting
• have only limited weight loss, muscle wasting, or edema
• display a pattern of regular and adequate meal intake
• verbalize having enough energy for activities of daily living.

Interventions

1. See the "Nutritional deficit" plan, page 80.

2. Administer medication to control nausea and vomiting, as needed and as ordered. Document administration and patient response. Provide small, frequent meals. Document dietary intake.

3. Collaborate with the doctor and nutritionist to design a high-carbohydrate diet that provides small quantities of high-quality proteins (containing essential amino acids); limits fluids, potassium, and sodium; and includes vitamin supplements.

4. Additional individualized interventions: _____

Rationales

1. General assessments and interventions are included in the "Nutritional deficit" plan. This nursing diagnosis focuses on information specific to ARF.

2. The patient with ARF commonly experiences nausea and vomiting because of uremia's effects on the GI system. Medication and smaller servings enhance tolerance to the diet.

3. A high-carbohydrate diet provides calories for energy while sparing proteins and preventing protein catabolism. Because the kidneys cannot excrete the waste products of protein metabolism, proteins are limited to easily used, high-quality proteins. The kidneys cannot regulate water balance, so fluids are limited. Electrolytes such as potassium are limited because the kidneys cannot excrete them. Sodium is limited to prevent volume overload. Dialysis may remove vitamins, requiring administration of supplements.

4. Rationales: _____

Renal disorders

Nursing diagnosis

Knowledge deficit (ARF and dialysis) related to lack of exposure to information on complex disease and its management

Nursing priority

Provide information on ARF and dialysis, as appropriate.

Patient outcome criteria

According to individual readiness, the patient will be able to relate on request:
• signs and symptoms, such as headache, nausea, and vomiting, to be reported to the nurse
• commitment to comply with treatments, including dialysis, dietary modifications, and activity restrictions.

Interventions

1. See the "Knowledge deficit" plan, page 72.

2. Provide, as appropriate, information about the complexity and life-threatening nature of ARF and dialysis, including:
• the common stages of ARF
• medications
• signs and symptoms that should be reported to the nurse, such as dizziness and nausea
• procedures, including hemodialysis or peritoneal dialysis
• dietary modifications
• activity restrictions.

3. Additional individualized interventions: _____

Rationales

1. General interventions appropriate for any patient are included in the "Knowledge deficit" plan. This plan contains information specific to ARF.

2. The acutely ill patient may not be receptive to extensive teaching. However, if appropriate, teaching may decrease anxiety and enhance recovery.

3. Rationales: _____

Discharge planning

Discharge checklist

Before discharge, the patient shows evidence of:
❏ stable vital signs and monitoring parameters
❏ absence of infection, hemorrhage, and major complications in all systems
❏ stabilized fluid and electrolyte status, including limited edema and appropriate potassium, calcium, sodium, phosphate, and magnesium levels
❏ stabilized BUN, creatinine, uric acid, and pH levels
❏ intact and healing dialysis access site
❏ stable nutritional status including a positive nitrogen balance and minimal weight loss
❏ therapeutic drug levels.

Teaching checklist

Document evidence that the patient and family demonstrate an understanding of:
❏ common stages of ARF and patient's current stage
❏ fluid and diet regimen, including limitations of proteins, electrolytes, and fluids
❏ rest and activity schedule
❏ medications, including action and adverse effects
❏ dialysis treatment if appropriate, including schedule and adverse effects
❏ signs and symptoms, including fever, pain, nausea, vomiting, and dizziness, to report to the nurse.

Documentation checklist

Using outcome criteria as a guide, document:
❏ clinical status on admission
❏ significant changes in status

❏ pertinent laboratory and diagnostic test findings, including serum drug levels
❏ dialysis access site condition and care
❏ urine characteristics and quantity, if appropriate
❏ I&O
❏ weights
❏ diet tolerance
❏ activity tolerance
❏ mentation status
❏ skin status
❏ pertinent procedures including dialysis.

ASSOCIATED PLANS OF CARE
Gastrointestinal hemorrhage
Knowledge deficit
Nutritional deficit

REFERENCES
Garret, B.M. "The Nutritional Management of Acute Renal Failure," *Journal of Clinical Nursing* 4(6):377-82, November 1995.
Kirby, S., and Davenport, A. "Haemofiltration/dialysis Treatment in Patients with Acute Renal Failure," *Care of the Critically Ill* 12(2):54, 56, 58, March-April, 1996.
LeMone, P., and Burke, K.M. *Medical-Surgical Nursing: Critical Thinking in Client Care.* Menlo Park, Calif.: Addison-Wesley-Longman Publishing Co., 1996.
Lewis, S.M., et al. *Medical-Surgical Nursing: Assessment and Management of Clinical Problems.* St. Louis: Mosby–Year Book, Inc., 1996.
Tressler, K.M. *Clinical Laboratory and Diagnostic Tests: Significance and Nursing Implications.* Stamford, Conn.: Appleton & Lange, 1995.

Renal disorders

Chronic renal failure

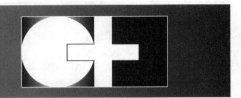

DRG information

DRG 316   Renal Failure.
           Mean LOS = 7.6 days
           Principal diagnoses include chronic renal
           failure.
DRG 317   Admit for Renal Dialysis.
           Mean LOS = 2.9 days
DRG 315   Other Kidney and Urinary Tract Operating
           Room Procedures.
           Mean LOS = 9.3 days
           Principal diagnoses include arteriovenosto-
           my for renal dialysis.

INTRODUCTION

Definition and time focus

Chronic renal failure (CRF) is a progressive, irreversible decrease in kidney function to the point where homeostasis can no longer be maintained. Usually slow and insidious, CRF eventually has consequences in all organ systems and physiologic processes. The final stage of CRF, when more than 90% of kidney function is permanently lost, is called end-stage renal disease (ESRD). During ESRD, chronic abnormalities occur, and patient survival depends on maintenance dialysis or kidney transplantation. This plan focuses on the ESRD patient receiving maintenance hemodialysis or peritoneal dialysis, who has been admitted for evaluation of the systemic consequences of CRF and the effectiveness of therapy.

Etiology and precipitating factors

• Untreated acute renal failure or poor response to treatment (for example, acute tubular necrosis)
• Diabetes mellitus (DM) leading to diabetic nephropathy
• Severe hypertension leading to hypertensive nephropathy
• Lupus erythematosus leading to lupus nephritis
• Recurrent glomerulonephritis, typically related to chronic streptococcal infection
• Pyelonephritis
• Polycystic kidney disease
• Chronic use of nephrotoxic drugs
• Frequent lower urinary tract infections (UTIs) with eventual kidney involvement
• Neoplasms (metastatic or primary)
• Developmental and congenital disorders
• Complications of pregnancy (for example, eclampsia, UTI, hemorrhage, or abruptio placenta)

• Sarcoidosis
• Amyloidosis
• Goodpasture's syndrome (autoimmune disease involving basement membrane of glomerular capillaries)

FOCUSED ASSESSMENT GUIDELINES

Nursing history (functional health pattern findings)

Health perception–health management pattern
• Signs and symptoms that cause the patient to seek health care vary widely and may include decreased urine output, edema, extreme fatigue, depression, loss of interest in environment, impotence, and flank pain
• Commonly has a history of acute or chronic renal problems and may be receiving treatment for acute renal failure, chronic renal insufficiency, hypertension, DM, generalized arteriosclerosis and atherosclerosis, lupus erythematosus, or other systemic diseases involving the kidneys

Nutritional-metabolic pattern
• Anorexia, nausea, and vomiting
• Weight loss related to decreased intake of nutrients or weight gain related to fluid retention
• Unpleasant taste in mouth

Elimination pattern
• Polyuria and nocturia if patient is in an early stage of CRF
• Oliguria (with polycystic kidney disease, urine output may be normal, or polyuria may occur), if patient is in advanced stage of CRF
• Diarrhea alternating with constipation

Activity-exercise pattern
• Fatigue, malaise, and decreased energy level

Sleep-rest pattern
• Extreme somnolence or insomnia and restlessness
• Sleep often interrupted by muscle cramps and leg pain

Cognitive-perceptual pattern
• Shortened attention span
• Memory loss
• Decreased ability to perform abstract reasoning or mathematical calculations
• Loss of interest in environment

Self-perception–self-concept pattern
• Depression or frequent mood swings
• Altered self-concept and body image
• Decreased self-esteem
• Reduced level of independence and self-care
• Sense of powerlessness and hopelessness

Role-relationship pattern
• Inability to work
• Inability to maintain spousal and parental roles
• Decrease in social contacts and activities

Sexuality-reproductive pattern
• Amenorrhea, infertility, decreased libido, and decreased or absent sexual expression in female patient
• Impotence, decreased libido, and decreased or absent sexual expression in male patient

Coping–stress tolerance pattern
• Ineffective individual and family coping patterns in response to changes caused by chronic catastrophic disease and its treatment
• Defense mechanisms (for example, denial, projection, displacement, or rationalization)

Value-belief pattern
• Loss of confidence in health care providers
• Questioning or reaffirming lifelong religious and philosophical values and beliefs

Physical findings
Integumentary
• Rough, dry skin
• Bronze-gray, pallid skin color
• Pruritus
• Ecchymoses
• Poor skin mobility and turgor (skin mobility is the ease with which it can be lifted between the fingers; turgor is the speed with which it resumes position)
• Excoriation
• Signs and symptoms of inflammation
• Thin, brittle nails
• Coarse and thinning hair

Cardiovascular
• Hypertension, or hypotension (uncommon)
• Orthostatic hypotension
• Pitting edema of feet, legs, fingers, and hands
• Periorbital edema
• Sacral edema
• Engorged neck veins
• Arrhythmias
• Pericardial friction rub (with pericarditis)
• Paradoxical pulse (with pericardial effusion or tamponade)
• Palpitations

Pulmonary
• Crackles
• Shortness of breath
• Coughing
• Thick, tenacious sputum
• Deep, rapid respirations (with acidosis)

Gastrointestinal
• Smell of urine and ammonia on the breath
• Gum ulcerations and bleeding
• Dry, cracked, bleeding mucous membranes and tongue
• Vomiting
• Bleeding from GI tract
• Constipation or diarrhea
• Weight loss related to decreased intake of nutrients masked by fluid retention (peripheral edema), leading to increase in overall body weight; after the patient receives appropriate treatment (fluid restriction and dialysis), excess fluid is decreased and weight loss is especially evident
• Liver enlargement
• Ascites

Neurologic
• Malaise, weakness, and fatigue
• Confusion and disorientation
• Memory loss
• Slowing of thought processes
• Changes in sensorium (somnolence, stupor, or coma)
• Seizures
• Changes in behavior (irritability, withdrawal, depression, psychosis, or delusions)
• Numbness and burning of soles of feet
• Decreased sensory perception
• Muscle cramps
• Restlessness of legs
• Diminished deep tendon reflexes
• Positive Chvostek's and Trousseau's signs (rare)

Musculoskeletal
• Muscle cramps (especially in the legs)
• Loss of muscle strength
• Limited range of motion in joints
• Bone fractures
• Lumps (calcium-phosphate deposits) in skin, soft tissues, and joints
• Footdrop with motor nerve involvement

Reproductive
• Amenorrhea (in females)
• Atrophy of testicles (in males)
• Gynecomastia

Diagnostic studies
• Blood urea nitrogen (BUN) levels — elevated
• Serum creatinine levels — elevated (see *Creatinine ranges in renal failure,* page 700.)
• Creatinine clearance — decreased by more than 90% in ESRD (see *Creatinine ranges in renal failure*, page 700.)
• Serum electrolyte levels — hypernatremia (common), hyperkalemia, hyperphosphatemia, hypocalcemia, elevated calcium-phosphate product, hypermagnesemia
• Venous carbon dioxide (comparable to arterial bicarbonate) levels — decreased
• Arterial blood gas levels — acid-base imbalance, typically metabolic acidosis
• Hemoglobin levels and hematocrit — decreased (hemoglobin usually 6 to 8 mg, hematocrit usually 20% to 25%)

Renal disorders

Creatinine ranges in renal failure

Renal function	Serum creatinine (approximate mg/100 ml)	Creatinine clearance (ml/min)
Normal	1.0 to 1.4	85 to 150
Mild failure	1.5 to 2.0	50 to 84
Moderate failure	2.1 to 6.5	10 to 49
Severe failure	> 6.5	< 10
End-stage failure	> 12	0

Source: Lancaster, L.E., ed. *Core Curriculum for Nephrology Nursing*, 3rd ed. Pitman, N.J.: American Nephrology Nurses' Association, 1995.

• Red blood cell (RBC) count — decreased
• Serum albumin and total protein levels — commonly decreased
• Alkaline phosphatase levels — may be elevated
• White blood cell count — may be elevated
• Electrocardiogram (ECG) — may show abnormal rhythms or altered wave form appearance
• Urinalysis — of minimal diagnostic value in ESRD
• Renal biopsy — indicates the nature and extent of renal disease; necessary to diagnose cause of CRF
• Radionuclide tests (renal scan and renogram) — may show abnormal renal structure and function
• Renal arteriogram — may identify narrowed, stenosed, missing, or misplaced blood vessels
• Plain X-ray of kidneys, ureters, and bladder — may indicate gross structural abnormalities
• Ultrasonography — may indicate gross structural abnormalities
• Computed tomography scan — may show renal masses, abnormal filling of the collecting system, or vascular disorders
   Note: Because CRF commonly coexists with other systemic diseases and because it affects all organ systems and physiologic processes, numerous additional laboratory tests and diagnostic procedures are commonly required to assess the other diseases and systemic consequences of CRF.

Potential complications
• Uncontrollable hypertension
• Hyperkalemia and related cardiac electrical conduction deficits
• Pericarditis, pericardial effusion, or pericardial tamponade
• Pulmonary edema

• Heart failure
• Osteodystrophy
• Metastatic calcium-phosphate calcifications
• Aluminum intoxication
• Profound neurologic impairment
• Profound psychosocial disequilibrium
• Abnormal protein, lipid, and carbohydrate metabolism
• Accelerated atherosclerosis
• Anemia

CLINICAL SNAPSHOT

CHRONIC RENAL FAILURE

Major nursing diagnoses and collaborative problems	Key patient outcomes
Risk for hyperkalemia	Maintain serum potassium levels within acceptable limits as specified by the doctor, ideally 3.5 to 5.5 mEq/L.
Risk for pericarditis, pericardial effusion, and pericardial tamponade	Display no signs of pericarditis, such as fever, chest pain, and pericardial friction rub.
Hypertension	Maintain blood pressure within acceptable limits as specified by the doctor.
Anemia	Maintain a stable hematocrit within a defined range, usually 20% to 25%.
Risk for osteodystrophy and metastatic calcifications	Exhibit serum calcium, phosphorus, alkaline phosphatase, aluminum, and calcium-phosphate product levels within an acceptable range.
Risk for nutritional deficit	Demonstrate ability to weigh self and to maintain weight and intake and output (I&O) records.
Risk for altered oral mucus membrane and unpleasant taste	Maintain clean, moist oral mucous membrane without ulcers, bleeding, or signs of infection.
Risk for peripheral neuropathy	Ambulate and carry out activities of daily living (ADLs) safely and comfortably.
Risk for impaired skin integrity	Maintain clean, intact, infection-free skin.
Risk for altered thought processes	Show no neurologic complications, such as seizures and encephalopathy.
Risk for noncompliance	Express commitment to comply with therapeutic regimen.
Risk for sexual dysfunction	Express concerns about sexual and reproductive functioning with spouse or partner.
Knowledge deficit (vascular access care)	Describe all protective measures appropriate to the vascular access.

Renal disorders

COLLABORATIVE PROBLEM

Risk for hyperkalemia related to decreased renal excretion, metabolic acidosis, excessive dietary intake, blood transfusion, catabolism, and noncompliance with therapeutic regimen

Nursing priorities
• Implement measures to prevent or treat hyperkalemia.
• Monitor their effectiveness.

Patient outcome criteria

• Within 2 hours after treatment is initiated, the patient will:
  – maintain serum potassium levels within acceptable limits as specified by the doctor, ideally 3.5 to 5.5 mEq/L
  – exhibit no signs of hyperkalemia on ECG
  – have an arterial pH of 7.35 to 7.45 and a venous carbon dioxide of 22 to 25 mEq/L (or as defined as acceptable for the patient).
• By the time of discharge, the patient will demonstrate ability to plan a 3-day diet incorporating potassium restrictions and other dietary requirements.

Interventions

1. Monitor serum potassium daily, and notify the doctor if the level exceeds 5.5 mEq/L.

2. Assess and report signs and symptoms of hyperkalemia — slow, irregular pulse; muscle weakness and flaccidity; diarrhea; and ECG changes (tall, tented T wave; ST-segment depression; prolonged PR interval; wide QRS complex; or cardiac standstill, indicating extreme hyperkalemia).

3. Implement measures to prevent or treat metabolic acidosis, as ordered, such as administering alkaline medications (for example, sodium bicarbonate) and maintenance dialysis.

4. If blood transfusions are necessary, administer fresh packed RBCs during dialysis, as ordered.

5. Decrease catabolism by encouraging the patient to consume prescribed amounts of dietary protein and carbohydrates, by treating infections, and by decreasing fever.

6. Encourage compliance with the therapeutic regimen.

7. Implement and evaluate therapy for hyperkalemia, as ordered:
• sodium bicarbonate I.V.

• hypertonic glucose and insulin I.V.

• calcium lactate or calcium gluconate I.V.

• cation-exchange resin (such as Kayexalate)

• dialysis.

Rationales

1. Hyperkalemia causes adverse and even lethal physiologic effects.

2. Cardiovascular signs and symptoms are the most important physiologic indicators of the effects of hyperkalemia.

3. In the acidotic state, hydrogen ions move into the cell to compensate for the acidosis to maintain electrochemical neutrality; potassium ions move out of the cell and into the plasma, producing hyperkalemia.

4. In fresh blood, fewer RBCs have hemolyzed and released potassium as compared with stored blood. Dialysis removes excess potassium.

5. Catabolism causes release of intracellular potassium into the plasma. Appropriate intake of dietary protein reduces breakdown of the body's cells. Infections and fever increase the metabolic rate and can lead to a catabolic state.

6. Dietary noncompliance can result in excessive potassium intake; noncompliance with the dialysis regimen causes hyperkalemia from decreased removal of potassium.

7. Rationales for hyperkalemia therapy include the following:
• Sodium bicarbonate helps correct acidosis and causes potassium to shift from the plasma back into the cells.
• Hypertonic glucose and insulin cause potassium to move from the extracellular to the intracellular space.
• Calcium antagonizes potassium and reduces its potentially deleterious effects on the cardiac conduction system.
• This medication exchanges sodium for potassium and increases potassium excretion through the intestines.
• Hemodialysis rapidly and efficiently removes potassium from the blood; peritoneal dialysis removes potassium at a much slower rate.

8. Monitor serial serum potassium levels and ECG readings for signs of hypokalemia during treatment.

9. Additional individualized interventions: _____

8. Overtreatment of hyperkalemia may result in hypokalemia.

9. Rationales: _____

COLLABORATIVE PROBLEM

Risk for pericarditis, pericardial effusion, and pericardial tamponade related to uremia or inadequate dialysis

Nursing priority

Detect complications and intervene promptly to maintain hemodynamic status.

Patient outcome criteria

With adequate treatment, the patient will exhibit relief of pericarditis (if present), maintenance of hemodynamic status, and prevention of complications as evidenced by:
• blood pressure within defined parameters
• strong, regular peripheral pulses
• normal heart sounds (strong, readily audible apical impulse without friction rub)
• normal temperature
• maintenance of alert and oriented (or usual) mental status
• maintenance of usual respiratory status
• absent or decreased peripheral edema
• ECG without evidence of pericarditis
• maintenance of usual energy level.

Interventions

1. Assess for signs and symptoms of pericarditis daily: fever, chest pain, and pericardial friction rub. Report their occurrence to the doctor.

2. If signs and symptoms of pericarditis are present, collaborate with the nephrology team to assess the adequacy of dialysis and increase frequency as necessary and as ordered.

3. If signs and symptoms of pericarditis are present, assess for signs and symptoms of pericardial effusion and tamponade every 4 hours, as follows:
• Palpate peripheral pulses for rate, quality, waxing, and waning.
• Assess for paradoxical pulse greater than 10 mm Hg.
• Assess for peripheral edema.
• Assess for decrease in sensorium.
• Assess for profound hypotension, narrow pulse pressure, weak or absent peripheral pulses, cold and poorly perfused extremities, rapid decrease in sensorium, and bulging neck veins (signs of rapidly occurring large tamponade).

Rationales

1. Of CRF patients on dialysis, 30% to 50% develop uremic pericarditis; the classic triad of fever, chest pain, and pericardial friction rub is the hallmark of this condition.

2. Inadequate dialysis, with subsequent uremic toxin accumulation, is one cause of pericarditis; intense dialysis therapy is the usual treatment.

3. Pericardial effusion is a common complication that can lead to tamponade, a life-threatening condition. Signs and symptoms vary from mild compromise of cardiac output with small effusion to severely compromised hemodynamic status in tamponade.
   To assess paradoxical pulse, place a blood pressure cuff on the patient's arm and instruct him to breathe normally. Inflate the cuff above the systolic level. Slowly deflate the cuff and note the systolic pressure on expiration. Wait, reinflate the cuff, and deflate it again, this time noting the systolic pressure on inspiration. The difference between the two readings is the paradoxical pulse. A paradoxical pulse of 10 mm Hg or less indicates a normal blood pressure response to inspiration. A value greater than 10 mm Hg indicates an exaggerated response to inspiration typical of cardiac tamponade.

Renal disorders

4. If tamponade develops, prepare the patient for emergency pericardial aspiration.

4. The mortality rate in tamponade is 95%. Immediate aspiration of fluid from the pericardial cavity is essential to restore cardiac function and hemodynamic status.

5. Encourage compliance with the therapeutic regimen.

5. Dialysis removes uremic toxins that can cause pericarditis. Dialysis combined with fluid restriction reduces the risk of effusion.

6. Additional individualized interventions: _____

6. Rationales: _____

_____

COLLABORATIVE PROBLEM

Hypertension related to sodium and water retention and malfunction of the renin-angiotensin-aldosterone system

Nursing priority

Implement the therapeutic regimen and patient teaching to control hypertension.

Patient outcome criteria

• Throughout the hospital stay, the patient will:
  – maintain blood pressure within acceptable limits
  – show no hypertensive complications.
• By the time of discharge, the patient will demonstrate ability to measure blood pressure and pulse rate.

Interventions

1. Administer antihypertensive medications, as ordered, and assess for desired and adverse effects. Reassure the patient that some adverse effects may decrease once the body adjusts to the medication.

2. With the doctor, determine an acceptable range for the patient's blood pressure. Measure blood pressure at various times of the day with the patient supine, sitting, and standing. Record blood pressure readings on a flow sheet to correlate the influence of time of day, positioning, medications, diet, and weight. Teach the patient to measure blood pressure and pulse rate.

3. Teach the patient how to avoid orthostatic hypotension by changing position slowly, such as sitting for 5 minutes when changing from a supine to a standing position.

4. Encourage compliance with therapy.

5. Instruct the patient to report any changes that may indicate fluid overload, hypertensive encephalopathy, or vision changes. These include periorbital, sacral, or peripheral edema; headaches; seizures; and blurred vision.

Rationales

1. Antihypertensive medications are an essential part of treatment of CRF. Antihypertensives act by vasodilation, beta-adrenergic blocking, angiotensin blocking, alpha$_1$-adrenergic receptor blocking, or calcium channel blocking. Reassurance helps prevent noncompliance because of initial adverse effects.

2. Blood pressure measurements commonly vary throughout the day and in relation to medication administration, diet, weight, and positioning. Excessive doses of antihypertensives or dehydration can cause orthostatic hypotension.

3. Orthostatic hypotension may cause falls and injuries. Medication noncompliance may result if the patient is unable to prevent orthostatic hypotension.

4. Dialysis removes sodium and water and controls vascular volume; diet restrictions prevent excessive sodium and fluid intake.

5. These signs and symptoms may indicate poor control of hypertension and the need to alter therapy.

6. Recognize the significance of funduscopic changes reported on medical or nursing examination: arteriovenous nicking, exudates, hemorrhages, and papilledema.

7. Additional individualized interventions: _____

6. These conditions suggest uncontrolled hypertension and the need to reevaluate the therapeutic regimen.

7. Rationales: _____

COLLABORATIVE PROBLEM

Anemia related to decreased life span of RBCs in CRF, bleeding, decreased production of erythropoietin and RBCs, and blood loss during hemodialysis

Nursing priorities

- Stabilize the RBC count.
- Maximize tissue perfusion.

Patient outcome criteria

Throughout the hospital stay, the patient will:
- maintain a stable hematocrit within a defined range, usually 20% to 25%
- exhibit symptomatic relief of the effects of anemia
- verbalize ways to protect self from trauma
- perform ADLs without undue fatigue.

Interventions

1. Assess daily the degree of anemia (as reflected by hemoglobin level, hematocrit, and RBC count) and its physiologic effects, such as fatigue, pallor, dyspnea, palpitations, ecchymoses, and tachycardia.

2. Administer the following as ordered, and assess for desired and adverse effects: iron and folic acid supplements, vitamin B complex, vitamin C, and epoetin alfa (Epogen). Do not administer folic acid and vitamins during dialysis or iron with phosphate binders.

3. Assist the patient to develop an activity and exercise schedule, with regular rest periods, to avoid undue fatigue.

4. Avoid taking unnecessary blood specimens.

5. Instruct the patient how to prevent bleeding: using a soft toothbrush, avoiding vigorous nose blowing, preventing constipation, and avoiding contact sports.

6. Administer blood transfusions as indicated and ordered.

7. Additional individualized interventions: _____

Rationales

1. The severity of anemia and its physiologic effects vary. The therapeutic plan is based on anemia's effects on the individual patient.

2. Iron, folic acid, and vitamins are required for RBC production, but are commonly deficient in the CRF patient's diet. Like endogenous erythropoietin, epoetin alfa (erythropoietin produced through recombinant DNA techniques) stimulates RBC production. However, the patient's iron stores must be adequate for epoetin alfa to be effective. Dialysis removes folic acid and vitamins. Phosphate binders decrease iron absorption.

3. Decreased hemoglobin decreases tissue oxygenation and increases fatigue. A carefully developed plan of activity and exercise can lessen fatigue and allow the patient to perform ADLs.

4. Frequent collection of blood specimens worsens anemia.

5. Bleeding from any site worsens anemia.

6. Blood transfusions are administered only when the patient becomes symptomatic with low hematocrit; frequent blood transfusions suppress RBC production even further. Fresh packed RBCs are administered during dialysis, as noted previously.

7. Rationales: _____

Renal disorders

COLLABORATIVE PROBLEM

Risk for osteodystrophy and metastatic calcifications related to hyperphosphatemia, hypocalcemia, abnormal vitamin D metabolism, hyperparathyroidism, and elevated aluminum levels

Nursing priority

Minimize bone demineralization and metastatic calcifications.

Patient outcome criteria

Throughout the hospital stay, the patient will:
• exhibit serum calcium, phosphorus, alkaline phosphatase, aluminum, and calcium-phosphate product levels within an acceptable range
• exhibit minimal bone demineralization on bone scan
• exhibit minimal calcium-phosphate deposits
• show no signs or symptoms of hypocalcemia, such as numbness or tingling fingertips and toes
• maintain a safe, painless level of activity.

Interventions

1. Administer phosphate binders, calcium supplements, and vitamin D supplements, as ordered, and assess their effects:
• Weekly, monitor serum levels of calcium, phosphate, alkaline phosphatase, aluminum, and calcium-phosphate product; report abnormal findings to the doctor.
• Monitor X-rays for bone fractures and joint deposits.
• Weekly, palpate joints for enlargement, swelling, and tenderness.
• Weekly, inspect the patient's gait, range of motion in joints, and muscle strength.

2. With the patient, develop an activity and exercise schedule to avoid immobilization.

3. Daily, question the patient about signs and symptoms of hypocalcemia: numbness, tingling, and twitching of fingertips and toes; carpopedal spasms; seizures; and confusion.

4. Monitor each ECG (or ECG report) for prolonged QT interval, irritable arrhythmias, and atrioventricular conduction defects.

Rationales

1. In renal failure, the decreased glomerular filtration rate causes phosphate retention and hyperphosphatemia; plasma calcium levels decrease to compensate. Decreased vitamin D metabolism by the kidneys decreases calcium absorption from the GI tract. The decrease in plasma calcium levels stimulates production of parathyroid hormone, which causes reabsorption of calcium and phosphate from the bones and eventual bone demineralization.

As plasma calcium and phosphate levels rise, the plasma calcium phosphate product level also rises; the excess calcium phosphate is deposited as metastatic calcifications in joints, soft tissue, eyes, heart, and brain. These metastatic calcifications decrease function of the involved organs. Administering phosphate binders, such as aluminum hydroxide (Amphojel), aluminum carbonate (Basaljel), calcium carbonate (BioCal), or calcium acetate (Phos-Lo), with meals binds phosphate in the GI tract and decreases its absorption. Calcium and vitamin D supplements help support normal plasma calcium levels.

Excess aluminum (absorbed from phosphate binders and from high levels of aluminum in water used to prepare dialysate) is deposited into the bones and exacerbates osteodystrophy.

2. Immobilization increases bone demineralization.

3. Hypocalcemia causes nervous system irritability and alters nerve conduction. The signs and symptoms listed indicate tetany, hypocalcemia's most obvious manifestation.

4. Hypocalcemia can alter normal cardiac electrical conduction.

5. Daily, assess for positive Chvostek's and Trousseau's signs. See Appendix C, Fluid and Electrolyte Imbalances, for details.

6. Encourage the patient to comply with therapy.

7. Additional individualized interventions: _____

_____

5. Positive Chvostek's and Trousseau's signs indicate hypocalcemia.

6. Dialysis, medications, and diet work together to maintain acceptable calcium-phosphate balance.

7. Rationales: _____

_____

NURSING DIAGNOSIS

Risk for nutritional deficit related to anorexia, nausea, vomiting, diarrhea, restricted dietary intake, GI inflammation with poor absorption, and altered metabolism of proteins, lipids, and carbohydrates

Nursing priority

Maintain acceptable nutritional status.

Patient outcome criteria

- During the hospital stay, the patient will:
  – maintain weight within 2 lb (5 kg) of ideal body weight
  – exhibit BUN, serum sodium, potassium, albumin, and total protein levels within acceptable limits
  – maintain preillness pattern of elimination.
- By the time of discharge, the patient will:
  – plan a 3-day dietary intake (including fluid)
  – demonstrate ability to weigh self and to maintain weight and I&O records.

Interventions

1. Assess nutritional status on admission by determining weight in relation to height and body build; serum albumin, protein, cholesterol, and transferrin values; triceps skinfold thickness; degree of weakness and fatigue; dietary intake; and history of anorexia, nausea, vomiting, and diarrhea.

2. Weigh the patient daily, comparing actual and ideal body weights. Be sure to consider the effect of excess fluid on actual weight by comparing the current weight with nonedematous weight (500 ml fluid = 1 lb body weight). Teach the patient to measure weight under consistent conditions, to maintain a weight record, and to maintain an I&O record.

3. Encourage the patient to eat the maximum amount of nutrients allowed. Encourage compliance with the dialysis regimen.

4. Encourage intake of foods high in calories from carbohydrates and low in protein, potassium, sodium, and water. Provide related teaching, including planning of food and fluid intake.

5. As necessary, consult with a dietitian to find ways to include the patient's preferences in the prescribed diet.

6. Implement interventions to reduce nausea and vomiting, diarrhea or constipation, and stomatitis.

Rationales

1. A baseline assessment is necessary to monitor progress and the need to modify the patient's diet.

2. Achieving ideal body weight is the goal. If the patient weighs less than the ideal body weight, additional calories may be added to the diet; if more, calorie restriction may be necessary.

3. Diet and dialysis must complement each other to minimize toxin accumulation and maintain fluid and electrolyte and acid-base balance.

4. High-carbohydrate foods provide calories for energy and allow storage of dietary proteins. Restriction of potassium, sodium, and water is necessary to prevent electrolyte imbalances and volume overload. Protein is restricted to control the degree of uremia.

5. Including preferred foods makes the diet more palatable and increases dietary compliance.

6. These conditions commonly result in anorexia or decreased GI absorption of nutrients.

Renal disorders

7. Monitor BUN, serum creatinine, sodium, potassium, albumin, and total protein levels as indicators of dietary adequacy and compliance with dietary restrictions. (Consult with the doctor regarding appropriate laboratory values for the patient.)

7. BUN levels may be elevated from excessive dietary protein; serum creatinine levels may be elevated from inadequate dietary protein and subsequent muscle breakdown; serum albumin levels are decreased in the malnourished patient; serum sodium and potassium levels are elevated by excessive intake. Appropriate laboratory values vary depending on the type of dialysis and other therapeutic measures, and so must be determined for the individual patient.

8. Additional individualized interventions: _____

8. Rationales: _____

NURSING DIAGNOSIS

Risk for altered oral mucous membrane and unpleasant taste related to accumulation of urea and ammonia

Nursing priorities
• Maintain intact oral mucous membrane.
• Relieve unpleasant taste.

Patient outcome criteria

Throughout the hospital stay, the patient will:
• maintain clean, moist oral mucous membrane without ulcers, bleeding, or signs of infection
• report pleasant taste and sensation in mouth.

Interventions

1. On admission, inspect oral mucous membrane for ulcers and bleeding.

2. Teach the patient an appropriate mouth care regimen that includes rinsing with a pleasant-tasting or dilute vinegar mouthwash as needed, using a soft toothbrush to clean teeth at least twice daily, sucking sour candies or lemon wedges as needed, and drinking cool liquids (within fluid restrictions).

3. Encourage the patient to comply with therapy.

4. Additional individualized interventions: _____

Rationales

1. Early detection and treatment can lessen consequences of severe stomatitis. (Excessive uremic toxins cause stomatitis.)

2. Mouthwash decreases unpleasant taste and halitosis. Vinegar achieves the same results by neutralizing ammonia. A soft toothbrush reduces the risk of bleeding, and frequent mouth care decreases bacterial growth and the chance of infection. Sour candies or lemon wedges improve taste in the mouth while decreasing thirst.

3. Dialysis removes uremic toxins, which are partly responsible for stomatitis.

4. Rationales: _____

COLLABORATIVE PROBLEM

Risk for peripheral neuropathy related to effects of uremia, fluid and electrolyte imbalances, and acid-base imbalances on the peripheral nervous system

Nursing priority

Ameliorate effects of peripheral neuropathy.

Patient outcome criterion

Throughout the hospital stay, the patient will ambulate and carry out ADLs safely and comfortably.

Interventions	Rationales
1. On admission, have a physical therapist assess muscle strength, gait, and degree of neuromuscular impairment.	**1.** A baseline assessment is essential for devising an individualized activity and exercise schedule.
2. In collaboration with a physical therapist, help the patient develop an activity and exercise regimen.	**2.** Regular activity and exercise prevent the hazards of immobility.
3. Guard against leg and foot trauma.	**3.** With decreased peripheral sensation, the patient may be unaware of impending trauma.
4. Administer analgesics as ordered and indicated; observe for desired effects.	**4.** Analgesics may be necessary for severe pain; if the medication ordered is excreted by the kidneys, observe for toxic effects.
5. Encourage the patient to comply with therapy.	**5.** Dialysis removes uremic toxins and improves fluid and electrolyte and acid-base balance.
6. Additional individualized interventions: _____	**6.** Rationales: _____

NURSING DIAGNOSIS

Risk for impaired skin integrity related to decreased activity of oil and sweat glands, scratching, capillary fragility, abnormal blood clotting, anemia, retention of pigments, and calcium phosphate deposits on the skin

Nursing priorities
• Maintain intact skin.
• Relieve dryness and itching.

Patient outcome criteria

Throughout the hospital stay, the patient will:
• maintain intact, clean, infection-free skin
• exhibit relief from dryness and itching.

Interventions	Rationales
1. On admission and twice daily, assess skin for color, turgor, ecchymoses, texture, and edema.	**1.** A baseline assessment is essential for developing an individualized plan of skin care. Regular follow-up assessments allow modification as necessary.
2. Keep the skin clean while relieving dryness and itching using superfatted soap, oatmeal baths, and bath oils; apply lotion daily and as needed, especially while the skin is still moist after bathing.	**2.** These measures help relieve dry skin. Applying lotion immediately after bathing helps the skin retain moisture. Itching decreases when the skin is kept moist; decreased itching prevents scratching and subsequent skin excoriation.
3. Keep the patient's nails trimmed.	**3.** Trimming prevents excoriation from scratching.
4. Monitor serum calcium and phosphorus levels weekly.	**4.** Excess calcium phosphate deposited in the skin causes dryness and itching.
5. Administer phosphate binders, as ordered.	**5.** These medications decrease serum phosphate levels and thus lessen irritating deposits in the skin.

6. Administer antipruritic medications as indicated and ordered; assess effects.

7. Encourage the patient to comply with therapy.

8. Additional individualized interventions: _____
_____

6. These medications are indicated in severe pruritus when other measures are not effective.

7. Dialysis removes uremic toxins that dry and irritate the skin and helps normalize serum calcium and phosphorus levels.

8. Rationales: _____
_____

NURSING DIAGNOSIS

Risk for altered thought processes related to the effects of uremic toxins, acidosis, fluid and electrolyte imbalances, and hypoxia on the central nervous system

Nursing priority

Protect the patient from neurologic complications.

Patient outcome criteria

By the time of discharge, the patient will:
• show improved memory and reasoning ability
• show an increased interest in ADLs
• show no neurologic complications, such as seizures and encephalopathy.

Interventions

1. On admission and daily, assess the patient's thought processes. With assistance from the family, compare current findings with premorbid intellectual status.

2. Alter communication methods as needed.

3. Minimize environmental stimuli. Alter the environment as needed to ensure the patient's safety.

4. Do not administer opiates or barbiturates.

5. Encourage the patient to comply with therapy, including following dietary restrictions, undergoing dialysis, and taking epoetin alfa as directed.

6. Additional individualized interventions: _____
_____

Rationales

1. The premorbid status provides guidelines for establishing realistic goals. Ongoing assessment allows prompt detection of any changes and modification of treatment as needed.

2. The patient will typically require short periods of simple communication, responding best to direct questions.

3. Excessive environmental stimuli may cause sensory overload and disorientation. The patient usually functions best in a consistently quiet, organized environment that is free from hazards.

4. Opiates and barbiturates have an increased half-life in renal failure. Mental status worsens as a result.

5. Dietary restrictions and dialysis are essential to control uremic toxin buildup and fluid and electrolyte and acid-base balance, and to reduce the risk of adverse effects on the central nervous system. Epoetin alfa enhances RBC production, increasing oxygen delivery to the brain.

6. Rationales: _____
_____

NURSING DIAGNOSIS

Risk for noncompliance related to knowledge deficit; lack of resources; adverse effects of diet, dialysis, and medications; denial; and lack of social support systems

Nursing priority

Help the patient make informed choices about compliance and noncompliance.

Patient outcome criteria

- Throughout the hospital stay, the patient will:
  - state knowledge of the therapeutic regimen
  - express commitment to comply with therapeutic regimen or a realistic treatment alternative more in keeping with personal beliefs and lifestyle.
- By the time of discharge, the patient will:
  - explain the cause and implications of the disease
  - name each medication and its dosage, interval, desired effects, and adverse effects
  - describe associated problems, how to manage them, and when to report them
  - explain the plan for follow-up care.

Interventions

1. Clarify the patient's understanding of the therapeutic regimen and the consequences of noncompliance.

2. Assess for physiologic, psychological, social, and cultural factors that could contribute to noncompliance. Explore ways to alter treatment to fit the patient's social and cultural beliefs.

3. Teach the patient about the therapeutic regimen, including medications, common problems related to CRF and their management, and plans for follow-up care. Clarify areas of misunderstanding in relation to the disease and therapeutic regimen. Allow the patient to make as many informed decisions and choices from as many alternatives as possible.

4. Additional individualized interventions: _____

Rationales

1. In many cases, noncompliance results from the patient's lack of understanding about the nature of the disease and the objectives of therapy.

2. Many patients deny that they have a chronic, irreversible illness. Compliance is more likely if treatment is congruent with the patient's beliefs.

3. The patient is more likely to comply if encouraged to participate in decision making and allowed maximum independence. Thus, each patient requires an individualized plan of care that considers physiologic, psychosocial, and cultural factors and the patient's desires.

4. Rationales: _____

NURSING DIAGNOSIS

Risk for sexual dysfunction related to the effects of uremia on the endocrine and nervous systems and to the psychosocial impact of CRF and its treatment

Nursing priority

Help the patient and spouse (or partner) achieve satisfying sexual expression.

Patient outcome criteria

Throughout the hospital stay, the patient will:
- express concerns about sexual and reproductive functioning with spouse or partner
- express satisfaction with sexual relationship with spouse or partner.

Interventions

1. Discuss with the patient and spouse (or partner) the meaning of sexuality and reproduction to them, how changes in sexual functioning affect masculine and feminine roles, and mutual goals for their sexual functioning.

2. Evaluate the couple's receptiveness to learning, and discuss alternative methods of sexual expression.

3. Emphasize the importance of giving and receiving love and affection as alternatives to intercourse.

4. Consult with the doctor about the appropriateness of a penile prosthesis for a male patient, if indicated.

5. Additional individualized interventions: _____
_____

Rationales

1. Sexuality and reproduction assume different levels of significance at various stages of maturity and at various times during CRF. Sex drive varies from person to person; therefore, sexuality and reproduction are very personal experiences. Sexual dysfunction affects sex role in many ways, based on past experiences and future expectations. Thus, the nurse must explore sexuality with the couple to establish baseline data and to determine their mutual goals.

2. If impotence or decreased libido is present or if intercourse causes fatigue, and if the couple is receptive to experimentation, then fellatio, cunnilingus, or mutual masturbation may provide sexual gratification.

3. Sexual intercourse and orgasm are not necessarily the goal of all meaningful intimate interactions: Love and affection are also important in strengthening a relationship.

4. If a male patient cannot achieve or maintain an erection, a penile prosthesis may provide a means for successful intercourse.

5. Rationales: _____
_____

NURSING DIAGNOSIS

Knowledge deficit (vascular access care) related to lack of exposure to information

Nursing priority

Teach the patient about care and precautions related to vascular access. (If the patient is receiving peritoneal dialysis, consult the "Peritoneal dialysis" plan, page 731.)

Patient outcome criteria

Throughout the hospital stay, the patient will:
• describe all protective measures appropriate to the vascular access
• correctly demonstrate the procedure for checking fistula patency
• describe specific measures to control bleeding
• state how to contact a nephrology professional.

Interventions

1. Emphasize the patient's crucial role in protecting the vascular access.

Rationales

1. The vascular access is essential for hemodialysis. Loss of access may disrupt the dialysis schedule and require surgery. Various vascular access methods may be used. The most common is the internal arteriovenous fistula, an internal surgical anastomosis of an artery and vein. It usually is placed in the nondominant forearm and requires 2 to 3 months for the venous wall to thicken and the fistula to distend. The major complications are occlusion and postdialysis bleeding.

2. Explain these activity restrictions for the affected extremity:
• Do not wear constrictive clothing or jewelry.
• Do not carry heavy objects.
• Do not allow blood pressure measurements.
• Do not allow venipunctures for I.V. fluids or laboratory blood specimens.
• Do not lie on the access.

3. Teach these additional measures to maintain fistula patency:
• Assess patency daily by feeling for pulsation at the anastomosis site.

• If pulsation is absent, contact a nephrology professional immediately.
• If a pressure dressing is applied after dialysis, remove it after 4 hours.

• Check needle insertion sites for bleeding for 4 hours after dialysis, or longer if bleeding occurs.

4. Additional individualized interventions: _____

2. These activities threaten the integrity of the vascular access and may cause occlusion, dislodgment, or infection.

3. These interventions protect the patency of the internal fistula:
• Because the fistula is internal, patency cannot be determined visually. Pulsation is caused by the surge of arterial blood into the vein to which the artery has been anastomosed.
• Loss of pulsation implies impending loss of patency. A clotted fistula may require surgery.
• Direct pressure on the venipuncture sites is necessary to control bleeding. Usually 10 minutes of firm finger pressure is sufficient, but at times a pressure dressing may be applied. If left on too long, a pressure dressing may cause occlusion.
• Because the patient is heparinized during hemodialysis, bleeding may occur after dialysis.

4. Rationales: _____

DISCHARGE PLANNING

Discharge checklist
Before discharge, the patient shows evidence of:
❑ ability to perform care of the fistula
❑ vital signs within expected parameters
❑ stable nutritional status
❑ intact skin
❑ ability to control pain using oral medications
❑ acceptable hemoglobin levels
❑ absence of pulmonary complications
❑ absence of cardiovascular complications
❑ ability to comply with and tolerate diet and fluid restrictions
❑ weight within expected parameters
❑ home support adequate to ensure compliance with therapy or appropriate referrals made for follow-up care
❑ appropriate activity tolerance
❑ absence of fever and other signs of infection
❑ ability to manage ADLs.

Teaching checklist
Document evidence that the patient and family demonstrate an understanding of:
❑ cause and implications of renal failure
❑ purpose of dialysis

❑ all discharge medications' purpose, dosage, administration schedule, desired effects, and adverse effects (usual discharge medications include antihypertensives, phosphate binders, calcium, vitamin D, folic acid, iron, vitamins B and C, and others, depending on patient's response to the disease)
❑ recommended diet and fluid modifications
❑ common problems related to CRF and their management
❑ care of the fistula (if receiving hemodialysis)
❑ how to obtain and record weights
❑ how to measure and record blood pressure and pulse rate
❑ how to maintain an I&O record
❑ problems to report to health care provider
❑ financial and community resources to assist with treatment of CRF
❑ dialysis schedule, location of dialysis facility, and day and time of appointments
❑ resources for counseling
❑ how to contact the doctor or nephrology nurse.

Documentation checklist
Using outcome criteria as a guide, document:
❑ clinical status on admission
❑ significant changes in status
❑ pertinent laboratory and diagnostic test findings

Renal disorders

❏ response to medication
❏ physical and psychological response to dialysis
❏ nutritional intake
❏ activity and exercise tolerance
❏ ability to perform self-care
❏ compliance with therapy
❏ patient and family teaching
❏ discharge planning (postdischarge referrals and plans for long-term and follow-up care).

ASSOCIATED PLANS OF CARE

Anemia
Dying
Grieving
Ineffective individual coping
Knowledge deficit
Pain
Peritoneal dialysis

REFERENCES

Brundage, D.J. *Renal Disorders.* St. Louis: Mosby–Year Book, Inc., 1992.

Greenberg, A., ed. *Primer on Kidney Diseases.* San Diego: Academic Press, 1994.

Ignatavicius, D.D., et al. *Medical-Surgical Nursing: A Nursing Process Approach.* Philadelphia: W.B. Saunders Co., 1995.

Lancaster, L.E., ed. *Core Curriculum for Nephrology Nursing*, 3rd ed. Pitman, N.J.: American Nephrology Nurses' Association, 1995.

McCance, K.L., and Huether, S.E. *Pathophysiology: The Biologic Basis for Disease in Adults and Children*, 2nd ed. St. Louis: Mosby–Year Book, Inc., 1994.

Ileal conduit urinary diversion

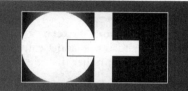

DRG information
DRG 303   Kidney, Ureter, and Major Bladder Procedure for Neoplasm.
Mean LOS = 10.2 days
DRG 304   Kidney, Ureter, and Major Bladder Procedure for Nonneoplasm with Complication or Comorbidity (CC).
Mean LOS = 10.3 days
DRG 305   Kidney, Ureter, and Major Bladder Procedure for Nonneoplasm without CC.
Mean LOS = 4.9 days

INTRODUCTION

Definition and time focus
An ileal conduit urinary diversion, also known as a urostomy or Bricker procedure, is the most common urinary diversion procedure for adults. It is usually performed with a cystectomy and involves isolating a 6½″ to 8½″ (15 to 20.5 cm) segment of the terminal ileum, with its mesentery intact, then reanastomosing the GI tract. The proximal end of the isolated ileal segment is sutured closed, and the distal end of the ileal segment is brought out through the right lower abdominal quadrant and everted to form a stoma. The ureters are implanted into the body of the ileal segment, which then becomes a conduit for urine. Other segments of the small or large intestine can be used as conduits for urinary diversion, especially if the ileum has been damaged by radiation.

Ileal conduit urinary diversion is most commonly performed for transitional cell cancer of the bladder; however, in rare instances, it may also be done for other conditions requiring total cystectomy, such as severe trauma to the bladder or persistent, severe urinary tract infections. This plan focuses on the immediate preoperative and postoperative care of a patient undergoing ileal conduit diversion for transitional cell cancer of the bladder.

Etiology and precipitating factors
• Transitional cell carcinoma, accounting for 90% of bladder cancers that require cystectomy — that is, lesions unresponsive to conservative treatment, lesions found at or near the bladder neck in the female, or deep infiltrating tumors that may involve the lymphatic system

FOCUSED ASSESSMENT GUIDELINES

Nursing history (functional health pattern findings)
Health perception–health management pattern
• Sudden onset of gross painless hematuria, which may be intermittent
• Treatment for transitional cell carcinoma of the bladder (being followed by cystoscopy every 3 to 6 months)
• History of intravesical instillations of chemotherapeutic agents, such as thiotepa (Thioplex), mitomycin-C (Mutamycin), or doxorubicin (Adriamycin), after transurethral resection of a bladder tumor, or may have received intravesical bacillus Calmette-Guérin (BCG; TheraCys) as prophylactic treatment against tumor recurrence
• Preoperative radiation therapy to shrink the tumor and reduce spread at the time of surgery
• Fluorouracil (5-FU) use for recurrent or progressive invasive bladder cancer
• Photodynamic techniques, which cause cancer cells to retain toxic chemicals
• Limited information received from doctor about upcoming urinary diversion surgery and its effects on activities of daily living (ADLs)
• Increased risk if patient is between ages 50 and 70
• Cigarette smoker (increases risk of bladder cancer)
Elimination pattern
• History of urinary urgency or frequency for 3 to 8 months before diagnosis of transitional cell carcinoma of bladder
• Cystitis as an adverse effect of intravesical chemotherapy
Sleep-rest pattern
• Sleep disturbances from nocturia
Self-perception–self-concept pattern
• Expressed negative feelings about self, along with anger; disappointment; fear of pain, mutilation, and loss of control; and distaste for altered bodily functions
Role-relationship pattern
• Occupational exposure to dust and fumes from dyes, rubber, leather, leather products, paint, or organic chemicals (increases risk of bladder cancer)
• Concern about spouse's or partner's adjustment to ostomy and possibility that ostomy may change that person's feelings toward the patient
• Concerns about sexual dysfunction following cystectomy

Coping–stress tolerance pattern
• With recent diagnosis of bladder cancer, concern about cancer treatment rather than the creation of an ostomy

Value-belief pattern
• Delay in seeking medical attention because of fear combined with embarrassment over the intimate nature of problem

Physical findings
Transitional cell carcinoma may be asymptomatic except for the following genitourinary symptoms.

Genitourinary
• Gross hematuria
• Urgency, frequency, and dysuria unrelieved by antibiotics

Diagnostic studies
• Complete blood count — drop in hematocrit and hemoglobin level may indicate internal bleeding; elevated white blood cell count may signify beginning of infection or abscess
• Electrolyte panel — monitors fluid status and acid-base balance
• Serum creatinine and blood urea nitrogen levels — used to monitor renal function
• Preoperative excretory urography — helpful in evaluating upper urinary tract functioning; size and location of kidneys, filling of the renal pelvis, and outline of ureters
• Postoperative conduitogram or loopogram — assesses length and emptying ability of the conduit along with the presence or absence of stricture, reflux, angulation, or obstruction
• X-ray of kidneys, ureter, and bladder — indicates structural changes in the urinary tract along with presence or absence of stool or gas in GI tract

Potential complications
• Peritonitis
• Leakage at point of GI anastomosis
• Leakage at proximal end of the conduit
• Ureteral-ileum anastomotic leakage
• Abscess formation
• Thrombophlebitis
• Stoma necrosis
• Ureteral obstruction from edema or mucus
• Wound dehiscence
• Small-bowel obstruction
• Pneumonia
• Ileus
• Atelectasis
• Wound infection
• Mucocutaneous separation around stoma

CLINICAL SNAPSHOT

ILEAL CONDUIT URINARY DIVERSION

Major nursing diagnoses and collaborative problems	Key patient outcomes
Preoperative knowledge deficit (care of an ileal conduit)	On request, express understanding of upcoming surgery and its expected effects.
Risk for postoperative peritonitis	Show no signs of peritonitis.
Risk for stoma ischemia and necrosis	Have a viable stoma with red, moist mucosa.
Risk for stoma retraction and mucocutaneous separation	Have a healed mucocutaneous border around a budded stoma.
Altered urinary elimination	Describe normal stoma and urine characteristics after creation of an ileal conduit.
Body image disturbance	Express feelings about the ostomy.
Postoperative knowledge deficit (care of the ileal conduit)	Change the pouch two to three times with minimal assistance from the nurse.
Risk for sexual dysfunction	Ask questions about impact on sexual function or agree to appropriate referrals.

NURSING DIAGNOSIS

Preoperative knowledge deficit (care of an ileal conduit) related to lack of exposure to information

Nursing priority

Prepare the patient physically and emotionally for upcoming urinary tract alterations.

Patient outcome criterion

Before surgery, the patient will express understanding of upcoming surgery and its expected effects.

Interventions

1. Assess what the patient already knows about the upcoming cystectomy and creation of an ileal conduit from information the doctor has provided or from someone who has had an ostomy.

2. Assess the patient's ability to learn. Check occupation, level of education, and hobbies, and note if the patient may have difficulty learning.

3. Assess the patient's manual dexterity and visual acuity, and determine if any sensory deficits are present. Enlist the help of a family member, if possible and appropriate. Allow the patient to see and handle a pouch at eye level before surgery.

4. Inquire about the patient's past and recent fluid intake habits, especially quantity and preferred types of fluids.

5. Describe construction of the conduit, bowel preparation, and normal stoma characteristics.

6. Anticipate problems with pouch use. Assess the patient for allergies or sensitivity to tape or adhesives.

7. Request a doctor's order for an enterostomal (ET) nurse to mark the stoma site before surgery. This mark should place stoma away from old scars, dimples, the umbilicus, belt line, fat folds, and skin creases, and within the rectus muscle in a spot the patient can see. The stoma may be placed above the umbilicus in an obese patient or one who uses a wheelchair.

8. If the patient is male, discuss what effect the cystectomy may have on sexual functioning. Explain that a urologist or sexual therapist can give him more information in the future.

9. Additional individualized interventions: _____

Rationales

1. The patient may have received limited or confusing information from the doctor. If the patient has known anyone with an ostomy, impressions gained from that person will strongly influence personal expectations of surgery and adaptation to the ostomy.

2. Learning difficulties, especially reduced reading ability, will affect the strategy and literature used to teach ostomy care.

3. Degree of dexterity will affect the patient's ability to care for the stoma and apply a pouch effectively. If the patient cannot care for the stoma, a family member is the best substitute. Handling the pouch before surgery increases later adaptation.

4. Inadequate fluid intake may cause odor problems from urine concentration and peristomal skin problems from dehydration.

5. The patient should know that an ileal conduit is not a substitute bladder. Bowel preparation usually consists of 1 to 2 days of a clear liquid diet, a bowel-cleansing oral liquid such as polyethylene glycol and electrolyte solution the day before surgery, and then nothing by mouth after midnight the night before surgery.

6. Any allergy to these products suggests a need to patch-test the patient for sensitivity before selecting ostomy equipment.

7. The stoma should be marked where the pouch will have an optimal seal, giving the patient some sense of control. Placing the stoma within the rectus muscle reduces the risk of hernia or prolapse. To achieve independence, the patient must be able to see the stoma.

8. Informed legal consent includes the male patient's understanding that erectile dysfunction can be expected along with ejaculatory incompetence. It is important to give the patient "permission" to discuss sexual concerns.

9. Rationales: _____

COLLABORATIVE PROBLEM

Risk for postoperative peritonitis related to GI or genitourinary anastomosis breakdown or leakage

Nursing priority

Prevent and assess for signs of peritonitis.

Patient outcome criteria

- Within 1 to 2 days after surgery, the patient will:
  – have stabilized urine output
  – have no gross hematuria.
- Within 4 to 5 days after surgery, the patient will:
  – pass flatus
  – have normal bowel sounds
  – be afebrile
  – show no signs of peritonitis.

Interventions

1. Monitor and document nasogastric (NG) tube patency, NG output, abdominal pain and distention, bowel sounds, and appearance of and drainage from the abdominal incision.

2. Evaluate for signs of GI anastomosis leakage and peritonitis, such as paralytic ileus and abdominal pain with muscle rigidity, vomiting, and leukocytosis.

3. Monitor for signs of urine leakage. Assess carefully for pouch leakage to allow for accurate output measurement. Document characteristics of urine output and presence of ureteral stents or catheters. When changing pouch (if necessary because of leakage), observe that urine is dripping from *each* stent. Also note abdominal wound drainage, abdominal tenderness or distention, bowel sounds, and temperature.

4. Additional individualized interventions: _____

Rationales

1. Adynamic ileus usually resolves within 72 hours after surgery. Changes in NG output, rapid abdominal distention, and crampy pain with hyperactive and tinkling bowel sounds may indicate small-bowel obstruction. Obstruction increases pressure on newly anastomosed sites.

2. A GI anastomosis is weakest until the fourth day after surgery. Leakage of intestinal secretions may result in peritonitis. I.V. fluids, electrolyte replacement, intestinal decompression, and appropriate I.V. antibiotic therapy are indicated if peritonitis is present.

3. Urine should be blood-tinged for only 1 to 2 days after surgery. Improper pouch fit or application can cause ongoing stomal bleeding. Ureteral stents prevent ureteral obstruction from edema or mucus; it is normal for urine to flow out around the stents. Signs of urine leakage may include a sudden decrease in urine output with a corresponding increase in drainage from the wound or a drain. Abdominal distention, an increase in abdominal pain, prolonged ileus, and fever may also indicate urine leakage. Small leaks may seal themselves within 8 to 12 hours; otherwise, surgery is needed.

4. Rationales: _____

COLLABORATIVE PROBLEM

Risk for stoma ischemia and necrosis related to vascular compromise of conduit

Nursing priority

Monitor stoma viability.

Patient outcome criterion

Immediately postoperatively and then continuously, the patient will have a viable stoma with red, moist mucosa.

Interventions

1. Apply a disposable transparent urinary pouch, as ordered, and attach the pouch to a bedside drainage bag.

2. Observe the stoma for color changes every 4 hours and as needed.

3. Report color change of stoma (to purple, brown, or black) immediately to the doctor.

4. To differentiate superficial ischemia from necrosis, insert a small, lubricated test tube about ½″ (1.3 cm) into the stoma, then shine a flashlight into the lumen of the test tube. Observe for red, moist mucosa indicating that the body of conduit is viable.

5. Additional individualized interventions: _____

Rationales

1. A transparent pouch with continual bedside drainage allows visualization of the stoma.

2. Color changes reflect adequacy of perfusion. Stoma should stay red or pink.

3. Color changes may imply ischemia leading to a necrotic, nonviable stoma. A necrotic stoma can develop from tension on the mesentery, possibly from abdominal distention; from twisting of the conduit during surgery; or from arterial or venous insufficiency. A necrotic stoma requires surgery.

4. If the inner lumen of conduit is viable, the stoma may be showing only minimal ischemia from edema; the stoma may then change color and appear viable. A dusky stoma may slough its outer layer during the next 5 to 7 days.

5. Rationales: _____

COLLABORATIVE PROBLEM

Risk for stoma retraction and mucocutaneous separation related to peristomal trauma or tension on the intestinal mesentery

Nursing priorities

- Monitor the mucocutaneous border.
- Minimize the risk of separation.
- Encourage healing.

Patient outcome criterion

By 5 to 7 days after surgery, the patient will have a healed mucocutaneous border around a budded stoma.

Interventions

1. Apply a pouch with an antireflux valve, as ordered. Make sure the opening of the adhesive barrier is 12″ (3 mm) larger than the diameter of the stoma.

2. If compatible with the pouch barrier, use a skin sealant under the pouch to protect and waterproof peristomal skin.

Rationales

1. An antireflux valve promotes healing by preventing urine from pooling on the stoma and mucocutaneous border. An opening that is too small can compromise circulation to the stoma at the mucocutaneous junction or lacerate the stoma.

2. Protecting and waterproofing the peristomal skin by routinely applying a skin sealant encourages healing of the mucocutaneous border and minimizes trauma when removing the pouch.

3. If mucocutaneous separation occurs, protect the separated area and take measures to encourage granulation. Fill the mucocutaneous separation with desiccated hydrocolloid starch powder; then apply stoma adhesive paste and a properly sized skin barrier and pouch. Notify the surgeon of the separation.

4. Additional individualized interventions: _____

3. Mucocutaneous separation does not usually require surgery. The measures described increase the rate of healing and provide additional support for the stoma. If, however, the stoma retracts through the fascia into the peritoneum, peritonitis may develop and surgery is essential.

4. Rationales: _____

NURSING DIAGNOSIS

Altered urinary elimination related to creation of an ileal conduit

Nursing priorities

• Protect peristomal skin and contain urine.
• Teach the patient the conduit's function and purpose.

Patient outcome criteria

Within 3 days after surgery, the patient will:
• have intact skin around the stoma
• describe normal stoma and urine characteristics after creation of an ileal conduit.

Interventions

1. Maintain a good pouch seal, and protect peristomal skin with sealants.

2. Review the construction and function of the conduit, assuring the patient of GI tract continuity. Use diagrams and pictures.

3. Describe and show normal urine and stoma characteristics. Explain the following: The conduit and stoma are made from the GI tract, so they have the same red, moist lining as the mouth. The stoma has no sensory nerve endings, so it is insensitive to pain. Without a sphincter, voluntary control of urination is gone. The stoma is vascular and may bleed when cleaned. The GI tract makes mucus, so mucus in the urine is to be expected.

4. Additional individualized interventions: _____

Rationales

1. Urine can irritate and macerate the skin after prolonged contact.

2. Reviewing preoperative teaching after surgery reinforces information the patient may have forgotten or misunderstood. The patient should understand the nature of the surgery and its anatomical effects. The patient may mistakenly expect the ileal conduit to act as a substitute bladder.

3. The patient needs to know what is now normal. Blood in the urine can result from stomal bleeding. Urine will flow continuously from the stoma. There will be a greater amount of mucus in the urine during the early postoperative period, when oral intake is low, or when a urinary infection is present. The patient may mistake mucus for pus.

4. Rationales: _____

NURSING DIAGNOSIS

Body image disturbance related to urinary diversion

Nursing priorities

• Minimize damage to self-concept.
• Promote a healthy body image.

Patient outcome criteria

Within 2 to 4 days after surgery, the patient will:
• express feelings about the ostomy
• demonstrate ability to empty pouch in bathroom
• express confidence about ability to care for self.

Interventions

1. Encourage the patient to express feelings and beliefs about the diagnosis, surgery, and stoma.

2. Allow for privacy when teaching ostomy care.

3. Have the patient empty the pouch in the bathroom.

4. Suggest a visit from a United Ostomy Association (UOA) visitor (may also be helpful before surgery). The local chapter will be listed in the telephone directory's white pages.

5. Show an accepting, tolerant attitude when performing or teaching ostomy care. Explain that wearing gloves is necessary to comply with standard precautions.

6. Additional individualized interventions: _____

Rationales

1. The patient may feel fear or isolation or may harbor misconceptions. Expression of feelings is the first step in the coping process.

2. Privacy encourages the patient to ask questions and facilitates learning.

3. Mimicking normal bathroom behavior minimizes feelings of being disabled or different.

4. The UOA provides the patient with fellowship, information, and support from others with ostomies. Seeing a well-adjusted person with an ostomy can encourage hope and provide a positive role model for the patient.

5. The nurse's acceptance and tolerance reassure the patient and facilitate advancement to complete self-care. The patient may perceive the nurse's gloves as a sign of unacceptance of or disgust for the new stoma.

6. Rationales: _____

Nursing diagnosis

Postoperative knowledge deficit (care of the ileal conduit) related to lack of exposure to information

Nursing priority

Encourage independence in caring for the ileal conduit.

Patient outcome criteria

• Within 5 days after surgery, the patient will display learning readiness, such as looking at the stoma or holding wicks (rolled-up gauze or tampons).
• By the time of discharge, the patient will change the pouch two or three times with minimal assistance from the nurse.

Interventions

1. Instruct the patient how to empty the pouch when it is one-third to one-half full. Demonstrate the emptying procedure using a pouch the patient is not wearing. (A female can sit on the toilet to empty; a male can stand.)

Rationales

1. Emptying is usually taught first because it is done most often. A too-full pouch may pull away and have to be changed. Opening and closing the spout is easier to practice on a pouch the patient can hold out and see. Mimicking normal toileting behavior facilitates the patient's adjustment.

Renal disorders

2. Demonstrate the use and care of the nighttime bedside drainage bag. Run tubing from the drainage bag down the patient's pajama leg, or attach it to the leg with a Velcro strap. Attach the pouch, with urine in it, to the drainage bag. Explain that the drainage bag is easily cleaned with white vinegar and water or a commercial cleaner.

3. Encourage the patient to change the pouch by giving step-by-step written instructions, teaching the use of wicks, having the patient practice on a stoma model, explaining that the patient should clean urine and mucus from stoma and skin with warm water only, using a mirror if necessary to help the patient see the underside of the stoma, and having the patient apply the pouch while standing.

4. Teach the patient how to treat minor peristomal skin irritations using karaya powder and a skin sealant. Explain that momentary stinging may result if desiccated hydrocolloid starch powder or sealant is applied to denuded skin, but they should be used to prevent more serious peristomal skin complications.

5. Explain fluid intake requirements. Demonstrate pH testing of urine. Check pH routinely on the first few drops of urine in a freshly changed pouch. Warn against touching nitrazine paper to the skin or stoma. Explain why the patient should not drink more than 3 or 4 glasses of citrus juice or milk per day.

6. List recommended ways to control urine odor through diet. Explain that pouches are odor-proof except during emptying and changing.

7. Define routine follow-up care, and explain the rationale for it.

8. Address any special concerns the patient has about living with an ostomy. Consult an enterostomal nurse for specialized ostomy care.

9. Additional individualized interventions: _____

---

2. A bedside drainage bag prevents pouch overfilling and leakage at night. Attaching a partially filled pouch prevents suction vacuum, which can lead to overfilling and leakage. Cleaning keeps the drainage bag free from odor and urine sediment or crystals.

3. Written instructions promote continuity of care. Wicks are placed on the stoma to absorb urine and keep the peristomal skin dry so the pouch can seal. Practicing on a stoma model decreases fear and allows for repetition. Water is used for cleaning because soap can leave a film on the skin and disrupt the pouch seal. The patient needs to monitor the condition of the peristomal skin during each pouch change. Standing minimizes abdominal creases, which predispose the pouch to leakage.

4. Routinely applying a skin sealant before pouch application protects skin from adhesives and urine. Treating minor skin irritations with karaya powder and sealant minimizes the risk of serious complications requiring surgery. Intact, healthy skin increases a pouch's wearing time and prevents unexpected leaks.

5. Normal urine is acidic in a well-hydrated adult. Touching nitrazine paper to the skin or stoma will yield inaccurate results. The patient may need to drink 10 to 12 glasses of fluid daily to keep urine acidic; drinking large amounts of citrus juice or milk will negate this effect and make urine alkaline. Alkaline urine predisposes the patient to foul-smelling urine, urinary infections, peristomal skin irritations, stomal stenosis, increased mucus production from the conduit, urine crystals and calculi, and pyelonephritis.

6. Increased urine odor is associated with eating fish, eggs, asparagus, onions, and spicy foods.

7. The patient will see the urologist routinely every 6 to 12 months. Routine follow-up includes urine culture and sensitivity testing to rule out or detect infection, plus excretory urography or a renal scan to check upper urinary tract function and evaluate for recurrent tumor. The stoma and skin should be checked and pouch problems evaluated.

8. Enterostomal nurses are specially trained to teach, counsel, and help rehabilitate the ostomy patient. They are knowledgeable about the newest pouch supplies and can assist the patient in coping with problems of daily living.

9. Rationales: _____

NURSING DIAGNOSIS

Risk for sexual dysfunction: Male erectile dysfunction related to cystectomy and possible ejaculatory incompetence with prostatectomy

Nursing priorities

• Help the patient maximize remaining sexual function.
• Provide information or referrals as needed.

Patient outcome criterion

During the postoperative teaching phase, the patient will ask questions about impact on sexual function or agree to appropriate referrals.

Interventions

1. Assess the patient's readiness to discuss sexual matters. If the patient is not ready, arrange for outpatient follow-up.

2. Describe the separate nerve pathways for sexual excitement, erection, ejaculation, and orgasm. Explain which ones may be affected by surgery and why.

3. If indicated, mention alternatives, such as a penile prosthesis or external devices that aid erection. Refer the patient to the urologist or enterostomal nurse for details.

4. Additional individualized interventions: _____

Rationales

1. The patient may deny interest in resumption of sexual activity at first, while learning to cope with the ostomy and the diagnosis of cancer.

2. Cystectomy may only affect the patient's ability to experience erection or ejaculation, or it may affect both.

3. The patient may need specific suggestions for resumption of fulfilling sexual activity. A urologist may surgically implant a penile prosthesis. The enterostomal nurse can counsel the patient on alternatives, help obtain information on external devices, and suggest ways to minimize the ostomy's presence during sex.

4. Rationales: _____

DISCHARGE PLANNING

Discharge checklist

Before discharge, the patient shows evidence of:
❒ a viable stoma
❒ stable vital signs
❒ stable nutritional status
❒ absence of pulmonary or cardiovascular complications
❒ adequate support system for postdischarge assistance and ability to perform stoma care
❒ referral to home care if indicated by lack of a home support system or inability to perform ADLs and stoma care
❒ absence of fever
❒ ability to control pain using oral analgesics
❒ no need for I.V. support (discontinued for at least 24 hours before discharge)
❒ bowel sounds
❒ healing incision with no redness or other sign of infection
❒ ability to ambulate at preoperative level.

Teaching checklist

Document evidence that the patient and family demonstrate an understanding of:
❒ extent of tumor and resection
❒ nature of urinary diversion and its construction
❒ incision care (if not healed)
❒ procedure for emptying and changing pouch
❒ use and cleaning of bedside drainage system
❒ treatment of minor peristomal skin irritations
❒ written list of supplies and suppliers, with doctor's prescription to facilitate insurance payment
❒ chemotherapy (if needed) and its expected adverse effects
❒ availability of support groups such as UOA and the American Cancer Society (list their telephone numbers)
❒ amount and types of fluids preferred, along with any dietary considerations such as avoiding odor-causing foods
❒ signs and symptoms to report to the doctor, such as fever, flank pain, or hematuria

❏ concerns to report to the enterostomal nurse, such as pouch problems and skin or stoma problems
❏ signs and symptoms of urinary tract infection
❏ considerations in resuming sexual activity
❏ date and time of follow-up appointments
❏ how to contact the doctor
❏ how to contact the enterostomal nurse.

Documentation checklist

Using outcome criteria as a guide, document:
❏ clinical status on admission
❏ significant changes in status
❏ pertinent laboratory and diagnostic test findings
❏ preoperative marking of stoma site
❏ preoperative teaching
❏ bowel preparation
❏ UOA visitor recommendation (if appropriate)
❏ stoma viability
❏ mucocutaneous border and sutures
❏ urine characteristics
❏ patient's response to ostomy
❏ fluid intake and output
❏ presence of stents
❏ GI status
❏ incision status
❏ patient's progress in learning ostomy care
❏ patient and family teaching
❏ discharge planning.

ASSOCIATED PLANS OF CARE

Grieving
Ineffective family coping: Compromised
Ineffective individual coping
Knowledge deficit
Surgery

REFERENCES

Beardsky, T. "Testing, Testing," *Scientific American* 274(6):38-39, June 1996.
Dickson, C. "The Bladder: Cystectomy and Ileal Conduit to Treat Bladder Cancer," *Nurse Times* 91(42):34-35, October 18, 1995.
Kelly, L., and Miaskowski, C. "Overview of Bladder Cancer: Treatment and Nursing Implications," *Oncology Nurse Forum* (3):459-70, April 23, 1996.

Nephrectomy

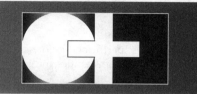

DRG information

DRG 303   Kidney, Ureter, and Major Bladder Procedures for Neoplasm.
Mean LOS = 10.2 days

DRG 304   Kidney, Ureter, and Major Bladder Procedures for Nonneoplasms with Complication or Comorbidity (CC).
Mean LOS = 10.3 days

DRG 305   Kidney, Ureter, and Major Bladder Procedures for Nonneoplasms without CC.
Mean LOS = 4.9 days

INTRODUCTION

Definition and time focus

Kidney removal may be necessary for various reasons. The reason for the excision dictates the surgical approach. The flank or lumbar approach, the traditional approach through the retroperitoneum, is indicated in inflammatory renal disease, calculi, perinephric abscess, hydronephrosis, and renal cystic disease. The transabdominal approach allows easy access to the renal vessels, as is required in renal tumors, trauma, or renal vascular disease. Either approach may be used to remove a kidney for transplantation.

This plan focuses on the immediate preoperative and postoperative care for the patient undergoing nephrectomy. Refer to the "Surgery" plan, page 103, for more detailed information on preoperative and postoperative care.

Etiology and precipitating factors

• Renal tumors (benign or malignant)
• Obstructive uropathy (intrinsic or extrinsic), including renal calculi, vascular lesions (such as abdominal aortic aneurysm), pelvic disorders (such as endometriosis), GI disorders (such as Crohn's disease), retroperitoneal disorders (such as tumor or abscess), or effects of radiation therapy
• Blunt or penetrating trauma
• Kidney donation

FOCUSED ASSESSMENT GUIDELINES

Nursing history (functional health pattern findings)

Health perception–health management pattern
• History of concomitant health problems if the patient is older (such as diabetes mellitus, hypertension, hyperparathyroidism, or vascular disease) that contributed to need for nephrectomy
• Concerns or fears about maintaining normal kidney function after surgery
• Concerns about diet and activity restrictions and need for adjuvant therapies after surgery
• History of contact with nephrotoxic substances

Activity-exercise pattern
• Fatigue

Nutritional-metabolic pattern
• Anorexia, nausea or vomiting, or weight loss

Self-perception–self-concept pattern
• Anxiety or depression

Physical findings

Cardiovascular
• Hypertension
• Tachycardia
• Edema
• Ecchymosis at injury site (with trauma)
• Hypotension (primarily with trauma)
• Signs of fluid overload (such as peripheral edema and distended neck veins)

Pulmonary
• Tachypnea
• Crackles

Genitourinary
• Dysuria
• Hematuria
• Oliguria
• Polyuria

Musculoskeletal
• Pain with movement
• Ecchymosis
• Muscle spasm (rarely)

Integumentary
• Diaphoresis
• Pallor

Diagnostic studies

Diagnostic studies, performed before surgery, may reveal no significant abnormalities initially, unless related to a coexisting condition.

• complete blood count — establishes baseline; may reveal preexisting disorder (such as anemia) or extent of blood loss from injury; white blood cell count may be elevated in response to injury

• blood typing and crossmatching — allows blood replacement during surgery

• chemistry panel — establishes baseline and reveals imbalances that may be related to renal dysfunction or that may affect care during surgery (such as potassium, calcium, or phosphate imbalances that may cause cardiac irritability during anesthesia); blood urea nitrogen and creatinine levels evaluate renal function

• prothrombin time/international normalized ratio (PT/INR) and activated partial thromboplastin time (APTT) — establishes baseline; some patients (older, obese, or with prosthetic valves) may receive anticoagulant therapy after surgery to minimize the risk of thromboembolism complications

• urinalysis — establishes baseline and evaluates for presence of infection

• chest X-ray — rules out preexisting conditions that may affect care during surgery

• 12-lead electrocardiography — establishes baseline and identifies preexisting cardiac abnormalities or pericardial effusion

Potential complications

• Shock
• Hemorrhage
• Pulmonary embolism
• Pulmonary edema
• Atelectasis
• Pneumonia
• Wound infection, dehiscence, and evisceration
• Thrombophlebitis
• Paralytic ileus
• Acute renal failure

CLINICAL SNAPSHOT

NEPHRECTOMY

Major nursing diagnoses and collaborative problems	Key patient outcomes
Knowledge deficit (perioperative procedures)	Verbalize understanding of perioperative procedures.
Pain	Rate pain (while using pain medication) as less than 3 on a 0 to 10 pain rating scale.
Risk for fluid and electrolyte imbalance	Have a urine output of 60 ml/hour or better.
Risk for atelectasis	Display ABG levels within normal limits: pH, 7.35 to 7.45; $Paco_2$, 35 to 45 mm Hg; HCO_3^-, 23 to28 mEq/L; or Sao_2, greater than 90%.
Risk for postoperative paralytic ileus or intestinal obstruction	Have regular bowel movements.

NURSING DIAGNOSIS

Knowledge deficit (perioperative procedures) related to lack of exposure to information

Nursing priority

Prepare the patient for perioperative procedures.

Patient outcome criteria

Before surgery, the patient will:
• verbalize understanding of perioperative procedures
• demonstrate ability to perform coughing and deep-breathing exercises, use the incentive spirometer, splint the incision, and perform leg exercises.

Interventions

1. See the "Knowledge deficit" plan, page 72.

2. See the "Surgery" plan, page 103.

3. Tell the patient where the incision will be made (flank or abdomen), whether to expect a chest tube (for a flank incision) or a drain (for an abdominal incision), and the potential effects of positioning during surgery.

4. Additional individualized interventions: _____

Rationales

1. General interventions related to patient teaching are included in the "Knowledge deficit" plan. This plan presents additional information about the nephrectomy patient's learning needs.

2. General interventions related to perioperative procedures are included in the "Surgery" plan.

3. Knowing what to expect decreases the patient's anxiety and increases the likelihood of compliance after surgery.

4. Rationales: _____

NURSING DIAGNOSIS

Pain related to tissue injury, edema, or spasm after surgery

Nursing priority

Prevent or reduce pain.

Patient outcome criteria

Within 1 hour of pain onset, the patient will:
• rate pain (while using pain medication) as less than 3 on a 0 to 10 pain rating scale
• maintain vital signs within normal limits, typically with heart rate of 60 to 100 beats/minute, systolic blood pressure 90 to 140 mm Hg, and diastolic blood pressure 50 to 90 mm Hg.

Interventions

1. See the "Pain" plan, page 88.

2. Teach the patient about postoperative analgesia administration (injection, patient-controlled analgesia pump, or epidural infusion), potential adverse effects, and the importance of requesting medication before pain becomes severe.

3. Additional individualized interventions: _____

Rationales

1. The "Pain" plan contains general interventions regarding pain management.

2. The patient is more likely to comply with postoperative care if pain is controlled.

3. Rationales: _____

Renal disorders

COLLABORATIVE PROBLEM

Risk for fluid and electrolyte imbalance related to decreased renal reserve and third-space fluid shifting immediately after surgery

Nursing priority

Prevent fluid and electrolyte imbalance.

Patient outcome criteria

• Within 1 day after surgery, the patient will:
  – have urine output of 30 ml/hr or greater
  – have adequate I.V. or oral fluid intake
  – exhibit normal electrolyte levels.
• By the time of discharge, the patient will have urine output of 60 ml/hr or greater.

Interventions

1. See Appendix C, Fluid and Electrolyte Imbalances.

2. Preserve and protect the remaining kidney.
• Maintain adequate hydration. Monitor urine output, color, and specific gravity, as ordered.
• Avoid or minimize use of nephrotoxic agents, such as aminoglycoside antibiotics and chemotherapeutic agents.

3. Additional individualized interventions: _____

Rationales

1. The Fluid and Electrolyte Imbalances appendix contains detailed information on these imbalances.

2. Removal of one kidney makes preservation of remaining renal function imperative.
• Appropriate hydration preserves renal function and promotes efficient removal of metabolic wastes.
• Nephrotoxic agents can damage the remaining kidney.

3. Rationales: _____

COLLABORATIVE PROBLEM

Risk for atelectasis related to anesthesia, immobility, pain, presence of chest tube, and location of incision

Nursing priorities

• Maintain adequate oxygenation.
• Prevent pulmonary complications.

Patient outcome criteria

After surgery, the patient will:
• display ABG levels within normal limits: pH, 7.35 to 7.45; $PaCO_2$, 35 to 45 mm Hg; HCO_3^-, 23 to28 mEq/L; or SaO_2, greater than 90%
• have deep, unlabored respirations
• manifest audible, clear breath sounds in all lobes.

Interventions

1. Implement interventions listed under "Risk for post-operative atelectasis" in the "Surgery" plan, page 106. As needed, check pulmonary status frequently, help the patient to perform incentive spirometry, encourage frequent position changes, and promote early and progressive ambulation.

2. Additional individualized interventions: _____
_____

Rationales

1. In addition to the risk of atelectasis inherent to general anesthesia, the patient with a lumbar or flank incision is at increased risk because the intercostal muscles must be spread and the 12th rib may be removed. The resulting pain limits deep inspiration. If not detected and treated aggressively, atelectasis can lead to pneumonia. The "Surgery" plan contains measures to prevent this complication.

2. Rationales: _____
_____

COLLABORATIVE PROBLEM

Risk for postoperative paralytic ileus or intestinal obstruction related to surgical manipulation, anesthesia, and immobility

Nursing priority

Promptly detect abnormal GI function.

Patient outcome criteria

By the time of discharge, the patient will:
• have normal, active bowel sounds
• tolerate a regular diet
• have regular bowel movements.

Interventions

1. Implement measures listed under "Risk for postoperative paralytic ileus" in the "Surgery" plan, page 111. As appropriate, assess the abdomen frequently, monitor nasogastric tube drainage, administer fluids, provide a diet appropriate to peristaltic activity, and encourage early and frequent ambulation.

2. Additional individualized interventions: _____

Rationales

1. Bowel manipulation during nephrectomy increases the risk of paralytic ileus, the most common GI complication. Significant manipulation increases the risk of intestinal obstruction. The "Surgery" plan details related interventions and their rationales.

2. Rationales: _____
_____

Renal disorders

DISCHARGE PLANNING

Discharge checklist

Before discharge, the patient shows evidence of:
❏ stable vital signs
❏ absence of cardiovascular or pulmonary complications
❏ absence of fever
❏ healing wound without signs or symptoms of infection (swelling, inflammation, tenderness, or drainage)
❏ ability to tolerate oral intake

❏ ability to ambulate and perform activities of daily living same as before surgery
❏ ability to void and have bowel movements same as before surgery
❏ ability to control pain using oral medications
❏ adequate home support system or referral to home health agency or nursing home, if indicated.

Teaching checklist

Document evidence that the patient and family demonstrate an understanding of:
❏ plan for resuming normal activity, with restrictions

❏ dietary recommendations
❏ wound care
❏ signs of wound infection or other complications
❏ all discharge medications' purpose, dosage, administration, and adverse effects requiring medical attention (discharge medications may include analgesics and antibiotics)
❏ necessary home care and referrals for follow-up care
❏ when and how to contact the doctor
❏ date, time, and place of follow-up appointments.

Documentation checklist

Using outcome criteria as a guide, document:
❏ clinical status on admission
❏ preoperative assessment and treatment
❏ preoperative teaching and its effectiveness
❏ preoperative checklist (usually includes documentation of operative consent, pertinent laboratory test results, skin preparation, voiding on call from the operating room, and removal of nail polish, jewelry, dentures, glasses, hearing aids, and prostheses — check hospital's specific requirements)
❏ postoperative assessment and treatment
❏ amount and character of drainage on dressing and through drains
❏ patency of I.V. lines, nasogastric tube, indwelling urinary catheter, and drains
❏ pulmonary hygiene
❏ pain-relief measures
❏ activity tolerance
❏ nutritional intake and tolerance
❏ fluid intake and output
❏ bladder and bowel function
❏ pertinent laboratory findings
❏ patient and family teaching
❏ discharge planning.

ASSOCIATED PLANS OF CARE

Acute renal failure
Hypovolemic shock
Knowledge deficit
Pain
Surgery

REFERENCES

Lewis, S., et al. *Medical-Surgical Nursing: Assessment and Management of Clinical Problems,* 4th ed. St. Louis: Mosby–Year Book, Inc., 1997.
Thompson, J., et al. *Mosby's Clinical Nursing,* 4th ed. St. Louis: Mosby–Year Book, Inc., 1997.

Peritoneal dialysis

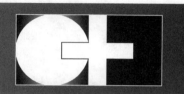

DRG information

DRG 316   Renal Failure.
               Mean LOS = 7.6 days
               Principal diagnoses include:
                • acute renal failure
                • chronic renal failure.

DRG 449   Poisoning and Toxic Effects of Drugs with Complication or Comorbidity (CC); Age 17+.
               Mean LOS = 4.5 days
               Principal diagnoses include drug overdose.

DRG 450   Poisoning and Toxic Effects of Drugs without CC; Age 17+.
               Mean LOS = 2.3 days

DRG 451   Poisoning and Toxic Effects of Drugs; Ages 0 to 17.
               Mean LOS = 2.1 days

DRG 205   Disorders of the Liver except Malignancy, Cirrhosis, and Alcoholic Hepatitis with CC.
               Mean LOS = 7.3 days
               Principal diagnoses include hepatic coma.

DRG 206   Disorders of the Liver except Malignancy, Cirrhosis, and Alcoholic Hepatitis without CC.
               Mean LOS = 4.7 days

Peritoneal dialysis is used to treat numerous disorders. Therefore, the diagnosis necessitating its use determines the DRG assigned. Examples of diagnoses for peritoneal dialysis are listed above.

INTRODUCTION

Definition and time focus

Peritoneal dialysis (PD) indirectly removes excess water, solutes, and toxins from the blood by using the peritoneal membrane as a dialyzing membrane. Solution (dialysate) is instilled into the peritoneal cavity through a catheter and remains for a prescribed period of time, usually 15 minutes to 4 hours. During that time (dwell time), substances in the blood and in the dialysate equalize across the membrane, moving from areas of higher concentration to areas of lower concentration. The solution is then allowed to flow out (drain time), removing excess water and waste products. PD is contraindicated with:
• recent abdominal, retroperitoneal, or chest surgery
• abdominal drains
• preexisting peritonitis

• diaphragmatic tears
• paralytic ileus
• diffuse bowel disease
• respiratory insufficiency.
   This plan focuses on the patient receiving PD for the first time and then regularly (at least three times weekly).

Etiology and precipitating factors

PD is indicated to treat chronic renal failure, acute renal failure, drug overdose, and hepatic coma. The patient awaiting hemodialysis whose vascular access device is not yet operable may receive PD temporarily. Because PD is not a diagnosis but a procedure, this plan does not address specific illnesses. Refer to plans for specific disorders for more information.

FOCUSED ASSESSMENT GUIDELINES

Nursing history (functional health pattern findings)

Health perception–health management pattern
• History of chronic or acute renal failure
• Inadequate or exhausted venous access
• Treatment for diabetes mellitus
• History of drug overdose or drug intolerance
• History of a clotting disorder or cardiovascular disease

Nutritional-metabolic pattern
• Anorexia, nausea, or vomiting
• Weight loss or diet intolerance

Elimination pattern
• Diminished urine output
• Constipation

Role-relationship pattern
• Inability to work or maintain usual roles because of chronic, disabling illness, treatment regimen, or both

Self-perception–self-concept pattern
• Verbalized decreased sense of self-worth

Coping–stress tolerance pattern
• Denial, anger, or depression over condition and needed treatment

Activity-exercise pattern
• Fatigue
• Shortness of breath or other signs of exercise intolerance

Value-belief pattern
• Religious or personal beliefs that do not allow blood transfusions

Physical findings

Cardiovascular
- Hypertension
- Periorbital, ankle, or sacral edema

Pulmonary
- Crackles
- Dyspnea

Gastrointestinal
- Nausea
- Anorexia
- Hiccoughs
- Constipation
- Stomatitis

Neurologic
- Lethargy
- Confusion
- Shortened attention span
- Restlessness

Integumentary
- Fragile skin
- Dry, flaky skin
- Yellow-gray skin hue
- Ecchymoses or purpura
- Poor skin turgor

Musculoskeletal
- Impaired mobility
- Bone deformities

Diagnostic studies

- Creatinine clearance — determines glomerular filtration rate, which directly reflects renal function
  - normal, 85 to 150 ml/minute
  - mild renal failure, 50 to 84 ml/minute
  - moderate renal failure, 10 to 49 ml/minute
  - severe renal failure, less than 10 ml/minute
  - end-stage renal failure, 0 ml/minute

- Serum creatinine levels — determine renal function (normal is 1.0 to 1.4 mg/dl; elevation indicates renal impairment; see the "Chronic renal failure" plan, page 698)
- Arterial blood gas (ABG) levels — determine acid-base abnormalities (normal pH is 7.35 to 7.45; the patient in renal failure is usually acidotic)
- serum electrolyte levels — usually show hyperkalemia (greater than 5 mEq/L)
- Sodium level — may be low (less than 120 mEq/L) because of kidney's inability to conserve sodium
- Phosphate and calcium levels — commonly show hypocalcemia and hyperphosphatemia
- Blood urea nitrogen levels — elevated in renal failure, reduced in severe liver damage
- Complete blood count — hemoglobin level may be reduced from decreased erythropoietin production
- Erythrocyte sedimentation rate — increased if infection present
- Serum drug levels — determine degree of overdose
- Culture and sensitivity of PD drainage — identifies causative organism and appropriate antibiotic for peritoneal infection
- Chest X-ray — rules out heart failure

Potential complications

- Peritonitis
- Respiratory distress
- Cardiac arrhythmias
- Hypovolemia or hypervolemia
- Hyperglycemia
- Electrolyte imbalance
- Bowel or bladder perforation

CLINICAL SNAPSHOT

PERITONEAL DIALYSIS

Major nursing diagnoses and collaborative problems	Key patient outcomes
Risk for injury: Bleeding, perforation, or ileus	Produce his usual amount of urine and stool.
Ineffective breathing pattern	Show no dyspnea.
Risk for fluid and electrolyte imbalance	Have a dialysate deficit less than 500 ml.
Risk for infection	Have no exudate, edema, redness, or leakage at the catheter site.
Pain	Rate pain as less than 3 on a 0 to 10 pain rating scale.
Nutritional deficit	Tolerate oral intake of at least 0.5 g/kg of ideal weight daily and 45 to 50 kcal/kg/day.

NURSING DIAGNOSIS

Risk for injury: Bleeding, perforation, or ileus related to catheter insertion or irritation from dialysate

Nursing priority

Prevent or promptly detect and report injuries related to PD.

Patient outcome criteria

- After catheter insertion, the patient will:
  - have no unusual urge to void or defecate
  - produce his or her usual amount of urine and stool
  - have dialysate returns free from fecal material or blood.
- Throughout the hospital stay, the patient will:
  - have normal bowel sounds
  - maintain a normal bowel elimination pattern
  - show no abdominal distention and tenderness.

Interventions

1. Have the patient void before catheter insertion.

2. During dialysate infusion, observe for indications of bladder or bowel perforation, such as an extreme urge to urinate or defecate; large urine output; fecal color, odor, or material in returned dialysate; and liquid or watery stools. If any occur, stop the infusion and notify the doctor immediately.

3. Report persistently blood-tinged dialysate.

4. Auscultate bowel sounds every 4 hours.

5. Inspect and palpate the abdomen every 8 hours between dialysate infusions.

6. Monitor the patient's appetite and sense of well-being.

7. Encourage ambulation.

8. Apply warm compresses to the abdomen.

9. Additional individualized interventions: _____

Rationales

1. The catheter is inserted with a trocar near the bladder. Bladder distention increases the risk of perforation.

2. Bowel or bladder perforation may lead to severe peritonitis unless detected. Surgical repair and prompt antibiotic therapy are indicated. The signs listed appear when dialysate leaks into the bladder or bowel.

3. Slight bleeding may be normal after catheter insertion, but the fluid should clear rapidly. Persistent bleeding or gross blood in the return flow requires prompt evaluation.

4. Diminished or absent bowel sounds may suggest ileus or bowel obstruction from bowel injury or irritation from catheter placement or dialysate.

5. Abdominal distention and tenderness may indicate ileus.

6. Anorexia, nausea, vomiting, and malaise can be signs and symptoms of ileus.

7. Ambulation stimulates peristalsis.

8. Heat increases peristalsis.

9. Rationales: _____

Renal disorders

NURSING DIAGNOSIS

Ineffective breathing pattern related to elevation of diaphragm during PD exchanges and reduced mobility

Nursing priority

Prevent respiratory distress and pulmonary complications during PD exchanges.

Patient outcome criteria

During PD treatment, the patient will:
• show no dyspnea
• have minimal or no crackles
• perform pulmonary hygiene measures effectively.

Interventions

1. Elevate the head of the bed during exchanges.

2. Administer oxygen, as ordered.

3. Assess for possible causes of pain or discomfort. Administer analgesics, as ordered.

4. Encourage deep-breathing and coughing exercises during PD exchanges, hourly while awake. Teach and promote hourly incentive spirometer use, as ordered.

5. Auscultate the patient's lungs every hour, assessing for and reporting crackles or other abnormal findings.

6. Turn and reposition the patient at least every hour.

7. Perform chest percussion every 2 hours.

8. Additional individualized interventions: _____

Rationales

1. Elevating the head of the bed minimizes pressure on the diaphragm and allows fuller chest expansion.

2. Hypoventilation related to pressure on the diaphragm reduces partial pressure of arterial oxygen.

3. Pain may prevent effective breathing. Rapid inflow of dialysate, patient position, and air in the system can all cause discomfort; possible causes should be investigated before analgesics are given.

4. Good pulmonary hygiene helps prevent fluid accumulation in the lungs and air passages by promoting full chest expansion and preventing collapse of alveoli.

5. Crackles suggest pulmonary complications related to fluid retention.

6. Changing position promotes full chest expansion and optimal drainage of dialysate.

7. Percussion helps loosen secretions.

8. Rationales: _____

COLLABORATIVE PROBLEM

Risk for fluid and electrolyte imbalance related to dialysis and underlying disease or disorder

Nursing priority

Maintain normal fluid and electrolyte balance.

Patient outcome criteria

During PD exchanges, the patient will:
• show no distended neck veins
• have a decrease in peripheral edema
• have blood pressure within the normal range: typically, systolic pressure, 90 to 140 mm Hg and diastolic pressure, 50 to 90 mm Hg
• have a dialysate deficit less than 500 ml.

Interventions

1. See Appendix C, Fluid and Electrolyte Imbalances. Closely monitor vital signs, observing for tachycardia or orthostatic changes.

2. Monitor serum potassium levels, as ordered, to help determine appropriate additions to the dialysate.

3. Maintain accurate fluid intake and output records. Notify the doctor if the fluid return deficit exceeds 500 ml.

4. Additional individualized interventions: _____

Rationales

1. The Fluid and Electrolyte Imbalances appendix provides detailed information on the fluid and electrolyte disturbances seen in the patient receiving PD.

2. Dialysate normally contains no potassium. This is desirable for the hyperkalemic patient, but it may cause hypokalemia in others.

3. Normally, return should be equal to or slightly greater than the amount infused. A persistent deficit that is not corrected by position changes may indicate fluid retention.

4. Rationales: _____

Nursing diagnosis

Risk for infection related to invasive procedure

Nursing priority

Prevent infection.

Patient outcome criteria

By the time of discharge, the patient will:
• be afebrile for 24 hours
• have no exudate, edema, redness, or leakage at the catheter site
• show no signs or symptoms of peritonitis, such as abdominal pain or rebound tenderness
• have clear return drainage.

Interventions

1. Use strict aseptic technique for all aspects of PD, including daily dressing changes.

2. Maintain a sterile, closed system during exchanges.

3. Observe for and report leakage around the catheter.

4. Observe the catheter site for redness, exudate, and edema.

5. Observe the outflow for cloudiness, sediment, and odor. Observe the patient for signs or symptoms of peritonitis, such as abdominal pain, guarding, rigidity, and rebound tenderness.

6. Take and record the patient's temperature at least every 8 hours.

Rationales

1. Introduction of pathogens through the catheter may cause peritonitis.

2. Airborne bacteria can cause infection if introduced into the peritoneal cavity.

3. Further securing the catheter at the entry site and reducing the amount or rapidity of the infusion may control leakage. Moisture around the catheter provides a pathway for microorganisms and increases the risk of infection.

4. These are signs of infection.

5. Fluid appearance and odor may indicate peritonitis. Physical signs result from peritoneal inflammation.

6. Temperature elevation is a sign of infection.

Renal disorders

7. Administer systemic or local antibiotics, as ordered. Add antibiotics to the dialysate using the two-needle technique (one needle used to draw up the medication, another to inject it into the dialysate).

8. Additional individualized interventions: _____

7. Antibiotics prevent the growth and reproduction of bacteria. The two-needle technique reduces the risk of contamination.

8. Rationales: _____

NURSING DIAGNOSIS

Pain related to dialysate temperature or rapid inflow

Nursing priority

Minimize discomfort during fluid exchanges.

Patient outcome criterion

During PD treatment, the patient will rate pain as less than 3 on a 0 to 10 pain rating scale.

Interventions

1. Warm the dialysate to body temperature before beginning the infusion.

2. Change the patient's position every 1 to 2 hours.

3. Slow the infusion rate by lowering the bottle and by clamping the tubing as needed.

4. Prevent air from entering the catheter.

5. Assess pain level using a 0 to 10 pain rating scale. Notify the doctor if pain persists.

6. See the "Pain" plan, page 88.

7. Additional individualized interventions: _____

Rationales

1. Cold dialysate causes vasoconstriction (which interferes with circulation to the peritoneal membrane) and discomfort.

2. Frequent position changes improve dialysate drainage.

3. Reducing bottle height decreases the infusion rate and reduces pressure during fill time.

4. Air introduced into the abdominal cavity causes distention and pain, sometimes referred to the shoulder area. Air in the tubing may also create an air lock, preventing adequate dialysate flow.

5. Persistent pain may indicate peritonitis.

6. The "Pain" plan contains further details related to pain management.

7. Rationales: _____

NURSING DIAGNOSIS

Nutritional deficit related to anorexia, abdominal distention, stomatitis, or nausea

Nursing priority

Promote adequate nutritional intake.

Patient outcome criteria

- During PD, the patient will:
  - participate in dietary planning
  - perform oral hygiene before and after meals
  - eat adequate amounts of protein-rich foods.
- By the time of discharge, the patient will:
  - retain food for at least 12 hours
  - tolerate oral intake of at least 0.5 g/kg of ideal weight daily and 45 to 50 kcal/kg/day.

Interventions

1. With the dietitian and patient, plan a menu that incorporates personal preferences, increased nutrient needs, and any restrictions related to the underlying disorder.

2. Offer snacks and supplements between meals, providing plenty of high-protein foods unless contraindicated. Avoid foods high in potassium if hyperkalemia is a problem. See the "Chronic renal failure" plan, page 698, for more information.

3. Encourage frequent oral hygiene.

4. Offer small, frequent meals.

5. Avoid manipulating equipment or emptying drainage bags at mealtime.

6. Drain the peritoneal cavity before meals. If possible, allow 1 to 2 hours between a meal and the next dialysate infusion.

7. If the patient cannot tolerate adequate oral intake, discuss enteral or parenteral feedings with both the patient and doctor.

8. Additional individualized interventions: _____

Rationales

1. The dietitian's expertise may be helpful in selecting food for optimal nutritional value. When the patient's appetite is decreased, considering individual preferences is essential to promote adequate intake.

2. PD can cause weekly protein losses of 30 to 70 g. The adult dialysis patient requires 45 to 50 kcal/kg daily. Hyperkalemia is common in renal failure. The "Chronic renal failure" plan contains specific interventions related to diet planning.

3. Good oral hygiene decreases unpleasant odors and tastes in the mouth that can decrease appetite.

4. Large amounts of food may seem overwhelming and unappetizing. The patient may complain of being too full to eat because of pressure from peritoneal fluid.

5. Unpleasant sights and odors may cause nausea and vomiting.

6. Draining peritoneal fluid decreases intra-abdominal pressure and may enable the patient to eat and retain food more easily.

7. During acute illness, enteral or parenteral nutrition may be indicated.

8. Rationales: _____

DISCHARGE PLANNING

Discharge checklist

Before discharge, the patient shows evidence of:
- ❏ vital signs stable and within expected parameters
- ❏ electrolyte, ABG, and hemoglobin levels within acceptable parameters
- ❏ absence of drainage, redness, and edema at catheter site
- ❏ absence of cardiovascular and pulmonary complications
- ❏ absent or minimal peripheral edema
- ❏ ability to tolerate adequate nutritional intake, as ordered
- ❏ absence of abdominal distention and tenderness
- ❏ absence of nausea and vomiting
- ❏ normal bowel and bladder function
- ❏ stabilizing weight
- ❏ ability to control pain using oral medications
- ❏ ability to ambulate and perform activities of daily living independently or with minimal assistance
- ❏ adequate home support system or referral to home care or a nursing home as indicated by inadequate home support system, frequency of and tolerance to PD, and inability to care for self.

Additional information: For long-term PD, the patient typically receives treatments at home with the assistance of home health nurses. The number of treatments needed and the patient's ability to perform treat-

Renal disorders

ments at home are essential in determining where the patient will be discharged. Long-term PD treatments create financial problems for most patients. For this reason, a referral to the social services department should be an automatic part of discharge planning.

Teaching checklist

Document evidence that the patient and family demonstrate an understanding of:

☐ renal failure (pathophysiology, signs and symptoms, and implications)
☐ concepts of PD treatment
☐ importance of aseptic technique during treatment
☐ dietary modifications (sodium restrictions and high protein intake)
☐ all discharge medications' purpose, dosage, administration schedule, and adverse effects requiring medical attention (discharge medications vary, depending on underlying disorder)
☐ catheter care between treatments
☐ activity restrictions (usually only contact sports and swimming are prohibited)
☐ importance of a daily weight record
☐ changes in condition to report to the doctor
☐ date, time, and location of next treatment
☐ community resources
☐ how to get help in an emergency.

Documentation checklist

Using outcome criteria as a guide, document:

☐ clinical status at beginning of treatment, including vital signs and weight
☐ significant changes in clinical status
☐ appearance of catheter site
☐ time each exchange begins and ends
☐ fluid intake and output
☐ color, odor, and character of dialysate return
☐ care of catheter site
☐ weight at end of treatment
☐ nutritional intake
☐ pertinent laboratory and diagnostic test findings
☐ bowel status
☐ patient and family teaching
☐ discharge planning.

ASSOCIATED PLANS OF CARE

Acute renal failure
Chronic renal failure
Knowledge deficit
Liver failure
Pain
Total parenteral nutrition

REFERENCES

Alfaro, R. *Applying Nursing Diagnosis and Nursing Process,* 3rd ed. Philadelphia: Lippincott-Raven Pubs., 1994.
Nettina, S. *The Lippincott Manual of Nursing Practice,* 6th ed. Philadelphia: Lippincott-Raven Pubs., 1996.
Nursing Procedures, 2nd ed. Springhouse, Pa.: Springhouse Corp., 1996.

Urolithiasis

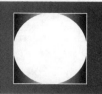

DRG information
DRG 323   Urinary Stones with Complication or Comorbidity (CC) or Treatment with Extracorporeal Shock-wave Lithotripsy.
Mean LOS = 3.6 days

DRG 324   Urinary Stones without CC.
Mean LOS = 2.1 days

DRG 304   Kidney, Ureter, and Bladder Procedures for
Nonneoplasm with CC.
Mean LOS = 10.3 days

DRG 305   Kidney, Ureter, and Bladder Procedures for
Nonneoplasm without CC.
Mean LOS = 4.7 days

DRG 310   Transurethral Procedures with CC.
Mean LOS = 4.6 days

INTRODUCTION

Definition and time focus
Urolithiasis is the formation of mineral crystals (renal
calculi or stones) around organic matter in the urinary
tract. Calcium oxalate and calcium phosphate calculi
are the most common. Calculi in the renal pelvis usually cause no symptoms until they pass into a ureter,
where they commonly obstruct urine flow and cause severe pain, bleeding, and infection. This plan focuses on
the patient admitted for treatment of upper urinary
tract calculi by percutaneous nephrolithotomy with ultrasonic lithotripsy. In this procedure, a nephroscope is
passed through a small incision into the kidney. The
calculi are then fragmented with ultrasonic waves,
flushed, and aspirated by suction or grasped and removed with forceps or special baskets.

Etiology and precipitating factors
• Urinary tract infection (UTI), which increases the alkalinity of the urine and causes calcium and other substances to precipitate and form renal calculi
• Immobility, dehydration, and urinary obstruction or
stasis, increasing likelihood that calculus-forming substances will precipitate
• Metabolic or dietary changes, such as hyperthyroidism; bone disease; corticosteroid use; excessive vitamin A and D intake; diet high in calcium or purine; or
other factors increasing calcium, phosphorus, uric acid,
and other calculus-forming substances in the blood or
urine
• More common in males ages 30 to 50

FOCUSED ASSESSMENT GUIDELINES

Nursing history (functional health pattern findings)
Health perception–health management pattern
• Severe pain is typical: If calculi are in the pelvis, patient reports dull constant pain, usually over costovertebral angle; if in a ureter, patient reports intermittent, ex-
cruciating pain radiating anteriorly down to vulva (female) or testes (male); in some cases, patient may not
report pain or may report abdominal pain
• History of UTI or previous calculus formation and
treatment (a history of calculi increases the risk of recurrence)
Nutritional-metabolic pattern
• Nausea, vomiting, diarrhea, and abdominal discomfort
• Diet high in calcium (milk, cheese, beans, nuts, cocoa), purine (fish, fowl, meat, organ meat), oxalate
(spinach, parsley, rhubarb, cocoa, instant coffee, tea), or
vitamins A and D
• Decreased fluid intake
Elimination pattern
• History of UTI or urinary tract obstruction
• Blood in urine (hematuria)
• Cloudy, odorous urine (indicates infection); painful,
urgent, and frequent urination; and decreasing urine
output
Activity-exercise pattern
• Sedentary occupation or recent increased need for
bed rest
Cognitive-perceptual pattern
• Difficulty understanding metabolic influences on cal-
culus formation and the new treatment options avail-
able (percutaneous ultrasonic lithotripsy, extracorporeal
shock-wave lithotripsy, electrohydraulic lithotripsy, and
laser lithotripsy)
Role-relationship pattern
• Family history of renal calculi, gout, or other renal
problems
Sexuality-reproductive pattern
• Sexual dysfunction related to UTI and pain
Coping–stress tolerance pattern
• Anxious appearance and obvious distress

Physical findings
Genitourinary
• Calculi in urine

- Costovertebral tenderness
- Hematuria
- Pyuria
- Oliguria
- Urinary frequency

Gastrointestinal
- Vomiting
- Abdominal tenderness
- Diarrhea
- Abdominal distention
- Absent bowel sounds

Integumentary
- Warm, flushed skin or chills and fever
- Pallor
- Diaphoresis

Diagnostic studies
- Urinalysis — commonly shows red blood cells, white blood cells (WBCs), crystals, casts, minerals, and pH changes
- Urine culture — commonly shows presence of bacteria
- 24-hour urine study — commonly shows high levels of calcium, phosphorus, uric acid, creatinine, oxalate, or cystine
- Renal calculus analysis — shows mineral composition of stones

- Blood studies — may show high serum levels of calcium, protein, electrolytes, uric acid, phosphates, blood urea nitrogen, creatinine, or WBCs
- Serum and urine creatinine tests — may show renal dysfunction (creatinine levels high in serum, low in urine)
- Kidney-ureter-bladder (KUB) X-ray — commonly shows calcium calculi and gross anatomical changes, such as distortions or enlargement (uric acid calculi cannot be visualized)
- I.V. urography (excretory urography or retrograde pyelogram) — commonly shows anatomical abnormalities, obstruction, and outlines of radiopaque calculi
- Computed tomography scan, with or without dye — commonly shows calculi, masses, or other abnormalities
- Ultrasound (kidney sonogram) — shows size, density, and perfusion
- Cystoscopy — commonly shows obstruction or other problems

Potential complications
- Bleeding (may be acute or delayed for 1 to 2 weeks)
- Sepsis
- Renal pelvis perforation and loss of irrigating fluid into retroperitoneal area
- Nonremovable calculi
- Loss of calculus fragments into retroperitoneum

CLINICAL SNAPSHOT

UROLITHIASIS

Major nursing diagnoses	Key patient outcomes
Pain	Rate pain as less than 3 on a 0 to 10 pain rating scale.
Risk for altered urinary elimination patterns: Dysuria, oliguria, pyuria, or frequency	Void more than 200 ml of clear amber urine per attempt.
Knowledge deficit (potential causes of calculus formation)	On request, express understanding of dietary restrictions, the need for increased fluid intake, the recommended activity level, the need to monitor such metabolic problems as gout, and the signs and symptoms of a recurrence.

NURSING DIAGNOSIS

Pain related to procedural manipulation, incision, and passage of calculus fragments

Nursing priority

Relieve pain.

Patient outcome criterion

Within 24 hours of the procedure, the patient will rate pain (with pain medication) as less than 3 on a 0 to 10 pain rating scale.

Interventions

1. See the "Pain" plan, page 88.

2. Assess and document pain episodes, asking the patient to rate pain on a scale of 0 to 10.

3. Medicate with analgesics and antispasmodics, as ordered. Narcotic analgesics are usually necessary.

4. Apply heat to painful areas, as ordered, for 15 to 20 minutes every 2 hours as needed.

5. Administer antiemetics as ordered and needed.

6. Encourage activity, as allowed. (The patient with an indwelling ureteral catheter may be on bed rest to prevent dislodgment.)

7. Additional individualized interventions: _____

Rationales

1. General interventions for pain are included in that plan.

2. Pain may indicate calculus movement. Persistent pain may indicate obstruction or perforation. Sudden absence of pain may indicate calculus passage. Increased ureteral pressure may cause abdominal pain from extravasation of urine into perirenal spaces.

3. These medications reduce pain, relax tense muscles, and reduce reflex spasms. Narcotic analgesics are warranted because of the pain's severity.

4. Heat relaxes tense muscles and diminishes reflex spasms.

5. Nausea and vomiting are commonly associated with renal pain from shared nerve pathways.

6. Activity prevents urine stasis, helps retard calculi formation, aids passage of calculus fragments, and promotes return of urinary tract function.

7. Rationales: _____

NURSING DIAGNOSIS

Risk for altered urinary elimination patterns: Dysuria, oliguria, pyuria, or frequency related to calculus fragment passage, obstruction, hematuria, or infection

Nursing priorities

• Prevent urinary tract complications.
• Promote return of normal urinary function.

Patient outcome criteria

Within 3 days of surgery, the patient will:
• void more than 200 ml of clear amber urine per attempt
• have no infection
• have no hematuria
• show a reduced amount of calculus fragments in the urine
• have catheters removed without problems
• show adequate hydration
• maintain vital signs within normal limits: typically, heart rate, 60 to 100 beats/minute; systolic blood pressure, 90 to 140 mm Hg; and diastolic blood pressure, 50 to 90 mm Hg.

Renal disorders

Interventions

1. Measure each voiding and note urine characteristics. Monitor fluid intake and output every 4 to 8 hours, more frequently if the patient is oliguric. Alert the doctor if urine output is less than 30 ml/hour.

2. Monitor the patency of an indwelling ureteral catheter or indwelling urinary catheter every hour.

3. Strain all urine for calculi and calculus fragments. Send any calculi for laboratory analysis. Notify the doctor of calculi passage and document your observations.

4. Observe for signs or symptoms of ureteral obstruction (increased flank pain and oliguria) or urethral obstruction (bladder distention and suprapubic pain), and report any that occur.

5. Observe for signs of dehydration, such as dry skin and mucous membranes, thirst, poor skin turgor, low urine output, decreased blood pressure, tachycardia, and weight loss.

6. Encourage intake of twelve to seventeen 8-oz (240-ml) glasses of fluid daily. Document intake.

7. Give antibiotics every 4 to 8 hours, as ordered.

8. Monitor and document vital signs every 2 to 4 hours, as ordered.

9. As ordered, irrigate the catheter with acid or alkaline solutions, depending on calculus composition.

10. Additional individualized interventions: _____

Rationales

1. Urine characteristics may indicate such complications as infection (cloudy, odorous urine) and hemorrhage. Some hematuria is expected for 1 to 2 days after surgery, but bright red blood may indicate hemorrhage. Adequate fluid intake is necessary to flush calculi through the kidneys, prevent further calculus formation, and prevent tissue damage. Adequate urine output indicates proper kidney function. Calculi may increase the frequency and urgency of urination as they near the ureterovesical junction.

2. If present, a ureteral catheter aids passage of calculus fragments and prevents obstruction of urine flow. A patent urinary catheter aids in monitoring urine output and assessing calculus passage. Calculus fragments can easily obstruct catheters.

3. The type and amount of calculi passed may influence the treatment used to prevent recurrence.

4. Calculi are most likely to lodge in a ureter or the urethra.

5. Dehydration concentrates urine, increasing the risk of calculus formation and infection.

6. Fluids enhance passage of calculus fragments and help prevent obstruction and infection.

7. UTI is a major predisposing factor for urolithiasis. UTI provides organic material and alkalizes urine, precipitating minerals and causing calculi formation. Antibiotics are commonly given to prevent infection and recurrence.

8. Changes in vital signs may indicate infection or other complications. Fever is common.

9. Catheter irrigations with acid or alkaline solutions promote acidification or alkalinization of the urine and help prevent further calculus formation.

10. Rationales: _____

NURSING DIAGNOSIS

Knowledge deficit (potential causes of calculus formation) related to lack of exposure to information

Nursing priority

Promote understanding of the medical regimen to prevent calculi recurrence.

Patient outcome criteria

By the time of discharge, the patient will:
• on request, express understanding of the need for increased fluid intake, the recommended activity level, the need to monitor such metabolic problems as gout, and the signs and symptoms of recurrence
• demonstrate accurate testing and interpretation of urine pH.

Interventions

1. See the "Knowledge deficit" plan, page 72.

2. Provide information, reinforcing as necessary, and document teaching regarding:
• dietary limitations for calcium calculi (dairy products and green leafy vegetables), uric acid calculi (meats, legumes, and whole grains), and oxalate calculi (chocolate, caffeinated beverages, beets, and spinach)
• need for regular activity

• need for adequate fluid intake

• need to maintain desired urine pH with medications and regular urine pH testing, according to the doctor's recommendations

• need to monitor and treat metabolic and other conditions (such as gout) that predispose the patient to calculus formation
• signs and symptoms of recurrence, such as pain, hematuria, oliguria.
3. Additional individualized interventions: _____

Rationales

1. The "Knowledge deficit" plan contains general information on patient teaching. This plan contains additional information specific to urolithiasis.

2. The patient needs accurate information to comply with the preventive regimen.
• Limiting foods rich in calculus-forming substances may inhibit recurrence. (A dietitian can provide details about specific diets, which vary considerably.)

• Activity decreases urine stasis and the risk of calculus formation.
• Fluids flush calculus fragments and help prevent recurrence.
• Depending on their composition, calculi may form in either acid or alkaline urine. The goal of treatment is to prevent calculus formation by maintaining the urine at the desired pH using appropriate medications.
• Treating underlying conditions such as gout (uric acid accumulation) is necessary to prevent calculus formation.
• The incidence of recurrence is high.

3. Rationales: _____

DISCHARGE PLANNING

Discharge checklist

Before discharge, the patient shows evidence of:
❏ absence of gross hematuria
❏ absence of fever
❏ healing incision with no redness or other signs of infection
❏ absence of pulmonary or cardiovascular complications
❏ ability to tolerate and follow dietary and fluid regimen
❏ ability to perform activities of daily living independently
❏ ability to ambulate same as before hospitalization
❏ ability to perform pH monitoring
❏ ability to control pain using oral medications
❏ absence of infection or appropriate antibiotic prescribed

❏ stable vital signs
❏ absence of indwelling ureteral or urinary catheter or, if urinary catheter is present, ability to perform appropriate catheter care
❏ referral to home care if catheter is in place or if the patient's home support system is inadequate.

Teaching checklist

Document evidence that the patient and family demonstrate an understanding of:
❏ care of incisions, drains, or catheters
❏ activity precautions
❏ dietary modifications
❏ desired fluid intake

❏ all discharge medications' purpose, dosage, administration schedule, and adverse effects requiring medical attention; usual medications include ascorbic acid (to increase urine acidity), ammonium chloride (for phosphate calculi), sodium or potassium phosphate (to decrease urine calcium for calcium calculi), sodium bicarbonate, acetazolamide (Diamox) and allopurinol (Lopurin) (for uric acid calculi), and antibiotics
❏ signs and symptoms of recurring calculi
❏ urine pH testing
❏ need for follow-up laboratory tests
❏ need for follow-up visits with the doctor
❏ need for follow-up diagnostic tests
❏ date, time, and location of next appointment
❏ how to contact the doctor.

Documentation checklist
Using outcome criteria as a guide, document:
❏ clinical status on admission
❏ significant changes in status
❏ pertinent laboratory and diagnostic test findings
❏ renal pain episodes
❏ pain-relief measures
❏ passage of renal calculi fragments
❏ fluid intake
❏ urine output and characteristics
❏ other therapies
❏ nutritional intake
❏ patient and family teaching
❏ discharge planning.

ASSOCIATED PLANS OF CARE

Knowledge deficit
Pain
Surgery

REFERENCES

LeMone, P., and Burke, K.M. *Medical-Surgical Nursing: Critical Thinking in Client Care*. Menlo Park, Calif.: Addison-Wesley-Longman Publishing Co., 1996.

Lewis, S.M., et al. *Medical-Surgical Nursing: Assessment and Management of Clinical Problems*. St. Louis: Mosby–Year Book, Inc., 1996.

Lingeman, J.E. "Lithotripsy and Surgery," *Seminars in Nephrology* 16(5):487-98, September 1996.

Tressler, K.M. *Clinical Laboratory and Diagnostic Tests: Significance and Nursing Implications*. Stamford, Conn.: Appleton & Lange, 1995.

Part 12

Hematologic and immunologic disorders

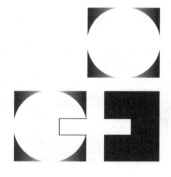

Acquired immunodeficiency syndrome
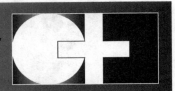

DRG information

DRG 488   HIV with Extensive Operating Room Procedure.
Mean LOS = 20.5 days

DRG 489   HIV with Major Related Condition.
Mean LOS = 10.7 days

DRG 490   HIV with or without Other Related Condition.
Mean LOS = 6.6 days

Additional DRG information: To ensure maximum reimbursement, document all complications of acquired immunodeficiency syndrome (AIDS).

INTRODUCTION

Definition and time focus

AIDS is a progressive, chronic disorder of cell-mediated and humoral immunity caused by the human immunodeficiency virus (HIV), a retrovirus previously referred to as the human T-lymphotropic virus type III or the lymphadenopathy-associated virus. HIV is a ribonucleic acid (RNA) virus that selectively infects human cells marked with a CD4 surface antigen and, when stimulated, rapidly produces additional HIV, destroying and killing the human cell. Although T4 lymphocytes are most commonly infected, any cell with the CD4 surface antigen is vulnerable to infection, including monocytes, macrophages, bone marrow progenitors, and glial, gut, and epithelial cells. HIV infection renders the patient immunodeficient and susceptible to opportunistic infections, unusual cancers, and other characteristic abnormalities.

The Centers for Disease Control and Prevention (CDC) first described AIDS in 1981. The 1993 modification of its case surveillance definition includes HIV-infected youths and adults with CD4 counts of less than 200 cells/µl or total lymphocytes of less than 14%. HIV infection is seen as a continuum of disease, ranging from being asymptomatic to causing multiple opportunistic infections.

The current definition of AIDS includes three categories for CD4 counts and three clinical categories, allowing the patient with HIV to be placed into one of nine mutually exclusive categories. See *CD4 lymphocyte categories* for an illustration of the three CD4 categories. The three clinical categories (A, B, and C) range from least to most severe. A patient in category A is an adolescent or adult with documented HIV infection who does not have any of the conditions included in categories B or C but does have one or more of the following:

• asymptomatic HIV infection
• persistent generalized lymphadenopathy
• acute (primary) HIV infection with accompanying illness or history of acute HIV infection.

A patient in category B is an HIV-infected adolescent or adult with one or more of the following symptomatic conditions (the patient may also have other symptomatic conditions not listed below):

• bacillary angiomatosis
• candidiasis (thrush), oropharyngeal
• candidiasis, vulvovaginal; persistent, frequent, or poorly responsive to therapy
• cervical dysplasia, cervical carcinoma in situ
• hairy leukoplakia, oral
• herpes zoster (shingles), involving at least two distinct episodes or more than one dermatome
• idiopathic thrombocytopenic purpura
• listeriosis
• pelvic inflammatory disease, particularly if complicated by tubo-ovarian abscess
• peripheral neuropathy.

A category B patient also does not have any condition listed in category C, and his conditions (1) are attributed to HIV infection or indicate a defect in cell-mediated immunity or (2) are considered by the doctor to have a clinical course or to require management that is complicated by HIV infection. For classification purposes, category B conditions take precedence over category A conditions. An HIV-positive patient who has been treated and has not developed a category C condition and is asymptomatic is classified as category B.

A patient in category C has one or more of the conditions listed in *Diagnostic criteria for AIDS*, page 749.

CD4 lymphocyte categories

Below are CD4 lymphocyte categories

CD4 T-cell category	CD4 cells/µl	CD4 percentage
1	500	≥ 29
2	200 to 499	14 to 28
3	< 200	< 14

For classification purposes, once the patient has developed one of these conditions, he remains classified as category B. These guidelines may change with further study and developments in clinical practice.

Two disorders commonly linked with AIDS are *Pneumocystis carinii* pneumonia (PCP) and Kaposi's sarcoma (KS). PCP, the most common opportunistic infection present at diagnosis, is a protozoal pneumonia. KS is a malignant neoplasm that begins as reddish or purplish skin lesions with variable distribution that may gradually spread, involving internal organs, mucous membranes, and lymph nodes. Various other conditions may present with AIDS, including infections related to cytomegalovirus (CMV), *Mycobacterium avium* complex (MAC; also known as *Mycobacterium avium-intracellulare [MAI]*), *Mycobacterium intracellulare*, *Cryptococcus*, *Candida*, or herpesvirus.

AIDS currently has no cure, and the prognosis for long-term survival is unknown. The introduction in 1996 of protease inhibitors has greatly improved the projected life expectancy for patients with HIV. The so-called AIDS cocktail typically is made up of three drugs, one of which is a protease inhibitor. To keep the virus suppressed, the patient must take 20 pills each day on a strict dosing schedule that must continue indefinitely; the individual immune response seems to play a role in survival. Some patients cannot comply with this strict regimen, and others cannot tolerate the adverse effects of treatment. The cost of the treatment is prohibitively expensive for many developing nations as well as for those who are poor or uninsured in developed nations. The number of inpatient hospitalizations has decreased since the advent of this treatment. This plan focuses on the patient admitted for diagnosis and treatment of one or more HIV-related conditions.

Etiology and precipitating factors

• Sexual transmission or artificial insemination (via semen, seminal fluid, or vaginal secretions)
• Blood-borne transmission from I.V. drug use, multiple blood transfusions (especially before 1985), blood product transfusions (including clotting factors), organ transplants, or cuts or sticks from needles or other sharp instruments that may be contaminated
• High-risk groups include homosexual and bisexual men, I.V. drug users, recipients of contaminated blood or blood products, sexual partners of those considered at high risk, and neonates born to mothers who were HIV-positive during pregnancy

Focused assessment guidelines

Nursing history (functional health pattern findings)

Health perception–health management pattern
• Asymptomatic or mononucleosis-like symptoms reported by patient for 3 to 6 weeks after initial exposure
• Weeks to months of fatigue, malaise, low-grade fever, drenching night sweats, anorexia, sore throat, upper respiratory disorder that lingers, cough, or shortness of breath
• History of recurrent infections (including sexually transmitted diseases [STDs]), amebiasis, or herpes simplex infections
• Known exposure to HIV
• Self-identification for high risk, such as a male homosexual or bisexual, I.V. drug user, or recipient of blood products
• History of multiple blood transfusions
• Sexual partner of someone at high risk

Nutritional-metabolic pattern
• Anorexia or dysphagia
• Episodic oral candidiasis (thrush), which may interfere with eating and taste
• Weight loss greater than 10 lb (4.5 kg) in 1 month

Elimination pattern
• Persistent diarrhea, even with treatment
• Incontinence (from myopathy)

Activity-exercise pattern
• Severe exertional shortness of breath (with pulmonary involvement)
• Dry mouth
• Displayed lack of energy and malaise
• Leg weakness (from myopathy) or pain and numbness (from neuropathy)

Sleep-rest pattern
• Drenching night sweats
• Erratic sleep patterns because of other symptoms

Cognitive-perceptual pattern
• Forgetfulness, depression, mental dullness or lability, difficulty concentrating, or other changes in mental status
• Headache
• Pain from tumor invasion, fever, or neurogenic causes

Role-relationship pattern
• Close friends or sexual partners who have died from AIDS
• Expressed anxiety over potential loss of social contact if diagnosis becomes known to others or expressed distress over actual losses

Sexuality-reproductive pattern
• Sexual activity with multiple partners
• Previous infection with other STDs

Coping–stress tolerance pattern
• Young to middle-age, previously healthy person who reports little experience with illness or death
• Delayed pursuit of medical attention until symptoms became severe because of fear, denial, lack of information, or low self-esteem
• Extreme anxiety and uncertainty expressed regarding diagnosis, current status, and prognosis
• Denial as initial coping behavior
• Signs of depression
• Suicidal thoughts expressed
• Fear regarding lifetime antiretroviral and prophylaxis treatment regimen expressed

Value-belief pattern
• Belief that illness is punishment for previous behavior
• Survivor guilt experienced by patient

Physical findings
Pulmonary
• Shortness of breath
• Dry cough
• Crackles
Gastrointestinal
• Diarrhea
• Hepatomegaly
• Splenomegaly
• Diffuse abdominal tenderness
• Thrush
• Mucosal lesions
• Oral hairy leukoplakia
Neurologic
• Anxiety
• Decreased mental acuity (as shown by slowed speech or impaired memory)
• Tendency to not initiate conversation
• Impaired sense of position or vibration
• Weakness
• Paresthesia or paralysis
• Hyperreflexia
• Retinal abnormalities
• Diffuse retinal hemorrhage or exudates
• Positive Babinski's sign
Integumentary
• Drenching night sweats
• In KS, reddish or purplish lesions varying in size from a few millimeters to a few centimeters across; may be macules or papules, usually appearing first on the head and neck or mucous membranes
• Dermatitis
• Lymphadenopathy
• Herpes zoster or simplex
• Anal warts
• Diffuse dry skin
• Butterfly rash on nose or cheeks
• Tinea
• Edema (with advanced KS)

• Hypersensitivity to light touch
• Molluscum contagiosum
Musculoskeletal
• Weakness
• Pain
• Stiff neck

Diagnostic studies
The following are HIV antibody tests:
• enzyme-linked immunosorbent assay (ELISA) — identifies HIV antibody (In the asymptomatic person, the ELISA is not diagnostic for AIDS: An individual may have a positive test without subsequently developing signs or symptoms. In addition, the ELISA may be falsely negative if performed too soon after exposure to the virus, or falsely negative or falsely positive if the person has had influenza or another viral illness recently. A positive ELISA in a patient who exhibits one or more indicator diseases, such as PCP, KS, emaciation, or dementia, can be considered diagnostic. A positive result is usually followed by a Western blot assay for a more definitive diagnosis. Consult current CDC guidelines.)
• Western blot assay — uses electrophoretically marked proteins to distinguish and differentiate antibodies; used with ELISA to confirm diagnosis
• radioimmunoprecipitation assay — more costly, time-consuming, and labor-intensive than the Western blot assay; generally used in cases that are hard to diagnose
• anonymous home testing kit — manufactured by Home Access and approved by the Food and Drug Administration (FDA) in 1996, this test provides results in 3 to 7 days along with pretest and posttest counseling (1-800-HIV-TEST)
• salivary testing (OraSure) — approved by the FDA in 1994, its use is limited to extreme cases in Africa where tribesmen cannot return for test results
• urine testing for HIV antibodies — approved by the FDA in August of 1996, this test has a false-positive rate of 1 to 2/100 and is thus usually followed by the Western blot assay for a more definitive diagnosis.

Viral load tests detect changes in viral load, referred to in "logs." A significant change is > 0.5 log. These tests are used to decide when to initiate or change treatment in an attempt to keep the viral load below detectable levels. However, these tests are limited because they cannot reveal viral levels in reservoirs where the virus may be hiding, such as the brain. Such tests include the following:
• polymerase chain reaction technique — amplifies target deoxyribonucleic acid (DNA) to estimate the virion population to levels as low as 20 copies/ml, considered "undetectable"
• branched-chain DNA amplification technique — provides an estimate of HIV RNA levels and can measure levels as low as 500 copies/ml

Diagnostic criteria for AIDS

According to the Centers for Disease Control and Prevention (1993), a patient who tests positive for human immunodeficiency virus and who has a CD4 count less than 200 cells/μl or who has one or more of the following diseases is diagnosed as having acquired immunodeficiency syndrome (AIDS).

Viruses
• Herpes simplex virus that causes a mucocutaneous infection of more than 1 month; or bronchitis, pneumonitis, or esophagitis
• Cytomegalovirus in an organ other than the liver, spleen, or lymph nodes
• Papovavirus such as progressive multifocal leukoencephalopathy

Bacteria
• Mycobacterium that causes disease outside the lungs, skin, or cervical or hilar lymph nodes
• *Salmonella* infection that causes recurrent, nontyphoidal septicemia
• *Mycobacterium tuberculosis* at any site
• Recurrent bacterial pneumonia

Fungi
• Candidal infection that causes disease in the esophagus, trachea, bronchi, or lungs
• Cryptococcosis that causes extrapulmonary disease
• Histoplasmosis or coccidioidomycosis that causes disease outside the lungs and cervical and hilar lymph nodes
• Disseminated coccidioidomycosis

Protozoa
• *Pneumocystis carinii* pneumonia
• Toxoplasmosis of the brain
• Cryptosporidiosis or isosporiasis that causes diarrhea for more than 1 month

Cancer
• Kaposi's sarcoma
• Primary lymphoma of the brain
• Other malignant lymphomas, such as B cell or unknown immunologic phenotype, small noncleaved lymphoma, and immunoblastic lymphoma
• Invasive cervical cancer

Other
• Wasting syndrome that causes unexplained weight loss of more than 10% and diarrhea or fever that lasts for more than 1 month
• Dementia that causes cognitive or motor dysfunction and interferes with work or activities of daily living
• HIV-related encephalopathy

• nucleic acid sequence-based assay — quantifies HIV RNA in blood plasma; more commonly used in Europe
• genotypic antiretroviral resistance testing — used to detect mutations in reverse transcriptase and protease genes associated with resistance to antiretroviral agents; used to determine what medication is likely to be most effective.

The following laboratory findings represent characteristic values in patients with AIDS but are not specific to or diagnostic of AIDS:
• complete blood count (CBC) — reveals leukocytopenia and anemia
• total T-cell count — reduced; CD4 cell count commonly less than 400 cells/μl

• CD4 to CD8 cell ratio — low; decrease depends on patient's status, usually less than 1.0 (CD4 cells also are known as helper or inducer T cells; CD8 cells also are known as cytotoxic or suppressor T cells)
• immunoglobulin (Ig) levels — usually elevated, especially IgG and IgA
• platelet count — shows thrombocytopenia
• absolute neutrophil count — may be low because of a reaction to a drug, underlying opportunistic infection, or disease progression; calculated by adding the percentage of bands and neutrophils and then multiplying by the total number of white blood cells (WBCs)
• skin test antigen studies — reveal anergy

• aspartate aminotransferase level — may be elevated (associated with hepatitis)
• lactate dehydrogenase level — may be elevated in PCP
• serum cholesterol level — may be low
• serum iron level — may be low
• hepatitis screen — may demonstrate carrier state or active disease (hepatitis A, B, C, and others)
• stool culture and examination — may reveal parasites or infection (such as cryptosporidiosis, salmonellosis, acid-fast bacilli, microsporidiosis, *Clostridium difficile*, MAC, *Isospora belli,* or *Giardia lamblia*)
• serum albumin and protein levels — may be low in emaciation
• blood urea nitrogen (BUN) level — may be elevated in emaciation.
   The following diagnostic procedures may be ordered for patients with AIDS:
• bronchoscopy — to diagnose PCP or other disorders, by transbronchial lung biopsy (to examine tissue) or by bronchoalveolar lavage to obtain a specimen containing PCP cysts, fungus, CMV, or KS
• chest X-ray — may reveal diffuse interstitial infiltrates (associated with PCP); however, may not be diagnostic even in active PCP
• colonoscopy and endoscopy — used to visualize and take a biopsy of the site for diagnosis of KS and other tumors
• culture of lesions — may demonstrate *Candida* or other organisms
• biopsy of lesions — may demonstrate KS, toxoplasmosis, or other complications
• gallium scan — may show radio-labeled gallium accumulation in WBCs of infected areas; used to help establish early diagnosis of PCP, although test is nonspecific
• blood cultures — may identify pathogen if bacteremia is present
• lumbar puncture — results vary; may reveal cryptococcal meningitis; culture of spinal fluid may reveal HIV; results may be inconclusive for CMV infection
• sputum test for acid-fast bacillus — may indicate *Mycobacterium*
• computed tomography scan or magnetic resonance imaging (MRI) — may identify lesions for later biopsy; MRI may be the only means to detect progressive multifocal leukoencephalopathy
• bone marrow aspiration — may reveal hypoplasia.

Potential complications

For a list of potential complications, see *Diagnostic criteria for AIDS*, page 749.

CLINICAL SNAPSHOT

ACQUIRED IMMUNODEFICIENCY SYNDROME

Major nursing diagnoses and collaborative problems	Key patient outcomes
Risk for infection	Maintain antiretroviral regimen.
Risk for ineffective individual coping	Identify specific personal stressors.
Risk for hypoxemia	Exhibit oximeter or arterial blood gas (ABG) measurements improved from baseline.
Sensory or perceptual alteration	Take appropriate precautions to prevent injury.
Social isolation	Contact support and resource persons, as appropriate.
Impaired physical mobility	Engage in physical activity as tolerated.
Nutritional deficit	Take food orally without excessive nausea or vomiting *or* state and demonstrate understanding of outpatient or home total parenteral nutrition therapy, if appropriate.
Risk for fluid volume deficit	Maintain normal fluid and electrolyte balance.
Altered oral mucous membrane	Perform or receive oral care at least four times daily.
Risk for impaired skin integrity	Maintain clean, dry, intact skin.
Risk for sexual dysfunction	Share sexual concerns with partner, friends, or staff members.
Risk for knowledge deficit (symptoms of disease progression, risk factors, transmission of disease, home care, and treatment options)	List precautionary measures to avoid infections.

COLLABORATIVE PROBLEM

Risk for infection related to immunosuppression (low CD4 lymphocyte count, low CD4-CD8 ratio, or neutropenia)

Nursing priorities
• Prevent or promptly treat new infections.
• Minimize effects of associated hyperthermia.

Patient outcome criteria
Throughout the hospital stay, the patient will:
• maintain antiretroviral regimen
• display no unanticipated medication adverse effects
• exhibit no signs or symptoms of dehydration.

Hematologic and immunologic disorders

Interventions

1. Provide continuous protection against infection. Implement CDC and institution precautions for the immunosuppressed patient, including meticulous hand washing before entering the patient's room and after leaving, providing only cooked or well-washed foods, prohibiting standing water in the room (such as in flower vases), protecting the patient from visitors with infections, and preventing the patient from handling live flowers or plants.

2. Monitor vital signs, including temperature, at least every 4 hours. Report fever onset or temperature spikes immediately.

3. Monitor CBC daily and report increasing leukopenia or neutropenia.

Rationales

1. The immunosuppressed patient is at risk for infection from any source, even those considered benign to a healthy person, such as raw fruits and vegetables. Such precautions minimize the patient's exposure to infectious organisms. Hand washing is the primary infection-control measure for any patient. Gloves are recommended along with protective gowns and eyewear, as indicated, to guard against exposure to HIV-contaminated blood or secretions. (See *Protecting yourself against HIV infection* for more information on infection control.) Raw produce may harbor gram-negative bacilli; standing water provides a medium for microorganisms, particularly *Pseudomonas*. Visitors may transmit organisms through direct contact or airborne bacteria. Plants and soil may harbor fungi.

2. Fever is the body's response to pyrogens released from invading microorganisms. The increase in metabolic rate is accompanied by a corresponding increase in the heart and respiratory rates. In the severely immunocompromised patient, however, the usual response mechanisms may fail, and sepsis may occur in the absence of fever. For this reason, careful, frequent observation to detect subtle changes in the patient's condition is essential.

3. These changes indicate further compromise of the body's ability to resist or fight infection.

Protecting yourself against HIV infection

When caring for patients with human immunodeficiency virus (HIV), health care providers are themselves at risk for infection because of exposure to infected waste, blood, body fluids, and needle-stick injury. Prevention of exposure to HIV and other infectious diseases should be the goal of all health care providers.

Take preventive measures
The Centers for Disease Control and Prevention (CDC) recommends that health care providers participate in in-service programs on current standard blood and body fluid precautions and body substance isolation. These techniques should be implemented to prevent the spread of HIV, hepatitis, and other contagious diseases.

Respond to exposure
If a needle-stick injury or exposure to infected waste, blood, or body fluid occurs, the health care worker will receive appropriate counseling with the options of testing and treatment. If an accidental injury or exposure occurs, follow your facility's policies and procedures, such as:
• wash the wound thoroughly and report the incident to the nursing supervisor
• seek counseling, including updated information on confidential testing and treatment.
The risk of seroconversion from a needle stick is 0.3%; the CDC recommends testing for HIV infection after the exposure and then at 6 weeks, 12 weeks, and 6 months.

Seek medication
Research shows that zidovudine may help prevent seroconversion if treatment starts within 1 hour after exposure. If the blood exposure came from a person known to have been using protease inhibitors, current clinical practice guidelines recommend the use of multiple antiretroviral agents within 1 hour or no more than 3 days after exposure to help prevent seroconversion.

4. Monitor potential sites of infection daily. Check I.V. and injection sites, mucous membranes (including the rectum and vagina), and any wounds or skin breaks for changes in color, texture, or sensation; swelling; pain; induration; purulent drainage; or other abnormalities. If the patient is alert, discuss the importance of ongoing monitoring and early reporting of signs and symptoms of infection to medical personnel.

5. Be alert for signs and symptoms of neurologic infection, including stiff neck, headache, visual or motor abnormalities, memory impairment, and altered level of consciousness (LOC). Compare new findings with baseline neurologic or mental status findings, and report abnormalities to the doctor immediately. Consult with the doctor about the need for a lumbar puncture or MRI series.

6. Monitor for evidence of new pulmonary infections, checking breath sounds at least every 8 hours. Report crackles, decreased breath sounds, or other abnormal findings promptly.

7. Obtain cultures, as ordered, from blood, stool, urine, sputum, or wound drainage. Evaluate sensitivity results and verify appropriateness of antibiotic therapy.

4. The skin is one of the body's most important barriers against infection, and any break in the skin provides an entry point for microorganisms. Classic signs and symptoms of infection may be masked or delayed in the immunocompromised patient, so regular, careful observation for any changes is essential. For example, dysphagia may indicate esophagitis, while white patches in the mouth may signal candidiasis (both are common in AIDS). Any suspicious area warrants prompt investigation because even benign microorganisms can cause life-threatening illness in a patient with AIDS.

5. Neurologic abnormalities are common in AIDS. Encephalitis, a common neurologic complication, may be caused by various microorganisms, including CMV, *Toxoplasma gondii*, or HIV. Progressive multifocal leukoencephalopathy, another common finding, is usually detectable only by MRI scanning. Early detection and treatment of neurologic infection is crucial; once such involvement is advanced, the patient's prognosis is poor.

6. The most common AIDS-related pulmonary infection is PCP, but others — including tuberculosis (TB) and fungal infections — may occur. Although the effectiveness of current pharmacologic treatment for PCP is related to individual response, prompt treatment of other pulmonary infections may be lifesaving for the immunocompromised patient.

7. If a new infection is suspected, immediate cultures will identify causative organisms. Sensitivity results guide antibiotic therapy.

Hematologic and immunologic disorders

8. Watch closely for signs and symptoms of systemic, skin, mucocutaneous, hematologic, ophthalmologic, oral cavity, esophageal, GI, pulmonary, and central nervous system opportunistic infections. Administer antibiotics and anti-infectives, as ordered. Once treatment begins, look for indications of adverse effects and report your findings. Consult current guidelines because recommendations may change with further research and clinical practice:

• MAC: ethambutol (Myambutol), clarithromycin (Biaxin), azithromycin (Zithromax), clofazimine (Lamprene), and ciprofloxacin (Cipro). Potential adverse effects include nausea, uveitis, neutropenia, thrombocytopenia, anemia, flulike syndrome, and hepatitis.

• TB: Active TB is treated with isoniazid, rifampin, pyrazinamide (PZA), ethambutol, and streptomycin. Potential adverse effects include aminotransferase elevations and hepatitis, peripheral neuropathy, and drug interactions.

• PCP: sulfamethaxole-trimethoprim (SMZ-TMP septra), pentamidine isethionate (Pentam), clindamycin (Cleocin), primaquine, dapsone, and trimetrexate. Potential adverse effects include anaphylaxis, severe rashes, Stevens-Johnson syndrome, fever, pancreatitis, and renal, hematologic, and GI reactions.

• CMV: ganciclovir, foscarnet, and cidofovir (Vistide) given indefinitely to prevent recurrence of retinitis. Potential adverse effects include anemia, leukopenia, nephrotoxicity, neuropathy, fever, rash, proteinuria, tremors, headaches, granulocytopenia, and penile ulceration.

• histoplasmosis and coccidioidomycosis: amphotericin B (Fungizone) and itraconazole (Sporanox). Potential adverse effects include nausea, vomiting, adrenal insufficiency, and drug interactions.

9. If the patient is on a prophylactic antiretroviral regimen (as most patients are), keep up-to-date with the specific drugs the patient is taking. Maintain the strict schedule of every 8 hours for protease inhibitors. Consult current guidelines for treatment. Have the pharmacy run a drug interaction chart to help prevent interactions and to optimize timing and use of medications. Experimental drugs include the following:

8. Depending on the organism, therapy may involve several drugs simultaneously. Antibiotics may also be ordered prophylactically. Specific acute and prophylactic drug treatment may vary with the patient, depending on the effectiveness of the medication and the patient's tolerance. Prophylactic treatment reduces the risk of developing an opportunistic infection and helps prevent a recurrence of an infection. More than any other intervention, this approach can improve the quality of life for an AIDS patient and increase his life span. Effectiveness varies, particularly in a second episode of PCP, which has a mortality rate of approximately 60%. If CMV is also involved, the mortality rate is higher.

9. Specific medications the patient takes may change while the patient is hospitalized. If protease inhibitors are not taken on a strict schedule, resistance and mutations may rapidly occur. Treatment guidelines change with advances in research and clinical practice. Drug interactions are common with anti-HIV medications and other drugs the patient may need during hospitalization.

It is rare for any of these agents to be used alone, with the exception of zidovudine, didanosine, and stavudine. Combination therapy affects the virus at the integration and budding stages, decreasing the number of mutations and keeping the virus at undetectable levels. The patient needs close monitoring for drug interactions.

• nucleoside reverse transcriptase inhibitors (NRTIs): zidovudine (Retrovir, AZT, ZDV), didanosine (Videx, ddI), zalcitabine (HIVID, ddC), stavudine (Zerit, d4T), and lamivudine (Epivir, 3TC); experimental drugs that are not FDA approved include carbovir. Adverse effects of zidovudine include anemia, granulocytopenia, myositis, and myopathy; didanosine can cause pancreatitis, hepatotoxicity, and peripheral neuropathy; zalcitabine can cause peripheral neuropathy, pancreatitis, esophageal or mouth ulcers, cardiomyopathy, and anaphylaxis; stavudine can cause anemia, hepatotoxicity, neutropenia, and peripheral neuropathy; and lamivudine can cause headache, myalgia, pancreatitis, and peripheral neuropathy.

• nonnucleoside reverse transcriptase inhibitors (NNRTIs): nevirapine (Viramune) and delavirdine (Rescriptor).

• protease inhibitors: indinavir (Crixivan), ritonavir (Norvir), saquinavir (Invirase), and nelfinavir (Viracept). Adverse effects of saquinavir include abdominal discomfort, diarrhea, nausea, and photosensitivity; ritonavir can cause nausea and diarrhea; indinavir can cause kidney stone formation and hyperbilirubinemia; and nelfinavir can cause abdominal discomfort and diarrhea.

10. If fever is present, administer acetaminophen, as ordered. Consult the doctor about alternating doses of acetaminophen with aspirin, naproxen (Naprosyn), or ibuprofen (Motrin) for persistent fever. Check platelet count and bleeding time before giving aspirin or ibuprofen, and withhold medication if clotting is prolonged.

11. Institute the following measures for fever, as ordered and appropriate: administering antipyretics, using a hypothermia blanket, monitoring for signs of dehydration, and replacing fluids as needed. See Appendix C, Fluid and Electrolyte Imbalances.

12. Additional individualized interventions: _____

• NRTIs inhibit reverse transcriptase action. They impede binding and entry of the virus into the host CD4 cell, resulting in DNA chain termination.

• NNRTIs also inhibit reverse transcripterase action. These drugs are still under study and are used only in combination with NRTIs and protease inhibitors.

• Protease inhibitors are active in late stages of HIV replication. Protease is needed for budding, and protease inhibitors render the virions ineffective.

10. Acetaminophen, aspirin, and ibuprofen inhibit the effects of pyrogens on the thermoregulatory center, thereby reducing fever. Aspirin and acetaminophen may impair zidovudine metabolism, resulting in toxicity; alternating antipyretics may avoid this effect. Aspirin and ibuprofen may decrease platelet adhesion, prolonging clotting time.

11. A hypothermia blanket may be necessary to reduce body temperature if aspirin and acetaminophen are ineffective or contraindicated. Prolonged fever increases the metabolic rate and promotes diaphoresis, contributing to dehydration and electrolyte imbalances. The Fluid and Electrolyte Imbalances appendix contains detailed information on these imbalances.

12. Rationales: _____

NURSING DIAGNOSIS

Risk for ineffective individual coping related to potentially life-threatening illness, decisions regarding treatment, or potentially uncertain prognosis for long-term survival

Nursing priority

Promote positive coping behaviors.

Hematologic and immunologic disorders

Patient outcome criteria

Throughout the hospital stay, the patient will:
• use positive coping behaviors, such as relaxation and verbalization of feelings
• display awareness of legal rights and available support, if appropriate to condition
• have opportunities to address issues of grieving and dying
• identify specific personal stressors
• identify resources and begin mobilizing them.

Interventions

1. Assess for excessive anxiety. Note signs and symptoms, such as poor eye contact, agitation, or restlessness.

2. Introduce yourself and other staff members. Provide continuity of caregivers; minimize use of unfamiliar staff whenever possible. Demonstrate acceptance by touching, making eye contact, and listening actively.

3. Implement measures to promote physical relaxation, as indicated, including progressive relaxation or controlled breathing techniques, therapeutic use of heat or massage, environmental modifications (such as reducing noise, heat, light, and other stimuli), physical therapy, and providing familiar articles brought from home.

4. Encourage verbalization of feelings. Anticipate fear, guilt, and anger, and accept such expressions as normal. If uncomfortable discussing explicit issues, arrange for another nurse to care for the patient. Whenever possible, refer the patient at the time of diagnosis to a mental health professional who can provide ongoing counseling.

5. Identify and discuss unhealthy coping behaviors. Teach the patient about the effects of alcohol or drug abuse on immune function.

Rationales

1. Prolonged or excessive anxiety may have negative psychological and physiologic effects. Anxiety interferes with the ability to learn, make decisions, and mobilize resources. Anxiety also increases sympathetic nervous system activity, increasing metabolic and cardiac demands and placing further stress on the body.

2. Consistency in staffing facilitates development of trust. Unfamiliar staff members may increase the patient's anxiety. Demonstrating acceptance promotes a therapeutic relationship. Patients with AIDS commonly report "feeling like lepers"; touch reduces this sense of isolation.

3. The patient may be unaware of physical tension and its contribution to anxiety. Physical relaxation promotes restoration of psychological equilibrium.

4. Some patients receive their HIV diagnosis at the same time as their first inpatient hospitalization. The diagnosis of AIDS carries an enormous psychosocial impact that may overwhelm the patient initially. The patient is typically unable to utilize usual defenses and resources; for example, denial may be impossible because of the media's coverage of AIDS, and friends or family may abandon the patient once the diagnosis is confirmed. If the disease was contracted through sexual contact, the patient may experience guilt over unresolved issues, anxiety or anger toward previous partners, or ambivalence about past or future desires or behaviors. The diagnosis requires that the patient immediately rethink relationships and commonly involves a loss of intimacy at a time when the patient needs support. Multiple referrals may lead to fragmented care; consistency in follow-up promotes optimal use of resources.

5. The patient may use alcohol or illegal drugs to avoid painful realities. If the disease was contracted through I.V. drug use, the underlying dependency must be addressed when planning care. Alcohol and drug abuse can compromise immune activity. The harm-reduction model can lead to safer behaviors. Include referral to counseling or rehabilitation program in discharge.

6. Help the patient identify and list specific fears and concerns contributing to anxiety. Focus on modifiable factors.

7. Help the patient identify and activate resources, considering inner strengths, coping ability, and such external supports as friends, family, and a spiritual advisor. See the "Ineffective individual coping" plan, page 67.

8. Assess the patient's knowledge about HIV, and teach him about anti-HIV medications. Explain the use of the mediset (daily or weekly medication box) and timer.

9. Acknowledge the unknowns of AIDS. Answer questions honestly and accurately. Accept the patient's response to losses. See the "Dying" and "Grieving" plans, pages 20 and 44, respectively.

10. Additional individualized interventions: _____

_____

6. Anxiety increases when fears seem overwhelming and all-encompassing. Identifying specific concerns helps quantify feelings and allows the patient to begin planning a coping strategy. Focusing on modifiable factors may increase the patient's sense of control.

7. Initial anxiety may be so overwhelming that the patient is unable to mobilize usual coping methods. The "Ineffective individual coping" plan provides specific interventions for the patient experiencing anxiety.

8. The regimen for taking medications is complex and the patient must take up to 20 pills a day, some with food and some fasting, on a strict schedule. If the patient must also take prophylactic drugs, he will need careful teaching to understand his schedule and the rationale behind treatment, including a written schedule, mediset, and timer.

9. Acknowledging unknowns reassures the patient that the caregiver understands and is sensitive to the profound changes AIDS implies. Reminding the patient that emotional reactions are a normal response to a realistic threat may reduce anxiety and facilitate coping. The "Grieving" and "Dying" plans provide further interventions related to psychosocial adjustment to illness and the losses illness entails.

10. Rationales: _____

_____

COLLABORATIVE PROBLEM

Risk for hypoxemia related to pneumonia, respiratory failure, or ventilation-perfusion imbalance

Nursing priority

Promote oxygenation.

Patient outcome criteria

Within 2 days of admission, the patient will:
• exhibit decreased dyspnea
• exhibit oximeter or ABG measurements improved from baseline
• cough and deep-breathe effectively
• initiate a plan for energy conservation.

Interventions

1. Assess continually for signs of hypoxemia, such as tachycardia, restlessness, anxiety, tachypnea, irritability, and pallor or cyanosis. Monitor oxygenation with an oximeter or take ABG measurements, as ordered and needed for increasing dyspnea or inadequate respiratory effort. Report abnormal findings immediately, and prepare the patient for ventilatory support, as condition indicates. Administer corticosteroids, colloids, and crystalloids, as ordered.

2. Administer oxygen therapy via nasal cannula, face mask, nonrebreather mask, or continuous positive airway pressure mask according to unit protocol or as ordered.

3. Perform airway clearance measures, as needed:
• If the patient is cooperative, teach coughing and deep-breathing exercises, and encourage hourly use of the incentive spirometer, as ordered.
• If the patient is uncooperative, perform artificial sighing and coughing with a handheld resuscitation bag hourly. Suction as needed if the patient is unable to cough effectively, as indicated by noisy respirations or gurgles auscultated over the large airways. Use supplemental oxygen before, during, and after airway clearance procedures.

4. Observe for complications of bronchoscopy; report any bleeding, anxiety, or unusual findings.

5. Evaluate and document the following every 8 hours and as needed: presence or absence of an effective cough, sputum character and color, respiratory effort, skin color, breath sounds, and activity tolerance. Be alert for changes in LOC, and report promptly any that occur.

6. If narcotic analgesics are used to control pain, be alert for signs of respiratory depression after analgesic administration. Report an excessively slowed respiratory rate, frequent sighing, decreased alertness, or any other indications of inadequate respiratory effort.

Rationales

1. PCP causes hard cysts to form in the interstitial spaces of the lungs, displacing surfactant and decreasing diffusion across the alveolar-capillary membrane. As partial pressure of arterial oxygen (PaO_2) levels decrease, the sympathetic nervous system attempts to compensate by increasing the heart rate. Progressive deterioration in ventilatory status in moderate to severe PCP may lead to respiratory failure — a common cause of death in AIDS-related illness. Ventilatory support may be required to maintain oxygenation. Routine use of corticosteroids, which may blunt the inflammatory reaction resulting from antipneumocystis treatment, has significantly decreased the need for mechanical ventilation. Corticosteroids also protect the pulmonary parenchyma from accelerated injury. Colloids and crystalloids may reduce the risk of overhydration and alveolar flooding.

2. Supplemental oxygen elevates arterial oxygen content and decreases hypoxia.

3. The patient may be unable to clear the airway effectively because of general debilitation and weakness. Deep breathing helps expand the lungs fully and prevents areas of atelectasis associated with pneumonia and bed rest. Incentive spirometry and coughing also promote lung expansion; however, exercise caution because coughing and positive-pressure breathing may cause alveolar rupture secondary to decreased surfactant in PCP. All airway clearance procedures may reduce PaO_2 levels. Supplemental oxygen may be provided through nasal prongs during suctioning.

4. Irritation from the bronchoscope may cause bleeding, further decreasing oxygenation and threatening airway patency.

5. Careful serial observations of respiratory status are essential to detect subtle changes that may indicate the need to reevaluate therapy. The patient with PCP may require multiple antibiotics if other infections occur simultaneously. Changes in LOC may signal impending respiratory failure.

6. Narcotics cause central nervous system depression and may impair respiratory center function.

7. Assist with self-care activities as needed (see the "Impaired physical mobility" nursing diagnosis in this plan). Teach energy conservation measures, such as using a shower chair, organizing activities and grouping procedures, using large muscles, avoiding activities that involve raising the arms over the head, and scheduling rest periods between activities.

7. Because activity increases oxygen demand, hypoxemia may worsen with exertion. Sitting requires less energy than standing. Organizing and grouping procedures reduce unnecessary exertion. Large-muscle groups are more efficient. Raising the arms over the head rapidly causes fatigue.

8. Additional individualized interventions: _____

8. Rationales: _____

NURSING DIAGNOSIS

Sensory-perceptual alteration related to neurologic involvement

Nursing priority

Minimize effects of neurologic changes.

Patient outcome criteria

Throughout the hospital stay, the patient will:
• use cues for reorientation
• take appropriate precautions to prevent injury
• acknowledge limitations appropriate to neurologic deficits.

Interventions

1. Assess the patient's mental and neurologic status on admission and at least daily thereafter, including LOC, orientation, long-term and recent memory, ability to follow directions and think abstractly, speech, pupillary responses, and strength and sensation in arms and legs.

2. Evaluate the patient's emotional state, considering the effects of depression, anxiety, grief, or other emotions on mental status findings. Also be alert to the possibility that medications may cause confusion, memory impairment, or other unusual findings.

3. Assess for possible visual impairment by using an eye chart, if possible. If the patient has significant visual impairment, prevent injury by placing items within easy reach and ensuring that side rails are always up.

4. If confusion is present, provide cues for reorientation, such as identifying yourself when entering the room, putting identifying signs on doors and objects, providing a large calendar and clock, discussing the day's events, and encouraging frequent visits, if possible, from family and friends.

Rationales

1. Baseline and ongoing mental and neurologic assessments allow early detection of neurologic involvement, a common and usually ominous finding in the patient with AIDS. Such disorders range from encephalopathies and neuropathies, occurring in 8% of patients, to less specific manifestations such as headache, occurring in up to 45% of patients. Delirium and seizures may also occur, impairing cognitive function.

2. Emotional responses and medication adverse effects may contribute to reduced alertness, confusion, withdrawal, hyperactivity, anxiety, or other mental status changes.

3. CMV infection of the optic nerve can cause blindness. Vision changes may be particularly frightening and difficult for the patient to accept. Precautionary interventions, particularly if confusion is also a factor, reduce the risk of injury.

4. Reorientation may help decrease anxiety, reduce the risk of injury, and facilitate coping.

Hematologic and immunologic disorders

5. Explain neurologic symptoms to the patient and to family and friends. Emphasize supportive behaviors, such as using humor, changing the subject if repetitive or irrational behaviors are present, providing gentle reminders of appropriate behavior, and listening actively.

6. Provide a safe and supportive environment, instituting safety measures appropriate to the patient's deficits.

7. Observe for involuntary movements, paresthesia, numbness, pain, weakness, and atrophy of extremities. Consult the doctor regarding treatment, if needed, and institute measures to protect the extremities if sensation is impaired.

8. Additional individualized interventions: _____

5. Explanations may help the patient feel less isolated and anxious about mentation changes. Family members and friends may be more supportive if they understand that mentation changes may be related to disease progression.

6. Confusion, disorientation, and loss of function are emotionally devastating. Because the disoriented patient is at increased risk for injury, safety measures must be instituted.

7. Distal symmetrical sensorimotor neuropathy is a common peripheral nerve complication in AIDS. The cause is unknown. Although a relatively benign condition, it may cause significant discomfort. Treatment may include heat, range-of-motion exercises, and electrical stimulation.

8. Rationales: _____

Nursing diagnosis

Social isolation related to communicable disease, associated social stigma, and fear of infection from social contact

Nursing priority

Minimize feelings of social isolation.

Patient outcome criteria

Throughout the hospital stay, the patient will:
• express feelings related to social losses
• express and receive affection
• contact support and resource persons, as appropriate.

Interventions

1. Assess the patient's support system, such as family, partner, and friends. Ask the patient and others in the support system about any recent losses in their lives, any recent change in the patient's living situation, and attitudes of family and friends toward the disease.

2. Provide opportunities for the patient and family to express their feelings.

3. Provide an atmosphere of acceptance. Encourage staff, family, and friends to touch and hug the patient.

Rationales

1. The patient's and others' lack of accurate knowledge as well as the social stigma associated with AIDS may diminish the patient's social contacts. In addition, the patient may isolate self from fear of contracting infections from others. Assessing the patient's social support system helps identify resources and may allow the nurse to correct misconceptions about the disease.

2. Expressing feelings helps decrease the sense of isolation.

3. Physical contact decreases feelings of isolation and demonstrates caring. Family and friends may need gentle reminders that such contact does not transmit the virus. The nurse can be a good role model for family and friends.

4. Teach family and friends about ways the AIDS virus is *not* transmitted, including the following: toilet seats and bathroom fixtures, swimming pools, dishes, furniture, handshakes, hugging, social (dry) kissing and other nonsexual physical gestures of affection, pets (although pets may carry microorganisms threatening to the patient), doorknobs, or casual social contact. Saliva, tears, and coughing are not considered sources of transmission. If an opportunistic infection is present, family members should observe the usual precautions, including hand washing, good health habits, and avoiding contact with contaminated secretions. Provide audio or written materials to reinforce these points.

5. Provide the patient and family with telephone numbers of available resources for counseling, support, and information. Check with the local public health department for resources in your area. See *AIDS resource numbers and Web sites* for more information. Refer the patient to the social services department for help with financial concerns.

6. Additional individualized interventions: _____

4. The "worried well" (those who are healthy but worried about contracting AIDS) may be torn between their desire to support the patient and their concern for personal health. Education may help reduce their conflicts and encourage normal interaction with the patient. The AIDS virus does not survive on inanimate objects and is killed by soap and hot water. Opportunistic infections can be transmitted to others, but healthy individuals are at no greater risk than usual. Audio or written materials reinforce oral teaching and provide a source for future reference.

5. Ongoing support is essential for the AIDS patient and the family throughout the illness. Support groups offer understanding, practical advice, and the latest information on new developments, which may surpass the support clinicians can provide. In addition, such groups may provide enriching relationships that enhance the patient's ability to cope with the disease. Referral to a social services department is essential because treatment is expensive and the patient may have special housing needs.

6. Rationales: _____

AIDS resource phone numbers and Web sites

Centers for Disease Control and Prevention (CDC)
1-800-342-AIDS
http://www.cdc.gov

CDC in Spanish
1-800-344-7432

CDC National AIDS Clearinghouse
1-800-458-5231 or
http://www.cdcnac.org/nacdb.html

UCSF Center for AIDS Prevention Studies
http://hivinsite.ucsf.edu/medical

AIDS Foundation
(415) 487-3000

National AIDS Clinical Trials
1-800-874-2572

Trial Search
http://www.cmegate.com/choice/ucsf

AIDS Knowledge Base (an on-line textbook for providers edited by Cohen, P., et al.) http://hivsite.ucsf.edu/akb/

AIDS articles in *JAMA*
http://www.amaassn.org/special/hiv/library/libhome.htm

Hematologic and immunologic disorders

NURSING DIAGNOSIS

Impaired physical mobility related to fatigue, weakness, hypoxemia, depression, altered sleep patterns, medication adverse effects, and orthostatic hypotension

Nursing priorities

• Promote maximum physical mobility.
• Prevent complications associated with decreased mobility.

Patient outcome criteria

Throughout the hospital stay, the patient will:
• appear rested
• verbalize adequacy of rest
• call for assistance as appropriate
• experience no falls or other injuries related to weakness
• engage in physical activity as tolerated
• develop no complications from impaired mobility.

Interventions

1. Provide standard nursing care for decreased mobility. Refer to the "Impaired physical mobility" plan, page 50.

2. Assist with activities of daily living (ADLs) as necessary. Anticipate the patient's needs. Assess the patient's neurologic status (see the "Sensory-perceptual alteration" nursing diagnosis in this plan).

3. Assess the need for sedatives, administer medications as ordered, and monitor their effects.

4. Encourage the patient experiencing weakness or orthostatic hypotension to use the call light, ask for assistance when standing and walking, and leave belongings within reach.

5. Additional individualized interventions: _____

Rationales

1. The "Impaired physical mobility" plan provides general nursing interventions for this condition. This plan supplies additional information specific to the AIDS patient.

2. The patient may never have been sick or hospitalized before and may feel uncomfortable asking for help. The "Sensory-perceptual alteration" diagnosis provides interventions and rationales for this diagnosis.

3. Anxiety and worry commonly interrupt sleep in the patient with AIDS. Rest is essential for healing.

4. The patient may have never been this weak or dizzy before and may need reminders to ask for assistance.

5. Rationales: _____

NURSING DIAGNOSIS

Nutritional deficit related to nausea, vomiting, diarrhea, anorexia, medication adverse reactions, or decreased nutrient absorption secondary to the disease

Nursing priority

Promote adequate nutritional intake.

Patient outcome criteria

• Throughout the hospital stay, the patient will maintain adequate oral intake of food *or* tolerate enteral or parenteral feedings without complications.
• By the time of discharge, the patient will:
  – exhibit BUN values decreased since admission
  – take food orally without excessive nausea or vomiting *or* state and demonstrate understanding of outpatient or home total parenteral nutrition (TPN) therapy, if appropriate.

Interventions

1. Provide typical assessments and interventions for nutritional status. Refer to the "Nutritional deficit" plan, page 80, for information.

2. Administer appetite stimulants (such as megestrol [Megace] and dronabinol [Marinol]), as ordered, to help stimulate the patient's appetite. Thalidomide, oxandrolone, nandrolone, and human growth hormone are all being used to combat HIV wasting; watch for adverse effects, including neutropenia. Keep in mind that the goal of therapy is to increase lean body mass. Consult current guidelines for use of appetite stimulants to combat HIV wasting. Refer to the "Altered oral mucous membrane" diagnosis in this care plan for information on fungal infections.

3. Administer antiemetics, as ordered, if nausea and vomiting are present.

4. Consult the doctor about nasogastric (NG) feedings or TPN if the patient is unable to tolerate adequate oral intake or has severe chronic diarrhea. See the "Total parenteral nutrition" plan, page 527, for further information.

5. Additional individualized interventions: _____

Rationales

1. The "Nutritional deficit" plan discusses general interventions for this condition. This plan contains additional information pertinent to AIDS.

2. First used in pregnant women to stimulate appetite, megestrol works well for some HIV patients. Dronabinol can stimulate appetite and decrease nausea. Thalidomide is thought to decrease the tumor necrosis factor, making it easier for the patient to gain weight. Human growth hormone and anabolic drugs (oxandrolone, nandrolone) promote muscle development and may prevent wasting. Long-term use of hormone stimulation is uncertain at this time. A weight gain from water retention or an increase in fat does not improve the patient's well-being. Guidelines for use of appetite stimulants may change with advances in research and clinical practice. The "Altered oral mucous membrane" diagnosis provides interventions for fungal infections.

3. Chemotherapeutic agents administered for infections commonly cause nausea and vomiting. Antiemetics block stimulation of the vomiting center.

4. NG feedings provide nutrients without as many associated complications as TPN. However, severe diarrhea from cryptosporidiosis, salmonellosis, or intestinal KS lesions may reduce GI absorption, making TPN necessary.

5. Rationales: _____

NURSING DIAGNOSIS

Risk for fluid volume deficit related to chronic, persistent diarrhea associated with opportunistic infection

Nursing priority

Maintain optimal fluid status.

Patient outcome criterion

Throughout the hospital stay, the patient will maintain normal fluid and electrolyte balance.

Interventions

1. To rehydrate the patient, encourage fluids by mouth, administer parenteral fluids, as ordered, or both. Monitor intake and output. See Appendix C, Fluid and Electrolyte Imbalances.

2. As ordered, administer antidiarrheal agents, such as loperamide (Imodium), diphenoxylate (Lomotil), or opium tincture.

3. Additional individualized interventions: _____

Rationales

1. Diarrhea is one of the most problematic signs for the AIDS patient. Various microorganisms contribute to the problem, while rectal mucosal lesions, hemorrhoids, and nutritional deficit exacerbate it further. Fever increases the potential for dehydration. The Fluid and Electrolyte Imbalances appendix provides further guidelines for monitoring fluid and electrolyte status and intervening to maintain optimal hydration and metabolic balance.

2. Many anti-HIV drugs and opportunistic infections can cause diarrhea, although many patients adjust to the diarrheal effects of drugs over time. Because a patient can have up to 20 stools per day, antidiarrheal medications are important to prevent dehydration.

3. Rationales: _____

NURSING DIAGNOSIS

Altered oral mucous membrane related to infections or masses

Nursing priority

Reduce discomfort and prevent further damage to the mucous membrane.

Patient outcome criteria

Throughout the hospital stay, the patient will:
• perform or receive oral care at least four times daily
• have oral mucous membrane lesions (if present) treated promptly.

Interventions

1. Assess the patient's mouth at least twice daily for signs and symptoms of thrush, lesions, or bleeding.

2. Ensure that the patient receives or completes mouth care after meals and at bedtime. Provide the following instructions:
• Use a soft toothbrush or swabs.
• Use dilute hydrogen peroxide or toothpaste.

3. Apply lubricant to the lips as needed.

4. Obtain cultures from suspicious oral lesions, as ordered.

Rationales

1. Candidiasis is extremely common in AIDS and has even been considered a harbinger of the disease. Lesions may occur as a medication adverse effect or from changes in normal oral flora.

2. Mouth care helps reduce the risk of infection by maintaining circulation to the mucous membrane and by decreasing bacteria in the mouth. Vigorous brushing is discouraged because it may cause bleeding and injure the mucous membrane, providing a place of entry for pathogens.

3. Lubricant helps prevent dry and cracked lips.

4. Culture results guide therapy.

5. Administer medications to treat the underlying diseases that can cause oral lesions as well as antifungal medications. Thalidomide is used for aphthous ulcers. Protease inhibitors cause mouth lesions associated with KS to recede, although some lesions only recede with the use of chemotherapeutic agents or radiotherapy. Antifungal agents used to treat thrush include clotrimazole (Mycelex), fluconazole, and itraconazole. Watch for adverse effects from treatments. No known treatment exists for hairy leukoplakia. Consult current treatment guidelines for oral lesions.

6. Avoid using alcohol, lemon-glycerin swabs, and commercial mouthwashes.

7. Assess for and report inflammation or ulceration of the oral mucosa, leukoplakia, pain, dysphagia, or voice changes.

8. Additional individualized interventions: _____
_____

5. Treatments that decrease oral lesions lessen discomfort and irritation, improving the patient's ability to swallow. Treatment guidelines may change with advances in research and clinical practice.

6. These products contain alcohol, which may dry and irritate mucous membranes.

7. Stomatitis, pharyngitis, and esophagitis are common AIDS-related infections. Initial signs and symptoms include inflammation of the mucous membranes, voice changes, and difficulty swallowing (if the inflammation involves the esophagus or larynx).

8. Rationales: _____

NURSING DIAGNOSIS

Risk for impaired skin integrity related to effects of immobility, disease, medications, or poor nutritional status

Nursing priority

Prevent skin breakdown.

Patient outcome criterion

Throughout the hospital stay, the patient will maintain clean, dry, intact skin.

Interventions

1. Implement usual measures to detect and prevent skin breakdown, such as inspection, frequent turning, and skin care.

2. If a pressure ulcer develops, institute therapeutic treatment, as ordered. This may include:
• cleaning or debriding agents (according to facility protocol or the doctor's recommendations)

• topical antibiotics

• blow-drying after bathing or treatments (follow facility policy)
• positioning to avoid pressure on the lesion, using foam or other padding as needed.

Rationales

1. Immunosuppression makes effective treatment of pressure ulcers difficult. Preventive care is essential.

2. Prompt treatment is essential to prevent further complications.
• Agent selection depends on the patient's status and the doctor's preference. Half-strength povidone-iodine solution (Betadine) is commonly used.
• The choice of prophylactic antibiotic (which varies) should be reevaluated if infection develops.
• A blow-dryer may be useful for certain areas such as the anus.
• Additional pressure leads to further tissue breakdown.

Hematologic and immunologic disorders

3. Observe for urticaria, maculopapular rash, pruritus, or other allergic reactions.

4. Provide appropriate patient teaching related to the above measures.

5. Additional individualized interventions: _____

3. Medications commonly used to treat opportunistic infections may cause skin irritation. Additionally, HIV infection itself may result in skin abnormalities.

4. For the able patient, such knowledge promotes self-care and a sense of increased control and self-esteem. For the patient unable to perform self-care, such knowledge promotes understanding of frequent interventions.

5. Rationales: _____

NURSING DIAGNOSIS
Risk for sexual dysfunction related to fatigue, depression, fear of rejection, and fear of disease transmission

Nursing priorities
- Promote a positive sexual self-concept.
- Teach safer sex practices.

Patient outcome criteria
By the time of discharge, the patient will:
- list safer sex measures
- exchange affection with loved ones
- share sexual concerns with partner, friends, or staff members.

Interventions

1. Determine if the patient is currently involved in a sexual relationship by asking direct questions in a non-judgmental manner. If you are uncomfortable discussing sexuality, refer the patient to another professional or an AIDS counselor.

2. Encourage open discussion and sharing of feelings between the patient and partner. Provide accurate information.

3. Encourage expression of affection and nonsexual touching, such as hugging, massaging, and holding hands.

4. Discuss safer sex practices. Refer to current CDC guidelines for detailed, up-to-date recommendations. Teach the patient and spouse or partner to observe the following guidelines:

- Abstain from sex or engage in a mutually monogamous relationship.

Rationales

1. Because the disease may be transmitted through sexual contact, assessing sexual relationships is essential. Many patients with AIDS are abandoned by their partners after diagnosis. If the patient is a homosexual, the high incidence of AIDS among homosexual males may add to the anxiety of both the patient and partner. This is especially true if the patient's sexual orientation is not known or accepted by family or friends.

2. Sharing of feelings may help the couple maintain closeness and offer mutual support. Accurate information helps dispel fears based on misunderstandings about AIDS.

3. Liberal use of touch reduces feelings of shame and abandonment.

4. Safer sex guidelines may help reduce the likelihood of disease transmission. CDC guidelines are revised frequently, so nurses should consult current information before providing specific teaching. The harm-reduction model encourages less risky sexual activities, decreasing the risk of sexual transmission.
- Multiple sexual contacts are associated with an increased risk of HIV transmission.

• Avoid exchange of blood or body fluids, including swallowing semen.
• Use sexual techniques that do not involve exchange of body fluids, such as mutual masturbation and fantasy.
• Avoid sex practices classified as "unsafe," such as intercourse without a condom, oral sex without a condom, and inserting objects into the rectum.
• Maintain safe sexual practices throughout life.

5. Additional individualized interventions: _____
_____

• The virus is transmitted through such exchanges.

• Alternative techniques may provide sexual satisfaction without the risk of disease transmission.
• Unsafe practices are associated with disease transmission.

• Even after AIDS education and years of safe sexual practices, the patient may relapse to unsafe behaviors.

5. Rationales: _____
_____

NURSING DIAGNOSIS

Risk for knowledge deficit (symptoms of disease progression, risk factors, transmission of disease, home care, and treatment options) related to lack of exposure to information

Nursing priority

Provide the patient and family with complete and accurate information.

Patient outcome criteria

By the time of discharge, the patient will:
• list precautionary measures to avoid infections
• list symptoms that may indicate infections or other complications
• discuss appropriate home care and waste disposal guidelines
• list precautions to prevent disease transmission
• verbalize awareness of legal rights.

Interventions

1. See the "Knowledge deficit" plan, page 72.

2. Teach the patient and loved ones about infection prevention measures, including:
• regular cleaning of bathrooms and kitchen

• avoiding crowds and persons with known or suspected infections; using good hand-washing techniques
• avoiding touching fish tanks, animal waste, or birdcages
• consulting the doctor before obtaining pets
• thoroughly washing all raw fruits and vegetables and avoiding raw and undercooked meat, seafood, and eggs and unpasteurized milk
• smoking cessation, as indicated

• consulting the doctor about vaccines

• following dietary recommendations, including high-protein, high-calorie intake

Rationales

1. The "Knowledge deficit" plan contains detailed interventions for patient and family teaching. This plan contains additional information pertinent to AIDS.

2. Infection control is essential to minimize the risk of further complications.
• Moisture in bathrooms and kitchen may facilitate fungal growth.
• Immunosuppression renders the patient extremely susceptible to infections.
• Animal waste harbors microorganisms.

• Pets may carry intestinal protozoa.
• These may be sources of microorganisms.

• Smoking increases the incidence of respiratory infections.
• The immunosuppressed patient may not be able to manufacture appropriate antibodies and may develop the disease the vaccine would normally protect against.
• Malnutrition predisposes the patient to infection.

• eliminating sources of standing water

• practicing good health habits, such as getting adequate rest and regular exercise, and avoiding steroids or recreational drugs that may further decrease immune function.

3. Discuss signs and symptoms that may indicate AIDS-related complications. These include night sweats, chest pain, shortness of breath, swollen glands, persistent fever, weight loss, diarrhea, weakness, purplish blotches on the skin, white patches or ulcerations in the mouth, difficulty swallowing, dry cough, headache, confusion, easy bruising, and skin lesions. Emphasize the importance of promptly reporting signs and symptoms to health care providers.

4. Review with the family recommendations for home care and waste disposal:
• Wash hands thoroughly before touching the patient and after contact with blood or secretions.
• Use 1:10 bleach-in-water solution for cleaning blood spills and washing soiled bedding, medical equipment, bedpans or commodes, and soiled surfaces.
• Dispose of contaminated waste carefully. Flush body fluids, blood, and used tissues down the toilet. Place needles in a puncture-proof container; when full, seal and dispose of it in the trash. Double-bag nonflushable items soiled with secretions in plastic bags, tie closed, and dispose of in the trash.
• Use masks only when suctioning or performing other measures that may allow direct contact with secretions, or to protect the patient from the caregiver's infection.
• Wear gloves when handling body fluids or blood.
• Wash dishes and utensils in hot, soapy water.

5. Teach the patient and loved ones how the AIDS virus may be spread: by sexual activity or by direct contact of an infected person's blood or body fluids with the broken skin or mucous membrane of an uninfected person. Discuss such precautionary measures as:
• avoiding sharing personal toiletry items (such as razors and toothbrushes) and needles (including piercing and tattoo needles)
• not donating blood or organs

• obtaining pregnancy counseling

• using safer sex practices (see the "Risk for sexual dysfunction" nursing diagnosis in this plan for details).

• Standing water provides a medium for microbial growth.
• Overall health maintenance maximizes immune response.

3. Early reporting of new signs and symptoms, and prompt treatment of complications, may prolong active life.

4. Thorough, specific teaching reduces anxiety for family members and promotes safe and effective care. Current evidence does not suggest any danger of HIV transmission from casual contact. The CDC recommends that caregivers use blood and body fluid precautions.

5. Awareness of transmission factors may help the patient avoid spreading the disease to others.

• Sharing these items may permit transmission of the virus.

• The virus has been transmitted through blood transfusions and transplanted organs.
• The AIDS Clinical Trial Group study number 076 has demonstrated that when mothers are treated with AZT, the transmission rate from mother to child is 8.3%, compared to 25.5% in the group receiving placebos. The worldwide transmission rate varies from 8.3% to 45%. Increasingly, the use of AZT and other antiretrovirals is becoming the standard of care to decrease HIV transmission from mother to child.
• Sexual activity is a major method of HIV transmission.

6. Provide information regarding the patient's legal rights, including privacy and confidentiality of medical records, laws protecting against discrimination in housing and employment, and the right to choose treatment and participate in research studies, as appropriate. If unable to provide such information yourself, refer the patient to an AIDS support group or AIDS hotline as appropriate.

6. Because of the widespread fear of AIDS, the patient may encounter discrimination. Knowledge of legal rights and options may help prevent further losses.

7. Encourage the patient to explore treatment options with the doctor, including new or experimental medications and alternatives to traditional medicine (such as acupuncture, visualization, nutritional therapy, and stress control).

7. At this time, no cure for AIDS exists; however, new or alternative therapies may offer as-yet-undocumented benefits. In addition, such therapies may offer the patient hope, energy, and an increased sense of wellness.

8. Additional individualized interventions: _____

8. Rationales: _____

DISCHARGE PLANNING

Discharge checklist
Before discharge, the patient shows evidence of:
❏ stable vital signs
❏ absence of cardiovascular and pulmonary symptoms
❏ absence of skin breakdown
❏ stabilizing weight
❏ ability to tolerate adequate nutritional intake
❏ ability to control pain and nausea using oral medications
❏ ability to transfer, ambulate, and perform ADLs independently or with minimal assistance
❏ absence of bowel or bladder dysfunction
❏ mentation indicating an ability for continued independent self-care
❏ adequate home support system or referral to home care or hospice if indicated by disease stage, inadequate home support system, or inability to manage ADLs and care independently.

Teaching checklist
Document evidence that the patient and family demonstrate an understanding of:
❏ disease and its implications
❏ the purpose, dosage, administration schedule, and adverse effects requiring medical attention for all discharge medications
❏ community resources available for emotional support, financial counseling, grief counseling, and individual and family counseling
❏ treatment options, including investigational studies and compassionate-use medications
❏ resources for long-term care or terminal care, such as hospice or home care
❏ signs and symptoms of opportunistic infection or complications

❏ ways to prevent HIV transmission
❏ ways to decrease risk of new infection
❏ symptoms to report to the health care provider
❏ importance of keeping follow-up appointments
❏ how to contact the doctor
❏ legal rights and resources.

Documentation checklist
Using outcome criteria as a guide, document:
❏ clinical status on admission
❏ significant changes in mental and physical status
❏ pertinent laboratory and diagnostic test findings
❏ occurrence of opportunistic infections
❏ treatment decisions
❏ nutritional program and support
❏ breathing patterns
❏ sleep patterns
❏ emotional coping
❏ support from family and friends
❏ patient and family teaching
❏ discharge planning.

ASSOCIATED PLANS OF CARE

Dying
Grieving
Impaired physical mobility
Ineffective family coping: Compromised
Ineffective individual coping
Knowledge deficit
Lymphoma
Nutritional deficit
Pain
Pneumonia
Total parenteral nutrition

Hematologic and immunologic disorders

REFERENCES

Baker, R., ed. "Guidelines for the Use of Antiretroviral Agents in HIV-Infected Adults and Adolescents," *Bulletin of Experimental Treatments for AIDS (BETA)* 11-22, June 1997.

Bower, M. "Blood Tests," *Bulletin of Experimental Treatments for AIDS (BETA)* 16-20, December 1996.

Centers for Disease Control and Prevention, "1993 Revised Classification System for HIV Infection and Expanded Surveillance Case Definition for AIDS Among Adolescents and Adults," *Morbidity and Mortality Weekly Report* 44(RR-17):1-9, 1992.

Chaisson, R.E. "1997 Revisions to Guidelines for Prevention of Opportunistic Infections," *The Johns Hopkins AIDS Service: Hopkins HIV Report* 9(3):1-4, May 1997.

Cohen, P., et al., eds. *The AIDS Knowledge Base*. Waltham, Mass.: Medical Publishing Group, 1994.

Deeks, S.G., ed. "Genotypic Resistance Assays and Antiretroviral Therapy," *Lancet* 349(9064):1489-90, May 24, 1997.

Elsner, L.G., ed. "AIDS Treatment Information Service (ATIS) Marks Second Anniversary," *CDC: Centers for Disease Control and Prevention: HIVAIDS Prevention* 10-12, December 1996.

Elsner, L.G., ed. "AIDS Deaths Decline While Decreases are Noted in Perinatally Acquired Cases," *CDC: Centers for Disease Control and Prevention: HIVAIDS Prevention* 11, March 1997.

Flaskerud, J., and Ungvarski, P. *HIV/AIDS: A Guide to Nursing Care*, 3rd ed. Philadelphia: W.B. Saunders Co., 1995.

Goldschmidt, R.H., and Dong, B.J. "Current Report — HIV: Treatment of AIDS and HIV-Related Conditions — 1996 Treatment of AIDS," *Journal of American Board of Family Practice* 9(2):125-48, March-April 1996.

Kaplan, J., et al. "USPHS/IDSA Guidelines for the Prevention of Opportunistic Infections in Persons Infected with Human Immunodeficiency Virus: A Summary," *Morbidity and Mortality Weekly Report* 44(44-8):1-33, 1995.

Lefkowitz, M. "Pain Management for the AIDS Patient," *Journal of the Florida Medical Association* 83(10):701-704, December 1996.

McMahon Casey, K., et al., eds. *ANAC's Core Curriculum for HIV/AIDS Nursing*. Philadelphia: Nursecom, Inc., 1996.

"New Information About Treatments for HIV 1997-1998," Treatment Education and Advocacy Department of the San Francisco AIDS Foundation *Bulletin of Experimental Treatments for AIDS (BETA)* 36, January 1998.

Phillips, K.D. "Protease Inhibitors: A New Weapon and a New Strategy Against HIV," *Journal of the Association of Nurses in AIDS Care* 7(5):57-71, September-October 1996.

Porche, D.J. "Treatment Review: Postexposure Prophylaxis after an Occupational Exposure to HIV," *Journal of the Association of Nurses in AIDS Care* 8(1):83-87, January-February 1997.

Price, R.W. "Neurological Complications of HIV Infection," *Lancet* 348(9025):445-52, August 1996.

Sabo, C.E., and Carwein, V.L. "Women and HIV/AIDS," *Journal of the Association of Nurses in AIDS Care* 5(3):15-21, May-June 1994.

Sande, M.A., and Volberding, P.A. *Medical Management of AIDS*, 5th ed. Philadelphia: W.B. Saunders Co., 1997.

Stephenson, K. "Open Clinical Trials for HIV/AIDS Treatments," *Bulletin of Experimental Treatment for AIDS (BETA)* 61-63, January 1998.

Anemia

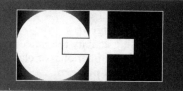

DRG information
DRG 395   Red Blood Cell Disorder; Age 17+.
          Mean LOS = 5.4 days
          Principal diagnoses include:
          • acquired hemolytic anemia
          • iron-deficiency anemia
          • aplastic anemia
          • other.
DRG 396   Red Blood Cell Disorder; Ages 0 to 17.
          Mean LOS = 3.8 days

INTRODUCTION

Definition and time focus
Anemia is not a disease but a laboratory diagnosis comprising a constellation of physiologic symptoms. These symptoms result from an inadequate number of circulating red blood cells (RBCs) or from a decreased hemoglobin level. The primary function of the RBC is to carry oxygen from the lungs to the tissues; anemia reduces the blood's oxygen-carrying capacity and produces signs and symptoms of tissue hypoxia.

Anemia occurs in three situations:
• life-threatening conditions, such as massive hemorrhage or bone marrow depression
• life-threatening complications, such as arrhythmias, angina, or pulmonary edema
• as a complication of another disease such as lymphoma.

Anemia may be classified by cause or by RBC morphology; both classifications are discussed in the appropriate sections below. This plan focuses on the newly diagnosed anemic patient with hemorrhagic or dietary deficiency anemia, the most common types. The principles of care can be generalized to other types of anemia but would be supplemented with condition-specific care, such as discontinuing medication (in toxic hemolytic reactions) or offering genetic counseling (in sickle cell disease).

Etiology and precipitating factors
• Excessive bleeding (acute or chronic)
• Decreased RBC production, caused by:
  – dietary deficiencies of iron, folic acid, or vitamin B_{12} (cobalamin)
  – damaged bone marrow (aplastic anemia) from medications, such as chloramphenicol (Chloromycetin) or sulfonamides; from chemotherapy with alkylating and antimetabolite agents; or from radiation

– impaired production of erythropoietin (in kidney disease)
  – defective hemoglobin synthesis (as in sickle cell disease and thalassemia)
  – decreased metabolic oxygen demand (as in hypothyroidism)
• Increased RBC destruction (hemolytic anemia), caused by:
  – hereditary disorders (such as sprue, sickle cell disease, or thalassemia)
  – autoimmune hemolytic reactions (such as from transfusions or lupus erythematosus)
  – toxic drug reactions (such as from penicillin, methyldopa [Aldomet], quinine [Quinine Sulfate], quinidine [Duraquin], or sulfonamides)
  – trauma (such as burns and crush injuries)
  – systemic diseases (such as Hodgkin's disease and lymphomas)

FOCUSED ASSESSMENT GUIDELINES

Nursing history (functional health pattern findings)
Not all of the following signs and symptoms are present in all anemias. Because of the many types of anemias, symptoms vary widely. The symptoms also vary with the anemia's severity. The patient with mild anemia (hemoglobin level greater than 10 g/dl) is usually asymptomatic at rest but is symptomatic with exertion. The patient with moderate anemia (hemoglobin level 6 to 10 g/dl) is chronically fatigued as well as symptomatic on exertion. The patient with severe anemia (hemoglobin level less than 6 g/dl) is exhausted, cold, and symptomatic even at rest.

Health-perception–health-management pattern
• Fatigue, headaches, dizziness, irritability, sensation of being cold, or palpitations at rest
• History of bleeding (such as from ulcers or hemorrhoids), renal disease, liver disease, cancer, chronic infections, angina (especially in older patients), or inflammation
• Current or recent use of medications (see list above) that affect RBC production (rare)
• Recent exposure to a chemical or a myelotoxic substance (such as benzene or a benzene derivative) or to large doses of radiation (rare)
• Family history of a disease such as sickle cell anemia, thalassemia major, or hereditary spherocytosis (all rare)

Activity-exercise pattern
• Fatigue, decreasing activity tolerance, weakness, shortness of breath, palpitations, or claudication
Cognitive-perceptual pattern
• Dizziness, headache, numbness, tingling of fingers and toes, or difficulty concentrating
Nutritional-metabolic pattern
• Weight loss, anorexia, nausea, indigestion, pruritus, or soreness of mouth, esophagus, or tongue (all rare)
Elimination pattern
• Tarry stools, constipation, diarrhea, or flatulence (all rare)
• Brown, hazy urine (rare)
• Gross blood in excretions (rare)
Sexuality-reproductive pattern
• Loss of libido, irregular menstruation or amenorrhea (if female), or impotence (if male)

Physical findings
Cardiovascular
• Tachycardia
• Cardiac enlargement (less common)
• Murmurs (less common)
• Dependent edema (less common)
• Vascular bruits (less common)
• Bounding arterial pulses (less common)
Pulmonary
• Dyspnea on exertion
• Tachypnea
• Orthopnea (less common than other signs)
Integumentary
• Pallor of skin and mucous membranes
• Diaphoresis
• Delayed wound healing
• Purpura (less common than other signs)
• Jaundice (less common than other signs)
• Spider angiomas (less common than other signs)
• Koilonychia (spoon nails) — late sign of iron deficiency

Diagnostic studies
• Hemoglobin level — may be decreased with iron-deficiency, pernicious, hemolytic, and hemorrhagic anemias
• Hematocrit — may be low
• RBC count — may be below normal
• Microscopic evaluation of peripheral blood (performed by a hematologist) — reveals size, shape, color, and number of RBCs; useful in diagnosing the specific type of anemia
  Note: The morphologic classification of anemias is based on structural changes seen in RBCs, which are classified by size and hemoglobin content:
    –Normocytic (normal size) and normochromic (normal color) RBCs are associated with anemias of sudden blood loss; pregnancy; chronic disease such as

cancer, kidney disease, or chronic infection; and some hemolytic anemias.
    –Macrocytic (abnormally large) and normochromic RBCs are associated with pernicious anemia, folic acid anemia, vitamin B_{12} deficiency, and some hemolytic anemias.
    –Microcytic (abnormally small) and normochromic RBCs are associated with anemias of chronic disease.
    –Microcytic and hypochromic (pale-colored) RBCs are associated with iron-deficiency anemia and thalassemia.
• Erythrocyte indices — use the RBC count, hemoglobin level, and hematocrit to define the size, hemoglobin weight, and hemoglobin concentration of a typical RBC; mean corpuscular volume (MCV) gives the average cell size; mean corpuscular hemoglobin gives the average hemoglobin weight; and mean corpuscular hemoglobin concentration (MCHC) identifies the average hemoglobin volume. Low MCV and MCHC indicate microcytic, hypochromic anemia (such as iron-deficiency anemia and thalassemia); a high MCV suggests macrocytic anemia (such as folic acid anemia or vitamin B_{12} deficiency).
• Reticulocyte count — if low, may indicate hypoplastic or pernicious anemia; if high, may indicate bone marrow response to anemia resulting from blood loss or hemolysis
• Erythrocyte fragility test — if low, may indicate thalassemia, iron-deficiency anemia, or sickle cell disease; if high, may indicate spherocytosis (hereditary disorders associated with autoimmune hemolytic anemia)
• Direct Coombs' test — positive response may indicate autoimmune hemolytic anemia (idiopathic, drug-induced, or caused by an underlying disease such as cancer or lupus erythematosus)
• Hemoglobin electrophoresis — identifies hemoglobin types by measuring the degree of negative charge
• Sickle cell test — identifies sickle cell disease and trait (hemoglobin electrophoresis is then needed to differentiate the two disorders)
• Serum iron and total iron-binding capacity (TIBC) levels — serum iron level decrease and TIBC increase indicate iron-deficiency anemia
• Serum folic acid levels — low levels may indicate megaloblastic anemia
• Serum vitamin B_{12} levels — low levels could indicate inadequate dietary intake of vitamin B_{12} or a malabsorption disorder
• Bone marrow aspiration and biopsy — histologic examination and differential count with erythroid-to-myeloid ratio useful for differential diagnosis of aplastic, hypoplastic, or pernicious anemia
• Liver-spleen scan — can detect splenomegaly associated with hereditary spherocytosis
• Chest X-ray — may show cardiac enlargement

Potential complications
- Hemorrhagic shock
- Angina pectoris
- Heart failure
- Pulmonary edema
- Renal damage
- Arrhythmias

CLINICAL SNAPSHOT

ANEMIA

Major nursing diagnoses and collaborative problems	Key patient outcomes
Hypoxemia	Maintain stable vital signs: typically, heart rate, 60 to 100 beats/minute; systolic blood pressure, 90 to 140 mm Hg; and diastolic blood pressure, 50 to 90 mm Hg.
Nutritional deficit	Follow the recommended diet.
Risk for impaired skin integrity	Maintain dry, intact skin.
Activity intolerance	Perform simple activities of daily living (ADLs) independently without reporting fatigue.
Hopelessness	Identify pertinent community resources.

COLLABORATIVE PROBLEM

Hypoxemia related to decreased oxygen-carrying capacity of RBCs

Nursing priority

Prevent or promptly relieve hypoxemia.

Patient outcome criteria

Throughout the hospital stay, the patient will:
- maintain vital signs within normal limits: typically, heart rate, 60 to 100 beats/minute; systolic blood pressure, 90 to 140 mm Hg; and diastolic blood pressure, 50 to 90 mm Hg
- have no palpitations or chest pain
- maintain usual mental status, ideally alert and oriented
- display arterial blood gas (ABG) levels within normal limits: pH, 7.35 to 7.45; PCO_2, 35 to 45 mm Hg; HCO_3^-, 23 to 28 mEq/L
- show normal skin color
- have clear breath sounds
- maintain acceptable hemoglobin level and hematocrit (as determined by the doctor)
- have no complaints of feeling cold.

Note: The expected outcomes for a patient with newly diagnosed anemia vary, depending on the type of anemia, its severity, its chronicity, the treatment selected, and the underlying disease. Therefore, these outcome criteria are general; more specific outcomes may need to be determined for each patient.

Hematologic and immunologic disorders

Interventions

1. Elevate the head of the bed.

2. Monitor for and report signs of hypoxemia, such as restlessness, irritability, and confusion. Observe oral mucosa, fingernail beds, palmar creases, and conjunctivae for pallor or cyanosis.

3. Monitor respirations before and after activity. Assess breath sounds at least every 8 hours and report crackles, gurgles, or decreased breath sounds to the doctor promptly.

4. Monitor the patient's pulse, noting strength and rate. Report a pulse that does not fall within normal limits for the patient.

5. Note chest pain or palpitations.

6. Monitor ABG measurements as ordered, and report results to the doctor.

7. Administer oxygen, as ordered.

8. Administer whole blood or packed RBCs, as ordered.

9. Monitor hemoglobin level and hematocrit.

10. Maintain a warm room temperature. Provide extra blankets if the patient desires.

11. Additional individualized interventions: _____

_____

Rationales

1. This position allows for greater lung expansion, promoting alveolar gas exchange.

2. Baseline and serial assessments of these signs of hypoxemia help individualize care. Neurologic signs reflect cerebral ischemia. Skin color changes are observed best in unpigmented sites. Because cyanosis indicates the presence of 5 g/dl or more of desaturated hemoglobin and hemoglobin levels may be so depressed that the patient cannot accumulate 5 g/dl of desaturated hemoglobin without decompensating, cyanosis may be absent or a late sign.

3. Dyspnea and tachypnea may be present in mild to moderate anemia. The exact cause of dyspnea is unclear. One hypothesis suggests that decreased oxygen pressure plays an important role. Heart failure may develop with severe anemia if the heart is unable to handle the increased cardiac output necessary to compensate for the lower oxygen saturation of the blood.

4. To compensate for the decreased hemoglobin level, cardiac rate and output increase. Pulse weakness, threadiness, and rapidity are more pronounced as anemia becomes more severe.

5. Angina pectoris may develop in severe anemia from ischemia of the heart muscle. Palpitations reflect increased myocardial irritability secondary to hypoxemia.

6. ABG measurements document the degree of hypoxemia. Inadequate hemoglobin saturation decreases the oxygen-carrying capacity of the blood.

7. Supplemental oxygen helps prevent tissue hypoxia by elevating the arterial oxygen content.

8. Transfusions elevate the RBC count, hemoglobin level, and hematocrit. An increased hemoglobin level improves arterial oxygen content, lessening signs and symptoms of hypoxemia.

9. These tests provide objective evidence of the degree of anemia and the efficacy of treatment.

10. The body compensates for chronic hypoxemia by lowering the metabolic rate and shunting blood to vital organs, making the patient more sensitive to cold. A cold room temperature induces vasoconstriction, which further impairs the release of oxygen to tissues.

11. Rationales: _____

_____

NURSING DIAGNOSIS

Nutritional deficit related to stomatitis, glossitis, anorexia, fatigue, lack of knowledge, or sociocultural factors

Nursing priority

Maintain adequate nutritional intake.

Patient outcome criteria

By the time of discharge, the patient will:
• show signs of improving nutritional deficiencies (manifested by improved hematocrit and hemoglobin level, serum albumin, and folic acid levels)
• have less tongue, mouth, and esophagus soreness
• increase weight toward normal for age, height, and body type
• have increased energy level
• follow the recommended diet
• verbalize ability to obtain recommended diet after discharge or have appropriate referrals made.

Interventions

1. Provide mouth care before and after meals, or assist the patient in performing mouth care. (Use a soft or sponge toothbrush to minimize trauma to the gums.)

2. Observe for soreness of the tongue, mouth, and esophagus.

3. Recommend a bland diet (avoidance of hot, spicy, or acidic foods).

4. Serve six small meals a day, providing foods that appeal to the patient and meet specific dietary needs. Consult the dietitian for a specific diet. Specific needs vary with the type of anemia and may include the following:
• for iron deficiency — red meat, organ meats, green vegetables, and enriched breads and cereals
• for vitamin B_{12} deficiency — meat, chicken, liver, shellfish, dairy products, egg yolks, and legumes
• for folic acid deficiency — green and leafy vegetables, fruits, meats, and whole grain breads and cereals
• for vitamin C deficiency — citrus fruits and juices.

Rationales

1. A patient with pernicious anemia or severe iron-deficiency anemia may have a sore mouth, tongue, or esophagus. Mouth care soothes and refreshes irritated tissues and can stimulate the patient's appetite. Frequent mouth care also decreases bacterial growth, thereby decreasing the risk of infection.

2. Stomatitis and glossitis may be present in pernicious anemia.

3. Spicy and acidic foods can further irritate the mouth, tongue, and esophagus. Hot foods have stronger odors than cold foods and may not appeal to the patient with a poor appetite.

4. Small portions require less energy to consume and digest. Large meals shunt blood to the GI tract, further contributing to fatigue. Foods that appeal to the patient are more likely to be eaten. The dietitian is best qualified to plan a diet that meets the patient's needs.

Hematologic and immunologic disorders

5. Administer vitamins and minerals, as ordered (for example, iron preparations, vitamin B_{12}, folic acid, and vitamin C). Use the Z-track method to administer I.M. iron. If parenteral iron is ordered, a test dose must be given to screen for allergies. Be alert for adverse effects of parenteral iron. If oral iron is prescribed, monitor the patient and teach these precautions:
• Take iron with meals.
• Avoid taking iron with dairy products, eggs, coffee, tea, or antacids.
• Increase vitamin C intake.
• If iron is in liquid form, dilute it, drink it through a straw, and rinse the mouth afterward.

6. Teach the patient the importance of a well-balanced diet, including specific dietary needs. Emphasize the importance of adequate intake. Relate dietary recommendations to the patient's signs and symptoms.

7. Document the patient's food intake.

8. Weigh the patient daily or as ordered.

9. If the patient's nutritional needs are not met by dietary intake, consult the doctor about enteral or parenteral feeding.

10. Before discharge:
• assess the patient's understanding of the importance of proper nutrition
• evaluate the patient's ability to obtain the prescribed diet and medications
• make referrals to social services or community agencies as indicated.

11. Additional individualized interventions: _____

5. Iron, vitamin B_{12}, and folic acid are needed to synthesize hemoglobin. The patient taking either folic acid or vitamin B_{12} may have allergic signs and symptoms of wheezing and itching. Possible adverse reactions to parenteral iron can include tachycardia, muscle pain, chest pain, backache, headache, chills, dizziness, fever and nausea. The Z-track method minimizes leakage of iron into surrounding tissues (thus minimizing pain) or out through the injection site (thus minimizing medication loss and tissue staining). Precautions for oral iron maximize absorption and minimize gastric distress and tooth staining. Vitamin C promotes iron absorption and influences folic acid metabolism.

6. Lack of knowledge can contribute to poor dietary intake. Stressing the importance of diet may enlist the patient's cooperation despite fatigue or discomfort. Using personal examples makes recommendations more meaningful.

7. Accurate documentation helps determine daily calorie needs.

8. The patient's weight can be used as part of the ongoing nutritional assessment and can help monitor fluid status.

9. Tube feedings or total parenteral nutrition may be indicated to improve nutritional status.

10. Poor nutrition may result from ignorance, poverty, or limited ability to shop for food, as in the debilitated older person who depends on public transportation.

11. Rationales: _____

NURSING DIAGNOSIS

Risk for impaired skin integrity related to tissue hypoxia, decreased mobility, and bed rest

Nursing priority

Maintain skin integrity.

Patient outcome criterion

Throughout the hospital stay, the patient will maintain dry, intact skin.

Interventions

1. Assess the patient's skin, including bony prominences, for redness and induration at every position change.

2. Keep the skin clean and dry; keep the bed linen dry and wrinkle-free.

3. Reposition the patient at least every 2 hours. Apply lotion to and massage pressure points. Increase the frequency of position changes if redness or induration occurs. Avoid weight bearing on reddened areas.

4. Teach active range-of-motion (ROM) exercises, and instruct the patient to do them hourly while awake, if tolerated. (If the patient cannot tolerate active ROM exercises, substitute passive ones.)

5. Assess the patient's need for a pressure-relieving device, such as a foam mattress or alternating pressure mattress, and obtain the device if indicated. (A doctor's order may be required to ensure insurance reimbursement.)

6. Additional individualized interventions: _____

Rationales

1. Mechanical pressure and decreased hemoglobin availability increase the risk of tissue hypoxia and cell damage. Abnormally red skin, especially over a pressure point, may indicate reactive hyperemia after relief of pressure-induced ischemia. Induration results from cellular changes that occur with ischemia.

2. The skin is the first line of defense against infection. Moisture provides a good medium for bacterial growth and can lead to maceration. Wrinkle-free linens distribute pressure evenly over the skin.

3. Hypoxemia increases the risk of tissue breakdown. Frequent turning relieves pressure and reestablishes blood flow. Massaging pressure points with lotion keeps the skin soft and increases circulation. Redness results from reactive hyperemia when pressure is relieved. Weight bearing on reddened areas may worsen ischemia.

4. Movement stimulates circulation and maintains muscle tone and joint mobility.

5. Pressure-relieving devices eliminate, change, or decrease the amount of pressure on the skin, improving or maintaining circulation.

6. Rationales: _____

NURSING DIAGNOSIS

Activity intolerance related to weakness and fatigue

Nursing priority

Increase the patient's independence in ADLs while minimizing weakness and fatigue.

Patient outcome criteria

By the time of discharge, the patient will:
• perform simple ADLs, such as eating, washing face and hands, and toileting, independently without reporting fatigue
• identify priority tasks on which to expend energy.

Interventions

1. Provide rest periods between activities and an environment that promotes rest. Get a description of the patient's room at home, and try to simulate it if possible. Teach the importance of rest.

Rationales

1. Rest decreases oxygen demand. Simulating features of the patient's room at home contributes to relaxation.

2. Assess the patient's normal ADLs, and offer help in prioritizing them. Help the patient establish a realistic activity level. Teach the patient to:
• avoid energy-taxing activities
• eliminate nonessential activities
• perform priority and necessary activities at times when the patient has the most energy.

3. Help the patient ambulate. Observe for and teach signs and symptoms of activity intolerance, such as dizziness, fainting, shortness of breath, chest pain, and worsened fatigue. Monitor orthostatic vital signs.

4. Allow as much self-care as possible, and assist as needed.

5. Place personal items (such as a water pitcher and tissues) within the patient's reach.

6. Additional individualized interventions: _____

2. Initially, the patient may need to limit activities to a few. Involving the patient in selecting these activities gives a sense of self-control.

3. Orthostatic hypotension may aggravate cerebral ischemia or cardiac ischemia. The patient may need encouragement to change position slowly and to pace activities according to tolerance.

4. Self-care encourages independence and helps promote and maintain self-esteem.

5. Placing personal items within the patient's reach encourages independence while conserving energy.

6. Rationales: _____

NURSING DIAGNOSIS

Hopelessness related to chronic fatigue, activity intolerance, and lack of independence

Nursing priority

Provide emotional support and guidance in solving practical problems.

Patient outcome criteria

By the time of discharge, the patient will:
• identify personal support systems
• identify pertinent community resources.

Interventions

1. Actively listen while the patient expresses personal feelings and frustrations.

2. Identify and assess the patient's personal resources. Assist with problem solving.

3. Provide information about available community agencies and the services offered by each. With the patient's consent, make appropriate referrals.

4. Additional individualized interventions: _____

Rationales

1. Active listening provides empathic support.

2. The patient's participation in identifying personal resources represents a significant step in actively coping with problems.

3. The patient may require help to meet basic needs. Community assistance may be available for preparing meals, performing light household duties, assisting with ADLs, and counseling.

4. Rationales: _____

DISCHARGE PLANNING

Discharge checklist

Before discharge, the patient shows evidence of:
- ❏ stable vital signs
- ❏ absence of fever
- ❏ hemoglobin level and hematocrit within acceptable parameters
- ❏ ABG measurements within normal parameters
- ❏ absence of cardiovascular and pulmonary complications, such as dyspnea and angina
- ❏ ability to tolerate adequate nutritional intake
- ❏ stabilizing weight
- ❏ ability to obtain recommended diet
- ❏ ability to perform ADLs and ambulate the same as or better than before hospitalization
- ❏ adequate home support system or referral to home care (as indicated by lack of home support system, inability to follow diet and medication regimen, or inability to perform ADLs and tolerate moderate activities).

State professional review organizations have specific parameters for acceptable hemoglobin levels upon discharge. Parameters vary by state. A hospital can receive a citation for discharging a patient whose hemoglobin is less than 10 g/dl, especially if the patient is readmitted within 15 days of discharge. Therefore, the patient's blood work results should be examined closely at discharge, and any abnormal findings should appear in the discharge summary.

Teaching checklist

Document evidence that the patient and family demonstrate an understanding of:
- ❏ type of anemia and its implications
- ❏ all discharge medications' purpose, dosage, administration schedule, and adverse effects requiring medical attention
- ❏ special dietary needs
- ❏ community resources
- ❏ signs and symptoms indicating need for medical attention
- ❏ dates, times, and location of follow-up appointments
- ❏ how to contact the doctor.

Documentation checklist

Using outcome criteria as a guide, document:
- ❏ clinical status on admission
- ❏ significant changes in clinical status
- ❏ pertinent laboratory and diagnostic test findings
- ❏ nutritional intake
- ❏ activity tolerance
- ❏ patient and family teaching
- ❏ discharge planning.

ASSOCIATED PLANS OF CARE

Geriatric care
Ineffective individual coping
Knowledge deficit
Pain

REFERENCES

Erickson, J. "Anemia," *Seminars in Oncology Nursing* 12(1):2-14, February 1996.

Torrance, C., and Jordan, S. "Bionursing: Signs of Iron Deficiency," *Nursing Standard* 10(12-14):29-31, December 1995.

Hematologic and immunologic disorders

Disseminated intravascular coagulation

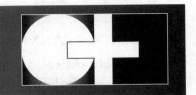

DRG information
DRG 397   Coagulation Disorders.
Mean LOS = 5.5 days
Principal diagnoses include all types of co-
agulation defects or disorders, including
disseminated intravascular coagulation.

INTRODUCTION

Definition and time focus
Disseminated intravascular coagulation (DIC) is a complex, acquired hematologic disorder characterized by a
paradoxical blend of coagulation and hemorrhage. One
or more procoagulants — such as bacterial toxins, exposure of collagen in damaged blood vessel walls, or
tissue fragments — provoke uncontrolled microcirculatory coagulation through the intrinsic clotting pathway,
extrinsic clotting pathway, or both.

The explosive production of thrombin causes widespread microcirculatory deposition of fibrin and rapid
consumption of clotting factors. It also triggers the
body's fibrinolytic system, a homeostatic mechanism
that limits coagulation. Fibrin split products, a by-prod-
uct of fibrinolysis, exacerbate bleeding because they
function as anticoagulants. Because of the anticoagulants and the scarcity of clotting factors, the patient cannot form stable clots and bleeding occurs throughout
the body. This plan focuses on the patient in the critical
care unit with acute DIC.

Etiology and precipitating factors
• Shock
• Cardiac arrest and cardiopulmonary resuscitation
• Adult respiratory distress syndrome (ARDS)
• Septicemia
• Neoplasms
• Transfusion reactions or other hemolytic conditions
• Trauma, lengthy cardiopulmonary bypass operations,
or other tissue injury
• Tissue necrosis
• Fat or amniotic fluid emboli

FOCUSED ASSESSMENT GUIDELINES

Nursing history (functional health pattern findings)
Health perception–health management pattern
Patient reports are relatively unimportant in diagnosis
of DIC. Usually, the patient is too ill from the primary
disorder to be aware of or report subjective manifesta-
tions. Even if the patient is alert, the widespread mani-
festations of DIC may cause variable, nonspecific symp-
toms.
Nutritional-metabolic pattern
• Nausea or vomiting
Activity-exercise pattern
• Dyspnea
• Fatigue or weakness
Cognitive-perceptual pattern
• Confusion, headache, or sudden localized pain

Physical findings
Physical findings vary greatly, depending on the under-
lying disorder, degree of organ involvement, and stage
of DIC.
Cardiovascular
• Blood oozing from multiple sites, such as I.V. inser-
tion sites, incisions, and nasal mucosa around endotra-
cheal or nasogastric tubes
• Repeated episodes of minor bleeding
• Frank hemorrhage
• Hypotension
• Tachycardia
Integumentary
• Acral cyanosis (irregularly shaped, patchy cyanosis of
fingers, toes, or ears), considered diagnostic of DIC
• Petechiae
• Purpura
• Ecchymoses
• Hematomas
• Necrosis over digits, nose, or genitals
Pulmonary
• Tachypnea or dyspnea or both
• Epistaxis or hemoptysis
Gastrointestinal
• Hematemesis
• Melena
Neurologic
• Coma
• Seizures
• Altered mentation or sensory-motor function

Renal
- Hematuria
- Oliguria or anuria

Diagnostic studies

DIC is a laboratory diagnosis based on a characteristic pattern of abnormal values.
- prothrombin time/international normalized ratio — prolonged, indicating dysfunction of the extrinsic clotting pathway
- activated partial thromboplastin time (APTT) — prolonged, indicating dysfunction of the intrinsic clotting pathway
- fibrinogen level — decreased because of fibrinogen consumption
- platelet count — diminished because of platelet consumption
- fibrin split products — increased because of fibrinolysis
- antithrombin III levels — decreased, indicating consumption by excessive thrombin formation
- d-dimer — increased, indicating excessive breakdown of fibrin bonds; highly predictive of DIC
- peripheral blood smear — reveals large platelets, reflecting rapid platelet usage, and red blood cell (RBC) fragments, reflecting damage during RBC passage through fibrin webs

Potential complications
- Organ necrosis
- Acute renal failure
- ARDS

CLINICAL SNAPSHOT

DISSEMINATED INTRAVASCULAR COAGULATION

Major nursing diagnoses and collaborative problems	Key patient outcomes
Risk for hemorrhage	Maintain stable vital signs: typically, heart rate, 60 to 100 beats/minute; systolic blood pressure, 90 to 140 mm Hg; and diastolic blood pressure, 50 to 90 mm Hg.
Ischemia	Produce more than 60 ml/hour of urine.
Risk for hypoxemia	Maintain arterial blood gas (ABG) values within normal limits: pH, 7.35 to 7.45; PCO_2, 35 to 45 mm Hg; and HCO_3^-, 23 to 28 mEq/L.
Impaired skin integrity	Maintain warm, dry, intact skin.
Pain	State that pain (with pain medication) is less than 3 on a 0 to 10 pain rating scale.

COLLABORATIVE PROBLEM

Risk for hemorrhage related to consumption of clotting factors, increased fibrinolysis, and presence of endogenous anticoagulants

Nursing priority

Control clotting and bleeding.

Patient outcome criteria

Within 72 hours of the onset of bleeding, the patient will:
- have no further episodes of oozing or frank hemorrhage
- maintain vital signs within normal limits: typically, heart rate, 60 to 100 beats/minute; systolic blood pressure, 90 to 140 mm Hg; and diastolic blood pressure, 50 to 90 mm Hg
- exhibit coagulation laboratory values within normal limits.

Hematologic and immunologic disorders

Interventions

1. Collaborate with the doctor to identify and treat the cause of DIC; for example, administer I.V. fluids to correct hypovolemia or antibiotics to combat sepsis, as ordered.

2. Monitor the presence and degree of hemorrhage. Observe for persistent oozing of blood at multiple sites, petechiae, purpura, ecchymoses, and hemorrhagic gingivitis. Note bleeding from wounds, drains, and chest tubes. In the female patient, check for vaginal bleeding. Test all drainage for occult blood.

3. Monitor trends in coagulation panels, as ordered.

4. Administer heparin, if ordered. Monitor the APTT, as ordered, and report values exceeding two times normal.

5. Administer transfusion therapy, as ordered, typically fresh whole blood, fresh frozen plasma, platelet concentrate, cryoprecipitate, or antithrombin III. Monitor trends in blood values, and anticipate the need for replacement blood products.

6. Monitor vital signs. Report systolic blood pressure below 90 mm Hg or a heart rate above 100 beats/minute.

7. Maintain a normal blood pressure by giving fluid and medications, as ordered.

8. Monitor for fluid overload. Observe for crackles, neck vein distention, or increased pulmonary artery (PA) and wedge pressures. If indicated, collaborate with the doctor to reduce fluid volume, such as by administering diuretics.

9. Additional individualized interventions: _____

_____

Rationales

1. Removing or controlling the underlying cause of DIC is essential to effective treatment.

2. The presence and degree of bleeding provide a rough indicator of the severity of DIC.

3. Coagulation values document the degree of DIC. They may be abnormal even if the patient does not show clinical signs of the disorder.

4. Heparin disrupts the vicious cycle of clotting and bleeding in DIC. Although it cannot lyse existing clots, it can prevent further clot formation. Heparin therapy during intense bleeding is controversial; however, it may be indicated when signs of thrombosis are present and blood component therapy is underway. Heparin inhibits thrombin (therefore limiting platelet aggregation and conversion of fibrinogen to fibrin) and factor X (therefore blocking both intrinsic and extrinsic pathways that lead to thrombin formation). Monitoring the APTT allows the doctor to adjust the heparin dose to maintain a therapeutic blood level.

5. Transfusion therapy replaces depleted clotting factors. Some doctors order it only after initiating heparinization, theorizing that replacing factors before interrupting the clotting cycle will only potentiate DIC. Antithrombin III inhibits the thrombin activation that triggers fibrin deposits.

6. Hypotension and tachycardia signal blood loss, requiring such interventions as fluid or blood replacement or medications to maintain blood pressure.

7. Both hypotension and hypertension are detrimental to the DIC patient. Hypotension contributes to the disease, while hypertension can dislodge precarious blood clots and initiate fresh bleeding.

8. The patient with DIC usually receives large amounts of fluid and frequent transfusions in an attempt to maintain optimal blood volume and cardiac output. Also, pulmonary capillary fragility increases the risk of interstitial edema. Untreated, fluid overload can progress to pulmonary edema.

9. Rationales: _____

COLLABORATIVE PROBLEM

Ischemia related to microcirculatory thrombosis

Nursing priority

Restore tissue perfusion.

Patient outcome criteria

Within 72 hours, the patient will:
• produce more than 60 ml/hour of urine
• exhibit a balanced fluid intake and output
• maintain vital signs within normal limits: typically, heart rate, 60 to 100 beats/minute; systolic blood pressure, 90 to 140 mm Hg; and diastolic blood pressure, 50 to 90 mm Hg.

Interventions

1. Evaluate status of organ systems at least every 4 hours by assessing:
• neurologic function, including level of consciousness, pupils, and sensorimotor function of the arms and legs
• cardiovascular function, including heart rate and volume, blood pressure, strength and symmetry of peripheral pulses (strength and symmetry), electrocardiogram pattern, and PA and wedge pressures
• GI function, including bowel sounds and abdominal girth
• skin condition (especially fingers and toes), looking for petechiae, bruising, and necrosis.

2. Monitor renal function closely. Document hourly urine output, noting and reporting any decreasing trend. Summarize fluid intake and output every 8 hours, noting and reporting undesirable fluid retention.

3. As ordered, implement measures (such as fluid administration) to treat the underlying cause of tissue ischemia.

4. Additional individualized interventions: _____

Rationales

1. Tissue ischemia and necrosis can occur in any body system from the widespread deposition of thrombi in the microcirculation. In addition, hypotension activates the complement system, resulting in increased vascular permeability and blood cell lysis, and the kallikrein system, resulting in increased vascular permeability and vasodilation. The net results are arteriolar vasoconstriction, capillary dilation, and arteriovenous shunting. Stagnant blood accumulates in the dilated, bypassed capillaries and becomes acidotic, further damaging tissue and contributing to clotting.

2. The renal system is most likely to suffer from thrombosis, resulting in acute tubular necrosis. Decreasing hourly urine outputs or oliguria may reflect this development. Because oliguria may also reflect other factors common in DIC, such as hypotension, cardiac failure, or hypovolemia, it must be interpreted in the context of the patient's overall condition.

3. Tissue ischemia is best treated by attacking its causes, such as hypovolemia.

4. Rationales: _____

COLLABORATIVE PROBLEM

Risk for hypoxemia related to increased pulmonary shunting, anemia, and acidosis

Nursing priority

Optimize oxygenation.

Hematologic and immunologic disorders

Patient outcome criteria

Within 72 hours, the patient will:
• display ABG levels within normal limits: pH, 7.35 to 7.45; PCO_2, 35 to 45 mm Hg; HCO_3^-, 23 to 28 mEq/L
• display a eupneic respiratory pattern
• have a respiratory rate between 18 and 24 breaths/minute
• display pink nail beds and buccal mucosa.

Interventions

1. Monitor ABG values, as ordered, for hypoxemia and acidosis. Monitor oxygen saturation, interpreting the percentage in relation to the current hemoglobin level; do not use the oxygen saturation percentage as the sole indicator of oxygenation.

2. Assess physical indicators of pulmonary status at least every 4 hours. Note increasing respiratory rate, abnormal respiratory rhythm, and crackles or other abnormal breath sounds. Observe nail beds and buccal mucosa for pallor and central cyanosis.

3. Administer supplemental oxygen, positive end-expiratory pressure (PEEP), or mechanical ventilation, as ordered.

4. Additional individualized interventions: _____

Rationales

1. Ischemic damage to the pulmonary parenchyma increases pulmonary shunting, impairing oxygen uptake in the lungs. RBC destruction produces a hemolytic anemia. These factors lessen arterial oxygen content. Also, acidosis and decreased tissue perfusion impair oxygen delivery to the tissues. Oxygen saturation measures only the percentage of available hemoglobin that is saturated with oxygen. The bleeding in DIC lowers hemoglobin levels, decreasing oxygen delivery to tissue even when hemoglobin is fully saturated.

2. The respiratory rate accelerates to compensate for hypoxemia. Rhythm changes may reflect medullary hypoxemia. Adventitious breath sounds may reflect alveolar accumulation of fluid as the heart fails from ischemia. Pallor and cyanosis reflect arterial oxygen desaturation.

3. Supplemental oxygen alone may be insufficient to raise low arterial oxygen content from pulmonary shunting. PEEP and mechanical ventilation may be necessary to improve functional residual capacity enough to combat hypoxemia.

4. Rationales: _____

NURSING DIAGNOSIS

Impaired skin integrity related to capillary fragility

Nursing priority

Prevent further bleeding.

Patient outcome criteria

Within 72 hours of onset of DIC, the patient will:
• have no new hematoma formation
• maintain warm, dry, intact skin.

Interventions

1. Avoid needle punctures, whenever possible. If a needle puncture is essential, use the smallest gauge needle possible and apply pressure to the site for 10 minutes afterward. Whenever possible, administer medications I.V., as ordered.

2. Handle the patient gently. Be particularly careful to avoid disturbing healing areas. Provide meticulous skin care.

3. Use an air flotation bed or cushioning and pressure-relieving devices, such as sheepskin. Pad the bed rails.

4. Provide gentle mouth care with swabs and diluted mouthwash.

5. Additional individualized interventions: _____

Rationales

1. These measures may help reduce hematoma formation. In addition, because of poor tissue perfusion, medication deposited I.M. may be absorbed erratically, if at all. Administering medications I.V. promotes absorption and avoids creating a puncture site from which the patient may bleed.

2. Gentle handling minimizes skin trauma. Being particularly careful around healing sites minimizes the risk of dislodging unstable clots.

3. These devices decrease pressure and the risk of trauma and minimize the risk of hematoma development from extreme capillary fragility.

4. A toothbrush may damage fragile capillaries and result in gingival bleeding.

5. Rationales: _____

NURSING DIAGNOSIS

Pain related to tissue ischemia, hematomas, or bleeding into organ or joint capsules

Nursing priority

Relieve pain.

Patient outcome criteria

Within 1 hour of pain onset, the patient will:
• have a relaxed facial expression and body posture
• if able to communicate, rate pain (with pain medication) as less than 3 on a pain rating scale of 0 to 10.

Interventions

1. Assess for pain frequently. Use various pain-relieving measures, such as ice packs for hematomas or soothing music. Promote rest and provide emotional support. Consult the "Pain" plan, page 88, for details.

2. Administer pain medications I.V.; if the patient's pain lasts for most of a 24-hour period, give him around-the-clock medication.

3. Additional individualized interventions: _____

Rationales

1. The "Pain" plan contains additional interventions for any patient in pain. This plan contains interventions specific to DIC. Soothing music helps relieve tension and lessen pain perception.

2. DIC may cause erratic absorption of I.M. medications. Around-the-clock administration can provide better pain control.

3. Rationales: _____

Hematologic and immunologic disorders

DISCHARGE PLANNING

Discharge checklist
Before discharge, the patient shows evidence of:
- ❏ stable vital signs
- ❏ laboratory coagulation panel within normal limits
- ❏ no bleeding episodes for at least 24 hours.

Teaching checklist
Document evidence that the patient and family demonstrate an understanding of:
- ❏ basic pathophysiology and implications of DIC
- ❏ rationale for therapy
- ❏ pain-relief measures.

Documentation checklist
Using outcome criteria as a guide, document:
- ❏ clinical status on admission
- ❏ significant changes in status
- ❏ pertinent diagnostic test findings
- ❏ bleeding episodes
- ❏ transfusion and fluid replacement therapy
- ❏ pain-relief measures
- ❏ patient and family teaching
- ❏ discharge planning.

ASSOCIATED PLANS OF CARE

Acute renal failure
Adult respiratory distress syndrome
Cardiac surgery
Hypovolemic shock
Impaired physical mobility
Ineffective individual coping
Liver failure
Major burns
Mechanical ventilation
Multiple trauma
Nutritional deficit
Pain
Septic shock

REFERENCES

Bell, T.N. "Disseminated Intravascular Coagulation: Clinical Complexities of Aberrant Coagulation," *Critical Care Nursing Clinics of North America* 5(3):389-410, September 1993.

Corbett, J.V., and Fonteyn, M.E. "Pharmacopeia. Treating Disseminated Intravascular Coagulation," *MCN: American Journal of Maternal Child Nursing* 20(5):290, September-October 1995.

Dressler, D.K. "Disseminated Intravascular Coagulation: Coping with a Paradoxical Crisis," *Nursing* 26(11):32aa-ff, November 1996.

Dressler, D.K. "Patients with Coagulopathies," in *Critical Care Nursing*, 2nd ed. Edited by Clochesy, J.M., et al. Philadelphia: W.B. Saunders Co., 1996.

Epstein, C., and Bakanauskas, A. "Clinical Management of DIC: Early Nursing Interventions," *Critical Care Nurse* 11(10):42-43, 45-53, November-December 1991.

Huston, C.J. "Disseminated Intravascular Coagulation," *AJN* 94(8):51, August 1994.

Rutherford, I.A. "Haemostasis and Disseminated Intravascular Coagulation," *Intensive and Critical Care Nursing* 12(3):161-67, June 1996.

Leukemia

DRG information

DRG 403   Lymphoma or Non-Acute Leukemia with Complication or Comorbidity (CC).
Mean LOS = 9.3 days

DRG 404   Lymphoma or Non-Acute Leukemia without CC.
Mean LOS = 5.1 days

DRG 405   Acute Leukemia without Major Operating Room (OR) Procedure; Ages 0 to 17.
Mean LOS = 4.9 days

DRG 473   Acute Leukemia without Major OR Procedure; Age 17+.
Mean LOS = 14.7 days

DRG 409   Chemotherapy with Acute Leukemia as Secondary Diagnosis.
Mean LOS = 17.4 days

These DRGs are used for the patient with leukemia admitted for either radiation or chemotherapy treatment.

INTRODUCTION

Definition and time focus

Leukemia is the proliferation and accumulation of abnormal blood cells in the bone marrow or lymph tissue. The malignant cells prevent normal hematopoiesis in the blood marrow, and migrate to other organs and tissues, causing the disease's symptoms. The leukemias may be classified according to several criteria, such as the cell and tissue type involved, the duration and course of the disease, or the number of leukocytes in the blood and bone marrow.

Leukemia is classified as *acute* if the bone marrow is infiltrated with undifferentiated, immature cells (blasts) and as *chronic* if the cells are primarily differentiated and mature. The most common types of leukemia involve abnormalities of white blood cells (WBCs), specifically granulocytes and lymphocytes.

Acute monoblastic leukemia is characterized by increased monoblasts (monocyte precursors). Adults with monoblastic leukemia have a poor prognosis, surviving about 1 year.

Acute myeloblastic (granulocytic) leukemia (AML) involves uncontrolled proliferation of myeloblasts, the precursors of granulocytes. The incidence of AML increases with age. The overall prognosis is poor, with a high mortality rate from infection and hemorrhage, usually within 1 year.

In *acute lymphoblastic leukemia (ALL)*, immature lymphocytes proliferate in the bone marrow. ALL is primarily a children's disease, with peak incidence between ages 2 and 4. Approximately 50% to 60% of patients survive 5 years.

Chronic granulocytic (myelogenous) leukemia (CGL) shows abnormal development of granulocytes in the bone marrow, blood, and tissues. An initial chronic phase is followed by an acute phase known as the blastic crisis. The disease occurs most commonly in patients ages 30 to 50. Patients survive 2 to 4 years after the initial phase but live only 3 to 6 months once the blastic crisis phase starts.

Chronic lymphocytic leukemia is the production and accumulation of functionally inactive but long-lived and mature-appearing lymphocytes. Patients (usually ages 50 to 70) typically survive 2 to 10 years.

This plan focuses on the adult patient admitted for diagnosis and treatment of leukemia.

Etiology and precipitating factors

The exact cause of leukemia is not known. Possible causes include:
• exposure to carcinogenic chemicals, such as benzene, alkylating agents, or chloramphenicol
• ionizing radiation
• viruses such as the Epstein-Barr virus
• familial tendency, congenital disorders such as Down syndrome, chromosomal abnormalities, ataxia-telangiectasia, and congenital immune deficiencies.

FOCUSED ASSESSMENT GUIDELINES

Nursing history (functional health pattern findings)

Health perception–health management pattern
• Gradual or sudden onset of fever, fatigue, weakness and lassitude, or headache
• Evidence of bleeding tendencies related by patient, such as gingival bleeding, purpura, petechiae, ecchymoses and easy bruising, epistaxis, and prolonged menstruation
• Identification as a monozygotic (identical) twin
• Positive family history for leukemia or chromosomal abnormalities
• Exposure to carcinogenic agents or ionizing radiation

Nutritional-metabolic pattern
• Nausea, anorexia, or weight loss
• Complaints of sore throat or dysphagia

Elimination pattern
- Blood in urine
- Tarry stools

Activity-exercise pattern
- Fatigue and weakness
- Dyspnea and palpitations on exertion
- Diminished activity because of bone and joint pain
- Abnormal bruising after minor trauma

Sleep-rest pattern
- Increased desire or need for sleep and rest

Cognitive-perceptual pattern
- Discomfort from mouth ulcers; abdominal, bone, and joint pain; and chills

Role-relationship pattern
- Verbalized difficulty in maintaining role function because of fatigue

Sexuality-reproductive pattern
- Decreased libido secondary to extreme fatigue
- Menorrhagia, if female

Coping–stress tolerance pattern
- Initial denial of diagnosis

Value-belief system
- Diagnosis of cancer as punishment
- Passive, fatalistic philosophy of life and death

Physical findings
General
- Elevated temperature
- Fatigued appearance

Cardiovascular
- Tachycardia
- Systolic ejection murmur

Respiratory
- Labored breathing
- Rapid breathing
- Wheezing
- Gurgles
- Decreased breath sounds
- Nosebleeds

Gastrointestinal
- Gingival hypertrophy or bleeding
- Mouth ulcers
- Hepatosplenomegaly
- Increased abdominal girth
- Vomiting
- Oral or rectal mucosal ulceration

Neurologic
- Confusion
- Visual changes

Integumentary
- Pallor
- Purpura
- Petechiae
- Pale mucous membranes
- Ecchymoses
- Erythema
- Rash
- Poor turgor

Genitourinary
- Hematuria

Lymphoreticular
- Lymphadenopathy

Musculoskeletal
- Joint swelling
- Decreased exercise tolerance

Diagnostic studies
- Complete blood count (CBC) — reflects bone marrow suppression by WBC infiltration
  - WBC count usually greater than 50,000/µl but may be low
  - differential shows increased number of lymphocytes or increased number of polymorphonuclear cells
  - red blood cell (RBC) count, hemoglobin level, and hematocrit below normal; platelet count very low, may be less than 50,000/mm^3
- Prothrombin time/international normalized ratio and activated partial thromboplastin time — may be prolonged
- Histochemistry — specific chemistry tests for leukemia show Sudan black or peroxidase; stains are positive in AML
- Uric acid and lactate dehydrogenase levels — elevated in acute leukemia; may indicate extensive bone marrow infiltration
- Liver enzyme levels — may be elevated, showing hepatic infiltration
- Leukocyte alkaline phosphatase levels — may be decreased
- Blood cultures — may show general sepsis
- Urinalysis — may show bacteria and WBCs (indicating infection) or RBCs (indicating bleeding)
- Blood urea nitrogen and creatinine levels — may be elevated in renal infiltration and failure
- Bone marrow aspiration — shows domination by leukemia blast cells of the affected cell line, may show abnormalities specific to leukemia, such as Auer bodies; shows decreased RBC levels and decreased platelet formation
- Lumbar puncture — may detect central nervous system (CNS) infiltration and meningeal irritation
- Liver-spleen scan — shows hepatosplenomegaly and enlarged abdominal lymph nodes
- Chest X-ray — may show lung infiltration, infection, or mediastinal adenopathy
- Computed tomography (CT) scan — may show enlarged lymph nodes or areas of consolidation
- Chromosome analysis — may help in the classification of leukemia by showing abnormal, translocated, extra, or missing chromosomes (such as the Philadelphia chromosome in CGL) in the patient's blood cells

Potential complications
- Infection, including sepsis
- Hemorrhage, especially of the CNS
- Immunosuppression
- Meningeal irritation
- Cardiotoxicity secondary to chemotherapy
- Hyperuricemia
- Mouth ulcers
- Constipation or diarrhea secondary to chemotherapy
- Arrhythmias secondary to electrolyte imbalance
- Malnutrition, including protein-calorie imbalances

CLINICAL SNAPSHOT

LEUKEMIA

Major nursing diagnoses and collaborative problems	Key patient outcomes
Knowledge deficit: Therapeutic modality and choice and care of vascular access device	State understanding of and correct response to vascular access device complications.
Risk for infection	Maintain stable WBC count and absolute neutrophil count.
Risk for hemorrhage	Maintain stable vital signs: typically, heart rate, 60 to 100 beats/minute; systolic blood pressure, 90 to 140 mm Hg; and diastolic blood pressure, 50 to 90 mm Hg.
Activity intolerance	Ambulate 20% further each day.
Nutritional deficit	Retain 75% or more of food intake.
Altered oral mucous membrane	Have no frank bleeding from gums.
Altered protection	Remain free from infection.
Risk for ineffective individual coping	Express feelings, if desired.

NURSING DIAGNOSIS

Knowledge deficit: Therapeutic modality and choice and care of vascular access device related to lack of exposure to information

Nursing priority

Teach the patient and family about the different types of vascular access devices, including how to care for the device and the site and how to identify complications.

Patient outcome criteria
- Within 3 days of admission, the patient will:
  - identify the type of vascular access device selected
  - state understanding of the rationale for using the device
  - state understanding of insertion procedure.
- Within 5 days of admission, the patient and family will state and demonstrate site care and basic technique for flushing the device.
- Within 7 days of admission, the patient and family will state the correct responses to vascular access device complications, including catheter occlusion, site infection, catheter damage or dislodgment, and infiltration or extravasation of I.V. fluids.

Interventions

1. Explain the rationale for and the different types of vascular access devices available for the patient with leukemia.

2. Assess the functional abilities, competency level, dexterity and coordination, visual acuity, motivation, and anxiety level of the patient and family.

3. Provide care for the vascular access device, and teach the patient and family how to care for it and the site and recognize and manage complications. Refer to the "Lymphoma" plan, page 804, for more information.

4. Additional individualized interventions: _____

Rationales

1. Treatment of leukemia requires ongoing antineoplastic chemotherapy, I.V. antibiotics, fluids and nutrition, I.V. infusions, blood and blood product transfusions, and venous blood sampling. Therapy is ongoing, and chemotherapy can have potentially devastating effects on the skin and vasculature, so a vascular access device, such as a tunneled catheter (Hickman, Groshong) or an implanted port (Port-A-Cath, Groshong), is inserted. This device consists of a vascular catheter whose tip is placed in the superior vena cava, allowing delivery of medication, blood and blood products, and parenteral nutrition. It avoids the irritating effects these substances would have if peripheral veins were used and allows for rapid absorption and higher blood concentrations.

2. After discharge, the patient and family will need to take responsibility for the device, including flushing the catheter and caring for the site. To prevent such complications as infection and catheter occlusion, they must be capable of performing the necessary level of care. Your assessment helps determine their capabilities.

3. Teaching helps prepare the patient and family to care for the vascular access device. The "Lymphoma" plan provides interventions and rationales for teaching the patient and family about vascular access devices..

4. Rationales: _____

NURSING DIAGNOSIS

Risk for infection related to incompetent bone marrow and immunosuppressive effects of chemotherapy treatment

Nursing priorities

• Recognize early signs of infection.
• Minimize local and systemic infection.

Patient outcome criteria

• Within 8 hours of admission, the patient will:
  – have potential sites of infection identified and monitored
  – present a temperature below 100° F (37.8° C)
  – exhibit pulse and respirations within normal limits.
• Within 1 day of admission, the patient will increase fluid intake to at least eight 8-oz (240-ml) glasses daily.
• Within 3 days of admission, the patient will:
  – exhibit no septicemia
  – exhibit no dysuria
  – have normal breath sounds.
• Within 7 days of admission, the patient will:
  – have intact oral mucous membranes
  – have no skin or rectal abscesses
  – maintain a stable WBC count and absolute neutrophil count (ANC)
  – maintain normal temperature
  – display negative urine, vaginal, blood, and sputum cultures.

Interventions

1. Assess the CBC, noting a WBC count below 2,000/µl and any sudden rise or fall in neutrophil level. Calculate the ANC using the formula

ANC = total WBC count × (% polys + % bands)

where polys are polymorphonuclear neutrophils and bands are immature neutrophils.

2. Place the patient in a private room or in protective isolation, according to protocol and the patient's condition. Maintain the immediate environment free from bacterial contamination, disinfect or sterilize equipment, keep equipment at the bedside, and do not use such items for other patients. Prohibit visitors or staff with known infections, such as a cold or influenza, from the room.

3. Monitor, report, and document any sign or symptom of infection: temperature above 100.4° F (38° C) lasting longer than 24 hours; chills; pulse above 100 beats/minute; crackles or gurgles; cloudy, foul-smelling urine; urgency or burning upon urination; redness; swelling; drainage from any orifice; perineal, rectal, or vaginal pain or discharge; and painful skin lesions.

4. Monitor and record fluid intake and output. Encourage fluid intake of up to twelve 8-oz (240-ml) glasses daily, unless contraindicated.

5. Use strict aseptic technique when starting an I.V. or accessing the patient's vascular access device. Consult the facility's policy manual for the frequency of and procedure for I.V. site, I.V. tubing, peripheral site, and central line dressing changes.

6. Provide a low-bacteria diet. Avoid raw fruits and vegetables, and use only cooked and processed or pasteurized foods.

7. Take measures to prevent respiratory tract infections. Instruct the patient to turn, cough, deep-breathe, and use the incentive spirometer every 2 hours. Document respiratory assessment every 4 hours.

8. Avoid invasive procedures, such as urinary catheterization, injections, and venipunctures, when possible. Examine the sites of earlier invasive procedures (such as bone marrow aspiration or venipuncture) for signs of inflammation.

Rationales

1. A decreased WBC count places the patient at increased risk for infection, a major cause of morbidity and mortality in the immunosuppressed patient. Such a decrease in WBC count results from both the disease and chemotherapy. A sudden change in the neutrophil level indicates impending infection. The largest component of granulocytes, neutrophils are responsible for the body's early response to infection, especially bacterial infection. Because the patient can have neutropenia even when the WBC count is normal, the ANC must be calculated to show the number of WBCs that are actually mature and able to fight infection. If the ANC is < 1,000/µl, the patient has neutropenia.

2. The patient must be protected from potential sources of infection.

3. An elevated temperature unrelated to drug or blood product administration indicates infection in about 80% of patients with leukemia. The immunosuppressed patient is unable to mount a normal response to infection, so an infection that would be harmless in a patient with a normal WBC count can cause septicemia in the leukopenic patient. Early treatment of any infection is essential to prevent complications and death.

4. Adequate fluid balance is essential to prevent dehydration from fever and fluid shift in septic shock.

5. Strict aseptic technique and following infection-control guidelines minimize the risk of bacterial contamination of the system and possible sepsis. The dressings on nontunneled central venous catheters are typically changed every 48 to 72 hours; dressings on tunneled catheters, every 5 to 7 days. Implanted ports do not need a dressing unless a continuous or intermittent infusion device is accessing the port.

6. These measures minimize potential sources of bacterial contamination from food.

7. Immobility promotes stasis of respiratory secretions, increasing the risk of pneumonia and atelectasis.

8. Any invasive procedure is a potential source of bacterial invasion. Take care to minimize trauma to the skin because of impaired healing abilities.

Hematologic and immunologic disorders

9. Provide meticulous skin care, paying close attention to any alteration in skin integrity. Wash the skin at least twice daily with antibacterial solutions. Monitor and document skin condition every shift.

10. Avoid trauma to the rectal mucosa; take the patient's temperature orally, and prevent constipation by ensuring adequate hydration and administering stool softeners, as ordered.

11. Observe for and report clinical signs of septicemia, such as tachycardia, hyperventilation, hypotension, or subtle mental changes. Obtain cultures and institute I.V. antibiotic therapy with cephalosporins (as ordered) within 1 hour of identifying signs and symptoms. Monitor fibrin degradation product (FDP) levels if the patient is septicemic.

12. Reduce temperature higher than 100° F (37.8° C). Administer acetaminophen (Tylenol) 650 mg every 4 hours, as ordered. Use tepid sponge baths, remove unnecessary clothing and linens, and apply a hypothermia blanket, as ordered. Prevent chilling and encourage oral fluid intake.

13. Prepare the patient for granulocyte transfusion if the WBC count is consistently below 500/µl and the patient has signs of infection. Infuse granulocytes slowly over 2 to 4 hours, as ordered. Observe for and document signs of a serious transfusion reaction, such as hypotension, allergic response, or wheezing. Discontinue the transfusion and notify the doctor immediately if a reaction occurs.

14. Administer sargramostim (granulocyte-macrophage colony-stimulating factor [Leukine]) or filgrastim (granulocyte colony-stimulating factor [Neupogen]) subcutaneously or I.V. when ordered for neutropenia. Watch for adverse effects. Report and document any that occur.

15. Additional individualized interventions: _____
_____

9. The skin is the body's first line of defense against infection. Any break in skin integrity is a source of potentially lethal bacterial contamination. The leukemic patient is as susceptible to infection from normal flora as from outside contamination. Frequent skin care minimizes the possibility of superficial skin breakdown and resultant infection.

10. Damage to rectal mucosa from frequent rectal temperatures or hard, dry stools may cause rectal abscesses.

11. Septicemia may occur without fever. Symptoms reflect initial stages of insufficient tissue perfusion. Prompt recognition and treatment of septic shock are crucial to prevent irreversible hypovolemia and decreased cardiac output. The septicemic patient is at increased risk for disseminated intravascular coagulation (DIC). Elevated FDP levels are seen in DIC.

12. Several measures may be necessary to reduce fever to a manageable level in the immunosuppressed patient. Untreated, high temperatures contribute to fluid imbalance, discomfort, and CNS complications.

13. Granulocyte transfusions are usually effective in the patient with granulocytopenia and progressive infections that do not respond to antibiotics or in the patient whose bone marrow does not recover after chemotherapy. Granulocytes are slightly contaminated with RBCs from the donor, so granulocyte transfusions must be ABO compatible to the recipient. Febrile reactions— shaking chills and temperature elevations—are not considered serious reactions to a WBC transfusion and should not prompt discontinuation of the transfusion. WBC transfusion can cause pulmonary symptoms, transmit cytomegalovirus, and contribute to the development of graft-versus-host disease.

14. Sargramostim and filgrastim are naturally occurring glycoproteins that increase granulocyte production. The usual dosage of sargramostim is 250 mcg/m^2 of body surface area daily for up to 21 days. The usual dosage of filgrastim is 5 mcg/kg daily for up to 14 days. Common adverse effects include flulike symptoms, generalized rash, and bone and muscle pain.

15. Rationales: _____
_____

COLLABORATIVE PROBLEM

Risk for hemorrhage related to incompetent bone marrow and the immunosuppressive effects of chemotherapy

Nursing priority

Minimize the potential for life-threatening hemorrhage.

Patient outcome criteria

- Within 1 day of admission, the patient will:
  - exhibit a platelet count above 50,000/mm^3
  - maintain stable vital signs: typically, heart rate, 60 to 100 beats/minute; systolic blood pressure, 90 to 140 mm Hg; and diastolic blood pressure, 50 to 90 mm Hg.
- Within 3 days of admission, the patient will:
  - exhibit no frank bleeding in stool, urine, vomitus, or sputum
  - present minimal extension of ecchymoses
  - present minimal bleeding from puncture sites, gums, and nose
  - have stable or improved hemoglobin level, hematocrit, and platelet count
  - exhibit minimal or no restlessness, confusion, lethargy, or other CNS symptoms.

Interventions

1. Monitor, report, and document signs and symptoms of bleeding problems:
- platelet count less than 50,000/mm^3
- petechiae, especially on distal portions of upper and lower extremities
- ecchymotic areas
- bleeding gums
- prolonged oozing from minor cuts or scratches
- frank or occult blood in urine, stool, vomitus, or sputum
- prolonged heavy menstruation
- decline in hematocrit and hemoglobin level
- narrowing pulse pressure with increased pulse rate
- restlessness, confusion, or lethargy.

2. Implement measures to prevent bleeding during invasive procedures:

- Use the smallest gauge needle possible when performing venipuncture or giving injections. Apply firm, direct pressure to the injection site for 3 to 5 minutes after the injection. If bleeding does not stop after 5 minutes, apply a sandbag to the site and notify the doctor.
- Monitor and document the condition of old puncture sites (such as from venipuncture, lumbar puncture, or I.V. infusion).

3. Provide a soft, bland diet, avoiding foods that are thermally, mechanically, or chemically irritating. Use only a soft-bristle or sponge toothbrush and an alcohol-free mouthwash (such as normal saline) every 4 to 8 hours.

Rationales

1. Normal platelet levels are required to maintain vascular integrity, platelet plug formation, and stabilized clotting. A decrease leads to local or systemic hemorrhage. With a platelet count of less than 20,000/mm^3, the patient is prone to spontaneous life-threatening bleeding. The patient with leukemia is prone to platelet deficiency because of the proliferation of WBCs, which interfere with normal platelet production, and because of the immunosuppressive effects of drug treatment.

2. Even minor invasive procedures can cause excessive bleeding, especially when the platelet count falls below 50,000/mm^3.
- The patient with thrombocytopenia may continue to bleed excessively even after minor invasive procedures. Firm pressure minimizes further blood loss and hematoma formation. Pressure dressings may be necessary if bleeding continues.
- Spontaneous bleeding from old puncture sites may occur at platelet levels below 20,000/mm^3.

3. The oral mucous membrane is very delicate in the leukemic patient and prone to hemorrhage with even minor irritation. Minimizing irritation decreases bleeding and promotes comfort.

Hematologic and immunologic disorders

4. Administer docusate sodium (Colace) or another stool softener daily, as ordered. Monitor and document the frequency of bowel movements. Avoid using enemas, suppositories, harsh laxatives, and rectal thermometers.

5. Instruct the patient to avoid activities that may cause bleeding, such as forcefully blowing the nose, using a straight-edged razor, cutting nails, and wearing tight, restrictive clothing.

6. Prepare the patient for a platelet transfusion, as ordered, when platelet counts drop below 20,000/mm^3. Obtain baseline vital signs before initiating the transfusion. Infuse each unit over approximately 10 minutes. Observe, report, and document signs and symptoms of transfusion reactions: nausea, vomiting, fever, chills, urticaria, or wheezing. Discontinue the transfusion immediately if symptoms develop, keep the vein open with normal saline, and notify the doctor. Be prepared to administer diphenhydramine (Benadryl), hydrocortisone (SoluCortef), or acetaminophen, as ordered.

7. Monitor hemoglobin level and hematocrit and test stools, urine, and sputum for occult blood, noting and reporting positive findings.

8. Avoid administering aspirin, anticoagulants, indomethacin (Indocin), and medications containing alcohol. Give phenothiazines cautiously.

9. Force fluid intake of eight to twelve 8-oz (240-ml) glasses daily, if tolerated. Check for elevated uric acid levels and acidic urine. Administer acetazolamide (Diamox), sodium bicarbonate, and allopurinol (Lopurin), as ordered. Monitor and record fluid intake and output. Provide appropriate patient teaching for measures to be continued after discharge.

10. Additional individualized interventions: _____

4. Constipation and straining during defecation must be avoided to prevent trauma to the rectal mucosa as well as increased intracranial pressure, which could cause spontaneous CNS bleeding. Rectal bleeding may develop with minimal trauma.

5. The patient may be unaware that some common actions can be dangerous when platelet counts are severely decreased.

6. Platelet transfusions reduce the risk of hemorrhage. A platelet transfusion can be made up of platelets taken from random donors or from a single donor. A random-donor platelet transfusion increases the risk of antibody development and sensitization reactions; a transfusion from a single donor decreases the chance of sensitivity and transfusion reactions. Special leukocyte reduction filters should be used for patients at risk for or with a history of febrile nonhemolytic reactions. If a transfusion reaction occurs, the doctor must evaluate the patient. If diphenhydramine and acetaminophen adequately control signs and symptoms, the remaining platelets can be transfused.

7. Decreasing hemoglobin level and hematocrit indicate hemorrhage. Occult bleeding must be detected and monitored to prevent hypovolemia.

8. These medications induce or prolong bleeding.

9. Hyperuricemia can result from rapid chemotherapy-induced leukemic cell lysis. Proper hydration and medication therapy are essential to prevent obstruction of the renal pelvis and ducts and subsequent renal failure. Acetazolamide is a diuretic, sodium bicarbonate maintains alkaline urine pH, and allopurinol inhibits uric acid synthesis.

10. Rationales: _____

NURSING DIAGNOSIS

Activity intolerance related to fatigue secondary to rapid destruction of leukemic cells, tissue hypoxia secondary to anemia, and depressed nutritional status

Nursing priorities

- Minimize energy-depleting activities.
- Maximize energy resources.
- Decrease tissue hypoxia.

Patient outcome criteria

• Within 1 day of admission, the patient will exhibit no adverse effects or toxic effects of blood transfusion, such as elevated temperature or urticaria.
• Within 3 days of admission, the patient will:
 – show improved ability to participate in self-care, bathing, and hygiene measures
 – sleep 1 hour before and after treatments
 – sleep 8 hours at night
 – ambulate 20% farther each day
 – participate in diversionary activities, such as reading, doing puzzles, and watching television
 – maintain hemoglobin level at 8 g/dl or higher
 – maintain hematocrit at 25% or higher.

Interventions

1. Assess, monitor, and document the cause, pattern, and impact of fatigue on the patient's ability to engage in activities of daily living (ADLs).

2. Monitor and document the degree of anemia present. Assess for pallor, weakness, dizziness, headache, and dyspnea. Evaluate and report hemoglobin level, hematocrit, and RBC count, especially a significant or consistent drop in hemoglobin (below 8 g/dl) or hematocrit (below 25%). Prepare for a blood transfusion, as ordered.

3. Monitor and document vital signs before, during, and after blood transfusion. Use a 19G or larger needle and tubing with a standard blood filter. Use standard Y-tubing with normal saline solution, filling the entire surface area of the filter with blood. Use a leukocyte reduction filter if the patient has a history of febrile nonhemolytic reactions.

4. Infuse blood slowly (20 drops/minute) for 15 minutes. Complete the transfusion within 1½ to 2 hours if the patient's condition remains stable.

5. Stop the transfusion at the first sign or symptom of a transfusion reaction: fever, chills, headache, low back pain, urticaria, wheezing, or hypotension. Keep the vein open with normal saline, and notify the doctor.

6. Implement measures to improve activity tolerance, such as the following:
• Provide uninterrupted rest periods before and after meals, procedures, and diagnostic tests.
• Instruct the patient to sit rather than stand when performing hygiene and daily care.
• Limit the number of visitors.
• Minimize environmental activity and noise.
• Assist the patient with activities.
• Keep supplies and personal articles within easy reach.

Rationales

1. Causes of fatigue in the patient with leukemia commonly have an additive effect. To treat the problem effectively, the nurse must use a holistic approach.

2. The degree of anemia significantly affects the level of fatigue. Decreased RBC count and the resulting decrease in the blood's oxygen-carrying ability cause severe weakness, exhaustion, and inability to mobilize energy. The values given indicate severe anemia and require therapy with blood transfusions.

3. Knowledge of baseline and ongoing vital signs is imperative to monitor for signs and symptoms of transfusion reaction. A large needle allows a suitable flow rate and prevents clumping and destruction of RBCs. The filter screens fibrin clots and particulate matter. Normal saline is the only solution suitable for use with RBCs because dextrose solutions cause hemolysis.

4. Blood is administered slowly during the first 15 minutes because transfusion reactions typically occur during this time. A slow rate minimizes the volume of cells transfused. However, blood should be transfused within 4 hours after leaving the blood bank, to prevent bacterial proliferation and RBC hemolysis.

5. Transfusion reactions must be recognized immediately to prevent death or organ damage.

6. Quiet, restful periods before and after meals, procedures such as chemotherapy, and diagnostic procedures help increase activity tolerance and promote a rested feeling. Conserving energy and improving activity tolerance usually help the patient participate more actively in care and treatment.

Hematologic and immunologic disorders

7. Assess, report, and document the patient's tolerance for progressive activity. Stop activity if the patient's pulse rate increases more than 20 beats/minute above the resting rate, if the blood pressure increases more than 40 mm Hg systolic or 20 mm Hg diastolic, or if dyspnea, chest pain, dizziness, or syncope occurs.

8. Reassure the patient that fatigue is an expected effect of chemotherapy.

9. Additional individualized interventions: _____

_____

7. The patient's response should guide any plan of progressive activity. The cited changes in baseline vital signs indicate that the patient is being pushed beyond therapeutic levels, and activity should be stopped.

8. The patient may fear that fatigue is related to extension of the disease. The patient should be reassured that fatigue is common after chemotherapy and does not necessarily reflect disease extension.

9. Rationales: _____

_____

NURSING DIAGNOSIS

Nutritional deficit related to anorexia, nausea, vomiting, taste perception changes, and alterations in cellular metabolism secondary to disease and chemotherapy

Nursing priorities

- Maximize oral intake of foods and fluids.
- Minimize catabolism and protein and vitamin deficiencies.

Patient outcome criteria

Within 3 days of admission, the patient will:
- exhibit no weight loss
- maintain serum electrolyte levels within normal limits
- tolerate nutritional supplements between meals
- maintain intake equal to output
- have no nausea or vomiting
- retain 75% or more of food intake.

Interventions

1. Provide standard nursing care related to nutritional deficit. Refer to the "Nutritional deficit" plan, page 80, for details.

2. Provide high-calorie, high-protein snacks, such as milk shakes, puddings, and eggnog.

3. Provide nutritional supplements between meals, as ordered. Serve them cold in a glass or other container, not in the can. Observe for and document undesirable adverse effects, such as gastric distention, cramping, or diarrhea.

Rationales

1. The "Nutritional deficit" plan presents general nursing care for this problem. This plan presents additional information related to leukemia.

2. Protein-calorie malnutrition is common in leukemia. Increased protein intake facilitates repair and regeneration of cells, and increased calories help fight the body's tendency toward cancer-induced catabolism.

3. Oral supplements are high in protein and are a valuable supplement to nutritious food. Many patients experience a metallic taste secondary to leukemia, and the sight of the can may aggravate this feeling. The adverse effects listed result from the high osmolality of supplemental liquids.

4. Take steps to decrease or prevent nausea and vomiting. Obtain a history of the patient's susceptibility to nausea and vomiting and determine the potential emetic effects of the chemotherapeutic agents prescribed. Administer antiemetics before the chemotherapy infusion begins. Antiemetics include benzodiazepines (such as lorazepam), butyrophenones (such as droperidol), cannabinoids (such as dronabinol), phenothiazines (such as prochlorperazine), substitute benzamides (such as metoclopramide), steroids (such as dexamethasone), antihistamines (such as diphenhydramine), and serotonin inhibitors (such as ondansetron or granisetron). Begin therapy 30 minutes to 2 hours before chemotherapy and continue for 24 to 72 hours, as ordered. Monitor the patient, and report and document the effectiveness of the therapy

4. Antiemetic medications block stimulation of the true vomiting center and the chemoreceptor trigger zone in the brain, thus decreasing nausea and vomiting and promoting relaxation. Because they have different mechanisms of action, antiemetics are often given in combination to enhance their effectiveness. Benzodiazepines depress the CNS and help treat anticipatory nausea and vomiting. Butyrophenones work as dopamine antagonists in the chemoreceptor trigger zone, thereby reducing the nausea and vomiting stimulus. Cannabinoids are believed to act by suppressing pathways to the vomiting and higher CNS centers. Phenothiazines block dopamine receptors in the chemoreceptor trigger zone and inhibit the vomiting center activities. Substitute benzamides work as dopamine antagonists at the chemoreceptor trigger zone and help suppress nausea by stimulating the motility of the GI tract. Steroids enhance the effectiveness of the other antiemetics and decrease the effects of prostaglandin activity. Antihistamines block neurotransmitters in the chemoreceptor zone. The recently approved serotonin inhibitors work as selective antagonists of the 5-hydroxytryptamine$_3$ serotonin receptors in the chemoreceptor trigger zone and have been successful as part of the new protocols for nausea and vomiting. To maintain a therapeutic blood level, antiemetic medications must be given around the clock rather than as needed.

5. Additional individualized interventions: _____

5. Rationales: _____

NURSING DIAGNOSIS

Altered oral mucous membrane related to decreased nutrition and immunosuppression secondary to disease and cytotoxic effects of chemotherapy

Nursing priorities
• Minimize pain and discomfort from stomatitis.
• Prevent further trauma to and infection of the oral mucous membrane.

Patient outcome criteria
• Within 3 days of admission, the patient will:
  – have no frank bleeding from gums
  – show improved ability to swallow
  – have decreased viscosity and improved amount of saliva.
• Within 5 days of admission, the patient will:
  – exhibit decreased number of oral open ulcers
  – exhibit decreased number of oral white patches.

Interventions

1. Assess for signs and symptoms of stomatitis, such as dry and ulcerated oral mucosa, pain, viscous saliva, or difficulty swallowing. Document and report the condition of the oral mucous membrane — including the lips, tongue, and gums — on a scale of 1 to 4, with 1 being normal and 4 being ulcerated, bleeding, irritated, and infected.Observe the amount and viscosity of saliva. Obtain a culture of suspicious lesions; note results.

2. Teach an appropriate mouth care regimen.

• If platelet levels are above 40,000/mm³ and leukocyte levels above 1,500/µl, recommend the following: Brush the teeth with a soft, nylon-bristle toothbrush 30 minutes after meals and every 4 hours while awake. Place the brush at a 45-degree angle between the gums and the teeth, and move it in short, horizontal strokes. Floss between teeth twice daily.

• If platelet or leukocyte levels are below the parameters specified, recommend rinsing only (using water or saline) until the values return to safer levels.

3. Provide hydrogen peroxide and water solution (1:2 or 1:4), baking soda and water (1 tsp to 500 ml), or normal saline to rinse the mouth during and after brushing.

4. Administer lidocaine (Xylocaine) viscous solution as needed, 1 tsp swished in the mouth every 3 to 4 hours, or acetaminophen with codeine elixir as needed, as ordered.

5. Lubricate lips with petroleum jelly or water-soluble lubricant (K-Y Lubricating Jelly), lip balm (ChapStick), or mineral oil. Use gauze with petroleum jelly to protect the lips when the patient drinks from a cup.

6. Encourage use of an artificial saliva product (Ora-Lub, Salivart, Xero-Lube).

7. Monitor, report,.and document the appearance of white patches on the tongue and oral mucosa. Administer nystatin (Mycostatin) oral suspension or a gentian violet preparation, as ordered. Document the patient's response.

8. Apply a substrate of magnesium hydroxide (Milk of Magnesia) or a kaolin preparation (Kaopectate) with a swab or a gauze-covered tongue blade. (To prepare the substrate, allow the bottle to stand for several hours; then pour off the supernatant liquid.) Rinse with normal saline after 15 minutes.

9. Additional individualized interventions: _____

Rationales

1. Stomatitis is both a sign of decreased immunocompetence and an adverse effect of chemotherapy that develops 7 to 10 days after treatment begins. Objective assessment is imperative for early identification of stomatitis so that appropriate therapy can be instituted.

2. Preventing accumulation of food debris and bacteria is essential to preventing breakdown of the oral mucous membrane.
• Take care to observe specified laboratory values because even this regimen will cause severe bleeding if platelet counts are low. If the WBC count is low, mouth care could cause local infection.

• For the patient with low platelet or leukocyte levels, this regimen removes debris while minimizing the risks of bleeding or infection.

3. Many commercial mouthwashes contain alcohol, which dries and irritates the oral mucosa.

4. Lidocaine is a topical anesthetic that relieves pain from mouth ulcers. Acetaminophen with codeine works systemically to control pain, and the elixir is easily swallowed.

5. Severe dryness, sores, and ulcers on the lips cause pain when the patient drinks from a cup or glass. This pain further discourages the patient from drinking adequate fluids and maintaining an adequate fluid balance.

6. Severe dryness of the oral mucous membrane increases risk of tissue breakdown and impairs optimal nutritional intake. Artificial saliva eases dryness, buffers acidity, and lubricates and soothes mucous membranes.

7. These white patches indicate yeast infection. (The immunosuppressed patient is prone to opportunistic infections such as candidiasis.) Prompt treatment of oral infection will prevent undue discomfort.

8. Topical protective agents soothe irritated areas and promote healing.

9. Rationales: _____

NURSING DIAGNOSIS

Altered protection related to severe immunosuppression associated with bone marrow transplantation (BMT) or peripheral stem cell transplantation protocol

Nursing priority

Assess, prioritize, and intervene in problems related to transplantation procedures.

Patient outcome criteria

- Within 7 days of transplantation, the patient will:
  - have stable liver function tests
  - maintain vital signs within normal limits: typically, heart rate, 60 to 100 beats/minute; systolic blood pressure, 90 to 140 mm Hg; and diastolic blood pressure, 50 to 90 mm Hg
  - respond positively to symptom management and comfort measures.
- Within 14 days of transplantation, the patient will:
  - be able to take foods and fluids by mouth
  - obtain relief from nausea and vomiting
  - maintain a stable body weight and a balanced intake and output
  - remain free from infection
  - have no signs of stomatitis, such as ulcerated or bleeding lips, tongue, and gums
  - have no evidence of veno-occlusive disease, such as right upper quadrant pain or jaundice.

Interventions

1. Reinforce the doctor's explanation for BMT or peripheral stem cell transplantation.

2. Explain the difference between BMT and peripheral stem cell transplantation, including the implications of each treatment.

Rationales

1. Because these treatments have been considered experimental and have commonly resulted in poor outcomes, the patient and family may be anxious about their effectiveness. Reinforcement that these treatments are becoming increasingly viable options, especially for AML, ALL, and CGL, helps allay anxiety.

2. BMT can be either allogenic (from another person) or autologous (from the patient's own bone marrow). In allogenic transplantation, a human leukocyte antigen (HLA) test is performed on the patient and family members to find a compatible bone marrow donor. Because of the complexity of the HLA system, which is composed of more than 100 antigens, a compatible family member may not be found. If so, the patient may register with the National Bone Marrow Donor Registry to find a compatible donor. The process of finding such a donor can be expensive, time consuming, and stressful.
　　Autologous BMT involves aspirating large volumes of the patient's own bone marrow for purging and then reinfusing. Peripheral stem cell transplantation involves transplantation of blood-forming components taken from the peripheral blood, not the bone marrow. The patient himself is usually the source of the stem cells, eliminating the need for a donor. Autologous BMT may cause relapses in the disease because reinfused marrow may contain residual tumor cells. Bone marrow (hematopoetic progenitors that restore blood function) is stored and reinfused after chemotherapy.

Hematologic and immunologic disorders

3. Help the patient through the extensive diagnostic and psychosocial evaluation that takes place before transplantation, providing teaching and emotional support.

4. Explain to the patient and family the rationale for and implications of preparations for transplantation, adverse effects of chemotherapy, symptom management, neutropenic precautions, care of the vascular access device, and comfort measures.

5. As ordered, administer antipyretics (such as acetaminophen), diuretics (such as mannitol), antihistamines (such as diphenhydramine), and corticosteroids (such as dexamethasone) before gravity or I.V. push infusion of bone marrow or peripheral stem cells. Check the patient's vital signs every 5 minutes during the infusion, and watch for and report such adverse effects as elevation in temperature or pulse and hypertension or hypotension.

6. Watch for, report, document, and treat complications of bacterial, fungal, or viral infections that occur during the acute phase of BMT. Maintain strict neutropenic precautions in a protective environment. Monitor and report results of chest X-rays, blood counts, and blood, tissue, urine, stool, wound, and sputum cultures.

3. Transplantation is an aggressive treatment that has potentially life-threatening complications and requires vigorous physical and diagnostic evaluation before the procedure. The patient must undergo extensive laboratory testing; tissue typing; evaluation of renal, hepatic, cardiovascular, and respiratory function; bone marrow studies to determine the stage of the disease; CT scans, magnetic resonance imaging, and bone scans; lumbar puncture; gynecologic examination (if the patient is female); and dental examination. The patient and family must also undergo fertility counseling (if appropriate) and comprehensive psychological evaluation to determine if the patient has sufficient support systems and coping mechanisms. All this is physically and emotionally exhausting for the patient, who already has symptoms of the disease; waiting for the results of tests adds to the patient's and family's stress. Teaching and emotional support play a crucial role in helping the patient and family cope.

4. The patient and family need to understand that, for transplantation to be successful, all malignant cells must be killed. The patient's immune system must be suppressed, and space in the bone marrow must be created for the new cells. The patient must undergo high-dose, disease-specific chemotherapy with such drugs as cyclophosphamide (Cytoxan), busulfan, or cytosine arabinoside; the patient who needs an allogenic transplant must also undergo total body irradiation. Specific interventions for managing adverse effects, neutropenic precautions, vascular access device care, and comfort measures are given in previous nursing diagnoses.

5. The most common adverse effects of bone marrow or stem cell transfusion include fever, chills, shortness of breath, rash, pruritus, hives, and hypertension or hypotension. Premedication can help combat these effects. Patients who receive autologous BMT or peripheral stem cell transplantation may also experience a bitter taste and an odd smell. These result from the chemical dimethylsulfoxide, used as a preservative in these transplant procedures.

6. The patient's immune system is wiped out, so he is at risk for overwhelming, life-threatening infection. From days 0 to 30, the patient needs close monitoring for signs of gram-negative and gram-positive bacterial, fungal, and herpes infections of the GI system, oropharynx, lungs, skin, and indwelling catheter sites. From days 30 to 90, the patient is at risk for cytomegalovirus and fungal, gram-positive bacterial, and *Pneumocystis carinii* infections.

7. Watch for, report, document, and treat complications of transplantation, including bleeding tendencies, hepatic dysfunction, cutaneous problems, GI problems, renal insufficiency, pulmonary toxicity, and acute graft-versus-host (GVH) disease. Monitor laboratory test results, especially hematocrit; platelet count; hemoglobin, creatinine, BUN, and bilirubin levels; liver enzymes; and chest X-rays.

7. Because of the intense nature of this aggressive therapy, failure to recognize the start of complications can be life-threatening. Active or occult bleeding episodes and signs of anemia may require blood or blood product transfusions. Veno-occlusive disease — as evidenced by hepatomegaly, elevated serum bilirubin levels, right upper quadrant pain, jaundice, and encephalopathy — can occur as a complication of treatment-induced (radiation or chemotherapy) liver damage; treatment is symptomatic. Stomatitis, mucositis, nausea, vomiting, or diarrhea may lead to malnutrition, fluid and electrolyte imbalance, and skin breakdown.

Renal complications can result from nephrotoxicity caused by certain transplantation drugs, hypovolemic states, infection, or hemorrhagic cystitis from high-dose cyclophosphamide administration. Symptoms of renal complications include anuria, elevated creatinine levels, and electrolyte and fluid imbalance.

Pulmonary complications from bacterial, viral, or fungal pneumonias; interstitial pneumonia; or fibrotic changes may occur in the acute or later phases after BMT. These complications result in a high incidence of morbidity and mortality. Signs and symptoms include cough, shortness of breath, and fever.

GVH disease occurs in allogenic BMT when the donor T lymphocytes attack the recipient's cells and organs. Acute GVH disease affects the patient's integumentary and GI systems and liver and causes effects that range from mild to life-threatening; symptoms include erythematous maculopapular rash; intense, watery diarrhea; and altered liver function (jaundice, ascites, and increased liver enzymes).

8. Throughout the transplantation process, provide ongoing emotional support and education about the complications and long-term implications for the patient and family.

8. Although the complications from autologous stem cell transplantation are less severe than those from allogenic BMT, every patient needs intensive education and emotional support to learn how to manage self-care. Education includes prevention and recognition of infection, comfort measures, nutrition guidelines, body-image management and self-concept alterations, concerns about sexuality, and role changes. Follow-up care includes weekly laboratory testing, throat and urine cultures, and chest X-rays and periodic pulmonary function tests, bone marrow studies, skin biopsies, and lumbar puncture.

9. Additional individualized interventions: _____

_____

9. Rationales: _____

_____

NURSING DIAGNOSIS

Risk for ineffective individual coping related to uncertain prognosis and multiple disease- and treatment-induced losses

Hematologic and immunologic disorders

Nursing priority

Promote healthy coping behavior.

Patient outcome criteria

Throughout the hospital stay, the patient will:
• use healthy coping behaviors
• express feelings, if desired.

Interventions

1. See the "Dying," "Grieving," and "Ineffective individual coping" plans, pages 20, 44, and 67, respectively.

2. Additional individualized interventions: _____

_____

Rationales

1. The patient with leukemia suffers multiple losses, and self-care ability, social contact, and energy level are reduced. Additionally, adverse effects from chemotherapy may cause body-image changes that are difficult to accept. Weakness, dependence on others, and an uncertain prognosis may create anxiety or contribute to depression. The plans listed provide specific interventions helpful in dealing with the psychosocial aspects of caring for a patient with leukemia.

2. Rationales: _____

_____

DISCHARGE PLANNING

Discharge checklist

Before discharge, the patient shows evidence of:
❏ absence of fever
❏ absence of cardiovascular or pulmonary complications such as crackles, gurgles, arrhythmias, or atelectasis
❏ stabilizing weight
❏ WBC count greater than 2,000/µl
❏ platelet count greater than 50,000/mm^3
❏ hemoglobin level above 8 g/dl
❏ hematocrit above 25%
❏ absence of signs and symptoms of infection
❏ ability to tolerate adequate nutritional intake
❏ absence of gingival bleeding and sores
❏ absence of hematuria or other bladder or bowel dysfunction
❏ ability to control pain using oral medications
❏ ability to manage care of vascular access device
❏ ability to follow BMT or peripheral stem cell transplantation protocol
❏ ability to perform ADLs, transfers, and ambulation independently or with minimal assistance
❏ adequate home support system or referral to home care or nursing home if indicated by an inadequate home support system or the patient's inability to perform ADLs, transfer, ambulate, and follow medication regimen.

Note: All patients with leukemia must be referred to the social service department. Leukemia is a financially draining disease, commonly requiring long-term and expensive treatment, so the patient is likely to have financial concerns. For terminal leukemia, refer the patient for hospice care.

Teaching checklist

Document evidence that the patient and family demonstrate an understanding of:
❏ diagnosis and course of treatment
❏ all discharge medications' purpose, dosage, administration schedule, and adverse effects requiring medical attention (Usual chemotherapy medications include alkylating agents, such as busulfan [Myleran] and chlorambucil [Leukeran]; antibiotics, such as daunorubicin [Cerubidine] and doxorubicin [Adriamycin]; antimetabolites, such as methotrexate and 6-mercaptopurine [Purinethol]; and plant alkaloids, such as vincristine [Oncovin] and vinblastine [Velban].)
❏ ways of preventing and identifying infections
❏ appropriate modifications of activity-rest patterns
❏ proper care of vascular access device
❏ ways of preventing, identifying, and reporting abnormal bleeding tendencies
❏ techniques to control nausea, vomiting, and anorexia
❏ recommended dietary modifications
❏ techniques to prevent urinary calculi formation

- ❏ appropriate oral hygiene techniques and procedures
- ❏ signs and symptoms indicating relapse or exacerbation of disease
- ❏ frequency of follow-up laboratory tests
- ❏ schedule for future diagnostic tests, chemotherapy administration, and appointments with health care providers
- ❏ how to contact the doctor
- ❏ community resources for home management, lifestyle modifications, and support
- ❏ emotional response to chronic or terminal illness
- ❏ changes in family role patterns.

Documentation checklist
Using outcome criteria as a guide, document:
- ❏ clinical status on admission
- ❏ significant changes in status, especially development of CNS symptoms and septicemia
- ❏ pertinent laboratory and diagnostic test findings
- ❏ response to chemotherapy treatments
- ❏ management of chemotherapy adverse reactions
- ❏ response to transfusions of RBCs, WBCs, or platelets
- ❏ nutritional intake
- ❏ fluid-electrolyte balance
- ❏ activity-rest pattern
- ❏ emotional coping patterns
- ❏ condition of skin and mucous membranes
- ❏ signs and symptoms of infection or bleeding tendencies
- ❏ I.V. line patency, condition of veins, and status of vascular access device
- ❏ tolerance of diagnostic procedures
- ❏ response to anti-infection measures
- ❏ patient and family teaching.

Associated plans of care
Anemia
Disseminated intravascular coagulation
Dying
Grieving
Ineffective individual coping
Lymphoma
Nutritional deficit
Septic shock
Total parenteral nutrition

References
Buchsel, P., et al. "Delayed Complications of Bone Marrow Transplantation: An Update," *Oncology Nursing Forum* 23(8):1267-91, September 1996.

Carpenito, L. *Handbook of Nursing Diagnosis*, 7th ed. Philadelphia: Lippincott-Raven Pubs., 1997.

Chanock, S., and Pizzo, P. "Infectious Complications of Patients Undergoing Therapy for Acute Leukemia: Current Status and Future Prospects," *Seminars in Oncology* 24(1):132-40, February 1997.

Gordon, M. *Manual of Nursing Diagnoses: 1995-1996*. St. Louis: Mosby–Year Book, Inc., 1995.

Groenwald, S., et al. *Cancer Nursing Principles and Practice*, 3rd ed. Boston: Jones & Bartlett Pubs., Inc., 1993.

Hadaway, L. "Comparison of Vascular Access Devices," *Seminars in Oncology Nursing* 11(3):154-66, August 1995.

Holland, J., et al. *Cancer Medicine*, Volume II, 4th ed. Baltimore: Williams & Wilkins Co., 1997.

Miaskowski, C. *Oncology Nursing: An Essential Guide for Patient Care*. Philadelphia: W.B. Saunders Co., 1996.

Nettina, S. *The Lippincott Manual of Nursing Practice*, 6th ed. Philadelphia: Lippincott-Raven Pubs., 1996.

Polaski, A., and Tatro, S. *Luckmann's Core Principles of Medical-Surgical Nursing*. Philadelphia: W.B. Saunders Co., 1996.

Smeltzer, S., and Bare, B. *Brunner and Suddarth's Textbook of Medical-Surgical Nursing*, 8th ed. Philadelphia: Lippincott-Raven Pubs., 1996.

Weinstein, S. *Plumer's Principles and Practice of Intravenous Therapy*, 6th ed. Philadelphia: Lippincott-Raven Pubs. 1996.

Winslow, M., et al. "Selection of Vascular Access Devices and Nursing Care," *Seminars in Oncology Nursing* 11(3):167-73, August 1995.

Hematologic and immunologic disorders

Lymphoma

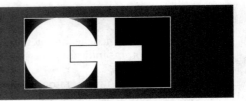

DRG information

DRG 400   Lymphoma or Leukemia with Major Operating Room (OR) Procedure.
          Mean LOS = 10.4 days
          Major OR procedures include biopsy, excision, or incision.

DRG 401   Lymphoma or Non-Acute Leukemia with Other OR Procedure with Complication or Comorbidity (CC).
          Mean LOS = 12.4 days

DRG 402   Lymphoma or Non-Acute Leukemia with Other OR Procedure without CC.
          Mean LOS = 4.7 days

DRG 403   Lymphoma or Non-Acute Leukemia with CC.
          Mean LOS = 9.3 days

DRG 404   Lymphoma or Non-Acute Leukemia without CC.
          Mean LOS = 5.1 days

Additional DRG information: After hospitalization for the staging workup and initial course of therapy, the patient would most likely receive ongoing chemotherapy as an outpatient.

INTRODUCTION

Definition and time focus
Lymphoma is the abnormal, malignant proliferation and enlargement of lymph nodes, spleen, and other lymphoid tissue, resulting in impaired cellular and humoral immunity, obstruction and infiltration of adjacent structures, and systemic involvement. Lymphomas are classified as Hodgkin's (commonly called Hodgkin's disease) or malignant.

Hodgkin's disease is characterized by contiguous node involvement. Extranodal spread at the time of diagnosis is uncommon. Staging is important in Hodgkin's disease, as in other cancers, because it helps determine treatment and estimate prognosis. (See *Staging classification [Ann Arbor] for Hodgkin's disease* for staging and treatment guidelines.) Commonly, the disease is localized; fever, weight loss, and night sweats (termed "B" symptoms in staging classification) are seen in about 40% of patients at presentation. Hodgkin's disease occurs most commonly between ages 15 and 35, with a second peak between ages 50 and 75.

Malignant lymphomas comprise many histologic variations. They are characterized by noncontiguous nodal spread, commonly with extranodal involvement in the GI tract, testes, central nervous system (CNS), or bone marrow. The disease is usually disseminated; "B" symptoms occur in only about 20% of patients. Malignant lymphoma is three times more common than Hodgkin's disease in the United States and can occur at any age.

Both types of lymphoma are more common in males than in females, and males tend to have a worse prognosis.

Hodgkin's disease and malignant lymphoma are considered together here because their clinical presentations, diagnostic workups, treatments, and nursing management are similar. This plan focuses on the undiagnosed, symptomatic patient with lymphoma who is admitted for a staging workup and initial therapy.

Etiology and precipitating factors
• Viral etiology (suggested for some lymphomas; may involve a herpeslike virus related to the Epstein-Barr virus)
• Family history (increased incidence among family members suggests genetic and environmental factors)
• Environmental exposure to certain herbicides (such as phenoxyacetic acid) linked to increased risk of malignant lymphoma

FOCUSED ASSESSMENT GUIDELINES

Nursing history (Functional health pattern findings)
Health perception–health management pattern
• Fever — highest in the afternoon; twice-daily peaks greater than 101° F (38.3° C) are common
• Drenching night sweats
• Pruritus — more intense at night, worse with bathing
• General malaise and fatigue
• Painless, swollen lymph nodes (typically in the cervical chain)

Nutritional-metabolic pattern
• Unexplained weight loss
• Anorexia
• Pain in nodes immediately after drinking alcohol (cause unknown)

Activity-exercise pattern
• General fatigue: "I'm unable to do the things I want to do"
• Shortness of breath if ascites, pleural effusion, or anemia is present

Sleep-rest pattern
• Sleep disturbances due to night sweats
Self-perception–self-concept pattern
• Fear regarding prognosis and progression of disease
• Difficulty coping with changes in lifestyle, self-esteem, and body image
Cognitive-perceptual pattern
• Interest or disinterest in knowing prognosis and expected progression of disease
Role-relationship pattern
• Concern regarding role reversals at home and inability to fulfill previous roles
Sexuality-reproductive pattern
• Concern regarding adverse effects of chemotherapy on fertility and sexual performance
• Decreased libido from chemotherapy, radiation, or general fatigue
Coping–stress tolerance pattern
• Increased anxiety

Physical findings
Lymphoreticular
• Lymphadenopathy
• Tonsillar enlargement
• Edema and cyanosis of face and neck (rare)
Pulmonary
• Shortness of breath (rare)
• Cough (rare)
• Stridor (rare)
• Signs of pleural effusion (rare)
Gastrointestinal
• Splenomegaly
• Hepatomegaly
• Ascites (uncommon)
• Jaundice (rare)

Diagnostic studies
Extensive testing is necessary to diagnose and stage lymphoma.
• Complete blood count and platelet count — may reveal neutrophilic leukocytosis and mild normochromic anemia, lymphopenia, or increased eosinophil sedimentation rate
• Serum alkaline phosphatase values — increased values indicate liver or bone involvement
• Direct Coombs' (antiglobulin) test — detects autoimmune hemolytic anemia (more common in malignant lymphoma)
• Immunoglobulin studies — may show overproduction of immunoglobulin by proliferating B-cell lymphocytes
• Lymph node biopsy (performed on the most central node of the involved group) — Hodgkin's disease shows Reed-Sternberg cells and malignant lymphoma reveals destruction of lymph node architecture; normal

Staging classification (Ann Arbor) for Hodgkin's disease

Stage	Description
I	Nodal involvement within one region
IE	Single extralymphatic organ or site
II	Nodal involvement within two or more regions, limited by the diaphragm
II E	Localized extranodal site and nodal involvement within one or more regions, limited by the diaphragm
III	Nodal involvement of regions above and below the diaphragm
III E	With localized extralymphatic site
III S	With spleen involvement
III ES	Localized extralymphatic site with spleen involvement
IV	Diffuse or disseminated involvement of one or more extralymphatic organs or tissues, with or without lymph node involvement

E = Extralymphatic involvement
S = Spleen involvement
ES = Both extralymphatic and spleen involvement

From Carbone, P., et al. "Report of the Committee on Hodgkin's Disease Staging," *Cancer Research* 31:1860, 1971. Adapted with permission.

cellular elements are replaced by increased lymphocytes and lymphoblasts
• Excretory urography — detects unsuspected renal involvement and ureteral deviation and obstruction by involved nodes
• Chest X-ray — with computed tomography (CT) scan, may reveal hilar lymphadenopathy; mediastinal masses in lymphoma usually appear as a dense rounded mass (occurring as commonly in the anterior mediastinum as in the middle mediastinum)
• Lymphangiography — may show enlarged, foamy-looking nodes (number of nodes affected, unilateral or bilateral involvement, and extent of extranodal involvement help determine stage); less useful in malignant lymphoma because does not visualize mesenteric nodes, which are usually involved; occasionally, nodes are so enlarged they cannot be visualized
• Abdominal CT scan — may detect intra-abdominal, intrapelvic nodal involvement as well as liver involvement
• Bone scan — used to detect bone involvement
• Bone marrow aspirate and biopsy — elevated lymphocyte values indicate bone marrow involvement,

more common in malignant lymphoma
• Bilateral bone marrow biopsies — commonly performed because of spotty bone marrow involvement; chances of identifying bone marrow involvement are increased by 15% to 20% with bilateral procedure
• Laparotomy and splenectomy — undertaken only if outcome will affect a therapeutic decision; may detect splenic involvement

Potential complications
• Intestinal obstruction and perforation
• Ureteral obstruction
• Sepsis (treatment-related)
• Anemia
• Thrombocytopenia (treatment-related)
• Hyperuricemia (treatment-related)
• Superior vena cava syndrome (airway occlusion related to edema from impaired superior vena cava drainage)
• Spinal cord compression (rare)
• Hypercalcemia (rare)
• Sterility (treatment-related)
• Secondary cancers (treatment-related)
• Pleural, pericardial, or abdominal effusions

CLINICAL SNAPSHOT

LYMPHOMA

Major nursing diagnoses and collaborative problems	Key patient outcomes
Risk for hypoxemia	Demonstrate effective, regular use of breathing techniques.
Risk for infection	Show no signs of systemic or localized infection.
Pruritus	List three self-care measures to reduce pruritus.
Risk for hemorrhage	Show no signs or symptoms of hemorrhage.
Risk for nutritional deficit	Participate in planning and implementing a dietary regimen.
Knowledge deficit (self-care)	List three possible complications of a vascular access device and identify appropriate interventions for each.
Risk for body-image or self-esteem disturbance	List measures to minimize effects of chemotherapy and radiation therapy.

COLLABORATIVE PROBLEM

Risk for hypoxemia related to enlarged mediastinal nodes, pulmonary compression and, for malignant lymphoma only, superior vena cava syndrome

Nursing priority

Optimize alveolar ventilation.

Patient outcome criteria

Within 48 hours of admission, the patient will:
• demonstrate effective, regular use of breathing techniques
• rate pain as less than 3 on a 0 to 10 pain rating scale
• tolerate increased activity level
• show relaxed posture and facial expression
• exhibit no head or neck cyanosis.

Interventions

1. Position the patient comfortably when short of breath: Elevate the upper torso at least 45 degrees, tilt the shoulders forward, support the arms away from the sides, and support the feet.

2. Teach and supervise therapeutic breathing techniques:
• pursed-lip breathing

• abdominal breathing.

3. Limit activity according to respiratory capabilities.

4. Plan activities to allow minimal energy expenditure and adequate rest periods: provide bed baths, assist the patient with meals as needed, and limit visitors.

5. Decrease anxiety associated with dyspnea: Explain all procedures in a calm, supportive manner; provide a quiet environment to promote adequate rest; and use relaxation techniques, music, and other diversionary activities.

6. Control pain with analgesics, as ordered. Use non-pharmacologic pain-control techniques as appropriate. See the "Pain" plan, page 88.

7. Monitor for signs and symptoms of superior vena cava syndrome, as follows:
• early — thoracic and neck vein distention (especially on arising), change in collar size, and headache
• advanced — progressive periorbital and facial edema, dizziness, cough, stridor, dysphagia, and dyspnea. Report such findings to the doctor immediately, and transport the patient to the radiation therapy department, as ordered, if superior vena cava syndrome is identified.
   After radiation therapy, assess for indications of improvement: reduced edema, increased ease in swallowing, and improved respiratory parameters.

8. Administer tranquilizers, as ordered.

Rationales

1. This position promotes maximum aeration by taking weight off the shoulders and arms, allowing the accessory muscles to be used solely for breathing.

2. Breathing techniques minimize respiratory impairment.
• Pursed-lip breathing has two benefits: It creates back pressure, holding the airways open, and the prolonged expiration time slows the flow of air, preventing premature closure of the airways and allowing more complete emptying of the lungs.
• The abdominal muscles can aid the diaphragm during expiration. As the patient inhales, the abdominal muscles relax. During expiration, they contract and help the diaphragm move upward to expel air.

3. Decreased activity decreases the need for oxygen.

4. Fatigue is both a symptom of hypoxemia and a cause of increased dyspnea. As respiratory muscles tire, respiratory excursion and alveolar ventilation drop, worsening hypoxemia and reinforcing the vicious circle of fatigue and dyspnea.

5. Anxiety and fear increase the heart rate, increasing the need for oxygen.

6. Pain may be present if enlarged nodes are compressing adjacent structures or nerve roots. Pain control will help decrease anxiety, thereby reducing associated shortness of breath. The "Pain" plan contains specific information and detailed interventions.

7. In superior vena cava syndrome, enlarged nodes press on the superior vena cava, impairing normal venous drainage from the head and neck. The resulting progressive edema may lead to tracheal deviation and airway occlusion. Rapid onset of superior vena cava syndrome is considered an oncologic emergency. Radiation therapy is the treatment of choice: immediate therapy of 300 to 400 rads daily for 3 to 4 days, then a full course of 3,000 to 6,000 rads. In most patients, symptoms should decrease rapidly, usually within a few days.

8. Physiologic reactions to anxiety include stimulation of the autonomic nervous system, such as increased heart and respiratory rates. Tranquilizers relieve anxiety without inducing sleep. The benzodiazepines appear to depress the CNS at the limbic and subcortical levels of the brain, producing sedation and relaxing skeletal muscles.

Hematologic and immunologic disorders

9. Additional individualized interventions: _____

9. Rationales: _____

Nursing diagnosis

Risk for infection related to leukopenia, lymphopenia from bone marrow involvement, chemotherapy, and radiation therapy effects

Nursing priorities

Prevent or promptly detect and treat superinfection.

Patient outcome criteria

After a full course of antibiotic therapy (5 to 10 days) and return of adequate immunity, or 14 days after completion of the chemotherapy cycle, the patient will:
• be afebrile
• show no signs of systemic or localized infection.

Interventions

1. Prioritize patient care assignments. Care for the neutropenic patient first.

2. Observe good hand-washing technique.

3. Monitor daily white blood cell (WBC) counts and differentials. Inform the patient and doctor of results.

4. Take protective precautions when the patient's absolute granulocyte count is dangerously depressed, typically when less than 1,000/µl. Protective measures should include:
• serving only cooked foods
• avoiding raw, unpeeled fruits and vegetables
• removing sources of standing water (such as vases of flowers)
• not handling live flowers or plants.
Institute further protective measures according to facility protocol, as appropriate to the patient's condition.

5. Assess actual and potential infection sites at least every 8 hours, including the lungs, mouth, rectum, I.V. sites, vagina, and surgical incisions. Monitor urine culture results. Observe carefully for subtle changes in skin and mucous membrane color, texture, or sensation. Note new complaints of pain.

Rationales

1. This minimizes the risk of cross-contamination by the caregiver.

2. The most important way to protect against infection is meticulous hand washing. Improper or infrequent hand washing is a well-known contributor to cross-contamination.

3. The degree of granulocytopenia indicates the patient's susceptibility to infection and is the most important factor in determining the risk of sepsis.

4. The risk of infection increases significantly when the absolute granulocyte count ranges from 500 to 1,000/µl and persists for more than a few days. The absolute granulocyte count indicates the number of mature WBCs (the cells most effective in fighting infection). To calculate the absolute granulocyte count, add the percentage of polys (mature neutrophils) to the percentage of bands (slightly immature neutrophils); multiply the result by the WBC count. Protective precautions may decrease the number of pathogenic organisms the immunosuppressed patient contacts. Raw fruits and vegetables are sources of gram-negative bacilli; live plants and soil are sources of fungi. Standing water may provide a medium for microorganisms, particularly *Pseudomonas*.

5. Early detection may prevent serious complications and spread of infection. In the immunocompromised patient, however, an altered inflammatory response complicates early detection. Classic signs and symptoms of infection (such as erythema, pus, and fever) may be masked in a neutropenic patient or in a patient taking steroids (a factor in many lymphoma protocols). Localized pain may indicate a site of infection.

6. Screen and limit visitors. Prohibit visits by those with recent or current infections.

7. Institute an appropriate oral hygiene protocol. Monitor for oral herpes lesions and *Candida* stomatitis.

8. Avoid invasive measures, such as injections, enemas, rectal temperatures, suppositories, and indwelling urinary catheters whenever possible.

9. Measure the patient's temperature at least every 4 hours; if it is higher than 101.3° F (38.5° C) and the patient develops signs and symptoms of septic shock (tachycardia, tachypnea, restlessness, confusion, cough, decreased pulse pressure, and cool extremities), notify the doctor.

10. Obtain blood, urine, throat, and sputum cultures, using correct technique, as ordered. Ensure that cultures are obtained before antibiotic therapy begins.

11. Report all positive blood cultures, even if the patient is already taking antibiotics.

12. Administer antibiotics only after obtaining blood and urine cultures, ideally within 60 minutes of detecting sepsis. Give subsequent doses on time.

13. Additional individualized interventions: _____

_____

6. Minimizing the patient's exposure to microorganisms may help avert sepsis.

7. The patient with lymphoma is at increased risk for viral and fungal infections because of impaired cell-mediated immunity. (T lymphocytes protect against viruses, fungi, and parasites.)

8. Intact skin is the body's first line of defense. Sweat glands and sebaceous glands keep bacteria under control. Lysozymes, enzymes secreted by the sweat glands, attack the cell walls of bacteria. Sebum, secreted by the sebaceous glands, has antifungal and antibacterial properties. Skin and blood infections may occur when invasive measures damage the skin.

9. Septic shock (a medical emergency) is reversible in its early stages. Massive infection, usually from gram-negative bacteria, causes septic shock. As the body fights the infection, the bacteria die, releasing endotoxins that in turn impair cell metabolism and damage surrounding tissue. Lysozomal enzymes, bradykinin, and histamine cause peripheral vasodilation and increased capillary permeability, resulting in peripheral blood pooling, inadequate venous return, and severely reduced cardiac output.

10. Cultures must be uncontaminated to permit accurate diagnosis. Current culture results determine appropriate antibiotic therapy.

11. When specific organisms are identified, therapy should be modified according to antibiotic sensitivity.

12. Prompt, timely administration of antibiotics increases the survival rate in neutropenic patients. Therapeutic blood levels of medication must be maintained to treat sepsis effectively.

13. Rationales: _____

_____

COLLABORATIVE PROBLEM

Pruritus related to histamine or leukopeptidase release from WBCs and to effects of radiation therapy

Nursing priorities

• Relieve discomfort.
• Prevent or minimize skin injury.

Patient outcome criteria

Throughout the hospital stay, the patient will:
• present intact skin
• verbalize reduced discomfort
• on request, list three self-care measures to minimize pruritus.

Hematologic and immunologic disorders

Interventions

1. Promote adequate hydration: twelve 8-oz (240-ml) glasses of fluid daily, unless contraindicated.

2. Use emollient creams on the skin (if allowed during radiation therapy).

3. Provide tepid, cooling baths.

4. Keep the patient's fingernails short. Provide clean cotton gloves at night.

5. Use soap designed for sensitive or dry skin.

6. Administer antihistamines, antibiotics, tar extracts, or chemotherapeutic agents, as ordered.

7. Instruct the patient to avoid harsh cold and wind.

8. Remove excessive clothing or bedding; instruct the patient not to wear restrictive clothing.

9. Launder the patient's clothing with a nondetergent cleanser, and rinse thoroughly.

10. Additional individualized interventions: _____

Rationales

1. Adequate hydration is essential to minimize skin dryness.

2. Emollient creams are oil-in-water emulsions. Water keeps the skin moist while the oil creates a film that slows normal evaporation.

3. Regular bathing helps protect the immunosuppressed patient from infection. Additionally, tepid water promotes vasoconstriction. Proteases are sensitive to heat, and the cutaneous nerve endings that mediate the scratch impulse are made more sensitive by vasodilation.

4. These measures may prevent damage to the skin if the patient cannot control scratching.

5. Soaps for sensitive skin have a large proportion of emollient oils and contain no detergents or dyes to strip the skin. They liquefy instantly and leave no irritating residue.

6. Antihistamines will help if the underlying cause of pruritus is increased histamine release. Tar extracts and topical steroids may inhibit protease release. If infection is the underlying cause, antibiotics are indicated. If a tumor is releasing enzymes, chemotherapy may shrink the tumor and proportionately reduce enzyme release.

7. Exposure to cold and wind dries the skin.

8. A cool environment promotes vasoconstriction. Restrictive clothing may irritate the skin.

9. These precautions help prevent chemical irritation of the skin.

10. Rationales: _____

COLLABORATIVE PROBLEM

Risk for hemorrhage related to decreased platelet count secondary to chemotherapy or radiation therapy effects

Nursing priority

Maximize the patient's available protective mechanisms.

Patient outcome criteria

Throughout the hospital stay, the patient will:
• have regular, soft, formed stools
• show no signs or symptoms of hemorrhage.

Interventions

1. Do not administer aspirin or aspirin-containing products.

2. Administer stool softeners, as ordered, and monitor the frequency of stools to detect constipation.

3. Avoid such invasive measures as I.M. injections, enemas, and rectal suppositories.

4. Use an electric razor when shaving the patient. Avoid activities with the potential for physical injury.

5. Administer steroids, as ordered, with milk products or antacids.

6. Maintain optimal nutritional status, encouraging protein intake.

7. Test all stool, vomitus, and urine for occult blood.

8. Apply direct pressure to venipuncture sites for at least 5 minutes.

9. Administer platelet infusions, as ordered.

10. Use a soft-bristle toothbrush, and avoid flossing the patient's teeth.

11. Instruct the patient to avoid strenuous activity, Valsalva's maneuver, and lifting heavy objects.

12. Teach the patient self-protection measures related to the above interventions, such as avoiding aspirin, taking stool softeners, and using an electric razor.

13. Additional individualized interventions: _____

Rationales

1. The acetyl group in the aspirin compound inhibits platelet aggregation, thereby impairing fibrin strand formation. A single dose of aspirin produces an effect that remains for days, long after the aspirin has been metabolized and excreted.

2. Straining at stool produces excessive pressure on the anal orifice; the rectal area is highly vascular and can hemorrhage.

3. Intact skin reduces the risk of bleeding. A decreased platelet count means that even minor trauma may result in significant bleeding.

4. These measures minimize the risk of skin trauma.

5. Coating the stomach helps prevent gastric irritation.

6. Protein is needed to produce megakaryocytes, precursors of platelets.

7. Early detection of bleeding promotes early and effective treatment.

8. Decreased platelet levels delay clot formation.

9. A platelet count below $20,000/mm^3$ increases the risk of spontaneous hemorrhage. Active bleeding is an indication for platelet administration.

10. These measures decrease the risk of physical irritation to oral mucous membranes.

11. These activities increase intracranial pressure and may cause cerebrovascular hemorrhage.

12. The knowledgeable patient's active involvement in self-care minimizes the risk of hemorrhage, especially after discharge.

13. Rationales: _____

NURSING DIAGNOSIS

Risk for nutritional deficit related to anorexia, taste alterations, fatigue, nausea and vomiting, and altered oral mucous membrane

Nursing priority

Promote adequate nutrition to enhance response to therapy and prevent complications.

Patient outcome criteria

Throughout the hospital stay, the patient will:
• participate in planning and implementing a dietary regimen
• maintain an adequate nutritional status to facilitate therapy, as evidenced by stable weight, nonemaciated appearance, and nutrition-related laboratory values within normal limits.

Hematologic and immunologic disorders

Interventions

1. Arrange for a dietary consultation to address the patient's calorie and protein needs. Explore the patient's food preferences and attempt to obtain the foods requested. Explain prescribed dietary recommendations and help the patient set goals for meeting them. Consult the "Nutritional deficit" plan, page 80.

2. Offer sandwiches and other cold foods.

3. Avoid giving liquids with meals.

4. Avoid offering favorite foods during peak periods of nausea and vomiting or while the patient is receiving chemotherapy.

5. Offer salty foods (such as broth or crackers) and tart foods (such as lemons or dill pickles) unless the patient has stomatitis.

6. Offer small, frequent meals, and encourage the patient to eat and drink slowly.

7. Avoid offering greasy foods.

8. Provide mouth care before meals and after vomiting episodes.

9. If taste alterations are present, consult with the dietary department and advise the patient to:
• use plastic utensils instead of metal silverware
• eat protein in the form of eggs, cheese, beans, and peanut butter instead of meat
• experiment with spices and flavorings to enhance taste sensation (such as mint, vanilla, lemon, and basil), unless contraindicated by stomatitis.

10. Advise the patient to increase intake of sugar and sweet foods.

11. Teach the patient how to use viscous lidocaine (Xylocaine) to reduce stomatitis pain (swish and swallow 15 ml 15 minutes before or after meals). If ineffective, try dyclonine (Dyclone).

12. Offer soft, moist foods, such as custards, ice cream, gelatins, cottage cheese, and ground meats with sauces and gravies.

Rationales

1. The dietitian's expertise may be helpful in planning a diet that meets the patient's needs while incorporating the patient's preferences. Including the patient in planning and goal-setting enhances compliance and promotes a sense of self-control. The "Nutritional deficit" plan contains detailed information on assessing and managing the problem. This plan provides additional information pertinent to lymphoma.

2. The odor of hot foods commonly aggravates nausea.

3. Fluids contribute to gastric distention and may reduce intake of solid foods.

4. The patient can develop an aversion to foods served during periods of nausea and vomiting. During anorexic periods, favorite foods may supply the patient's only intake, so maintaining positive associations is essential.

5. These foods increase salivation and stimulate the taste buds. In the patient with stomatitis, however, salt and acidity will further irritate open mucous membranes.

6. Small meals and slow eating minimize gastric distention and help prevent early satiety.

7. High-fat foods prolong gastric emptying time, causing feelings of overfullness and distention.

8. Regular mouth care refreshes the mouth and enhances the flavor of foods.

9. The presence of actively dividing cells in the oral mucous membrane that excrete amino acid–like substances enhances the bitter taste sensation. Large tumor mass also increases the degree and duration of any taste sensation. Beef and pork have high amino acid levels. A negative nitrogen balance also decreases the patient's threshold for the bitter taste sensation. Certain chemotherapy agents used in lymphoma protocols, specifically mechlorethamine (Mustargen), cyclophosphamide (Cytoxan), vincristine (Oncovin), and dacarbazine (DTIC-Dome) contribute further to taste alterations.

10. Taste alterations associated with the disease and chemotherapy commonly include decreased sensitivity to sweetness, although this is sometimes accompanied by an aversion to sweet foods. Increased sugar also boosts caloric intake.

11. A topical anesthetic decreases sensitivity to pain, enabling the patient to eat without discomfort. Using the anesthetic after meals decreases food-induced discomfort.

12. Soft foods minimize mechanical irritation to the oral mucous membrane and are easier to swallow.

13. Encourage the patient to eat liquid and pudding supplements.

14. Consult the doctor regarding temporary enteral or parenteral feedings if other interventions are ineffective.

15. Additional individualized interventions: _____

_____

13. High-calorie supplements may compensate for decreased intake.

14. The patient may need a temporary alternative to oral nutrition to prevent severe malnutrition, which may affect the outcome of therapy.

15. Rationales: _____

_____

NURSING DIAGNOSIS

Knowledge deficit (self-care of vascular access device, including peripherally or centrally inserted venous catheters or subcutaneous [S.C.] ports) related to lack of exposure to information

Nursing priority

Teach self-care techniques and measures for home management of the vascular access device.

Patient outcome criteria

By the time of discharge, the patient will:
• list signs of infection
• demonstrate dressing change and irrigation techniques as taught
• list three possible complications of a vascular access device and identify appropriate interventions for each.

Interventions

1. Teach the patient the name of the catheter or port and its purpose and anatomic placement.

2. Teach the patient how to change dressings at home (usually a clean, occlusive dressing changed when wet or soiled, or according to protocol). Have the patient demonstrate the proper technique before discharge; arrange for home care follow-up. If the patient has an S.C. port, explain that a dressing is not necessary because the device is completely under the skin.

3. Teach the patient to identify early signs and symptoms of local or generalized infection, such as redness, swelling, purulent drainage, fever, increased fatigue, and malaise.

4. Teach the patient the importance of proper irrigation technique, including frequency and solution used, specified by the manufacturer and agency policy.

Rationales

1. Central venous catheters or S.C. ports may be used to administer chemotherapy. The patient who is knowledgeable about all aspects of care is better prepared to use good judgment in decision making and to teach others about care needs. Assuming greater responsibility for the device helps the patient develop an increased sense of control, easing incorporation of the device into the patient's body image.

2. Because the catheter exit site is a break in skin integrity, the risk of opportunistic infections increases. A clean occlusive dressing can decrease the potential for microbial contamination. The frequency of dressing changes varies among institutions.

Anxiety may interfere with learning by decreasing the patient's ability to concentrate. Written materials and home care follow-up reinforce earlier learning and allow the patient to learn in a less-threatening environment.

3. Early detection of infection results in more timely and effective treatment.

4. Although catheters and S.C. ports are in place continuously, chemotherapy administration is intermittent. Catheter or port patency must be maintained for the device to function. Proper technique decreases the risk of contamination.

Hematologic and immunologic disorders

5. Inform the patient of potential complications and appropriate interventions, as follows:

• clot formation (catheter will not irrigate): Avoid forcing irrigation if resistance is felt. Contact the doctor.
• catheter displacement (catheter pulled out): Apply a pressure dressing and call the doctor. If bleeding is present, apply direct manual pressure until it stops.

6. Give the patient the names and telephone numbers of appropriate resource persons, such as the doctor, emergency squad, and the home health nurse.

7. Additional individualized interventions: _____

5. Recognizing complications may prevent a potentially hazardous situation, such as infection, tissue damage, catheter migration, or loss of the device.
• Forcing irrigation may push a clot out the end of the catheter and into the circulatory system.
• Pressure controls bleeding if the catheter is accidentally removed.

6. A health care provider can speed resolution of a patient problem or concern. Knowing how and where to contact resource persons may help decrease anxiety and promote a sense of control.

7. Rationales: _____

NURSING DIAGNOSIS

Risk for body-image or self-esteem disturbance related to effects of chemotherapy or radiation therapy

Nursing priorities
• Prepare the patient for therapy.
• Promote a positive self-concept.

Patient outcome criteria
• Throughout the hospital stay, the patient will:
 – verbalize feelings freely, if desired
 – participate in decision making related to care.
• By the time of discharge, the patient will:
 – identify personal concerns that may affect self-concept
 – identify personal or external resources to deal with concerns
 – list measures to minimize effects of chemotherapy or radiation therapy.

Interventions

1. Inform the patient of anticipated adverse effects of chemotherapy or radiation that will affect body image and role performance. Suggest measures to prevent or lessen their impact (see *Suggestions for minimizing chemotherapeutic adverse effects*).

2. Inform the male patient of the availability of sperm banking before beginning chemotherapy.

3. Provide adequate time to discuss the patient's concerns and feelings. Strive to maintain a nonjudgmental attitude. See the "Grieving," "Ineffective family coping: Compromised," and "Ineffective individual coping" plans, pages 44, 63, and 67, respectively.

Rationales

1. Chemotherapy protocols for lymphoma are aggressive and cause many adverse effects. Radiation therapy may also cause severe adverse effects. Teaching the patient about specific preventive or palliative measures before therapy begins increases the patient's sense of control, decreases powerlessness, and promotes self-image.

2. Because the peak incidence of Hodgkin's disease corresponds with peak childbearing years, fertility is a major concern. Chemotherapy may cause permanent sterility. For a male patient, sperm banking can help offset this adverse effect of treatment. The well-informed patient is able to base decisions on sound judgment after considering available options.

3. The patient is more likely to discuss personal concerns if a trusting relationship is developed. Judgmental responses that reflect the caregiver's personal biases may inhibit open discussion. These plans provide interventions helpful in addressing emotional needs.

Suggestions for minimizing chemotherapeutic adverse effects

Alopecia
- Shampoo only one or two times weekly.
- Use a mild, protein shampoo.
- Avoid using an electric hair dryer or electric curlers.
- Avoid using hair spray or other drying products.
- Try a satin pillowcase to minimize tangling.
- Avoid excessive hair brushing or combing.
- Use a wide-toothed comb.
- Avoid using scalp hypothermia devices, which may reduce flow of medication to the head.

Weight gain
- Exercise regularly.
- Follow prescribed dietary guidelines.
- Select flattering, loose-fitting clothing.

Nausea and vomiting
- Avoid fatty, salty, or spicy foods.
- Use diversionary activities.
- Avoid eating or drinking for at least 1 hour before and after chemotherapy.
- Use a sedative that has an amnesic effect, such as lorazepam (Ativan), before chemotherapy, if prescribed.
- Suggest that family members avoid perfumes, aftershaves, and other aromatic toiletries.

Constipation
- Maintain a diet high in fiber, bulk, and fluids.
- Exercise regularly.
- Use stool softeners.

Diarrhea
- Try adding nutmeg to foods.
- Avoid milk or milk products (except yogurt, which may be helpful).
- Ensure adequate replacement of fluid and potassium.

Depression
- Understand that this is normal and usually temporary.
- Identify and use resources for emotional support.

Sore throat or dysphagia
- Observe self closely while eating for sore throat or difficulty swallowing.
- Eat soft foods.
- Use topical anesthetics as prescribed.

Dermatitis
- Avoid using deodorants, cosmetics, or creams, unless prescribed.
- Avoid hot baths or use of heat.

4. Include the patient in decision making. Allow the patient to plan the day's events (within facility limitations).

5. Instruct the patient and spouse (or partner) on specific sexual adverse effects of chemotherapy and radiation therapy: for example, decreased libido, decreased vaginal lubrication, and temporary impotence. Provide written material for specific interventions related to each. Encourage the couple to share concerns and ask questions. Refer them to the social services department or other resources for ongoing counseling and support, if needed.

4. Promoting maximum patient participation in care planning conveys respect and increases the patient's sense of control.

5. The couple may be comforted to know that many adverse effects of therapy are temporary. Fatigue, fear, anxiety, and lack of privacy may also contribute to problems. Many patients (and many health care professionals) are not well educated about sex or are uncomfortable discussing sexual problems. Written information is a less threatening but effective means of providing this information. Sharing concerns may reduce the couple's anxiety.

Hematologic and immunologic disorders

6. Additional individualized interventions: _____
_____

6. Rationales: _____
_____

DISCHARGE PLANNING

Discharge checklist

Before discharge, the patient shows evidence of:
- ❏ stable vital signs
- ❏ absence of fever
- ❏ absence of cardiovascular or pulmonary complications
- ❏ ability to control pain using oral medications
- ❏ absence of bowel or bladder dysfunction
- ❏ WBC count within expected parameters
- ❏ absence of signs and symptoms of infection
- ❏ ability to tolerate adequate nutritional intake
- ❏ ability to perform activities of daily living and to ambulate independently or with minimal assistance
- ❏ ability to care appropriately for VAD, if present
- ❏ adequate home support system or referral to home care or a nursing home if indicated by inadequate home support system or the patient's inability to care for self.

Teaching checklist

Document evidence that the patient and family demonstrate an understanding of:
- ❏ disease and its progression
- ❏ signs and symptoms of infection and preventive measures
- ❏ all discharge medications' purpose, dosage, administration schedule, and adverse effects requiring medical attention (usual discharge medications may include antineoplastics, analgesics, stool softeners, antiemetics, and others, depending on symptoms)
- ❏ purpose and results of radiation therapy, schedule for future treatments, and management of anticipated adverse effects
- ❏ maintenance of a VAD
- ❏ indications for seeking emergency medical care
- ❏ services available from local American Cancer Society chapter
- ❏ availability of home health care and ancillary support services
- ❏ date, time, and location of next scheduled appointment
- ❏ how to contact the doctor.

Documentation checklist

Using outcome criteria as a guide, document:
- ❏ clinical status on admission
- ❏ significant changes in clinical status

- ❏ teaching about and response to diagnostic and staging workups
- ❏ chemotherapy administration — I.V. line patency and site status, name of medication, dosage, and response (include teaching about protocol and the patient's response)
- ❏ skin integrity over irradiated areas
- ❏ transfusion therapy and response or reactions
- ❏ nutritional status
- ❏ status and maintenance of VAD
- ❏ referrals initiated
- ❏ patient and family teaching
- ❏ discharge planning.

ASSOCIATED PLANS OF CARE

Dying
Grieving
Ineffective family coping: Compromised
Ineffective individual coping
Knowledge deficit
Nutritional deficit
Pain

REFERENCES

Campbell, K. "Lymphomas: Aetiology, Classification, and Treatment." *Nursing Times* 92(9):44-45, February 28-March 5, 1996.

DeVita. V., et al. *Cancer Principles and Practices of Oncology*, 5th ed. Philadelphia: Lippincott-Raven Pubs., 1997.

Dodd, M. *Managing the Side Effects of Chemotherapy and Radiation Therapy*, 3rd ed. San Francisco: UCSF Press, 1996.

Groenwald, S., et al. *Cancer Nursing: Principles and Practices*, 4th ed. Boston: Jones & Bartlett Pubs., Inc., 1997.

McCorkle, R., et al. *Cancer Nursing: A Comprehensive Textbook.* 2nd ed. Philadelphia: W.B. Saunders Co., 1996.

Miaskowski, C. *Oncology Nursing: An Essential Guide for Patient Care.* Philadelphia: W.B. Saunders Co., 1996.

Murphy, G.P., et al. *American Cancer Society Textbook of Clinical Oncology*, 2nd ed. Atlanta, Ga.: American Cancer Society, 1995.

Nettina, S. *The Lippincott Manual of Nursing Practice*, 6th ed. Philadelphia: Lippincott-Raven Pubs., 1996.

Persson, L., et al. "Survivors of Acute Leukemia and Highly Malignant Lymphoma — Retrospective Views of Daily Life Problems During Treatment and When in Remission." *Journal of Advanced Nursing* 25(1):68-78, January 1997.

Warmkessel, J. "Caring for Patients with Non-Hodgkin's Lymphoma." *Nursing97* 27(6):48-49, June 1997.

Part 13

Reproductive disorders

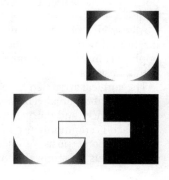

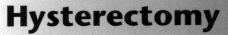

Hysterectomy

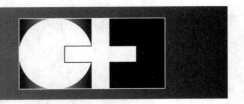

DRG information
DRG 353   Pelvic Evisceration, Radical Hysterectomy, and Radical Vulvectomy.
            Mean LOS = 8.3 days
DRG 354   Uterine and Adnexa Procedure for Non-Ovarian, Adnexal Malignancy with Complication or Comorbidity (CC).
            Mean LOS = 6.3 days
DRG 355   Uterine and Adnexa Procedure for Non-Ovarian, Adnexal Malignancy without CC.
            Mean LOS = 3.9 days
DRG 357   Uterine and Adnexa Procedures for Ovarian or Adnexal Malignancy.
            Mean LOS = 9.8 days
DRG 358   Uterine and Adnexa Procedures for Non-Malignancy with CC.
            Mean LOS = 4.8 days
DRG 359   Uterine and Adnexa Procedures for Non-Malignancy without CC.
            Mean LOS = 3.3 days

INTRODUCTION

Definition and time focus
Hysterectomy is the surgical removal of the uterus. Several surgical variations exist. Subtotal hysterectomy, seldom performed, is the surgical removal of the corpus (body) of the uterus, leaving the cervical stump in place. Total hysterectomy is the surgical removal of the uterus and cervix. Total hysterectomy or simple hysterectomy with bilateral salpingo-oophorectomy is the surgical removal of the uterus, cervix, uterine (fallopian) tubes, and ovaries. (Salpingectomy is the surgical removal of the uterine tube or tubes; oophorectomy is the removal of an ovary or ovaries.) Radical hysterectomy is the surgical removal of the uterus, cervix, upper portion of the vagina, connective tissue, and lymph nodes.

All hysterectomy procedures result in permanent sterilization. If performed in conjunction with bilateral oophorectomy in the premenopausal woman, abrupt menopause results.

The surgical approach for a hysterectomy may be vaginal or abdominal. The vaginal approach is used for cervical cancer and uterine prolapse. The abdominal approach is commonly used for pelvic exploration for cancer, endometriosis, or infection; removal of an enlarged uterus; or removal of tubes and ovaries.

This plan focuses on preoperative assessment and postoperative care for a patient undergoing total abdominal hysterectomy.

Etiology and precipitating factors
• Recent diagnosis of cervical, endometrial, or ovarian cancer
• Irreparable rupture or perforation of the uterus
• Severe (life-threatening) pelvic infection
• Myoma or nonmalignant tumor of the uterus (fibroid)
• History of endometriosis
• Hemorrhage, metrorrhagia (dysfunctional uterine bleeding), postmenopausal bleeding, perimenopausal menometrorrhagia (excessive, prolonged vaginal bleeding at irregular intervals), menorrhagia (excessive uterine bleeding occurring during regular menstruation), or postcoital bleeding with pelvic pain

FOCUSED ASSESSMENT GUIDELINES

Nursing history (functional health pattern findings)
Health perception–health management pattern
• Postmenopausal with sudden uterine bleeding
• Abnormal Papanicolaou (Pap) test results in the past (if cervical or endometrial cancer is present)
• History of prolonged postmenopausal estrogen replacement therapy (if endometrial cancer present)
• History of prolonged, heavy, or painful menstruation (if uterine myoma, endometriosis, or endometrial cancer is present)
• History of fibroids (myomas) in the uterus
Nutritional-metabolic pattern
• Obesity
Elimination pattern
• Pattern of frequent urination related to presence and proximity of tumor
Activity-exercise pattern
• Fatigue-related decrease in activity level if excessive vaginal bleeding has caused anemia
Sleep-rest pattern
• Sleep disturbance related to nocturia
• Sleep disturbance related to emotional stress of planned hospital stay and surgery
Cognitive-perceptual pattern
• History of abdominal, pelvic, back, or leg pain
• Fear of anticipated discomfort and pain from abdominal incision

Self-perception–self-concept pattern
- Concerns expressed about abdominal scar and removal of uterus
- Concerns expressed about femininity
- Concerns expressed about infertility

Role-relationship pattern
- Concerns expressed about spouse's or partner's acceptance of infertility

Sexuality-reproductive pattern
- Concerns expressed about resuming sexual intercourse after surgery

Value-belief pattern
- Delay in seeking medical attention if perimenopausal (because irregular menses are normal during early menopause)

Physical findings

Gastrointestinal
- Lower abdominal distention (with ovarian cancer)
- Abdominal discomfort (with uterine myoma)
- Adnexal mass (with ovarian cancer)

Genitourinary
- Leukorrhea (with infection)
- Vaginal bleeding (with uterine myoma)

Musculoskeletal
- Leg edema (less common)

Diagnostic studies

- Hemoglobin level — may reveal decreased hemoglobin concentration, indicating anemia
- Hematocrit — may reveal a decrease in volume percentage of red blood cells in whole blood, indicating blood loss

- White blood cell (WBC) count — may be elevated because of severe pelvic infection
- D&C (cervical dilatation and fractional curettage) and four-quadrant endometrial biopsy — provides endometrial tissue for a histopathologic study, which may reveal endometrial cancer
- Wedge biopsy or conization biopsy of the cervix (removal of tissue for microscopic examination) — may reveal cervical cancer
- Pap test (removal of exfoliated cervical cells) — may reveal cellular dysplasia
- Colposcopy (visualization of the cervix with a colposcope) — may identify abnormal cell growth
- Schiller's test (staining of the cervix with iodine) — identifies abnormal cells
- Ultrasound or computed tomography scan — may reveal size and location of mass

Potential complications

- Hemorrhagic shock
- Peritonitis
- Emboli
- Pneumonia
- Perforated bladder
- Ligation of ureter
- Wound infection
- Atelectasis
- Thrombophlebitis
- Urine retention
- Urinary tract infection (UTI)

CLINICAL SNAPSHOT

HYSTERECTOMY

Major nursing diagnoses and collaborative problems	Key patient outcomes
Risk for thromboembolic and hemorrhagic complications	Show no signs or symptoms of thromboembolic or hemorrhagic complications.
Risk for postoperative infection	Have clean, dry, intact wound.
Risk for urine retention	Void at least once (greater than 100 ml) within 8 hours after catheter removal.
Pain	Rate pain as less than 3 on a pain rating scale of 0 to 10.
Risk for body-image disturbance	Verbalize beginning acceptance of possible alterations in body appearance and function.
Risk for sexual dysfunction: Decreased libido or dyspareunia	Verbalize strategies to manage temporary alteration in sexual functioning.

COLLABORATIVE PROBLEM

Risk for thromboembolic and hemorrhagic complications related to immobility, venous stasis, pelvic congestion, or possible predisposing factors

Nursing priority

Prevent or promptly treat thromboembolic and hemorrhagic complications.

Patient outcome criteria

Throughout the hospital stay, the patient will:
• show no signs or symptoms of significant postoperative bleeding such as tachycardia, hypotension, or pallor
• show no signs or symptoms of thromboembolic complications, such as calf pain or swelling or difficulty breathing.

Interventions

1. Monitor for signs of bleeding. Check vital signs and the surgical site according to standard postoperative protocol (see the "Surgery" plan, page 103, for details), and report tachycardia, dropping blood pressure, increasing drainage, restlessness, pallor, diaphoresis, or any other sign of hemorrhage immediately. Institute fluid replacement therapy, as ordered (see the "Hypovolemic shock" plan, page 432, for details).

2. Institute measures to prevent and assess for thromboembolic phenomena: Help the patient change position frequently, avoid using the knee gatch, tell the patient to avoid prolonged sitting, apply antiembolic hose or pneumatic compression devices, and assist the patient with range-of-motion exercises. Administer anticoagulant medication, as ordered. (See the "Surgery" and "Thrombophlebitis" plans, pages 103 and 468, respectively, for further details.)

3. Before discharge, instruct the patient to promptly report any bleeding and to avoid heavy lifting, prolonged sitting, and wearing constrictive clothes.

4. Additional individualized interventions: _____

Rationales

1. The proximity of the surgical site to large vessels may increase the risk of significant postoperative bleeding. Additionally, a patient with a presurgical diagnosis of cancer may have clotting factor abnormalities that increase the risk of hemorrhage. Untreated, such bleeding rapidly progresses to hypovolemic shock; death may result. The "Surgery" plan provides further details about standard postoperative monitoring, while the "Hypovolemic shock" plan covers assessment and management of that complication.

2. The postoperative patient is always at increased risk for thromboembolic complications because of circulatory disruption, immobility, and edema. The posthysterectomy patient may be at additional risk because of pelvic congestion. The "Surgery" and "Thrombophlebitis" plans contain further details regarding this potential postoperative problem.

3. Postoperative hemorrhage may occur as late as 14 days after surgery. Avoiding activities that put stress on the operative site or cause venous stasis or pelvic congestion helps minimize the risk of bleeding or thromboembolic phenomena after discharge.

4. Rationales: _____

NURSING DIAGNOSIS

Risk for postoperative infection related to abdominal incision, urinary tract proximity, contamination of peritoneal cavity, hypoventilation, anesthesia, or preoperative infection

Nursing priority

Prevent or promptly detect and treat infection.

Patient outcome criteria

Throughout the postoperative period, the patient will:
• have clean, dry, intact wound
• perform pulmonary hygiene measures correctly and regularly
• show no symptoms of peritonitis, such as abdominal pain and rigidity
• show no signs of UTI, such as cloudy, foul-smelling urine.

Interventions

1. Monitor for signs and symptoms of peritonitis, such as a significant increase in abdominal pain or a change in pain quality, abdominal rigidity or tenderness, nausea and vomiting, absent bowel sounds, or tachycardia. Report abnormal findings to the doctor immediately.

2. Implement standard postoperative nursing measures to prevent or detect other infections:

• atelectasis and pneumonia

• UTI

• incisional infection.
See the "Surgery" plan, page 103, for further details.

3. Before discharge, teach the patient about signs and symptoms indicating infection, such as cough or respiratory congestion; urinary pain or burning, or cloudy urine; or redness, swelling, or purulent wound drainage. Emphasize the importance of promptly reporting such findings to the doctor.

4. Additional individualized interventions: _____

Rationales

1. The uterus is a peritoneal organ, so tissue oozing after its removal drains into the peritoneal cavity. Significant contamination from tissue, bleeding, or infection may result in potentially life-threatening peritonitis if not promptly treated.

2. The hysterectomy patient may be at increased risk for infection compared to other surgical patients because of the surgery site and the predisposing factors that may be involved.
• Ciliary depression from anesthesia, decreased mobility, and hypoventilation from abdominal incision pain contribute to stasis of pulmonary secretions, thus increasing the risk of infection.
• The urinary tract's proximity to the surgical area makes it prone to surgical trauma, edema, and resultant urine retention, which may predispose the patient to infection.
• Wound infection can be a complication of any surgery, but if the hysterectomy is performed because of cancer, the patient's immune response may be impaired, further increasing the risk.
  Nursing measures related to these problems are standard postoperative interventions.

3. Prompt detection facilitates early treatment.

4. Rationales: _____

Nursing diagnosis

Risk for urine retention related to decreased bladder and urethral muscle tone from anesthesia and mechanical trauma

Nursing priority

Promote optimal urine elimination.

Patient outcome criteria

Within 8 hours after catheter removal, the patient will:
• void at least once
• produce adequate output (at least 100 ml per voiding)
• evidence clear, pale yellow urine.

Interventions

1. Monitor for signs of urine retention after catheter removal, such as small, frequent voidings; bladder distention; intake greater than output; or restless behavior.

2. Implement measures to resolve retention, if it occurs. Encourage voiding. Obtain an order for catheterization if no voiding occurs within 8 hours after surgery. (See the "Surgery" plan, page 103, for details.)

3. Additional individualized interventions: _____
_____

Rationales

1. Small, frequent voidings (less than 100 ml) may indicate urine retention, possibly related to edema, decreased muscle tone, or nerve damage to the bladder or urethra during surgery. Urine retention appears most commonly during the first 24 hours after surgery or catheter removal.

2. The "Surgery" plan contains specific information about this common postoperative problem.

3. Rationales: _____
_____

Nursing diagnosis

Pain related to abdominal incision and distention

Nursing priority

Minimize and relieve abdominal pain.

Patient outcome criteria

• Within 1 hour of pain onset, the patient will:
  – report pain level as less than 3 on a scale of 0 to 10 with pain medication
• Within 3 days after surgery, the patient will:
  – need analgesics less frequently or in lower doses
  – pass flatus.

Interventions

1. Implement measures for pain control. See the "Pain" and "Surgery" plans, pages 88 and 103, respectively.

2. Offer application of heat to the abdomen 48 hours after surgery, as ordered.

3. Additional individualized interventions: _____
_____

Rationales

1. These plans contain measures applicable to any patient in pain.

2. Heat increases the elasticity of collagen tissue; lessens pain; relieves muscle spasms; helps resolve inflammatory infiltration, edema, and exudates; and increases blood flow. Heat applied less than 48 hours after surgery may cause undesirable edema.

3. Rationales: _____
_____

NURSING DIAGNOSIS

Risk for body-image disturbance related to changes in body appearance and function as a result of surgery

Nursing priority

Assist the patient in recognizing and accepting possible alteration in body appearance and function.

Patient outcome criteria

By the time of discharge, the patient will:
• verbalize understanding of body changes
• verbalize ability to cope with possible alterations in body appearance and function.

Interventions

1. Assess the patient's level of understanding regarding hysterectomy and the recovery period.

2. Acknowledge the patient's feelings of loss and dependency and fears of complications. Provide reassurance that these concerns are normal.

3. Provide opportunities, every shift, for the patient to discuss concerns about symptoms associated with recovery. Encourage discussion of possible fatigue, wound problems, discomfort, urinary problems, and weight gain. Clarify misconceptions of such posthysterectomy myths as growing fat and flabby, developing facial hair, becoming wrinkled or masculine in appearance, or becoming depressed and nervous.

4. Encourage the patient to discuss plans for recovery at home.

5. Additional individualized interventions: _____

Rationales

1. Evaluating the patient's level of understanding allows the caregiver to individualize patient teaching according to the patient's preexisting knowledge base.

2. Loss of the uterus commonly triggers grief over lost fertility and concerns about femininity. Acknowledgment validates the patient's feelings and encourages communication to alleviate fears and anxieties.

3. Frequent, short teaching sessions enhance learning through repetition and by preventing information overload. Factual discussion prepares the patient to accept common symptoms. Such information does *not* act as a self-fulfilling prophecy. Clarifying misconceptions and myths reduces fears and anxiety during the recovery period.

4. Such discussion allows the patient to make plans incorporating appropriate limitations in physical activities. It also demonstrates the patient's acceptance and understanding of physical abilities.

5. Rationales: _____

NURSING DIAGNOSIS

Risk for sexual dysfunction: Decreased libido or dyspareunia related to fatigue, pain, grieving, altered body image, decreased estrogen levels, loss of vaginal sensations, sexual activity restrictions, or concerns about acceptance by spouse or partner

Nursing priority

Facilitate healthy coping with sexual alterations.

Patient outcome criterion

By the time of discharge, the patient will verbalize strategies to manage temporary alteration in sexual functioning.

Interventions

1. Encourage the patient to explore perceptions of how surgery will affect sexual function. Listen sensitively.

2. Discuss the potential impact of surgery on sexuality by explaining:
• the predictability of temporarily decreased libido

• the temporary nature of loss of vaginal sensations and of activity restrictions (sexual intercourse is discouraged for 4 to 6 weeks, then may be resumed gradually); also explain that return to full function is likely in approximately 4 months
• the rationale for avoiding douching during the recovery.

3. Explain that decreased libido and vaginal dryness may result from hormone loss and that hormone replacements are available.

4. Suggest ways to ease sexual adjustment during the immediate postoperative period, such as holding hands, kissing, massage, and other methods of expressing love and sexuality.

5. Discuss options for conserving energy and preventing discomfort during return to sexual functioning, such as using a vaginal lubricant, scheduling sex for periods of peak energy, and avoiding positions that put pressure on the incision.

6. Encourage the patient and spouse or partner, if present, to share concerns and feelings with each other.

7. Additional individualized interventions: _____

Rationales

1. Identifying current perceptions is the first step in coping with concerns. Sensitive listening allows the caregiver to identify appropriate and inappropriate perceptions.

2. Providing factual information clarifies misconceptions and reduces fears of sexual loss.
• Abdominal hysterectomy is major surgery that can have profound emotional implications. Fatigue, pain, and grieving may require so much coping energy that little remains for dealing with sexuality. The patient may need gentle "permission" to allow time to recover.
• Vaginal sensory loss from surgical trauma resolves typically over a period of weeks to months. Activity restrictions allow time for tissues to heal.

• Douching may increase the risk of infection or bleeding.

3. The patient may not recognize that changes in sexual feelings and function can have a physiologic basis.

4. Continued physical affection provides reassurance that a spouse's or partner's sexual interest continues after the hysterectomy.

5. Sexual activity during the recovery period may be modified temporarily, but return to full sexual function is expected.

6. Mutual loving support is a positive factor in the couple's adjustment to sexual alterations.

7. Rationales: _____

Discharge planning

Discharge checklist
Before discharge, the patient shows evidence of:
❏ stable vital signs
❏ hemoglobin level and WBC count within normal parameters
❏ absence of cardiovascular and pulmonary complications
❏ bowel function same as before surgery
❏ absence of dysuria, hematuria, pyuria, burning, frequency, or urgency
❏ absence of fever
❏ absence of signs and symptoms of infection

❏ ability to control pain using oral medications
❏ ability to ambulate and perform activities of daily living (ADLs) same as before surgery
❏ healing surgical incision without redness, inflammation, or drainage
❏ ability to perform wound care independently or with minimal assistance
❏ ability to tolerate adequate nutritional intake
❏ adequate home support, or referral to home care if indicated by inadequate home support system or inability to perform ADLs and wound care.

Teaching checklist

Document evidence that the patient and family demonstrate an understanding of:

❏ implications of total abdominal hysterectomy
❏ all discharge medications' purpose, dosage, administration schedule, and adverse effects requiring medical attention
❏ incision care (aseptic technique, dressing changes, irrigations, cleaning procedures, hand-washing technique, and proper disposal of soiled dressings)
❏ signs and symptoms of possible infection
❏ dietary requirements and restrictions, if any
❏ activity and exercise restrictions
❏ date, time, and location of follow-up appointment
❏ how to contact the doctor.

Documentation checklist

Using outcome criteria as a guide, document:
❏ clinical status on admission
❏ postoperative clinical assessment
❏ significant changes in status
❏ appearance of incision and wound drainage
❏ I.V. line patency and condition of site
❏ assessment of pain and relief measures
❏ nutritional intake
❏ fluid intake and output
❏ patient and family teaching
❏ discharge planning.

ASSOCIATED PLANS OF CARE

Grieving
Ineffective individual coping
Knowledge deficit
Pain
Surgery
Thrombophlebitis

REFERENCES

Bran, D.F., et al. "Outpatient Vaginal Hysterectomy as a New Trend in Gynecology." *AORN Journal*, 62(5):810-12, 814, November 1995.

Common Uterine Conditions: Options for Treatment. AHCPR Publication #98-0003. Rockville, Md.: Agency for Health Care Policy and Research, December 1997. (http://www.ahcpr.gov/consumer/uterine1.htm)

Gorman, L.M. *Davis's Manual of Psychosocial Nursing in General Patient Care*. Philadelphia: F.A. Davis Co., 1996.

Kramer, M., and Reiter, R. "Hysterectomy: Indications, Alternatives and Predictors." *American Family Physician* 55(3):827-34, February 15, 1997.

Lambden, M., et al. "Women's Sense of Well-Being Before and After Hysterectomy." *Journal of Obstetric, Gynecologic and Neonatal Nursing* 26(5):540-48, September-October 1997.

Nettina, S. *The Lippincott Manual of Nursing Practice*, 6th ed. Philadelphia: Lippincott-Raven Pubs., 1996.

Polaski, A.L., and Tatro, S.E. *Luckman's Core Principles and Practice of Medical-Surgical Nursing*. Philadelphia: W.B. Saunders Co., 1996.

Read, C. "Early Discharge Schemes for Hysterectomy Patients." *Nursing Standard* 10(42):43-45, July 1996.

Segal, S. "Nursing Rounds. Postoperative TAH/BSO...Total Abdominal Hysterectomy/Bilateral Salpingoophorectomy." *American Journal of Nursing*, 96(1): Continuing Care Extra Edition: 45, 47, January 1996.

Sparks, S.M., and Taylor, C.M. *Nursing Diagnosis Reference Manual*, 4th ed. Springhouse, Pa.: Springhouse Corp., 1997.

Mastectomy

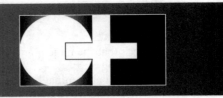

DRG information

DRG 257   Total Mastectomy for Malignancy with
Complication or Comorbidity (CC).
Mean LOS = 3.4 days
Principal diagnoses include:
- carcinoma in situ, breast
- neoplasm, breast, malignant, secondary
- neoplasm, breast, uncertain behavior
- neoplasm, female
- male breast, malignant (primary)
- neoplasm, skin, malignant, secondary

DRG 258   Total Mastectomy for Malignancy without
CC.
Mean LOS = 2.5 days

DRG 259   Subtotal Mastectomy for Malignancy with
CC.
Mean LOS = 3.5 days

DRG 260   Subtotal Mastectomy for Malignancy without CC.
Mean LOS = 1.9 days

INTRODUCTION

Definition and time focus

Mastectomy is the surgical removal of mammary tissue
and, in some cases, the pectoral muscles. Although usually used to treat breast cancer, subcutaneous mastectomy (with preservation of chest muscles, skin, nipple,
and areola) may be appropriate in male gynecomastia
and severe fibrocystic breast disease requiring multiple
biopsies. Subcutaneous mastectomy may also be performed to prevent breast cancer in women at increased
risk. Mastectomy commonly is followed by chemotherapy or radiation therapy. However, if the tumor is large
or the cancer is advanced (with skin or chest wall involvement), such treatments may be administered before surgery.

Breast tissue is affected by several cancers, including
carcinoma of the secreting glands (ductal carcinoma),
carcinoma of the glandular epithelium (breast adeno-
mas), breast sarcomas, and lymphomas. Infiltrating in-
traductal carcinoma accounts for 80% of all breast cancers; it has a poor prognosis. Breast cancer is responsible for 36% of all new cancer cases and 18% of all
cancer deaths in women; the high mortality rate has not
changed significantly in 60 years.

The mastectomy performed depends on tumor size,
nodal involvement, and evidence of metastasis. The pa-

tient's age and desire for breast reconstruction is also
considered. Procedures include:
- lumpectomy — a complete excision of the tumor
(usually followed by local irradiation to destroy microscopic cancer cells)
- partial (segmental) mastectomy — removal of tumor
and adjacent tissue, leaving nipple, areola, and remaining breast tissue intact
- total (simple) mastectomy — removal of all breast
and mammary tissue; pectoral muscles remain intact
- subcutaneous mastectomy — a variation of simple
mastectomy in which the skin, nipple, areola, and chest
muscles are preserved in preparation for breast reconstruction
- modified radical mastectomy (Patey method) — removal of all breast tissue, overlying skin, nipple and
areola, minor pectoral muscle, and samples of adjacent
and axillary lymph nodes
- radical mastectomy (Halsted method) —removal of
tissue as in the modified radical mastectomy plus removal of the major pectoral muscle (rarely performed
in the United States).

This plan focuses on the care of the female breast
cancer patient before and after mastectomy.

Etiology and precipitating factors

Although the exact cause of breast cancer is unknown,
risk factors have been identified.

Factors associated with greatest risk
- Age — only 15% of cases occur before age 40; the
greatest percentage occur between ages 45 and 60
- Personal history of previous breast cancer
- Family history of breast cancer — risk is 3 to 5 times
higher if mother, sister, or daughter had the disease
- Hormones — peak incidence between ages 45 and 49
probably related to ovarian estrogen problems; between
ages 65 and 69, probably related to adrenal estrogen
problems
- Gene defect — a mutation or injury to the BrCA 1
gene or mutation of the p53 gene (located on chromosome 17) may increase a woman's risk of developing
breast cancer with metastasis; 13% of breast cancers are
thought to be from genetic defects

Factors associated with increased risk
- History of breast cancer in a maternal or paternal
grandmother or aunt
- Personal history of endometrial, ovarian, or colon
cancer
- History of fibrocystic breast disease
- Nulliparity

• Birth of first child after age 30
• Early onset of menstruation and late menopause
• Estrogen replacement therapy
• Culture — at increased risk if white in the upper socioeconomic levels of a Western society
• Obesity
• Diet high in animal fats
• Daily alcohol consumption
• Exposure to ionizing radiation — radon or naturally occurring nuclear fallout; excessive medical or dental X-rays; previous radiation therapy or fluoroscopy examinations (1% increase in risk per rad)

FOCUSED ASSESSMENT GUIDELINES

Nursing history (functional health pattern findings)

Health perception–health management pattern
• Painless, firm to hard lump or nodule that has indistinct boundaries and is not easily movable; may be found anywhere in breast tissue or axilla but most commonly in the left breast, upper outer quadrants, or just below the nipple
• Delay in seeking treatment after tumor discovery
• Focal, constant pain unrelated to menstrual cycle (advanced disease)
• Spontaneous discharge of bloody, clear, or milky secretions from nipple or nipple inversion, retraction, elevation, ulceration, or scaliness (advanced disease)

Nutrition-metabolic pattern
• Weight loss, anorexia, early satiety, and taste alterations, such as reduced sensitivity to sweetness or decreased desire for beef, pork, chocolate, coffee, and tomatoes (related to cancer or protein-calorie malnutrition)
• Nausea, vomiting, stomatitis, and mucositis (related to chemotherapy or radiation therapy)

Elimination pattern
• Constipation (related to anorexia, depression, immobility, or narcotic administration)
• Diarrhea (related to increased bacterial growth from decreased GI tract motility)

Activity-exercise pattern
• General malaise
• Weariness, weakness, or lack of physical energy
• Physical and emotional withdrawal related to depression
• Complaints of shoulder and arm immobility related to pain

Sleep-rest pattern
• Insomnia from pain, anxiety, or fear of cancer or the unknown
• Increased desire for sleep (withdrawal behavior)

Self-perception–self-concept pattern
• Grief related to perceived or actual loss

• Body-image disturbance related to impending loss of breast or lymphedema
• Guilt, anger, hostility, or denial related to diagnosis
• Breast loss with loss of femininity, desirability, and maternal instincts
• Self-concept problem related to hair loss (if alopecia is present)

Role-relationship pattern
• Hostility toward health care providers as a result of anger over role loss or sense of injustice
• Withdrawal from family and friends to avoid anticipated rejection
• Inability to assume family or work roles

Sexuality-reproductive pattern
• Concern over need for additional surgery (hysterectomy with oophorectomy or adrenalectomy) if the tumor is estrogen receptive
• Concern over adverse effects of androgenic drugs, including excessive facial hair (hirsutism), male pattern baldness, deepening voice, or increased libido

Coping–stress tolerance pattern
• Anxiety, fear, restlessness, and depression related to unknown extent of tumor and resulting prognosis
• Need for counseling
• Dependency
• Extreme independence related to fears of becoming dependent or a burden to others
• Financial, child care, and job concerns, especially if a single parent
• Demonstrated depression and despondency

Value-belief pattern
• Social conditioning leads patient to believe that personal worth and value are measured by the size and shape of breasts
• Adoption of a fatalistic attitude, equating cancer with death
• Disease perceived as punishment for past actions or indiscretions or fear passing cancer to the next generation
• Belief that external factors control personal life
• Feelings of being forsaken by source of spiritual strength

Physical findings

Integumentary
• Painless tumor, mass, lesion, thickening, or unusual growth in breast tissue
• Palpable medial, supraclavicular, cervical or axillary nodes; isolated skin nodules; solitary, unilateral lesions; purplish color; heat and redness; ulcerations with secondary infection; or peau d'orange (skin of the orange) appearance resulting from lymphatic invasion and edema (advanced disease)
• Alopecia (from chemotherapy)

(Text continues on page 830.)

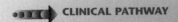 **CLINICAL PATHWAY**

Managing mastectomy

DRG: 257, 258

Patient problem	Preadmission teaching	Early morning admission (EMA)

Cardiopulmonary
• Altered hemodynamics related to surgery
• Increased risk of atelectasis related to surgery
• Increased risk for deep vein thrombosis (DVT) & pulmonary embolism (PE)
	• Goal: Normal sinus rhythm (NSR) on ECG.
	  – Assess cardiopulmonary (C/P) status. ECG if > 40 yr & not done in past 30 days. CBC, survey 27, chest X-ray.
	• Goal: Verbalizes understanding of postop pulmonary toilet regimen.
	  – Instruct on turning, coughing, and deep breathing (T, C, DB).
	• Goal: Verbalizes understanding of thromboembolitic disease (TED) stockings and sequential compression device (SCD).
	  – Instruct on TEDS & SCD.
		• Goal: NSR on ECG.
		  – Assess C/P status. ECG if > 40 yr & not done. in past 30 days. Instruct re T, C, DB.
		• Goal: Maintains adequate venous return.
		  – Apply TEDS. Apply SCD per doctor's order.

Fluid balance
• Risk for altered fluid balance or diet
	• Goal: Verbalizes understanding of preop NPO instructions.
	  – Instruct re NPO.
	• Goal: Verbalizes understanding postop diet progression.
	  – Instruct re postop diet regimen.
		• Goal: Compliance with NPO preop status.
		  – NPO.

Pain
• Alteration in comfort related to surgery
	• Goal: Verbalizes understanding of pain management.
	  – Discuss pain management vs. absence of pain.
		• Goal: Verbalizes understanding of pain management.
		  – Discuss pain management vs. absence of pain.

Integumentary
• Potential for infection at operative site or drain site
	• Goal: Verbalizes understanding of incision location & purpose of drains.
	  – Instruct re: surgical incision & postop drains.
		• Goal: Verbalizes understanding of incision location & purpose of drains.
		  – Reinforce preop instruction.

Activity • Alteration in mobility related to surgical procedure • Self-care deficit related to decreased mobility and pain with movement	• Goal: Verbalizes understanding of postop activity progression & restrictions. – Instruct re plan of postop activity/mobility restrictions with progression.	

Psychosocial/spiritual
• Fear related to cancer diagnosis and future implications
• Fear related to change in sexual self-concept
	• Goal: Verbally acknowledges feelings of anxiety related to surgery.
	  – Encourage expression of feelings. Assess patient and family support system. Discuss available services (social service, pastoral care).
		• Goal: Verbally acknowledges feelings of anxiety related to surgery.
		  – Encourage expression of feelings.
		  – Pastoral care visit.

Knowledge deficit
• R/T surgical procedure
• R/T preop preparation
• R/T acquisition of prosthesis
• R/T discharge/home care
	• Goal: Verbalize understanding of EMA admitting process & surgical procedure.
	  – Instruct re admission process, preop procedures, and use of home meds.
	• Goal: Verbalize understanding of plan for prosthesis acquisition.
	  – Notify Reach for Recovery, Breast Care Team.
	  – Instruct re available resources
		• Goal: Verbalizes understanding of EMA admitting process & surgical procedure.
		  – Reinforce instructions.

Day of surgery	Postoperative day 1	Postoperative day 2

• Goal: SBP>90, DBP>50, HR>50, R>12
  – VS q 15 min X 4 q 30 min X 2, q 1 hr X 4, q 4 hr
• Goal: Clear bilateral breath sounds
  – Auscultate lungs q 8 hr
  – Assist with T, C, DB q 2 hr x 4
• Goal: No s/s of DVT or PE
  – Apply TEDS; SCD per doctor's order.
  – Assess left extremity for temp, redness, & calf tenderness q 8 hr
  – Dangle legs & out of bed with help 4-6 hr postop
	• Goal: SBP>90, DBP>50, HR>50, R>12
	  – VS q 4 hr
	• Goal: Clear bilateral breath sounds
	  – Auscultate lungs q 8 hr
	• Goal: No s/s of DVT or PE
	  – Remove TEDS for bath; then reapply
	  – Maintain SCD when in bed
	• Goal: Independent ambulation q.i.d.
	  – Assist with first walk in hall then amb q.i.d.
		• Goal: SBP>90, DBP>50, HR>50, R>12.
		  – VS q 8 hr
		• Goal: No s/s of DVT or PE
		  – Remove TEDS for bath; then reapply
		  – Discontinue SCD
		• Goal: Compliance with ambulation
		  – Up ad lib; assess compliance

• Goal: Tolerates 500 ml P.O. 8 hr, postop without nausea and vomiting.
  – Sips of clear liquid; advance diet as tol
  – Measure & record amt q 8 hr
  – Heplock I.V. or maintain I.V. KVO if PCA
• Goal: Voids freely, urine output of 250 ml q 8 hr for 24 hr.
  – Measure & record urine output q 8 hr
	• Goal: Tolerates regular diet
	  – Regular diet; record % taken
	  – Encourage 6-8 glasses fluids per 24 hr
	• Goal: Voids freely, urine output of 250 ml q 8 h 24 hr
	  – Measure & record urine output q 8 hr
		• Goal: Tolerates regular diet
		  – Regular diet; record % taken
		  – Encourages 6-8 glasses fluids per 24 hr
		• Goal: Voids freely, urine output of 250 ml q 8 hr for 24 hr
		  – Measure & record urine output q 8 hr

• Goal: Pain controlled at level <7
  – Assess pain level q 4 hr
  – Reinforce instructions R/T PCA pump mgt if ordered
  – Elevate arm on operative side on 1-2 pillows
	• Goal: Pain controlled with P.O. meds & without adverse drug reactions
	  – Assess pain level q 4 hr
	  – Offer P.O. analgesics p.r.n.
	  – Discontinue PCA pump if ordered
	  – Elevate arm on operative side on 1-2 pillows
		• Goal: Pain controlled with P.O. meds & without adverse drug reactions
		  – Assess pain level q 4 hr
		  – Offer p.c. analgesics p.r.n.
		  – Elevate arm on operative side on 1-2 pillows

• Goal: Dressing dry & intact
  – Assess dressing q 4 hr; reinforce p.r.n.
• Goal: Drains patent & compressed.
  – Assess drains for patency and compression q 2 hr X 4
  – Measure & record drainage q 8 hr & p.r.n.
	• Goal: Dressing dry & intact
	  – Assess dressing q 4 hr. Reinforce p.r.n.
	• Goal: Drains patent & compressed
	  – Assess drains for patency and compression q 2 hr X 4
	  – Measure & record drainage q 8 hr & p.r.n.
		• Goal: Wound & s/s of infection
		  – Dressing change per doctor
		• Goal: Drains patent & compressed
		  – Measure and record drainage q 8 hr & p.r.n.
		• Goal: Describe s/s of infection
		  – Instruct re s/s of infection with patient & significant other

• Goal: Compliant with activity restrictions
  – Encourage arm activity within levels of comfort or as ordered per doctor
	• Goal: Compliant with postmastectomy exercise regimen
	  – Instruct re limitations & restrictions
	• Goal: Participates in self-care activities
	  – Assess need for assistance with bath
		• Goal: Compliant with postmastectomy exercise regimen
		  – Reinforce instructions
		• Goal: Perform ADLs with minimal assistance
		  – Assess need for assistance with bath

• Goal: Verbalizes thoughts/feelings re surgery & future implications
  – Encourage expression of thoughts & feelings
  – Assess need for inpt. support services
	• Goal: Verbalizes thoughts/feelings re surgery & future implications
	  – Encourage expression of thoughts & feelings
	  – Assess need for inpt support services
		• Goal: Verbalizes thoughts & feelings re surgery & future implications
		  – Encourage expression of thoughts & feelings; assess need for inpt support services
		• Goal: Verbalizes feelings of self-worth
		  – Actively listen; provide positive reinforcement; instruct re postop support services

• Goal: Decreased anxiety related to postop process & procedures	• Goal: Verbalizes understanding of postop drain management
	  – Instruct & demonstrate drain management
	• Goal: Verbalize understanding of breast self exam (BSE) postop
	  – Instruct re BSE of operative site
		• Goal: Patient or significant other demonstrates ability to manage drain
		  – Reinforce instructions of POD 1; provide measuring cup; observe technique
		• Goal: Verbalize understanding of plan for medical follow-up
		  – Review discharge instructions

• Scalded skin syndrome (a debilitating condition in the immunosuppressed patient in which a *Staphylococcus aureus* infection produces epidermolytic toxins)

Hematologic
• Hypercalcemia
• Thromboembolic infarction related to hypercoagulability from cancer and tumor lysis

Cardiovascular
• Hypertension related to effect of hypercalcemia on smooth muscle
• Bradycardia or premature ventricular contractions caused by digitalis toxicity from increased calcium level
• Compensatory tachycardia with decreasing blood pressure
• Distended neck veins
• Peripheral edema

Neurologic
• Confusion, restlessness, or disorientation (resulting from serum calcium level above 15 mg/dl)
• Muscle weakness and proximal myopathy
• Diminished deep tendon reflexes

Renal
• Polyuria or renal calculi, if hypercalcemia is present

Gastrointestinal
• Polydipsia from polyuria
• Nausea, vomiting, and anorexia as a result of hypercalcemia, chemotherapy, or radiation therapy

Musculoskeletal
• Pathologic fractures with bony metastases

Diagnostic studies
• Hemoglobin level and hematocrit — if low, may be related to anemia or blood loss during surgery; before surgery, the patient should donate 2 to 3 units of blood which later can be transfused to maintain postoperative hemoglobin level and hematocrit and to aid healing
• Serum calcium level — level above 11 mg/dl indicates hypercalcemia, a common complication of cancer
• Serum phosphate level — hypophosphatemia is commonly associated with hypercalcemia
• Platelet counts, prothrombin time/international normalized ratio (PT/INR), and activated partial thromboplastin time (APTT) — a depressed platelet count, PT/INR, and APTT may indicate disseminated intravascular coagulation (DIC)
• Carcinoembryonic antigen titer — increases 75% with metastatic disease
• Human chorionic gonadotropin — presence in blood or urine of nonpregnant females indicates cancer; declining amounts indicate treatment effectiveness
• Serum ferritin level — may be low, indicating anemia
• Serum albumin level — may be low from fluid shifting to interstitial spaces
• Serum alkaline phosphatase level — if elevated, may indicate metastatic activity in bone and liver

• Flow cytometry studies (cellular deoxyribonucleic acid content) — identify the 40% to 50% of patients at risk for recurrence
• Estrogen receptor assay — estrogen-sensitive tumors are more susceptible to hormone therapy; non-estrogen-sensitive tumors have a low response rate to hormonal manipulation and a high recurrence rate
• Mammography — may detect nonpalpable lesions (80% to 90% accurate); 50% of breast cancers appear as a cluster of microcalcifications
• Magnetic resonance imaging — differentiates benign and malignant lesions; accurately identifies premalignant tissue changes; detects tumors in dense breast tissue; is unique in defining tumor extent; also used for staging for treatment planning
• Breast-specific positron emission tomography
• Ultrasound — differentiates fluid from solid tumor; cannot detect very small tumors
• Open biopsy — surgery differentiates benign from malignant lesions
• Closed biopsy — image-guided needle biopsy (for women with nonpalpable lesions) and fine needle aspiration biopsy (for women with palpable lesions) differentiates fluid-filled cyst from solid tumor
• Liver and bone scans (indicated if liver chemistries are elevated) — may reveal metastatic disease
• Electrocardiography (ECG) — T-wave changes, bundle-branch block, P-wave notching, or other abnormalities may result from chemotherapy

Potential complications
From breast cancer
• Hypercalcemia
• Lymphedema
• Hypophosphatemia
• Thrombophlebitis
• DIC

From metastasis
• Pathological fractures
• Obstructive uropathy
• Metabolic acidosis (lactic acid increase)
• Thrombocytopenia
• DIC
• Superior vena cava syndrome
• Spinal cord compression
• Meningeal carcinomatosis
• Intracerebral metastasis
• Pleural effusion
• Pulmonary embolism
• Spontaneous pneumothorax

From metastasis or radiation therapy
• Inflammatory constrictive pericarditis
• Pericardial effusion and tamponade
• Scalded skin syndrome

From chemotherapy
• Alopecia

- Anaphylaxis
- Amyloidosis
- Hyperuricemia
- GI hemorrhage
- Paralytic ileus
- Cardiomyopathy or cardiotoxicity
- Neurotoxicity

- Pulmonary toxicity
- Sepsis
- Bone marrow suppression
- Renal tubular necrosis

Other
- Reactive depression
- Suicidal ideation

CLINICAL SNAPSHOT

MASTECTOMY

Major nursing diagnoses and collaborative problems	Key patient outcomes
Risk for lymphedema	Display circumference equal in both arms.
Body-image disturbance	Be able to touch and look at the wound.
Risk for hypercalcemia	Maintain a serum calcium level of 8.5 to 10.8 mg/dl.

COLLABORATIVE PROBLEM

Risk for lymphedema related to interrupted lymph circulation from axillary node dissection during mastectomy

Nursing priority

Prevent or minimize lymph stasis.

Patient outcome criteria

By the time of discharge, the patient will:
- list signs and symptoms of lymphedema and appropriate response to them
- demonstrate exercises to promote lymph circulation and minimize postoperative lymphedema
- display circumference equal in both arms
- remain free from infection and injury
- demonstrate increased mobility from range-of-motion (ROM) exercises.

Interventions

1. Determine if the patient is to have a radical or modified radical mastectomy.

Rationales

1. Radical mastectomy and modified radical mastectomy are the major cause of secondary lymphedema. During axillary node dissection, lymph channels are blocked or removed, shifting lymph fluid to soft tissue and decreasing lymphatic circulation.

2. Before surgery, measure and record the circumference of each arm 2 ¼" (6 cm) above and below the elbow. After surgery, repeat measurement each morning until discharge.
• If lymphedema is noted, obtain an antiembolism sleeve for the patient to wear from morning to night (some patients wear the sleeve only at night).
• If lymphedema is severe, consult the doctor about using a mechanical pressure pump every 2 to 3 hours, as needed.

3. Immediately after mastectomy, position the affected arm on a pillow with the elbow higher than the shoulder, and the wrist and hand higher than the elbow.

4. Protect the affected arm from injury.

• Place the patient on an air mattress or sheepskin pad; pad the side rails.
• Keep the patient's fingernails short and smooth.
• Do not allow the patient to wear a name band, watch, or similar items on the affected arm.

5. Monitor laboratory data. Alert the doctor to deviations from these normal ranges:
• serum albumin level — 3.5 to 5 g/dl
• serum sodium level — 135 to 145 mEq/L
• white blood cell (WBC) count — 4,500 to 11,500/µl

6. Check peripheral pulses daily.

7. Inspect the skin for color, translucency, temperature, or breakdown daily.

8. Assess the arm for edema daily by pressing a thumb into the tissue for 5 to 10 seconds and observing for a depression after removing thumb.

9. Administer diuretics and salt-poor albumin, as indicated.

10. Elevate and massage the affected arm daily with lotion, beginning at the wrist and advancing to the shoulder.

11. Administer pain medication 30 to 45 minutes before beginning exercises.

2. Baseline measurements allow for later comparison. Lymphedema is present if the circumference of the affected arm is 1 ½" (4 cm) larger than the unaffected arm.
• Compression of vein walls increases tissue perfusion and prevents venous stasis and edema.

• A mechanical pressure pump stimulates circulation more aggressively.

3. Positioning the arm above the apex of the heart facilitates lymph and blood movement by gravity flow.

4. Eliminating possible sources of trauma decreases the risk of infection.
• Padding cushions the affected arm.

• Short fingernails are less likely to damage the skin.
• Removing constricting bands prevents ischemia.

5. A low serum albumin level promotes lymphedema. A high serum sodium level promotes fluid retention. An abnormal WBC count may indicate infection (lymph node dissection increases the risk of infection).

6. A pulse deficit may occur in the edematous arm.

7. Lymph stasis promotes infection and decreases arterial and venous circulation.

8. Arm lymphedema usually presents as indurated (hardened) skin and, except in the early phase, is non-pitting.

9. Diuretics promote fluid excretion. Albumin maintains osmotic pressure and prevents fluid shifting to the interstitial spaces of soft tissue.

10. Elevation and compression increase lymph flow.

11. Pain relief promotes exercising.

12. Instruct the patient to elevate the affected arm for 30 to 45 minutes every 2 hours for 2 to 3 weeks after discharge, then 2 to 3 times daily for 6 weeks.
One day after surgery, have the patient perform the following exercises as often as the surgeon recommends:
• ball squeezing
• making a tight fist and then flexing and extending the fingers.
Two to three days after surgery, have the patient perform the following exercises as often as recommended:
• raising the affected arm to a 45- to 90-degree side angle
• walking the fingers up a wall to move the arm and shoulder
• bending over at the waist and letting the affected arm dangle, making small circular motions from the shoulder
At discharge, provide a copy of the American Cancer Society pamphlet *Reach to Recovery, Exercises After Mastectomy: Patient Guide.*
Suggested postdischarge exercises include but are not limited to:
• rope pulley — Toss a rope over the top of a door. Sit with both legs bent at the knees and feet planted firmly on the floor. Hug both sides of the door with the knees. Holding the ends of the knotted rope, slowly raise the affected arm as far as comfortable by pulling down on the rope with the unaffected arm. Keeping the raised arm close to the head, reverse the motion; rest and repeat as tolerated.
• elbow pull — Stand with arms extended sideways at shoulder level. With bent elbows, clasp the fingers at the back of the neck and pull the elbows in toward each other until they touch. Relax, rest, and repeat as tolerated.

13. Refer the patient to Reach to Recovery or a similar support group.

14. Teach the patient and family the signs and symptoms of lymphedema and when it is most likely to occur. Advise the patient to seek medical care if any of the following occur in the affected arm:
• pain
• tingling or tightness
• loss of sensation
• increased circumference
• muscle weakness.

12. Exercise is essential to prevent muscle deformities, shortening, contractures, stiffness, and "frozen shoulder." Specific postoperative exercises depend on the extent of the surgery and whether skin grafting was necessary. Exercise regimens must have the surgeon's approval.

13. Reach to Recovery volunteers have experienced breast cancer. Their "I've been there" approach aids the mastectomy patient's rehabilitation. They encourage the patient to use the affected arm and shoulder, and can facilitate psychological and emotional adaptation to the diagnosis of cancer, loss of a breast, and changes in body image and interpersonal relationships.

14. The knowledgeable patient is more likely to obtain early treatment. Acute lymphedema occurs 4 to 6 weeks after surgery, can be transient, and is usually self-limiting; chronic lymphedema may occur weeks, months, or years after surgery.

15. Teach the patient how to maintain lymphatic circulation in the affected arm and prevent infection and injury. Reinforce teaching with written instructions.
• Use padded mitts around the oven, grill, or fireplace. Limit skin exposure to the sun and use a strong sunscreen when outdoors.
• Carry purses, packages, luggage, and other heavy objects on the unaffected side.
• Stop smoking.
• Avoid clothes with elastic or tight sleeves. Never allow blood pressure to be taken on the affected arm.
• Do not allow injections to be given in or blood to be drawn from the affected arm.

15. Maintaining effective lymphatic circulation and preventing infection and injury require the patient's active participation.
• These measures prevent burns.

• Carrying heavy items with the affected arm creates pressure that can lead to lymph stasis.
• Smoking constricts vessels.
• Tight sleeves and constricting bands impede lymph flow.
• Such measures prevent irritation and injury.

Nursing diagnosis

Body-image disturbance related to loss of a body part

Nursing priority

Assist patient to cope with the loss of a breast.

Patient outcome criteria

According to individual readiness, the patient will:
• be able to touch and look at the wound
• participate in decision making
• verbalize loss and work through the grief of an altered body image
• seek out community resources as necessary
• be able to talk about changes that impact sexuality with her partner
• experience no complications if choosing reconstruction
• agree to share information about reconstruction with at least two friends or a group of women, if the patient desires.

Interventions

1. Provide empathetic emotional support. Encourage the patient to express feelings. Listen actively, use therapeutic touch, and be available to sit with the patient as needed. Also refer to the "Grieving" plan, page 44.

2. Assess the patient's feelings about the mastectomy.

3. Monitor the patient's comments about and willingness to look at and touch the incision site. Be alert for mood swings, continued tearfulness, expressions of overwhelming sadness, or withdrawal from family or friends.

4. Counsel the spouse or partner to hold and touch the patient.

Rationales

1. The patient is experiencing a time of intense personal crisis, and grieving is a normal part of emotional adjustment. Empathetic emotional support can facilitate healthy grieving and crisis resolution. The diagnosis of cancer, hospitalization, and surgery all present losses the patient may need to grieve for. The "Grieving" plan contains interventions helpful for any patient experiencing grief.

2. Attitudes, values, and beliefs influence physical and psychological adjustment.

3. Comments and behaviors can help the nurse assess the patient's level of acceptance.

4. The patient with a recent mastectomy has altered tactile perception over the operative site and over part of the upper arm. Touching creates intimacy and affirms that she is loved and lovable.

5. Encourage the patient to wear makeup (if appropriate), nightgowns, and soft, front-closing brassieres (if dressings do not interfere).

6. Offer to refer the patient to a mastectomy support group, a member of the clergy, a social worker, or a psychiatric or oncology clinical nurse specialist.

7. Assess the patient's suitability for reconstructive surgery.

8. If reconstruction is an option, support the patient in the decision-making process.
• Encourage the patient to share thoughts and feelings related to breast reconstruction.

• Teach the patient about reconstruction procedures, the need for skin or muscle flap grafting, and the possibility of nipple and areolar reconstruction. Help the patient obtain information about the procedure's cost and the likelihood of insurance coverage. If possible, provide a copy of the American Cancer Society pamphlet *Breast Reconstruction Following Mastectomy from Cancer.*
• Validate the patient's decision even if you believe it would not be appropriate for you.

9. If reconstruction is not an option or will be delayed, provide information about external breast prostheses when the patient asks about them.

10. After reconstruction, provide appropriate interventions to preserve the reconstructed breast.

• Assess the incision site. Note its appearance and the presence of any pain or tenderness to touch. Monitor WBC counts as ordered. If the suture line does not appear to be healing by primary intention, request a WBC count from the surgeon. Assess surgical drains daily.

5. Some women adjust to breast surgery immediately; others need weeks or months. Attention to appearance may be a sign of recovering self-worth. The nurse's affirmation of the patient's continued femininity may bolster a shaky self-concept.

6. Other patients and professionals can help the patient accept an altered body image and return to wellness. However, such referrals should supplement nursing interventions, not substitute for the nurse's caring and empathy.
    The American Cancer Society offers services to patients and their families, including "I Can Cope," an 8-week group program on learning how to live with cancer, and "I Can Surmount," a support group facilitated by trained patients with cancer. Other local support groups facilitated by professionals also are available. Information about these services is available at all local offices of the American Cancer Society as well as through community hospitals.

7. Contraindications to reconstructive breast surgery include inflammatory carcinomas, high-dose radiation therapy, extensive systemic metastases, and unrealistic attitudes and expectations regarding the surgery's outcome.

8. The nurse can help the patient make an informed decision.
• Some patients immediately accept reconstruction, while others may believe a desire for reconstruction is vain.
• Reconstruction is an accepted option in the management of breast cancer. The patient should have the opportunity to talk and read about breast reconstruction.

• Clarifying and validating feelings conveys respect for the patient's values and beliefs.

9. Queries indicate emotional readiness to focus on this area. A breast prosthesis may boost the patient's self-esteem by providing a natural-appearing substitute for the lost breast.

10. Loss of the reconstructed breast will provide a further blow to the patient's body image and jeopardize emotional recovery.
• Drainage, a darkening suture line, pain and tenderness to touch, and a WBC count over 11,000/µl indicate infection. Infection prolongs healing and promotes dependency on family members and health care professionals, which may result in decreased self-esteem and depression.

• Be alert to pallor, cyanosis, coolness, or increased capillary refill time at the surgical site. If these occur, notify the doctor promptly. Protect the reconstructed breast from pressure. Assess the tightness of the dressing.
• Elevate the head of the bed to Fowler's or semi-Fowler's position.
• Monitor the patient's verbal comments and willingness to look at and touch the reconstructed breast.
• Provide psychological support. Encourage the patient to wear make-up (if appropriate), nightgowns, and soft, front-closing brassieres (if dressings do not interfere).

• Counsel the patient's spouse or partner about the importance of expressing satisfaction with the reconstructed breast.
• Instruct the patient to begin daily, vigorous massage of the implant or graft 6 weeks after surgery.
• Educate the patient about the value of sharing information about reconstruction with other women.

11. Encourage the patient to talk about sexual concerns. Suggestions to initiate conversation may include, "Tell me about any sexual concerns you might have as a result of your mastectomy." Or, "Some women have anxiety and fears about their sexual relationships following a mastectomy. Is there something you would like to discuss, or questions I might help you with?" Or, "Some women have anxiety about their sexual relationships following this surgery. I will be happy to talk with you now, or later if you prefer. Here is my card with my phone number if you need to get in touch with me at another time."

12. Maintain a hopeful and positive outlook when discussing sexuality. Clarify any misconceptions. Encourage the patient to talk with members of mastectomy support groups.

13. A few weeks after discharge, make a home call. Inquire about visits the patient has made away from home, and the resumption of social activities as well as physiological status. Reintroduce the subject of sexuality and ask about concerns the woman might have encountered since surgery.

14. Additional individualized interventions: _____

_____

• These signs may indicate inadequate blood flow. If circulation is not restored, graft or implant rejection or flap necrosis may occur. Preventing pressure at the site promotes adequate blood flow.
• Elevating the head of the bed reduces edema and stress on the reconstructed breast.
• Comments and behaviors can help the nurse evaluate the patient's acceptance of the reconstructed breast.
• Some women adjust to a reconstructed breast immediately; others need weeks or months. Attention to appearance may be a sign of recovering self-worth. The nurse's affirmation of the patient's continued femininity may bolster a shaky self-concept.
• The spouse's or partner's attitude plays a powerful role in the patient's acceptance of the reconstructed breast.

• Massage helps prevent capsular contraction, maintain breast softness, and permit a more natural contour.
• If women are aware that reconstruction is an option, they may seek help when a lump or abnormality is first discovered, rather than delaying diagnosis and treatment for fear of disfigurement.

11. Body image is intimately related to sexuality. Breast cancer patients require continuing education, support, and encouragement in dealing with the emotional trauma and sexual sequelae of treatment. Many patients will desire information but will not initiate the discussion with a doctor or nurse. Such information is essential to emotional healing.

12. Maintaining a positive outlook conveys hope. Clarifying misconceptions (such as a mastectomy destroying sexual attractiveness) can gently challenge beliefs that otherwise might become self-fulfilling prophecies. Women who have "been there" may provide more credible reassurance than a health professional.

13. Some patients remain at home to avoid their friends and hesitate to resume social activities. Reasons for withdrawal may include fear of rejection by others. Fear of rejection from a spouse or significant other commonly manifests in withdrawal. Home calls provide an excellent opportunity for the nurse to ask questions about sex or sexuality and allow the patient to share any fears, concerns, or questions that might have arisen since discharge.

14. Rationales: _____

_____

COLLABORATIVE PROBLEM

Risk for hypercalcemia related to abnormal calcium transport or skeletal metastases

Nursing priority

Maintain normal serum calcium levels and prevent complications of hypercalcemia.

Patient outcome criteria

• Within 48 hours, calcium levels of 12 mg/dl or more will decrease to 8.5 to 10.8 mg/dl.
• By the time of discharge, the patient with controllable hypercalcemia and family will verbalize signs and symptoms of blood calcium increase and appropriate interventions.

Interventions

1. Monitor for hypercalcemia (serum calcium level greater than 11 mg/dl). Early signs and symptoms include nausea, vomiting, and anorexia.

2. Monitor blood pressure and heart rate every 2 hours.

3. Auscultate for heart sounds and rhythms in four sites and record daily.

4. Assess ECG changes. Observe for prolonged PR intervals, lengthening QT intervals, lengthening and widening T waves, atrioventricular (AV) block, and asystole.

5. If the patient is receiving a digitalis glycoside, measure the apical pulse rate before administering; if below 60 beats/minute, withhold the drug and check with the doctor.

6. Assess the patient's level of consciousness every 4 to 8 hours. Assess for confusion, restlessness, disorientation, drowsiness, profound weakness, and personality changes. Orient to time, place, and person. Elevate and pad side rails, as indicated.

7. Document fluid intake and output every 2 hours to monitor fluid balance. Obtain baseline weight on admission. Weigh daily thereafter.

8. Assess amount and color of urine, and note specific gravity (normal range is 1.010 to 1.035).

9. Assess for flank pain and strain all urine for calculi.

10. Anticipate I.V. administration of saline, 250 to 300 ml/hour, and a loop diuretic such as furosemide (Lasix), 80 to 100 mg every 2 hours, as tolerated.

Rationales

1. Hypercalcemia, a metabolic complication, develops in 10% to 20% of all cancer patients; in breast cancer with metastasis, the incidence increases to 50%. Although the majority of patients with hypercalcemia have skeletal metastases, not all patients with metastases develop hypercalcemia.

2. Increased calcium levels can affect smooth muscle, causing hypertension.

3. Hypercalcemia may cause arrhythmias or extra heart sounds.

4. Changes in PR or QT intervals or T-wave configuration indicate a serum calcium level of 16 mg/dl or more. AV block and asystole may occur at serum calcium levels of 18 mg/dl.

5. Increased serum calcium levels enhance the action of digitalis glycosides, possibly causing toxicity; the doctor may withhold the drug to prevent bradycardia, premature ventricular contractions, or paroxysmal atrial tachycardia.

6. If serum calcium levels are 15 mg/dl or more, central nervous system depression may alter mental status or thought processes, creating a risk for injury.

7. Effects of hypercalcemia include defective water conservation, leading to dehydration, sodium excretion, potassium wasting, and severe weight loss.

8. Hypercalcemia may interfere with antidiuretic hormone, limiting the kidney's ability to concentrate urine and resulting in polyuria.

9. Hypercalcemia may cause renal calculi to form.

10. Saline and furosemide diuresis usually causes calcium excretion, decreasing the serum calcium level.

11. Anticipate administration of calcitonin (Calcimar), glucocorticoids, phosphates, plicamycin (Mithracin), or gallium nitrate (Ganite). Be alert to adverse reactions, which may include headache, anorexia, nausea and vomiting, hepatic and renal impairment, and hemorrhage from thrombocytopenia.

11. These drugs may increase urinary calcium excretion and decrease intestinal calcium absorption by inhibiting bone resorption or inhibiting tumor production of prostaglandins.

12. Apply an ice collar to the patient's neck if nauseated. Administer an antiemetic, if appropriate.

12. Both hypercalcemia and the drugs used to treat it can cause nausea and vomiting through vagal nerve stimulation in the upper GI tract or through activation of the brain's chemoreceptor trigger zone. Vagal nerve stimulation produces vasodilation; an ice collar causes vasoconstriction, providing temporary relief from nausea. Antiemetics inhibit stimulation of the chemoreceptor trigger zone.

13. Provide mouth care every 4 hours, after vomiting, and before meals. Clean the teeth daily with baking soda and hydrogen peroxide or a similar solution.

13. Oral cleaning and antiseptics refresh the mouth. Baking soda and hydrogen peroxide neutralize mouth acids.

14. Auscultate for bowel sounds daily in four quadrants and record changes in pitch and frequency. Be alert to high-pitched, diminished, or absent sounds. Increase fluid intake to four 8-oz (240-ml) glasses every 8 hours, as tolerated.

14. Hypercalcemia depresses smooth-muscle contractility, delays gastric emptying, and decreases intestinal motility, leading to constipation, obstipation, and paralytic ileus. Dehydration exacerbates obstipation and paralytic ileus.

15. In the first weeks of androgen therapy, monitor serum calcium levels.

15. Endocrine therapy may precipitate hypercalcemia in premenopausal or early menopausal women.

16. Teach the patient and family signs and symptoms of hypercalcemia and appropriate interventions.

16. Hypercalcemia may recur. Being aware of its signs and symptoms may cause the patient and family to seek early medical intervention.

17. If hypercalcemia does not respond to interventions, alert the family and help them prepare for the patient's death.

17. Uncontrollable hypercalcemia is a sign of impending death.

18. Additional individualized interventions: _____

18. Rationales: _____

DISCHARGE PLANNING

Discharge checklist
Before discharge, the patient shows evidence of:
- ❑ hemoglobin level and hematocrit within normal limits
- ❑ serum calcium and serum phosphate levels within normal limits
- ❑ platelet count, PT/INR, and APTT within normal limits
- ❑ ferritin levels within normal limits
- ❑ serum albumin–serum globulin ratio normal (1.5:1)
- ❑ normal total protein values
- ❑ absent or low serum levels of carcinoembryonic antigen
- ❑ absence of HCG in serum or urine
- ❑ absence of metabolic complications
- ❑ absence of cardiac arrhythmias, and neuromuscular, renal, and GI complications
- ❑ absence of secondary lymphedema
- ❑ arms equal in circumference
- ❑ radial pulses equal bilaterally
- ❑ affected arm free from injury
- ❑ ability to perform ROM exercises
- ❑ absence of "frozen shoulder"
- ❑ support from family and spouse or partner
- ❑ referral to other health care professionals, if indicated.

Teaching checklist

Document evidence that the patient and family demonstrate an understanding of:

❏ nature of cancer and its implications — patients and families need to be alert to signs and symptoms of ovarian and bowel cancers; there is a moderate association between breast cancer and cancers of the ovary and bowel (fiber-optic colonoscopy aids in early detection of bowel cancer)
❏ signs and symptoms of oncologic emergencies
❏ importance of support for the patient's decision regarding reconstructive surgery
❏ signs and symptoms of graft rejection
❏ activity recommendations and limitations
❏ community or professional resources and support groups
❏ need for follow-up appointments
❏ need for long-term emotional support as a result of cancer diagnosis.

Documentation checklist

Using outcome criteria as a guide, document:

❏ clinical status on admission
❏ changes in status
❏ presence of adequate support systems
❏ need for knowledge of endocrine therapies
❏ activity and exercise tolerance and recommendations
❏ patient and family teaching
❏ discharge planning.

ASSOCIATED PLANS OF CARE

Dying
Grieving
Ineffective family coping: Compromised
Ineffective individual coping
Lung cancer
Pain
Surgery

REFERENCES

"Improving Imaging Methods for Breast Cancer Detection and Diagnosis," *CancerNet News From the National Cancer Institute*. World Wide Web site (http://cancernet.nci.nih.gov) and Gopher server (gopher://gopher/nih.gov).

Clark, J. "Psychosocial Responses of the Patient," in *Cancer Nursing—Principles and Practice*, 3rd ed. Edited by Groenwald, S., et al. Boston: Jones & Bartlett, Pubs., Inc., 1993.

Crane, R. "Breast Cancer," in *Oncology Nursing*, 2nd ed. Edited by Otto, S. St. Louis: Mosby–Year Book, Inc., 1994.

Goodman, M., and Chapman, D. "Breast Cancer," in *Cancer Nursing—Principles and Practice*, 3rd ed. Edited by Groenwald, S., et al. Boston: Jones & Bartlett Pubs., Inc.,1993.

Lang-Kummer, J. "Hypercalcemia," in *Cancer Nursing—Principles and Practice*, 3rd ed. Edited by Groenwald, S., et al. Boston: Jones and Bartlett Pubs., Inc., 1993.

Parker, S., et al. "Cancer Statistics, 1997," *Ca — A Cancer Journal for Clinicians* 47(1):5-27, 1997.

Pfeifer, K. "Surgery," in *Oncology Nursing*, 2nd ed. Edited by Otto, S. St. Louis: Mosby–Year Book, Inc., 1994.

Price, J., and Purtell, J. "Prevention and Treatment of Lymphedema After Breast Cancer," *AJN* 97(9):34-37, 1997.

Schafer, S. "Oncologic Complications," in *Oncology Nursing*, 2nd ed. Edited by Otto, S. St. Louis: Mosby–Year Book, Inc., 1994.

Prostatectomy

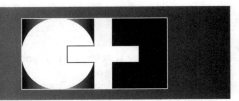

INTRODUCTION

Definition and time focus
Prostatectomy is the surgical removal of the prostate, a
gland (in males) located in line with the urethra and
positioned between the bladder and rectum. There are
three types of prostatectomies: a partial resection removes only enlarged tissue, a simple prostatectomy removes the prostate and its capsule, and a radical prostatectomy removes the prostate, its capsule, the seminal
vesicles, and a portion of the bladder neck.

Four surgical approaches are used: transurethral,
suprapubic, retropubic, and perineal (see *Surgical approaches to prostatectomy*). The surgery's extent and approach depend on the patient's general condition and
the specific problem requiring treatment. The
transurethral approach is suitable for a partial resection;
the suprapubic for a simple prostatectomy; and the
retropubic and perineal for simple and radical prostatectomies.

Transurethral resection of the prostate (TURP), in
which prostatic tissue is removed through the urethra,
is performed most commonly. It is indicated for benign
prostatic hyperplasia that can no longer be managed
medically and for small cancerous lesions. Because this
approach requires a lithotomy position, it is not suitable
for the patient with a hip problem or prior surgery of
the hip joint.

The suprapubic approach involves a lower abdominal
suprapubic incision and then a bladder incision. It is
indicated for prostatic obstruction and removal of bladder calculi or diverticula.

In the retropubic approach, the gland is entered directly through an abdominal incision, without an incision into the bladder. It is used to remove a gland too
large for a TURP, to remove large cancerous lesions, and
for the patient who cannot tolerate a lithotomy posi-

tion. A nerve-sparing technique may be used to prevent
or minimize impotence.

With the perineal approach, an incision is made in
the perineum, the area between the scrotum and anus.
This approach is used for removal of a large gland when
an abdominal approach is contraindicated, such as in
an obese patient.

TURP usually has the shortest recovery period; the
suprapubic approach, somewhat longer; and the retropubic and perineal approaches, the longest.

This plan focuses on preoperative and postoperative
care for the patient undergoing prostatectomy.

Although the collaborative problems and nursing diagnoses discussed in this plan apply to all types of
prostatectomies, their relative importance varies with
the specific surgical approach, as indicated in each
problem.

Etiology and precipitating factors
• Age — men age 50 and over usually experience some
prostate enlargement
• Benign prostatic hyperplasia — usually associated
with hormonal changes of aging
• Prostate cancer — unknown cause; most common tumor is adenocarcinoma. Risk factors include:
   – age (peak incidence averages at age 65)
   – race (progresses faster in black men)
   – marital status (lowest incidence in single men)
   – occupation (increased incidence among workers
     employed in the rubber and cadmium industries)
   – hormonal factors (altered androgen and estrogen
     metabolite levels may contribute)

FOCUSED ASSESSMENT GUIDELINES

Nursing history (functional health pattern findings)
Health perception–health management pattern
• Preexisting cardiac or pulmonary disorders or dia-
betes
• Preoperative urinary tract infection (UTI) and bladder
outlet obstruction
• Antibiotics taken for UTIs
Nutritional-metabolic pattern
• Weight loss, nausea and vomiting, or anorexia (from
impaired renal function because of obstruction or
chronic UTI)

Surgical approaches to prostatectomy

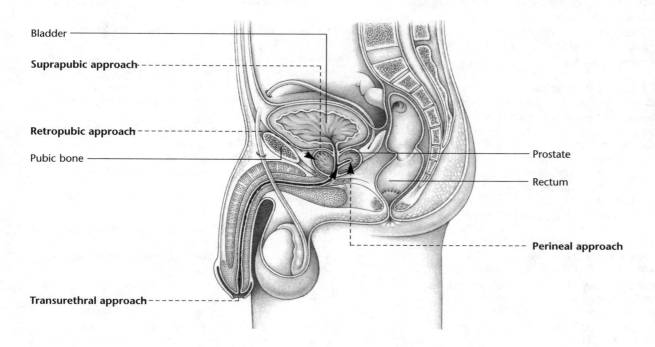

Bladder

Suprapubic approach

Retropubic approach

Pubic bone

Prostate

Rectum

Perineal approach

Transurethral approach

Transurethral approach: Instrument inserted into the urethra for prostate resection — no visible scar

Suprapubic approach: Incision made into lower abdomen and bladder neck

Retropubic approach: Incision made into lower abdomen; bladder neck not resected

Perineal approach: Incision made anterior to rectum

Elimination pattern
• Urine retention, dysuria, frequency, hesitancy, nocturia, urgency, decreased stream, postvoid dribbling, urinary incontinence; or hematuria (rare)
• Constipation or epigastric discomfort (from pressure of the bladder on the GI tract)

Activity-exercise pattern
• Decreased activity coinciding with pain
• Fatigue and weakness from anorexia or nocturia, with associated sleep deprivation
• Preexisting age-related cardiopulmonary disorders influencing exercise tolerance

Sleep-rest pattern
• Sleep pattern disturbances from pain, nocturia, frequency, or urinary incontinence

Cognitive-perceptual pattern
• Lack of knowledge about disease (benign prostatic hyperplasia or cancer) or surgical procedure and expected outcomes

Self-perception–self-concept pattern
• Fears and anxieties about alterations in body image, retrograde ejaculation, or impotence from nerve transection or injury
• Feelings of hopelessness, powerlessness, and lowered self-esteem associated with diagnosis of cancer

Role-relationship pattern
• Disturbed role performance
• Fear of social isolation associated with diagnosis of cancer
• Experiences of family or friends who died from cancer or during surgery reported by patient

Sexuality-reproductive pattern
• Preexisting impotence as adverse effect of cardiac medications
• Concerns about possible impotence expressed by patient
• Spouse or sexual partner may express concerns about postoperative sexual performance

Coping–stress tolerance pattern
• Fears and anxieties associated with diagnosis of cancer
• Appearance of depression

Value-belief pattern
• Disbelief (denial) about diagnosis of cancer
• Increased reliance on spiritual support system as coping mechanism

Physical findings
Patients with localized prostatic cancer commonly have no signs or symptoms; signs and symptoms indicate advanced disease.

Genitourinary
• Enlarged prostate on rectal examination
  – smooth, elastic, nonfixed gland suggests benign prostatic hyperplasia
  – hard, irregular, fixed nodule suggests cancer
• Postvoid dribbling or incontinence
• Urine retention
• Hematuria (rare)

Cardiovascular
• Peripheral edema (in renal failure or in hydroureteronephrosis from obstruction)

Pulmonary
• Pulmonary edema (in renal failure or in hydroureteronephrosis from obstruction)

Musculoskeletal
• Costovertebral angle tenderness (in renal failure)
• Back pain or stiffness (with bony metastasis)

Diagnostic studies
• White blood cell (WBC) count and sedimentation rate — increase with inflammation and infection (preoperative values for this laboratory test should be within normal limits)
• Hemoglobin level, hematocrit, and platelet count — decrease with hemorrhage (preoperative values for this laboratory test should be within normal limits)
• Prothrombin time/international normalized ratio (PT/INR) and activated partial thromboplastin time (APTT) — increase with hemorrhage (preoperative values for this laboratory test should be within normal limits)
• Blood typing and crossmatching — may be done in case transfusion is needed (preoperative values for this laboratory test should be within normal limits)
• Acid phosphatase — increases in about 25% of patients with early prostatic cancer when total serum level is measured and in the majority of patients when specific enzymes are used
• Prostate-specific antigen (PSA) — increases in about 73% to 96% of patients with prostate cancer but may also be elevated in 55% to 80% of patients with benign prostatic hyperplasia; useful in monitoring patients for cancer metastasis after radical prostatectomy
• Digital rectal examination — early screening examination for prostate cancer; performed in conjunction with PSA
• Alkaline phosphatase level — increases when cancer metastasizes to bone
• Blood urea nitrogen and creatinine levels — increase may indicate renal failure
• Urinalysis — increase in WBCs suggests infection; increase in red blood cells indicates hematuria, which may delay surgery
• Culture and sensitivity testing — defines microorganisms responsible for UTIs or other infections
• Cystoscopy — evaluates degree of prostate gland fixation, especially when cancerous; evaluates bladder problems and allows direct assessment of obstruction
• Prostate biopsy — provides differential diagnosis of cancer
• Excretory urography — helps determine presence and severity of kidney obstruction
• Chest X-ray — indicates lung status before surgery, may reveal lung metastasis
• Electrocardiography — indicates preoperative cardiac status; used as baseline for comparison if changes occur
• Bone scan — aids in detecting bony metastasis
• Transrectal ultrasound — determines internal prostatic anatomy and its related pathology; guides biopsies

Potential complications
• Hemorrhage
• Hypovolemic or septic shock
• Infection
• Epididymitis
• Rectal perforation during surgery
• Pulmonary embolism
• Atelectasis
• Bowel incontinence with perineal prostatectomy (rare)

CLINICAL SNAPSHOT

PROSTATECTOMY

Major nursing diagnoses and collaborative problems	Key patient outcomes
Risk for hypovolemia	Show stable vital signs: typically, heart rate, 60 to 100 beats/minute; systolic blood pressure, 90 to 140 mm Hg; and diastolic blood pressure, 50 to 90 mm Hg.
Risk for postoperative infection	Present a clean, dry incision with well-approximated edges.
Pain	Rate pain as less than 3 on a pain rating scale of 0 to 10.
Risk for urine retention	Have no suprapubic distention.
Urge incontinence	Have no postvoid residual volume.
Altered sexuality patterns: Decreased libido, infertility, or impotence	Identify available community resources to help with altered sexuality patterns.
Self-esteem disturbance	Participate in activities of daily living (ADLs).

COLLABORATIVE PROBLEM

Risk for hypovolemia related to prostatic or incisional bleeding after surgery

Nursing priority

Prevent or promptly detect internal or external bleeding.

Patient outcome criteria

- Within 24 hours after surgery, the patient will:
  - show stable vital signs: typically, heart rate, 60 to 100 beats/minute; systolic blood pressure, 90 to 140 mm Hg; and diastolic blood pressure, 50 to 90 mm Hg
  - have normal laboratory values.
- Within 3 days after surgery, the patient will:
  - have regular bowel movements
  - avoid straining the abdominal and perineal muscles.

Interventions

1. Monitor and document the amount of blood collecting on incisional dressings and in the urinary drainage system hourly for the first 12 to 24 hours after surgery, then every 4 hours. Typical drains and catheters include the following:
• for TURP, a urethral catheter
• for the suprapubic approach, a urethral catheter, a suprapubic tube, and an abdominal drain
• for the retropubic approach, a urethral catheter and an abdominal drain
• for the perineal approach, a urethral catheter and a perineal drain.
Observe the frequency of clots in the urine. Use standard precautions. Consult the surgeon concerning the amount of bleeding anticipated. Alert the surgeon if any of the following occur:
• bright red drainage
• persistent burgundy-colored drainage
• persistent clot formation.

2. Evaluate and document pulse rate, blood pressure, respirations, skin color, and level of consciousness according to unit protocol — typically every 4 hours for 24 hours or until stable, then every 8 hours.

3. Monitor hemoglobin level, hematocrit, platelet count, and coagulation studies daily. Compare current values with preoperative values. Alert the doctor to abnormal values. Administer blood transfusions as ordered, using standard precautions.

4. Consult the surgeon about applying traction to the catheter or preparing the patient for surgery if bleeding persists.

5. Teach the patient to avoid straining during bowel movements. Avoid using rectal thermometers or tubes or giving enemas.

6. Administer and document stool softeners and laxatives, as ordered. Use alternatives, such as increased fiber, fluids, and prune juice in the diet. Monitor the frequency and consistency of bowel movements.

Rationales

1. The amount of bleeding expected after surgery varies with the reason for and extent of the surgery. Heavy bleeding is expected for the first 24 hours after a TURP or a suprapubic or retropubic prostatectomy. Minimal bleeding is expected with the perineal approach.
Blood loss from incisional drainage usually is minimal, while blood loss through the urinary catheter may range from minimal to life-threatening. Bright red blood indicates arterial bleeding; dark blood suggests venous bleeding.
   Hemorrhage may occur with any surgical approach, but it is a particular problem with TURP. Venous bleeding during the early postoperative period is common. If necessary, traction may be placed on the catheter for 6 to 8 hours.
   Hemorrhage may occur with a suprapubic or perineal approach, but usually it is not a major problem. With the retropubic approach, the risk of hemorrhage usually is minimal because this approach affords better control of bleeding.
   Blood volume loss may decrease cardiac output, arterial and venous blood pressure, and hemoglobin level, decreasing the blood's oxygen-carrying capacity. A blood volume loss of 20% or more can cause hypovolemic shock.
   Expected removal times for urinary catheters are discussed later in this plan; abdominal drains are usually removed after 4 to 7 days (occasionally after 10 days with a radical perineal prostatectomy).

2. An increased pulse rate, a blood pressure 20 mm Hg below normal or 80 mm Hg or less, rapid and deep respirations, cold and clammy skin, pallor, and restlessness indicate shock.

3. A sudden decrease in hemoglobin level, hematocrit, and platelet count or an increase in PT or APTT may indicate the need for a transfusion.

4. Applying traction pulls the catheter balloon against the bladder neck. The resulting pressure compresses bleeding vessels in the prostatic fossa. For prolonged or excessive bleeding, sutures or cauterization may be necessary.

5. Straining to defecate or introducing objects into the rectum may cause bleeding, especially after the retropubic or perineal approach for radical prostatectomy.

6. Preventing constipation is important to decrease the risk of bleeding or rectal tearing.

7. Teach the patient to avoid lifting heavy objects for 6 to 8 weeks after surgery to allow time for internal and external wound healing.

8. Additional individualized interventions: _____
_____

7. Undue strain on the abdominal and perineal muscles places stress on the bladder and prostate and may cause bleeding.

8. Rationales: _____

Nursing diagnosis

Risk for postoperative infection related to preoperative status or urinary catheter or abdominal drain placement

Nursing priority

Prevent or promptly detect infection.

Patient outcome criteria

• Within 24 hours after surgery, the patient will:
  – have no fever
  – have no urinary clots
  – ambulate.
• Within 3 days after surgery, the patient will:
  – present a clean, dry incision with well-approximated edges
  – have clear urine.

Interventions

1. Monitor and record vital signs according to unit protocol, typically every 4 hours for 24 hours or until stable, then every 8 hours. Notify the doctor of significant changes from the patient's baseline values.

2. Monitor the incision site daily for induration, erythema, and purulent or odorous drainage. Document all findings. Send drainage samples for culture and sensitivity testing, as ordered.

3. Monitor drains and catheters for patency, and irrigate as ordered, using standard precautions.

4. Provide and document meticulous urinary catheter care at least once daily. Send urine samples for culture and sensitivity testing, as ordered, using standard precautions.

5. Administer I.V. fluids, as ordered. Beginning on the first postoperative day, encourage oral fluid intake of eight to twelve 8-oz (240-ml) glasses daily (unless contraindicated) to maintain a urine output of at least 1,500 ml daily. Record fluid intake and output.

6. Encourage the patient to ambulate the day after surgery.

Rationales

1. The risk of infection varies with the procedure used. The risk is high with the suprapubic approach, in which a bladder incision can allow urine to leak into surrounding tissue. The presence of catheters or drains also increases the risk of infection. Sudden fever, chills, hypotension, and tachycardia are signs and symptoms of septic shock, a particular risk after prostatectomy.

2. The skin is the first line of defense against infection. Testing drainage samples will identify the causative microorganism.

3. Catheter obstruction commonly occurs from blood clots at the tip of the indwelling urinary catheter. This may cause urine retention, stasis, and infection. Irrigation usually relieves obstruction.

4. Although questioned by some, most authorities believe that cleaning with soap and water is essential to prevent microbial growth. Analysis of urine samples will identify any microorganisms.

5. Adequate hydration promotes renal blood flow and flushes out bacteria in the urinary tract. The I.V. line is usually removed on the first postoperative day if the patient is tolerating oral fluids.

6. Immobility contributes to urinary stasis and creates a reservoir for microorganisms.

7. Administer and document prophylactic antibiotics, as ordered.

8. If the patient is discharged to home with a catheter in place, consider a home health referral.

9. Additional individualized interventions: _____

7. Antibiotics combat and control microbial growth. They are ordered prophylactically because of the high risk of infection with prostatectomy.

8. Providing support services after discharge allows follow-up and continuation of care.

9. Rationales: _____

Nursing diagnosis

Pain related to urethral stricture, catheter obstruction, bladder spasms, or surgical intervention

Nursing priority

Relieve pain.

Patient outcome criteria

- Within 30 minutes after surgery, the patient will:
  - have stable vital signs: typically, heart rate, 60 to 100 beats/minute; systolic blood pressure, 90 to 140 mm Hg; and diastolic blood pressure, 50 to 90 mm Hg
  - have no urinary obstruction.
- Within 1 hour after surgery, the patient will:
  - rate pain as less than 3 on a scale of 0 to 10, with pain medication
  - find a relaxed position in bed.

Interventions

1. See the "Pain" plan, page 88.

2. Observe for signs and symptoms of bladder spasms, such as sharp intermittent pain, a sense of urgency, or urine around the catheter.

3. Irrigate, using standard precautions, and check the urinary catheter and tubing for kinks, blood clots, and mucus plugs, as needed.

4. Assess for incisional pain. Have patient rate pain on a scale of 0 to 10, with 0 indicating no pain, and 10 indicating severe pain.

5. For severe or persistent pain, administer analgesics or antispasmodics such as oxybutynin chloride (Ditropan). Administer medication at the pain's onset. Monitor vital signs before and after administering medication, and evaluate pain relief after 30 minutes.

Rationales

1. General interventions for pain management are included in the "Pain" plan. Measures specific to prostatectomy are covered below.

2. Bladder spasms occur when catheter placement or surgical manipulation irritate the bladder stretch receptors. Pain from bladder spasms can be severe in the transurethral and suprapubic approaches, in which the bladder is entered surgically. Spasm-induced pain is minimal with the retropubic and perineal approaches because they do not involve a bladder incision.

3. Urine retention from catheter obstruction causes abdominal distention and pain, and may trigger bladder spasms. When the patient complains of suprapubic pain, this intervention usually is all that is needed.

4. Incisional pain usually is moderate with the suprapubic and retropubic approaches; with the perineal approach, it usually is mild. Using a pain scale helps monitor the patient's perception of the pain.

5. Early medication administration prevents severe pain. Oxybutynin directly relaxes smooth muscle and inhibits acetylcholine's parasympathetic-stimulating action on the bladder.

6. Provide alternative pain-relief measures and teach them to the patient. If appropriate, help the patient take a sitz bath and apply heat to the rectal area with a heat lamp after a perineal prostatectomy. Position the patient comfortably.

7. Additional individualized interventions: _____
_____

6. Alternative pain-relief measures may enhance relief in conjunction with analgesics. Heat application reduces inflammation. Proper positioning may decrease discomfort from the urinary catheter.

7. Rationales: _____
_____

NURSING DIAGNOSIS

Risk for urine retention related to urinary catheter obstruction

Nursing priority

Prevent or minimize urine retention.

Patient outcome criteria

- Within 24 hours after surgery, the patient will:
  - have no urinary clots
  - show approximately equal fluid intake and output
  - have no suprapubic distention.
- Within 48 hours after surgery, the patient will have stable weight.

Interventions

1. Monitor and record continuous bladder irrigation, as ordered. Adjust the irrigating solution's flow rate, as ordered, to maintain pink-tinged urine.

2. If the patient is not on continuous bladder irrigation, irrigate the urinary catheter with 30 to 60 ml of normal saline solution every 3 to 4 hours or as needed and as ordered, using gentle pressure. Use aseptic technique and standard precautions.

3. Monitor and document fluid intake and output. Encourage fluid intake of eight to twelve 8-oz (240-ml) glasses daily.

4. Weigh the patient daily. Compare with preoperative weight, and document.

5. Observe for suprapubic distention and discomfort every 4 hours while the patient is awake. If a suprapubic catheter is in place, monitor and record urine outflow. Use standard precautions.

6. Additional individualized interventions: _____
_____

Rationales

1. Continuous irrigation dilutes blood clots and decreases obstruction. Urine normally remains pink-tinged for 3 to 4 days.

2. Blood clots or mucus plugs may adhere to the tip of the catheter and obstruct urine flow. This occurs most commonly when continuous irrigation is not used.

3. Hydration increases urine flow. Urine output less than 60 ml/hour suggests obstruction or decreased renal perfusion.

4. Increasing weight suggests urine retention.

5. Increased distention may signal urine retention. A suprapubic catheter is commonly placed after suprapubic prostatectomy or urethral trauma or stricture.

6. Rationales: _____
_____

NURSING DIAGNOSIS

Urge incontinence related to urinary catheter removal, trauma to the bladder neck, or decrease in detrusor muscle or sphincter tone

Nursing priority

Relieve or minimize incontinence.

Patient outcome criteria

Within 24 hours after surgery, the patient will:
• exercise perineal muscles as instructed
• void no more than once every 2 hours
• have no postvoid residual volume
• present a clean, dry perineal area.

Interventions

1. Before surgery, teach the patient to tighten buttock and perineal muscles for 5 to 10 seconds, then relax them, repeating 10 to 20 times/hour. Instruct the patient to perform this exercise before and after surgery.

2. Monitor and document the patient's urination pattern after catheter removal. Instruct the patient to void with each urge, but no more than once every 2 hours during the first 24 hours after surgery and no more than once every 4 hours subsequently.

3. If a suprapubic catheter is present after the urethral catheter is removed, measure residual volume after each voiding, using standard precautions. Alert the doctor if the residual volume exceeds 50 ml.

4. Obtain one urine sample with each voiding during the first 24 hours after catheter removal, and note its color, amount, and specific gravity. Use standard precautions.

5. Provide absorbent incontinence pads. Keep the perineal area clean and dry. Condom catheters may be used to promote dryness, especially at night.

6. Additional individualized interventions: _____

Rationales

1. Urinary incontinence is more common with perineal incisions and takes longer to resolve. With a TURP, temporary incontinence results from trauma to the urinary sphincter. With the suprapubic approach, temporary incontinence may result from the bladder neck incision. Strengthening the bladder sphincter promotes bladder control after urinary catheter removal. Normal urinary function usually returns in 2 to 3 weeks, although complete urinary control may take as long as 6 months to return after a perineal incision.

2. Catheter removal occurs 3 to 5 days after TURP and as long as 12 days after other procedures. Voiding with each urge prevents urine retention, and spacing voidings aids in bladder retraining.

3. When urethral and suprapubic catheters are present, the urethral catheter usually is removed on the first postoperative day to minimize the risk of stricture formation. The suprapubic catheter usually is clamped for 24 hours before removal 7 to 10 days after surgery. If the residual volume exceeds 50 ml, the catheter may be left in until complete emptying is achieved through the urethra.

4. Analysis of a urine specimen helps indicate renal function. Hematuria should gradually decrease, and volume should increase. Specific gravity reflects urine concentration.

5. Keeping the perineal area clean and dry promotes comfort and reduces the risk of infection.

6. Rationales: _____

NURSING DIAGNOSIS

Altered sexuality patterns: Decreased libido related to fear of incontinence and decreased self-esteem; infertility related to retrograde ejaculation (from TURP and suprapubic prostatectomy); or impotence related to parasympathetic nerve damage (from radical prostatectomy)

Nursing priority

Prevent or minimize impact of altered sexuality patterns.

Patient outcome criteria

Within 24 hours before discharge, the patient will:
• identify impact of surgery or disease on sexuality
• express feelings about masculinity and changes in sexuality
• verbalize understanding of anticipated sexual capacity
• identify available community resources.

Interventions

1. Teach the patient before surgery, and reinforce after surgery, the expected effects of prostatectomy on sexual functioning. Include the patient's spouse or partner in the discussion.

2. Encourage the patient and spouse or partner to verbalize feelings of loss, grief, anxiety, and fear.

3. Encourage the patient and spouse or partner to discuss feelings about and expectations of the sexual relationship.

4. Provide information about a penile prosthesis, if appropriate.

Rationales

1. Providing correct information may decrease threats to the patient's sexual self-esteem and body image by clarifying misconceptions. TURP and suprapubic prostatectomy will produce some degree of retrograde ejaculation secondary to opening of the bladder neck during surgery: Seminal fluid flows into the bladder and is excreted in the urine. Retrograde ejaculation does not interfere with sexual activity but does cause infertility. Ejaculation should return to normal within a few months. Sexual function is unaffected by suprapubic prostatectomy; a patient with erectile capability can usually resume intercourse in 4 to 6 weeks. Impotence always results from a radical prostatectomy because perineal nerves are cut.

2. Loss of the prostate gland commonly causes feelings of loss and grief similar to those women experience after hysterectomy. The patient with prostate cancer may also fear transmitting cancer to his sexual partner. Some men feel that impotence and sterility make them less manly. Verbalizing these feelings decreases anxiety and may assist in identifying ways to deal with losses.

3. Promoting open communication between sexual partners may prevent misunderstandings, enhance the relationship, and increase the patient's feelings of self-worth.

4. A penile prosthesis restores erectile capacity and may increase the patient's feelings of self-worth and sexual self-esteem after radical prostatectomy, which causes impotence, unless a nerve-sparing surgical approach is used. The patient should be totally healed (2 to 3 months after prostatectomy) before pursuing prosthetic surgery.

5. Provide information and refer the patient for sexual counseling, as needed after surgery.

6. Additional individualized interventions: _____

5. The patient may need a sexual counselor if the prostatectomy exacerbates preexisting sexual problems. Follow-up may be needed after discharge.

6. Rationales: _____

Nursing diagnosis

Self-esteem disturbance related to incontinence, potential impotence, or sexual alterations

Nursing priority

Maximize feelings of self-esteem.

Patient outcome criteria

By the time of discharge, the patient will:
• identify effective coping behaviors
• express satisfaction with personal appearance
• express positive feelings of self-worth
• participate in daily care and ADLs.

Interventions

1. Encourage the patient to verbalize feelings about postoperative changes in body functioning and how these changes will affect lifestyle.

2. Assist the patient in identifying and using effective coping behaviors. If problems arise, see the "Ineffective individual coping" plan, page 67. Patients experiencing prostate cancer may benefit from local community support groups (such as those sponsored by various cancer support services).

3. Encourage the patient to continue perineal and buttock exercises to decrease incontinence. Reassure the patient that incontinence is temporary. Instruct the patient to use absorbent pads to prevent embarrassment.

4. Compliment the patient on personal appearance. Instruct the spouse or partner and family to provide compliments and positive feedback to the patient.

5. Encourage the patient to participate in ADLs and in decisions affecting care.

6. Additional individualized interventions: _____

Rationales

1. As with sexual alterations discussed in the previous problem, verbalizing feelings about other changes in body function is the first step in identifying healthful coping methods.

2. Promoting positive coping behavior increases adaptation to change and also increases self-esteem.

3. Incontinence may cause the patient to avoid social activities and neglect self-care. See the "Urge incontinence" nursing diagnosis in this entry.

4. Knowledge that a person is perceived by others as attractive and sexually desirable fosters self-esteem. Positive feedback reinforces a positive self-image.

5. Participating in care activities fosters independence. Decision making increases self-control and self-confidence.

6. Rationales: _____

DISCHARGE PLANNING

Discharge checklist

Before discharge, the patient shows evidence of:
- ❏ absence of urinary obstruction
- ❏ absence of urine retention
- ❏ urine output of at least 800 ml for the past 24 hours
- ❏ absence of gross hematuria or large clots
- ❏ absence of infection
- ❏ absence of pulmonary complications
- ❏ absence of cardiovascular complications (including thrombophlebitis)
- ❏ stable vital signs (oral temperature below 100° F [37.8° C] for the past 24 hours without antipyretics, and blood pressure within preoperative limits)
- ❏ ability to control pain using oral medications
- ❏ ability to perform ADLs independently
- ❏ ability to perform catheter care
- ❏ ability to tolerate diet
- ❏ adequate home support or referral to home health agency or extended care facility.

Teaching checklist

Document evidence that the patient and family demonstrate an understanding of:
- ❏ surgical outcome and disease
- ❏ all discharge medications' purpose, dosage, administration schedule, and adverse effects requiring medical attention (usual discharge medications include analgesics, antispasmotics if a urinary catheter is present, and antibiotics)
- ❏ urinary catheter care techniques and supplies
- ❏ signs and symptoms indicating obstruction, bleeding, or infection
- ❏ supplies to manage incontinence
- ❏ exercises to regain urinary control
- ❏ common postoperative feelings
- ❏ appropriate activity level to prevent muscle straining
- ❏ resumption of sexual activity and community resources for sexual counseling
- ❏ community or interagency referral
- ❏ need for consultation with an oncology specialist (if the diagnosis of cancer is confirmed)
- ❏ availability of cancer support groups
- ❏ date, time, and location of follow-up appointments
- ❏ how to contact the doctor.

Documentation checklist

Using outcome criteria as a guide, document:
- ❏ clinical status on admission
- ❏ significant changes in status after surgery
- ❏ pertinent laboratory and diagnostic test findings
- ❏ episodes of hemorrhage
- ❏ transfusion with blood products
- ❏ infection and treatment

- ❏ fluid intake and output
- ❏ urinary obstruction episodes
- ❏ urine retention
- ❏ urinary incontinence
- ❏ patient and family teaching
- ❏ discharge planning
- ❏ community or interagency referral.

ASSOCIATED PLANS OF CARE

Grieving
Ineffective family coping: Compromised
Ineffective individual coping
Pain
Septic shock
Surgery
Thrombophlebitis

REFERENCES

Cumes, D. "Transurethral Prostate Resection: A Frustration-Free Surgical Method," *AORN Journal* 58(2):302, 304-08, 311, August 1993.

Groenwald, S., et al. *Cancer Nursing Principles and Practice,* 4th ed. Boston: Jones & Bartlett Pubs., Inc., 1998.

Maxwell, M. "Cancer of the Prostate," *Seminars of Oncology Nursing* 9(4):237-51, November 1993.

McNally, J., et al. *Guidelines for Cancer Nursing Practice*, 2nd ed. Philadelphia: W.B. Saunders Co., 1991.

Raiwet, C., et al. "Care Maps Across the Continuum — To Standardize the Care of TURP Patients," *Canadian Nurse* 93(1): 26-30, January 1997.

Ronk, L., and Kavitz, J. "Perioperative Nursing Implications of Radical Perineal Prostatectomy," *AORN Journal* 60(3):438-41, 443-46, September 1994.

Radioactive implant for cervical cancer

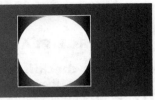

DRG information

DRG 357   Uterine and Adnexa Procedures for Ovarian or Adnexa Malignancy.
Mean LOS = 9.8 days

DRG 363   Dilatation and Curettage (D&C), Conization, and Radio-Implant for Malignancy.
Mean LOS = 3.5 days
Many patients now receive radioactive implants as outpatients, although in the past such patients were routinely hospitalized. A patient who receives an implant during removal of the malignant neoplasm is always hospitalized.

INTRODUCTION

Definition and time focus

The primary treatment for cervical cancer, radiation therapy usually combines internal irradiation (given as inpatient therapy) with external irradiation (usually given as outpatient therapy). This plan focuses on inpatient management of the patient receiving a radioactive implant for cervical cancer. Cancers of the vagina and endometrium may also be treated in this manner with a similar nursing plan of care.

The implant may be inserted before, during, or after external radiation therapy. With the patient in the operating room and anesthetized, an applicator is inserted into the vagina. The stainless steel applicator consists of a central hollow tube, passed through the cervical os into the uterine cavity, and two hollow ovoids, placed in the vagina next to the cervix. After correct placement is confirmed by X-ray, the patient is brought back to a private room on the unit, where the doctor threads the radioactive material (radium or cesium is most common) into the central cylinder and ovoids to radiate the cervix and the paracervical tissue, the usual area into which cervical cancer spreads.

During implant therapy, radiation exposure of the nursing staff is minimized by efficiently organizing care, wearing radiation monitoring devices, rotating staff assignments, and not allowing pregnant staff to care for these patients.

The implant stays in place for 2 to 4 days. Computer calculations determine the radiation dose to the tumor and the dose absorbed by normal tissues, such as the bladder and rectum. After the dose has been delivered, the doctor removes the radioactive material and then the applicator. An analgesic or sedative may be required before removal.

Etiology and precipitating factors

Risk factors associated with the development of squamous cell carcinoma of the cervix include:
- early age of first intercourse
- multiple sexual partners
- multiparity
- history of human papillomavirus infection (condylomata or genital warts)
- cigarette smoking
- history of an abnormal Papanicolaou (Pap) test.

Most of these risk factors are related to early or repeated exposure of the cervix to an oncogenic virus that is probably transmitted sexually.

FOCUSED ASSESSMENT GUIDELINES

Nursing history (Functional health pattern findings)

Health perception–health management pattern
- Abnormal vaginal bleeding, commonly occurring after intercourse or douching
- History of an abnormal Pap test that was never adequately evaluated

Nutritional-metabolic pattern
- Unexplained weight loss (not usually seen with early cancers)

Elimination pattern
- Feelings of pelvic pressure with resulting constipation or frequent urination
- Decreased urine output if the tumor has caused ureteral obstruction
- Incontinence of stool or urine if rectovaginal or vesicovaginal fistulae are present

Activity-exercise pattern
- Weakness or fatigue, especially if anemic from vaginal blood loss

Cognitive-perceptual pattern
- Pelvic pain or pressure, sometimes experienced as low back pain
- Leg or hip pain as the tumor encroaches on nerve roots

Self-perception–self-concept pattern
- Anxiety or depression over the diagnosis of cancer and perceived threat of death

Role-relationship pattern
- Isolation from family, friends, or coworkers

Sexuality-reproductive pattern
• Fear of sexual intercourse because of bleeding or concern about transmitting cancer to partner
• Grief related to loss of reproductive function

Coping–stress tolerance pattern
• Feelings of powerlessness and decreased ability to cope with other stresses
• Need for education and support from community resources

Value-belief pattern
• Guilt over delaying early detection behaviors (regular Pap tests) or evaluation of early symptoms

Physical findings

Reproductive
• Vaginal bleeding
• Cervical tumor that may:
  – be exophytic (growing outward on the cervix) or endophytic (growing inside the endocervical canal, making the cervix barrel shaped)
  – extend down the vagina
  – extend to the pelvic side wall
  – invade the bladder or rectum

Gastrointestinal
• Constipation
• Passage of stool through vagina (rare)

Urinary
• Frequent urination
• Decreased urine output or anuria (rare)
• Passage of urine through vagina (rare)

Diagnostic studies
Initial laboratory data may reflect no significant abnormalities.
• Blood urea nitrogen and creatinine levels — may be elevated, indicating ureteral obstruction and diminished renal function
• Hemoglobin level and hematocrit — may be lowered if vaginal bleeding has been heavy
• Excretory urography — may show ureteral obstruction by pelvic tumor
• Cystoscopy — may show bladder wall invasion by tumor
• Barium enema or proctoscopy — may show extrinsic pressure by pelvic tumor or invasion into rectal wall
• Lymphangiogram or computed tomography scan — may indicate spread of tumor outside the pelvis to para-aortic lymph nodes or other organs

Potential complications
• Deep vein thrombosis or pulmonary embolus
• Peritoneal perforation by the implant apparatus
• Hemorrhage
• Atelectasis or pneumonia

CLINICAL SNAPSHOT

RADIOACTIVE IMPLANT FOR CERVICAL CANCER

Major nursing diagnoses	Key patient outcomes
Risk for injury	Show no signs or symptoms of perforation, such as abdominal pain.
Risk for disuse syndrome	Show no signs of pulmonary or vascular complications of bed rest, such as calf or chest pain.
Social isolation	Encourage visitors' compliance with radiation safety principles.
Altered sexuality patterns	Verbalize on request purpose and methods of maintaining vaginal patency.

NURSING DIAGNOSIS

Risk for injury related to dislodgment of the implant

Nursing priority

Minimize risk of dislodgment and resulting perforation and peritonitis.

Patient outcome criteria

- While the implant is in place, the patient will:
  - have no bowel movements
  - show no signs or symptoms of perforation.
- After the implant is removed, the patient will have normal bowel movements.

Interventions

1. Administer preoperative laxatives or enemas, as ordered. Document your actions.

2. Provide a low-residue diet with adequate fluid intake.

3. Administer medications as ordered to decrease peristalsis, such as diphenoxylate hydrochloride (Lomotil), loperamide hydrochloride (Imodium), or codeine.

4. Document the presence and position of the implant. When the patient returns from the operating room, place a small ink mark on the leg at the bottom of the applicator as a baseline indicator in case the applicator is dislodged. Also note the position of the handles on the applicator (vertical, horizontal, or oblique).

5. Assess for signs and symptoms of perforation, including vaginal bleeding, abdominal pain or distention, fever, nausea, and vomiting. Notify the doctor immediately.

6. Document placement of an indwelling urinary catheter (may be done at the time of implant insertion) and connection to bedside drainage; record output.

7. Raise the head of the bed slightly (usually no more than 45 degrees); place a trapeze bar over the bed. Limit side-to-side movement.

Rationales

1. Evacuating the lower colon minimizes the likelihood that stool will contaminate the field during the insertion procedure. Bowel movements or bedpan placement while the implant is in place may dislodge it or cause perforation by the implant apparatus.

2. Low-residue foods minimize bulk formation in the colon. Adequate oral fluid intake lessens the need for I.V. hydration.

3. Medications that slow bowel function induce the constipation necessary for optimal placement and effectiveness of the implant.

4. Accurate ongoing assessment of the implant's position detects dislodgment, which may lead to uterine perforation.

5. The uterine cavity may be perforated at the time of insertion or with considerable pelvic movement. Prompt medical intervention is required because perforation can lead to peritonitis.

6. Continuous urinary drainage allows the patient to keep the hips positioned as recommended and avoids the movement necessary for bedpan use. The catheter also helps decrease the risk of bladder injury during the procedure.

7. Because the implant apparatus may protrude slightly from the vagina, raising the patient's head more than 45 degrees may change the angle of her hips and could dislodge the implant. Changing the angle of her head will allow the patient to sleep, eat, or read more comfortably. A trapeze bar may allow the patient to move her upper body more easily. Side-to-side movement may dislodge the implant.

8. Encourage the patient to perform grooming and personal hygiene activities. Do not change bed linen unless necessary.

9. After the implant is removed, administer (and document the use of) laxatives or enemas, begin regular diet, and discontinue constipating medications.

10. Additional individualized interventions: _____

8. Self-care increases the patient's involvement and decreases the caregiver's radiation exposure. Changing linens may cause pelvic movement that could dislodge the implant.

9. Normal bowel function is restored after the implant is removed so that the patient can be discharged with normal functions intact.

10. Rationales: _____

NURSING DIAGNOSIS

Risk for disuse syndrome related to imposed bed rest

Nursing priority

Minimize risks of bed rest.

Patient outcome criteria

• While the implant is in place, the patient will:
 –exercise lower extremities every 2 hours while awake
 –perform deep-breathing exercises every 2 hours while awake.
• Throughout the hospital stay, the patient will show no signs of pulmonary or vascular complications of bed rest, such as calf pain, chest pain, or dyspnea.

Interventions

1. Attach a footboard to the foot of the bed; teach foot and leg exercises, and encourage the patient to perform them every 2 hours while awake to increase blood flow; and apply antiembolism stockings.

2. Assess for signs and symptoms of thromboembolic phenomena, including calf pain, redness, and warmth; positive Homans' sign; and sudden onset of chest pain and dyspnea. See the "Thrombophlebitis" plan, page 468, for details. Report abnormalities promptly.

3. Administer anticoagulants as prescribed; monitor for excessive bleeding around the implant.

4. Teach deep-breathing exercises and encourage the patient to perform them every 2 hours while awake.

5. Assess for signs and symptoms of lung infection every shift, such as crackles, bronchial breath sounds, fever, productive cough, and pleuritic chest pain. Report abnormalities.

6. Additional individualized interventions: _____

Rationales

1. Deep vein thrombophlebitis or pulmonary embolism may occur in the patient on bed rest. The patient with gynecologic cancer is at increased risk from the pressure of the pelvic tumor on large vessels. Measures to decrease venous pooling lessen this risk.

2. These signs and symptoms reflect inflammation of the vein wall and clot formation. The "Thrombophlebitis" plan contains detailed information on thromboembolic phenomena.

3. Anticoagulants, such as heparin or warfarin (Coumadin), inhibit blood clotting, thus decreasing the risk of a thromboembolic event but increasing the risk of hemorrhage.

4. Bed rest contributes to poor lung expansion. Stasis of secretions leads to airway obstruction and atelectasis and provides a medium for bacterial growth. Deep-breathing exercises prevent pooling of secretions.

5. Systematic assessment improves the likelihood of prompt detection and treatment of developing infection.

6. Rationales: _____

Nursing Diagnosis

Social isolation related to implant radioactivity

Nursing priority

Minimize feelings of social isolation while the radioactive implant is in place.

Patient outcome criteria

While the implant is in place, the patient will:
• encourage visitors' compliance with radiation safety principles
• verbalize understanding of why nursing time must be limited
• pass time with diversionary activities.

Interventions

1. Explain to the patient and family the reasons for isolation from other patients and the nursing staff. Limit time spent with the patient and remind the family to remain behind the lead shields as much as possible. Limit the number of visitors, and do not allow children or pregnant women into the room.

2. Organize patient care into multiple short interactions instead of spending a lot of time in the room. Arrange the room so that items are within the patient's reach. Check on the patient frequently from the door.

3. Encourage diversionary activities, such as reading, handwork, talking on the phone, or watching television.

4. Additional individualized interventions: _____

_____

Rationales

1. Time, distance, and lead shielding are the three components of safe care for a patient with a radioactive implant. The areas of lowest radiation levels are at the foot and the head of the bed, and the lead shields are placed at the patient's sides where the radiation dose is higher.

2. Limiting time spent near the implant, maximizing distance from the implant, and staying behind the lead shields when providing bedside care will protect the nurse from excessive radiation exposure. Because of the limited number of visitors permitted, the patient will welcome frequent contact with the nurse.

3. A patient with cancer commonly experiences social isolation. Add to this mandatory physical isolation, and the patient may feel disoriented, with lowered self-esteem. Performing meaningful activities will help the patient pass the time and lend some sense of normalcy to the situation. Support and encouragement from the nurse may boost the patient's spirits.

4. Rationales: _____

Nursing Diagnosis

Altered sexuality patterns related to vaginal tissue changes or fear of radioactivity

Nursing priority

Minimize the physical and psychosexual effects of a vaginal implant.

Patient outcome criteria

By the time of discharge, the patient will:
• on request, verbalize awareness of potential problems after radioactive implant removal
• on request, verbalize purpose and methods of maintaining vaginal patency.

Interventions

1. Allow the patient to explore concerns and fears about the radioactive implant and resumption of sexual activity. Reassure the patient that once the implant has been removed, the tissues do not retain any radioactivity and, therefore, cannot harm anyone.

2. Discuss with the patient and spouse or partner (if present) the value of resuming intercourse (if the patient has a partner) or use of vaginal dilators when postimplant discomfort has abated (usually after 2 to 4 weeks).

3. Discuss with the patient and spouse or partner (if present) fears and concerns related to pain and bleeding during intercourse. Encourage use of lubrication during intercourse.

4. Additional individualized interventions: _____

Rationales

1. The patient (and her partner) may be concerned with the risk of radiation exposure during intercourse.

2. Radiation can cause scarring, narrowing, or fibrosis of the vaginal tissues. Regular dilation of the vagina through intercourse or the use of dilators will help minimize these effects. Vaginal flexibility facilitates vaginal examination and the taking of Pap smears to monitor the disease.

3. Atrophy and the resulting dryness of the vaginal tissues can occur after radioactive implant insertion. Tissues may be thin and easily traumatized, leading to pain or bleeding. Lubrication with a water-soluble lubricant may make the patient and partner more comfortable. Do not recommend petroleum-based products; they are too thick and may cause greater irritation.

4. Rationales: _____

DISCHARGE PLANNING

Discharge checklist

Before discharge, the patient shows evidence of:
- ☐ ability to perform activities of daily living (ADLs) independently
- ☐ ability to ambulate same as before surgery
- ☐ absence of dysuria
- ☐ stable vital signs
- ☐ absence of pulmonary or cardiovascular complications
- ☐ ability to have a bowel movement
- ☐ absence of infection
- ☐ ability to control pain with oral medications
- ☐ no need for I.V. support (preferably discontinued for at least 24 hours)
- ☐ hemoglobin level within expected parameters
- ☐ minimal vaginal discharge and absence of gross bleeding
- ☐ knowledge of how to contact a cancer support group
- ☐ adequate home support, or referral to home care if indicated by an inadequate home support system or inability to perform ADLs.

Teaching checklist

Document evidence that the patient and family demonstrate an understanding of:
- ☐ the cancer and its implications
- ☐ treatment administered

- ☐ all discharge medications' purpose, dosage, administration schedule, and adverse effects requiring medical attention (generally, medications are not ordered routinely, but pain medication, antibiotics, or medications for constipation or diarrhea may be prescribed, depending on special problems)
- ☐ need to call the doctor if abdominal pain or temperature above 100° F (37.8° C) develops
- ☐ likelihood of weakness or fatigue for 7 to 10 days after discharge
- ☐ likelihood of vulvovaginal discomfort for a few days
- ☐ possibility of some discharge (possibly bloody) for up to 2 weeks (Tell the patient to call the doctor if bleeding becomes heavy, requiring one or more pads every hour. Tampons are usually discouraged because of the increased risk of toxic shock syndrome.)
- ☐ ability to resume intercourse after tenderness and discharge decrease
- ☐ community resources for cancer education and support
- ☐ date, time, and location of follow-up appointments
- ☐ how to contact the doctor.

Documentation checklist

Using outcome criteria as a guide, document:
- ☐ clinical status on admission
- ☐ significant changes in clinical status
- ☐ pertinent laboratory and diagnostic test findings
- ☐ preimplant patient teaching
- ☐ results of preimplant laxatives or enemas

❑ application of antiembolism stockings and teaching
  of lower extremity exercises
❑ function of indwelling urinary catheter
❑ head of bed elevated no more than 45 degrees
❑ correct placement of radioactive implant
❑ nutritional intake
❑ teaching of deep-breathing exercises
❑ results of postimplant laxatives or enemas
❑ patient and family teaching
❑ discharge planning.

ASSOCIATED PLANS OF CARE

Grieving
Ineffective family coping: Compromised
Ineffective individual coping
Knowledge deficit
Pain
Thrombophlebitis

REFERENCES

Cook, R.V., et al. "Radiotherapy," in *Women and Cancer: A Gyneco-logic Oncology Nursing Perspective*. Edited by Moore, G.J. Boston: Jones & Bartlett Pubs., Inc., 1997.

Hilderly, L.J., and Hassey Dow, K. "Radiation Oncology," in *Cancer Nursing: A Comprehensive Textbook*, 2nd ed. Edited by Mc-Corkle R., et al. Philadelphia: W.B. Saunders Co., 1996.

Holmes, S. "Making Sense of Radiotherapy: Delivery and Safety," *Nursing Times* 92(27):42-43, July 1996.

Nag, S., et al. "Comprehensive Surgical Radiation Oncology," *AORN* 60(1):27-37, July 1994.

Appendices and Index

Appendix A: Monitoring standards

Monitoring of clinical signs and symptoms, laboratory tests, and diagnostic procedures is presented within specific plans of care in this text. This appendix outlines generally accepted standards for implementing selected hemodynamic monitoring techniques for critically ill patients. It should be individualized according to a specific patient's needs and unit protocol. For all monitoring techniques, remember that the trend of values is more significant than isolated readings.

Electrocardiography (ECG) monitoring
• Monitor ECG continuously. Observe for arrhythmias, ST-segment changes, and T-wave abnormalities.
• Monitor in MCL_1 or MCL_6 whenever possible, because they best differentiate ectopy from aberrancy. Monitor in Lead II for atrial arrhythmias.
• Keep rate alarms on at all times.
• Mount rhythm printouts in the patient's record routinely every 8 hours and as needed for significant arrhythmias.
• Evaluate and document atrial and ventricular rate, rhythm, PR interval, QRS duration, QT interval, and appearance of P waves, QRS complex, ST segment, and T waves at least once every 8 hours and as needed for significant changes.

Vital sign monitoring
• Monitor apical pulse, blood pressure, and respiratory rate every 15 minutes until stable, then every 1 to 2 hours.
• Monitor temperature at least every 4 hours.

Intake and output (I&O) monitoring
• Monitor hourly and 8-hour or 24-hour cumulative intake and output levels.
• Besides standard nursing I&O measures (for example, including gelatin in intake total), record the amount of all I.V. flush solutions administered.
• Measure urine specific gravity hourly or as indicated.
• Measure fingerstick blood glucose levels every 6 hours in diabetic patients, patients on total parenteral nutrition, postoperative cardiac surgery patients, and others, as indicated.

Arterial pressure monitoring
• Monitor arterial pressure continuously in patients with arterial lines.
• Keep pressure alarms on at all times.

• Keep all connections in constant view; the patient can exsanguinate in a matter of minutes if a disconnection occurs.
• Balance and calibrate the transducer according to the manufacturer's directions at least every 8 hours to negate the influence of atmospheric pressure on readings and to confirm the measuring accuracy.
• Use a constant low-flow closed heparinized flush solution to maintain patency.
• Periodically observe for the characteristic arterial waveform on the oscilloscope; investigate damping or abnormal appearance promptly.
• Compare to sphygmomanometer pressure every 8 hours; investigate significant discrepancies between the two.
• Check pulse, skin temperature, and skin color distal to the insertion site at least every 2 hours.

Pulmonary artery (PA) monitoring
• Measure right atrial pressure (central venous pressure) and PA systolic, diastolic, and mean pressures every hour or as needed.
• Use consistent baseline position for obtaining readings.
• Level the transducer's air-fluid interface with the phlebostatic axis.
• Follow unit protocol for removing patients from ventilators to record readings. If recording pressures while the patient is on the ventilator, read pressures at end-expiration to minimize respiratory influences on hemodynamic values. Document whether pressures are recorded when the patient is on or off the ventilator.
• Balance and calibrate the transducer according to the manufacturer's directions at least every 8 hours to negate the influence of atmospheric pressure on readings and to confirm accuracy of measurement.
• Use a constant low-flow closed heparinized flush solution to maintain patency.
• Before readings, confirm patency by observing the oscilloscope for characteristic PA waveforms.
• Usually, when the above standards are followed, regard a change in values of more than 5 mm Hg as clinically significant.

Pulmonary artery wedge pressure (PAWP) monitoring
• Measure PAWP as ordered.
• To read PAWP, inflate the balloon until the characteristic PAWP waveform appears, using no more than the specified amount of air for that size balloon. After reading the pressure, be sure the balloon is deflated by re-

moving the syringe used for inflation, releasing the lever if used to lock air in the balloon for the reading, and confirming on the oscilloscope the return to the usual PA waveform.

• To avoid frequent wedging, which damages the balloon and can cause pulmonary infarction, and to monitor left ventricular filling pressure constantly, consider continuous monitoring of PA diastolic pressure. Verify correlation with PAWP every 4 to 8 hours by confirming that the pressures are within 5 mm Hg of each other.

Cardiac output (CO) monitoring

• Measure CO as ordered.

• Obtain at least three readings at a time. Discard any readings that deviate significantly from each other and average the remaining readings.

• Use injectate at room temperature. Use iced injectate if room temperature injectate readings consistently deviate more than 15% from each other.

• Monitor cardiac index electronically or by dividing CO by the patient's body surface area, obtainable from a DuBois nomogram.

• Monitor systemic vascular resistance electronically or by dividing CO into mean arterial pressure (MAP) minus mean right atrial pressure.

Intracranial pressure (ICP) monitoring

• Monitor ICP continuously in patients with ICP monitoring catheters.

• Use a consistent baseline position for obtaining readings, usually a 20- to 30-degree elevation of the head of the bed.

• Level the air-fluid interface of the transducer with the reference point for the foramen of Monro, usually considered to be the outer corner of the eye, top of the ear, or the external auditory meatus.

• Verify patency of the line by observing the characteristic waveform on the oscilloscope.

• Do not read pressures while the patient is moving, coughing, or has the head turned to one side or the other; all will falsely elevate pressures.

• Never aspirate an ICP line; doing so may draw brain tissue into the catheter or screw.

• Do not flush an ICP line unless specifically ordered to do so by the patient's doctor.

• Monitor cerebral perfusion pressure by subtracting ICP from MAP.

• Balance and calibrate the transducer at least every 8 hours.

References

Chulay, M., et al. *AACN Handbook of Critical Care Nursing.* Stamford, Conn.: Appleton & Lange, 1997.
Clochesy, J.M., et al. *Critical Care Nursing,* 2nd ed. Philadelphia: W.B. Saunders Co., 1996.
Ruppert, S.D., et al. *Dolan's Critical Care Nursing: Clinical Management through the Nursing Process,* 2nd ed. Philadelphia: F.A. Davis Co., 1996.

Appendices

Appendix B:
Acid-base imbalances

Imbalance	ABG findings	Pathophysiology	Possible causes	Signs and symptoms	Compensatory mechanisms
Respiratory acidosis	• Decreased pH • Increased $Paco_2$ • Compensatory decrease in HCO_3^-	Decreased alveolar ventilation, which leads to retention of carbon dioxide	• Depression of medullary respiratory center from drugs, injury, or disease • Pulmonary diseases • Inadequate tidal volume or respiratory rate on ventilator	• Decreased mentation • Restlessness • Combativeness • Headache • Diaphoresis • Anxiety • Tachycardia	Renal compensation via HCO_3^- retention, acid elimination, and increased ammonia production
Respiratory alkalosis	• Increased pH • Decreased $Paco_2$ • Compensatory decrease in HCO_3^-	Increased alveolar ventilation, which results in a loss of carbon dioxide	• Hyperventilation from anxiety, pain, or excessive tidal volume or respiratory rate on ventilator • Respiratory-center stimulation by drugs, injury, or disease • Fever or high ambient temperature • Sepsis	• Increased rate and depth of respirations • Numbness and tingling • Light-headedness, syncope • Anxiety	Renal compensation via HCO_3^- elimination, acid retention, and decreased ammonia production
Metabolic acidosis	• Decreased pH • Decreased HCO_3^- • Compensatory decrease in $Paco_2$	• Loss of HCO_3^- • Increased acid formation	• Diarrhea • Diabetes • Shock • Renal failure • Azotemia • Small-bowel fistulas	• Increased rate and depth of respirations • Fatigue • Lethargy • Acetone odor to breath • Unconsciousness	Rapid pulmonary compensation via hyperventilation, renal metabolic compensation (except in renal failure) by HCO_3^- retention, acid elimination, increased ammonia production
Metabolic alkalosis	• Increased pH • Increased HCO_3^- • Compensatory increase in $Paco_2$	• Increased HCO_3^- retention • Loss of acids or potassium	• Vomiting • Gastric suctioning • Prolonged use of diuretics • Excessive HCO_3^- ingestion	• Decreased rate and depth of respirations • Hypertonicity • Twitching, tetany • Seizures • Irritability • Restlessness • Combativeness • Unconsciousness	Rapid pulmonary compensation via hypoventilation, renal metabolic compensation by HCO_3^- elimination, acid retention, decreased ammonia production

Appendix C: Fluid and electrolyte imbalances

Imbalance	Possible causes	Signs and symptoms	Laboratory results	Treatment
Hypovolemia	• Hemorrhage • Diabetes insipidus (DI) • Renal disease • Vagal stimulation • Drug reactions • Hyperosmolar hyperglycemic nonketotic syndrome	• Tachycardia • Weak pulse • Hypotension • Oliguria • Pallor • Decreased level of consciousness (LOC)	• Decreased central venous pressure (CVP) • Decreased hematocrit and hemoglobin	• Correct the underlying cause. • Administer appropriate I.V. fluids.
Hypervolemia	• Excessive I.V. fluid administration	• Hypertension • Edema • Bounding pulse • Pulmonary edema • Venous distention	• Increased CVP • Decreased hemoglobin and hematocrit • Decreased blood urea nitrogen (BUN)	• Treat with diuretics and dialysis as ordered. • Keep in mind that no treatment may be needed and that prevention is the best treatment.
Intravascular to interstitial shift	• Hemorrhage • Decreased water intake • Concentrated tube feedings • Vomiting • Diarrhea • Burns • Prolonged gastric suctioning • Soft-tissue injury • Intestinal obstruction • Fever	• Shock state • Tachycardia • Weak pulse • Oliguria • Dry mucous membranes • Hypotension	• Decreased LOC • Increased hemoglobin and hematocrit • Increased BUN	• Correct the underlying cause. • Administer appropriate I.V. fluids.
Interstitial to intravascular shift	• Burns • Soft-tissue injury • Excessive colloid or hypertonic I.V. administration	• Hypertension • Bounding pulse • Venous distention • Weakness • Hyponatremia	• Increased CVP • Decreased hemoglobin and hematocrit • Decreased BUN	• No treatment is usually needed for otherwise healthy patients. • Administer diuretics to patients with abnormal heart, liver, or kidney function.
Hyponatremia	• Excessive sweating or water intake • Decreased salt intake • Heart failure • Renal failure • Diuretic therapy • Fresh water near drowning • Vomiting • Diarrhea • Burns	• Confusion • Headache • Abdominal cramps • Apathy • Hypotension • Weakness • Hyperactive reflexes • Seizures • Oliguria	• Decreased serum sodium • Decreased chloride • Decreased urine specific gravity	• Decrease water intake or increase sodium intake.

(continued)

Imbalance	Possible causes	Signs and symptoms	Laboratory results	Treatment
Hypernatremia	• Decreased water intake • Increased sodium intake • Prolonged watery diarrhea • Prolonged hyperventilation • Salt water near drowning • DI	• Dehydration • Thirst • Dry mucous membranes • Weakness • Fever • Warm, flushed skin • Muscle pain	• Increased serum sodium level • Increased serum chloride level • Increased urine specific gravity	• Correct the underlying cause, if possible. • Restrict sodium intake. • Increase fluid intake.
Hypokalemia	• Decreased potassium intake • Diuretics • Vomiting or diarrhea • Burns • Heart failure • Fistulas • Colitis • Steroids	• Diminished reflexes • Irregular pulse • Thirst • Hypotension • Electrocardiography (ECG) changes • Muscular weakness or irritability	• Decreased serum potassium level • Decreased serum chloride level	• Increase dietary potassium intake. • Administer P.O. or I.V. potassium supplements.
Hyperkalemia	• Increased potassium intake • Burns • Soft tissue injury • Advanced kidney disease • Adrenal insufficiency • Hemorrhagic shock • Excessive I.V. administration • Irritability	• Nausea • Diarrhea • Confusion • Flaccid muscles • ECG changes • Hypotension • Abdominal cramping	• Increased serum potassium level	• Decrease dietary potassium intake. • Treat with dialysis. • Administer a sodium polystyrene sulfonate enema. • Administer sodium bicarbonate, glucose, and insulin together I.V.
Hypocalcemia	• Diarrhea • Burns • Renal failure • Draining wounds • Citrated blood administration • Overcorrection of acidosis • Vitamin D deficiency	• Carpopedal spasms • Tetany • Seizures • Tingling in fingers, toes, lips • Muscle cramps • ECG changes	• Decreased serum calcium level	• Administer calcium P.O. or I.V.
Hypercalcemia	• Vitamin D overdose • Renal disease • Excessive antacid use • Excessive calcium intake	• Pathologic fractures • Deep-bone or flank pain • Lethargy • Nausea • Vomiting • ECG changes • Osteoporosis • Kidney stones • Kidney infections	• Increased serum calcium level	• Correct the underlying cause. • Administer disodium phosphate, sodium sulfate, and diuretics.

Imbalance	Possible causes	Signs and symptoms	Laboratory results	Treatment
Hypomagnesemia	• Alcohol abuse • Vomiting • Decreased intake • Malnutrition • Diuretics • Prolonged GI suctioning • Diarrhea • Pancreatitis • Kidney disease	• Tetany • Lethargy • Nausea • Vomiting • Tachyarrhythmias • Hypotension • Confusion • Hyperactive reflexes	• Decreased serum magnesium level	• Increase dietary magnesium intake. • Administer I.V. magnesium.
Hypermagnesemia	• Excessive magnesium intake • Kidney disease • Severe dehydration • Repeated magnesium-containing enemas • Magnesium antacids in renal failure	• Lethargy • Flushing • Depressed respirations • Hypotension • Flaccid muscles or paralysis • Arrhythmias	• Increased serum magnesium level	• Decrease dietary magnesium intake. • Administer I.V. 10% calcium gluconate. • Treat renal failure patients with dialysis.

Appendices

Appendix D: Nursing diagnostic categories

This list represents nursing diagnostic categories approved by the North American Nursing Diagnosis Association (NANDA) for clinical use and testing as of 1996. Numbers correlate with NANDA's placement of diagnoses under the unitary man schema.

Health perception-health management pattern

1.6.1	Risk for injury
1.6.1.1	Risk for suffocation
1.6.1.2	Risk for poisoning
1.6.1.3	Risk for trauma
1.6.1.4	Risk for aspiration
1.6.1.5	Risk for disuse syndrome
5.2.1	Ineffective management of therapeutic regimen (individual)
5.2.1.1	Noncompliance (specify)
5.2.2	Ineffective management of therapeutic regimen: families
5.2.3	Ineffective management of therapeutic regimen: community
5.2.4	Effective management of therapeutic regimen: individual
5.4	Health-seeking behaviors (specify)
6.4.2	Altered health maintenance

Nutritional-metabolic pattern

1.1.2.1	Altered nutrition: more than body requirements
1.1.2.2	Altered nutrition: less than body requirements
1.1.2.3	Altered nutrition: risk for more than body requirements
1.2.1.1	Risk for infection
1.2.2.1	Risk for altered body temperature
1.2.2.2	Hypothermia
1.2.2.3	Hyperthermia
1.2.2.4	Ineffective thermoregulation
1.2.3.1	Dysreflexia
1.4.1.1	Altered tissue perfusion (specify type: renal, cerebral, cardiopulmonary, gastrointestinal, peripheral)
1.4.1.2.1	Fluid volume excess
1.4.1.2.2.1	Fluid volume deficit
1.4.1.2.2.2	Risk for fluid volume deficit
1.4.2.1	Decreased cardiac output*
1.6.2	Altered protection
1.6.2.1	Impaired tissue integrity
1.6.2.1.1	Altered oral mucous membrane
1.6.2.1.2.1	Impaired skin integrity*
1.6.2.1.2.2	Risk for impaired skin integrity

1.7.1	Decreased adaptive capacity: intracranial
6.5.1	Feeding self-care deficit
6.5.1.1	Impaired swallowing
6.5.1.2	Ineffective breast-feeding
6.5.1.2.1	Interrupted breast-feeding
6.5.1.3	Effective breast-feeding
6.5.1.4	Ineffective infant feeding pattern

Elimination pattern

1.3.1.1	Constipation
1.3.1.1.1	Perceived constipation
1.3.1.1.2	Colonic constipation
1.3.1.2	Diarrhea
1.3.1.3	Bowel incontinence
1.3.2	Altered urinary elimination
1.3.2.1.1	Stress incontinence
1.3.2.1.2	Reflex incontinence
1.3.2.1.3	Urge incontinence
1.3.2.1.4	Functional incontinence
1.3.2.1.5	Total incontinence
1.3.2.2	Urinary retention

Activity-exercise pattern

1.5.1.1	Impaired gas exchange
1.5.1.2	Ineffective airway clearance
1.5.1.3	Ineffective breathing pattern
1.5.1.3.1	Inability to sustain spontaneous ventilation
1.5.1.3.2	Dysfunctional ventilatory weaning response
6.1.1.1	Impaired physical mobility
6.1.1.1.1	Risk for peripheral neurovascular dysfunction
6.1.1.1.2	Risk for perioperative positioning injury
6.1.1.2	Activity intolerance
6.1.1.2.1	Fatigue
6.1.1.3	Risk for activity intolerance
6.3.1.1	Diversional activity deficit
6.4.1.1	Impaired home maintenance management
6.5.2	Bathing/hygiene self-care deficit
6.5.3	Dressing/grooming self-care deficit
6.5.4	Toileting self-care deficit
6.6	Altered growth and development
6.8.1	Risk for disorganized infant behavior
6.8.2	Disorganized infant behavior
6.8.3	Potential for enhanced organized infant behavior

Sleep-rest pattern

6.2.1	Sleep pattern disturbance

Cognitive-perceptual pattern

7.2	Sensory or perceptual alteration (specify: visual, auditory, kinesthetic, gustatory, tactile, olfactory)
7.2.1.1	Unilateral neglect
8.1.1	Knowledge deficit (specify)
8.2.1	Impaired environmental interpretation syndrome
8.2.2	Acute confusion
8.2.3	Chronic confusion
8.3.1	Impaired memory
8.3	Altered thought processes
9.1.1	Pain
9.1.1.1	Chronic pain

Self-perception–self-concept pattern

7.1.1	Body-image disturbance
7.1.2	Self-esteem disturbance
7.1.2.1	Chronic low self-esteem
7.1.2.2	Situational low self-esteem
7.1.3	Personal identity disturbance
7.3.1	Hopelessness
7.3.2	Powerlessness
9.3.1	Anxiety
9.3.2	Fear

Role-relationship pattern

2.1.1.1	Impaired verbal communication
3.1.1	Impaired social interaction
3.1.2	Social isolation
3.1.3	Risk for loneliness
3.2.1	Altered role performance
3.2.1.1.1	Altered parenting
3.2.1.1.2	Risk for altered parenting
3.2.1.1.2.1	Risk for altered parent/infant/child attachment
3.2.2	Altered family processes
3.2.2.1	Caregiver role strain
3.2.2.2	Risk for caregiver role strain
3.2.2.3.1	Altered family process: alcoholism
3.2.3.1	Parental role conflict
9.2.1.1	Dysfunctional grieving
9.2.1.2	Anticipatory grieving
9.2.2	Risk for violence: self-directed or directed at others

Sexuality-reproductive pattern

3.2.1.2.1	Sexual dysfunction
3.3	Altered sexuality patterns

Coping–stress-tolerance pattern

5.1.1.1	Ineffective individual coping

5.1.1.1.1	Impaired adjustment
5.1.1.1.2	Defensive coping
5.1.1.1.3	Ineffective denial
5.1.2.1.1	Ineffective family coping: disabling
5.1.2.1.2	Ineffective family coping: compromised
5.1.2.2	Family coping: potential for growth
5.1.3.1	Potential for enhanced community coping
5.1.3.2	Ineffective community coping
5.3.1.1	Decisional conflict (specify)
6.7	Relocation stress syndrome
9.2.2.1	Risk for self-mutilation
9.2.3	Post-trauma response
9.2.3.1	Rape-trauma syndrome
9.2.3.1.1	Rape-trauma syndrome: compound reaction
9.2.3.1.2	Rape-trauma syndrome: silent reaction

Value-belief pattern

1.8	Energy field disturbance
4.1.1	Spiritual distress (distress of the human spirit)
4.2	Potential for enhanced spiritual well-being

* The author believes these diagnoses represent renaming of commonly accepted medical terms and recommends that they not be used for nursing diagnoses guiding independent nursing care. Interdependent nursing care related to these problems is included in the collaborative problems in this book and labeled with familiar terms (such as shock and ischemia).

Appendices

Functional health patterns adapted from Gordon, M. *Nursing Diagnosis: Process and Application.* St. Louis: Mosby–Year Book, Inc., 1993. Used with permission. The adaptation for this book uses the patterns to organize subjective data and groups historical data under the health perception–health management pattern.

Appendix E: Critical care transfer criteria guidelines

Although the decision to transfer a patient is a medical one, the critical care nurse commonly has input in the decision. This appendix presents general criteria for transferring a patient from a critical care unit to a telemetry unit or a medical-surgical unit. These transfer criteria guidelines should be individualized according to the patient's needs and unit protocol. (Additional disease-specific criteria are presented within the plans in this text.)

General considerations
• Patient no longer requires constant surveillance.
• Resuscitation status is specified in medical order.
• Discharge planning has been initiated (with assessments made of patient's living arrangements before admission, discharge prognosis, anticipated length of stay, ability to perform activities of daily living, educational goals, and family or friend's ability and willingness to assist the patient after discharge).
• Referrals to appropriate ancillary services have been initiated.

Neurologic system
• Level of consciousness and other neurologic vital signs have improved or remained stable for 12 hours.
• Patient does not require intracranial pressure monitoring line.

Pulmonary system
• Pulmonary status has been stable for 12 hours.
• If patient still requires mechanical ventilation, he is stable and being transferred to caregivers experienced with this therapy.
• Pao_2 is greater than 80 mm Hg (except in chronic obstructive pulmonary disease).
• $Paco_2$ is less than 10 mm Hg above patient's normal value.

Cardiovascular system
• Patient no longer needs I.V. therapy requiring continuous cardiac monitoring.
• Blood pressure is within 20 mm Hg of patient's normal value (or has an otherwise acceptable value) for 12 hours, without I.V. drugs, such as inotropes, vasodilators, or vasoconstrictors; or mechanical assist devices, such as intra-aortic balloon pump.
• Patient does not require an arterial line or pulmonary artery catheter.

Renal system
• Urine output is at least 0.5 ml/kg/hour, except in chronic renal failure.
• If patient is receiving concentrated potassium infusion greater than 20 mEq/hour, transfer him to a monitored bed.

Index

A

Abdominal aortic aneurysm repair, 330-337
  bleeding and, 334-335
  cardiac decompensation and, 333
  complications of, 331
  definition of, 330
  diagnostic studies for, 331
  discharge checklist for, 337
  documentation checklist for, 337
  DRG information for, 330
  hypercapnia and, 333-334
  hypoxemia and, 333-334
  injury and, 335-336
  knowledge deficit and, 332
  pain and, 336
  teaching checklist for, 337
Abdominal trauma, 604. *See also* Trauma, multiple.
Accessibility of health care, 2
Acetaminophen overdose, 152t
Acid-base imbalances, 862t
Acidosis, DKA and, 670-671
Acquired immunodeficiency syndrome, 746-769
  altered oral mucous membrane and, 764-765
  CD4 lymphocyte categories for, 746, 746t
  clinical categories for, 746-747
  complications of, 749
  definition of, 746-747
  diagnostic criteria for, 749
  diagnostic studies for, 748-750
  discharge checklist for, 769
  disorders associated with, 747
  documentation checklist for, 769
  DRG information for, 746
  etiology of, 747
  fluid volume deficit and, 763-764
  hypoxemia and, 757-759
  impaired physical mobility and, 762
  impaired skin integrity and, 765-766
  ineffective individual coping and, 755-757
  infection and, 751-755
  knowledge deficit and, 767-769
  nursing history for, 747-748
  nutritional deficit and, 762-763
  physical findings in, 748
  resources for, 761
  sensory-perceptual alteration and, 759-760
  sexual dysfunction and, 766-767
  social isolation and, 760-761
  teaching checklist for, 769
Activated charcoal, 156

Activity intolerance
  anemia and, 777-778
  angina and, 372
  cardiogenic shock and, 399
  COPD and, 263-264
  heart failure and, 425-426
  leukemia and, 794-796
  lung cancer and, 278
  MI and, 356-358
  myasthenia gravis and, 207
Acupuncture, 94
Acute angle-closure glaucoma, 222. *See also* Glaucoma.
Acute idiopathic polyneuritis. *See* Guillain-Barré syndrome.
Acute renal failure, 686-697
  complications of, 688
  definition of, 686
  diagnostic studies for, 687-688
  discharge checklist for, 696
  documentation checklist for, 696-697
  DRG information for, 686
  electrolyte imbalance and, 689-690
  etiology of, 686
  fluid volume excess and, 690-691
  infection and, 694-695
  injury and, 692-694
  knowledge deficit and, 696
  nursing history for, 686-687
  nutritional deficit and, 695
  physical findings in, 687
  teaching checklist for, 696
Adult respiratory distress syndrome, 240-246
  complications of, 241
  definition of, 240
  diagnostic studies for, 241
  discharge checklist for, 246
  documentation checklist for, 246
  DRG information for, 240
  etiology of, 240
  hypoxemia and, 242-244
  ineffective family coping and, 245-246
  ineffective individual coping and, 245-246
  injury and, 244-245
  nursing history for, 241
  physical findings in, 241
  teaching checklist for, 246
Advanced practice nursing, opportunities in, 5
AIDS. *See* Acquired immunodeficiency syndrome.
Airway clearance, ineffective
  CVA and, 132-133
  drug overdose and, 154-155
  impaired physical mobility and, 52-54
  mechanical ventilation and, 289-291
  myasthenia gravis and, 206-207

Airway clearance, ineffective *(continued)*
  radical neck dissection and, 624
  seizures and, 215-216
Albumin level, nutritional assessment and, 81
Alcohol dependence, signs and symptoms of, 622
Alcohol overdose, 152t
Alcohol withdrawal syndrome, signs and symptoms of, 623
Alternative health care, 5
Alveolar ventilation, ineffective, mechanical ventilation and, 284-288
Alzheimer's disease, 118-126
  complications of, 119
  constipation and, 124-125
  definition of, 118
  diagnostic studies for, 119
  discharge checklist for, 126
  documentation checklist for, 126
  DRG information for, 118
  etiology of, 118
  impaired cognitive function and, 120-122
  ineffective family coping and, 125-126
  injury and, 123-124
  nursing history for, 118-119
  nutritional deficit and, 122-123
  physical findings in, 119
  stages of, 121t
  teaching checklist for, 126
Aminoglycosides, minimizing adverse effects of, 615t
Amputation, 568-576
  assessment guidelines for, 568
  body-image disturbance and, 574-575
  complications of, 569
  definition of, 568
  diagnostic studies for, 568-569
  discharge checklist for, 575
  disuse syndrome and, 572-574
  documentation checklist for, 575-576
  DRG information for, 568
  hemorrhage and, 569-570
  infection and, 571-572
  pain and, 570-571
  precipitating factors for, 568
  teaching checklist for, 575
Amrinone, 398
Anemia, 771-779
  activity intolerance and, 777-778
  chronic renal failure and, 705
  complications of, 773
  definition of, 771
  diagnostic studies for, 772
  discharge checklist for, 779
  documentation checklist for, 779
  DRG information for, 771
  etiology of, 771

C

Calcium channel blocker, 363t, 370
Cardiac contusion, 604
Cardiac decompensation, abdominal aortic aneurysm repair and, 333
Cardiac output, decreased
heart failure and, 422-424
mechanical ventilation and, 293
signs and symptoms of, 397
Cardiac output, inadequate, cardiogenic shock and, 397-399
Cardiac output monitoring, standards for, 861
Cardiac surgery, 376-391
arrhythmias associated with, 383t
assessment guidelines for, 377
clinical pathway for, 380-382t
complications of, 377
definition of, 376
diagnostic studies for, 377
discharge checklist for, 391
documentation checklist for, 391
DRG information for, 376
endocarditis and, 384-385
hypovolemia and, 386-388
hypoxemia and, 388-389
interstitial edema and, 385-386
knowledge deficit and, 390
low cardiac output syndrome and, 378-379, 383-384
precipitating factors for, 376
sensory-perceptual alteration and, 389
teaching checklist for, 391
Cardiogenic shock, 392-400
activity intolerance and, 399
complications of, 393
definition of, 392
diagnostic studies for, 392-393
discharge checklist for, 400
documentation checklist for, 400
DRG information for, 392
etiology of, 392
hemodynamic monitoring and, 395
hypoxemia and, 393-397
inadequate cardiac output and, 397-399
MI and, 340-341, 349
nursing history for, 392
pulmonary embolism and, 312-313
physical findings in, 392
teaching checklist for, 400
Care planning, 10
Carotid endarterectomy, 401-412
assessment guidelines for, 401-402
blood pressure lability and, 403-405
cerebral ischemia and, 405-406
complications of, 403
cranial nerve injury and, 407-408
definition of, 401
diagnostic studies for, 402
discharge checklist for, 411
documentation checklist for, 412
DRG information for, 401
hypoxemia and, 409-411
MI and, 409

Carotid endarterectomy *(continued)*
precipitating factors for, 401
teaching checklist for, 411
Cascade cough, 271
Cathartics, 156
Catheterization, postoperative, 111
Cephalosporins, minimizing adverse effects of, 615t
Cerebral circulation, factors that disrupt, 127
Cerebral injury, CVA and, 133-135
Cerebral ischemia
carotid endarterectomy and, 405-406
causative factors for, 127
craniotomy and, 144
increased intracranial pressure and, 171-174
Cerebral metabolism, increased, increased intracranial pressure and, 175-176
Cerebrospinal fistula, laminectomy and, 186-187
Cerebrovascular accident, 127-140
cerebral injury and, 133-135
complications of, 131
definition of, 127
diagnostic studies for, 131
discharge checklist for, 140
documentation checklist for, 140
DRG information for, 127
etiology of, 127
hemorrhage and, 134
impaired physical mobility and, 135-136
impaired verbal communication and, 137
ineffective airway clearance and, 132-133
knowledge deficit and, 138-139
nursing history for, 127, 130-131
occlusion and, 134
physical findings in, 131
sensory-perceptual alteration and, 136-137
signs and symptoms of, 139
teaching checklist for, 140
Cervical cancer, radioactive implant for, 852-858
altered sexuality patterns and, 856-857
assessment guidelines for, 852-853
complications of, 853
definition of, 852
diagnostic studies for, 853
discharge checklist for, 857
disuse syndrome and, 855
documentation checklist for, 857-858
DRG information for, 852
injury and, 854-855
precipitating factors for, 852
social isolation and, 856
teaching checklist for, 857
Chemotherapy, adverse effects of, 815
Chest drainage system, care of, 323-325

Chest pain
angina and, 369-370
MI and, 345-346
Chest splinting, postoperative atelectasis and, 106
Chest trauma, 604. *See also* Trauma, multiple.
Cholecystectomy, 542-550
altered oral mucous membrane and, 549
assessment guidelines for, 543
complications of, 543
definition of, 542
diagnostic studies for, 543
discharge checklist for, 550
documentation checklist for, 550
DRG information for, 542
hemorrhage and, 545
ineffective breathing pattern and, 547-548
nutritional deficit and, 548-549
pain and, 545-546
peritonitis and, 544-545
postoperative infection and, 546-547
precipitating factors for, 542-543
teaching checklist for, 550
Cholecystitis, 542-543. *See also* Cholecystectomy.
Cholelithiasis, 542, 543. *See also* Cholecystectomy.
Cholesterol level, nutritional status and, 82
Cholinergic crisis, 205
Chronic obstructive pulmonary disease, 255-267
activity intolerance and, 263-264
altered sexuality patterns and, 266
clinical pathway for, 258-260t
complications of, 257
definition of, 255
diagnostic studies for, 256-257
discharge checklist for, 266-267
documentation checklist for, 267
DRG information for, 255
etiology of, 255
ineffective breathing pattern and, 262
knowledge deficit and, 265-266
nursing history for, 255-256
nutritional deficit and, 262-263
physical findings in, 256
respiratory failure and, 257, 261
sleep pattern disturbance and, 264-265
teaching checklist for, 267
Chronic renal failure, 698-714
altered oral mucous membrane and, 708
altered thought processes and, 710
anemia and, 705
complications of, 700
creatinine ranges in, 700t
definition of, 698
diagnostic studies for, 699-700
discharge checklist for, 713
documentation checklist for, 713

Index

i refers to an illustration; t refers to a table.

Index

i refers to an illustration; t refers to a table.

Index

i refers to an illustration; t refers to a table.

i refers to an illustration; t refers to a table.